Essentials of Physiology

Essentials of Physiology

Second Edition

Edited by

Nicholas Sperelakis, Ph.D.

Joseph Eichberg Professor of Molecular and Cellular Physiology,
University of Cincinnati College of Medicine, Cincinnati

Robert O. Banks, Ph.D.

Professor of Molecular and Cellular Physiology, University of
Cincinnati College of Medicine, Cincinnati

Illustrations by
Kristen Wienandt, C.M.I.

Little, Brown and Company
Boston   New York   Toronto   London

Library of Congress Cataloging-in-Publication Data
Essentials of physiology / edited by Nicholas Sperelakis, Robert O.
   Banks.—2nd ed.
      p.   cm.
   Rev. ed. of: Physiology. 1st ed. c1993.
   Includes bibliographical references and index.
   ISBN 0-316-80628-5
   1. Human physiology.   I. Sperelakis, Nick, 1930–   .   II. Banks,
   Robert O.
      [DNLM: 1. Physiology.   QT   104 E781 1996]
   QP34.5.P4967   1996
612—dc20
DNLM/DLC
for Library of Congress   95-34889
                                                                     CIP

Printed in the United States of America
MV-NY   ⋒

Editorial: Evan R. Schnittman, Rebecca Marnhout
Production Services: Textbook Writers Associates
Copyeditor: James Madru
Indexer: Michael Loo
Cover Design: Hannus Design Associates
Cover Illustration: Kristen Wienandt

To all the physiologists who have, over many years, produced the facts and developed the principles that are presented herein. It was our job to chronicle and summarize their collective achievements as best we could.

Contents

Preface

A number of important changes and additions have been incorporated into the second edition of *Essentials of Physiology*. First and foremost is the inclusion of a complete section covering neurophysiology. As noted in the preface to our first edition, neurophysiology was omitted because the publisher had plans to present this material in a separate book on neuroscience. This decision was based on the fact that several medical and dental science programs have, in recent years, taught this subject in a separate neuroscience course. The exclusion of neurophysiology from the first edition precluded its adoption by a number of allied health programs, such as pharmacy, nursing, and physical therapy. We felt these programs would benefit from using our physiology text, and our revised text is now suitable for this larger audience.

To accommodate the relatively broad and important discipline of neurophysiology, virtually all the part editors deleted extraneous information to reduce their sections by 10% or more. Nonetheless, no key facts or principles were sacrificed, and, indeed, we believe that these changes actually render the book more readable for students in the health sciences.

Another major improvement is that almost all the figures have been drawn by artist Kristen Wienandt, using computer graphics. Artist Glenn Doerman at the University of Cincinnati College of Medicine also provided a few figures. Not only are the illustrations more uniform, they are also clearer and higher quality than those in the first edition.

We trust that students and faculty will find the second edition of *Essentials of Physiology* considerably improved over the first. Our goal remains the same—namely, to provide an intermediate-level coverage of basic facts, concepts, and principles in human physiology for students entering graduate programs in medicine, dentistry, and the medical sciences. We hope we have provided a useful textbook, one that can fill the gap between the overly simplistic, survey-type texts and the ultracomplex encyclopedic texts. We also wanted to provide a properly balanced text containing discussions of physiology at the molecular, cellular, organ, and whole-organism levels.

N. S.
R. O. B.

Contributing Authors

Douglas K. Anderson, Ph.D.
C. M. and K. E. Overstreet Professor of Neuroscience, University of Florida College of Medicine; Research Career Scientist, Medical Research Service, Veterans Affairs Medical Center, Gainesville, Florida

Gary L. Anderson, Ph.D.
Associate Professor of Physiology and Biophysics, University of Louisville School of Medicine, Louisville, Kentucky

Robert O. Banks, Ph.D.
Professor of Molecular and Cellular Physiology, University of Cincinnati College of Medicine, Cincinnati

Frank C. Barone, Ph.D.
Assistant Director, Department of Cardiovascular Pharmacology, SmithKline Beecham Pharmaceuticals, King of Prussia, Pennsylvania

Michael M. Behbehani, Ph.D.
Professor of Molecular and Cellular Physiology, University of Cincinnati College of Medicine, Cincinnati

Alvin S. Blaustein, M.D.
Associate Professor of Medicine, Baylor College of Medicine; Chief, Cardiac Non-Invasive Diagnostic Laboratory, Veterans Affairs Medical Center, Houston

Barbara N. Campaigne, Ph.D.
Director, Department of Research Development, American College of Sports Medicine, Indianapolis

Lawrence M. Dolan, M.D.
Associate Professor of Pediatrics, University of Cincinnati College of Medicine; Attending Physician, Department of Pediatrics, Children's Hospital Medical Center, Cincinnati

William C. Farr, M.D., Ph.D.
Lecturer, Department of Family and Community Medicine, University of Arizona College of Medicine, Tucson, Arizona

Donald G. Ferguson, Ph.D.
Associate Professor of Anatomy, Case Western Reserve University School of Medicine, Cleveland

Joseph D. Fondacaro, Ph.D.
Senior Research Scientist, Department of Preclinical Pharmacology, Hoechst Marion Roussel Inc., Cincinnati

Ernest C. Foulkes, Ph.D.
Interim Director, Department of Environmental Health, University of Cincinnati College of Medicine, Cincinnati

Lawrence A. Frohman, M.D.
Edmund F. Foley Professor and Chairman, Department of Medicine, University of Illinois College of Medicine at Chicago; Physician-in-Chief, Department of Medicine, University of Illinois at Chicago Medical Center, Chicago

John H. Galla, M.D.
Director, Division of Nephrology and Hypertension, and Professor of Medicine and Molecular and Cellular Physiology, University of Cincinnati College of Medicine; Director, Division of Nephrology and Hypertension, University Hospital, Cincinnati

Gunter Grupp, M.D., Ph.D.
Professor of Molecular and Cellular Physiology, University of Cincinnati College of Medicine, Cincinnati

Ingrid L. Grupp, M.D.
Professor of Pharmacology and Cell Biophysics, University of Cincinnati College of Medicine, Cincinnati

Patrick D. Harris, Ph.D.
Professor of Physiology and Biophysics and Senior Investigator, Center for Applied Microcirculatory Research, University of Louisville School of Medicine, Louisville, Kentucky

Judith A. Heiny, Ph.D.
Associate Professor of Molecular and Cellular Physiology, University of Cincinnati College of Medicine, Cincinnati

James E. Heubi, M.D.
Professor of Pediatrics, University of Cincinnati College of Medicine; Director, Clinical Research Center, and Staff Physician, Division of Gastroenterology and Nutrition, Children's Hospital Medical Center, Cincinnati

Robert F. Highsmith, Ph.D.
Associate Dean for Research, Office of the Dean, and Professor and Vice-Chairman, Department of Molecular and Cellular Physiology, University of Cincinnati College of Medicine, Cincinnati

Brian D. Hoit, M.D.
Associate Professor of Medicine, University of Cincinnati College of Medicine; Director, Department of Echocardiography, University Hospital, Cincinnati

Nelson D. Horseman, Ph.D.
Professor of Molecular and Cellular Physiology, University of Cincinnati College of Medicine, Cincinnati

James P. Hughes, Ph.D.
Professor of Life Sciences, Indiana State University, Terre Haute, Indiana

Harriet S. Iwamoto, Ph.D.
Associate Professor of Pediatrics and Molecular and Cellular Physiology, University of Cincinnati College of Medicine; Associate Professor, Division of Neonatology, Children's Hospital Medical Center, Cincinnati

Shahrokh Javaheri, M.D.
Professor of Medicine, University of Cincinnati College of Medicine; Director, Sleep Disorders Laboratory, Veterans Affairs Medical Center, Cincinnati

Ira R. Josephson, Ph.D.
Research Associate Professor of Molecular and Cellular Physiology, University of Cincinnati College of Medicine, Cincinnati

Andrew R. LaBarbera, Ph.D.
Professor of Obstetrics and Gynecology, University of Cincinnati College of Medicine; Director, Andrology Laboratory, University Hospital, Cincinnati

Richard J. Paul, Ph.D.
Professor of Molecular and Cellular Physiology, University of Cincinnati College of Medicine, Cincinnati

Robert W. Putnam, Ph.D.
Associate Professor of Physiology and Biophysics, Wright State University School of Medicine, Dayton, Ohio

Edward S. Redgate, Ph.D.
Associate Professor of Cell Biology and Physiology, University of Pittsburgh School of Medicine, Pittsburgh

R. John Solaro, Ph.D.
Professor and Chairman, Department of Physiology and Biophysics, University of Illinois College of Medicine at Chicago

Nicholas Sperelakis, Ph.D.
Joseph Eichberg Professor of Molecular and Cellular Physiology, University of Cincinnati College of Medicine, Cincinnati

Janusz B. Suszkiw, Ph.D.
Professor of Molecular and Cellular Physiology, University of Cincinnati College of Medicine, Cincinnati

Richard A. Walsh, M.D.
Stonehill Professor of Medicine, Division of Cardiology, University of Cincinnati College of Medicine; Director, Division of Cardiology and Cardiovascular Center, University Hospital, Cincinnati

Laura F. Wexler, M.D.
Professor of Medicine, University of Cincinnati College of Medicine; Chief, Cardiology Section, Veterans Affairs Medical Center, Cincinnati

I Cellular Physiology

Part Editor

Nicholas Sperelakis

Notice

The indications and dosages of all drugs in this book have been recommended in the medical literature and conform to the practices of the general medical community. The medications described do not necessarily have specific approval by the Food and Drug Administration for use in the diseases and dosages for which they are recommended. The package insert for each drug should be consulted for use and dosage as approved by the FDA. Because standards for usage change, it is advisable to keep abreast of revised recommendations, particularly those concerning new drugs.

1 Body Fluid Spaces and Osmotic Forces

Robert O. Banks and Richard J. Paul

Objectives

After reading this chapter, you should be able to

List the various fluid compartments of the body and their approximate relative sizes

Describe several methods for measuring each compartment and explain why operational definitions are used

State the major cations and anions of each compartment and their approximate concentrations

Define an *osmole* and *osmotic pressure* as well as how much pressure one osmole generates

Explain the difference between total osmotic pressure and effective osmotic pressure; explain the term *reflection coefficient*

Contrast hydrostatic pressure and osmotic (or effective osmotic) pressure

Explain why osmotic pressure is expressed in terms of solute rather than solvent (H_2O) concentration

Explain why only the number, not the kind, of particles is important in calculating osmotic pressure

Describe what the effective osmotic pressure is between the vascular compartment and the interstitial fluid space, and between the interstitial fluid space and the intracellular fluid space

Define *tonicity,* and describe how it is related to osmolarity

Summarize the forces that result in movement of water and electrolytes across biologic membranes

Explain the movements of fluid between the major compartments in conditions such as hemorrhage, sweating, and starvation, as well as other disturbances leading to hypoalbuminemia

---

Physiology is the study of organ systems and their role in the homeostatic mechanisms that attempt to maintain the internal environment of an organism in a steady state. This chapter focuses on the fluid compartments of the body, the composition of these compartments, the methods used to measure these fluid spaces, and the osmotic and hydrostatic forces that maintain a stable distribution of fluid among these fluid compartments.

Body Fluid Compartments

There are two major fluid compartments in most multicellular organisms: the **intracellular fluid** (ICF) **space** and the **extracellular fluid** (ECF) **space.** The ECF space can be divided functionally into the **plasma space** (the volume occupied by plasma) and the **interstitial fluid** (ISF) **space.** Normally, the fluid in the ISF space is an ultrafiltrate of plasma entrapped in minute spaces of a gel-like matrix composed of proteoglycan filaments. However, a number of pathologic conditions, particularly those characterized by low plasma protein concentrations, increased venous pressure, increased lymphatic pressure, or increased capillary permeability to plasma proteins, are characterized by marked expansion of the ISF space that results in a state known as *edema.* Some fluid spaces (e.g., ocular fluid, cerebrospinal fluid, intestinal fluid) are relatively small but unique ECF compartments and are referred to as *transcellular fluids.*

The total water content of the body, the ECF plus the ICF, constitutes approximately 45% to 60% of the body weight. As shown in Table 1-1, the fraction of body weight that is water varies with both age and gender of the individual. The difference in the fractional water composition between males and females is due to the fact that fat, which contains less water than other body tissues, represents a greater portion of the body weight in females.

In healthy individuals, the plasma volume, ISF volume, and ICF volume are approximately 5%, 15% to 25%, and 30% to 40% of the total body weight, respectively. Because the normal hematocrit, defined as the ratio of the red blood cell volume to the blood volume, is about 40%; the blood volume in a healthy individual is approximately 7% to 9% of body weight. The balance of body weight (i.e., 40%) is roughly composed of 18% proteins, 7% minerals, and 15% fat. Thus a healthy 20-year-old, 70-kg male contains about 42 liters of body water, of which 3.5 liters is plasma, 14 liters is ISF, and 24 liters is ICF. Blood volume is about 6 liters.

Volume Measurements of Biologic Compartments

Theory

Estimates of the size of body fluid spaces are based on the **dye** (indicator) **dilution principle,** which is based on conservation of mass and the relationship between concentration, volume, and mass, or:

(Concentration)(Volume) = Mass
(milligrams/milliliter or moles/liter) (milliliters or liters) = (milligrams or moles)

Following are two examples to illustrate the application of this principle to the measurement of fluid volumes.

Example 1
In the first example, consider one compartment with an unknown volume (V_2) to which samples are added or removed. If a relatively small volume (V_1) containing a

Table 1-1. Total-Body Water (percentage of body weight)

Age (years)	Male	Female
17–34	60%	55%
50–86	54%	46%

substance at a concentration C_1 is added to the unknown volume, then, following establishment of a **steady state** (a condition in which there is uniform mixing of the substance within V_2, and therefore the concentration does not change with time), V_2 can be calculated. Since conservation of mass must apply, it follows that

$$(C_1)(V_1) = (C_2)(V_2)$$

Since C_1 and V_1 are known and C_2 can be measured, then

$$V_2 = (C_1)(V_1)/C_2$$

Two requirements apply: (1) uniform mixing of substance in V_2 and (2) no loss or gain of substance in the unknown volume. If there has been loss or gain, then $(C_1)(V_1) = (C_2)(V_2)$ + amount lost or – amount gained.

Example 2
Add 0.1 ml of a solution containing 200 mg/ml of an indicator substance to an unknown volume (V_2). After mixing, the concentration of the indicator in V_2 is 0.2 mg/ml. V_2 is calculated as follows:

$$V_2 = (C_1)(V_1)/C_2 = \text{Amount added/Final conc.}$$
$$V_2 = (200 \text{ mg/ml})(0.1 \text{ ml})/0.2 \text{ mg/ml}$$
$$V_2 = 100 \text{ ml}$$

Three-Compartment Model

The body actually represents a complex communicating system of compartments. Nonetheless, a three-compartment analysis based on an ICF, ISF, and plasma space can be used to approximate the distribution of total body water. These three spaces are separated by the **capillary unit** and the **cell membrane.** For this analysis, samples of fluid can only be added to or extracted from the plasma compartment.

Idealized Analysis of a Three-Compartment System
Assume that three substances (*A, B,* and *C*) are injected into the plasma compartment, that none of these substances was present in the system before the injection, that the capillary unit is permeable to *B* and *C* but not to *A,* and that the cell membrane is permeable only to *C.*

Based on the information provided, the volume of distribution of *A* would be the plasma compartment, of *B* would be the ECF, and of *C* would be the total-body water space. Because substance C is distributed in the largest volume, the concentration of C would be the lowest of the three solutes.

Specific Substances for Measurement of Biologic Compartments

Plasma Volume

Proteins or substances that bind to plasma proteins and thus do not readily pass through the capillary membrane can be used to measure the **plasma volume.** For example, albumin, a plasma protein that can be labeled with radioactive iodine, or agents such as Evans blue, which bind to plasma proteins with high affinity, can be used. Red blood cells can be labeled with isotopes of chromium or iron and used to measure the vascular space. By determining the volume of distribution of these agents and the hematocrit (hct), where hct = red blood cell volume/blood volume, one can measure the plasma volume and blood volume. The red blood cell volume also can be measured if one neglects the small volume of other types of blood cells. Thus 1 – hct = plasma volume/blood volume.

ECF (ISF + Plasma Volume)

As noted above, the volume of the ECF space can be measured with substances that cross the capillary unit but do not enter the cells. Examples of such solutes are isotopes of sodium ions (Na^+), isotopes of chloride ions (Cl^-), sulfate, thiocyanate, and molecules such as inulin (a polymer of fructose). Because some of these molecules do enter cells (e.g., Na^+ and Cl^-) or can slowly penetrate the transcellular spaces, each molecule yields a slightly different value for ECF volume. Therefore, an **operational definition** is usually employed, meaning that an Na^+ space or an inulin space is reported rather than a value for the "ECF space." Estimates of most biologic variables are operationally defined because these values depend on the method selected.

Total-Body Water

Any substance that is uniformly distributed between the ECF and ICF spaces has a volume of distribution equivalent to the **total-body water.** A number of substances, including labeled water (^3H_2O or D_2O), urea, and various lipid-soluble (membrane permeable) molecules such as antipyrine, can be used.

Composition of Body Fluids

Mass, Amount, or Quantity

Quantities of solutes are usually expressed as grams (also as kilograms = 10^3 g, milligrams = 10^{-3} g, micrograms = 10^{-6} g, nanograms = 10^{-9} g, picograms = 10^{-12} g, or femtograms = 10^{-15} g), moles (also as millimoles), equivalents (also as milliequivalents), or osmoles (also as milliosmoles). Similarly, volumes are generally expressed in liters, milliliters (10^{-3}), and microliters (10^{-6}).

One **gram molecular weight** of a substance represents 1 mole of the substance and consists of approximately 6×10^{23} molecules. For example, the molecular weight of sodium chloride (NaCl) is 23 + 35.5 = 58.5; hence 1 mole of NaCl represents 58.5 g (1 mmole is 58.5 mg).

The concept of **equivalents** relates to the presence of an electric charge on the molecule. Thus one equivalent (eq) represents 1 mole of a substance divided by its valence. Since NaCl, for example, dissociates into two particles in solution, 1 mole of NaCl contains 1 eq (23 g) of Na^+ and 1 eq of Cl^- (35.5 g). By contrast, 1 eq of calcium (Ca^{2+}) is 40/2, or 20 g.

The concept of **osmoles** relates to the numbers of particles released into solution when the solute is dissolved. Thus 1 osmole is the **gram** molecular weight of the substance divided by the number of ionic species generated when the substance is dissolved in solution.

Mass Per Unit Volume

Concentration represents an amount (mass) per unit volume. Each of the units described in the preceding section (grams, moles, equivalents, or osmoles) can be used to express a concentration. When 1 mole or 1 osmole is dissolved in 1 liter of water, this gives a 1-molar or 1-osmolar solution. When 1 mole of a substance is dissolved in 1 kg of water, this gives a 1-mol*al* solution. The difference between molarity and molality is small.

A number of units can be used to express concentration, though moles or grams per liter and milliliter are often employed. In addition, many biologic concentrations are expressed as milligram percent (mg%), which indicates a mass (mg) per 100 ml, or deciliter. For example, the plasma glucose concentration is often expressed as mg% or as mg/dl.

Concentrations of Major Cations and Anions in Biologic Fluids

Most of the major **anions** and **cations** present in the ICF and ECF spaces are illustrated in Fig. 1-1 and Table 1-2 (a more detailed list is in Appendix 1). Some important facts to note are that Na^+ is the major ECF cation, K^+ is the major ICF cation, Cl^- is the major ECF anion, and inorganic PO_4 is the major ICF anion. Another important cation is Ca^{2+}.

A large difference in the protein concentration exists between the plasma space and ISF space. In addition, the **net charge** on most proteins is negative (e.g., the net negative charge on albumin is about 15), and thus some cations are bound to plasma proteins. For example, the total concentration of Ca^{2+} in plasma is about 2.5 mM (5.0 meq/liter), but 40% to 50% of the total plasma Ca^{2+} is bound to albumin and globulins.

Water Movement Across Biologic Membranes

Forces Involved

Two forces lead to the net movement of water across biologic membranes: (1) **hydrostatic** or **hydraulic pressure**

Table 1-2. Plasma Concentrations of Some Major Cations and Anions

Cations	Anions
Sodium = 135–145 meq/liter	Chlorine = 100–106 meq/liter
Potassium = 3.5–5.0 meq/liter	Bicarbonate = 24–30 meq/liter
Calcium = 4.3–5.3 meq/liter	Protein^{-15} = 6–8.4 g/dl

differences and (2) **osmotic pressure differences.** Both forces are physiologically important.

Hydrostatic and Hydraulic Pressure
Pressure within a fluid system has both a hydrostatic component, resulting from the gravitational force exerted on a column of fluid, and a hydraulic component, resulting, for example, from the action of a pump. Both forces are important when evaluating fluid movement in the cardiovascular system, both in the vascular space and between the plasma compartment and the ISF space. Water moves down a hydrostatic/hydraulic pressure gradient (i.e., from higher to lower pressure).

Osmotic Pressure
Osmotic pressure is one of the so-called colligative properties of solutions. To appreciate the contribution of osmotic pressure to net water movement across biologic membranes, one also must understand the distinction between the total or **calculated,** or **potential, osmotic pressure** and the physiologically important component, known as the **effective osmotic pressure.** The effective osmotic pressure is determined by the permeability properties of the membrane separating two solutions.

To illustrate the importance of the membrane as the determinant of the effective osmotic pressure of a solution, a simple experiment can be performed. A **semipermeable membrane** (a membrane that is not permeable to solute but is permeable to water) is attached to the end of a thistle tube and suspended in a beaker of water; alternatively, a **permeable membrane** (one that is freely permeable to both solute and water) is placed at the end of the tube. This experiment is illustrated in Fig. 1-2. If a solution of water plus solute is added to the inside of the tube with the semipermeable membrane (see Fig. 1-2A), a net flow of water will occur into the tube until the column of water (i.e., the hydrostatic pressure) offsets the osmotic pressure of the solution in the tube. Alternatively, if hydraulic pres-

Fig. 1-1. The ionic composition of body fluid spaces.

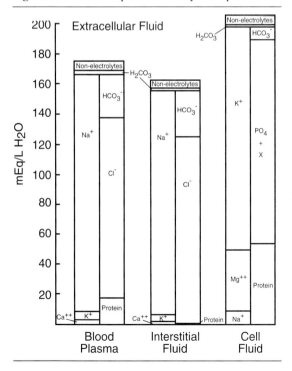

sure is applied to the solution inside the thistle tube, the amount of pressure necessary to prevent net water movement would be equal to the osmotic pressure. The reason why water enters the tube is that water, like solute (see Chap. 2), diffuses from regions of high concentration to regions of low concentration. The concentration of pure water is 55.5 M (the molecular weight of water is 18.02, and 1 liter of water weighs 1 kg; therefore, the concentration is 1000 g/18.02, or 55.5 M). The concentration of water following addition of solute is lowered in proportion to the amount of solute added. Thus a higher concentration of an impermeant solute on one side of a membrane will result in net diffusion of water into that solution. By contrast, if the same solution is added to the thistle tube with a solute-water–permeable membrane (see Fig. 1-2B), the solute will equilibrate across the membrane, and the effective osmotic pressure of the solution will be zero. Thus, if the membrane is as permeable to the solute as it is to water, no net water flow will occur, even though the theoretical osmotic pressure of the solution (calculated by the van't Hoff equation) is the same. Effective osmotic pressure is therefore dependent on the relative permeability of the membrane to the solute.

Osmotic pressure (π) can be calculated by the **van't Hoff equation:**

$$\pi = C_S RT$$

where C_S is the osmolar concentration of the solute, R is the universal gas constant, and T is the absolute temperature; at 0°C, RT has a value of 22.4 liter atm per osmole (at 37°C, RT = 25.4).

Osmolarity is defined as the number of moles per liter multiplied by the number of dissociating ions. Osmolarity must be used when considering osmotic pressure, since osmotic pressure depends on the number of nonpenetrating molecules. Thus

1 mole urea = 1 osmole
1 mole urea/liter = 1 osmolar solution
1 mole NaCl = 2 osmoles
1 mole NaCl/liter = 2 osmolar solution
1 mole $CaCl_2$ = 3 osmoles
1 mole $CaCl_2$/liter = 3 osmolar solution

Since the NaCl concentration in the ECF space is about 150 mM/liter, the osmolar concentration is about 300 mOsm/liter.

It is the total number of moles or particles in solution

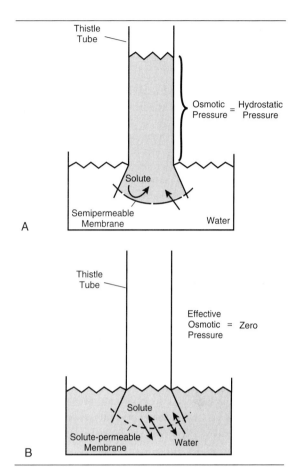

Fig. 1-2. (A) Measurement of osmotic pressure using a semipermeable membrane (i.e., a membrane that is only permeable to water). The addition of solute to the thistle tube results in a concentration gradient for water between the outside and inside of the tube; consequently, water diffuses into the tube until the height of the fluid column offsets this movement. (B) The permeability properties of the membrane determine the physiologically important component of the calculated osmotic pressure (i.e., the effective osmotic pressure). When the membrane is equally permeable to both water and solute, the solute equilibrates between the two solutions and no effective osmotic pressure is generated.

that is important in determining the osmotic pressure, not the kind of solute. The presence of solute lowers the mole fraction or concentration of water and creates the imbalance that drives water movement.

This is true for colligative properties in general, in that the number of particles is the critical factor in freezing-point depression or boiling-point elevation of water. However, when considering water flows in situations where solute flows also occur — across biologic membranes separating compartments — the kind of solute and its permeability across the membranes become major factors in the osmotic flow of water.

In general, biologic membranes show varying degrees of permeability to many substances. If both water and solute flows are taking place, an effective osmotic pressure is defined as $\pi \cong \sigma RTC$, where σ is the **reflection coefficient.** The reflection coefficient depends on the properties of both the membrane and solute and has a value that ranges from 0 to 1.

Osmotic Behavior of Cells

Water diffuses freely across cell membranes, whereas Na^+ ions, glucose, and large organic molecules do not. Thus **osmotic pressure** plays an important role in water movements across the cell membrane. This is particularly critical for animal cells, which, unlike plant cells, do not have a rigid cell wall and cannot withstand large osmotic forces.

Osmotic pressure is a very powerful driving force for water movement, and a small change in solute concentration can result in a large change in pressure. This can be illustrated as follows: If the concentration of osmotically active particles inside a cell is 0.3 Osm/liter, then a cell placed in pure water would experience an osmotic pressure:

π = (22.4 liter/atm/Osm) $\times$ 0.3 Osm/liter
   = 6.7 atm

Since 1 atm equals 760 mm Hg, the osmotic pressure is more than 5000 mm Hg. This is sufficient to support a column of water approximately 68 meters high (mercury is about 13 times heavier than water).

Oxygen, carbon dioxide, urea, and certain amino acids and fatty acids are relatively permeable to the plasma membrane and do not develop an osmotic pressure equal to their number of particles. Thus it is possible for cells placed in an isosmotic solution (one containing the same number of particles per volume as inside the cell) to gain water, depending on the effective osmotic pressure of the solution (which is dependent on the relative permeability of the solutes).

The **tonicity** of a solution is defined in terms of the water movement. Cells placed in an isotonic solution neither gain nor lose volume. Cells placed in a hypertonic solution shrink because of an osmotic loss of water. Conversely, cells placed in a hypotonic solution swell because water flows into the cell.

Osmotic equilibrium is achieved very rapidly through the flow of water across the cell membrane. Therefore, cells are always in osmotic equilibrium with plasma. If a red blood cell is placed in a hypotonic solution, its volume will increase until osmotic equilibrium is reached (osmotic uptake of water decreases the intracellular tonicity until it is isotonic with the originally hypotonic solution). Once osmotic equilibrium is reached, the volume of the cell, unless it ruptures, will remain constant. The volume changes of red blood cells in hypotonic and hypertonic solutions can thus be used to measure the tonicity of plasma. Plasma tonicity will be equal to that of a solution in which red blood cells have the same volume as they did in plasma (Fig. 1-3).

Utilizing the relationship between the relative red blood cell (RBC) volume and the osmolarity (of impermeant solute), as depicted in Fig. 1-3, at equilibrium, one gets:

$$Osm_{RBC} = Osm_{out} \quad \text{or} \quad \pi i_{RBC} = \pi_{soln}$$

Fig. 1-3. Osmotic behavior of red blood cells. The osmotic behavior of red blood cells can be measured easily, as shown. Red blood cells placed in various NaCl solutions shrink (or swell) due to water loss (or gain). This can be measured in terms of the volume of a fixed number of cells in a hematocrit tube. The relationship between red blood cell volume and the solution osmolarity is shown in the graph. As described in the text, the relative red blood cell volume is inversely proportional to the solution osmolarity.

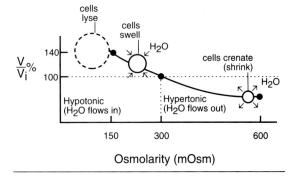

Thus, using the van't Hoff equation: $RTC_{RBC} = RTC_{soln}$ where:

$$C_{RBC} = \frac{n_{RBC}}{V_{RBC}}$$

and n_{RBC} is the number of moles of osmotically active particles inside the red blood cell, which is constant, and V_{RBC} is the red blood cell volume. Thus,

$$C_{RBC} = \frac{n_{RBC}}{V_{RBC}} = C_{soln}$$

Therefore, $V_{RBC} \sim 1/C_{soln}$ as shown in Fig. 1-3.

As already mentioned, a permeant solute represents a more complex situation. A solution containing only a penetrating solute, whether or not it is isosmotic with the cell interior, cannot be isotonic. In fact, from the definition of tonicity described previously, all solutions containing only penetrating solutes must be regarded as hypotonic, whatever their actual osmolarity may be. The rate of swelling (or the time required for hemolysis in red blood cells) in an isosmotic solution of a penetrating solute can be used as an index of its permeability.

As an example, consider the case of a red blood cell placed in a 300-mM urea solution. This solution is isosmotic but hardly isotonic, since the rapid hemolysis of the cell indicates a large inward flow of water (Fig. 1-4).

Therefore, in order to predict the tonicity of solutions, one has to know the permeability of the solutes, in addition to their concentration, and for electrolytes, the number of particles upon dissociation.

The **reflection coefficient** (σ) is used to modify the van't Hoff equation, to take into account the effects of permeant solutes. It is most simply defined as

$$\sigma = \frac{\pi_{meas}}{\pi_{expected}} = \frac{\pi_{meas}}{RTC}$$

In the example using urea, because hemolysis occurs rapidly, the effective osmotic pressure elicited by the urea solution is very small, and hence the reflection coefficient for urea must be near zero. To calculate the effective osmotic pressure of a solution containing many different solutes, the following equation is used:

$$\pi = RT \sum_i \sigma_i C_i = RT (\sigma_1 C_1 + \sigma_2 C_2 + \cdots)$$

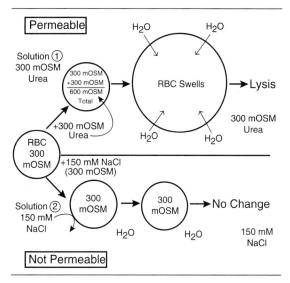

Fig. 1-4. Demonstration of the difference between osmolarity and tonicity. Red blood cells (*RBCs*) are exposed to solutions of 300 mM urea or 150 mM NaCl; both solutions are 300 mOsm. Cells in NaCl remain intact, whereas those in the urea solution lyse, due to an inward flow of water. Water flowing into the red blood cells in the urea solution is attributable to a larger number of particles inside the red blood cell than outside, due to the penetration of urea as shown. Thus the urea solution is hypotonic, though isosmotic.

Thus, to understand water flows across the cell membrane into or out of the ICF space, one must additionally understand the factors involved in solute transport across this barrier. Although this will be reviewed in Chap. 2, at this point it is instructive to consider the osmotic behavior of red blood cells with respect to various solutes. The term *permeable* is relative. For example, K^+, Cl^-, and glucose are considered "permeable." However, in terms of the consequential water flows, none is very permeable, as indicated by the time required for hemolysis to occur, as shown in Table 1-3. Cl^- is readily permeable, however, if its counterion, such as Na^+, is not, then Cl^- cannot move alone without violating electroneutrality. K^+ is not very permeable compared with water. The larger size of thiourea compared with urea causes a longer time for hemolysis. Ammonium chloride (NH_4Cl) appears to be highly permeable. NH_4Cl is always in equilibrium with ammonia, which is very lipid soluble and rapidly permeates biologic membranes. Glucose too is quite impermeable when compared with water. This is explained by the

Table 1-3. Properties of Various Solutes

Solute	Concentration (mM)	Osmolarity (mOsm/liter)	Tonicity	Time to Hemolysis (approximate)
Urea	300	300	Hypo	<1 sec
Urea	600	600	Hypo	<1 sec
Thiourea	300	300	Hypo	90 sec
Sodium chloride	150	300	Iso	∞
Ammonium chloride	150	300	Hypo	12 min
Potassium chloride	150	300	Approx Iso	>24 hr
Glucose	300	300	Approx Iso	8 hr
Sucrose	300	300	Iso	∞

fact that only relatively small amounts of glucose can penetrate cells via a saturable, carrier-mediated diffusion mechanism (see Chap. 2). Finally, sucrose, a disaccharide, is virtually impermeable and often used as a marker for the ECF space. When studying membrane transport in subsequent chapters, bear in mind the effects on the duration of time before red blood cell hemolysis of these various solutions in terms of their relative permeabilities and consequent water flows.

Fluid Movement Into and Out of the Capillary

If a membrane is equally permeable to water and solute, no effective osmotic pressure is realized. A good example of this relates to osmotic forces across the capillary wall. Na^+ and Cl^-, the major ECF ions, move rapidly between capillary plasma and ISF and therefore are not effective osmotic agents in that system. Conversely, plasma proteins are restricted primarily to the plasma compartment and are therefore the only effective osmotic agents mediating osmotic water flow between plasma and ISF. Thus the effective osmotic pressure difference between plasma and ISF is only a small fraction of the theoretical (potential) osmotic pressure. As noted previously, the potential osmotic pressure, as calculated from the total solute osmolar concentration, is more than 5000 mm Hg. By contrast, the effective osmotic pressure (due to plasma proteins) is about 25 mm Hg. This latter pressure is usually referred to as the **colloid osmotic pressure** or **plasma oncotic pressure.**

In the early 1900s, Starling was one of the first investigators to recognize the forces involved in fluid movement across the capillary and formulated what is generally referred to as **Starling's law of the capillary** (see Chap. 26).

Finally, it is important to understand the direction of fluid and water shifts that occur between the three major fluid compartments (the plasma, ISF, and ICF spaces) during various physiologic and pathophysiologic conditions. For example, during a hemorrhage, among the many events that occur is a decrease in blood pressure and a reflex increase in the activity of the sympathetic nervous system. Consequently, there is a decrease in capillary pressure and a shift in the balance of the Starling forces that favors net reabsorption of fluid from the ISF space into the plasma compartment. Because the reabsorbate does not contain protein, the plasma oncotic pressure falls after a hemorrhage. On the other hand, because the initial volume of blood lost during a hemorrhage is isosmotic, neither the total osmolarity of the ECF nor the volume of the ICF space changes as a consequence of bleeding.

During sweating, ICF is mobilized because sweat is hypotonic (the osmolarity is about 150 mOsm/liter). Therefore, during sweating, there is increased osmolarity of the ECF, bringing about extraction of water from the ICF space into the ECF space. Net fluid shifts out of the plasma space and into the ISF space (the formation of edema) occur whenever there are decreases in the plasma concentration of proteins (e.g., liver disease), during reduced protein intake, and during starvation.

Summary

Water constitutes 45% to 60% of body weight and is distributed among the three major fluid compartments: the plasma space (about 5%), the ISF space (about 15%), and the ICF space (about 40%). The nonwater components are fat, minerals, and proteins. Na^+ and Cl^- represent the primary osmotic components in ECF (the plasma space plus the ISF space), whereas K^+ and proteins account for the major elements in ICF. The size of these fluid spaces can be estimated using agents that, when injected into the vascular space, remain in plasma, distribute within the ECF space, or diffuse throughout the entire body fluid. Hydraulic and hydrostatic as well as osmotic pressures produce net water flow. Hydraulic and hydrostatic pressures are created through compression of fluid by a pump and by a column of fluid, respectively. Osmotic pressure is a property of solutions and can be calculated using the van't Hoff equation. The physiologically important component of the total osmotic pressure (i.e., the effective osmotic pressure) depends on the solute permeability of the membrane separating two solutions. If the membrane is not permeable to any of the solute, the effective osmotic pressure of the solution is equal to the calculated osmotic pressure. By contrast, as the solute permeability of the membrane increases, the effective osmotic pressure decreases.

Bibliography

Rose, B. D. *Clinical Physiology of Acid-Base and Electrolyte Disorders.* New York: McGraw-Hill, 1989.

Rhoades, R. A., and Tanner, G. A., *Medical Physiology.* Boston: Little, Brown, 1995.

2 Solute Movement Across Biologic Membranes

Robert W. Putnam

Objectives

After reading this chapter, you should be able to

Describe a cell membrane, including lipid bilayers and integral and membrane-associated proteins

Explain the forces that contribute to solute movement and what the electrochemical potential is

Describe the meaning of and how to calculate the Nernst potential

Describe the relationship between the diffusion coefficient and the permeability coefficient and define the partition coefficient

Describe the relationship between Nernst potential and the membrane potential and be clear about the sign of the membrane potential

Clearly distinguish and define *equilibrium* and *steady state*

Describe the various pathways for transmembrane movement of solutes, including channels versus carriers, facilitated diffusion, primary and secondary active transport, exchangers, and cotransporters

Differentiate electroneutral from electrogenic transport

Describe the general structure of transport proteins

The human body is designed to maintain a constant internal environment (**homeostasis**) for proper functioning, including constant temperature, supply of oxygen, salt and water contents, and energy supply. Cells within the body, in addition to their specialized functions, are designed to maintain a degree of cytoplasmic homeostasis. To accomplish this, the cells must exchange materials with the external solutions: the **extracellular fluid** (ECF), the **blood,** the **lymph,** and in the central nervous system, the **cerebrospinal fluid** (CSF). To understand this process, we must consider first the basic structure of a cell, the properties of solutions, the forces that control the movements of solutes, and the specialized molecules that often mediate solute movement into and out of cells. These processes underlie many of the functions of the cells in the body, and alterations of these processes result in a variety of pathologic conditions of medical significance.

Properties of Solutions

A solution is made up of two basic components: **solvent** and **solutes.** The solvent is the fluid into which the solutes are dissolved, and for virtually all biologic considerations, **water** is the main solvent. In considering the movement of solutes across the cell membrane, a **lipid** solvent (see below) also will have to be considered. Unless stated otherwise, water will be assumed to be the solvent.

Solutes are the substances dissolved in the solvent and can be broadly classed as **uncharged** (such as glucose, mannitol, and gases such as oxygen and carbon dioxide) or electrically **charged** (such as small inorganic **cations** like Na^+ and K^+ and **anions** like Cl^-, as well as organic anions like $lactate^-$ and $pyruvate^-$). Further, molecules such as NaCl or lactic acid, which dissociate into **ions** in solution (Na^+ and Cl^-, H^+ and $lactate^-$), are referred to as **elec-**

trolytes, whereas molecules such as glucose, which do not dissociate in solution, are referred to as **nonelectrolytes** (Fig. 2-1).

Several parameters can be used to describe a solution. The most common parameter is the **concentration** of a particular solute, which refers to the amount of solute dissolved in a given volume of solvent (**molality**) or volume of solution (**molarity**). Another parameter of importance to describe a solution is the **osmotic pressure,** which is the sum of the concentration of all the various solutes in the solution. **Ionic strength** describes the electrical properties of the solution and is defined as

$$\omega = \tfrac{1}{2}\Sigma C_j z_j^2 \qquad (2\text{-}1)$$

where ω is the ionic strength, C_j is the concentration of a particular solute (e.g., Na^+ or glucose), and z_j is the valence of that solute. Note that because uncharged solutes have a valence of 0, they do not contribute to ionic strength, only the ions do. Note also that polyvalent ions (ions with a charge of more than 1) will increase the ionic strength more than monovalent ions at the same concentration because the valence term is squared. The normal ionic strength for plasma is about 0.15 M. Finally, the amount of a given solute in a volume of the solution can be expressed as the **activity** of that solute and is defined by $\alpha_j - \gamma_j C_j$, where α_j is the activity of a given solute, and γ_j is the **activity coefficient** of that solute. The activity coefficient is a coefficient of proportionality relating the thermodynamic effect of a solute (its activity) to its concentration and, for ions, is related to the ionic strength of the solution. Values of the activity coefficient can vary from 0 to 1. It is generally assumed that dilute solutions of uncharged solutes have an activity coefficient of 1, and thus their activity is equal to their concentration. Ions, on the other hand, are affected by the concentration of the ions in solution (the ionic strength) and thus often have an activity that is less than their concentration. For example, a typical activity coefficient for K^+ inside cells is about 0.7, so if the cell $[K^+]$ is 140 mM, α_K is about 100 mM. **This distinction between activity and concentration is important because it is an ion's activity, not its concentration, that determines the driving force for its movement** (see below).

Cells and Cell Membranes

All cells are separated from the external medium by a **cell membrane,** or **plasmalemma.** The cell membrane serves several functions: (1) a **barrier** to the loss of needed cell components and the uptake of unwanted substances, (2) a **selectivity filter** that permits certain substances to enter and leave the cell, and (3) a **communication system,** interacting with external signals and transducing those signals into an internal message. The ability of a cell to control its internal environment is critically dependent on the transport of substances across the cell membrane, and thus the properties of the membrane and its transport characteristics have received a great deal of attention.

The cell membrane is composed predominantly of two components, **lipids** and **proteins.** The lipid portion of the membrane is formed by two layers called the **lipid bilayer** (Fig. 2-2). Each layer is composed of phospholipids, molecules that have a polar head group and two long tail groups composed of hydrophobic carbon chains (**fatty acyl chains**). The hydrophobic tails from each layer self-associate, with the polar head groups of the outer lipid layer facing the extracellular solution and the polar head groups of the inner lipid layer facing the cytoplasm. The lipids that make up the outer layer may differ from those which compose the inner layer, creating asymmetry of the bilayer. For instance, some lipids have sugar moieties attached (**glycolipids**), and these are restricted to the outer layer. The hydrophobic core of the liquid bilayer forms an effective barrier to the passage of water-soluble substances (e.g., organic ions, Na^+, K^+ and Cl^-). This barrier function allows ions to have different concentrations within the cell compared with the external solution, which is important for membrane transport and electrical phenomena (see below). The barrier function also allows the cell to retain

Fig. 2-1. Examples of electrolytes and nonelectrolytes in plasma.

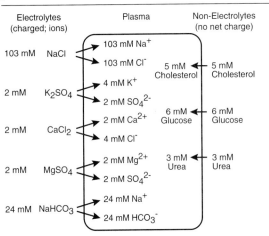

Electrolytes (charged; ions)	Plasma	Non-Electrolytes (no net charge)
103 mM NaCl	103 mM Na$^+$ 103 mM Cl$^-$	
	5 mM Cholesterol	5 mM Cholesterol
2 mM K$_2$SO$_4$	4 mM K$^+$ 2 mM SO$_4^{2-}$	
	6 mM Glucose	6 mM Glucose
2 mM CaCl$_2$	2 mM Ca^{2+} 4 mM Cl$^-$	
2 mM MgSO$_4$	2 mM Mg^{2+} 2 mM SO$_4^{2-}$	3 mM Urea
	3 mM Urea	
24 mM NaHCO$_3$	24 mM Na$^+$ 24 mM HCO$_3^-$	

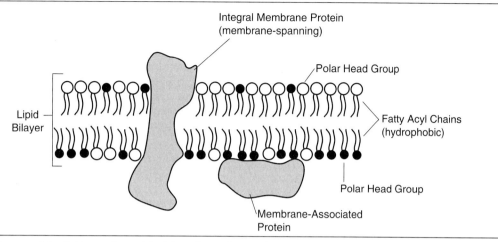

Fig. 2-2. Cartoon of the fluid-mosaic model of the cell membrane. The membrane includes the lipid bilayer, composed of two sheets made from various phospholipids that contain polar (hydrophilic) head groups and hydrophobic fatty acyl chains and associated proteins. Integral membrane proteins are embedded in the membrane and interact extensively with the bilayer, while membrane-associated proteins associate less extensively with the membrane.

water-soluble organic solutes that are essential for cellular metabolism.

The selectivity and communication functions of the cell membrane are largely mediated by the protein component, which consists of either **integral membrane proteins** or **membrane-associated proteins** (peripheral proteins). Integral membrane proteins lie within and often span the lipid bilayer and interact markedly with the lipids in the bilayer (see Fig. 2-2). Integral membrane proteins include such components as carriers, channels, and receptors. Membrane-associated proteins interact with the inner surface of the lipid bilayer (see Fig. 2-2). Examples of such proteins are protein kinase C and certain cytoskeletal proteins. This model of a membrane with proteins associated in a patchy fashion and a fluid lipid layer is referred to as the **fluid mosaic model** of membrane structure (see Fig. 2-2).

Solute Movement

Any molecule that is not at absolute zero temperature has kinetic energy and is thus constantly in motion and colliding with other molecules. This motion gives rise to **diffusion,** the random movement of single molecules. Even for solutions in two compartments that are at equilibrium, there will be diffusion of solutes between the compartments (Fig. 2-3). However, **there will be no net diffusion of solute;** i.e., the amount of solute diffusing in one direction will be equal to the amount of solute diffusing in the other direction (see Fig. 2-3). To have a net, directed movement of solute, there must be net forces acting on these molecules (see Fig. 2-3). The two main forces that promote net diffusion of solute molecules in solution are forces due to differences in **electrical potential** and to differences in **concentration.** A term μ_j, or **electrochemical potential,** can be assigned to any solute j, which includes these forces and is defined mathematically by the following equation:

$$\mu_j = \mu^0 + RT \ln(\alpha_j) + z_j F(V) \qquad (2\text{-}2)$$
$$\Delta\mu_j = RT \ln(\alpha_{j2}/\alpha_{j1}) + z_j F(V_2 - V_1) \qquad (2\text{-}3)$$

where μ^0 is an arbitrary standard value that is an unknown constant, α_j is the activity of species j, V is the electrical potential, z_j is the valence of species j, and R, T, and F have their usual meanings (see Chap. 3 for definitions). Equation (2-2) has a term for the concentration force (the first term on the right-hand side) and a term for the electrical force (the second term on the right-hand side). It is the difference in electrochemical potential between two regions, 1 and 2, that is of importance. This difference, $\Delta\mu_j$, is calculated by subtracting μ_j for region 1 from μ_j for region 2 (Eq. 2-3). Equation (2-3) is a valid description of the electrochemical potential difference between two different compartments, e.g., the cytoplasm versus the extracellular fluid. **The change in the electrochemical potential is re-**

No Net Diffusion

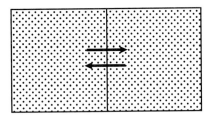

Net Diffusion to Right

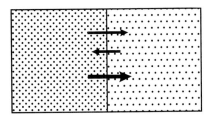

Fig. 2-3. Example of two solutions containing a solute separated by a membrane permeable to that solute. Upper panel: When both solutions have the same solute concentration, the diffusion of solute from right to left is the same as the diffusion of solute from left to right; there is no *net* diffusion. Lower panel: When the solution on the left has a higher solute concentration than the solution on the right, the diffusion of solute from left to right is higher than the diffusion from right to left; there is *net* solute diffusion from left to right *(large arrow).*

lated to the change in Gibbs free energy (**ΔG**), and thus $\Delta\mu_j$ has the same properties as ΔG. That is, when $\Delta\mu_j$ is 0, j in region 1 is at equilibrium with respect to j in region 2, and no net movement of solute j occurs. When $\Delta\mu_j$ is negative, the solute can move spontaneously from region 1 to 2, and when $\Delta\mu_j$ is positive, the solute can move spontaneously in the opposite direction, from region 2 to 1. Further, $\Delta\mu_j$ describes the maximum Gibbs free energy available when a mole of j moves to a region of lower electrochemical potential or, conversely, the cost of moving a mole of j to a region of higher electrochemical potential. Thus the change in the electrochemical potential is a work term, reflecting the amount of work that is needed (or is available) when solute molecules move.

A **gradient** is defined as the change in a parameter in a given direction, say x. Thus the electrochemical potential gradient is defined as $\Delta\mu_j/\Delta x$ (or the equivalent partial dif-

ferential form $\delta\mu_j/\delta x$). Since the electrochemical gradient includes all the forces that will cause a solute to move, $\Delta\mu_j/\Delta x$ is referred to as the **driving force** for the movement of j. The amount of solute that actually moves is often referred to as a **flux,** defined as the amount of solute that moves per unit surface area per unit time (often in units of moles per square centimeter per second). A general rule, of widespread application, is the relationship between the flux and the driving force:

$$\text{flux} = \frac{\text{driving force}}{\text{resistance}}$$

The most common starting point in discussions of **diffusion of charged solutes across a membrane** is the determination of equilibrium. As stated above, equilibrium occurs when $\Delta\mu_j$ (or ΔG) equals zero. Substituting 0 for $\Delta\mu_j$ in Eq. (2-3) and rearranging yields the **Nernst equation** (for a full discussion of the Nernst equation, see Chap. 3):

$$E_j = -(RT/z_jF)\ln(\alpha_{ji}/\alpha_{jo}) \tag{2-4}$$

where E_j is referred to as the Nernst potential **at equilibrium.** The Nernst potential is a **theoretical, calculated** value of membrane potential that must be achieved for ion j to be at equilibrium across a membrane. It can best be understood by realizing that for ion j to be at equilibrium, all the forces acting on it must equal 0. Thus a given concentration gradient of j across the membrane that creates a force for diffusion must be exactly counterbalanced by an electrical force in the opposite direction acting on j (Fig. 2-4, *middle panel*). **If the actual membrane potential (V_m) is equal to the calculated Nernst potential, j will be at equilibrium across the membrane, and no net flux of j will be observed** (since there is no driving force). On the other hand, if the actual membrane potential does not equal the Nernst potential, there will be a net flux of j across the membrane. The driving force for this flux will be the difference between the actual membrane potential and the Nernst potential, and the flux of the ion will result in a current, I_j, across the membrane:

$$I_j = g_j(V_m - E_j) \tag{2-5}$$

where g_j is the **membrane conductance** for j (the reciprocal of membrane resistance) (see Chap. 3 for further discussion). In Eq. (2-5), I_j represents the ionic flux, and $(V_m - E_j)$ is the driving force. Equation (2-5) shows that the

Concentration Force Bigger
Net Flux to Right

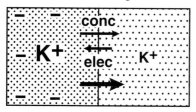

Equilibrium
No Net Flux

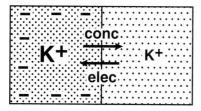

Electrical Force Bigger
Net Flux to Left

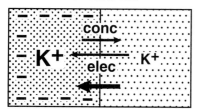

Fig. 2-4. Two compartments containing solutions with different concentrations of potassium ion (K+) are separated by a membrane permeable to K+. The left compartment has a negative membrane potential. In the top panel, the concentration force exceeds the electrical force, and there is a *net* driving force (and therefore net flux) to the right. In the middle panel, the two forces are equal; i.e., there is no net driving force on K+, and therefore, K+ is at equilibrium. In the bottom panel, the electrical force exceeds the concentration force, and there is a net driving force on K+ to the left; i.e., K+ diffuses to the left, against its concentration gradient but down its electrochemical gradient.

magnitude of passive ionic diffusion is directly related to the difference between V_m and the Nernst potential for that ion; the farther an ion is from equilibrium, the greater is its flux across the membrane. The **direction** of flux of an ion

is determined by the difference between V_m and E_j. If V_m is greater than E_j, the flux of j will be in one direction, but if V_m is below E_j, the flux will be in the opposite direction (see Fig. 2-4). **This implies that, depending on V_m, an ion could actually passively diffuse up its concentration gradient although always down its electrochemical gradient** (see Fig. 2-4, *bottom panel*). The ability of a potent electrical gradient to cause an ion to diffuse up a concentration gradient underscores the fact that the driving force for ions (the electrochemical gradient) is the sum of two separate forces.

The **flux of an uncharged solute** is also driven by the electrochemical potential gradient. Equation (2-2) is a description of the electrochemical potential for any solute. If **uncharged** solutes are considered, z_j is 0, and thus the electrical term drops out and γ_j becomes 1, leaving

$$\mu_j = \mu_j^0 + RT \ln(C_j) \qquad (2\text{-}6)$$

The flux of an **uncharged** solute j, J_j, driven by this gradient, is also proportional to the amount of solute present, and can be derived from Eq. (2-6). The resulting equation is **Fick's first law of diffusion** (the negative sign indicates that flux occurs in the direction of decreasing μ):

$$J_j = -U_j RT(dC_j/dx) = -D_j(dC_j/dx) \qquad (2\text{-}7)$$

where u_j is the **mobility** of j (its ease of movement through solution), and D_j is the **diffusion coefficient** of j. Fick's first law states that the flux of any uncharged solute is proportional to the driving force (dC/dx) and that D is the coefficient of proportionality:

$$D = U_j RT \qquad (2\text{-}8)$$

Thus D is directly related to the mobility of j and depends on temperature. D has units of square centimeter per second (cm^2/s).

When the flux of the uncharged solute occurs across a biologic membrane, Fick's first law can be written in a different form. Here, Δx is the thickness of the membrane, and ΔC_j is simply the difference in concentration of j across the membrane. Since the membrane is a lipid environment, it is the concentration difference **in the membrane** that is of importance in driving solute across the membrane. The concentration of j just inside the outer face of the membrane can be calculated as $\beta_j C_{jo}$, and that just inside the inner face of the membrane can be calculated as

$\beta_j C_{ji}$, where C_{jo} and C_{ji} are the concentrations of j in aqueous solution outside and inside the cell, respectively. The term β_j refers to the **partition coefficient** and is the ratio of the concentration of solute j in a lipid environment (usually olive oil) to the concentration of j in water. A high partition coefficient indicates a lipophilic substance, whereas a low value indicates a hydrophilic substance. Given these modifications, Eq. (2-5) can be rewritten for the flux of j across a biologic membrane:

$$J_j = -P_j(C_{ji} - C_{jo}) = P_j(C_{jo} - C_{ji}) \qquad (2\text{-}9)$$

where P_j is defined as the **permeability coefficient** of the membrane for j: $P_j = D_j\beta_j/\Delta x$. P_j will be high when D_j is high, when the substance is lipophilic (β_j is high), and when the membrane is thin (Δx is small). Note that the higher P_j is, the greater will be the flux of j across the membrane (given the same driving force). P_j has units of centimeters per second (cm/s). One of two main properties of a solute molecule will determine its permeability coefficient. Its lipid solubility is most important. If a solute molecule is lipophilic, it will have a large value of β and thus a large P_j, since lipophilic substances will be able to readily enter and move across the lipid bilayer. In addition, a larger molecule will have a lower diffusion coefficient, and thus lower P, than a smaller molecule.

Equation (2-9) indicates that the amount of uncharged solute entering or leaving a cell will be directly related to its **concentration** gradient across the membrane and its permeability coefficient. An influx of j is defined as a positive flux.

Membrane Potential

The movement of uncharged solutes across biologic membranes does not involve charge movement and therefore does not affect the electrical gradient across the membrane. In contast, the movement of ions does involve charge movement, and the current generated by ionic diffusion affects the membrane potential. In fact, **the membrane potential can be understood as the diffusion potential of permeable ions across a membrane.** All ions spontaneously seek equilibrium, and thus an ion whose E_j is different from V_m will move in such a way as to change V_m toward E_j. **For any cell that is permeable to only one ion, the membrane potential will be equal to the Nernst potential for that ion.** However, most cell membranes are permeable to more than one ion. **In a cell with multiple permeable ions, the actual membrane potential will be an intermediate between the Nernst**

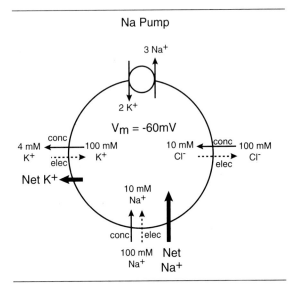

Na Pump

Fig. 2-5. A typical cell with a large $[K^+]_i$ and small $[Na^+]_i$ and $[Cl^-]_i$, with large $[Na^+]_o$ and $[Cl^-]_o$ and small $[K^+]_o$ ($E_K = -84$ mV; $E_{Na} = +60$ mV; $E_{Cl} = -60$ mV). In addition, this cell has a V_m of -60 mV. Under these conditions, there is a net driving force for Na^+ into the cell and for K^+ out of the cell. Cl^- is at equilibrium. The resulting net passive Na^+ influx and K^+ efflux are compensated by active K^+ influx and Na^+ efflux via the Na pump.

potentials of all the permeable ions (see Chap. 3 for a full discussion of membrane potential).

In a cell permeable to only one ion, the membrane potential will be equivalent to the Nernst potential of that ion, and the system will be at **equilibrium** with respect to that ion. A system at equilibrium will remain in that state over time unless acted on by some energy-requiring process. In contrast, in most cells, which are permeable to many ions, it is clear that all the ions cannot be at equilibrium at once. Therefore, whatever the membrane potential, ions will be moving passively across the membrane. This should cause the membrane potential to change over time as ion gradients are degraded. However, measurements show that membrane potential is usually constant over time. Any parameter (like V_m) that is not at equilibrium, but is stable over time, is referred to as being in **steady state.** In a typical cell, both K^+ and Na^+ are not at equilibrium, and there is a passive efflux of K^+ and influx of Na^+. The only way that V_m can remain constant is if some additional process results in a counterbalancing influx of K^+ and efflux of Na^+. In such a case, there would not be any total net currents. Since K^+ influx and Na^+ efflux are both **uphill** (i.e.,

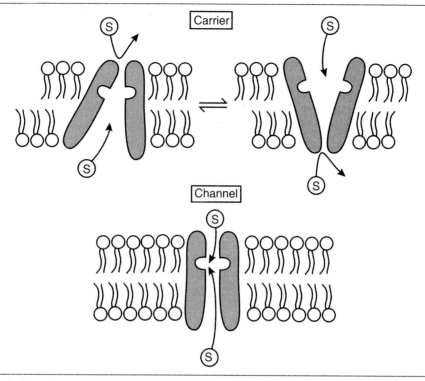

Fig. 2-6. A model of a carrier and a channel. The solute binding site within a *carrier* is accessible to solute molecules on only one side of the membrane at a time. In order for the binding site to be exposed to the solution on the other side of the membrane, the carrier must undergo a conformational change. In contrast, the solute (S) binding site within a *channel* is accessible to solute molecules from both sides of the membrane at the same time (see Chap. 4 for a discussion of channels).

resulting in movement up the electrochemical gradient), the transport that mediates such fluxes requires energy. These fluxes are meditated by the **Na+, K+-ATPase (the Na+ pump)**, which uses the energy from ATP hydrolysis to move K+ into the cell and Na+ out of the cell (Fig. 2-5). This combination of passive ion fluxes **(leaks)** counterbalanced by an energy-requiring transport **(pumps)** is a common way for a cell to maintain a steady state of ion concentrations and has been called, appropriately enough, the **pump-leak model.**

Pathways Responsible for the Transmembrane Movement of Solutes

There are two main ways in which solutes can cross a membrane: either through the lipid bilayer or in associa-

tion with integral membrane proteins. Less significant pathways for fluid and solute movement across membranes involve **exocytosis** and **endocytosis,** which will be discussed in detail later. Solute movement through the lipid bilayer is largely restricted to gases and uncharged lipophilic molecules. The main pathway for most types of solutes to cross cell membranes is in association with integral membrane proteins. These transport proteins are often broadly categorized into two types: **channels** and **carriers.** Both are integral membrane proteins that form a membrane-spanning pathway that allows movement of solute molecules across the membrane. Further, both these transport pathways exhibit a degree of **specificity,** allowing only certain solute molecules to pass. This specificity is generally attributed to a binding site for the particular solute molecule on the transport protein. Only solute molecules that can bind to this site are transported across the membrane. There are two main features that differentiate channels from carriers. The first is that this transport binding site is accessible to solute molecules from both sides of the membrane at the same time in a channel but accessible to only one side at a time in a carrier (Fig. 2-6). This implies that for a carrier to move a solute molecule across the membrane, it must undergo a molecular rearrangement, which requires time. This results in the second distinguishing feature of channels and carriers: Channels have a higher **turnover number** than carriers. The turnover number is the number of solute molecules moved per unit time and is quite high for channels (usually greater than 10^6 per second). For carriers, the turnover number is at most 10^5 per second and usually much lower (e.g., the Na^+ pump may have a turnover number as low as 20 per second).

Channels mediate only passive, downhill movement of solute molecules. While many of these channels may require ATP to function, the transport they mediate is not energy requiring. They include specific channels for K^+, Na^+ and Cl^- that mediate the establishment of membrane potential described above. In addition, voltage-gated channels for Na^+ confer the ability to generate action potentials in nerve and muscle cells, and voltage-gated channels for Ca^{2+} are involved in the prolonged action potential in heart muscle. Channels also play a major role in fluid secretion and absorption by the epithelia in various systems in the body, including the gastrointestinal tract, the kidneys, and the lungs.

Carriers can mediate both passive, downhill transport and uphill transport. Carrier-mediated passive transport is often called **facilitated transport, or facilitated diffusion.** In this type of transport, solute movement is only down the electrochemical gradient, but the carrier increases the rate of transport, i.e., facilitates it. An example of facilitated transport is the insulin-activated glucose carrier in skeletal muscle, which increases the entry of glucose into muscle in response to insulin stimulation.

Uphill transport is also called **active transport,** indicating the requirement for energy in order to move solute molecules up their electrochemical gradient. Active transport can be subdivided into **primary active transport** and **secondary active transport.** In primary active transport, the energy for uphill transport comes **directly** from ATP hydrolysis, and thus the proteins that mediate this transport are called **ATPases** (or pumps). Examples of such transporters include the H^+, K^+-ATPase that is responsible for acidification of the stomach, the Ca^{2+}-ATPase that is responsible for relaxation of muscle contraction, the H^+-ATPase that is responsible for acidification of intracellular vesicles, and the Na^+,K^+-ATPase discussed above.

Secondary active transport, as the name implies, depends only secondarily on the hydrolysis of ATP. In such transport, the uphill movement of one solute is achieved by the downhill movement of another solute. In mammalian cells, Na^+, moving down its gradient, is most commonly used to supply the energy for uphill movement of solute. If the two solutes move in opposite directions (one into the cell and the other out), the transport is called **exchange** (or **antiport**), whereas if the two solute molecules move in the same direction, it is called **cotransport** (or **symport**). Common examples of exchange include the Na^+/H^+ exchange, where the influx of a Na^+ is coupled to the efflux of an H^+; Na^+/Ca^{2+} exchange, where Na^+ influx is coupled to Ca^{2+} efflux; and Cl^-/HCO_3^- exchange (band 3 from red blood cells), which mediates the exchange of Cl^- for HCO_3^-. Common examples of cotransport include Na^+-glucose cotransport, which involves the downhill movement of Na^+ coupled with the marked uptake of glucose in the gastrointestinal tract, and Na^+-K^+-$2Cl^-$ cotransport, which mediates the uptake of Na^+, K^+, and Cl^- (often with water to reestablish cell volume). The downhill movement of other ions than Na^+ can power transporters. For example, K^+-Cl^- cotransport uses the energy obtained from K^+ efflux to move Cl^- out of the cell. This type of transport is referred to as secondary active transport because it depends on ATP hydrolysis only secondarily. Secondary active transport is powered directly by gradients, usually Na^+ or K^+ gradients. However, these gradients are established and maintained only by the consumption of ATP by the Na^+ pump, and thus this form of transport also depends on ATP hydrolysis ultimately.

These transport processes can be further characterized by their ability to generate a current. If transport involves no net current movement, it is called **electroneutral.** Examples of such transport are Na^+/H^+ exchange, where one positive ion enters the cell (Na^+) in exchange for a positive ion (H^+) leaving the cell, and K^+-Cl^- cotransport, where both a positive and negative ion enter the cell together. In contrast, transport processes that involve the movement of net charge are called **electrogenic.** The Na^+ pump is a good example of such a transporter. It mediates the efflux of three Na^+ for the entry of two K^+, thus resulting in the net exit of one positive charge. Likewise, Na^+/Ca^{2+} exchange is believed to involve the entry of three Na^+ for the exit of one Ca^{2+}, resulting in the net influx of one positive charge. These net ion fluxes result in small currents that have been measured and which can affect membrane voltage. For instance, the efflux of net positive charge by the Na^+ pump causes the membrane voltage to **hyperpolarize** (i.e., become more negative), while the net influx of positive charge on the Na^+/Ca^{2+} exchange causes membrane voltage to **depolarize** (i.e., become less negative).

Several membrane transport and channel proteins have been characterized, and certain properties of these proteins are becoming clear. These proteins vary from large to very large proteins, ranging in molecular weight (in daltons) from 80,000 to 110,000 for the Na^+/H^+ exchanger to over 2 million for the Ca^{2+} release channel from mammalian skeletal muscle. Many of the transporters, including the Na^+/H^+, the Na^+/Ca^{2+}, and the Cl^-/HCO_3^- exchangers and the Ca^{2+}-ATPase, have molecular weights between 100,000 and 200,000. Much of the protein is dedicated to helical stretches that are hydrophobic and span the membrane lipid bilayer. Most transport proteins have between 7 (bacteriorhodopsin) and 14 (Cl^-/HCO_3^- exchanger) **membrane-spanning helices** (e.g., see Fig. 4-15). It is believed that these spanning regions form a three-dimensional structure with an aqueous pore through the center. These spanning regions are connected by external and cytoplasmic loops (see Fig. 4-15). Some of these **cytoplasmic loops** are believed to be the sites of binding to cytoskeletal components, regulatory modification (e.g., phosphorylation sites), and binding sites for various components such as adenine nucleotides. The external loops may have sugar moieties bound (**glycosylation sites**) that are important for transport function in some proteins.

While some membrane transport proteins are believed to be a single unit (Na^+/H^+ and Cl^-/HCO_3^- exchangers), many consist of a variety of subunits. For example, Na^+, K^+-ATPase has two different subunits (alpha and beta), the skeletal muscle transverse tubular dihydropyridine-sensitive Ca^{2+} channel (the voltage sensor) has five subunits (two types of alpha, beta, gamma, and delta), and the mitochondrial H^+-ATPase has five distinct subunits (alpha, beta, gamma, delta, and epsilon). The skeletal muscle Ca^{2+} release channel (ryanodine receptor) has four subunits, but they are each identical. With multiple distinct subunits, many of the subunits have specialized functions. For instance, the alpha subunit of the Na^+ pump is the "catalytic" subunit, binding Na^+ and K^+ and mediating their transport. The function of the beta subunit is not as clear, but it is glyco-

sylated, appears to be involved in proper movement of the pump to the surface membrane, and may be involved in cell-cell adhesion.

Summary

The cytoplasm of a cell is separated from the external solution by a lipid bilayer that serves as a barrier to the movement of solutes, as a selectivity filter allowing only certain substances into or out of the cell, and as a communication system between the outside and inside of the cell. Within this lipid bilayer are proteins, some of which serve as pathways for solute movement across the membrane. The movement of uncharged solutes across the membrane is driven by the concentration gradient of the solute; the movement of charged solutes (ions) is driven by both concentration and electrical gradients (i.e., the electrochemical gradient). In fact, the membrane potential of a cell is due to concentration gradients of membrane-permeable ions. The movement of solutes across the membrane can be through channels (purely passive movement) or through mechanisms of active transport (pumps and carriers). These membrane transport proteins have helical regions that span the membrane. Several of these membrane-spanning regions associate in such a way as to form an aqueous pore through the membrane that serves as a pathway for solute movement across the membrane. Pathology results when these movements are abnormal.

Bibliography

Nobel, P. *Introduction to Biophysical Plant Physiology.* San Francisco: W. H. Freeman, 1974.

Schultz, S. G. *Basic Principles of Membrane Transport.* New York: Cambridge University Press, 1980.

Singer, S. J., and Nicholson, G. L. The fluid mosaic model of the structure of cell membranes. *Science* 175:720–731. 1972.

Stein, W. D. *Transport and Diffusion Across Cell Membranes.* New York: Academic Press, 1986.

3 Origin of the Resting Membrane Potential

Nicholas Sperelakis

Objectives

After reading this chapter, you should be able to

Describe the molecular structure and function of the membranes of cells at rest (i.e., not electrically excited)

Explain the maintenance of the cell's internal ion concentrations through the action of ion pumps and exchangers

Explain the production of voltages by separation of ionic charges

Describe the equilibrium potentials for ions distributed across the cell membrane

Identify the driving forces for ionic currents

Explain the meaning of permeability and ionic conductance

List the factors that determine the value of the resting potential

Explain why the resting potential decreases when the potassium ion concentration in the blood plasma is elevated above normal (life-threatening)

Describe the influence of electrogenic pump potentials on the resting potential

Explain how spontaneous pacemaker potentials develop in some cell types

---

The cell membrane exerts tight control over the contractile machinery of muscle cells during the process of **excitation-contraction** (electromechanical) **coupling.** Some drugs and toxins exert primary or secondary effects on the electrical properties of the cell membrane and thereby exert effects on automaticity, arrhythmias, conduction, and force of contraction. Therefore, for an understanding of the mode of action of toxins, therapeutic agents, neurotransmitters, hormones, and plasma electrolytes on the electrical activity of cells, it is necessary to understand the electrical properties and behavior of the cell membrane at rest and during excitation. The first step is to examine the electrical properties of nerve and muscle cells at rest, including the origin of the resting membrane potential, E_m. The resting potential, RP, and action potential, AP, result from properties of the cell membrane and the ion distributions across the cell membrane. The level of the RP has

profound effects on the APs, including amplitude, duration, rate of rise, and propagation velocity (see Chap. 4).

Passive Electrical Properties

Membrane Structure and Composition

The cell membrane is composed of a bimolecular leaflet of phospholipid molecules (e.g., phosphatidylcholine and phosphatidylethanolamine). The nonpolar hydrophobic tails of the phospholipid molecules project toward the middle of the membrane, and the polar hydrophilic heads project toward the edges of the membrane bordering on the water phases (see Fig. 2-1). This orientation is thermodynamically favorable. The lipid bilayer membrane is about 50 to 70 Å thick, and the phospholipid molecules are the right length (30 to 40 Å) to stretch across half the membrane thickness. Cholesterol molecules are highly concentrated in the cell membrane (of animal cells), yielding a phospholipid/cholesterol ratio of about 1.0; these molecules are inserted between the heads of the phospholipid molecules. Large protein molecules are also inserted in the lipid bilayer matrix. Some proteins protrude through the entire membrane thickness (e.g., the Na^+, K^+ -ATPase and the various ion channel proteins). These proteins "float" in the lipid bilayer matrix, and the membrane has fluidity (reciprocal of microviscosity) such that the protein molecules can move around laterally in the plane of the membrane. Thus these floating proteins do not appear to be anchored in one place in most cases.

The outer surface of the cell membrane is lined with strands of mucopolysaccharides (the cell coat, or glycocalyx) that endow the cell with immunochemical properties. The cell coat is highly negatively charged and therefore can bind cations such as Ca^{2+}.

Membrane Capacitance and Resistivity

Artificially made lipid bilayer membranes have a specific **membrane capacitance, C_m,** of 0.4 to 1.0 $\mu F/cm^2$, which is close to the value for biologic membranes. The capacitance of cell membranes is due to the lipid bilayer matrix. A capacitor consists of two parallel-plate conductors separated by a high-resistance dielectric material and has the ability to store electric charges across its two plates. The following equation defines membrane capacitance:

$$C_m = \frac{Q}{V}$$

where Q is the charge (in coulombs) and V is the potential (in volts or millivolts) across the membrane. The higher the dielectric constant,* the greater is the capacitance. As will be illustrated in Chap. 5, membrane capacitance is an important element in determining the velocity of propagation of APs.

The artificial lipid bilayer membrane has a specific resistance several orders of magnitude higher than that of the biologic cell membrane. The membrane resistance is greatly lowered, however, if the bilayer is treated with certain proteins. Therefore, the presence of proteins that span the thickness of the cell membrane must account for the relatively low resistance (high conductance) of the cell

---

*Dielectric constant is a measure of the ability of a material (e.g., lipid bilayer) to shield or reduce the force of interaction between electric charges.

---

membrane. These proteins include the voltage-dependent gated ion channels of the cell membrane.

Membrane Fluidity

The ion transport and electrical properties of the cell membrane are determined by the molecular composition of the membrane. The lipid bilayer matrix even influences the function of the membrane proteins (e.g., the Na^+, K^+-ATPase activity is affected by the surrounding lipid). A high cholesterol content lowers the fluidity of the membrane. The polar portion of cholesterol lodges in the hydrophilic part of the membrane, and the nonpolar part of the planar cholesterol molecule wedges between the fatty acid tails, thus restricting their motion and lowering fluidity. A high degree of unsaturation and branching of the tails of the phospholipid molecules raises the fluidity; chain length also affects fluidity. Phospholipids with unsaturated and branched-chain fatty acids cannot be packed tightly because of steric hindrance due to their greater rigidity; hence such phospholipids increase membrane fluidity.

Low temperature decreases membrane fluidity, as expected. Ca^{2+} and Mg^{2+} may diminish the charge repulsion between the phospholipid head groups; this allows the bilayer molecules to pack more tightly, thereby constraining the motion of the tails and reducing fluidity. Membrane fluidity changes occur in muscle development and in certain disease states, such as cancer, muscular dystrophy (Duchenne type), and myotonic dystrophy.

The hydrophobic portion of local anesthetic molecules may interpose between the phospholipid molecules. This further separates the acyl chain tails, thus reducing the van der Waals forces of interaction between adjacent tails and so increasing the membrane fluidity. The local anesthetics produce a nonselective depression of most conductances of the resting and excited membrane. Part of the depression of ion conductances and Na^+, K^+ -ATPase activity could arise indirectly from the anesthetics' effect on the fluidity of the lipid matrix.

Potential Profile Across Membrane

The cell membrane has **fixed negative charges** at its outer and inner surfaces. The charges are presumably due to acidic phospholipids in the bilayer and to protein molecules either embedded in the membrane or tightly adsorbed to the surface of the membrane. Most proteins have an acid isoelectric point, so they possess a net negative charge at a pH near 7.4. The charge at the outer surface of the cell membrane, with respect to the solution bathing the cell, is known as the **zeta potential.** This charge is responsible for the electrophoresis of cells in an electric field [i.e., the cells moving toward the anode (positive electrode)] because unlike charges attract. The **surface charge** affects the true potential difference across the membrane, as illustrated in Fig. 3-1. At each surface, the fixed charge produces an electric field that extends a short distance into the solution and causes each surface of the membrane to be slightly more negative (by a few millivolts) than the extracellular and intracellular solutions. The potential theoretically recorded by an ideal electrode as it is driven through the solution perpendicular to the membrane surface should become negative as the electrode approaches within a few Angströms of the surface. The potential difference between the membrane surface and the solution declines exponentially as a function of distance from the surface. The magnitude of the potential difference depends on the density of the charge sites (number per unit area); the number of charges is also affected by the ionic strength and pH.

The membrane potential, E_m, measured by an intracellular microelectrode is the potential of the outer solution (Ψ_o, the reference electrode) minus the potential of the inner solution (Ψ_i, the active microelectrode); thus $E_m = \Psi_o - \Psi_i$. The true potential difference across the membrane, E'_m, however, is really that which is directly across the membrane (see Fig. 3-1). If the surface charges at each surface of the membrane are equal, then $E'_m = E_m$.

If the outer surface charge is decreased by extra binding of protons or cations, then the membrane becomes slightly hyperpolarized ($E'_m > E_m$). This effect is not measurable by an intracellular microelectrode. Because the membrane ionic conductances are controlled by the potential difference directly across the membrane (i.e., by E'_m and not by E_m), changes in the surface charges (e.g., by drugs, ionic strength, or pH) can lead to apparent shifts in the threshold potential.

Maintenance of Ion Distributions

Resting Potentials and Ion Distributions

The transmembrane potential in resting nerve and muscle cells varies with cell type. In nerve cells, the **resting potential** (RP) is about –70mV, whereas in skeletal muscle fibers and myocardial cells, the RP is close to –80 mV. The RP or maximum diastolic potential in cardiac Purkinje fibers is somewhat greater (about –90 mV). In smooth muscle cells and nodal cells of the heart, the RP is lower (about –55 mV). The values of the RPs of some nerve and muscle cells are summarized in Table 3-1.

The total ion distributions are listed in Table 3-2. The ionic composition of the extracellular fluid bathing the cells is similar to that of the blood plasma. It is high in Na^+ (about 145 mM), and Cl^- (about 105 to 115 mM) but low in K^+ (about 4.5 mM). The Ca^{2+} concentration is about 2 mM. In contrast, the intracellular fluid has a low concentration of Na^+ (about 15 mM or less) and Cl^- (about 6 to 8 mM) but a high concentration of K^+ (about 140 to 150 mM). In smooth muscle cells, Cl^- concentration is higher (e.g., 30 mM). The free intracellular Ca^{2+} concentration ($[Ca]_i$) is about 10^{-7}M, but during contraction it may rise as high as 10^{-5}M. The total intracellular Ca^{2+} is much higher (about 2

Fig. 3-1. Potential profile across the cell membrane.

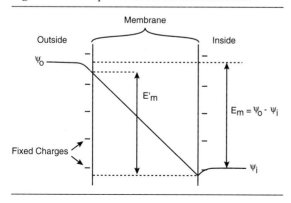

Table 3-1. Comparison of the Resting Potentials in Different Types of Cells

Cell Type	Resting Potential (mV)
Neuron	–70
Skeletal muscle (mammalian)	–80
Skeletal muscle (frog)	–90
Cardiac muscle (atrial and ventricular)	–80
Cardiac Purkinje fiber	–90
Atrioventricular nodal cell	–65
Sinoatrial nodal cell	–55
Smooth muscle cell	–55

Table 3-2. Summary of the Ion Distributions in Most Types of Cells and the Equilibrium Potential Calculated from the Nernst Equation

Ion	Extracellular Concentration (mM)	Intracellular Concentration (mM)	Equilibrium Potential (mV)
Na^+	145	15	+60
Cl^-	110	5.4*	−80
K^+	4.6	150	−92
Ca^{2+}	1.8	0.0001	+129
H^+	0.0001	0.0002	−18

*Assuming Cl^- is passively distributed and the resting potential is −70 mV.

mmol/kg), but most of this is bound to molecules such as proteins or is sequestered in compartments such as mitochondria and the sarcoplasmic reticulum. Most of the intracellular K^+ is free, and it has a diffusion coefficient only slightly less than K^+ in free solution.

Thus, under normal conditions, the cell maintains internal ion concentrations markedly different from those in the medium bathing the cells, and it is these ion concentration differences that create an RP. The existence of the RP enables APs to be produced in those types of cells which are excitable. The ion distributions and related pumps and exchange reactions are depicted in Fig. 3-2.

Inhibition of the Na^+-K^+ pump (e.g., by cardiac glycosides such as digitalis) gradually runs down (depletes) the ion concentration gradients. The cells lose K^+ and gain Na^+, and therefore, the K^+ (E_K) and Na^+ (E_{Na}) equilibrium

Fig. 3-2. Intracellular and extracellular ion distributions in vertebrate myocardial cells and skeletal muscle fibers. Arrows indicate direction of the net electrochemical gradient for each ion species. Phospholamban (PL) is depicted close to the Ca^{2+} pump of the SR and serves to regulate pump activity.

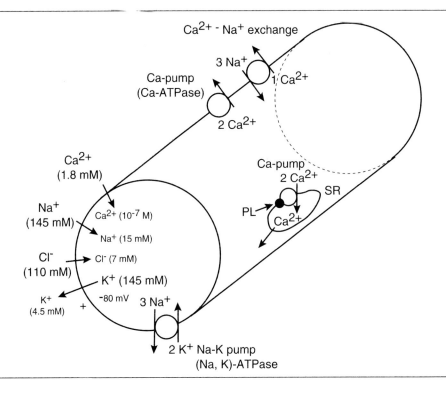

potentials become smaller (see "Equilibrium Potentials"). The cells thus become depolarized, which causes them to gain Cl⁻ (because the intracellular Cl⁻ concentration, $[Cl]_i$, was held low by the large RP) and therefore also water (cells swell) because of the resultant gain in intracellular osmotic strength.

Na⁺-K⁺ Pump

As noted in Chap. 2, the intracellular ion concentrations are maintained differently from those in the extracellular fluid by active ion transport mechanisms that expend metabolic energy to propel specific ions against their concentration or electrochemical gradients. These ion pumps are located in the cell membrane at the cell surface and probably also in the transverse tubular membrane in striated muscle cells. The major ion pump is the **Na⁺-K⁺–linked pump,** which transports Na⁺ out of the cell against its electrochemical gradient while simultaneously transporting K⁺ in against its electrochemical gradient (see Fig. 3-2). The coupling of Na⁺ and K⁺ pumping is obligatory, because if the extracellular K⁺ concentration, $[K]_o$, is zero, the Na⁺ can no longer be pumped out. The coupling ratio of Na⁺ pumped out to K⁺ pumped in is generally 3 : 2. The Na⁺-K⁺ pump is half-inhibited (Michaelis constant, K_m, value) when $[K]_o$ is lowered to about 2mM.

If the ratio were 3 : 3, the pump would be electrically neutral or nonelectrogenic: A potential difference across the membrane would not be produced directly because the pump would pull in three positive charges (K⁺) for every three positive charges (Na⁺) it pushed out. When the ratio is 3 : 2, the pump is electrogenic and directly produces a potential difference that causes E_m to be greater (more negative) than it would be otherwise, solely on the basis of the ion concentration gradients and relative permeabilities.

The driving mechanism for the Na⁺-K⁺ pump is a membrane ATPase, the Na⁺, K⁺-ATPase, which requires both Na⁺ and K⁺ ions for activation. ATP and Na⁺ are thus required at the inner surface of the membrane, and K⁺ is required at the outer surface. A phosphorylated intermediate of Na⁺, K⁺-ATPase occurs in the transport cycle, its phosphorylation being Na⁺ dependent and its dephosphorylation being K⁺ dependent. The pump enzyme usually drives three Na⁺ in and two K⁺ out for each ATP molecule hydrolyzed. Na⁺, K⁺-ATPase is specifically inhibited by the cardiac glycosides (digitalis) acting on the outer surface by competing with K⁺ for the K⁺-binding site. The pump enzyme is also inhibited by sulfhydryl reagents (such as mercurial diuretics).

For short periods, excitability is independent of active ion transport. However, over a period of many minutes, depending on the ratio of surface area to volume of the cell, the resting E_m slowly declines because of gradual dissipation of the ionic gradients. The progressive depolarization depresses the rate of rise of the AP and hence the propagation velocity, and eventually, all excitability is lost. Thus a large RP and excitability, although not immediately dependent on the Na⁺-K⁺ pump, are ultimately dependent on it.

The rate of Na⁺-K⁺ pumping in excitable cells must change with cell activity in order to maintain relatively constant intracellular ion concentrations. A higher frequency of APs results in a greater overall movement of ions down their electrochemical gradients, and these ions must be repumped to maintain the ion distributions. For example, the cells tend to gain Na⁺, Cl⁻, and Ca²⁺ and to lose K⁺. The factors that control the rate of Na⁺-K⁺ pumping include the intracellular Na⁺ concentration and $[K]_o$. In cells with a large surface-area-to-volume ratio (such as small-diameter nonmyelinated axons), $[Na]_i$ may increase by a relatively large percentage during a train of APs, and this would stimulate the pumping rate. Likewise, an extracellular accumulation of K⁺ occurs and also stimulates the pump.

Chloride Ion Distribution

In many invertebrate and vertebrate nerve or muscle cells, Cl⁻ does not appear to be actively transported; i.e., there is no Cl⁻ pump (no Cl⁻-ATPase). In such cases, Cl⁻ distributes itself passively (no energy used) in accordance with E_m: The Cl⁻ equilibrium potential (E_{Cl}) is equal to E_m in a resting cell. For example, in mammalian myocardial cells, Cl⁻ also seems to be close to passive distribution, because $[Cl]_i$ is at or only slightly above the value predicted from the resting E_m. When passively distributed, $[Cl]_i$ is low because the negative potential inside the cell (the RP) pushes out the negatively charged Cl⁻ (like charges repel) until the Cl⁻ distribution is at equilibrium with the resting E_m. Hence, for a resting E_m of –80 mV and an extracellular Cl⁻ concentration ($[Cl]_o$) of 110 mM, $[Cl]_i$ would be at 5.4 mM (see section on Nernst equation). However, during the AP, the inside of the cell goes in a positive direction, and a net Cl⁻ influx (outward Cl⁻ current) occurs and thus increases $[Cl]_i$. The magnitude of the Cl⁻ influx (I_{Cl}) depends on the Cl⁻ conductance (g_{Cl}) of the membrane (see "Membrane Ionic Currents"). Thus the average $[Cl]_i$ in excitable cells should depend on the frequency and duration of the AP, i.e, on the mean E_m averaged over many AP cycles. In those types of cells in which $[Cl]_i$ is much higher than the value predicted from passive distribution, this elevated $[Cl]_i$ may be due to an exchange carrier (e.g., Cl⁻/bicarbonate exchange) or cotransporter (e.g., Na⁺, K⁺-Cl₂).

Calcium Ion Distribution

Need for Calcium Pumps

For the positively charged Ca^{2+}, there must be some mechanism for removing Ca^{2+} from the cytoplasm. Otherwise, the cell would continue to gain Ca^{2+} until there was no electrochemical gradient for net influx of Ca^{2+}. Therefore, one or more **Ca^{2+} pumps** must be in operation. The sarcoplasmic reticulum membrane contains a Ca^{2+}-activated ATPase that actively pumps two Ca^{2+} from the myoplasm into the sarcoplasmic reticulum lumen at the expense of one ATP and is capable of reducing the $[Ca]_i$ to less than 10^{-7} M. The Ca-ATPase of the sarcoplasmic reticulum is regulated by an associated low-molecular-weight protein, **phospholamban.** Phospholamban is phosphorylated by cyclic adenosine 5'-monophosphate–dependent protein kinase and, when phosphorylated, stimulates the Ca-ATPase and Ca^{2+} pumping (by removing inhibition). The sequestration of Ca^{2+} by the sarcoplasmic reticulum is essential for muscle relaxation. However, the resting Ca^{2+} influx and the extra Ca^{2+} influx that occurs with each AP must be returned to the interstitial fluid. Mechanisms proposed for this include Ca-ATPase and the Ca^{2+}-Na^+ exchanger present in the sarcolemma. The Ca-ATPase in the sarcolemma actively transports two Ca^{2+} outward against an electrochemical gradient, utilizing one ATP in the process. Phospholamban is not associated with the sarcolemmal Ca-ATPase.

Ca^{2+}/Na^+ Exchange Reaction

The **Ca^{2+}/Na^+ exchange reaction** exchanges one internal Ca^{2+} for three external Na^+ via a membrane carrier molecule (see Fig. 3-2). This reaction is facilitated by ATP, but ATP is not hydrolyzed (consumed) in this reaction. Instead, the energy for the transport of Ca^{2+} against its large electrochemical gradient is derived from the Na^+ electrochemical gradient. That is, the uphill transport of Ca^{2+} is coupled with the downhill movement of Na^+. Therefore, the energy required for this Ca^{2+} movement is effectively derived from Na^+,K^+-ATPase. Thus the Na^+-K^+ pump, which uses ATP to maintain the Na^+ electrochemical gradient, indirectly helps to maintain the Ca^{2+} electrochemical gradient. Hence the inward Na^+ leak is greater than it would be otherwise.

The energy cost (in joules per mole) for pumping Ca^{2+} out of the cytoplasm is directly proportional to its electrochemical gradient, namely,

$$\Delta G_{Ca} = zF(E_m - E_{Ca})$$

where ΔG_{Ca} is the change in free energy for Ca^{2+}, and zF is coulombs per mole. The energy available from the Na^+ distribution is directly proportional to its electrochemical gradient:

$$\Delta G_{Na} = zF(E_m - E_{Na})$$

Depending on the exact values of $[Na]_i$ and $[Ca]_i$ at rest, the energetics would be about adequate for an exchange ratio of three Na^+ to one Ca^{2+}. An exchange ratio of 3 : 1 produces a small depolarization, because there is one net positive charge moving inward for every cycle of the carrier; i.e., a net inward current is produced.

The exchange reaction depends on relative concentrations of Ca^{2+} and Na^+ on each side of the membrane and on relative affinities of the binding sites to Ca^{2+} and Na^+. Because of this Ca^{2+}/Na^+ exchange reaction, whenever the cell gains Na^+, it also gains Ca^{2+}, because the Na^+ electrochemical gradient is reduced and the outward Ca^{2+} movement slows down. In addition, when the membrane is depolarized during the long-duration AP in cardiac cells, the exchange carriers exchange the ions in reverse (internal Na^+ for external Ca^{2+}) and thus increase Ca^{2+} influx. The net effect of both mechanisms is to elevate $[Ca]_i$. The Ca^{2+}/Na^+ exchange process has been proposed as the mechanism that stimulates contraction of the heart resulting from cardiac glycoside inhibition of the Na^+-K^+ pump.

Equilibrium Potentials and the Nernst Equation

For each ionic species distributed unequally across the cell membrane, an **equilibrium potential** (E_i), or battery, can be calculated for that ion from the Nernst equation (for 37°C):

$$E_i = \frac{-61\,mV}{z} \log \frac{C_i}{C_o}$$

where C_i is the intracellular concentration of the ion, C_o is the extracellular concentration, and z is the valence of the ion (with sign). The –61-mV constant (2.303RT/F) becomes –59 mV at 22°C [R is the gas constant (8.3 joules/mole·deg K), T is the absolute temperature (deg K = 273 + deg C), F is the Faraday constant (96,500 C/equiv; zF = C/mol), and 2.303 is the conversion factor for natural log to $\log_{10}$]. The Nernst equation defines the potential difference (electrical force) that would exactly oppose the concentration gradient (diffusion force). Only very small charge separation ([Q]) in coulombs) is required to build up a very large potential difference: $E_m = Q/C_m$, where C_m is the membrane capacitance. For the ion distributions given in Table 3-2, the approximate equilibrium potentials are E_{Na} = +60 mV, E_{Ca} = +129 mV, E_K = –92 mV, and E_{Cl} = –80 mV (Fig. 3-3). The sign of the equilibrium potential represents the inside of the cell with reference to the outside.

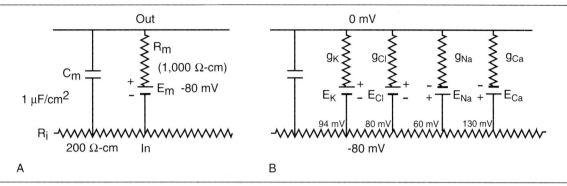

Fig. 3-3. Electrical equivalent circuits for a cell membrane at rest. (A) Simplified circuit of membrane. The membrane serves as a parallel resistance-capacitance circuit, the membrane resistance (R_m) being in parallel with the membrane capacitance (C_m). Resting potential (E_m) is represented by an 80-mV battery in series with the membrane resistance, the negative pole facing inward (R_i = internal longitudinal resistivity). (B) Expanded circuit. Membrane resistance is divided into four parts, one representing each of the four major ions of importance: K^+, Cl^-, Na^+, and Ca^{2+}. These ion resistances are depicted as their reciprocals, namely, ion conductances (g_K, g_{Cl}, g_{Na}, and g_{Ca}) and represent independent pathways for permeation of each ion through the resting membrane. Equilibrium potential for each ion, determined solely by the ion distribution in the steady-state and calculated from the Nernst equation, is shown in series with the conductance path for that ion. The resting potential is determined by the equilibrium potentials and by the relative conductances.

In a two-compartment system separated by a membrane, the side of higher concentration becomes negative for positive ions (cations) and positive for negative ions (anions). Any ion with an E_i different from the RP (e.g., –80 mV for a myocardial cell or skeletal muscle fiber) is off-equilibrium and therefore must effectively be pumped at the expense of energy. In a myocardial cell, only Cl^- appears to be at or near equilibrium, whereas Na^+, K^+, and Ca^{2+} are actively transported. Even H^+ is off-equilibrium E_H being closer to zero potential (see Table 3-2). If H^+ were passively distributed, the negative intracellular potential would cause the H^+ concentration ($[H]_i$) to be much greater, and therefore, the cell interior more acidic. The mechanism for development of the equilibrium potential is depicted in Fig. 3-4.

Fig. 3-4. (A) Illustration of the potential that develops across an artificial membrane containing negatively charged pores. The membrane is impermeable to Cl^- ions but permeable to cations such as K^+. The concentration gradient for K^+ causes a potential to be generated, the side of higher K^+ concentration becoming negative (see text for an elaboration of the Nernst equation). Continued on page 30.

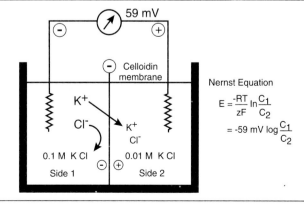

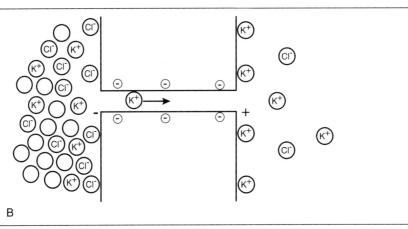

B

Fig. 3-4. (B) Expanded diagram of a water-filled pore in the membrane showing the permeability to K⁺ but lack of penetration of Cl⁻. The potential difference is generated by the charge separation, a slight excess of K⁺ being held close to the right-hand surface of the membrane; a slight excess of Cl⁻ ions is clustered close to the left-hand surface.

Electrochemical Driving Forces and Membrane Ionic Currents

The electrochemical driving force for each species of ion is the algebraic difference between its equilibrium potential (E_i) and E_m. The total driving force is the sum of two forces: an electrical force (the negative potential in a cell at rest tends to pull in positively charged ions because unlike charges attract) and a diffusion force (based on the concentration gradient) (Fig. 3-5). Thus, in a resting myocardial or skeletal muscle cell, the driving force for Na⁺ is $(E_m - E_{Na}) = -80$ mV $- (-60$ mV$) = -140$ mV. The negative sign means that the driving force is in the direction that brings about the net movement of Na⁺ inward. The driving force for Ca²⁺ is $(E_m - E_{Ca}) = -80$ mV $- (+ 129$ mV$) = -209$ mV. The driving force for K⁺ is $(E_m - E_K) = -80$ mV $- (-92$ mV$) = +12$ mV; hence the driving force for K⁺ is small and directed outward. For a cell at rest, and if Cl⁻ is distributed passively, the driving force for Cl⁻ is nearly zero: $(E_m - E_{Cl}) = -80$ mV $- (-80$ mV$) = 0$. However, during the AP, when E_m is changing, the driving force for Cl⁻ becomes large, and there is a net driving force for inward Cl⁻ movement (Cl⁻ influx is an outward Cl⁻ current). Similarly, the driving force for K⁺ outward movement increases during the AP, whereas those for Na⁺ and Ca²⁺ decrease.

The net current, I, for each ionic species is equal to its driving force times its conductance (g, reciprocal of the resistance) through the membrane. This is essentially Ohm's law, I = V/R = g • V, modified to reflect the fact that in an electrolytic system the total force acting to drive net movement of a charged particle must take into account both the

Fig. 3-5. Representation of the electrochemical driving forces for Na⁺, Ca²⁺, K⁺, and Cl⁻. The equilibrium potential for each ion was calculated from the Nernst equation for its extracellular and intracellular ion concentrations. The electrochemical driving force for an ion is the difference between its equilibrium potential and the membrane potential (E_m): $E_i - E_m$.

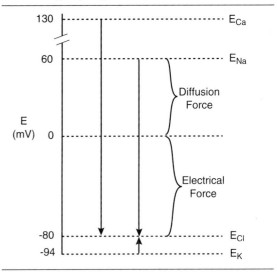

electric and the concentration (or chemical) force. Thus, for the four ions, the net current can be expressed as

$$I_{Na} = g_{Na} (E_m - E_{Na})$$
$$I_{Ca} = g_{Ca} (E_m - E_{Ca})$$
$$I_K = g_K (E_m - E_K)$$
$$I_{Cl} = g_{Cl} (E_m - E_{Cl})$$

In a resting cell, Cl^- and Ca^{2+} can be neglected, and the Na^+ current (inward) must be equal and opposite to the K^+ current (outward) in order to maintain a steady RP:

$$I_K = -I_{Na}$$

Thus, although the resting membrane has a driving force for Na^+ much greater than that for K^+, g_K is much larger than g_{Na}, so the currents are equal. Hence there is a continual leak of Na^+ inward and K^+ outward, and the system would run down even in a resting cell if active pumping were blocked. Because the ratio of the Na^+/K^+ driving forces (-140 mV/-12 mV) is about 12, the ratio of conductances (g_{Na}/g_K) is about 1 : 12. The fact that g_K is much greater than g_{Na} accounts for the RP being closer to the E_K than the E_{Na}.

The cell membrane of some cells (e.g., myocardial) has at least two separate voltage-dependent K^+ channels. One channel, the so-called **anomalous rectifier**, closes with depolarization. This channel is responsible for the rapid decrease in K^+ conductance upon depolarization. The second type of voltage-dependent K^+ channel, which is commonly found in excitable membranes, slowly opens (increasing total g_K) upon depolarization, the so-called **delayed rectifier**. This channel allows K^+ to pass outward down its electrochemical gradient. In cardiac muscle, this delayed rectifier channel turns on much more slowly than it does in nerve or skeletal muscle, and the activation of this current terminates the AP plateau.

Determination of Resting Potential

For given ion distributions, which normally remain nearly constant under usual steady-state conditions, the **resting potential** is determined by the relative membrane conductances (g) or permeabilities (P) for Na^+ and K^+. That is, the RP (about -80 mV in cardiac muscle and skeletal muscle) is close to the E_K (about -92 mV) because $g_K \gg g_{Na}$ or $P_K \gg P_{Na}$. (There is a direct proportionality between permeabilities and conductances at constant E_m and concentrations.) From simple circuit analysis (using Ohm's law and

Kirchhoff's laws), this can be proven true. Therefore, the membrane potential is always closer to the battery (E_i) having the lowest resistance (highest conductance) in series with it (see Figs. 3-3 and 3-5). In the resting membrane this battery is E_K, whereas in the excited membrane it will be E_{Na} (or E_{Ca}) because there is a large increase in g_{Na} (and/or g_{Ca}) during the AP.

Any ion that is passively distributed across the membrane cannot determine the RP; instead, the RP determines the distribution of that ion. Therefore, Cl^- is essentially not a factor in the RP for neurons, myocardial cells, and skeletal muscle fibers, because it seems to be nearly passively distributed. However, transient net movements of Cl^- across the membrane do influence E_m [e.g., washout of Cl^- (in Cl^--free solution) produces a transient depolarization, and reintroduction of Cl^- produces a hyperpolarization], and Cl^- movement is involved in production of some inhibitory postsynaptic potentials. Because of its relatively low resting conductance, the Ca^{2+} distribution has only a relatively small effect on the RP.

Therefore, a simplified version of the Goldman-Hodgkin-Katz **constant-field equation** can be given (for 37°C):

$$E_m = -61 \,\text{mV} \log \frac{[K]_i + \dfrac{P_{Na}}{P_K}[Na]_i}{[K]_o + \dfrac{P_{Na}}{P_K}[Na]_o}$$

This equation shows that for a given ion distribution, the resting E_m is determined by the P_{Na}/P_K ratio, or the relative permeability of the membrane to Na^+ and K^+. For myocardial cells and skeletal muscle fibers, the P_{Na}/P_K ratio is about 0.04, whereas for nodal cells of the heart and smooth muscle cells, this ratio is between 0.10 and 0.20. In the constant-field equation, the numerator of the log term will be dominated by the $[K]_i$ term, since the $(P_{Na}/P_K)[Na]_i$ term is very small. This relationship accounts for the deviation of the E_m versus log $[K]_o$ curve from a straight line (having a slope of 61 mV/decade) in normal Ringer's solution (Fig. 3-6). When $[K]_o$ is elevated ($[Na]_o$ reduced by an equimolar amount), the denominator becomes increasingly dominated by the $[K]_o$ term and decreasingly by the $P_{Na}/P_K [Na]_o$ term. Therefore, in bathing solutions containing high K^+ concentrations, the constant-field equation approaches the simple Nernst equation for K^+, and E_m approaches E_K. As $[K]_o$ is raised stepwise, E_K becomes correspondingly reduced because $[K]_i$ stays relatively constant; therefore, the membrane becomes increasingly depolarized (see Fig. 3-6).

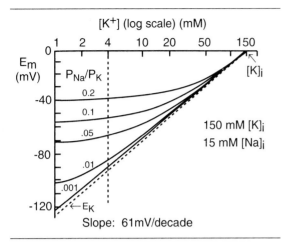

Fig. 3-6. Theoretical curves calculated from the Goldman-Hodgkin-Katz constant-field equation for the resting potential (E_m) as a function of the extracellular K^+ concentration ($[K]_o$). The family of curves is given for the various relative membrane permeabilities to Na^+ and K^+ (P_{Na}/P_K) (0.001, 0.01, 0.05, 0.1, and 0.2). E_K was calculated from the Nernst equation *(broken straight line)*. The curves were calculated for a $[K]_i$ of 150 mM and a $[Na]_i$ of 15 mM. Calculations made holding $[K]_o$ and $[Na]_o$ constant at 154 mM (i.e., as $[K]_o$ was elevated, $[Na]_o$ was lowered by an equimolar amount). The point at which E_m is zero gives $[K]_i$.

An alternative method of approximating the RP (E_m) is by the **chord-conductance equation:**

$$E_m = \left[\frac{g_K}{g_K + g_{Na}}\right]E_K + \left[\frac{g_{Na}}{g_K + g_{Na}}\right]E_{Na}$$

This equation can be derived for the condition when net current is zero ($I_{Na} + I_K = 0$) and again illustrates the important fact that the g_K/g_{Na} ratio determines the RP. When $g_K \gg g_{Na}$, E_m is close to E_K; conversely, when $g_{Na} \gg g_K$ (as during the AP spike), E_m shifts close to E_{Na} (or to E_{Ca} in the case of many smooth muscle cells).

Electrogenic Sodium Pump Potentials

Because two K^+ are usually pumped in for every three Na^+ pumped out, the pump is electrogenic; i.e., it produces a net current (and hence potential) across the membrane. If the Na^+-K^+ pump is inhibited for a short period, the RP is equal to the **net diffusion potential,** E_{diff}, as determined by the ion concentration gradients for K^+ and Na^+ and by the relative P_K and P_{Na}. However, a direct contribution of the pump to the resting E_m normally occurs. For example, if the Na^+-K^+ pump is blocked by ouabain, there usually is an immediate depolarization of between 2 and 16 mV, depending on the type of cell. The contribution of the electrogenic pump potential, V_p, to E_m (ΔV_p) is only a few millivolts in myocardial cells; the contribution is greater in smooth muscle (e.g., 8 mV) and even greater in mammalian skeletal muscle (e.g., up to 16 mV). Blockade of the Na^+-K^+ pump produces a small immediate depolarization of about 2 to 16 mV, depending on cell type, representing the contribution of V_p to E_m (ΔV_p). Thus, although the direct contribution of the V_p to the measured resting E_m is relatively small under physiologic conditions, it is very important, especially under nonphysiologic conditions. The electrogenic pump attempts to hold the RP constant despite dissipating ionic gradients. Thus the V_p delays depolarization under adverse conditions (e.g., ischemia and hypoxia) and speeds repolarization to the normal RP during recovery. It is crucial that the excitable cell maintains its normal RP as much as possible because of the effect of small depolarizations on AP rate of rise, conduction velocity, and rate of firing of pacemaker cells.

The relationship between RP and electrogenic pump current is

$$E_m = E_{diff} + R_m I_p$$
$$= E_{diff} + \Delta V_p$$

where I_p is the net pump current, and ΔV_p is the voltage contribution of the electrogenic pump to E_m. This equation states that E_m is the sum of E_{diff} and a voltage drop produced by the electrogenic pump current across the membrane resistance, R_m.

The density of Na^+-K^+ pump sites, estimated by specific binding of [^{3}H]ouabain, is usually about 700 to 1000/μm^2 (much greater than that of Na^+ and K^+ channels), and the turnover rate of the pump is 20 to 100 per second. The net pump current, I_p, is about 20 pmol/cm^2 • s or about 2 μA/cm^2 (20×10^{-12} mol/s • cm^2 x 0.965 x 10^5C/mol). If R_m were 1000 ohm • cm^2, the ΔV_p would be 2 mV.

Sinusoidal oscillations in the Na^+-K^+ pumping rate, produced by changes in $[Na]_i$, would cause oscillations in E_m that could exert important control over the spontaneous firing of the cell.

Pacemaker Potentials and Automaticity

To maintain a steady RP, the outward K^+ current (I_K) must be equal and opposite to the inward current, primarily Na^+ (I_{Na}) (but also Ca^{2+}), assuming Cl^- is passively distributed: $I_K = -I_{Na}$. If the inward current exceeds the outward current, then the membrane will depolarize along a certain time course (i.e., slope of the pacemaker potential), depending on the excess (or net) inward current. For the inward current to exceed the outward current (i.e., to achieve a net inward current), either the inward current can be increased or the outward K^+ current can be decreased. Both these mechanisms are used for genesis of **pacemaker potentials** (automaticity). For example, if an agent increases the resting g_K in cells, then the outward K^+ current is increased, the membrane hyperpolarizes, and the slope of the pacemaker potential decreases, thus reducing the frequency of firing. A prerequisite for automaticity is that the cells must have a relatively low g_{Cl}, as is the case with most types of heart cells and neurons. A high g_{Cl} clamps E_m, making it difficult for a pacemaker potential to develop.

The pacemaker depolarization in cells is usually linear (or a ramp). Accommodation does not occur in a pacemaker cell; the cell fires, no matter how slowly E_m is brought to the threshold potential. In any pacemaker cell, if the membrane is hyperpolarized by a current pulse, the frequency of spontaneous firing is slowed and stopped; i.e., automaticity is suppressed at high RPs. Conversely, application of depolarizing current increases the frequency of discharge. Thus the slope of the pacemaker potential is exquisitely sensitive to small changes in E_m.

Summary

Most of the factors that determine or influence the RP of cells have been discussed in this chapter. The structural and chemical composition of the cell membrane were correlated with the membrane's resistive and capacitive properties. The factors that determine the intracellular ion concentrations in cells were examined, including the Na^+-K^+ pump, the Ca^{2+}/Na^+ exchange/reaction, and a sarcolemmal Ca^{2+} pump. Na^+,K^+-ATPase requires both Na^+ and K^+ for activity and transports three Na^+ outward and usually two K^+ inward per ATP hydrolyzed. Cardiac glycosides are specific blockers of this transport ATPase. The Na^+-K^+ pump is only indirectly related to excitability, through its role in maintaining the Na^+ and K^+ concentration gradients. The carrier-mediated Ca^{2+}/Na^+ exchange reaction, which exchanges one internal Ca^{2+} for three external Na^+, is driven by the Na^+ electrochemical gradient (i.e., the energy for removing internal Ca^{2+} by this mechanism ultimately comes from Na^+,K^+-ATPase).

The mechanism whereby the ionic distributions give rise to diffusion potentials was discussed, as were the factors that determine the magnitude and polarity of each equilibrium potential (E_i). The E_i for any ion and the transmembrane potential determine the total electrochemical driving force for that ion. The product of this driving force and the membrane conductance for that ion determines the net ionic current or flux. The net ionic movement can be inward or outward across the membrane, depending on the direction of the electrochemical gradient. The key factor that determines the RP is the relative permeability of the various ions, particularly of K^+ and Na^+, i.e., the P_{Na}/P_K ratio (or g_{Na}/g_K ratio), as calculated from the Goldman-Hodgkin-Katz constant-field equation. In some cells Cl^- is distributed passively in accordance with the E_m; in other cells the $[Cl]_i$ is higher than that predicted from the E_m, thus giving an E_{Cl} value less than the RP. If Cl^- is passively distributed, it cannot determine the RP, but transient net movements of Cl^- (e.g., during the AP) can affect the E_m.

The degree of contribution of the Na^+-K^+ pump to the RP depends on the coupling ratio of Na^+ pumped out to K^+ pumped in, the turnover rate of the pump, the density of pump sites, and the magnitude of the membrane resistance. The rate of Na^+-K^+ pumping is controlled by $[Na]_i$ and by $[K]_o$. The contributions of the electrogenic pump current to the measured RP of myocardial cells and neurons is generally small. The electrogenic pump potential might be physiologically important under certain conditions that tend to depolarize the cells, such as transient ischemia or hypoxia; the actual depolarization produced may be less because of the pump potential.

Elevation of $[K]_o$ above the normal concentration of about 4.5 mM decreases E_K, as predicted from the Nernst equation, and depolarization is produced. Since the RP is the potential energy storehouse that is drawn on for production of APs, the rate of rise and propagation velocity of the APs are critically dependent on the level of the RP.

Bibliography

Sperelakis, N. Origin of the cardiac resting potential. In: R. M. Berne and N. Sperelakis, eds., *Handbook of Physiology, The Cardiovascular System*, Vol. 1: *The Heart.* Bethesda, Md.: American Physiological Society, 1979. Pp. 187–267.

Sperelakis, N. Basis of the resting potential. In: N. Sperelakis, ed., *Physiology and Pathophysiology of the Heart,* 3rd ed. Norwell, Mass.: Kluwer, 1994. Pp. 55–76.

Sperelakis, N. and Fabiato, A. Electrophysiology and excitation-contraction coupling in skeletal muscle. In: C. Roussos and P. Macklem, eds., *The Thorax: Vital Pump.* New York: Dekker, 1985. Pp. 45–113.

4 Basis of Membrane Excitability

Nicholas Sperelakis

Objectives

After reading this chapter, you should be able to

Describe the molecular structure and function of ion channels in the cell membrane

Explain how action potentials are generated

List the properties of the action potentials

Explain the importance of the resting potential on the action and its velocity of propagation

Explain why elevation of the potassium ion concentration above normal in the blood plasma has life-threatening consequences

---

Excitability is an intrinsic membrane property that allows a cell to generate an electric signal or action potential (AP) in response to environmental stimuli of sufficient magnitude. The highly elongated nerve axon transmits information over long distances in the form of APs. The AP mechanism is required in order to propagate a uniform depolarization in a nondecremental manner. In muscle cells, the AP spreads excitation rapidly over the entire cell surface and is involved in triggering contraction.

The energy source for the generation of the AP is stored in the excitable cell itself. The initial depolarization, caused by a given stimulus, merely triggers the intrinsic AP mechanism. The immediate source of energy (or battery) for the AP comes from the transmembrane ionic gradients for K^+ and Na^+. The K^+ concentration gradient is mainly responsible for generating the resting potential, which causes an excess of negative charge to be built up on the inner surface of the membrane. Upon depolarization to threshold, the Na^+ ion electrical and chemical driving forces, which are directed inward, cause a large and rapid inward Na^+ current that generates the AP upstroke. Over a longer time frame, the Na^+-K^+ pump is responsible for the generation and maintenance of the Na^+ and K^+ ionic gradients and for their restoration following prolonged repetitive AP activity. The Na^+-K^+ pump derives chemical energy from the hydrolysis of adenosine triphosphate (ATP).

Important technical developments have led to significant advances in the understanding of the basis of membrane excitability. In the early 1900s, Julius Bernstein proposed that at rest, the excitable cell membrane was selectively permeable to K^+ (hence the resting potential) and that during excitation the membrane became permeable to all ions. Several years earlier, Overton had demonstrated that Na^+ was essential for excitability. However, without a means to directly measure the transmembrane potential during excitation, Bernstein's and Overton's membrane hypothesis could not be tested. By the 1940s, improvements had been achieved in electronic instrumentation, and biophysicists began to study the squid giant axon (500–1000 µm in diameter), which permitted insertion of intracellular electrodes, yielding the first measurements of the true transmembrane potential (potential difference between an intracellular and an extracellular electrode). These findings were applied successfully to neurons from the vertebrate nervous system, whose much smaller diameter (1–20 µm) made direct experimentation difficult at that time.

The AP parameters, including **overshoot, duration,** and **rate of rise,** are characteristic for each type of excitable cell. For example, the duration of the AP of the squid giant axon is about 1.0 msec, whereas the cardiac AP lasts for over 100 msec. These differences in the APs subserve the functions performed by the different excitable tissues. The overshoot and a hyperpolarizing potential following the spike are illustrated in Fig. 4-1.

Fig. 4-1. Recording the transmembrane potential (E_m) of a squid giant nerve axon, measured as the difference in potential between the intracellular and extracellular electrodes. When the microelectrode is outside the axon, it measures 0 mV (segment a). As the electrode is advanced and crosses the membrane, the resting potential of –70 mV is measured (segment b). The cell membrane makes a tight seal around the glass electrode. Stimulation (*arrow*) elicits an AP with a hyperpolarizing afterpotential.

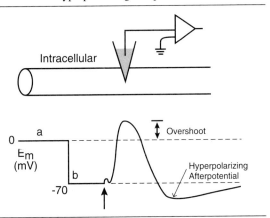

Action Potential Characteristics
Threshold and All-or-None Property

Nerve membrane responses near the site of application of brief current pulses vary depending on the magnitude and direction of the stimulating pulses (Fig. 4-2). Inward currents produce hyperpolarization, and outward currents produce depolarization. A **subthreshold** depolarization is defined as one that does not reach threshold and therefore does not elicit an AP. Subthreshold depolarizing responses are graded in magnitude according to the stimulus current intensity. However, a somewhat greater-intensity stimulating current produces a depolarizing response with a different waveform and a longer-lasting duration. This response is referred to as the **local excitatory state** (see Fig. 4-2). It occurs when a small area of the membrane near the stimulus electrode begins to become excited, but it is not yet sufficient to generate an AP. This local membrane activity is not propagated. A slightly greater stimulus is, however, sufficient to bring the membrane potential of a large enough membrane area to the **threshold potential,** thereby initiating an **all-or-none** AP. With regard to the applied stimulus, outward current depolarizes the membrane, whereas when threshold has been exceeded and an active excitatory response is in progress, inward currents are depolarizing.

Strength-Duration Curve

Whether the threshold potential is reached depends on the amount of charge transferred across the membrane.

Fig. 4-2. Initiation of the nerve impulse by membrane depolarization. (A) Membrane responses to depolarizing and hyperpolarizing current pulses are shown. The nonlinear local excitatory response occurs just below the threshold (V_{th}) for the all-or-none action potential. (B) Illustration of the local excitatory response (L.E.R.) obtained by subtraction of the membrane responses to hyperpolarizing current pulses from the responses to depolarizing pulses.

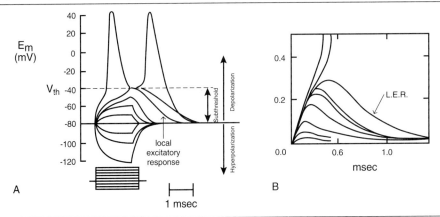

Figure 4-3 shows that the total charge transfer across the membrane necessary to produce excitation is approximately constant, since charge moved equals current times time ($Q = I \times T$). This relationship is known as the **strength-duration curve,** and it can be derived from the equation for the exponential charge of the membrane capacitance. The strength-duration curve deals only with the stimulus parameters (i.e., strength and duration of the applied current pulses) necessary to bring the membrane to threshold. It shows that the greater the duration of the applied pulse, the smaller is the current intensity required to just excite the fiber. The asymptote parallel to the X-axis is the **rheobase,** which is the lowest intensity of current capable of producing excitation, even when the current is applied for an infinite time (greater than 10 msec for myelinated nerve fibers). The asymptote parallel to the Y-axis is the **minimal stimulation time** and is the shortest duration of stimulation capable of producing excitation, even when huge currents are applied.

The rheobase is useless when comparing the excitability of one nerve with another because only the relative current intensity is meaningful. Furthermore, it is difficult to measure the stimulation time of a current of rheobasic strength because it is an asymptote. Thus a graphic measurement is made of the *time* during which a stimulus of double the rheobasic strength must act in order to reach threshold. This time is the **chronaxie.** Chronaxie values tend to remain constant regardless of the geometry of the stimulating electrodes. The shorter the chronaxie, the more excitable is the fiber. Some nerve disorders in humans can be detected early by changes observed in the chronaxies.

The membrane time constant τ_m is proportional to the chronaxie.

The strength-duration curve shows that current pulses of very short duration (e.g., <0.01 msec) are less effective for stimulation. Thus a sinusoidal alternating current (ac) at frequencies above 100,000 Hz is less capable of stimulation. Hence very high frequency ac has less tendency to electrocute, but the energy of such currents can be dissipated as heat in body tissues and thus formerly was used in diathermy for therapeutic warming of injured tissues.

Refractoriness

Once an AP is initiated, a characteristic time must elapse before a second AP can be generated. This time interval is called the **refractory period,** and its value depends on the type of excitable cell. Cells with long-duration APs (e.g., myocardial cells) have long refractory periods; cells with brief APs (e.g., neurons) have short refractory periods. That is, the refractory periods are proportional to the AP duration. Two types of refractory periods are usually defined: an **absolute refractory period** and a **relative refractory period** (Fig. 4-4.) The *absolute* refractory period denotes the interval during which a second AP cannot be elicited, regardless of the intensity of the applied stimulus. During the *relative* refractory period, a second AP may be elicited, provided that a greater-than-usual stimulus is applied; i.e., excitability is depressed. The second AP often is subnormal in amplitude and in rate of rise. Therefore, the physiologically important refractory period is the **functional refractory period,** or *effective* refractory period.

Fig. 4-3. Strength-duration curve for initiation of action potentials in excitable membranes. The intensity of stimulating pulses is plotted against their duration for stimuli that are just sufficient to elicit an action potential. The rheobase current and chronaxie (σ) are indicated.

Fig. 4-4. Refractory periods of a nerve action potential (without a hyperpolarizing afterpotential.) The absolute (ARP) and relative (RRP) refractory periods are labeled.

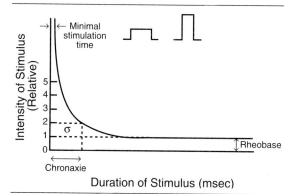

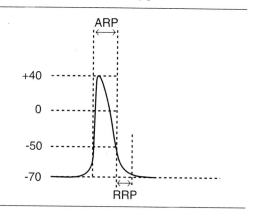

The functional refractory period encompasses all the absolute refractory period and part of the relative refractory period and is defined by the highest frequency of APs that the excitable cell (e.g., neuron) can propagate. For example, if a myelinated nerve axon can propagate impulses up to 1000/sec, the functional refractory period is 1.0 msec. The triggering of a second propagating impulse at a given point is limited by the amount of action current available (not like an electronic stimulator).

The absolute refractory period extends from when threshold is reached (at the initial portion of the rising phase of the AP) to when repolarization has reached about –50 mV. During further repolarization beyond –50 mV (e.g., to –70 mV), a larger and larger fraction of the fast Na$^+$ channels have recovered from inactivation (discussed later in this chapter) and so are again available to be reactivated to produce another AP. This is the period that inscribes the relative refractory period. The greater the degree of repolarization (toward the resting potential), the larger is the subsequent AP. Since both voltage and time are factors in the recovery of the ion channels, the relative refractory period actually exceeds the AP duration.

The afterpotentials that many cells exhibit also affect membrane excitability: Hyperpolarizing afterpotentials depress excitability (greater critical depolarization required to reach threshold), and depolarizing afterpotentials enhance excitability. The latter produces a **supernormal period of excitability,** and the former blends into and extends the relative refractory period. Propagation velocity is faster than normal during the supernormal period of excitability.

Accommodation

Accommodation, in physiologic terms, refers to the loss of sensitivity of a cell or tissue to an applied stimulus. Sensory organs exhibit the property of accommodation, as do many neurons and skeletal muscle fibers. For example, stretch receptors accommodate to a sustained stretch. When the stretch is first applied, there is a burst of APs, but the bursting frequency of discharge gradually slows down and then stops, even though the stretch is maintained.

When a rectangular (square wave) current pulse is used to depolarize a quiescent motor neuron (step depolarization) from the resting potential to the threshold potential or beyond, the neuron quickly responds with an all-or-none AP. However, if the applied pulse is ramp-shaped (triangular), depending on the slope of the ramp, the neuron may or may not respond, even if the normal threshold potential is exceeded. If the slope of the ramp is steep, the neuron

will respond, but at a higher threshold level (more critical depolarization is required). If the slope is shallow, the neuron will fail to fire an AP, regardless of what level it is depolarized to (Fig. 4-5A). This is accommodation. That is, when the membrane is depolarized gradually, the stimulus is ineffective in producing an AP response.

The explanation for this phenomenon of accommodation is as follows: As the membrane is slowly depolarized toward threshold, some of the fast Na$^+$ channels that are turned on (activated) spontaneously inactivate and are lost from the pool of available channels. If a critical number (critical mass) of fast Na$^+$ channels are not activated simultaneously, a regenerative AP is not produced. In addition, the delayed rectifier K$^+$ channels open during the slow depolarization, thus increasing K$^+$ conductance (g_K) and depressing excitability (because the outward K$^+$ current counteracts the inward Na$^+$ current.)

Such accommodation does not occur in pacemaker cells (see Fig. 4-5B). Such cells will discharge an AP no matter how gradually the membrane is brought to the threshold point. In fact, the pacemaker potential in cardiac nodal cells is of the ramp type, producing depolarization to

Fig. 4-5. The process of accommodation in response to a ramp stimulus in a motor neuron (A) and contrasted with the lack of accommodation in a nodal pacemaker cell from the heart (B). In (A) as the slope of the ramp stimulus is decreased (a→c), the action potential is delayed (b) and then fails completely (c) (E_m = membrane potential; V_{th} = threshold potential).

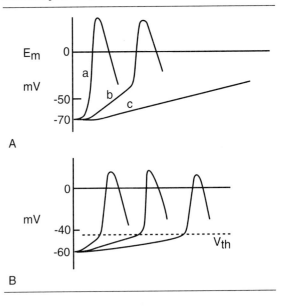

threshold over a period of about 200 to 800 msec. The lack of accommodation in automatic cells may be due to less spontaneous ion channel inactivation and less g_K increase during the ramp pacemaker potential. For example, in cardiac nodal cells, the inward current responsible for the rising phase of the AP is a slow Ca^{2+} current that inactivates very slowly, and the turn on of the delayed rectifier K^+ current is very slow.

Anodal-Break Excitation

Excitation occurs on the "make" (the beginning) of a square-wave depolarizing stimulus. If the applied stimulus duration is very long (relative to the AP duration), repetitive firing of APs will occur (if the membrane is nonaccommodating). If the membrane is accommodating, then only the initial AP is produced. If the cathode (negative) and anode (positive) electrodes are placed directly on an isolated single-nerve axon, then an AP will be triggered at the cathode region on the make of the stimulus. This happens because depolarization occurs under the cathode, whereas hyperpolarization occurs under the anode. However, under the anode, an AP is triggered on the "break" of the stimulating pulse. The excitability of that membrane region is transiently increased (lower threshold point) immediately following cessation of the applied pulse. The increase in excitability is due to depolarization caused by (1) an increase in Na^+ channel availability and (2) a decrease in K^+ channel availability. This is called **anodal-break excitation** and **postanodal enhancement of excitability.**

In contrast, under the cathode, after termination of the applied pulse, an opposite change occurs in excitability and E_m. The membrane is hyperpolarized transiently, and excitability is depressed. This is known as **postcathodal hyperpolarization** and **postcathodal depression of excitability.** This phenomenon is due to (1) a decrease in availability of fast Na^+ channels and (2) an increase in K^+ channel availability.

Electrogenesis of the Action Potential

During the AP, the membrane resistance (but not the capacitance) changes dramatically. The large **reduction in membrane resistance** that occurs during the AP results from a large increase in the ionic permeability of the membrane. To determine which ionic species are involved in generating the AP, the concentrations of the different ions bathing the axon can be varied. When the concentration of

Na^+ bathing an axon is lowered, the **overshoot** and the **rate of rise** of the AP decrease. These data demonstrate that the AP results from an increase in the membrane permeability to Na^+. This concept can be confirmed directly by the voltage-clamp method.

Voltage-Clamp Analysis

The membrane current I_m that generates the AP is composed of **ionic current** I_i and **capacitive current** I_c:

$$I_m = I_i + I_c$$

The flow of ionic currents across their respective resistive membrane pathways causes a change in the membrane potential (from Ohm's law: $V = IR$). The change in membrane voltage, in turn, causes a capacitive current to flow:

$$I_c = C_m \frac{dV}{dt}$$

where dV/dt is the rate of change of the AP. Because the membrane potential during an AP is constantly changing, it is difficult to separate the contributions of these interacting ionic and capacitive components. In addition, the total ionic current is composed of multiple individual currents carried by specific ions.

To analyze and separate the membrane currents into their capacitive and ionic components, a new and revolutionary method, called **voltage clamping,** was introduced in the early 1950s by Cole and Curtis and Hodgkin and Huxley. During a voltage-clamp experiment, the membrane potential is held constant ("clamped") by a **negative feedback amplifier,** and the amount of current that is necessary to perform this task is recorded. In the voltage-clamp technique, since the membrane potential V_m is held constant, the capacitive current is equal to zero, and hence $I_m = I_i$. The voltage-clamp technique identifies the magnitude and time course of the ionic currents that flow at a given clamp potential. By clamping the membrane to many different potentials, information is obtained about the flow of ionic currents and the underlying conductance changes that occur during the AP.

Another advantage of the voltage-clamp method is that the individual ion currents (such as Na^+, Ca^{2+}, or K^+ currents) can be isolated from the total ionic current and analyzed individually. For example, in the squid axon, the total ionic current consists of an early inward current followed by a delayed outward current (Fig. 4-6). By varying the external Na$^+$ concentration, it was shown that the early inward current is carried by Na$^+$. Similarly, by changing the K$^+$ concentration bathing the axon, one finds that the delayed outward current is carried by K$^+$.

The Na$^+$ and K$^+$ currents also can be separated by blocking their pathways through the membrane. Na$^+$ channels can be blocked with **tetrodotoxin** (TTX, derived from the ovaries of Japanese puffer fish), and delayed-rectifier K$^+$ channels can be blocked by several organic compounds, including tetraethylammonium ions (TEA$^+$). The remaining current can then be subtracted from the total ionic current to reveal the time course for the current that was blocked.

The **current-voltage relationship** is obtained by measuring the peak inward Na$^+$ current and peak outward K$^+$ currents during a series of voltage-clamp steps (Fig. 4-7). Depolarizing voltage steps to just above the resting potential produce a small outward current. In this voltage re-

Fig. 4-6. The ionic currents that flow when a squid giant axon is clamped from its resting potential (–70 mV) to a transmembrane potential of +20 mV. Trace A shows the net inward Na$^+$ current (I_{Na}) and outward K$^+$ current (I_K) in normal medium. Trace B shows the net ionic current when the axon is placed in artificial seawater with most of the Na$^+$ replaced by choline$^+$ (an impermeant cation) so that the intracellular and extracellular Na$^+$ concentrations are equal; this current is due to K$^+$ only. Trace C shows the difference between curves A and B, which represents I_{Na}. (Modified from: Hodgkin, A. L., and Huxley, A. F. Currents carried by sodium and potassium ions through the membrane of the giant axon of *Loligo. J. Physiol.* 116:449, 1952.)

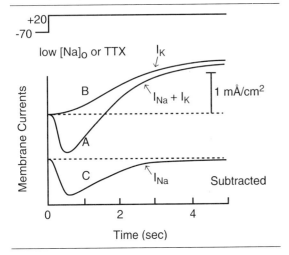

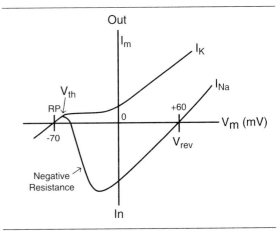

Fig. 4-7. Current/voltage relationship for the peak early inward current and delayed outward current obtained from a squid axon under voltage clamp. The inward current is carried by Na$^+$ (I_{Na}), the outward current by K$^+$ (I_K). The reversal potential (V_{rev}) for I_{Na} is the voltage at which the current changes from inward to outward. The region of the I_{Na} curve that has a negative slope is known as *negative resistance* (RP = resting potential; V_{th} = threshold; I_m = total membrane current; V_m = membrane potential).

gion, the membrane behaves in an ohmic fashion. With greater depolarization, the inward Na$^+$ current is activated, and the current-voltage relationship displays a negative slope or **negative resistance** region. A positive slope is seen at potentials above the peak of the current-voltage curve, and the current magnitude decreases as the Na$^+$ equilibrium potential E_{Na} is approached, actually becoming outward at voltages above E_{Na}. The voltage at which the current reverses in direction is the **reversal potential.** The reason that the current reverses at potentials above E_{Na} is that the net electrochemical driving force for Na$^+$ becomes outwardly directed, whereas the conductance for Na$^+$ remains constant over this entire voltage range. The outward K$^+$ current activates above –20 mV and increases with depolarization, as illustrated in Fig. 4-7.

Conductance Changes and Ionic Currents

The voltage-clamp experiments have revealed that the ionic conductances of excitable membranes are both **voltage-dependent** and **time-dependent.** The membrane conductance changes that occur during the AP are shown in Fig. 4-8. Both g_{Na} and g_K activate with depolarization, but with different time courses. The g_{Na} spontaneously turns off, or inactivates, with time (within 1–2 msec.) The in-

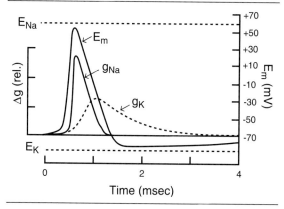

Fig. 4-8. The relative conductance for Na⁺ (g_{Na}) and K⁺ (g_K) during an action potential in nerve fibers. The rising phase of the action potential is caused by an increase in g_{Na}. The falling phase is due to the delayed rise of g_K and to the decrease in g_{Na}. The hyperpolarizing afterpotential is due to g_K remaining elevated for a short time following repolarization, tending to hold the membrane potential (E_m) near the K⁺ equilibrium potential (E_K) (E_{Na} = Na⁺ equilibrium potential; Δg = change in conductance). (Modified from: Hodgkin, A. L. *The Conduction of the Nervous Impulse.* Springfield, Ill.: Charles C Thomas, 1964.)

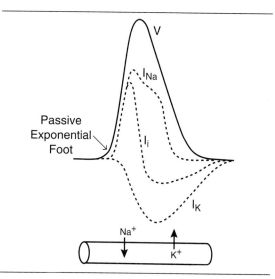

Fig. 4-9. Ionic currents that flow during the nerve action potential. The total current (I_i) is separated into an inward Na⁺ current (I_{Na}) and an outward K⁺ current (I_K). I_i is the algebraic sum of I_{Na} and I_K. A net inward Na⁺ flux occurs during the rising phase of the action potential, and a net K⁺ efflux occurs during the repolarizing phase. (Modified from: Hodgkin, A. L. and Huxley, A. F. Currents carried by sodium and potassium ions through the membranes of the giant axon of *Loligo. J. Physiol.* 116:449, 1952.)

ward Na⁺ current causes the regenerative depolarization of the AP (see Fig. 4-8). The depolarization is limited by the approach of the membrane potential toward E_{Na} and by the Na⁺ inactivation process. As the membrane is depolarized, both g_K and driving force for K⁺ current increase, and the outward K⁺ current repolarizes the membrane. The increase in g_K is self-limited, because the increase in g_K produces repolarization, which, in turn, shuts off the increase in g_K. The slow kinetics of the turnoff of g_K result in a transient hyperpolarization (the hyperpolarizing afterpotential), and the membrane potential is brought closer to the K⁺ equilibrium potential E_K than at rest (see Fig. 4-8).

The time course for the ionic currents during the nerve AP is shown in Fig. 4-9. The total ionic current I_i is separated into its two major components, I_{Na} and the K⁺ current I_K. Since I_K is slower to activate than I_{Na}, the inward I_{Na} predominates initially, giving rise to the upstroke of the AP. Later, I_K dominates, causing a net outward current that repolarizes the membrane.

The specific ionic currents are a product of the membrane conductance of the ionic species and the **electrochemical driving force** exerted on the ion. Thus

$$I_{Na} = g_{Na} (E_m - E_{Na})$$
$$I_K = g_K (E_m - E_K)$$

Since the membrane potential is constantly changing during the AP, the driving forces on Na⁺ and K⁺ continually change during the time course of the AP. At the resting potential, there is a large driving force for Na⁺ to flow into the cell because $E_m - E_{Na}$ is large. Conversely, at the peak of the AP, $E_m - E_{Na}$ is at its lowest value, and the driving force for Na⁺ entry is small. The driving force for K⁺ efflux is, however, largest at the peak of the AP, when $E_m - E_K$ is maximal. Since ionic current flow depends on both conductance and driving force, there is no net current if either factor is zero.

The biologic elements of the excitable membrane may be represented by an **electrical equivalent circuit,** as shown in Fig. 4-10. The conductances for Na⁺ and K⁺ are variable and depend on the transmembrane potential and time. Batteries, which are directed inwardly for Na⁺ and outwardly for K⁺, provide the driving force for ion flow. A passive leak conductance for Cl⁻ is also included in the

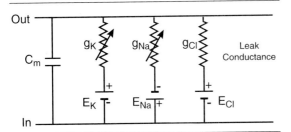

Fig. 4-10. Hodgkin-Huxley electrical equivalent circuit for the squid giant nerve axon. The K⁺ conductance (g_K) is in series with the K⁺ equilibrium potential (E_K), and the Na⁺ conductance (g_{Na}) is in series with the Na⁺ equilibrium potential (E_{Na}). The arrows indicate that g_{Na} and g_K vary with voltage and time. The low conductance for Cl⁻ (g_{Cl}) is termed the *leak conductance* (C_m = membrane capacitance; E_{Cl} = equilibrium potential for Cl⁻).

model. This model circuit will generate an AP if g_{Na} and g_K are varied appropriately.

Fast Na⁺ Channel Activation and Inactivation

The increase in g_{Na} during an AP is related to the membrane potential in a positive feedback fashion ("vicious cycle") (Fig. 4-11). That is, a small depolarization leads to an increase in g_{Na}, which allows a larger inward I_{Na} that causes further depolarization. This greater depolarization produces a greater increase in g_{Na}. This positive feedback process is an explosive one with a sharp trigger point (threshold), resulting from the exponential (positive) relationship between g_{Na} and E_m. It is this positive feedback relationship that accounts for the negative resistance (slope) in the current-voltage curve (see Fig. 4-7). g_{Na} reaches a maximum (saturates) at positive potentials that produce maximal activation of the population of fast Na⁺ channels.

The fast Na⁺ channels have a **double-gating mechanism,** consisting of an **activation gate** (A-gate) and an **inactivation gate** (I-gate) (Fig. 4-12). For a channel to be conducting, both the A-gate and I-gate must be open; if either is closed, the channel is nonconducting. The A-gate is located somewhere near the middle of the channel. The A-gate is closed at the resting E_m and opens rapidly upon depolarization. In contrast, the I-gate is open at the resting E_m and closes slowly upon depolarization.

A so-called **gating current** I_g has been measured that corresponds to the movement of the channel gates.* This

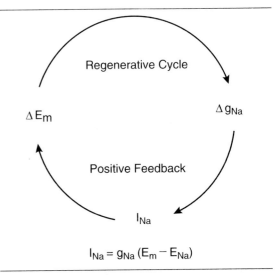

$$I_{Na} = g_{Na}(E_m - E_{Na})$$

Fig. 4-11. The positive feedback relationship between Na⁺ conductance (g_{Na}) and membrane potential (E_m) leading to the all-or-none action potential. The increase in g_{Na} allows an increase in the inward Na⁺ current: [$I_{Na} = g_{Na}(Em - E_{Na})$], which is depolarizing and so triggers a further increase in g_{Na}. This explosive feedback cycle is caused by the voltage dependency of the gated fast Na⁺ channels (I_{Na} = Na⁺ current; E_{Na} = Na⁺ equilibrium potential). (Modified from: Hodgkin, A. L. *The Conduction of the Nerve Impulse.* Springfield, Ill.: Charles C Thomas, 1964.)

outward current is very small in intensity and precedes the inward I_{Na}. TTX does not block I_g, although it does block I_{Na}. The gating current reflects the movement of the A-gates of the protein channels from the closed to the open configuration.

The I_{Na} lasts only for 1 to 2 msec because of the spontaneous inactivation of the fast Na⁺ channels. Inactivation of the fast Na⁺ channels is produced by the voltage-dependent closing of the inactivation gate (I-gate) (see Fig. 4-12). The I-gate is located near the inner surface of the membrane. The I-gate is presumably charged positively to allow it to move with changes in the membrane potential. At the normal resting potential, the I-gate is open. During

---

*In the Hodgkin-Huxley (1952) analysis, the opening of the A-gate requires simultaneous occupation of three negatively charged sites by three positively charged (m⁺) particles. If m, the activation variable, is the probability of one site being occupied, then m^3 is the probability that all three sites are occupied. Therefore, g_{Na} = max $g_{Na}m^3h$, where h is the inactivation variable and max g_{Na} is the maximum conductance.

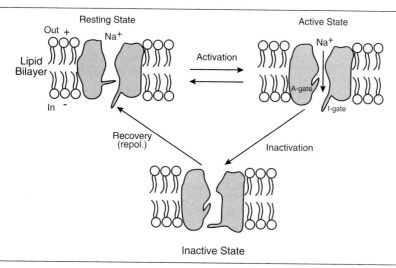

Fig. 4-12. Model of the three hypothetical states of the fast Na$^+$ channel. In the resting state, the activation gate (A) is closed and the inactivation gate (I) is open. Depolarization to the threshold activates the channel to the active state, the A-gate opening rapidly. The activated channel spontaneously inactivates to the inactive state due to delayed closure of the I-gate. The recovery process upon repolarization returns the channel back to the resting state, making it again available for reactivation. Na$^+$ is depicted as being bound to the outer mouth of the channel and poised for entry down its electrochemical gradient when both gates are open. The reaction between resting state and the active states is readily reversible. (Modified from: Hodgkin, A. L. *The Conductance of the Nervous Impulse.* Springfield, Ill.: Charles C Thomas, 1964.)

depolarization, the inside of the membrane becomes positive, and this causes the I-gate to close.

The voltage dependency of inactivation is given by the h_∞ versus E_m curve (Fig. 4-13). The inactivation variable (h, probability function) varies between 0 and 1.0 (reflecting occupation of a negatively charged site by a positively charged inactivation particle), and h_∞ is the value of the inactivation variable at infinite time (>10 msec) or at steady-state. When the inactivation variable is 1.0, the I-gates of all the fast Na$^+$ channels are open; conversely, when the inactivation variable is zero, all the I-gates are closed.* At the normal resting potential, h_∞ is nearly 1.0 and diminishes with depolarization, becoming nearly zero at about −50 mV. The decrease in g_{Na} is the cause of the decrease in the rate of rise of the AP (see Fig. 4-13). Therefore, depolarization by any means decreases max g_{Na} and excitability disappears at about −50 mV.

Any Na$^+$ channel that has been activated and then spon-

Fig. 4-13. Voltage inactivation of the fast Na$^+$ channels as a function of the membrane potential (E_m). h_∞ is plotted against E_m, where h_∞ is the inactivation factor of Hodgkin-Huxley. This graph illustrates that fast Na$^+$ channels begin to inactivate at about −80 mV, and nearly complete inactivation occurs at about −50 mV. Maximal rate of rise of the action potential (max dV/dt) as a function of resting E_m is also depicted. Since max dV/dt is a measure of the inward current intensity, which is dependent on the number of channels available for activation, max dV/dt decreases as h_∞ decreases (RP = resting potential).

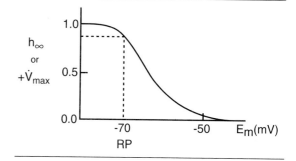

*Since the g_{Na} at any time is equal to the maximal value (max g_{Na}) times m^{3}h, when h = 0, g_{Na} = 0, and when h = 1.0, g_{Na} = max g_{Na} (if m = 1.0).

taneously inactivates must go through a **recovery process** before it can return to the resting state from which it can be **reactivated** (see Fig. 4-12). The recovery process depends on voltage and time. The membrane must be repolarized beyond –50 mV before the recovery process can begin. At any given E_m, it takes time for the recovery process to occur, namely, the time required for the charged A-gates and I-gates to be restored to their resting configuration (A-gate closed, I-gate open) with the electric field. The recovery process is fast for fast Na^+ channels.

Mechanisms of Repolarization

The AP is terminated primarily by the turn-on of the **delayed rectifier** g_K. It is called this because its turn-on is slower and delayed with respect to the turn-on of g_{Na}. The increase in g_K acts to bring E_m toward E_K (about –90 mV), because the membrane potential at any time is determined mainly by the ratio of g_{Na} to g_K (see Chap. 3). This type of g_K channel is activated by depolarization and turned off by repolarization. Therefore, this g_K is self-limiting, in that it is turned off as the membrane is repolarized by its action, as mentioned previously. The K^+ channel is generally believed not to have an I-gate, because it does not inactivate quickly.*

Contributing to repolarization is also turn-off of g_{Na}, which would occur for two reasons: (1) spontaneous inactivation of fast Na^+ channels that had been activated (i.e, closing of their I-gate) and (2) reversible shifting of activated channels directly back to the resting state (deactivation) because of the rapid repolarization occurring due to the g_K mechanism. Theoretically, it would be possible to have an AP that would repolarize (but slowly) even if there were no g_K mechanism, because the g_{Na} channels would inactivate spontaneously.

In skeletal muscle, there is an important third factor involved in repolarization of the AP. The Cl^- permeability and conductance (g_{Cl}) are very high in skeletal muscle, (about three times higher than that of K^+). As discussed in Chap. 3, although the Cl^- ion is passively distributed or nearly so, during AP depolarization, there is a larger and larger driving force for outward Cl^- current I_{Cl} (i.e., Cl^- influx) because $I_{Cl} = g_{Cl}(E_m - E_{Cl})$. In other words, the large electric field that was keeping Cl^- out diminishes during the AP, so Cl^- enters the fiber. This Cl^- entry is hyperpolarizing and so tends to repolarize the membrane more quickly than

would otherwise occur (i.e., repolarization is "sharpened"). Cl^- channels are known to be present in skeletal muscle fibers. In the disease known as **myotonia,** abnormally low Cl^- permeability in the skeletal muscle fibers causes slowed repolarization and repetitive firing of APs, thereby producing the muscle spasms characteristic of myotonia.

Molecular Basis of Excitability: Properties of Individual Ion Channels

A new electrophysiologic method, the **patch-clamp technique,** has enabled researchers to examine the basis of excitability at the molecular level. The method allows recording of the currents that flow through individual ion channels. By no other method available can the behavior of a single protein molecule be observed on a millisecond time scale. To record the channel currents, a small-tipped glass pipette is pressed against the cell membrane, and negative pressure is applied to draw a small "patch" of membrane into the tip of the pipette. A high-resistance seal [gigaohm (10^9)] spontaneously forms between the membrane and the glass, allowing the recording of the currents through a single channel, the so-called **cell-attached patch** mode (Fig. 4-14A). If one functioning channel resides in the patch of membrane, then the single-channel currents and their open (conducting) and closed times can be recorded by a high-gain amplifier.

The opening and closing of an individual channel, upon depolarization, appears to occur randomly in time (see Fig. 4-14B). If, however, the average behavior over time of a channel (or small group of channels) is considered, the random behavior becomes deterministic. For example, although the opening and closing of fast Na^+ channels or slow Ca^{2+} channels are random in each trial, the sum of the individual currents is similar to the time course for the whole-cell current (see Fig. 4-14B). The distribution of the individual open and closed times is characteristic of each type of channel.

Other information learned from single-channel recordings includes the single-channel conductance, which is characteristic of each channel type. The value [given in pS (picosiemens) or 10^{-12} S] reflects the maximal rate of ion flux through the channel.

The gating of ionic channels involved in generating the AP is voltage-dependent. This means that the channel protein contains a charged group or dipole that can sense the electric field across the membrane and respond to a change in the transmembrane voltage. When the gating region moves, it causes a shift in the overall conformation of the channel, which allows it to conduct ions. Most channels open, close, and reopen many times during long depolariz-

---

*In the Hodgkin-Huxley analysis of squid giant axon, the A-gate opens when four positively charged (n^+) particles simultaneously occupy four favorable positions (negatively charged sites). If n is the probability that one site is occupied, then n^4 is the probability that all four sites are occupied; therefore, $g_K = \max g_K n^4$.

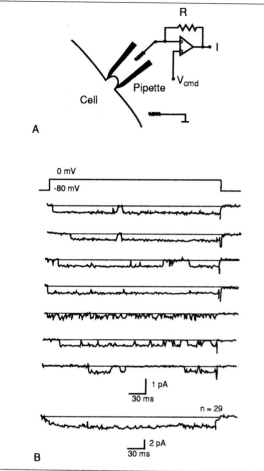

Fig. 4-14. Single-channel recording using the patch-clamp method. (A) The single-channel currents from the patch of membrane isolated by the pipette tip are amplified and recorded (R = feedback resistor; V_{cmd} = command voltage; I = current). (B) Current recordings from a cell-attached patch showing the activity of a slow Ca^{2+} channel in a single myocardial cell isolated from a 3-day-old embryonic chick heart. Single-channel currents were evoked by depolarizing voltage pulses (duration of 300 msec, 0.5 Hz) from a holding potential of –80 mV. Seven successive current recordings from the one patch are shown, and the ensemble-averaged currents from 29 such traces (n= 29) are shown at the bottom. The single-channel recordings appear as square steps of current as a channel opens, then closes, then reopens. Only one channel was present in this patch. (A: Modified from: Sigworth, F. J., and Neher, E. Single Na channel currents observed in cultured rat muscle cells. *Nature* 287:447, 1980; B: Modified from: Tohse, N., and Sperelakis, N. CGMP inhibits the activity of single calcium channels in embryonic chick heart cells. *Circ. Res.* 69:325, 1991.)

ing pulses, forming "bursts" of activity. The fast Na^+ channels inactivate (close) spontaneously during depolarization, without reopening. It is thought that inactivation is related to a specific region of the channel polypeptide, which resides on the inner (cytoplasmic) surface of the protein.

The amino acid sequences of Na^+, Ca^{2+}, and K^+ channels are known, and their putative tertiary structures have been suggested (Fig. 4-15). Na^+ and Ca^{2+} channels have several subunits: the ionophore itself and several regulatory subunits. Ca^{2+} channels have multiple sites for phosphorylation. Phosphorylation has been shown to alter the behavior of Ca^{2+} and K^+ channels. For example, in heart muscle, the Ca^{2+} channel activity is increased by phosphorylation (see Chap. 20).

As mentioned previously, the channel polypeptide contains specific charged residues that can "sense" the transmembrane electric field and actually move in response to changes in the electric field. The movement of the gating charge produces a small but measurable gating current. Gating currents have been recorded from Na^+, Ca^{2+}, and K^+ channels and provide information concerning the steps leading to channel opening.

A number of biologic toxins have been discovered that act on specific ion channels. For example, TTX (extracted from the ovary of the Japanese puffer fish) has a high affinity for the fast Na^+ channel of nerves and blocks the passage of Na^+ through the channel. Another type of toxin, batrachotoxin (BTX), prevents inactivation of the Na^+ channel so that the Na^+ currents continue during prolonged depolarization. Such toxins have proven to be valuable tools in understanding ion channel function because of their specific actions.

The macroscopic whole-cell current I is the product of the number of functional channels N, the probability that the "average" channel is open P_o, and the single-channel current i:

$$I = iNP_o$$

Single-channel recording allows direct measurement of these parameters (i.e., N, P_o, i), which were previously difficult to estimate indirectly from whole-cell recordings. In addition, the mechanism of action of channel regulatory agents can be examined at the level of the single channel. For example, epinephrine increases the Ca^{2+} current in heart cells by increasing the probability of opening.

Another discovery made using the patch-clamp method is that there are multiple subtypes of channels. For example, nerve cells possess three distinct types of Ca^{2+} channels having different conductances, kinetics, and voltage dependencies. In addition, Na^+ and Ca^{2+} channels have been shown to exhibit multiple modes of gating behavior, which can be elicited by certain drugs.

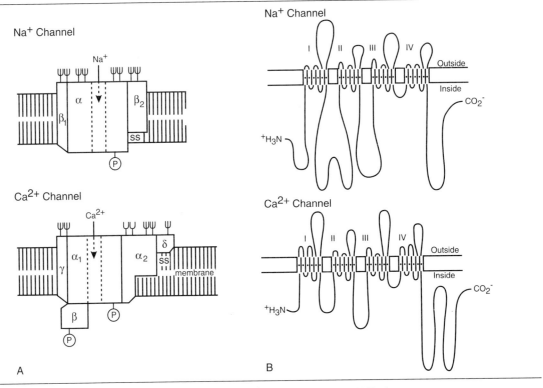

Fig. 4-15. Structural models of the fast Na^+ channel and the Ca^{2+} channel proteins. (A) Both Na^+ and Ca^{2+} channels have multiple protein subunits, labeled α, β, γ, and δ. The Ca^{2+} channel has two α subunits: α_1 and α_2. The α_1 subunit is the one that contains the water-filled pore through which Ca^{2+} passes. Two sites that can be phosphorylated by cyclic AMP–dependent protein kinase are present: one on the α_1 subunit and one on the β subunit. Only one α subunit exists in the Na^+ channel, but there are two β subunits: β_1 and β_2. The α subunit has a phosphorylatable site (SS = disulfide bond). (B) The structure of the central pore-forming α subunit for the Na^+ channel and Ca^{2+} channel. In each case, there are four homologous repeat domains, connected by intracellular polypeptide loops and arranged in a circular structure within the plane of the membrane to form a channel. Each domain consists of six segments that span the membrane, as depicted. (Modified from: Catterall, W. Structure and function of voltage-sensitive ion channels. *Science* 242:50, 1988.)

Effect of Resting Potential on Action Potential

Any agent that affects the resting potential has important repercussions on the AP. Depolarization reduces the rate of rise of the AP and thereby also slows its velocity of propagation. A slowed propagation through the nerve or muscle interferes with its ability to act effectively. For example, it would interfere with the heart's ability to act as an effective pump. This effect is progressive as a function of the degree of depolarization. If nerve, skeletal muscle fibers, or myo-

cardial cells are depolarized to about –50 mV, by any means, then the rate of rise goes to zero and all excitability (and contraction) is lost. The explanation for this is based on the sigmoidal h_∞ versus E_m curve (see Fig. 4-13).

Hyperpolarization usually produces only a small increase in the rate of rise. Large hyperpolarization may actually slow the velocity of propagation (because the critical depolarization required to bring the membrane to its threshold potential is increased), or it may cause propagation block.

The resting potential also affects the duration of the AP. When elevated extracellular K^+ levels are used to depolarize the cells, the AP is usually shortened. Agents or conditions that increase g_K, such as elevation of extracellular K^+ concentration, tend to shorten the duration. In contrast, agents that decrease g_K (or slow its activation) tend to lengthen the AP duration. Due to **anomalous rectification** (i.e., a decrease in g_K with depolarization), depolarization by applied current prolongs the AP and hyperpolarization shortens it. Agents that slow the closing of the I-gates of the fast Na^+ channels (such as veratridine) prolong the AP.

Electrogenesis of Afterpotentials

The APs of nerve and muscle cells usually consist of two components: an initial spike followed by an early afterpotential (Fig. 4-16). The afterpotentials may be of two types: depolarizing or hyperpolarizing. In addition, late afterpotentials may appear following a brief train of spikes.

Early Hyperpolarizing Afterpotentials

Neurons, heart pacemaker cells, and vascular smooth muscle cells often exhibit **early hyperpolarizing** ("positive") **afterpotentials** (see Fig. 4-16C). These are due to the delayed rectifier K^+ conductance increase (which terminates the spike) persisting after the spike, thereby bringing E_m closer to E_K. The maximum amplitude of the positive afterpotential is the difference between E_K and the normal resting potential. The time course of this afterpotential is determined by the decay of the K^+ conductance increase.

Late Hyperpolarizing Afterpotentials

Some cells, such as nonmyelinated neurons, exhibit **late hyperpolarizing afterpotentials** following a train of spikes (see Fig. 4-16D). These hyperpolarizing afterpotentials are due to the Na^+-K^+ pump, because inhibition of the pump by any means (such as ouabain or cold) abolishes it. Two mechanisms have been proposed for this phenomenon: (1) an increased electrogenic Na^+ pump potential stimulated by an increase in the intracellular Na^+ content (since these neurons are small in diameter and hence have a large surface-area-to-volume ratio) and by an increase in extracellular K^+ content (since these axons are surrounded by Schwann cells and hence a narrow intercellular cleft and restricted diffusion space) and (2) an increased E_K caused by K^+ depletion in the intercellular cleft due to the stimulated Na^+-K^+ pump overpumping the K^+ back in. It is generally believed that the first mechanism, namely, a larger pump potential, is the most probable, although it is difficult to distinguish between these two possibilities.

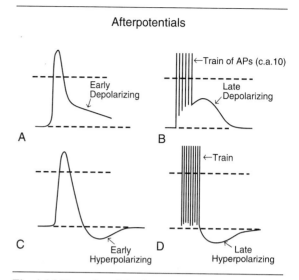

Fig. 4-16. Examples of the different types of afterpotentials. (A) Early depolarizing ("negative") afterpotential recorded after a single action potential in a skeletal muscle fiber. (B) Late depolarizing afterpotential recorded after a train (e.g., 10) of action potentials in a skeletal muscle fiber. (C) Early hyperpolarizing ("positive") afterpotential recorded after a single action potential in a nerve fiber. (D) Late hyperpolarizing afterpotential recorded following a train of action potentials in a nonmyelinated neuron.

Early Depolarizing Afterpotentials

The AP spike in skeletal muscle fibers is followed by a prominent depolarizing afterpotential (also called a **negative** afterpotential, based on the old terminology used when recording externally) that emerges from the spike (see Fig. 4-16A). The early afterpotential is due to a conductance change. The early depolarizing afterpotential of frog skeletal fibers is about 25 mV in amplitude, immediately after the spike component, and gradually decays to the resting potential over a period of 10 to 20 msec. It results from the fact that the delayed rectifier K^+ channel that opens during depolarization to terminate the spike is less selective for K^+ (the ratio of K^+ to Na^+ permeability is about 30 : 1) than is the K^+ channel in the resting membrane (P_K/P_{Na} about 100 : 1). Therefore, from the constant-field equation (see Chap. 3), one can predict that the membrane should be partly depolarized when the membrane is dominated by this K^+ conductance. Thus the early depolarizing afterpotential is due to the persistence of, and slow decay of, this less selective K^+ conductance.

Late Depolarizing Afterpotentials

In addition to the early afterpotential, there is a late depolarizing afterpotential that follows a tetanic train of spikes (e.g., 10 spikes) (see Fig. 4-16B). The electrogeneses of the early and the late afterpotentials are different. The late afterpotential results from accumulation of K^+ in the transverse (T) tubules (periodic invaginations of the surface membrane into the fiber interior, involved in excitation-contraction coupling). During the AP depolarization and turn-on of g_K (delayed rectifier), there is a large driving force for K^+ efflux from the myoplasm coupled with a large K^+ conductance, resulting in a large outward K^+ current $[I_K = g_K (E_m - E_K)]$ across all surfaces of the fiber, namely, the surface sarcolemma and T-tubule walls. The K^+ efflux at the fiber surface membrane can rapidly diffuse away and mix with the relatively large interstitial fluid volume, whereas the K^+ efflux into the T-tubules is trapped in this restricted diffusion space. The resulting high concentration of K^+ in the T-tubules decreases E_K across the T-tubule membrane and thereby depolarizes this membrane. Due to cable properties, part of this depolarization is transmitted to the surface sarcolemma and is recorded by an intracellular microelectrode. The K^+ accumulation in the T-tubules can only be dissipated relatively slowly by diffusion out of the mouth of the T-tubules and by active pumping back into the myoplasm across the T-tubule wall. Thus the decay of the late afterpotential is a function of these two processes. The amplitude and duration of the late depolarizing afterpotential of frog skeletal fibers are a function of the number of spikes in the train and their frequency. If the train consists of 20 spikes at a frequency of 50/sec, the amplitude of the afterpotential is about 20 mV. Another factor contributing to the late afterpotential may be the slow relaxation of a slow component of the K^+ conductance increase.

Importance of Afterpotentials

All afterpotentials have physiologic importance because they alter excitability and the propagation velocity of the cell. A depolarizing afterpotential should enhance excitability (lower threshold), and a hyperpolarizing afterpotential should depress excitability to a subsequent AP. This is so because the critical depolarization required would be decreased or increased, respectively. A large late depolarizing afterpotential can trigger repetitive APs under certain pathologic conditions. The effect of afterpotentials on the velocity of propagation is more complex because there are two opposing factors: (1) the change in critical depolarization required and (2) the change in the maximal rate of rise of the AP (h_∞ verses E_m curve).

Summary

Membrane excitability is a fundamental property of nerve cells and muscle cells (skeletal, cardiac, and smooth), as well as some endocrine cells. An excitable cell is one that, in response to certain environmental stimuli (electrical, chemical, or mechanical), generates an **all-or-none electrical signal** or **action potential** (AP). The AP is sometimes called an "impulse," as, for example, **nerve impulse**. The AP is triggered by depolarization of the membrane beyond threshold. The depolarization initates a large increase in the membrane permeability to Na^+, which then flows into the cell, causing a transient depolarization and reversal in the membrane potential. A slower increase in membrane permeability to K^+ contributes to the repolarization of the membrane, in addition to the spontaneous **inactivation** of the Na^+ channels. Some cells display **automaticity,** in that they produce APs spontaneously without any external stimulus.

The membrane currents that contribute to the AP can be studied by the voltage-camp method, which allows isolation and characterization of each membrane current as a function of membrane potential and time. Ionic currents flow across the membrane by means of numerous ion-specific protein **channels.** Each channel molecule has a region that senses the transmembrane potential and acts as a gate to open or close the channel to ion passage through its central pore.

Na^+ (and Ca^{2+}) channels have an additional gating system that closes (or inactivates) the channel during a maintained depolarization. The pattern of minute currents that flow through individual voltage-dependent ion channels can be studied using the **patch-clamp method.** Single-channel current measurement and channel protein structural information have provided a greater understanding of the molecular basis of membrane excitability.

The APs in vertebrate nerve fibers consist of a spike followed by a hyperpolarizing afterpotential. A large fast inward Na^+ current, passing through fast Na^+ channels, is responsible for electrogenesis of the spike, which rises rapidly (approximately 1000 V/sec). The nerve cell membrane has voltage-dependent K^+ channels that are responsible for repolarization. g_K increases more slowly than g_{Na} upon depolarization (called the **delayed rectifier**) and produces repolarization that terminates the AP.

The nerve AP amplitude is about 110 mV, from a resting potential of –70 mV to a peak overshoot potential of about 40 mV. The duration of the AP (at 50% repolarization) is about 1.0 msec. The threshold potential for triggering of the AP is about –55 mV; a critical depolarization of about 15 mV is required to reach threshold. The turn-on of the fast g_{Na} (fast I_{Na}) is very rapid (within 0.2 msec), and E_m is brought rapidly toward E_{Na}. There is an explosive (positive exponential initially) increase in g_{Na} caused by a positive feedback relationship between g_{Na} and E_m.

In certain nerve cells as well as muscle cells, as E_m depolarizes, it crosses the threshold potential (about –35mV) for the slow Ca^{2+} channels, turning on a slow inward Ca^{2+} current I_{Ca}. In some types of smooth muscle cells, the upstroke of the AP is produced by an inward slow Ca^{2+} current (rather than a fast Na^+ current) (see Chap. 20).

Bibliography

Hille, B. *Ionic Channels of Excitable Membrane.* Boston: Sinauer Associates, 1984.

Hodgkin, A. L. *The Conduction of the Nervous Impulse.* Springfield, Ill.: Charles C Thomas, 1964.

Katz, B. *Nerve, Muscle and Synapse.* New York: McGraw-Hill, 1966.

Sperelakis, N., and Fabiato, A. Electrophysiology and excitation-contraction coupling in skeletal muscle. In C. Roussos and P. Macklem, eds., *The Thorax: Vital Pump.* New York: Marcel Dekker, 1985. Pp. 45–113.

5 Cable Properties and Propagation Mechanisms

Nicholas Sperelakis

Objectives

After reading this chapter, you should be able to

Explain why a fast propagating electric signal, the all-or-none action potential, is required for rapid communication in the body

Describe the mechanism of propagation of the action potential

Describe the nature of saltatory conduction

List the factors that affect propagation velocity

Identify the type of records that are obtained on external recording of the action potentials from single fibers or a bundle of fibers

Now that we have considered the electrogenesis of the resting potential of cells (Chap. 3), which enables the electrogenesis of action potentials (APs) and excitability (Chap. 4), we will examine the mechanism for the propagation of APs and excitability from one part of a neuron or muscle fiber to a distal part. It is imperative that the body be able to transmit a very rapid signal from one point to another. The only way that this can be accomplished is through an electric mechanism. Blood flow and diffusion of signaling molecules are too slow to allow rapid signal-

ing. In contrast, electricity flows very quickly, at the speed of light (300,000,000 m/sec) in a copper wire and about one-ninth that in a water solution. Therefore, the body uses electricity for rapid signaling in the nervous system, skeletal muscle, and heart. Propagation velocity in our fastest nerve fibers is about 120 m/sec; it is about 6 m/sec in skeletal muscle, about 0.5 m/sec in cardiac muscle, and about 5 cm/sec in smooth muscle (Table 5-1).

As one example of the need for very fast communication or signaling, consider the process of walking. Very

Table 5-1. Conduction Velocity as a Function of Fiber Diameter in Various Nerve Axons and Muscle Fibers

Fiber Type	Fiber Diameter (μm)	Propagation Velocity (m/sec)	Velocity/Diameter (m/sec/μm)
Myelinated axons	20	120	6.0
	12	75	6.2
	5	30	6.0
Nonmyelinated axons	1.5	2.0	1.3
	1.0	1.3	1.3
Squid giant axons (20°C)	500	25	0.05
Skeletal muscle fibers	50	6.0	0.12
Cardiac muscle fibers	15	0.5	0.03
Smooth muscle fibers	5	0.05	0.01

rapid signals must travel from the motor cortex of the brain, down to the lower spinal cord region, and out the motor axons to the skeletal muscles of the lower extremities. In this process, the signal crosses one or more synapses, which are regions in which one neuron comes into close contact with another and in which a special chemical neurotransmitter signal is involved. At the termination of each branch of a motor nerve axon on the skeletal muscle fiber there is another synapse, known as the **neuromuscular junction** or **motor end-plate.** The signal crosses the neuromuscular junction and gives rise to an AP in the muscle fiber, which propagates in both directions from the motor end-plate. The muscle AP elicits contraction. Receptors in the muscles (e.g., stretch receptors) transmit information (in the form of propagating APs) back into the central nervous system (CNS). Thus, in walking, there is a continual rapid flow of information and instructions to the muscles in both directions: out of the CNS and into the CNS. Therefore, walking is not possible without a very rapid signaling system. In various demyelinating diseases (e.g., caused by some viruses, heavy metals, and autoimmune reactions), loss of the myelin sheath (around the myelinated nerve fibers) causes propagation to become

Fig. 5-1. A chemical excitatory synapse between two nerve fibers. An action potential (AP) in the presynaptic fiber on the left-hand side brings about release of the neurotransmitter at its nerve terminal. The transmitter molecules diffuse to the postsynaptic membrane and bind to receptor sites on ligand-gated nonselective (Na⁺, K⁺ mixed conductance) ion channels and open them. The associated synaptic current depolarizes the postsynaptic membrane, producing the excitatory postsynaptic potential (EPSP), and this depolarization spreads passively into the adjacent conductile membrane (excitable), thereby triggering one or more APs in the postsynaptic axon. The EPSPs are local, graded in amplitude, and nonrefractory, whereas the APs are all-or-none (maximal), refractory, and propagated actively. Thus the amplitude-modulated synaptic process gives rise to a frequency-modulated (or digital) signal.

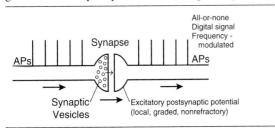

slowed and impaired in the affected nerve fibers, with associated incoordination and partial paralysis.

Since propagating all-or-none APs in a neuron are all very similar to each other (in shape, duration, amplitude, rate of rise, and propagation velocity), in order to make the signal stronger or weaker, the body increases or decreases the frequency of the APs accordingly. That is, the body uses a **frequency-modulated** system, rather than an amplitude-modulated system (Fig. 5-1). It is a **digital system** consisting of yes/no identical signals. At each synapse, the signal becomes **graded** in amplitude rather than all-or-none: The greater the amplitude and duration of the local postsynaptic potential, the higher is the frequency of APs triggered. The same is true of the local graded receptor potential generated at some sensory organs: Stronger signals translate into a higher frequency of impulses.

Cable Properties
Biologic Fiber as a Cable

An **electric cable** consists of two parallel conductors (e.g., copper) separated by insulation material (e.g., rubber). Usually one of the conductors is arranged as a tubular sleeve surrounding a central wire. The equivalent electric circuit for a cable consists of two parallel conductors (wires) separated by a transverse resistance distributed along the length of the cable. The resistance of the conductors is so small compared with the transverse insulation resistance that they are assumed to be zero. In the case of **biologic cable** (a long narrow nerve fiber or skeletal muscle fiber), one parallel conductor is the inside fluid (cytoplasm), and the other parallel conductor is the outside fluid surrounding (bathing) the cell (the interstitial fluid). Because the conductivity of biologic fluid is much less (i.e., much higher resistance) than that of copper wire, and because the cross-sectional area of the cell cytoplasm is so small, the inside longitudinal resistance is relatively high (Fig. 5-2). The outside longitudinal resistance is relatively small, as compared with the inside, because of the larger volume (cross-sectional area) of fluid available to carry the outside current; therefore, it is assumed to be negligible.

In addition, there is a **capacitance** distributed along the length of the cable (see Fig. 5-2), because a capacitance occurs when two parallel conductors ("plates") are separated by a high-resistance dielectric material. The **dielectric constant** of materials is related to vacuum (value of 1.000). Air has a value very close to vacuum; oils have a dielectric constant of 3 to 6. The biologic membrane, which has a matrix of phospholipid molecules, has a dielectric constant of about 5, typical of oils. The higher the

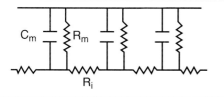

Fig. 5-2. Electrical equivalent circuit for a biologic cable. The outer conductor depicted has nearly zero resistance, and the transmembrane insulation resistance (R_m) is distributed along the length of the cable. The inner conductor is the cytoplasm (axoplasm or myoplasm), which is not of negligible resistivity, and therefore is depicted as R_i distributed along the length of the fiber. The transverse resistance is the cell membrane (R_m). The capacitance elements arise due to the lipid bilayer matrix of the cell membrane (C_m).

dielectric constant, the higher is the capacitance; the closer the parallel plates, the higher is the capacitance. Because the biologic membrane is so thin (approximately 70 Å, or 7 nm), its capacitance is relatively high: All cell membranes have a membrane capacitance of about 1.0 μF/cm² (F stands for farad).

Length Constant

In an electric cable, a voltage (or signal) applied at one end is transmitted to a distant end with little or no decrement (diminution or attenuation), and the so-called **length constant** is very long. In the biologic cable (see Fig. 5-2), however, a signal applied at one end rapidly falls off (decays) in amplitude as a function of distance, with a relatively short length constant λ. This decay in voltage is exponential (Fig. 5-3). An exponential process produces a straight line on a semilogarithmic plot (log V versus distance). In a cable, the relationship between the voltage at any distance x from the applied voltage V_o is

$$V_x = V_o e^{-x/\lambda}$$

$$(5\text{-}1)*$$

Thus, when x = λ, $V_x = V_o(1/e^1) = V_o(1/2.718) = 0.37 V_o$. Hence the distance at which the voltage decays to 37% of the initial value gives the length constant. In nerve fibers and skeletal muscle fibers, the length constant has a value of only about 1 to 3 mm. Therefore, the relatively short length constant, compared with the length of the neuron (e.g., 1.0 m for a lumbar motor neuron), means that a sig-

*The mathematical solution to Eq. (5-1) is

$$V_x = \text{anti-log}\left[\frac{(2.303 \log V_o - x/\lambda)}{2.303}\right].$$

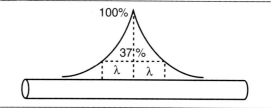

Fig. 5-3. Length constant (λ) of the biologic cable (fiber). An exponential decay of voltage on both sides of an applied current (voltage) occurs as a function of distance. The distance at which the voltage falls to 1/e (or 36.7%) of the voltage at the site of current injection gives the length constant.

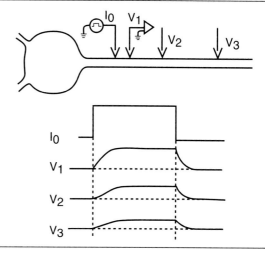

Fig. 5-4. Depiction of the manner in which a voltage signal would decay with distance if the neuron were only a passive cable (nonexcitable). The voltage traces illustrate the voltage signals that would be simultaneously recorded at three different points along the axon (V_1, V_2, and V_3) from the site of injection of a rectangular current pulse (I_0). As depicted, the amplitude of the steady-state voltage pulse rapidly falls off with distance, because the length constant of the biologic cable is short (e.g., 1 mm) compared with the length of the axon (e.g., 1000 mm). The voltage recorded at point V_1 also illustrates that the membrane potential changes in an exponential manner, both at the beginning of an applied rectangular current pulse and at the end, because of the membrane capacitance.

nal applied at one end (or midpoint) falls off very quickly over an increasing distance along the fiber (Figs. 5-3 and 5-4). If the length constant were 1.0 mm, the signal would become negligible at about 4 mm.

Hence the electric signal cannot be conducted passively in the biologic cable, because it would decrement and disappear over relatively short distances. The AP (signal) is amplified to a constant value at each point (or each node) in the membrane, as discussed in Chap. 4. That is, conduction is active, not passive, with energy being put into the signal at each point to prevent any decay of the signal.

The parameters of a cable that determine its length constant are the square root of the ratio of the transverse resistance (r_m in $\Omega \cdot cm$) to the sum of the inside (r_i in Ω/cm) and outside (r_o in Ω/cm) longitudinal resistances:

$$\lambda = \sqrt{\frac{r_m}{r_i + r_o}} \qquad (5\text{-}2)$$

where r_m, r_i, and r_o are the normalized resistances for a unit length (1 cm) of fiber. For surface fibers of a nerve or muscle bundle bathed in a large volume conductor, r_o is negligibly small, and Eq. (5-2) reduces to

$$\lambda = \sqrt{\frac{r_m}{r_i}} = \sqrt{\frac{R_m}{R_i} \frac{a}{2}} \qquad (5\text{-}3)$$

where a is the fiber radius (in cm) and R_m (in $\Omega \cdot cm^2$) and R_i (in $\Omega \cdot cm$) are the membrane resistance and cytoplasmic resistance, respectively, normalized for both length and cell diameter. Thus the greater the membrane resistance and the smaller the internal longitudinal resistance (larger cell diameter), the greater is the length constant value. We will see below that the propagation velocity is a function of the length constant and that myelination increases the effective membrane resistance and lowers the effective capacitance, thereby increasing propagation velocity.

Time Constant

Because of the large capacitance of the cell membrane, the membrane potential cannot change instantaneously upon application of a step-current pulse. Instead, the membrane potential changes in an exponential (negative) manner (see Fig. 5-4), both on the charge and the discharge. The membrane **time constant** τ_m defines the rate at which the membrane potential charges and is given by the product of the resistance R_m and capacitance C_m of the membrane:

$$\tau_m = r_m c_m = R_m C_m \qquad (5\text{-}4)$$

The **discharge** of the membrane capacitance (parallel RC network) is given by

$$V_t = V_{max} e^{-t/\tau} \qquad (5\text{-}5a)$$

where V_t is the voltage at any time t (at the site of current injection), and V_{max} is the final maximum voltage attained during the pulse. When $t = \tau$, $V_t = V_{max}(1/e^1) = V_{max}(1/2.718) = 0.37 V_{max}$. Hence the time at which the voltage decays to 37% of the initial (maximal) value gives the time constant. In nerve fibers and skeletal muscle fibers, the time constant is about 1.0 msec.

When the membrane is **charging**, there is a similar exponential (negative) process, with the identical time constant (see Fig. 5-4). The corresponding relationship is given by

$$V_t = V_{max}(1 - e^{-t/\tau}) \qquad (5\text{-}5b)$$

The time it takes for buildup of the voltage to 63% ($1 - 1/e = 1 - 0.37 = 0.63$) of the final voltage gives the time constant. Thus the time constant can be measured on the buildup (time to reach 63% of the final voltage) or on the decay of the pulse (time to reach 37% of the initial voltage).

Local Potentials

In contrast to the active propagation of APs, synaptic potentials and sensory receptor potentials are not actively propagated. Such potentials decay exponentially (from their source of initiation) along the cell cable, as already described. Therefore, synaptic and receptor potentials are **local potentials.** When local potentials are depolarizing, they can give rise to APs, which are propagated; when hyperpolarizing, they inhibit production of APs. These local potentials are similar to the **local excitatory response** (Chap. 4) in that both are confined to a local region, but the electrogenesis of the two is different. As stated previously, the neuromuscular junction is an excitatory type of chemical synapse and produces excitatory postsynaptic potentials, known here as **end-plate potentials.** Most **synaptic potentials** are **graded,** in that they can add on one another, both in time and space (temporal and spatial summation), to produce larger responses; larger synaptic potentials exert a greater stimulatory or inhibitory effect on the production of APs.

Conduction of Action Potentials
Local-Circuit Currents

This section examines the mechanism for the rapid propagation (conduction) of APs. Propagation occurs by means of the **local-circuit currents** that accompany the propagating APs (Fig. 5-5). Such currents exist because, when two points are at a different potential (voltage) in a conducting medium, current I will flow between the two points, as governed by Ohm's law ($I = V/R$). At the peak of the AP,

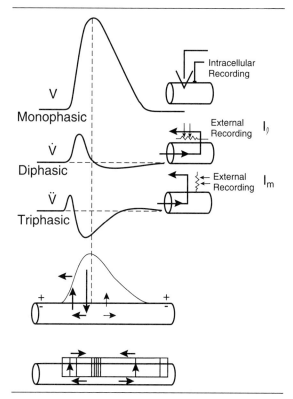

Fig. 5-5. The first ($\dot{V}$) and second ($\ddot{V}$) time derivatives of the action potential spike and the longitudinal (I_l) and radial currents associated with the propagating spike. The longitudinal (axial) current (I_l) is biphasic, having an intense forward phase and a less intense backward phase, as depicted in the diagram at the bottom. The radial transmembrane current (I_m) is triphasic, having a moderately intense initial outward phase, then a very intense inward phase (the current "sink"), followed by a less intense second outward phase, as depicted in the lower diagram. The arrows depict the three phases of the membrane current and the two phases of the axial current. The first derivative can be recorded externally by a pair of closely spaced (relative to the spike wavelength) electrodes arranged parallel to the fiber axis, and the second derivative, by a pair of electrodes arranged perpendicular to the fiber axis, as depicted.

the inside of the membrane at that region of the fiber becomes positive with respect to the outside. The inside is also positive with respect to the inside cytoplasm at a region downstream from the active region. Therefore, current flows through the cytoplasm from the active region (current source) to the adjacent inactive region, then out of the fiber across the cell membrane, then through the interstitial fluid back to the active region (current "sink"), and

finally through the membrane of the active region. This completes the closed loop for the current. The outward current through the membrane of the inactive region produces an IR voltage drop (Ohm's law), positive inside to negative outside, that depolarizes this region, because the polarity of the voltage drop is opposite to that of the resting potential (negative inside, positive outside). When the depolarization exceeds the threshold potential, an AP is triggered. Thus the inactive region is now converted to an active region. This process is repeated in each segment of fiber, resulting in movement (propagation) of the impulse sequentially down the fiber.

If we examine a propagating AP, we see that there is also a small backflow of current internally, coupled with a corresponding small forward flow externally, associated with the repolarizing phase of the AP (see Fig. 5-5). Thus, as the AP propagates down the fiber, from right to left, there is a simultaneous double flow of local-circuit current: clockwise flow associated with the rising phase of the AP and counterclockwise flow associated with the repolarizing phase of the AP. The internal longitudinal current, sweeping past a transverse plane of the fiber, has two phases: first forward (right to left) and then reverse (left to right). The external longitudinal current also has two phases: left to right and then right to left. The transverse membrane current, sweeping through a point in the membrane, has three phases: first outward (still passive membrane), then inward (active membrane), and finally outward again (still active membrane).

It is the local-circuit current flow that allows recording of the electrocardiogram (ECG) from the surface of the body, as well as the electromyogram (EMG) and electroencephalogram (EEG) from the body surface over the tissue of interest. The internal longitudinal current is confined to the cytoplasm of the fiber, but the external current can use whatever conducting fluid is available (i.e., current takes the path of least resistance). Thus this external local-circuit current causes the skin to be at different potentials, and these differences can be recorded by electrographs (see following section, "External Recording").

Propagation Velocity Determinants

The factors that determine active velocity of propagation include fiber diameter, length constant (λ), time constant (τ_m), local-circuit current intensity, threshold potential, and temperature. Some of these factors are interrelated, such as fiber diameter and length constant (since the length constant is proportional to the square root of fiber radius). Propagation velocity is directly proportional to the length constant and inversely proportional to the time constant.

Propagation velocity is directly proportional to the square root of fiber diameter or radius a and inversely proportional to membrane capacitance C_m. The larger the fiber diameter, the lower is the longitudinal resistance of the intracellular cytoplasm (law of resistors in parallel) and the greater is the length constant. For example, the larger the diameter of nerve fibers, the faster they propagate. If membrane capacitance can be reduced (by myelination), then propagation velocity increases (see section "Saltatory Conduction").

In addition, propagation velocity depends on the intensity of the local-circuit current and hence on the rate of rise of the AP. The greater the AP rate of rise (max dV/dt), the greater is the longitudinal current and the transmembrane capacitive current. Therefore, all other factors being constant, faster-rising APs propagate faster. As discussed in Chap. 4, the AP rate of rise depends on the density of the fast Na^+ channels that are available, on membrane capacitance, and on temperature. The max dV/dt decreases with increased membrane capacitance, with cooling, and with partial depolarization (due to voltage inactivation of fast Na^+ channels). Cooling slows the rate of all chemical reactions, especially those with a high activation energy, such as the ion conductance changes in activated membrane.

Finally, the threshold potential affects propagation velocity. If the threshold is shifted to a more positive voltage (more depolarized), it takes longer for a given point in the membrane to reach threshold (and explode) during propagation of an AP from upstream. A greater **critical depolarization** (difference between resting potential and threshold potential) is required to bring the membrane to threshold. Therefore, propagation velocity would be slowed.

The preceding discussion applies to nonmyelinated nerve axons and skeletal muscle fibers. In myelinated nerve fibers, propagation velocity is greatly increased by the myelin sheath.

Saltatory Conduction

The nerve cable has been vastly improved by the evolutionary development of myelination in vertebrates. The myelin sheath increases the effective membrane resistance about a hundredfold and decreases the effective membrane capacitance about a hundredfold. This increases the length constant while maintaining the time constant almost constant.

One consequence of myelination is that **propagation velocity** is greatly increased. A second consequence is that the **energy cost** of signaling is greatly decreased, because ion fluxes are restricted primarily to the small nodes of Ranvier, which are spaced relatively far apart: 0.5 to 2.0 mm internodal length. At each node, the length of exposed (naked) cell membrane is only a few micrometers. Therefore, the degree of energy-requiring active ion transport (Na^+-K^+ and Ca^{2+}) required to maintain the steady-state ion distributions and to keep the system in a state of high potential energy is greatly reduced. For example, the amount of Na^+ gained and K^+ lost per impulse is reduced as a result of myelination. The amount of oxidative metabolism in myelinated fibers reflects this lowered energy requirement.

The myelin sheath is produced by the Schwann cell, which is wrapped repeatedly in a spiral around the nerve fiber, forming 50 to 300 wrappings (we will assume an average of 100). The myelin sheath covers the nerve axon like a coat sleeve and is interrupted at each node. The cytoplasm of the Schwann cell is nearly completely extruded during formation of the myelin sheath, so the sheath essentially consists of 100 cell membranes in series. Because of the law of resistors in series, the effective transmembrane resistance is increased a hundredfold. Because of the law of capacitors in series, the effective capacitance is reduced a hundredfold. Since the length constant is directly proportional to the square root of the membrane resistance, the length constant is increased accordingly. As described previously, increasing the length constant and lowering membrane capacitance increase propagation velocity.

The node forms an annulus around the entire perimeter of the fiber. Myelinated nerves usually have an optimal amount of myelin such that the ratio of the diameter of axis cylinder (naked axon) to total fiber (including myelin sheath) is about 0.6 to 0.7.

In **saltatory** (L. *saltere,* "to jump") **conduction,** the impulse jumps from one node to the next. The internodal membrane does not fire an AP for two reasons: (1) the internodal membrane is much less excitable (e.g., much fewer fast Na^+ channels), and (2) the depolarization of the neuron cell membrane at the internodal region is only about 1/100 that at the node. The IR voltage drop across the internodal cell membrane is only 1/100 of that across the entire series of membranes (Kirchhoff's laws dealing with voltage drops across resistors in series). Therefore, the depolarization of the internodal membrane at the internode is only about 1 mV, which is well below threshold.

Although the cell membrane is fluid and proteins can diffuse (float) laterally in the lipid bilayer matrix, the fast Na^+ channel proteins remain confined, at high density, in the nodal region due to special anchoring proteins (e.g., anchorin) that tether the ion channel proteins to the cytoskeletal framework, thus preventing their lateral movement into the internodal membrane.

The myelin sheath makes propagation much faster. For

example, a 20-μm-diameter myelinated nerve fiber conducts even faster than a 1000-μm (1-mm)-diameter nonmyelinated nerve fiber (e.g., the giant axon in squid and lobster): 120 m/sec versus approximately 25 to 50 m/sec. Thus, for invertebrates to achieve fast conduction in some essential circuits, they have to resort to giant neurons, resulting in a lower longitudinal cytoplasmic resistance and hence fast conduction. Because of space and size limitations, only a few critical neurons can possess a giant diameter. In vertebrates, on the other hand, a large fraction of the nerve fibers in the peripheral nerves are myelinated for the purpose of fast propagation.

In myelinated axons, propagation velocity varies with the first power of the cell radius, because propagation velocity varies with the length constant squared. The dependence of conduction velocity on the diameter of myelinated and nonmyelinated fibers is summarized in Table 5-1.

Wavelength of Impulse

The **wavelength** of the AP, which is the length of the axon simultaneously undergoing some portion of the AP, is equal to the propagation velocity times the duration of the AP (APD_{100}). The wavelength in a large myelinated nerve axon is about 12 cm: 120 m/sec × 1.0 msec. In a skeletal muscle fiber, it is about 1.8 cm (6 m/sec × 3.0 msec), and in a smooth muscle bundle, it is only about 1.5 mm (5 cm/sec × 30 msec).

External Recording of Action Potentials

Monophasic, Biphasic, and Triphasic Recording

As discussed in the preceding section "Local-Circuit Currents," **local-circuit currents** accompany the propagating AP in each fiber. The local-circuit current has both longitudinal and radial (transverse) components and makes a complete circuit (Fig. 5-6). The intracellular and extracellular longitudinal currents are **biphasic** and are exactly equal in amplitude but flow in opposite directions; intracellularly, they travel in the forward direction and in the reverse direction. The forward-direction current is intense (high current density), and the reverse-direction current is weak (low current density). The transmembrane radial currents are **triphasic;** the first phase is outward (moderate intensity), the second phase is inward (high intensity), and

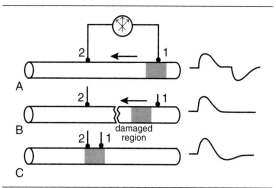

Fig. 5-6. The waveforms that would be recorded externally during propagation of an AP in a single fiber. (A) The two electrodes are far apart (relative to the AP wavelength), and so a biphasic recording is obtained, with the two phases symmetrical and separated by an isopotential segment. The two phases are due to the current flow through the voltmeter recorder traveling first in one direction and then in the opposite direction. (B) If the fiber between these two electrodes is damaged (e.g., by crushing) or depolarized (by elevating extracellular K^+ concentration) so that the AP cannot propagate to electrode 2, this second phase is prevented, and the recording is monophasic. (C) If the two electrodes are brought progressively closer, the isopotential segment depicted in (A) would shorten and disappear. If electrode 1 is brought very close to electrode 2 so that the interelectrode distance is short relative to the wavelength, then the second phase is smaller than the first phase, and the recording resembles the first derivative of the true AP.

the third phase is outward (low intensity). The first phase (outward) gives rise to the passive exponential foot of the AP and is due to the passive cable spread of voltage and current. The second phase (inward) corresponds to the large inward fast Na^+ current, which occurs during the later portion of the rising phase and peak of the AP. The third phase (outward) corresponds to the net outward current (K^+), which occurs during the repolarizing phase.

These longitudinal and radial currents can be recorded by suitably placed external electrodes. The extracellular **longitudinal currents** (axial) can be recorded by two electrodes (bipolar) placed close together along the length of the fiber. If the interelectrode distance is short (relative to the wavelength), an approximate first (time) derivative of the AP is obtained (see Fig. 5-5). The extracellular **radial currents** can be recorded by two electrodes placed close together in a plane perpendicular to the fiber axis, this giving an approximation of the second (time) derivative of the

AP (see Fig. 5-4). The internal axial currents are confined to the cytoplasm, whereas the external longitudinal currents can use the entire interstitial fluid space of the nerve bundle or muscle or even the entire torso (so-called **volume conductor**), since current takes the path of least resistance (law of resistors in parallel).

For biphasic recording in which the two phases are about equal, the two external electrodes can be placed far apart (with respect to the wavelength) along a nerve or muscle fiber (Fig. 5-6A). First the proximal electrode records the wave of negativity (associated with the propagating AP) and then returns to isopotential. When the wave reaches the second electrode, it is recorded in the reversed polarity (because current flow through the voltmeter is reversed). If the two electrodes are moved closer together, the isopotential region disappears, and the second phase of the AP becomes smaller, the shape approaching the first derivative of the AP. If the AP is prevented from reaching the second (distal) electrode by crushing this region of the fiber, a **monophasic recording** is obtained (Fig. 5-6B).

Compound Action Potential

When one records the APs of a nerve bundle externally, the records are **graded** and not all-or-none, as in the case of true APs recorded intracellularly from single fibers (see Chap. 4). That is, the recorded AP gets larger and larger, up to a maximum amplitude, as the intensity of stimulation is increased. This is the so-called **compound action potential.** It is graded because as an increasingly greater number of the fibers are activated, the external longitudinal currents associated with the all-or-none AP in each fiber cut across the recording electrodes and thereby produce a larger signal. The maximum amplitude occurs when all the individual fibers (capable of responding) are responding. The amplitude of the signal is determined by the resistance between the electrodes multiplied by the amount of current flowing through this resistance (V = IR).

The stimulus strength that just recruits all the axons in the bundle is known as the **maximal stimulus;** strength beyond that is known as **supramaximal stimulus.** In the graded region of the compound action potential, the stimulus strength is **submaximal,** and when the strength is insufficient to excite any of the fibers, it is **subthreshold.**

The compound action potential recorded from a nerve bundle often has a second smaller peak after the initial large peak; sometimes even a third tiny peak can be detected. The initial large peak reflects activation of the many large-diameter myelinated motor and sensory axons, which have a lower threshold (more excitable). The second smaller peak reflects activation of the fewer smaller-diameter myelinated fibers, which have a higher threshold (less excitable). The third peak represents activation of the small-diameter nonmyelinated axons. Propagation velocity is a function of axon diameter and myelination (see preceding section) such that the larger the diameter, the greater the velocity. Myelinated axons conduct much faster than nonmyelinated axons (see above). Therefore, the first peak in the compound action potential consists of the fast-propagating, low-threshold fibers. Like runners in a race, the slower runners cross the finish line later. Therefore, the slower-propagating, higher-threshold fibers compose the second peak.

The compound APs can be demonstrated by recording the EMG in a human subject with one electrode placed on the skin of the ventral forearm and the other (reference) electrode on the wrist of the same arm. As the subject voluntarily produces stronger and stronger contractions to flex the hand, the electric signals picked up become increasingly greater in amplitude and frequency. The amplitude gets larger because more muscle fibers are activated simultaneously. This is known as **fiber recruitment.** The frequency increases because the motor nerves fire at a higher frequency, causing the muscle fibers to fire at a higher frequency and thus producing more powerful tetanic contraction.

Summary

Although the biologic cable (i.e., nerve fiber or skeletal muscle fiber) is the best possible given the biologic circumstances, it is relatively poor compared with electric wires and cables. This is so because (1) the resistivity of the cytoplasm of nerve and skeletal muscle fibers is about 10^7 times that for copper wire, (2) the transverse membrane resistance is about 10^{-6} times that of a good insulator (like rubber) because it is so thin (approximately 70 Å, or 7 nm), and (3) the membrane has a high capacitance and therefore relatively long time constant. Because the biologic cable is poor, if the cable remained passive (no active impulse), there would be much signal loss in the transmission of information. Thus the signal would become greatly attenuated and distorted after traveling only a short distance. Therefore, for faithful and rapid signal transmission over long distances, energy must be introduced into the system at each point along the way. The system that has evolved consists of AP generation. APs are all-or-none signals of constant amplitude and constant propagation velocity with refractory periods and sharp thresholds. It is a frequency-modulated system, whereby an increase in frequency of the AP signals produces increasing strength of sensation or motor response.

AP propagation occurs by means of the local-circuit currents. The transmembrane current has three phases: outward, inward, and outward. The internal and external longitudinal currents have two phases: forward and backward (for internal) or backward and forward (for external). The external currents use the path of least resistance, enabling electrograms (e.g., ECG, EMG) to be recorded from the body surface. The compound AP is graded in amplitude, reflecting the summation of the external currents generated from each activated fiber: The more fibers activated simultaneously, the greater is the amplitude of the electrogram signal.

Propagation velocity is faster, the larger the fiber diameter, the longer the length constant, and the lower its time constant and capacitance. The myelin sheath in vertebrates enables much faster propagation velocity and at a lower energy cost. The resulting myelination increases the effective membrane resistance and lowers the effective capacitance, with excitability occurring only at the short nodes of Ranvier that uniformly interrupt the myelin sheath. There-fore, the AP signal jumps from node to node in a saltatory pattern of conduction.

Bibliography

Cole, K. C. *Membranes, Ions and Impulses: A Chapter of Classical Biophysics.* Berkeley: University of California Press, 1968.

Sperelakis, N. Origin of the cardiac resting potential. In R. M. Berne and N. Sperelakis, eds., *Handbook of Physiology: The Cardiovascular System,* Vol. I: *The Heart.* Bethesda, Md.: American Physiological Society, 1979. Pp. 187–267.

Sperelakis, N., and Fabiato, A. Electrophysiology and excitation-contraction coupling in skeletal muscle. In C. Roussos and P. Macklem, eds., *The Thorax: Vital Pump.* New York: Marcel Dekker, 1985. Pp. 45–113.

Taylor, R. E. Cable analysis. In W. L. Nastuck, ed., *Physical Techniques in Biological Research,* Vol. 6B. New York: Academic Press, 1963. P. 219.

Part I Questions: Cellular Physiology

1. A patient has 14 liters of ECF, 28 liters of ICF, and a plasma osmolarity of 270 mOsm/liter. If 100 ml of a 3000-mM urea solution were infused intravenously, which of the following is likely to occur (assume no loss through kidneys)?
   A. About 600 ml of water will move from the ICF to the ECF.
   B. The new steady-state plasma osmolarity will be 320 mOsm/liter.
   C. The new steady-state ICF volume will be about 28 liters.
   D. The plasma Na^+ concentration will decrease to 134 meq/liter.
   E. The plasma Na^+ concentration will increase to 146 meq/liter.

2. Which one of the following solutions of identical osmolarity is isotonic with respect to the red blood cell?
   A. 150-mM sucrose + 75-mM NaCl
   B. 150-mM urea + 75-mM NaCl
   C. 150-mM NH_4Cl
   D. 300-mM urea
   E. 150-mM urea + 75-mM NH_4Cl

3. Pathways for secondary active transport would include all of the following *except*
   A. Na/H exchanger.
   B. Na-glucose cotransporter.
   C. voltage-gated Na channel.
   D. Cl/HCO_3 antiporter.
   E. Na-K-2Cl symporter.

4. An example of an electrogenic transporter would be one that
   A. exchanges an internal Na^+ for an external K^+.
   B. cotransports an external Na^+ and Cl^- into the cell.
   C. transports a Na^+ and HCO_3^- ion into the cell in exchange for a Cl^- and H^+ ion.
   D. transports 3 Na^+ ions into a cell in exchange for a Ca^{2+} ion.
   E. uses the energy from ATP to move an H^+ out of the cell and a K^+ into the cell.

5. The resting potential E_m of a skeletal muscle fiber diminishes (membrane depolarizes) progressively as the $[K]_o$ in the bathing Ringer's solution is progressively elevated (K^+ substituted for Na^+ on an equimolar basis). When E_m passes (or extrapolates) to zero, this point indicates which one of the following?
   A. $[Na]_o$
   B. $[K]_1$
   C. $[Cl]_1$
   D. $[H]_1$
   E. E_{epp}

6. In a two-compartment system, with 100-mM potassium chloride on side no. 1 and 1.0-mM potassium chloride on side no. 2, the two solutions being separated by a thin membrane permeable to Cl^- but impermeable to K^+, the potential difference built up across the membrane (side no. 1 with respect to side no. 2) would be closest to (at 30°C)?
   A. −120 mV
   B. −60 mV
   C. 0 mV
   D. +60 mV
   E. +120 mV

7. *Threshold* for firing an action potential occurs when
   A. $I_{Na} < I_K$.
   B. I_{Na} inactivates.
   C. g_K increases.
   D. $I_{Na} > I_K$.
   E. None of the above

8. The fast Na^+ current
   A. activates after I_K.
   B. causes repolarization.
   C. turns on slowly.
   D. spontaneously inactivates.
   E. All of the above

9. Propagation velocity increases with which one of the following?
   A. Greater membrane capacitance

B. Greater membrane time constant
C. Cooling
D. Greater fiber diameter
E. Shorter length constant
F. More positive (higher) threshold potential

10. Which one of the following statements is true with respect to the myelin sheath?
    A. Increases the effective membrane capacitance
    B. Increases the effective membrane resistance
    C. Decreases the length constant
    D. Allows for smooth continuous conduction
    E. Has a large effect on the effective time constant

II Neurophysiology

Part Editors
Michael M. Behbehani
and Janusz B. Suszkiw

6 Synaptic Transmission

Janusz B. Suszkiw and Nicholas Sperelakis

Objectives

After reading this chapter, you should be able to

Describe the sequence of events in chemically mediated synaptic transmission

Explain the mechanism of transmitter release

Explain the mechanism of end-plate potential and action potential generation at the neuromuscular junction

Describe the effects and sites of action of drugs and toxins that affect neuromuscular transmission

Describe the actions of neurotransmitters at central excitatory and inhibitory synapses

Explain the integration of synaptic activity in brain synapses

Distinguish between postsynaptic and presynaptic inhibition

Transmission of signals between neurons and from neurons to muscle and gland cells takes place at specialized junctions called **synapses.** Synapses can be either **electrical** or **chemical.** At electrical synapses, transmission is accomplished through direct passage of current between the communicating cells. At chemical synapses, transmission is mediated by a chemical neurotransmitter substance. Although electrical synapses are relatively more common in lower animals, the synaptic transmission in higher vertebrates is predominantly chemical. The fundamental features of chemical transmission at the vertebrate neuromuscular junction and at central synapses are discussed in this chapter.

General Features of a Chemical Synapse

The structural and functional features of chemical synapses are illustrated in Fig. 6-1. The synaptic junction consists of presynaptic and postsynaptic elements that are separated by a 20- to 100-nm-wide extracellular gap, the **synaptic cleft.** The presynaptic element is usually an axon terminal, but it also may be formed by a dendrite or cell body of the transmitting neuron. The postsynaptic element is the chemosensitive portion of the receiving cell's membrane and contains specific receptors for the particular neurotransmitter that is released from the presynaptic neuron. Thus, depending on topographic relations between presynaptic and postsynaptic elements, synapses may be characterized by a variety of configurations, including axosomatic, axodendritic, dendrodendritic, and axoaxonic contacts. The synapses between neurons and peripheral effectors are commonly referred to as **neuroeffector junctions.** Owing to its morphologic appearance, the skeletal neuromuscular junction is commonly referred to as the **motor end-plate.**

Neurotransmitters are stored in **synaptic vesicles** and are released from the synaptic vesicles into the synaptic cleft by a Ca^{2+}-regulated exocytosis at specialized plas-

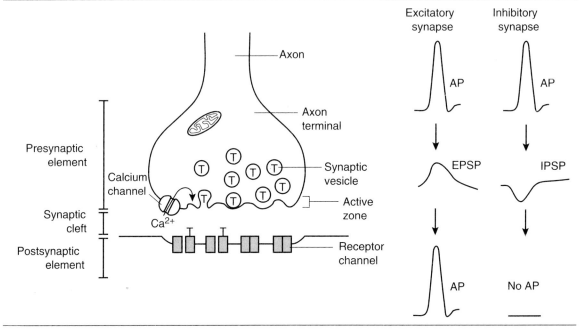

Fig. 6-1. Structural elements of a synapse (AP = action potential; EPSP = excitatory postsynaptic potential; IPSP = inhibitory postsynaptic potential; T = neurotransmitter).

malemmal release sites called the presynaptic **active zone.** The release of transmitter is initiated by a presynaptic action potential. The transmitter binds to specific receptors in the postsynaptic membrane causing a brief change in its ionic permeability and displacement of the membrane potential.

Synapses can be either **excitatory** or **inhibitory.** At excitatory synapses, transmitter-receptor interactions cause an increase in the postsynaptic membrane permeability to Na^+ and K^+ ions and a membrane depolarization called the **excitatory postsynaptic potential** (EPSP). This depolarization increases the likelihood of an action potential (AP) being fired in the postsynaptic cell. At inhibitory synapses, an increase in permeability of postsynaptic membrane to Cl^- and/or K^+ ions results in a membrane hyperpolarization referred to as the **inhibitory postsynaptic potential** (IPSP).

The synaptic action of transmitters is terminated through a rapid removal of the transmitter from the synaptic cleft by reuptake back into presynaptic terminal or glial cells or (in the case of acetylcholine) degradation to inactive components directly in the synaptic cleft.

Common identified transmitters and neuroactive peptides with transmitter functions are shown in Table 6-1. Glutamate and gamma-aminobutyric acid (GABA) are the

Table 6-1. Major Neurotransmitters and Neuroactive Peptides

Aminoacidergic	γ-Aminobutyric acid (GABA)
	Aspartic acid
	Glutamic acid
	Glycine
	Histamine
Cholinergic	Acetylcholine (ACh)
Monoaminergic	Dopamine (DA)
	Epinephrine (adrenaline)
	Norepinephrine (noradrenaline)
	Serotonin (5-HT)
Purinergic	Adenosine
	ATP
Neuroactive peptides	Cholecystokinin
	Enkephalin
	Neuropeptide Y
	Neurotensin
	Oxytocin
	Somatostatin
	Substance P
	Thyrotropin-releasing hormone (TRH)
	Vasoactive intestinal peptide (VIP)
	Vasopressin

major brain transmitters at excitatory and inhibitory synapses, respectively. Other transmitters may exert both excitatory and inhibitory actions, depending on the receptors with which they interact. For example, acetylcholine (ACh) acts on the nicotinic ACh receptors to transfer excitation at the skeletal neuromuscular junction but exerts an inhibitory effect in the heart by interacting with muscarinic ACh receptors. In addition to conventional fast synaptic actions, which occur in a millisecond time range, a number of neurotransmitters also may exert slow actions on the postsynaptic cells, lasting for seconds or longer. Some neuroactive peptides are costored and coreleased with conventional transmitters and exert slow synaptic actions.

The Skeletal Neuromuscular Junction

The skeletal neuromuscular junction, or the **motor end-plate** (Fig. 6-2), is an excitatory synapse designed to securely transfer action potentials from spinal motor neurons to skeletal muscle fibers. Owing to the discontinuity between the presynaptic and postsynaptic elements and the size mismatch of the nerve and muscle fibers, the current associated with the presynaptic action potential cannot depolarize the muscle membrane to a significant extent. The function of the synaptic transmitter acetylcholine is to amplify the presynaptic signal to ensure that threshold for generation of a muscle AP is reached. The motor end-plate is located near the middle of the long muscle fiber, so the muscle AP is initiated in this region and propagated in both directions down the muscle fiber. Some muscle fibers have a second motor end-plate nearby, the motor axon originating from an adjacent level of the spinal cord (thus providing some additional safety factor to ensure muscle activation).

Steps in Neuromuscular Transmission

Acetylcholine is synthesized in the nerve terminal cytoplasm by the enzyme cholineacetyltransferase and stored in the synaptic vesicles for subsequent release through the process of exocytosis. The process of synaptic transmission involves a sequence of steps as follows:

1. *ACh release from presynaptic axon terminal.* The arrival of a nerve AP depolarizes the nerve terminal and opens voltage-gated calcium channels in the presynaptic membrane, allowing an influx of Ca^{2+} into the terminal. The resulting transient increase in the intraterminal Ca^{2+} concentration triggers a nearly synchronous exocytosis of ACh from 100 to 300 synaptic vesicles.

2. *Generation of the end-plate potential (EPP).* The released ACh molecules diffuse quickly (about 10 μsec) over the short distance (approximately 50 nm) from the presynaptic terminal to the postsynaptic muscle membrane and combine with nicotinic ACh receptors (nAChR) that are an integral part of the ion channels. Binding of two ACh molecules to the receptor-channel complex induces a conformational change of the complex and opening of the channel for 1 to 2 msec, which in turn increases the permeability of the end-plate to Na^+ and K^+ about equally. That is, these channels are nonselective cation channels (anions like Cl^- are excluded). This synaptic channel is an example of ligand-gated ion channel, a subtype of receptor-operated ion channels. Such channels are not activated by voltage, i.e., depolarization.

Sodium ions flow in and potassium ions move out of the muscle cell through the receptor-gated synaptic channels in accordance with their respective electrochemical gradients. Since at the resting potential the electrochemical driving force for Na^+ influx is much greater than that for K^+ efflux, Na^+ ions will be the preponderant charge carrier through the synaptic channels, giving rise to a net inward synaptic current carried by Na^+ ions, which is called the **end-plate current.** The resulting depolarization of the end-plate is the **end-plate potential.**

3. *Initiation of the muscle action potential.* The synaptic current flows from the end-plate to the surrounding conductile membrane causing its depolarization. When the threshold potential of the conductile membrane is reached, a propagated muscle AP is fired. The EPP and muscle AP recorded from a frog nerve-muscle preparation in vitro are shown in Fig. 6-3. Note that the EPP is restricted to the end-plate region and is a nonpropagated, local potential. The sole function of the EPP is to depolarize the muscle membrane to threshold so that an AP is triggered, which then propagates simultaneously in both directions along the fiber.

4. *Termination of the synaptic action of ACh.* ACh released into the synaptic cleft is rapidly (within 1–2 msec) hydrolyzed to acetate and choline by the enzyme acetylcholinesterase (AChE), terminating its action on the postsynaptic receptors. The receptor-gated channels spontaneously reclose, and the end-plate potential decays to zero within a few milliseconds, in accordance with the membrane time constant τ_m.

Quantal Theory of Chemical Neurotransmission

The quantal theory of transmitter release was elaborated in the 1950s by Katz and associates in a series of elegant

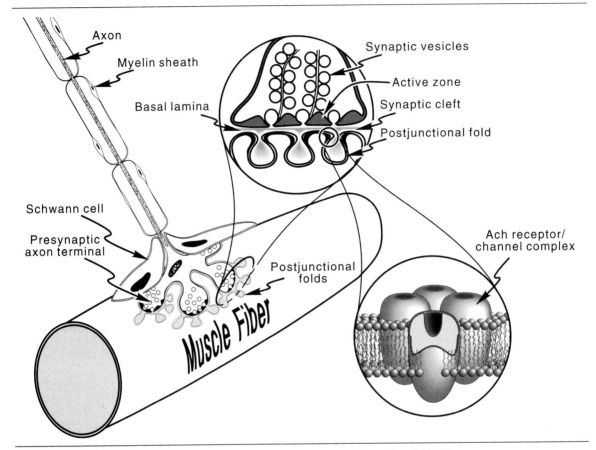

Fig. 6-2. Microanatomy of the skeletal neuromuscular junction. (Modified from: Sperelakis, N., ed. *Cell Physiology Source Book.* New York: Academic Press, 1995.)

electrophysiologic experiments on the frog neuromuscular junction. The essence of the theory is that acetylcholine release from the motor nerve endings occurs in discrete packets called **quanta.** A quantum is estimated to contain 1500 to 10,000 ACh molecules and likely represents the ACh content of a single synaptic vesicle. The smallest unit of quantal response is depolarization of the postsynaptic membrane by about 0.5 mV. These small depolarizations can be detected only at the end-plate region. They occur in a resting (i.e., in the absence of presynaptic APs) junctions at random intervals with a frequency of about 1/sec and are called **miniature end-plate potentials** (MEPP). A nerve impulse causes this activity to become enormously intensified for a very brief moment so that a few hundred quanta are released nearly synchronously within less than 1 msec, giving rise to a large depolarization of the end-plate, i.e., the end-plate potential (Fig. 6-4).

According to Katz, the quantal theory of synaptic transmission holds that the spontaneous MEPP and its underlying conductance change are the basic unit of transmitter action and that the large EPP evoked by a nerve impulse is composed of an integral multiple of such unit components. The quantal composition of the EPP is readily revealed in low-Ca^{2+} solutions. Calcium is an essential cofactor, and in the absence of Ca^{2+} in the external medium, depolarization of nerve terminals fails to increase the rate of ACh release. In low-Ca^{2+} solutions, the probability of transmitter release is reduced, and the EPPS evoked by nerve action potentials show a marked fluctuation in amplitude, which on average is a multiple integral of quantal MEPPs. In other words, the amplitudes of the EPPs do not vary continuously but rather occur in small, discrete quantal steps. Statistical analysis shows that the size of these steps corresponds to the size of a single MEPP, which is be-

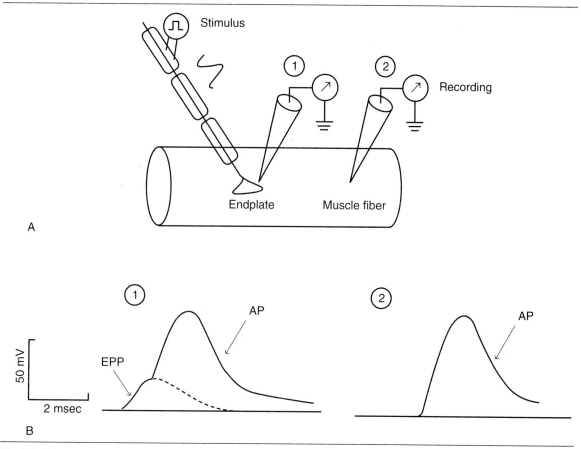

Fig. 6-3. Schematic representation of intracellular records from the muscle in response to presynaptic nerve stimulation. Presynaptic action potential is evoked by electrical pulse applied to the nerve. Postsynaptic membrane potentials are recorded with intracellular glass microelectrodes inserted at the end-plate (position 1) and some distance (2 mm) away from the end-plate (position 2). The records obtained with microelectrode 1 constitute the end-plate potential (EPP), which is largely masked by the action potential (AP) that it triggers but is evident as a step on the rising phase of the AP. In practice, EPP properties are studied in the presence of curare, which is used to depress the EPP to below the threshold for generation of the muscle AP so that EPP is revealed in its entirety (*dashed trace*). Due to decrement of the EPP within a short distance of the end-plate, only the propagated muscle AP is recorded by the microelectrode 2.

lieved to be produced by a quantum of ACh released from one synaptic vesicle. The statistical nature of transmitter release can be described by a simple equation:

$$m = n \cdot P \qquad (6\text{-}1)$$

in which m is the average number of quanta released by each nerve impulse, n is the number of quanta of ACh that are available for release, and P is the probability of any one quantum being released. The probability of transmitter release is a function of the Ca^{2+} concentration in the terminal. In resting preparations (in the absence of nerve impulses), the concentration of ionized Ca^{2+} in terminals is very low (about 10^{-7} M), and the probability of vesicle exocytosis is low. However, when the terminals are depolarized and Ca^{2+} enters into the terminal, the probability of vesicle exocytosis is greatly enhanced, resulting in a release of several hundred vesicles nearly simultaneously.

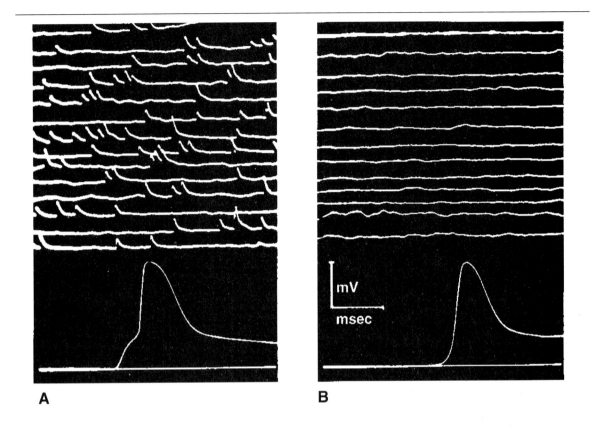

A   **B**

Fig. 6-4. Localization of end-plate potentials in the frog muscle. The records illustrated in (A)
are from the end-plate region and show spontaneously occurring miniature end-plate potentials (MEPPs) recorded at a resting junction (*upper trace*) and an EPP and the muscle action
potential triggered by it, recorded from active junction (*lower trace*). Note absence of MEPPs
or the EPP recorded from the same muscle fiber at a distance 2 mm from the end-plate (B).
Voltage and time scales: 50 mV and 2 msec for the lower part and 3.6 mV and 47 msec for the
upper part. (Modified from: Fatt, P., and Katz, B. Spontaneous subthreshold activity at motor
nerve endings. *J. Physiol.* 117:109, 1952.)

Mechanism of End-Plate Potential Generation

As indicated above, the EPP is a local depolarization that
is generated when ACh binds to its receptors and opens the
associated channels for 1 to 2 msec and then spontaneously recloses. During this time, Na$^+$ ions flow in and K$^+$
ions move out through the synaptic channels in accordance
with their respective electrochemical gradients. The resulting synaptic current I$_S$ can be thus expressed as the sum of
sodium (I$_{Na}$) and potassium (I$_K$) currents:

$$I_S = I_{Na} + I_K = g_{Na}(V_m - E_{Na}) + g_K(V_m - E_K) \qquad (6\text{-}2)$$

where g$_{Na}$ and g$_K$ are the Na$^+$ and K$^+$ ion conductances,
and E$_{Na}$ and E$_K$ are the Na$^+$ and K$^+$ equilibrium potentials,
respectively. Given the normal distribution of Na$^+$ and K$^+$
ions and the resting muscle membrane potential of about
−80 mV, the driving force for Na$^+$ ion entry is more powerful than for K$^+$ ion efflux. Therefore, there is a net inward
synaptic current I$_S$ that is carried by Na$^+$ ions, causing depolarization of the end-plate. It is evident from Eq. (6-2)
that as the membrane potential V$_m$ becomes depolarized,

the driving force $(V_m - E_{Na})$ acting on Na^+ ions to enter the cell decreases and the driving force $(V_m - E_k)$ acting on K^+ ions to exit the cell increases. At a certain membrane potential, the driving forces acting on Na^+ ions to flow in and K^+ ions to flow out of the end-plate will be equal in magnitude, that is,

$$g_{Na}(V_m - E_{Na}) = -g_K(V_m - E_K) \qquad (6\text{-}3)$$

The membrane potential V_m at which this occurs is called the **equilibrium potential** for the EPP (E_{EPP}), where

$$E_{EPP} = \frac{g_{Na}}{g_{Na} + g_K} E_{Na} + \frac{g_K}{g_{Na} + g_K} E_K \qquad (6\text{-}4)$$

E_{EPP} is the maximum theoretical potential to which the end-plate can be depolarized when all the receptor-gated channels are simultaneously activated by ACh.

The relationship between synaptic (end-plate) current flow and membrane depolarization can be analyzed in terms of an equivalent electric circuit consisting of parallel synaptic and nonsynaptic branches (Fig. 6-5). Since the sodium and potassium ions flow through the same synaptic channels at the end-plate, the conductance can be represented by single synaptic (end-plate) conductance g_S and synaptic current, expressed as

$$I_S = g_s(V_m - E_{EPP}) \qquad (6\text{-}5)$$

During the active phase, the synaptic current flows inward through the synaptic branch and outward through the parallel nonsynaptic branch, that is,

$$I_s = -(I_c + I_m) \qquad (6\text{-}6)$$

where I_c is the current flowing through the membrane capacitance, and I_m is the current flowing through the ionic channels in the nonsynaptic membrane. I_m is given by

$$I_m = g_m(V_m - E_m) \qquad (6\text{-}7)$$

where the conductance g_m is the reciprocal of muscle membrane resistance ($1/R_m$), and E_m is the resting potential. Once the membrane capacitance is discharged to its final value, the capacitive current I_c becomes zero and a steady-state (peak) membrane depolarization is reached at which $I_s = I_m$. Therefore,

$$I_s = g_m(V_m - E_m) \qquad (6\text{-}8)$$

The quantity $(V_m - E_m)$ is the amplitude of the end-plate potential V_{EPP} at the peak of synaptic activation. Thus

$$V_{EPP} = I_s R_m \qquad (6\text{-}9)$$

Equation (6-9) shows that V_{EPP} is a function of synaptic current I_s and resistance of the membrane. The higher the R_m, the greater is the depolarizing efficacy of the synaptic current. As indicated by Eq. (6-5), the magnitude of I_s is a function of the number of synaptic channels opened (g_s) and driving force $(V_m - E_{EPP})$. As the synaptic channels reclose within 1 to 2 msec, the synaptic current I_s rapidly decays to zero, and the membrane repolarizes to the resting value. The repolarizing phase of the EPP is passive and exponential and follows the membrane time constant, which varies between 2 and 10 msec (depending on species and type of muscle).

Effects of Drugs and Toxins on Neuromuscular Transmission

A number of drugs and toxins interfere with synaptic transmission by acting either on the nerve terminal or the postsynaptic process.

Presynaptic Actions

Inhibition of Precursor Uptake and Deficiency of Transmitter Synthesis. An example of this type of drug is provided by **hemicholinium-3** (HC-3), a potent competitive inhibitor of the high-affinity choline transport system that provides choline for the synthesis of ACh in nerve terminals. In the presence of HC-3, the supply of choline (and hence the synthesis of ACh) is depressed, and during repetitive stimulation, transmitter stores become depleted and synaptic fatigue ensues.

Disruption of Transmitter Packaging. Drugs such as D,1-2-(4-phenylpiperidino)cyclohexanol (Vesamicol) penetrate into presynaptic nerve terminals and block ACh uptake into synaptic vesicles. In presence of the drug, synaptic vesicles cannot be refilled with the transmitter even though ACh synthesis itself in the cytoplasm is not impaired. Ultimately, exhaustion of the releasable vesicular transmitter store leads to failure of neuromuscular transmission. **Alpha-latrotoxin,** a component of black widow spider venom, causes massive transmitter exocytosis and depletion of synaptic vesicles from terminals, thereby causing synaptic transmission to fail.

Interference with Exocytosis. Agents such as **botulin neurotoxins** produced by the microorganism

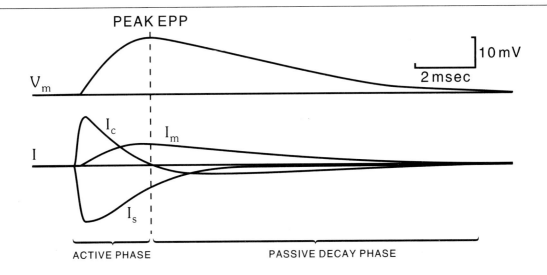

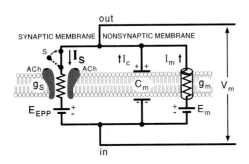 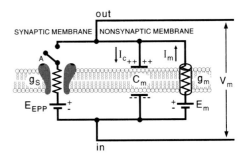

$$I_s = -(I_c + I_m)$$

$$I_s = 0 \quad I_c = -I_m$$

Fig. 6-5. Electrical equivalent circuit analysis of EPP. (*Top*) Time course of end-plate potential and the underlying membrane currents. (*Bottom*) the electric circuit description of current flow during EPP. At rest (absence of evoked ACh release), the synaptic switch is opened, and no current flows through the circuit. The resting membrane potential (Vm) measured between intracellular and extracellular electrodes would be equal to $E_M \approx -80$ mV. Activation of the ACh receptor-channel complex is equivalent to closing the synaptic switch. Current flows into the end-plate through the receptor gated channels (I_s) and out through the ionic channels (I_m) and capacitance (I_c) of the adjacent non-synaptic membrane. At the peak of EPP, $I_c = 0$, and $I_s = I_m$. The negative sign merely indicates the opposite directions of the current flow. As synaptic action of ACh is terminated by acetylcholinesterase, the receptor-gated channels reclose, and current no longer flows into the end-plate (synaptic switch open). The outward current diminishes in amplitude and returns through the capacitance to repolarize the muscle membrane. The EPP decay is determined by the RC properties of the muscle membrane. (Modified from: Kandel, E. R., Schwartz, J. H. and Jessell, T. M., *Principles of Neural Science,* 3rd ed. New York: Elsevier, 1991.)

Clostridium botulinum are responsible for the symptoms of food poisoning or botulism. The toxin's action is exerted following an internalization of its subunit into nerve terminals, where it blocks synaptic vesicle exocytosis irreversibly. This potent toxin is relatively specific for cholinergic nerve endings. **Heavy metals** such as Pb^{2+} and Cd^{2+} are potent antagonists of Ca^{2+} entry through the pre-synaptic voltage-gated Ca^{2+} channels and in submicro-molar concentration inhibit the evoked transmitter release.

Postsynaptic Actions

Neuromuscular Blockers. Nicotine, succinylcholine, and **decamethonium** are examples of drugs that bind reversibly to the receptor active site. Unlike ACh, these drugs are not inactivated by acetycholinesterase, and therefore, they cause persistent receptor activation that initially results in repetitive discharge of muscle action potentials, followed by block of neuromuscular transmission, probably due to inactivation of the muscle spiking mechanism (see Chap. 4), receptor desensitization, or both. The result is flaccid paralysis of the muscle.

Curare is a classic nicotinic ACh-receptor antagonist that prevents binding of ACh to the receptor. Increasing concentrations of curare at the neuromuscular junction cause progressive decrease in the amplitude and shortening of the EPPs. In severe curare poisoning, the EPPs are depressed to below the threshold potential and thus insufficient to initiate muscle action potentials. **Alpha-bungarotoxin** (a polypeptide component of the snake venom of the Formosan krait) combines essentially irreversibly with the receptor and, like curare, prevents its activation by ACh. As in the case of curare poisoning, the result is flaccid muscle paralysis.

Reversible neuromuscular blockers, such as succinyl-choline, are often used clinically to produce relaxation of skeletal muscle during surgery.

Anticholinesterases. As discussed previously, normally the action of ACh is terminated by its degradation by acetylcholinesterase (AChE) to inactive choline and acetate. When AChE is inhibited, ACh released into the synaptic cleft builds up in concentration and persists for a longer time. This results in increased and prolonged activation of the receptors by ACh and hence increased amplitude and duration of the EPP. As in the case of depolarizing blockers, after initial repetitive activation, the neuromuscular transmission is blocked, and a flaccid paralysis ensues. The inhibitors of AChE are of two types: slowly reversible (usually compounds that carbamylate the active site of the enzyme) or irreversible organophosphate anticholinesterases, which phosphorylate the active site of the enzyme. Since dephosphorylation is very slow ($t_{1/2}$ = days to weeks), the enzyme is essentially irreversibly inactivated. The classic example of an irreversible organophosphate anticholinesterase is **diisopropylfluoro-phosphate** (DFP) (originally developed as a nerve war gas). Currently, various anticholinesterases are employed as the principal component of some insecticides.

Diseases of the Neuromuscular Junction

Myasthenia Gravis (MG). The characteristic feature of this disease is muscle weakness, especially affecting cranial and upper limb muscles. There is a tendency for the weakness to vary in severity with remissions and exacerbations over longer periods of time. MG is a disorder caused by autoimmune response to ACh receptors, which leads to a reduction in the number of functional receptors and destruction of the postsynaptic membrane.

Lambert-Eaton Myasthenic Syndrome (LAMS). This disease is characterized by muscle weakness which, in contrast to MG symptoms, tends to improve with vigorous exercise. LAMS is associated with production of antibodies directed against the component(s) of the pre-synaptic active zone, most likely the voltage sensitive Ca^{2+} channels. The binding of antibodies leads to a reduction in Ca^{2+} entry and hence reduced probability of synaptic vesicle fusion and transmitter release.

Slow Channel Syndrome. This condition is hereditary (autosomal dominant) and is characterized by weakness, fatiguability, and atrophy of muscles. The syndrome is associated with an abnormally long ACh-gated channel open time. This results in prolongation of the end-plate potential, which in turn leads initially to discharge of multiple action potentials, followed by depolarizing block of transmission.

Congenital End-Plate Acetylcholinesterase Deficiency (CEPAD). The symptoms of this extremely rare condition are similar to those associated with slow channel syndrome and anticholinesterase poisoning. As might be expected, deficiency in cholinesterase results in buildup of ACh in the synaptic cleft and prolongation of ACh action on the receptors. This leads to prolongation of the EPP, which in turn causes multiple discharge of muscle APs and then depolarizing block of neuromuscular transmission and hence muscle weakness. As the disease progresses, there is significant atrophy of the muscles.

Effects of Denervation

Section of a nerve results in complete immediate flaccid paralysis of the muscle, since action potentials do not propagate past the site of section. The physiologic properties of the denervated muscle change over a period of days to weeks following the section: (1) the resting potential declines, (2) tetrodotoxin-insensitive Na^+ channels appear, (3) the muscle develops **denervation-supersensitivity,** which is associated with the appearance and spread of receptors in the extrajunctional muscle membrane, (4) during early stages, fibrillation (spontaneous twitching of individual muscle fibers) develops, and (5) the muscle atrophies. The effects of denervation on muscle are in part due to interruption in the supply of trophic factors by the nerve. Muscle inactivity appears to be an important factor in the establishment of denervation changes because direct stimulation of denervated muscles can slow down or even prevent the changes caused by severance of the nerve.

Properties of Synapses Between Neurons

In contrast to powerful single excitatory inputs received by the mammalian muscle fibers, central neurons usually receive multiple excitatory (E) and inhibitory (I) synaptic inputs. Since activation of any synapse alone produces a relatively small change in the membrane potential of the postsynaptic cell, several E-synaptic inputs must be active nearly simultaneously to bring the neuron to its threshold for firing an action potential. Furthermore, as will be discussed below, the effectiveness of the E-synaptic inputs can be diminished or nullified by activation of I-synaptic inputs. Thus, whereas the function of the skeletal neuromuscular junction is signal amplification to secure transmission of neural command signals to the muscle for the purpose of force generation, the function of central synapses is computational integration of many inputs converging onto the postsynaptic cell. At any instant, the postsynaptic cell integrates synaptic activity by adding and subtracting the E- and I-synaptic currents, and a propagated action potential is fired only if and when the net synaptic current causes sufficient depolarization to bring the postsynaptic neuron to its threshold.

Excitatory Postsynaptic Potentials

The ionic basis of EPSPs is analogous to that described for the EPP at the neuromuscular junction. EPSPs are generated when transmitter released from a presynaptic axon terminal acts on specific postsynaptic receptors to transiently increase membrane permeability to Na^+ and K^+ ions, giving rise to net inward synaptic current I_{EPSP}:

$$I_{EPSP} = g_{EPSP}(V_m - E_{EPSP}) \qquad (6\text{-}10)$$

which is carried by Na^+ ions and depolarizes the postsynaptic and adjacent conductile membrane of the neuron (Fig. 6-6A). The amplitude of the EPSP (V_{EPSP}) is a function of the size of I_{EPSP} and the neuronal membrane resistance, that is,

$$V_{EPSP} = I_{EPSP}R_m \qquad (6\text{-}11)$$

Unlike the large depolarization associated with the muscle EPP, the amplitudes of EPSPs generated at any single synapse are small, usually in the range of only 0.5 to 2 mV. Consequently, several EPSPs must summate in order to depolarize the membrane to the threshold potential for discharging the propagated AP.

Inhibitory Synaptic Potentials (IPSPs)

IPSPs (see Fig. 6-6) are generated when a transmitter increases conductance of the postsynaptic membrane to Cl^- or K^+ ions. Influx of Cl^- or efflux of K^+ ions gives rise to an outward current through the postsynaptic membrane and an inward current through the nonsynaptic, conductile membrane. The synaptic currents associated with Cl^- influx or efflux of K^+ ions produce a deficit of positive charges on the interior leaflet of the membrane and hence membrane hyperpolarization.

The inhibitory synaptic currents I_{IPSP} can be written in a fashion analogous to those for I_{EPSP}:

$$I_{IPSP} = g_{IPSP}(V_m - E_{IPSP}) \qquad (6\text{-}12)$$

where g_{IPSP} is the synaptic conductance (Cl^- or K^+), and E_{IPSP} is the equilibrium potential of the IPSP. Thus, during activation of chloride conductance, the membrane potential will tend to hyperpolarize toward the **chloride equilibrium potential** (E_{Cl} of about −80 mV). In the case of K^+ permeability change, the membrane potential will tend to hyperpolarize toward the **K^+ equilibrium potential** (E_K of about −90 mV).

The inhibitory effect of an IPSP on the cell's electrical excitability (e.g., spike generation) is not only due to

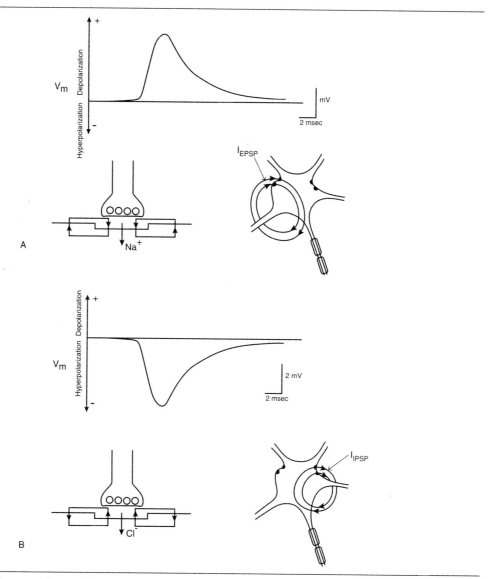

Fig. 6-6. Postsynaptic potentials at excitatory and inhibitory synapses in brain. (A) An EPSP is a depolarizing potential, a few millivolts in amplitude and a few milliseconds in duration. Current flow during the synaptic action of transmitter is inward through the synaptic membrane and outward through the nonsynaptic membrane. At the right is shown the distribution of currents over the entire area of the postsynaptic neuron, including the initial segment of the axon. (B) An IPSP is a hyperpolarizing potential, a few milliseconds in duration. Current flow during the synaptic action of transmitter at an inhibitory synapse is outward through the synaptic channels and inward through the nonsynaptic membrane. At the right is shown the distribution of currents over the entire area of the postsynaptic neuron. Compare the direction of current flow with that shown for activation of the excitatory synapse.

membrane hyperpolarization but also is related to the decrease in the cell's overall input resistance (R_m). The activation of inhibitory synapses and opening of the synaptic Cl^- or K^+ channels provide low-resistance conductance pathways for current flow out of the cell, thus reducing the EPSP.

Integration of Synaptic Inputs

Whether or not a neuron discharges a propagated AP is determined by integration of all synaptic inputs active at any given instant in time. Neurons integrate PSPs by algebraically summating all EPSPs and IPSPs at any instant in time. When and if the resulting potential reaches the threshold value, a propagated AP is triggered (Fig. 6-7). The AP is triggered usually at the **initial segment** of the axon, the short region between the axon hillock and the beginning of the myelin sheath. Since **summation of synaptic currents** at the initial segment is the principal determinant of whether or not a spike will be generated, the initial segment is referred to as the **integrative zone** of the neuron.

Integration of synaptic inputs occurs through **spatial summation** and **temporal summation.** Spatial summation occurs when two or more separate presynaptic inputs are activated nearly simultaneously so that the PSPs can summate (see Fig. 6-7A). The effectiveness of spatial summation is dependent on the membrane space constant. As discussed in Chap. 5, the membrane length (or space) constant is the distance at which electrotonic potentials decay to 1/e or 37% of the amplitude at the point of origin. Thus it is evident that synaptic inputs separated by a distance smaller than the length constant can summate more effectively than those which are separated by a distance exceeding the length constant. In other words, the larger the length constant, the greater is the cell's capability to summate the PSPs generated at various locations on the neuron.

Temporal summation occurs when APs in a single presynaptic neuron fire in rapid succession such that the interval between successive presynaptic APs is less than the duration of the PSP (e.g., 2–10 msec). In this case, the successive overlapping PSPs can summate, resulting in a larger overall PSP amplitude (see Fig. 6-7B). The effectiveness of temporal summation critically depends on the membrane time constant. As also discussed in Chap. 5, the membrane time constant determines the time required for an electrotonic potential to decay to 1/e or 37% of its peak value. The longer the time constant, the longer is the duration of the PSP, and thus the greater is the opportunity for

summation of successive PSPs. When and if the resulting potential reaches the threshold value, a propagated AP is triggered (see Fig. 6-7).

Presynaptic Inhibition

Besides postsynaptic inhibition, the probability of a postsynaptic neuron firing an AP may be decreased by **presynaptic inhibition.** Presynaptic inhibition is exerted at axoaxonic synapses formed by axon terminals of inhibitory neurons onto the axon terminals of excitatory neurons. Activation of this type of synapse results in a reduced quantity of excitatory transmitter release by the presynaptic AP in the excitatory neuron (Fig. 6-8). A decrease in the release of excitatory transmitter results in a smaller EPSP in the postsynaptic cell and thus a reduced effectiveness of the excitatory transmission.

Presynaptic inhibition tends to be found at sensory inflow points, where it presumably permits selective "switching off" of some inputs without affecting the responsiveness of the postsynaptic neuron to other synaptic inputs. In the spinal cord, presynaptic inhibition has been documented in the primary afferent fibers from the muscle stretch receptors and is exerted by other primary afferents or afferents from mechanoreceptors via spinal inhibitory interneurons. In this case, stimulation of afferents mediating presynaptic inhibition in the mammalian spinal cord causes a depolarization of the terminals of the excitatory primary afferent fibers (**primary afferent depolarization, or PAD).** Depolarization of presynaptic terminals reduces the quantity of transmitter released, probably because the presynaptic spike in the partially depolarized terminal is smaller and less effective in activating Ca^{2+} channels so that less Ca^{2+} enters into the terminal. Severe depolarization of the terminal arborizations also may block AP invasion into the terminals for a prolonged period. Unlike the direct fast postsynaptic IPSP, the presynaptic inhibition is of relatively long duration and may last up to several hundred milliseconds.

Modulation of Synaptic Transmission

The amount of transmitter released by each presynaptic action potential can be modified as a function of the pattern of impulse flow. When presynaptic APs are spaced sufficiently closely, the amount of transmitter released tends to increase with each succeeding impulse. This is reflected in a progressive increase in the amplitude of PSPs

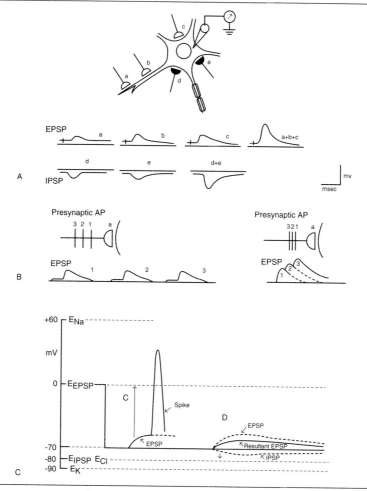

Fig. 6-7. Integration of postsynaptic potentials. A schematic of a postsynaptic neuron receiving excitatory (E-synapses a, b, and c) and inhibitory (I-synapses e and f) inputs. Activation of these synapses by presynaptic action potentials causes release of excitatory or inhibitory transmitters, respectively. Postsynaptic potentials are recorded with an intracellular electrode in the postsynaptic neuron. (A) *Spatial summation:* Activation of E-synapses (a, b, and c) individually results in EPSPs a, b, and c. Simultaneous activation of all three E-inputs results in algebraic summation of the EPSPs produced at each synapse, giving a summated EPSP$_{a+b+c}$. Similarly, spatial summation is illustrated for the activation of I-synapses located at different regions of the neuron. (B) *Temporal summation:* Application of sufficiently spaced (separated in time) stimuli (1 through 3) to the presynaptic neuron produces correspondingly spaced EPSPs in the postsynaptic neuron. When frequency of stimulation is increased so that presynaptic action potentials occur before the EPSPs have fully decayed, each succeeding EPSP adds to the preceding depolarization, thus giving a summated EPSP$_{1+2+3}$. (C) *Integration:* Diagram shows the equilibrium potentials for sodium (E_{Na}), potassium (E_K), and chloride (E_{Cl}) ions. The resting membrane potential (RMP) is at –70 mV, and the equilibrium potentials for IPSP and EPSP are given at –80 and 0 mV, respectively. The threshold for neuronal spike generation is at about –50. When the summated EPSP reaches the threshold membrane potential, an action potential is fired. If E- and I-synapses are activated approximately simultaneously, the IPSPs subtract from the EPSPs so that net membrane depolarization due to EPSP is reduced to below the threshold, and the action potential cannot be fired.

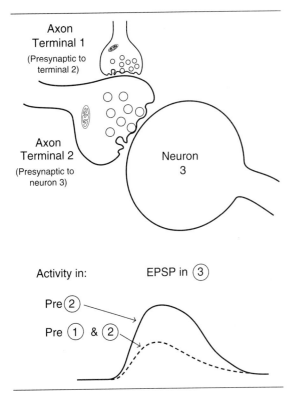

Fig. 6-8. Presynaptic inhibition at axoaxonic synapses. The presynaptic inhibitory terminal 1 forms an axoaxonic synapse with the terminal of neuron 2, which forms an excitatory synapse with the postsynaptic neuron 3. In the absence of activity in 1, activation of neuron 2 results in a normal EPSP in the postsynaptic neuron 3. However, when neuron 1 is activated shortly before or at about the same time as the neuron 2, the amount of transmitter released from the excitatory terminal 2 is reduced, and a correspondingly smaller EPSP is generated in the postsynaptic neuron 3. (Modified from: Sperelakis, N., ed. *Cell Physiology Source Book.* New York: Academic Press, 1995.)

and is termed **facilitation.** When the nerve is activated with a relatively prolonged high-frequency (tetanic) burst of impulses, the quantity of transmitter is increased upon subsequent stimulation even if there is a relatively long intervening rest period. This phenomenon is known as **posttetanic potentiation.** Facilitation and potentiation are thought to be associated with a transient buildup of ionized Ca^{2+} within the terminals, which in turn increases the probability of transmitter release. However, the two processes are kinetically distinct. Facilitation is relatively short-lived, whereas posttetanic potentiation may last for

minutes and sometimes hours, possibly indicating a long-term modification of presynaptic function secondary to the transient increase in the cytosolic Ca^{2+} levels.

During sustained high-frequency activation, the amplitudes of PSPs tend to progressively diminish and may fail altogether. This phenomenon is referred to as **synaptic depression or fatigue.** Synaptic depression is associated with a progressive reduction in the quantity of transmitter released per nerve impulse and presumably reflects a depletion of the transmitter stores when the rate of transmitter release exceeds the rate of replenishment of the transmitter store.

In addition to the presynaptic modulation, synaptic efficacy also can be altered by postsynaptic mechanisms that lead to short- or long-term modification of the excitability of the postsynaptic cell. An important example is the so-called **long-term potentiation** (LTP) in the hippocampus, which is thought to be a fundamental cellular process involved in learning and memory.

Summary

The transmission of signals at chemical synapses involves the transduction of an electrical signal (in the form of an AP) into release of chemical neurotransmitter substances that act on specific receptor-channel complexes to generate **postsynaptic potentials** (PSPs) in the receiving neuron or an effector cell, such as a skeletal muscle fiber. PSPs are electrotonic (nonpropagated) potentials that are elicited by a 1- to 2-msec change in the postsynaptic membrane permeability to select ions. The **excitatory postsynaptic potentials** (EPSPs) are associated with an increase in the postsynaptic membrane conductance to Na^+ and K^+ ions. The **inhibitory postsynaptic potentials** (IPSPs) are associated with an increase in postsynaptic membrane conductance to Cl^- or K^+ ions. The PSPs decay passively within 2 to 10 msec, depending on the membrane time constant, and decrement with distance, depending on the membrane length constant.

The excitatory postsynaptic potential at the skeletal neuromuscular junction is a large depolarization called the **end-plate potential** (EPP). EPP is generated when ACh released from the presynaptic motor neuron activates the postsynaptic nicotinic ACh receptors at the muscle endplate. Normally, every nerve AP always elicits an EPP of sufficient amplitude and duration to trigger one muscle AP. In abnormal states, when EPPs are reduced to below the threshold potential for firing muscle APs, neuromuscular transmission fails, causing muscle weakness and/or flaccid paralysis. These abnormal states may be brought about by drugs, neurotoxins, or diseases that cause a reduction in ACh release or interfere with ACh-receptor binding. Anticholinesterases that prolong the life of synaptically released ACh or drugs that act as nonhydrolyzable ACh-receptor agonists generate abnormally prolonged EPPs, resulting in a depolarizing block of neuromuscular transmission and muscle paralysis.

Neurons receive multiple excitatory and inhibitory synaptic inputs. Synaptic signals converging onto a neuron are integrated through algebraic summation of EPSPs and IPSPs, and the AP is triggered only if the summated voltage is sufficient to reach the threshold potential at the initial segment of the axon.

Efficacy of synaptic transmission can be modulated by the pattern of impulse flow and may be altered or impaired by drugs, neurotoxins, or diseases that interfere with the synthesis, formation, or release of presynaptic transmitters or modify their interaction with postsynaptic receptors.

Bibliography

Eccles, J. C. *The Physiology of Nerve Cells.* Baltimore: Johns Hopkins Press, 1957.

Kandel, E. R., Schwartz, J. H., and Jessell, T. M. *Principles of Neural Science,* 3rd ed. New York: Elsevier Science, 1991.

Katz, B. *Nerve, Muscle, and Synapse.* New York: McGraw-Hill, 1966.

7 Sensory Receptors and Somatosensory System

Michael M. Behbehani

Objectives

After reading this chapter, you should be able to

Describe the types of sensory receptors and their major functional properties

Describe the generator potential and its ionic basis

Describe the common characteristics of sensory receptors

Explain the properties of sensory nerves and their classification

List the components of the somatic sensory system

List the anatomic properties of the dorsal column–medial lemniscus system

Describe the properties of neurons in each major component of the dorsal column–medial lemniscus system

Describe the term *nociceptor,* and define the concept of adequate stimulus

List the types of chemicals that activate nociceptors and the sources of these agents

Describe the major neurotransmitters that mediate the interaction between nociceptive-related sensory nerves and the spinal cord

Explain the interactions that take place in the spinal cord between large and small fiber afferents and descending systems

Describe the anatomy of the pathways that conduct nociceptive information

Describe the major medullary sites involved in pain transmission and the characteristics of the cells in these areas

Describe the major pontine regions involved in pain processing and explain the functional properties of cells in these regions

Explain the properties of specific and nonspecific thalamic areas that process nociception

Describe the role of the cerebral cortex in the perception of pain

Describe the anatomic and functional characteristics of the descending pain inhibitory system

Describe the major transmitters that mediate the descending pain inhibitory pathway at the spinal dorsal horn and medullary and pontine levels

Introduction to the Sensory Systems

In order for an organism to function, it must be able to interact with its environment. This interaction requires perception of environmental factors and their relevance to the function of the organism. It is the function of the sensory systems to accomplish this task. Although there is a significant difference between the sensory systems, their general operational schema are very similar.

All sensory systems consist of a **receptor organ,** a **sensory nerve,** and several **central processing** networks. Receptor organs are physiologic transducers. They convert external energy into changes in the membrane potential that ultimately cause production of action potentials in the sensory nerve. Sensory nerves carry the message created by the receptors to the CNS. The integration of sensory information takes place within higher centers.

Sensory Receptors

In general, there are three types of sensory receptors. One class of receptors is called **extroceptors.** Examples of extroceptors are **photoreceptors,** which lead to sensation of vision, and **olfactory receptors,** which lead to sensation of smell. A second type of sensory receptor is the **proprioceptor,** which encodes muscle length and tension. The function of these receptors is to sense the position, tension, movement, and direction of movement. This information is relayed to the motor regions of the CNS and is crucial for control of motor function and balance. The third type of receptor is the **interoceptor.** Activation of this class of receptors does not lead to a conscious perception of the stimulus. Examples of these receptors are the sensory receptors that sense oxygen tension and those which sense blood pressure. Although there are significant differences between the three classes of sensory receptors, all receptors convert external energies into changes in membrane potential that, if large enough, can produce action potentials.

All sensory receptors produce a **generator potential.** The generator potential is a graded response, and its magnitude depends on the strength of the stimulus. As the strength of the stimulus increases, the amplitude of the generator potential increases (Fig. 7-1). In this respect, the generator potential is significantly different from the action potential. As you recall, the action potential is an all-or-none phenomenon, and when it is produced, its amplitude is independent of the intensity of the stimulus.

Generator potentials are produced by opening or closing of ion channels. In some receptors such as the **Pacinian corpuscle** that encodes the sense of vibration, mechanical pressure produces an opening of Na^+ and K^+ channels. In other receptors such as the vertebrate photoreceptors, absorption of light closes Na^+ channels. In general, the transduction can occur through activation of second messenger systems (such as Ca^{2+}, cAMP, or cGMP) or by direct coupling of the external energy to specific types of ion channels. For example, transduction in the photoreceptors and olfactory receptors involves cyclic GMP (cGMP). In the **stretch receptors,** on the other hand, stretching of the cell membrane opens Na^+ and K^+ channels without involvement of a second messenger.

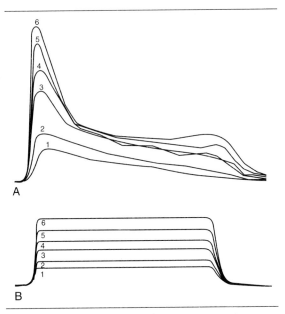

Fig. 7-1. The generator potential. The response of a pressure receptor to progressively larger pressure stimuli. Numbers denote intensity of stimulus. Note that the magnitude of the response increases as the intensity of stimulus increases, and the cell remains depolarized as long as the pressure is applied.

Common Operations of the Sensory Transduction Process. Transduction of sensory signals involves at least four operations: **detection, amplification, discrimination,** and **adaptation.** The first operation is detection. Sensory receptors operate at the low limit of their respective stimulus energy. For example, during the highly dark-adapted state, absorption of a single photon can activate **rod photoreceptors** and leads to the perception of light. Similarly, displacement of **hair cells** in the **organ of corti** by few nanometers can produce a significant change in the membrane potential and results in action potentials in the auditory nerve. Sensory receptors can be activated by a variety of stimuli; however, the threshold for each of these stimuli varies considerably. The stimulus for which a sensory receptor is most sensitive is called the **adequate stimulus.** For example, the adequate stimulus for the photoreceptors is photons. These receptors have a very low threshold for light, but they can be activated by other stimuli such as pressure. Although sensory receptors are highly sensitive to their adequate stimuli, the latency of their response is highly variable. In some mechanoreceptors such as hair cells in the cochlea, the latency can be as short as 10 μsec. On the other hand, the latency of the response of olfactory neurons to odorants can be several hundred milliseconds.

The second operation that is performed by sensory receptors is **signal amplification.** Several processes have been identified that lead to signal amplification. By far the most widely used mechanism involves activation of a second messenger in which production of a single molecule of an enzyme can cause alteration of several hundred molecules of the substrate. For example, in photoreceptors, absorption of a few photons can activate a few molecules of phosphodiesterase, which in turn hydrolyze several hundred molecules of cGMP. In this fashion, the absorption effect is amplified. Other amplification mechanisms include nonlinear voltage-gated channels and positive feedback.

The third operation is **discrimination** among several stimuli. In some receptors, the discrimination of quality depends on properties of receptor molecules. For example, in photoreceptors, color discrimination is due to presence of three different chromophores in the cone system. In other receptors, the physical location of the receptor determines its discrimination ability. For example, hair cells located at the tip of the basilar membrane of the organ of corti in the inner ear encode high-frequency auditory signals because of their physical location.

Adaptation is the fourth operation that all sensory receptors perform. Adaptation is defined as the reduction in the response of a sensory receptor to repeated or prolonged application of a stimulus. On the basis of their adapting properties, receptors can be classified as slowly adapting or rapidly adapting.

Rapidly adapting receptors encode sensations that change during a relatively short period of time. An example of the rapidly adapting receptor is the Pacinian corpuscle. This receptor encodes the sense of vibration. It is an ellipsoidal body composed of several concentric lamellae (Fig. 7-2A). A myelinated nerve fiber enters at one end, and the final node of Ranvier occurs within the corpuscle.

In an intact corpuscle, application of pressure leads to generation of an action potential when the stimulus is applied, and a second action potential is recorded when the pressure is removed (see Fig. 7-2B). If the lamellae of the Pacinian corpuscle are removed and a pulse of pressure is applied to the receptor, a generator potential is recorded as long as the pressure is applied (see Fig. 7-2C). This generator potential has no refractory phase and has spatial and temporal summation properties; i.e., the generator responses set up by two weak stimuli delivered sequentially at one spot or two different spots on the nerve terminal add

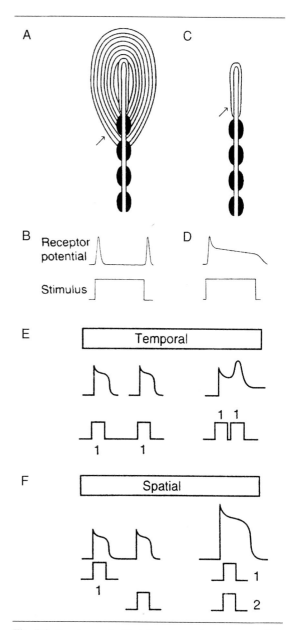

Fig. 7-2. Response of a Pacinian corpuscle to pressure. In an intact receptor (A), pressure causes production of a receptor potential (B) at the onset and offset of the stimulus. Removing the laminae (C) exposes the receptor terminal. Application of the stimulus to such a denuded receptor produces a depolarization that is maintained as long as the stimulus is applied (D). The generator potential does not have a refractory period and shows temporal (E) and spatial summation (F).

to produce a generator potential that is larger than the response of each stimulus alone (see Fig. 7-2D).

In the intact corpuscle, the laminated structure forms a mechanical filter and is responsible for the adaptive property of this receptor. If one records the action potential in a corpuscle in which the laminae have been removed, the application of pressure produces a generator potential that lasts as long as the stimulus. Nonetheless, only one or two action potentials are produced at the offset of the pressure.

Slowly-adapting receptors encode sensations that must be transmitted continuously for proper function of a system. An example of a slowly-adapting receptor is the **stretch receptor** (Fig. 7-3). Stretching this receptor produces a large generator potential shortly following application of the stretch; although the generator potential decreases slightly in amplitude, the depolarization is maintained for as long as the receptor is stretched.

Despite the fact that the processes leading to the initiation of generator potentials are different for different receptor types, most receptors utilize unique types of Na^+ and K^+ channels. These channels have very different properties compared with the channels that exist in nerve. Na^+ and K^+ channels in receptors are not voltage-sensitive. In addition, generator potentials can be readily initiated in a solution that contains tetrodotoxin, a poison that blocks the voltage-sensitive Na^+ channels involved in generation of action potentials in nerve (see Chap. 4).

Sensory Nerves

The depolarization produced in sensory receptors causes the generation of action potentials that travel through the sensory nerve axons. Each sensory receptor is the terminal region of the peripheral branch of a sensory neuron. Sensory neurons are bipolar cells with a peripheral branch and a central branch. The central branches of many axons form the sensory nerve. Just prior to entering the spinal cord, sensory nerves branch and form the primary afferents. The axons of sensory neurons have been classified according to their size and conduction velocity. There are two systems of classification. The axons that innervate sensory receptors have been classified as $A\alpha$, $A\beta$, $A\delta$, and C fibers. All A fibers are myelinated, whereas C fibers are unmyelinated. The sensory nerve axons that innervate muscle receptors have been classified as groups I, II, III, and IV. As shown in Table 7-1, both classifications are based on the size of the axons. As a general rule, the conduction velocity of a large or a medium-sized axon in meters per second is approximately six times its diameter in microns. For very small axons, the conversion factor is less.

The conduction velocity of a sensory nerve can be measured by recording extracellularly from it. These measurements can be used for the diagnosis of neuropathy. In isolated nerves, stimulation of the whole nerve produces a waveform that is called a **compound action potential**

Fig. 7-3. The generator potential of a stretch receptor. (A) The morphology of the cray fish stretch receptor. (B) Responses of the rapidly adapting (a) and slowly adapting (b) receptors to stretch (c).

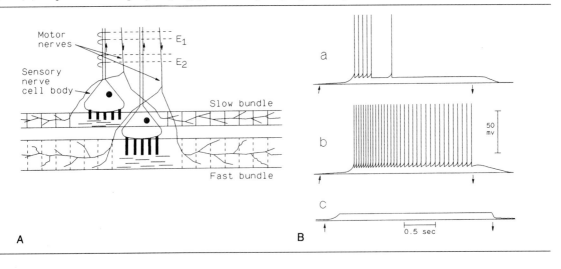

Table 7-1. Classification of Sensory Nerves

	Muscle Nerve	Cutaneous Nerve	Fiber Diameter (μm)	Conduction Velocity (m/sec)
Myelinated				
Large	I	Aα	13–20	80–120
Small	II	Aβ	6–12	35–75
Smallest	III	Aδ	1–5	5–30
Unmyelinated	IV	C	0.2–1.5	0.5–2

(Fig. 7-4). The compound action potential reflects conduction through all fiber sizes and conduction velocities within a nerve.

The Somatic Sensory System

The somatic sensory system processes sensations that arise from the skin. Three types of sensations are processed by this system: **touch, temperature, and pain.** Each of these modalities has submodalities; e.g., the sensations of light touch, pressure, and vibration are submodalities of touch that are clearly distinguished. Similarly, heat and cold are distinct sensations, and sharp and dull pain are separate

Fig. 7-4. Compound action potential of a sensory nerve recorded extracellulary. The A_{ALPHA} fibers produce the largest amplitude current that peaks at the shortest latency. A_{BETA} fibers produce less current than the A_{ALPHA} fibers, and their current reaches its peak at a later latency. A_{DELTA} fibers produce the smallest current, and the peak current occurs at the longest latency.

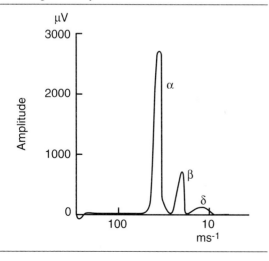

sensations. For each submodality there are specific receptors. The touch modality is encoded by encapsulated receptors (Fig. 7-5). The Meisner, Ruffini, Merkel, and Pacinian corpuscles encode sensations associated with touch. The **Ruffini** and **Merkel corpuscles** respond to skin indentation. Merkel corpuscles are located at the junction of the dermis and epidermis, and Meissner corpuscles are located in the epidermis; Ruffini corpuscles are located in the dermis and encode flutter (rapid small fluctuations). Finally, **Pacinian corpuscles** are located in the dermis and encode vibration. In addition to these receptors, in the hairy skin there are hair receptors that encode flutter. Heat and cold receptors are distinct receptors. Cold receptors respond to cooling the skin from 1 to 20°C below the normal skin temperature, and heat receptors respond to warming the skin by a similar temperature range. Nociceptors are naked nerve endings that are distributed in the dermis and epidermis.

Each receptor in the skin interacts with the CNS through a distinct pathway. Because of this arrangement, called the **labeled line,** activation of a sensory receptor produces the same sensation independent of the stimulus that activated the receptor. For example, heating a cold receptor produces the sensation of cold. Similarly, activation of small unmyelinated fibers that innervate the nociceptor by chemical or electrical stimulation leads to the sensation of pain.

Anatomy of the Somatic Sensory System

Somatosensory information is transmitted to the brain via three distinct systems: the **dorsal column medial lemniscus,** the **lateral columns,** and the **spinocervical system.** The dorsal column medial lemniscus system is involved in transmission to the brain of touch, vibration pressure, joint movement, and joint position. The central branches of the dorsal root ganglion cells that innervate the receptors for the preceding modalities enter the spinal cord and travel through the dorsal column. Afferents from the lumbar dor-

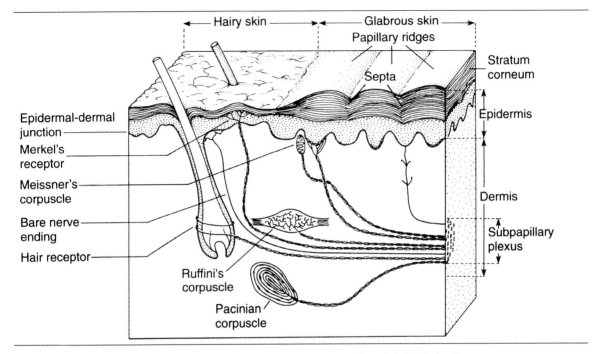

Fig. 7-5. The morphologic characteristics of mechanical receptors in the skin and their relative locations. The Pacinian and Meisner's corpuscles are encapsulated and encode vibration and light touch. Merkel's receptors are unincapsulated and encode pressure. Free nerve endings are the nociceptors. (Modified from: Light, A. R., and Perl, E. R. Reexamination of the dorsal root projection to the spinal dorsal horn including observations on the differential termination of coarse and fine fibers. *J. Comp. Neurol.* 186:117, 1979.)

sal roots travel through the fasciculus gracilus and synapse with cells in **nucleus gracilus.** The afferents from the cervical dorsal roots travel through the faciculus cuneatus and synapse with the **nucleus cuneatus.** The nucleus gracilus and the nucleus cuneatus are referred to as the **dorsal column nuclei.** Axons of the cells in the dorsal column nuclei cross the midline and form the medial lemniscus. These axons synapse with cells in the ventral posterior lateral (VPL) and ventral posterior medial (VPM) nuclei of the thalamus. Cells in these thalamic nuclei project to somatosensory area I in the cortex (Fig. 7-6).

Each cell in the somatosensory system has a **receptive field.** The receptive field of a cell is defined as the area in the skin where stimulation causes changes in the firing rate of the cell (Fig. 7-7). Because of convergence, the receptive field of neurons increases in size at each successive level of transmission. For example, the receptive field of dorsal root ganglion cells is smaller than the receptive field of dorsal column nuclei cells, and the receptive field of the dorsal column nuclei cells is smaller than the receptive

Fig. 7-6. Schematic of the dorsal column–medial lemniscus pathway that encodes vibration and touch.

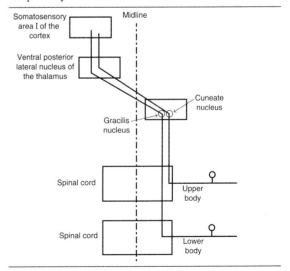

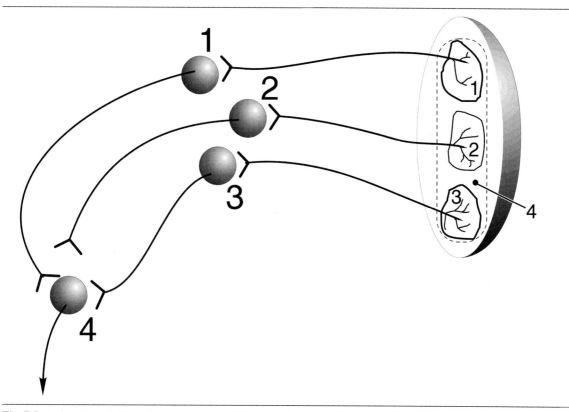

Fig. 7-7. A pictorial definition of the receptive field. The receptive fields of neurons 1, 2, and 3 are represented by areas 1, 2, and 3, respectively. The receptive field of neuron 4 is the combined areas 1+2+3.

field of the thalamic nuclei cells. The cells in the dorsal column medial lemniscus system have very small receptive fields. Usually these receptive fields include an area the size of a single phalange of the finger. In addition, the cells in the dorsal column medial lemniscus system are all modality-specific. Each cell responds to only a single modality. For example, a cell may respond to pressure applied to its receptive field but will not respond to vibration or heating of the same area. All nuclei of the dorsal column medial lemniscus system are topographically organized. An example of the organization of VPL is shown in Fig. 7-8, and the topographic organization of the somatosensory area I of the cortex is shown in Fig. 7-9. As can be seen in these figures, each region of the VPL or somatosensory area I is responsive to only a small region of the body. In addition, the regions of the body that are more sensitive to somatic stimulation are presented by larger areas in the cortex and thalamic nuclei. Because of this arrangement,

the map of the body presented on the cortex is highly distorted. The areas of the cortex devoted to processing information from the face and fingers are much larger than the areas that process information from the back or leg.

The highly topographic organization of the dorsal column medial lemniscus system allows this system to process information about the location of the stimulus that is applied to the body. Lesions of this system produce a reduction in the ability to discriminate tactile sensation and a loss of vibratory sensibility and joint position. Loss of sensibility is ipsilateral to the lesion site if the lesion is in the spinal cord.

Pain and Analgesia

Pain perception is affected by a variety of psychological factors such as mood and motivational state. For example,

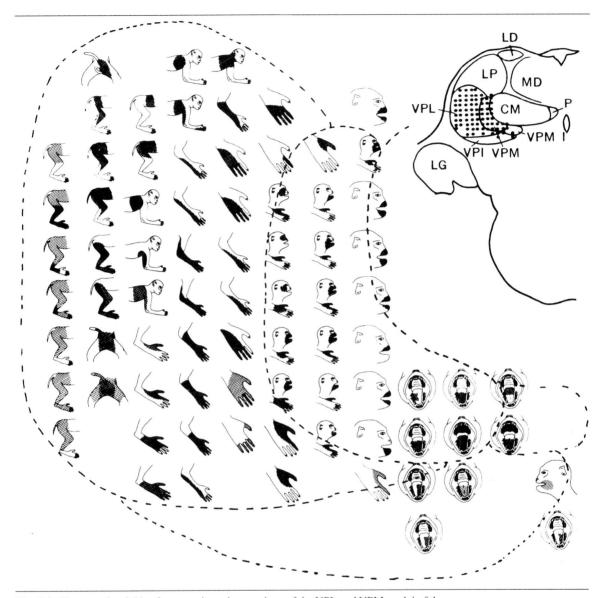

Fig. 7-8. The receptive fields of neurons in various regions of the VPL and VPM nuclei of the monkey thalamus. The VPM neurons respond to stimulation of specific regions of the face. The VPL neurons respond to stimulation of different regions of the body (CM = center median; LD = lateral dorsal; LP = lateral posterior; MD = medial dorsal; P = parafascicularis; VPI, VPL, and VPM = inferior, lateral, and medial divisions of the ventral posterior nucleus. (From: Mountcastle, V. B., and Henneman, E. The representation of tactile sensibility in the thalamus of the monkey. *J. Comp. Neurol.* 97:409, © 1952. Reprinted with permission of John Wiley & Sons, Inc.)

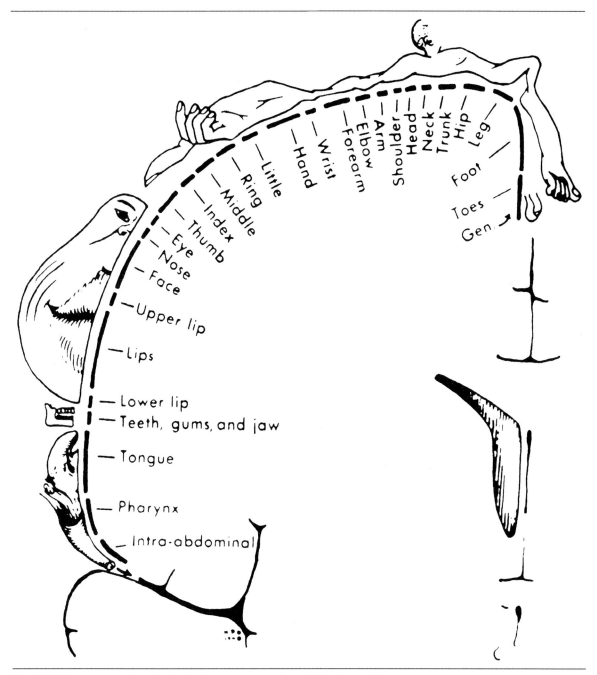

Fig. 7-9. The representation of the body in somatosensory area I. The lips and fingers occupy the largest areas, whereas the back and legs occupy the smallest areas of the cortex. (Modified from: Penfield, W., and Rasmussen, T. *The Cerebral Cortex of Man: A Clinical Study of Localization of Function.* New York: Macmillan, 1950.)

under "fight or flight" conditions, the threshold for pain increases such that stimuli that usually produce pain are not perceived as painful. Opposite phenomena also occur. For example, when a subject is anxious, a nonpainful stimulus may be perceived as painful. The pain system, however, follows a general pattern of other sensory systems, and as such, it consists of sensory receptors, sensory nerves that connect these receptors to the spinal cord, and several processing units.

Nociceptors

Noxious stimuli activate a class of receptors called the **nociceptors.** Nociceptors have very small diameters (<0.2 μm) and have multiple branches. They respond to noxious mechanical or thermal stimuli or to a variety of chemicals. Since these receptors respond to more than one modality, they are called **polymodal receptors.** There are two major classes of nociceptors: **A-mechano heat** (AMH) nociceptors and **C-mechano heat** (CMH) nociceptors.

The AMH receptors are innervated by Aδ or Aβ fibers. Information encoded by these receptors propagates at velocities that range between 15 and 55 m/sec and is involved in withdrawal reflexes. AMH receptors can be activated by temperatures >43°C and by mechanical stimuli that, if continued, would produce tissue damage.

CMH receptors respond to heat above 38°C and to mechanical stimuli that, if continued, would produce tissue damage. Perception of pain by human subjects closely matches the response of the C fibers innervating the skin. If a peripheral nerve is stimulated at an intensity that causes activation of C fibers, pain is perceived. In addition, individuals who lack C fibers are insensitive to pain.

In addition to conduction velocity and threshold, adaptation processes in CMH and AMH receptors are different. CMH receptors respond to continuous application of a noxious stimulus for a short time and then stop firing. On the other hand, AMH receptors begin firing after a delay, and their firing rate increases throughout the duration of stimulation. Another difference between the adaptive properties of these nociceptors is the phenomenon of sensitization. Following noxious thermal stimulation, the temperature at which a human subject perceives pain decreases.

Both AMH and CMH receptors are sensitive to a variety of substances. Among these, bradykinin, eicosenoids (arachidonic acid metabolites that include prostaglandins, thromboxanes, and leukotrienes), histamine, serotonin, substance P, and protons have been shown to either directly activate the nociceptors or increase their sensitivity to noxious stimuli. Many of these chemicals are released when tissue damage occurs. For example, cutting the skin can cause release of KCl from red blood cells, and histamine is released following ischemia.

Role of the Dorsal Horn in Pain

Axons of Aδ and C fibers enter the spinal cord and bifurcate. The branches of these axons ascend and descend in the spinal cord through the tract of Lissaur. These axons send collaterals that synapse with the neurons within the dorsal horn. Based on the cellular anatomy, the dorsal horn can be divided into six layers (Fig. 7-10). Layers I through VI are involved in the transmission and coding of nociception. Both small and large fibers synapse with cells in these layers.

Anatomically, the dorsal horn neurons can be classified as **projecting neurons** and **interneurons.** The projecting neurons have direct projections to thalamic nuclei and/or to the medullary and pontine areas. The interneurons have no direct projection to the brain, and they modulate and integrate activities within the dorsal horn. The largest number of projecting neurons are located in lamina I. In the monkey, approximately 40% of neurons in this region send direct projections to the ventral posterior thalamic nuclei; a smaller number of cells in lamina V are projecting neurons. Neurons in laminae II and III have few direct projections to the brain. Together these laminae are referred to as the **substantia gelatinosa,** and they play a major role in integration of ascending and descending pain-related information.

Functionally, the dorsal horn neurons have been classified as **nociceptive-specific** (NS) and **wide-dynamic-range** (WDR) neurons. NS neurons respond only to noxious mechanical and heat stimulation. The majority of cells in lamina I are NS type. WDR neurons respond to both noxious and innocuous stimulation. However, the magnitude and duration of their response increase as the intensity of the stimulus increases. The majority of WDR neurons are located in lamina V of the dorsal horn.

Visceral Pain

In humans, visceral pain is highly diffuse and poorly localized. In most cases, pain is associated with nausea. Nociceptive reflexes associated with visceral pain are slow in onset and have a long duration. In general, two types of pain localizations have been identified: **true visceral pain** and **referred pain.** True pain is perceived as arising from inside the body. For example, pain associated with appendicitis is initially felt in the midline, and as inflammation

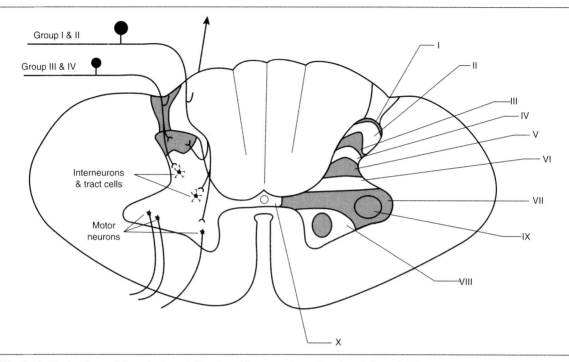

Fig. 7-10. The laminae of the spinal cord. The dorsal horn consists of laminae I through VI.

increases, pain is felt in the lower right quadrant. Referred pain is localized to superficial tissue that can be far from the affected organ. The somatic areas affected in referred pain enlarge as the intensity of pain increases. For example, following myocardial infarction, initially pain is perceived to arise from inside the chest. Within a few minutes, the pain is perceived in the chest and in the left shoulder. As the intensity of infarct increases, pain radiates into the arm. The somatic area involved in referred pain can become hyperalgesic, and tenderness develops in these areas; these events can last for an extended period of time.

The encoding of visceral pain is not the same in all organs. Stimulation (pressure, chemical, or cutting) of some visceral organs such as the lungs and the liver does not lead to pain sensation. Other organs, such as the bladder, are highly sensitive to pressure. Two types of stimuli can lead to visceral pain. The first stimulus is extension, which is encoded by mechanoreceptors that respond to stretch. The second type of stimulus is ischemia. During ischemia, algesic chemicals are generated and released. These agents act on the receptors or nerve fibers that innervate the visceral organs and cause pain. An example of a naturally occurring compound that activates visceral receptors and

causes pain is bradykinin, and its injection into the abdomen produces pain.

The encoding of noxious stimuli by the visceral organs is not identical to that of other organs. Three types of encoding processes have been postulated: the **specific nociceptors,** the **pattern of firing,** and **activation of silent receptors.**

The specificity mechanism requires the presence of receptors that only encode noxious stimuli. This type of receptor have been identified in the gallbladder and the heart. Recordings have been made from fibers that innervate the biliary system in the ferret. In this animal, there are fibers that have no spontaneous activity and only respond to distension caused by high pressure. Similar types of receptors have been identified in the heart.

The second encoding mechanism is related to the intensity of the stimulus that is encoded in the firing pattern of the receptor. This mechanism requires that receptors encode an innocuous as well as a noxious range of stimuli, a phenomenon that is accomplished by increasing their firing rate as the stimulus intensity increases. This type of firing pattern has been recorded from nearly all receptor organs. The nociceptive-specific and intensity-encoding mechanisms are mutually exclusive, and there is controversy about both mechanisms. In some organs such as the esophagus, there are both nociceptive-specific and intensity-encoding receptors. However, because of the methodologic differences that laboratories have employed to investigate these events, there is no consensus regarding specific mechanisms.

The third encoding mechanism is activation of silent receptors or synapses. According to this hypothesis, the visceral organs have receptors that under normal physiologic conditions do not produce responses. This can occur where receptors are not sensitive to any stimuli or if the synapses they form with the spinal cord neurons are ineffective. When tissue is injured or inflamed, these receptors become either sensitive to pressure, or their synaptic interactions within the dorsal horn neurons begin to encode extension and pressure. This type of encoding has been observed in the bladder and esophagus. In both organs, there are receptors that are normally silent but, following inflammation of the organ, respond to extension.

Recently, a model for encoding nociception by the visceral organs that includes all three types of mechanisms has been proposed. According to this model (Fig. 7-11), there are two types of encoding systems. One system is operational under normal physiologic conditions and encodes the internal pressure changes that do not lead to the sensation of pain. The second system, when activated, produces the sensation of pain. The first system receives inputs from low-threshold receptors; the second system obtains information from high-threshold receptors and from silent receptors. During normal function, the low-threshold receptors are active, and their activity is sufficient to excite the nonpain system but is not sufficient to activate the pain system. When a transient intense stimulation is applied, the low-threshold receptors and high-threshold receptors are activated, resulting in activation of the pain system. When the tissue is inflamed, the silent receptors become active and cause sensitization of the pain system. Because of this sensitization, the pain system can be activated by the low-threshold receptors, with the result that the normal physiologic activity of the organ can lead to the sensation of pain.

Afferents from visceral receptors travel with sympathetic and parasympathetic nerves and enter the spinal cord at the sacral, upper lumbar, and thoracic levels. Following entry, these fibers bifurcate and travel through the Lissaur tract and terminate in dorsal horn at all levels. For this reason, the afferents from the viscera have a wide terminal distribution. For example, afferents from the pelvic nerve enter at the sacral level but synapse with neurons at

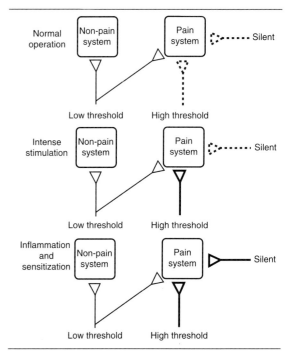

Fig. 7-11. A model for the function of visceral pain (see text for details). (Modified from: Cervero, F. Visceral pain. In: Wall, P. D., and Melzack, R., eds. *Textbook of Pain.* Edinburgh, New York: Churchill Livingstone, 1994.)

the lumbar enlargement (L4). The majority of visceral afferents synapse with neurons in laminae I and V; very few visceral afferents synapse with laminae II and III neurons. Many neurons in lamina V receive both somatic and visceral afferents and respond to stimulation of both regions. Convergence of these afferents on the same cell is the basis of referred pain.

Transmitters Involved in the Interactions Between Sensory Nerves and Dorsal Horn Neurons

The major neurotransmitters in this system are substance P (SP) and calcitonin gene–related peptide (CGRP). Both peptides are released from the terminals of the small fibers and cause depolarization of dorsal horn neurons. The effects of these peptides last for several seconds. In a significant number of primary afferent terminals, SP and CGRP are colocalized in the same terminal. In addition to these peptides, primary afferents also contain vasoactive intestinal peptide, somatostatin, galanin, and glutamic acid. Depletion of SP (e.g., by injection of capsaicin) can produce prolonged analgesia.

Integration of Afferent Signals Within the Dorsal Horn

The interaction within the dorsal horn of afferent signals is the major modulation site for pain processing in the CNS, and the outcome of these integration events will determine the perception of pain. As mentioned earlier, there are situations that result in a lack of pain response to noxious stimulation. Several theories have been proposed to explain this phenomenon. One theory is called the **gate theory,** and it is illustrated in Fig. 7-12. This theory proposes that both large and small fibers have an excitatory effect on cells in lamina V of the dorsal horn (the T cells). The large fibers excite cells in laminae II and III (substantia gelantinosa, SG), whereas small fibers inhibit the cells in the SG region. The SG cells in turn inhibit the T cells by making mostly presynaptic inhibitory synapses with the terminals of both the large and small fibers of the T cells. Neurotransmitters are involved in pain processing in the dorsal horn.

The major excitatory transmitters within the dorsal horn

Fig. 7-12. The gate-control theory. Large and small fibers excite a lamina V neuron that projects to the brain. Neurons in the substantia gelatinosa (SG) inhibit transmission between large fibers and lamina V cells and those from small fibers and lamina V cells. Activation of large fibers excites SC cells and therefore increases their inhibitory effect on the lamina V cells and closes the gate. Activation small fibers inhibits SG neurons and removes their inhibitory effect on the lamina V neurons and therefore opens the gate. (Modified from: Melzak, R., and Wall, P. D. Pain mechanisms: A new theory. *Science* 150:971, 1965.)

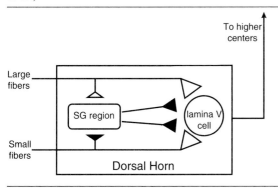

are SP, CGRP, and glutamic acid. Unlike the excitatory pathways that originate from the primary afferents, the major inhibitory systems within the dorsal horn are networks of intrinsic neurons. The major transmitters in this system are GABA, glycin, and enkephalin. The activities of the intrinsic neurons are modulated by both sensory afferents and descending systems. In addition to these transmitter systems, many neurons within the dorsal horn and in the dorsal root ganglion contain nitric oxide synthase and can synthesize nitric oxide (NO). Nitric oxide acts as a second messenger that can readily penetrate the cell membrane. As a result, NO can act both presynaptically and postsynaptically. The current hypothesis regarding the functional role of NO in the dorsal horn is that glutamic acid released from the primary afferents acts on N-methyl-D-aspartic acid receptors and thereby causes an increase in the intracellular calcium, which in turn causes release of NO. NO then diffuses and reaches presynaptic terminals of the primary afferents and enhances the release of neurotransmitters.

Pathways That Conduct Nociceptive Information to the Brain

There are four tracts that convey pain messages to the brain. The **spinothalamic tract** (STT) includes both the lateral (Fig. 7-13A) and ventral spinothalamic tracts. The origin of neurons in this tract are in laminae I and V of the dorsal horn. Axons of these cells cross the spinal cord at the midline, travel through the anterolateral white matter, and terminate in the ventral posterior lateral (VPL) and ventral posterior medial (VPM) thalamic nuclei. The VPL nucleus receives afferent information from the body, and the VPM nucleus receives afferent input from the face.

The second pathway that conveys nociceptive information is the **spinoreticular tract** (see Fig. 7-13B). The cells of origin of this pathway are located in laminae VII and VIII of the spinal cord and respond to pressure and noxious mechanical stimulation. The majority of their axons cross the midline and travel through the anterolateral column. However, some of the fibers do not cross but travel through the anterolateral column ipsilateral to the location of their cell bodies. Unlike the spinothalmic tract, the axons of the spinoreticular tract terminate in both the reticular formation and the thalamus.

The third tract is the **spinomesencephalic tract.** The cells of origin of this tract are located in laminae I and V and include both nociceptive-specific and wide-dynamic-range neurons. The axons of this tract terminate in the

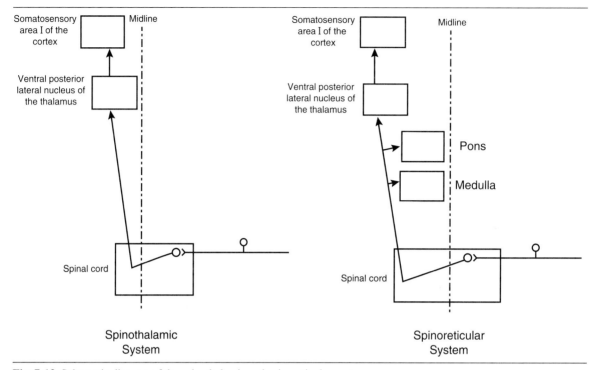

Fig. 7-13. Schematic diagram of the spinothalamic and spinoreticular systems.

mesencephalic reticular formation and the lateral region of the periaqueductal gray matter.

The **spinocervical tract** is the fourth tract that transmits pain information. Neurons of origin of this tract are located in laminae III and IV. Although the majority of these cells respond to innocuous stimuli, some neurons respond to noxious stimuli as well. The axons of these cells travel through the dorsolateral funiculus and terminate in the lateral cervical nucleus. The axons of cells in this nucleus cross the midline and travel in the medial lemniscus and terminate in the VPL and posterior nuclei of the thalamus.

Major Medullary Sites Involved in Pain Transmission

A large portion of the reticular formation is involved in pain processing. Among the medullary sites that have been studied, the nucleus gigantocellularis, the paragigantocellularis, the nucleus raphe magnus, the parabrachial nucleus, and the locus coeruleus have been shown to modulate pain. For example, stimulation of some of the nuclei in the gigantocellularis tract produces an escape behavior. Stimulation of other regions, such as the locus coeruleus, produces anxiety. Neurons in these nuclei have very large receptive fields and are of the WDR type. These neurons project to other medullary and pontine reticular formations and to the interlaminar thalamic nuclei. In the pontine reticular formation, the periaqueductal gray matter and the nucleus cuneiformis play an important role in pain processing.

Processing of Nociceptive Information by the Thalamus

The thalamic nuclei involved in processing of nociception can be divided functionally into two general classes: specific and nonspecific nuclei. The **specific thalamic nuclei** are the VPL, VPM, and posterior nuclei. The VPL and VPM together are referred to as the **ventrobasal complex.** The receptive fields of VPL and VPM neurons are small and located on the contralateral side of the body. Although VPL and VPM cells receive afferents from the lateral spinothalamic tract and from the dorsal column medial lemniscus system, the majority of VPL and VPM cells are modality-specific and respond to only one modality. That is, a cell in these regions can respond to light touch or to noxious pressure but not to both types of stimuli. In addition to somatic stimulation, neurons in the VPL cells also respond to visceral stimuli. Because of their modality specificity and their small receptive fields, it is believed that VPL and VPM neurons are involved in encoding fast pain such as that caused by a pin prick; these can be very accurately localized.

The nonspecific thalamic nuclei include the posterior, centralis lateralis, submedius, center median (CM), and parafascicularis (Pf) groups. Functionally, the CM and Pf neurons are very similar, and together these areas are referred to as **CM-Pf complex.** Neurons in the nonspecific thalamic regions have very large receptive fields that can encompass half the body. Neurons in these regions are not modality-specific. For example, neurons in the CM-Pf complex respond to noxious somatic and visceral stimuli as well as to touch. Some cells in these regions even respond to light and sound. An interesting property of nonspecific thalamic neurons is that their responses are highly sensitive to the state of arousal and vary with the sleep-wakefulness cycle. In addition, the responses of these cells are drastically affected by anesthesia. Because of these properties, it has been suggested that nonspecific thalamic cells are involved in the encoding of aching pain that is not well localized and varies with the state of arousal.

Cortical Areas Involved in Pain Processing

The somatosensory areas that are involved in pain processing are the primary (SI) and secondary (SII) somatosensory cortex. Neurons in the VPL and VPM nuclei project to the primary somatosensory cortex. Neurons in the SI region have small receptive fields and are modality-specific. Some of these cells show graded responses to mechanical and thermal stimuli in the noxious range. Neurons in the SII region have much larger receptive fields than those in SI. Some of the SII neurons also respond to noxious mechanical and thermal stimuli. Although both areas of the somatosensory cortex receive nociceptive information, there is controversy concerning the role of these areas in pain perception. In rats, cats, and monkeys, ablation of SI, SII, or both areas does not change the perception of pain. Recent studies in the human using combined MRI and PET imaging have shown that SI and SII areas contralateral to the stimulation site show significant increases in the metabolic rate following painful thermal stimulation.

In addition to the somatosensory cortex, the anterior cingulate gyrus contains neurons that are activated by noxious thermal stimulation. This area receives afferents from VPL and VPM neurons and from the CM-Pf complex. The cingulate gyrus is believed to be involved in the emotional aspect of pain processing; in patients with intractable pain, a bilateral lesion of this area reduces the emotional aspect of pain without altering the perception of pain intensity.

Descending Pain Inhibitory Systems

The background activity of dorsal horn neurons and their responses to peripheral and visceral stimuli are strongly influenced by a supraspinal mechanism. Anatomically, this system includes the hypothalamus, prefrontal cortex, amygdala, periaqueductal gray matter, parabrachial area, locus coeruleus, rostral ventral medulla, dorsolateral funiculus, and dorsal horn. Although stimulation of many brain areas can alter pain perception, the analgesia produced by stimulation of the midbrain periaqueductal gray (PAG) matter has been studied in great detail. In all species including the human, stimulation of the PAG and its rostral regions, the periventricular gray (an area that surrounds the third ventricle), produces strong and long-lasting analgesia. In addition, injection of variety of neurotransmitters including enkephalin, neurotensin, and glutamic acid into the PAG produces analgesia. Our current understanding of PAG mediated analgesia is that activation of PAG excites cells in the rostral ventral medulla (RVM), in particular those in the raphe magnus. Axons of the RVM cells project through the dorsal lateral funiculus and form inhibitory synapses with dorsal horn nociceptive neurons (Fig. 7-14).

A major unanswered question regarding the natural function of the descending pain modulatory system is how this system is activated. The consensus among investigators in this field is that the activity of the system is the basis for the emotional aspect of pain modulation. The PAG which is a major component of this system, has reciprocal connections with the amygdala. Since all these regions are components of the limbic system, their interaction with the PAG can lead to pain modulation.

Neurotransmitters of the Descending Pain Modulatory System

A large number of neurotransmitters are involved in the interactions between different regions of the descending pain modulatory pathway. The major classic neurotransmitter is glutamic acid and is involved in the interaction between the insular cortex and PAG and the prefrontal cortex and PAG. In addition, glutamic acid is involved in the interaction between the PAG and the RVM. The major classic inhibitory transmitter is gamma-aminobutyric acid (GABA).

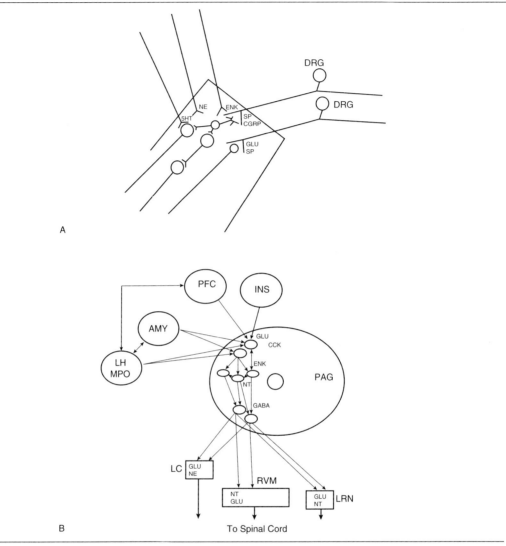

Fig. 7-14. Schematic model of a descending pain inhibitory pathway. (A) The spinal cord dorsal horn neurons receive excitatory inputs from dorsal root ganglion cells (DRG) that innervate nociceptors. These primary afferents release substance P (SP), calcitonin gene–related peptide (CGRP), and glutamic acid (GLU). The primary afferents synapse with interneurons and projecting neurons within the spinal cord. The dorsal horn neurons are inhibited by afferents from the brainstem and the midbrain that release serotonin (5HT), norepinephrine (NE), and enkephalin (ENK). (B) The PAG-RVM pain inhibitory pathway. The periaqueductal gray (PAG) receives afferents from the insular cortex (INS), the prefrontal cortex (PFC), the amygdala (AMY), and the lateral hypothalamus and medial preoptic nuclei (LH/MPO). The cortical structures have numerous connections with each other and form the limbic influence on the PAG network. The major cortical afferents to the PAG uses glutamic acid as a neurotransmitter. Within the PAG matter there is a tonically active GABAergic network (GABA) that is modulated by enkephalin (ENK). Neurotensin, cholecystokinin, and serotonin are also involved in the functions of PAG matter neurons. The output of PAG matter interacts with cells in the locus ceruleus (LC), RVM, and LRN. The major transmitters in this pathway are glutamic acid, neurotensin, and norepinephrine.

This transmitter acts on GABA-A and GABA-B receptors and is the major neurotransmitter of the interneuronal pools within the PAG, the RVM, and the spinal cord. In the spinal cord, GABA acts on both GABA-A and GABA-B receptors and inhibits nociceptive dorsal horn neurons. Serotonin (5-HT), acetylcholine, norepinephrine, and epinephrine are also involved in this system. The major peptides involved in the descending system are beta-endorphin, enkephalin, neurotensin, and tyrotropin-releasing hormone (TRH). Beta-dynorphin and enkephalins (both met- and leu-enkephalin) act on opioid receptors and produce analgesia.

Summary

The somatic sensory system processes information about touch, vibration, heat and cold, position of joint, joint movement, and pain. For each modality there is a specific receptor within the skin. Myelinated and moderately fast conducting fibers transmit touch, vibration, and joint information to the brain through the dorsal column medial lemniscus system. Pain and temperature information is transmitted via small-diameter and unmyelinated fibers through the anterolateral system to the brain. The dorsal column medial lemniscus system contains cells with small receptive fields that are modality-specific and is topographically organized. The dorsal horn of the spinal cord integrates and modulates pain processing. At this level there are interactions between large and small fibers as well as between ascending and descending pathways. The thalamic nuclei, VPL and VPM, process tactile and pain information. The centermedian and parafascicularis thalamic nuclei process dull pain. The somatosensory areas in the cortex are area I and area II and receive afferents from the thalamus and from the cortical sites that process somatic sensation. Pain transmission can be inhibited by activation of descending systems. An important descending system is the periaqueductal-RVM-spinal system.

The pharmacology of the pain system is complex. At the receptor level, prostaglandins, substance P, KCl, and bradykinin are among the most active substance that excite or sensitize the receptor. In the spinal cord, the excitatory transmitters are substance P, CGRP, and glutamic acid, and inhibitory transmitters are GABA, glycin, and enkephalin. These inhibitory transmitters, as well as norepinephrine and serotonin, are involved in the descending inhibition of pain.

Bibliography

Cervero, F., and Janig, W. Visceral nociceptors: A new world order. *Trends Neurosci.* 15:374, 1992.

Kandel, E. R., Schwartz, J. H., and Jessell, T. M. *Principles of Neural Science.* Norwalk, Conn.: Appleton & Lange, 1991.

Light, A. R., and Perl, E. R. Reexamination of the dorsal root projection to the spinal dorsal horn including observations on the differential termination of coarse and fine fibers. *J. Comp. Neurol.* 186:117, 1979.

Meyer, R. A., Campbell, J. N., and Srinivasa, N. R. Peripheral neural mechanisms of nociception. In Wall, P. D., and Melzack, R., Eds., *Textbook of Pain.* Edinburgh: Churchill-Livingstone, 1994. Pp. 13–34.

Mountcastle, V. B., and Henneman, E. The representation of tactile sensibility in the thalamus of the monkey. *J. Comp. Neurol.* 97:409–423, 1952.

8 Vision

Michael M. Behbehani

Objectives

After reading this chapter, you should be able to

Describe the anatomic structure of the eye

Name the muscles that move the eye, and describe their functions

Describe the anatomy of the retina, and explain the blood supply to the retina

Describe the functions of the pigment epithelium

Describe the process of phototransduction and spectral sensitivity of the photoreceptors

Explain how each cell type in the retina responds to light

Explain how the function of the retina can be tested and what is the physiologic basis for these tests

Describe color vision and its physiologic basis

Describe the anatomy of the central visual pathway

Explain how cells in the lateral geniculate and visual cortex respond to visual stimulation

The Eye

The visual system is one of the most complex sensory organs. It is designed for detection of form, color, and movement. The human eye is sensitive to a portion of the electromagnetic spectrum with wavelengths between 400 and 700 nm. The process of vision begins by transmission of light through the eye and the retina and its absorption by the photoreceptors. The eye (Fig. 8-1) is a spherical structure that consists of three layers. The first layer includes the **cornea,** a transparent structure, and the **sclera,** an opaque structure. These structures are joined together at the **limbus.** The second layer includes the **iris,** the **ciliary body,** and the **lens,** which is held in place behind the iris by transparent ligaments. The third layer of the eye consists of the **retina.** The eye also contains two fluid-filled chambers called the **anterior** and **posterior chambers.** The fluid that fills the posterior chamber is called the **aqueous humor** and has an ionic composition similar to cerebrospinal fluid. The anterior cavity behind the lens is filled with a viscous fluid called the **vitreous humor.** The aqueous humor is continuously secreted into the posterior chamber by epithelial cells covering the ciliary body. Fluid leaves this chamber through an opening called **Schlemm's canal.** As long as the fluid can drain easily, the pressure in the eye is less than 18 mmHg. If Schlemm's canal is blocked, the pressure increases and produces a potentially blinding disease called **glaucoma.**

Light enters the eye through an opening in the iris referred to as the **pupil.** Since the cornea is curved and has a different refractive index than air, the rays of light bend. After passing through the pupil and the anterior chamber, light goes through the lens, which focuses the light on the retina. Since the thickness of the lens can be controlled, the refractive power can be changed. In young individuals, the refractive power of the lens can be changed by as much as 10 diopters. With age, the ability of the lens to change its thickness decreases, and focusing at near distances becomes difficult. This condition is called **presbyopia.**

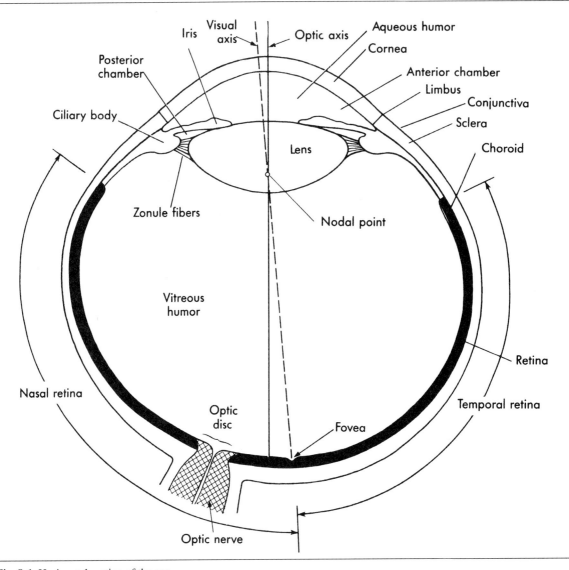

Fig. 8-1. Horizontal section of the eye.

Muscles of the Eye

The operation of the eye is controlled by two sets of muscles called the **intrinsic** and **extrinsic ocular muscles.** The intrinsic muscles are smooth muscles that control the opening diameter of the pupil and the thickness of the lens. Two groups of muscles control the pupil size. The sphincter of the iris is innervated by parasympathetic nerves, and when activated, these nerves cause constriction of the pupil (miosis). Dilation of the iris is controlled by the sympathetic nervous system, and its activation causes dilation of the pupil (mydriasis). The thickness of the lens is controlled by several layers of muscles within the ciliary body. These muscles are innervated by parasympathetic nerves. When these muscles contract, there is a reduction in the tension applied to the suspensory ligaments on the lens; consequently, the lens passively assumes an oval shape. This causes an increase in the thickness of the lens and adds positive diopter power to the lense, allowing accommodation for near vision. Relaxation of the ciliary muscles flattens the lens and allows accommodation to far vision.

The extrinsic muscles of the eye determine the position of the eye within the orbit and control the eyelid. Altogether there are six muscles that control the movement of the eye. These include the superior, inferior, lateral, and medial rectus muscles and the superior and inferior oblique muscles. These muscles are striated. The superior oblique and the lateral rectus muscles are innervated by the trochlear and abducens nerves, respectively, and the remaining muscles are innervated by the oculomotor nerve. Three muscle groups control the elevation of the eyelid: the levator palpebra, the superior tersa, and the orbicularis oculi muscles. The levator palpebra and superior tersa are smooth muscles and are innervated by the sympathetic nervous system. The orbicularis oculi are innervated by the facial nerve, and its activation causes closure of the eyelid.

Activation of striatal muscles depends on the position of the gaze direction. When the line of gaze is horizontal, the lateral and medial rectus muscles produce temporal and nasal deviation, respectively. When the gaze is temporal, the eye can be elevated by activation of the superior oblique and can be depressed by activation of the inferior oblique muscles. If the eye is deviated nasally, the superior oblique muscle causes elevation of the eye, and the inferior oblique causes a downward movement of the eye.

The Retina

Anatomy

The retina contains five types of neurons and one type of glial cell. The neurons are photoreceptors (rods and cones) and bipolar, horizontal, amacrine, and ganglion cells. The Müller cell is the only glial cell. The axons of the ganglion cells form the optic nerve. The photoreceptors-bipolar-ganglion cell connections form the input-output direction. Horizontal and amacrine cells are involved in lateral transmission of information. Most bipolar cells receive activity from a number of photoreceptors via the horizontal cells. Ganglion cells receive activity from a number of bipolar cells via the amacrine cells.

Blood Supply to the Retina

The retina is supplied by two separate circulation systems: the **retinal circulation** and the **choroidal circulation.** The retinal circulation consists of the central retinal artery, which enters the eye at the optic disc, and the central retinal vein, which leaves the eye at the optic disc. The choroidal circulation consists of vessels that penetrate the sclera and form a capillary plexus. This plexus lies immediately against the basement membrane of the pigment epithelium and forms Bruch's membrane. The choroidal circulation serves the receptors and the pigment epithelium. The cells of the ganglionic and inner nuclear layers are served by the retinal circulation.

Pigment Epithelium

The pigment epithelium is an important structure of the retina. It has three major functions: (1) it absorbs the light that has not been absorbed by the photoreceptors and thereby prevents reflection and interference, (2) it nourishes the photoreceptors, and (3) it phagocytizes the debris generated by renewal processes in the photoreceptors. If this function of pigment epithelium becomes defective, a disease that results in blindness called **retinitis pigmentosa** results.

Photoreceptors

Photoreceptors contain the machinery to transduce light into changes in the membrane potential. There are two types of photoreceptors: **rods** and **cones.** In the human retina there are approximately 100 million rods and 6 million cones. Both types of photoreceptors contain three regions, the **outer segment,** the **inner segment,** and the **synaptic foot.** The outer segment of the rod photoreceptors is composed of discs that contain the photon-absorbing pigment called **rhodopsin.** These discs regenerate; they are formed at the base of the outer segment and are pushed to the tip by the newly formed discs. The outer segment is connected to the inner segment by a structure called the **connecting celium.** The inner segment is connected to the synaptic foot region, which in turn contains synaptic vesicles. The cone system does not have separate discs, but the photopigments are embedded in the foldings of the outer segment membrane. In cones, the membrane regions that contain photopigments regenerate, but the rate of regeneration is significantly slower than that of the discs in the rod photoreceptors. In addition to these differences,

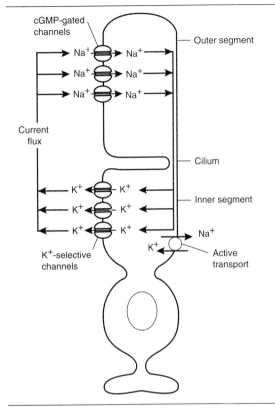

Fig. 8-2. The ionic basis of dark current of the photoreceptors. In the dark, the cGMP-gated Na$^+$ channels in the membrane of the outer segment of the photoreceptors are kept open by elevated cGMP level. This allows current flow from the inner segment to the outer segment and maintenance of a low membrane potential across the photoreceptor membrane. Absorption of light by rhodopsin increases a phosphodiestrase that breaks down cGMP and reduces its level. This causes closure of the cGMP-gated Na$^+$ channels and hyperpolarization of the cell membrane.

there is a significant difference in the response of these receptors to light: Rods are more sensitive to light than cones, and cones have color vision but rods do not.

Spectral Absorption

Biochemistry of Vision

The discs in the outer segment of rods contain a photopigment called **rhodopsin** that consists of a specific type of protein called **opsin** and a chromophore called **retinal.** Retinal is an aldehyde of vitamin A$_1$. In the dark, retinal is in its most unstable configuration, which is the 11-cis

form. Light causes a change in conformation of retinal from the 11-cis to an all-trans form, which is the most stable molecular structure. The following reactions take place following the absorption of light:

Rhodopsin $\longrightarrow$ prelumirhodopsin $\longrightarrow$

    lumirhodopsin $\longrightarrow$ metarhodopsin I $\longrightarrow$

    metarhodopsin Ii $\longrightarrow$ all-trans retinal + opsin

Resynthesis of rhodopsin occurs in the following manner:

$$\text{All-trans retinal} \xrightarrow{\text{dark}} \text{vitamin A}$$

$$\text{All-trans} \xrightarrow{\text{energy}} \text{11-cis retinal}$$

11-cis retinal + opsin $\longrightarrow$ rhodopsin + energy

Photoexcitation

In the dark, the membrane potential of the photoreceptors is around –40 mV. Absorption of photons by the visual pigment leads to **hyperpolarization** of the membrane of the photoreceptors. The resistance of the membrane increases during light response. The reason for the low membrane potential of the photoreceptor in the dark is that in dark the concentration of cyclic guanosine monophosphate (cGMP) in the outer segment is high, and there are cGMP-coupled Na$^+$ channels that are maintained in the open state as long as the cGMP concentration is high. These channels allow a current to flow from the inner segment into the outer segment (Fig. 8-2) called the **dark current.** A highly active Na$^+$-K$^+$ pump, located in the inner segment, continuously pumps out Na$^+$. When light is absorbed, this current stops. The transduction process occurs in several steps (Fig. 8-3): (1) absorption of light activates a G-protein called **tranducin,** (2) transducin activates cGMP phosphodiesterase, which is associated with the rhodopsin-containing discs, (3) cGMP phosphodiesterase hydrolyzes cGMP to 5'-GMP and lowers cGMP concentration in the rod cytoplasm, and (4) reduction of cGMP level causes Na$^+$ channels to close, and this leads to hyperpolarization of the membrane. This system can significantly amplify the transduction process. Because alteration of rhodopsin from the 11-cis to the all-trans conformation activates several hundred molecules of tranducin, and each phosphodiesterase molecule can hydrolyze thousands of cGMP molecules per second, the absorption of a single photon can be detected.

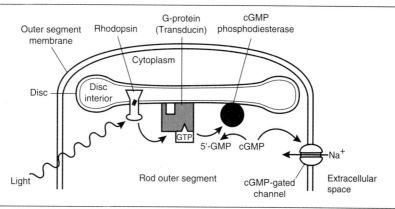

Fig. 8-3. The cascade of second messenger systems that are activated when light is absorbed by rhodopsin.

Electrical Signaling by Cells in the Retina

The absorption of photon is signaled by hyperpolarization of the photoreceptors in a graded fashion (i.e., the more intense the light, the higher is the amplitude of hyperpolarization). Although both rod and cone photoreceptors respond by hyperpolarization, the time course of their responses differs. Following stimulation, the membrane potential of cones returns to baseline faster than that of rods. This difference in response time causes differences in fusion frequency between the rod and cone systems. The **fusion frequency** is the frequency at which a flickering light is perceived to be on all the time. For the rod system, the fusion frequency is around 20 Hz. For the cone system, however, the fusion frequency is around 50 Hz. Fusion frequency is important because the majority of artificial light sources are powered by alternating current, which causes the light to be turned on and off. In the United States, the frequency of power lines is 60 Hz, which means that lights flicker 60 times per second. If the fusion frequency did not exist, we would not be able to use incandescent lights. In addition, the fusion frequency allows us to see movies. Movie frames are projected around 24 frames per second, a frequency that is slightly higher than the fusion frequency of the rod system. Because of fusion, we see movies as continuous images.

In addition to the photoreceptors, the horizontal and bipolar cells also respond in a graded fashion by hyperpolarization. The amacrine and ganglion cells respond by generating action potentials (Fig. 8-4). As noted earlier, the receptor, bipolar, and ganglion cells constitute the input-output (IO) pathway. The horizontal and amacrine cells are lateral interneurons. They receive signals from cells that precede them in the IO pathway and can transmit the signal back to the cell from which it came, across to the neighboring cells, or to next IO cell. In this way, horizontal cells can modify the signal transmitted by the photoreceptor and by the bipolar cells; the amacrine cell can modify the signal transmitted by ganglion cells and by bipolar cells.

Receptive Field Properties of the Retinal Neurons

All neurons in the retina have a circular receptive field organization (see Fig. 8-4). The horizontal cells have center-surround organization. Stimulation of the surround decreases the response amplitude of the horizontal cells. Bipolar cells have the same type of organization. Stimulation of the surround not only can decrease the amplitude of the response but also can change the polarity of the response. The amacrine cell responds by generating action potentials, and they also have a center-surround organization. There are two types of ganglion cells: **sustained** and **transient.** The sustained type responds to light by producing action potentials as long as the stimulus is on. The transient type only responds to the onset and to the offset of a stimulus. Based on their morphologic and response properties, ganglion cells have been classified as M (magnocellular) and P (parvocellular) cells. P cells are smaller than the M cells, have a small dendritic field, and are more numerous in the retina. They respond best to small objects and have a smaller receptive field compared with M cells. P cells are involved in color vision. It is believed that P cells are also involved in the analysis of fine detail in the visual image. By contrast, M cells are large, have a large

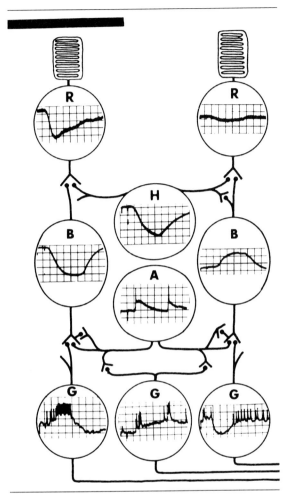

Fig. 8-4. The types of responses of each cell in the retina. Photoreceptors, horizontal cells, and bipolar cells respond by graded change in their membrane potential. Amacrine and ganglion cells respond by action potentials. The horizontal and amecrine cells have inhibitory influence on their surrounding cells. For this reason, activation of the center of the receptive field produces excitation, and activation of surround receptive field inhibits the ganglion cells that are the output of the retina. (From: Dowling, J. E. Organization of vertebrate retinas. *Inv. Ophthalmol.* 9:655–680, 1970.)

dendritic field, and have a large receptive field. They respond to visual stimuli by transient discharge. These cells are very responsive to movement and are believed to be involved in the analysis of form and movement.

Clinical Testing of Retinal Functions

A test that is used to determine the function of the retina is the **electroretinogram** (ERG). In this test, a recording electrode is positioned on the cornea, and the difference in potential between the cornea and an indifferent electrode positioned on another part of the body is measured. When the eye is stimulated, a waveform is obtained that is the ERG (Fig. 8-5). The ERG has three components, the **a wave,** the **b wave,** and the **c wave.** The a wave results from the responses of photoreceptors to light. The b wave results from activity of the Müller cells but also reflects the activities of the ganglion cells. The c wave reflects the activity of the pigment epithilium cells. Because of these properties, an ERG is useful for the diagnosis of damage to the retina. For example, in retinitis pigmentosa, the rod cells are affected early in the disease, but the cone cells remain intact for a longer time. The first sign of this disease is night blindness. In these patients, stimulation of the eye in a dark-adapted condition produces an ERG with either a small or absent a wave.

Color Vision

Color is subjective. Three parameters define color: **hue, saturation,** and **brightness.** Hue is exemplified by the color of the object, such as red or green. Saturation is a measure of the purity of the color. Addition of white to a given color causes it to be less saturated. Brightness is measured by the number of photons the source emits per unit area per second. Two theories have been proposed for color vision: (1) the first theory, the **Young-Helmholtz theory,** is based on the presence of three types of cone photoreceptors, blue, green, and red, and (2) the second theory, proposed by Hering, is referred to as the **opponent theory** and assumes that three types of receptors exist, a red-green, a blue-yellow, and a white-black. According to the opponent theory, an opposite, mutually exclusive response is produced by each type of receptor to the stimulation of its two colors.

Both theories are correct. The Young-Helmholtz theory describes color vision at the photoreceptor level, where there are three types of cones (Fig. 8-6); blue cones have a maximum absorption efficiency at 445 nm, green cones have a maximum absorption efficiency at 535 nm, and the maximum absorption efficiency of the red cones is at 570 nm. As shown in Fig. 8-6, there is a significant overlap in the spectral sensitivity of these receptors. Therefore, any

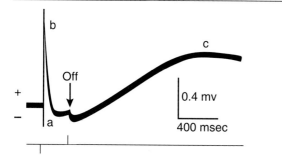

Fig. 8-5. The electroretinogram of the cat. The a wave occurring at approximately 19 msec is due to the photoreceptor activity. The b wave occurring at approximately 90 msec reflects the activity of the ganglion cells, and the c wave represents recovery of the photoreceptors. (Modified from: Brown, K. T. The electroretinogram: Its components and origins. *Vision Res.* 8:633, 1968.)

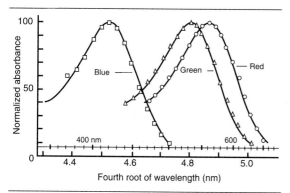

Fig. 8-6. The spectral absorption of human cone photoreceptors. The peak absorption of blue cones is at 445 nm, of green cones is at 535 nm, and of red cones is at 570 nm. Note that at wavelengths between 450 and 670 nm, light is absorbed by more than one type of cone. (Modified from: Dartnall, H. J., Bowmaker, J. K., and Mollon, J. D. Microspectrophotometry of human photoreceptors. In: Mollon, J. D., and Sharpe, L. T., eds. *Color Vision: Physiology and Psychophysics.* New York: Academic Press, 1983. Pp. 69-80.)

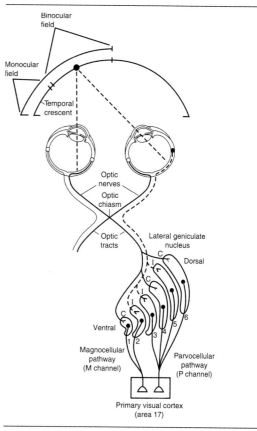

Fig. 8-7. Schematics of the projection pathway from the retina to the lateral geniculate nucleus (LGN). Note that each lateral geniculate nucleus receives input from both eyes, but each layer of LGN receives input from only one eye. Layers 1 and 2 comprise the magnocellular pathway, and layers 3, 4, 5, and 6 form the parvocellular pathway. (Modified from: Dartnell, H. J., Bowmaker, J. K., and Mollon, J. D. Microspectrophotometry of human photoreceptors. In: Mollon, J. D., and Sharpe, L. T., eds. *Color Vision: Physiology and Psychophysics.* New York: Academic Press, 1983. Pp. 69–80.)

given light activates more than one type of photoreceptor. Hering's theory describes color vision at the ganglion cell–lateral geniculate level. Cells in these regions respond to color by excitation or inhibition. For example, a red-green cell responds by excitation if the center of its receptive field is illuminated by a green light and by inhibition if it is illuminated by a red light.

Color Blindness

There are three types of color blindness: **protanopia, deuteranopia,** and **tritanopia.** In addition, a monochromatic defect exists, but this is a rare disorder.

Protanopia

In protanopia, there are no red cones. A photopic luminosity curve, which quantitates the brightness of each object as determined by the absorption of light by blue, red, and green receptors shows a deficit in the red range. Individuals with protanopia perceive objects that look dimmer compared with a normal individual. A protanopic individual has a **neutral point,** which is the wavelength at which the person obtains a perfect match against a neutral white light simply by making a brightness match. Protanopes confuse objects of a particular shade of green with objects of a particular shade of red as well as objects in the blue and violet region.

Deuteranopia

Unlike protanopia, deuteranopia is not characterized by a deficit system. Deuteranopes have a normal or above-normal luminosity curve. In these individuals, the red and green pigments have combined to form a yellow-absorbing pigment. These individuals also have a neutral point, at which a perfect match to a white color can be made by addition of only two colors. They confuse red-green shades with each other, but these shades are different from those that protanopes confuse. The same is true for colors in the blue and violet region.

Tritanopia

There are two kinds of tritanopia, **natural** and **acquired.** Acquired tritanopia usually occurs in almost any kind of retinitis and in retinal detachment. Individuals with tritanopia always see only red at wavelengths down to a normal's yellow locus, at which point they would see no hue. At wavelengths shorter than yellow, the spectrum would again present only one hue, which the individual may call blue-green, green, or even blue. Two primary lights, a red and a blue, would suffice for all color matching. In natural tritanopia, the center of the fovea is blue blind. These individuals have the same type of color blindness as those with acquired blue blindness.

Central Visual Pathways

The axons of ganglion cells form the optic tract that projects to the lateral geniculate of the thalamus. This projection is highly organized, and each eye projects to both the right and left lateral geniculate nuclei (Fig. 8-7). From the lateral geniculate, the visual signals are projected to the visual cortex and to other brain regions associated with processing of visual signals. A large number of areas in the brain are involved in processing visual information. The physiologic properties of these components are discussed below.

Lateral Geniculate Nucleus (LGN)

The LGN contains six layers and receives inputs from both eyes (see Fig. 8-7). However, each layer receives input from one eye only. The left visual field projects to the right LGN, and the right visual field projects to the left LGN. Layers 1 and 2 are called the **magnocellular layers,** and layers 3 to 6 are called the **parvocellular layers.** Layers 2, 3, and 5 receive inputs from the ipsilateral eye; layers 1, 4, and 6 receive inputs from the contralateral eye. The magnocellular regions encode brightness information and have poor acuity, but fast responses. These cells are functionally very similar to the M cells of the retina. Cells in the parvocellular regions have fine discrimination capability, interpret color, and have a sustained response. The visual field of these cells are similar to the visual fields of the P cells in the retina. In these visual fields, each color cell is antagonized by the complementary color—i.e., if red stimulates a cell in the center, then green in the periphery will inhibit it. This phenomena is called **center-surround antagonism,** red versus green and blue versus yellow.

In addition to these differences, in a given column, all cells respond to the same visual field; i.e., there is a topographic map such that each on-cell in a given path is receiving information from the same spot in the viewing field. Comparing the activity of one cell with that of the cell above it (i.e., comparing layer 1 with layer 2), indicates that the activity is slightly different because eyes are spaced slightly differently. This contributes to depth perception.

Connections of the Visual System in the Ascending Pathway

The retina projects to the LGN. The magno- and parvocellular layers project to the primary visual area of the cortex (area 17). Area 17 in turn projects to visual areas 2 and 3 in the cortex. Visual area 3 projects to area 3A (area 18), and 3A projects to V4 (area 18), which then projects to the inferior temporal area (areas 20 and 21), the posterior parietal area (area 7), and the frontal eye fields (area 8). Each of these areas extracts different information from the visual input, and every projection line has another projection line going in the opposite direction; i.e., if visual area 3A can project to 3B, then 3B can in turn project to 3A.

Receptive Field Properties of the Cortical Cells

Based on their receptive field characteristics, the cells in the primary visual cortex have been classified as **simple cells** and **complex cells**. The simple cells (Fig. 8-8) have receptive fields that are rectangular with a specific axis of orientation. For example, a cell can have a receptive field that is oriented vertically (from 12 to 6 o'clock). This cell will be excited by a vertical bar of light, and this excitatory zone will be flanked by two surrounding inhibitory zones. If the orientation of the stimulus is changed to the horizontal position (from 3 to 9 o'clock), this cell will not respond to the same stimulus. Other cells may have different orientation preferences and may respond by excitation to a bar of darkness. The complex cells also have rectangular receptive fields and are orientation-specific (Fig. 8-9). However, these receptive fields are larger than the receptive fields of the simple cells and do not have clearly defined on or off zones.

Columnar Organization of the Cortex

The visual cortex is organized in columns that run perpendicular to the brain surface. Each column is about 20 to 100 μm wide and 2 mm deep. Each column contains sim-

Fig. 8-8. (A) Receptive field characteristics of a simple cell in the visual cortex. This cell responds best when the stimulus has a vertical orientation and does not respond when the stimulus is oriented horizontally. (B) The receptive field characteristic of the simple cell can be synthesized by convergence of inputs of several LGN cells onto a single cortical simple cell. (Modified from: Hubel, D. H., and Wiesel, T. N. Receptive field binocular interaction and functional architecture of the cat's visual cortex. *J. Physiol. (Lond.)* 160:106, 1962.)

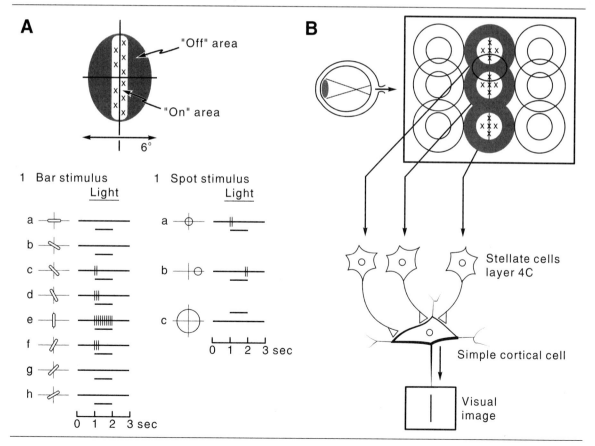

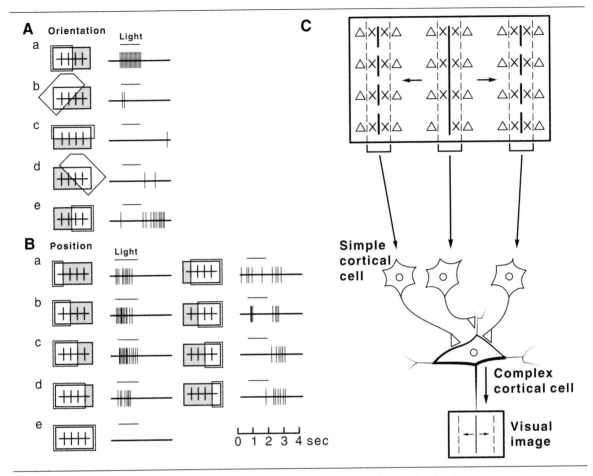

Fig. 8-9. Receptive field of a complex cell in the visual cortex. This cell responds to a stimulus that is oriented vertically (A) and is positioned such that only half the receptive field is stimulated (B). When the stimulus is oriented horizontally or positioned such that all the receptive field is stimulated, the cell will not respond. (C) The receptive field of the complex cell can be synthesized by convergence of several simple cells onto a single complex cell in the visual cortex. (Modified from: Hubel, D. H., and Wiesel, T. N. Receptive field binocular interaction and functional architecture of the cat's visual cortex. *J. Physiol. (Lond.)* 160:106, 1962.)

ple and complex cells, and all cells in a given column have the same axis of orientation. These columns are interrupted by a region called the **blob** or **peg region.** Cells in the blob region have a receptive field that is similar to the receptive field of the LGN cells. These cells are concerned with color processing. In addition to these columns, the primary visual cortex contains **ocular dominance** columns. Cells in these columns respond either to stimulation of the right or the left eye (Fig. 8-10).

Effect of Lesions in the Visual Pathway

Lesions of different regions of the visual pathway produce different types of field defects (Fig. 8-11). Prechiasmic lesions result in complete loss of vision in one eye (see Fig. 8-11A). Chiasmic lesions result in hemianopia. In this type of lesion, both eyes show a temporal field defect (see Fig. 8-11B). Lesions of the optic tract produce a field loss on the temporal side, contralateral to the lesion, and a field

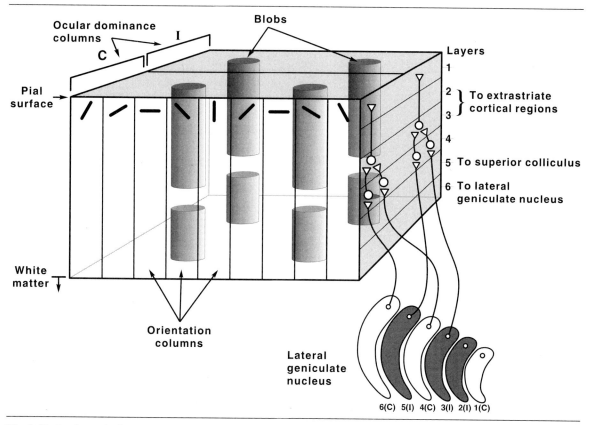

Fig. 8-10. A schematic diagram showing the microstructure of the primary visual cortex. The cortex is organized in columns. All types of cells (simple and complex) in one column have the same orientation sensitivity. The cortex is divided into ocular dominance sections. Cells in these sections are more responsive to stimulation of one eye than the other. The columns are separated by columns of cells that have receptive field characteristics that resemble the receptive field characteristics of the LGN cells. These are the blob or peg columns. (Modified from: Hubel, D. H., and Wiesel, T. N. *Brain Mechanisms of Vision.* New York: Scientific American Library, 1979.)

loss on the nasal side of the ipsilateral eye (see Fig. 8-11C). Lesions of the optic radiation or the visual cortex produce incomplete or quadratic field defects (see Fig. 8-11D, E, F).

Summary

The visual system is a highly organized, parallel processor. It has three parallel systems, each best suited to analyze one aspect of visual tasks: detection of color, form, and movement. The retina contains the photoreceptors that tranduce light into changes in the membrane potential.

Photoreceptors and horizontal and bipolar cells produce generator potentials rather than action potentials. The generator potential is a graded response, and its magnitude changes with the intensity of light. The amacrine and ganglion cells produce action potentials. The retina cells and the lateral geniculate cells have circular receptive fields with center-surround opposition. The cortical cells have rectangular receptive fields with highly organized orientation axes. The visual cortex is organized in columns. Some columns contain cells that have linear receptive fields, other columns contain cells that have circular receptive fields, and still other columns contain cells that are activated by stimulation of only one eye. Lesions

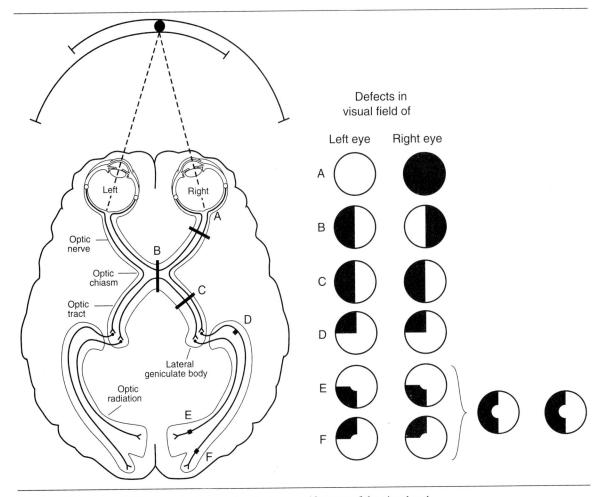

Fig. 8-11. The types of field losses that are produced when specific parts of the visual pathway are lesioned.

of the visual pathway produce distinct patterns of field loss.

Bibliography

Dowling, J. E. *The Retina: An Approachable Part of the Brain.* Cambridge, Mass.: Belknap Press, 1987.

Gouras, P. The perception of colour. In Cronly-Dillon, J., ed., *Vision and Visual Dysfunction,* Vol. 6. London: Macmillan, 1991.

Hubel, D. H., and Wiesel, T. N. Functional architecture of macaque monkey visual cortex. *Proc. R. Soc. Lond. [B]* 1981:1, 1977.

Stryer, L. Cyclic GMP cascade of vision. *Annu. Rev. Neurosci.* 9:87, 1986.

9 Hearing and Equilibrium

Michael M. Behbehani

Objectives

After reading this chapter, you should be able to

Describe the anatomy of the ear

Describe the units used to measure the intensity of sound, and explain the range of hearing in humans and how it varies with age

Explain the transduction of sound by the hair cells

Describe the anatomy of the auditory system

Explain the functional characteristics of neuronal elements in each component of the auditory system

Describe the anatomy of the vestibular system

Explain how each component of the vestibular system responds to changes in the position of the head

Describe the anatomic characteristics of the central vestibular pathway

Describe the functional characteristics of cells in the vestibular pathway

Hearing

Anatomy of the Outer and Middle Ear

Before hearing can take place, the vibration produced by sound must pass through the outer ear and the middle ear and generate a pressure wave within the cochlea that acts on the hair cells located in the inner ear. The outer ear consists of the **external meatus,** which is about 2.5 cm long and ends at the **tympanic membrane** (the ear drum). The tympanic membrane and three small bones called the **ossicles** form the middle ear. The tympanic membrane is connected to the three ossicles: the **malleus, incus,** and **stapes.** The handle of the malleus is attached to the tympanic membrane, and the head of the malleus is attached to the incus by ligaments. The incus articulates with the stapes. The stapes rests on the oval window of the cochlea (Fig. 9-1). Sound vibrates **Reissner's membrane** and the **basilar membrane.** There are two small muscles, the **tensor tympani** and the **stapedius,** that are located in the middle ear and are attached to the tympanic membrane and to the stapes. When they contract, they act to attenuate sound by about 20 dB. At one time these muscles were thought to be responsible for protecting the ear from extremely loud sounds. Since it takes at least 15 to 20 msec for these muscles to contract, loud sounds that last only for 2 to 3 msec are not attenuated by contraction of these muscles. However, these muscles can serve as protective elements for prolonged loud sounds. In addition, these two muscles contract and attenuate the sound of our own voices and are reflexively activated when we walk. The reason for the latter reflex is not entirely clear, but it is thought that this action protects the tympanic membrane and the stapes.

Anatomy of the Inner Ear

The inner ear consists of a highly specialized and complex structure called the **cochlea.** The cochlea is a spiral organ

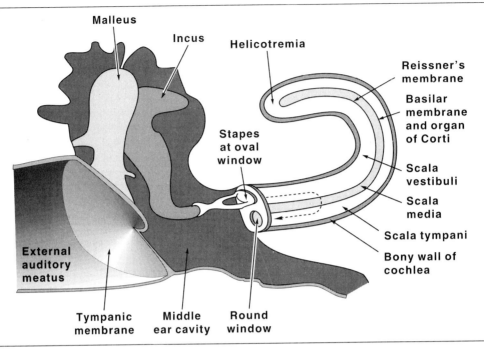

Fig. 9-1. Schematic diagram of the ear with the cochlea uncoiled. The external ear ends at the tympanic membrane. Vibration of the tympanic membrane is transmitted to the malleus and incus and finally to the stapes, which is connected to the oval window and causes its movement. Vibration of the oval window sets up a wave that propagates through the scala tympany and scala vestibuli, which are connected at heliotrema. The vibration causes movement of the hair cells located in the organ of Corti. The pressure wave is relieved through the round window.

with two and one-half turns. At one end, there are two windows called the **oval window** and the **round window.** The body of the cochlea is divided into three compartments, the **scala vestibuli,** the **scala media,** and the **scala tympani.** These compartments are divided by two membranes called **Reissner's membrane** and the **basilar membrane.** The scala vestibuli and the scala tympani are connected at the tip of the cochlea by a structure called the **helicotrema.** The compartments of the cochlea are filled with a solution that has the same constituents as the extracellular fluid and is called **perilymph.** The prelymph contains a high concentration of Na (approximately 150 mM) and a low concentration of KCl (approximately 5 mM). The scala media is completely enclosed on the side near the scala vestibuli by Reissner's membrane and on the side next to the scala tympani by the basilar membrane. The scala media contains a solution called **endolymph** that has the ionic concentration of the intracellular fluid with a high concentration of K (approximately 135 mM KCl) and a low Na concentration (approximately 15 mM).

The **organ of Corti** rests on the basilar membrane (Fig. 9-2). This structure consists of receptor cells called the **inner** and the **outer hair cells.** The mammalian organ of Corti contains approximately 3500 inner hair cells and 20,000 outer hair cells. These cells are innervated by the axons of the cochlear division of the eighth cranial nerve. The cell bodies of these nerves are located in the spiral ganglion. Hair cells have a diameter of 8 to 12 μm. The tip of the hair cells contains a very thin hair (0.1 μm in diameter and 4 μm long) that is embedded in a membrane called the **tectorial membrane.** The tectorial membrane is connected at one end to the limbus and at the other to the organ of Corti. When sound pressure moves the stapes, it applies pressure to the oval window and causes a pressure wave to propagate through the scala vestibuli and then to the scala media, causing the basila membrane to move downward. This movement causes the hair cells embedded in the tectorial membrane to bend. The pressure wave is also transmitted to the scala tympani, causing the round window to move outward into the middle ear. There is a

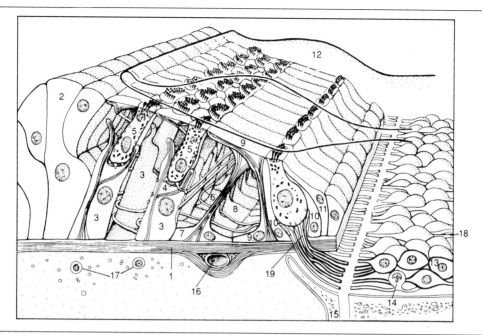

Fig. 9-2. Magnified image of the organ of Corti showing the morphologic characteristics of the hair cells in relation to the basilar and tectorial membranes (1, basilar membrane; 2, Hensen's cells; 3, Deiter's cells; 4, synaptic contact between hair cells and spiral afferent fibers; 5, outer hair cells; 6, outer spiral fibers; 7, outer pillar cells; 8, tunnel of Corti; 9, inner pillar cells; 10, inner phalageal cells; 11, boarder cells; 12, tectorial membrane; 13, type I spiral ganglion cell; 14, type II spiral ganglion cell; 15, bony spiral lamina; 16, nerve bundle). (From: Kandel, E. R., Schwartz, J. H., and Jessell, T. M. *Principles of Neural Science,* 3rd ed. New York: Elsevier, 1991.)

significant reduction in the surface area between the larger tympanic membrane, which is 50 to 60 mm^2, and the smaller oval window (3–4 mm^2) through which the stapes will transfer the sound to the inner ear. This reduction in surface area leads to a 15- to 20-fold amplification of the sound waves. This amplification is important in the maintenance of the pressure wave as it leaves the air-filled middle ear and enters the fluid-filled inner ear.

Hearing Range

The human range of hearing frequencies is about 20 to 20,000 Hz. At about age 20, the ability to hear high frequencies decreases to 16,000 Hz. The optimal hearing (lowest threshold) occurs at frequencies of 1000 to 3000 Hz. This is the frequency of most voices and represents a range of frequencies that is far less likely to be lost with age. Figure 9-3 illustrates how sound perception changes with age. A contributing factor in age-dependent hearing loss is that the elasticity of the tympanic membrane and oval and round windows decreases with age.

The unit of measurement of sound intensity is the decibel (dB), named after Alexander Graham Bell. The decibel is defined as

$$N_{dB} = 20 \log(E_2/E_1)$$

where N_{dB} is the intensity level of the sound in decibels, E_1 is the reference sound energy, and E_2 is the sound source. The reference energy is 0.0002 dyn/cm^2. This sound pressure is approximately the intensity of a sound at 1000 Hz, which is just detectable by young human observers. Since we can hear sounds over a 10-million-fold range of intensities, a logarithmic scale is simpler to use than a linear scale. Note that the threshold of hearing is at 0 dB, normal conversation is at 70 dB, and sound becomes uncomfort-

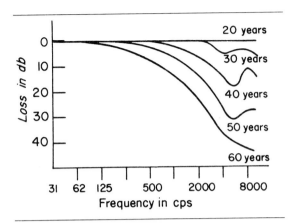

Fig. 9-3. Variation of hearing with age. (Modified from: Licklider, J. C. R. Basic correlate of auditory stimulus. In: Stevens, S. S., ed. *Handbook of Experimental Psychology*. New York: Wiley, 1951. Pp. 985–1093.)

able and then painful at between 120 and 140 dB. Sound intensities above 140 dB damage the auditory system.

Transduction Mechanism

The transduction of sound to changes in the membrane potential and ultimately to action potentials takes place by movement of the **hair cells** in the **organ of Corti.** The pressure wave–induced movement of the **basilar membrane** causes the hair cells to move relative to the fixed tectorial membrane at their apex. As the basilar membrane moves, the stereocilia on the hair cells must bend. This bending causes a change in the permeability of the hair cell membrane to ions. Unlike the transduction mechanism in other systems, the hair cells can hyperpolarize or depolarize. The hair cells send a signal through the afferent nerve fibers of the cochlear ganglion.

The basilar membrane is narrow (100 μm) and stiff near the **oval window** but becomes wider (500 μm) and more flaccid as it approaches the apex. These important changes in both width and rigidity are functionally significant. The initial segment of the membrane is highly responsive to high-frequency vibration, whereas the apical portion of the membrane is responsive to low-frequency vibration, with a gradual transition occurring between the two ends. In addition to the characteristic changes in the basilar membrane, there are also characteristic changes between the inner and outer hair cells.

For many years it was thought that when a sinusoidal wave propagates through the cochlear duct, different parts of the basilar membrane would respond to a specific fre-

quency. A more recent study using laser refractometry has shown that in actuality, almost the entire membrane moves but that there are segments that move maximally. The area of maximal movement occurs near the initial segment for high-frequency sounds and near the apex for lower-frequency sounds. This arrangement allows the basilar membrane and its associated hair cells to experience maximal displacement in one area for a particular frequency and gradually less displacement for adjacent cells (Fig. 9-4). Therefore, the auditory system acquires information relating to the overall pattern of firing. As shown in

Fig. 9-4. Pattern of the vibration envelope at various frequencies as a function of distance from stapes. (Modified from: Von Békésy, G. *Experiments in Hearing*. E. G. Wever, ed. and trans. New York: McGraw-Hill, 1960.)

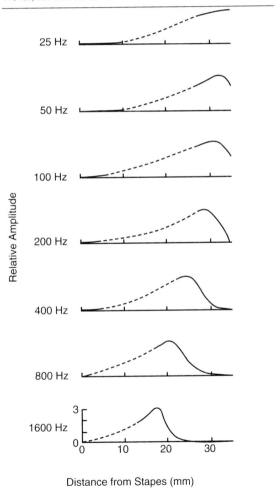

Fig. 9-4, at low frequencies (25 Hz), most of the cells are activated by movement of nearly all regions of the basilar membrane. At higher frequencies (1600 Hz), a smaller region of the basilar membrane undergoes movement; however, the cells in this small region of the membrane are displaced maximally.

Although the overall shapes of the hair cells are similar, there is a considerable difference in both the mechanical and electrical properties of hair cells in different regions of the organ of Corti. Hair cells that are located at the base of the basilar membrane (next to the oval window) are short and have stiff stereocilia. In contrast, hair cells located at the apex of the basilar membrane are more than twice as long as those in the base of the membrane and have a very flexible stereocilia. Because of these properties, hair cells near the apex show mechanical resonance.

The membrane potential of hair cells oscillates. The oscillatory response is due to movement of calcium into and out of the cell, which causes depolarization (Fig. 9-5). Calcium entry causes activation of two types of potassium currents, a calcium-activated potassium current and a voltage-sensitive delayed potassium current. These two potassium currents cause hyperpolarization of the hair cell. As calcium is sequestered inside the cell, the membrane po-

tential returns to the resting level, at which the magnitude of potassium currents is reduced. These events allow calcium entry to depolarize the cell in a cyclic manner.

Critical Frequency

Recording the response of a cochlear nerve to a tone illustrates that the **absolute threshold** (i.e., the least intensity to make the cells fire) occurs over a broad range of frequencies. However, the minimal threshold has a **characteristic** or **critical frequency** (CF) that occurs at a very discrete value (Fig. 9-6A). Different cells have different critical frequencies. The audiogram is obtained by using sound at different frequencies and is a composite of all critical frequencies of the hair cells.

Nerve Signal Transmission

There are more neurons in the spiral ganglion than there are hair cells; each hair cell is innervated by at least five nerves. This multiple innervation increases the speed and sensitivity of the auditory system. The auditory nerve fibers have spontaneous activity of about 100 Hz. For this reason, the inhibition can be detected accurately. The rapid transduction, the spontaneous activity, and the high propagation velocity of the auditory system are critical to our ability to localize sound. In order to be able to locate the source of a sound, the auditory system must be able to distinguish latency differences on the order of 1 msec. To ac-

Fig. 9-5. The types of currents that are activated by bending of a hair cell.

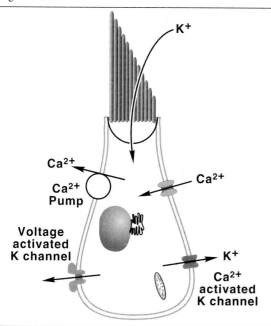

Fig. 9-6. Tuning curves of neurons located in the coclear nerve (A), inferior colliculus (B), trapezoid body (C), and medial geniculate body (D). The complete auditory response curve is a combination of many tuning curves (solid line in B.) (From: Katsuki, Y. Neural mechanism of auditory sensation in cats. In: Rosenlith, W. A., ed. *Sensory Communication*. Cambridge: MIT Press, 1961.)

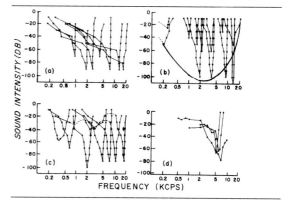

complish this sound localization, there are areas in the inferior colliculus, medical geniculate, and auditory cortex that are tuned to very small differences in latency and sound intensity between the two ears. In order to detect these differences, the system must be able to respond very quickly. If the system were not already spontaneously oscillating, it would take a few microseconds to initiate transduction, and the ability to distinguish differences would be blurred.

Anatomy of the Central Auditory Pathway

Auditory nerve fibers in the eighth nerve synapse with neurons in the **cochlear nucleus.** This nucleus is divided into dorsal and ventral divisions. Neurons in the dorsal cochlear nucleus cross the midline and reach the inferior colliculus. This pathway is predominantly a crossed pathway. In addition to its main projection site, some of the axons of the dorsal cochlear nucleus branch and send afferents to the contralateral reticular formation, the superior olivary complex and the nuclei of the lateral lemniscus. The axons of cells in the ventral cochlear nucleus cross beneath the inferior cerebellar peduncle and terminate bilaterally in the superior olivary complex. These axons also send collaterals bilaterally to the reticular formation. Superior olivary axons form the lateral lemniscus and project either directly to the inferior colliculus or relay at the nucleus of the lateral lemniscus. Cells in the inferior colliculus send ipsilateral projections to the medial geniculate nucleus of the thalamus. This nucleus projects ipsilaterally to the primary auditory cortex (Fig. 9-7).

Characteristics of Central Auditory Neurons

Neurons in all regions of the auditory pathway have specific **critical frequencies** (see Fig. 9-6). Cells in the cochlear nuclei have response characteristics that are very similar to the response of the auditory nerve. These cells have tuning curves and a critical frequency. However, unlike the auditory nerve, cells in the cochlear nuclei can be inhibited. Usually stimuli at frequencies on either side of the tuning curve of a cell cause inhibition of these cells. This inhibition process is used to sharpen the tuning curve and produce an increase in the signal-to-noise ratio of these cells. Neurons in the superior olivary complex also show a critical frequency. As will be discussed later, these cells are involved in sound localization. Cells

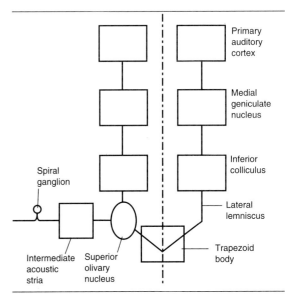

Fig. 9-7. Schematic diagram of propagation of auditory signal from the spiral ganglion neurons to the auditory cortex.

in the medial geniculate and cortex are tonotropically organized. **Tonatropic organization** refers to the fact that in the auditory cortex, all cells located in a single column respond to one sound frequency; if a recording is made from cells in the adjacent columns, they are tuned to a different frequency. In addition to tonotropic organization, the **auditory cortex** contains summation and supression columns. Cells in a summation column respond to stimulation of both ears better than to stimulation of only one ear. Cells in a supression column respond better to sound from one ear.

Sound Localization

Humans can distinguish sounds that originate from sources that are separated by as little as 1 degree. The first central site where localization of sound is processed is the **superior olivary complex** (SOC). This complex receives inputs from cochlear nuclei on both sides. SOC cells show significantly different responses to stimulation of one ear as compared with biaural stimulation. Some SOC cells are excited when one ear is stimulated but are inhibited when the other ear is stimulated. In addition, SOC neurons are very sensitive to the phase of the sound. If the phase of the sound in one ear leads that of the other ear, the cell may fire at a higher rate than when the phase of the sound is the same for both ears.

Noise Damage

Following exposure to loud noises over even relatively short periods of time (e.g., 2000 Hz at 120 dB for 16 minutes), there is a 40-dB loss in responsiveness to higher frequencies beginning at 2000 Hz. This deficit persists long after the stimulus is stopped. Even 3 days later, there is some slight residual hearing deficit. Prolonged exposure to loud noise permanently damages the auditory system.

Testing Auditory Function

The conduction portion of the auditory system can be tested by two types of tests, one is called the **Weber** test and the other the **Rinne** test. In the Weber test, the base of a tuning fork that vibrates at 256 Hz is placed on the middle of the forehead, and the subject is asked to localize the sound. If the person has some form of conduction deficit, such as a ruptured tympanic membrane, otosclerosis, or fluid in the middle ear, the sound is localized to the deaf ear because sound is propagated through the bone and reaches the cochlea. The reason that sound is not localized to the normal ear is because the normal ear is also activated by ambient noise that masks the sound of the tuning fork. In the Rinne test, the base of a vibrating tuning fork is placed on the mastoid process, and the subject is asked to indicate when the sound is no longer heard. At that time, the tuning fork is removed from the bone and is placed near the external auditory meatus. If the subject hears the sound again, then the conduction pathway is intact.

Equilibrium

The sense of balance is of critical importance in maintenance of posture and targeting of the eye. Unlike the activity of other sensory modalities, the sense of balance is not perceived at the conscious level. However, any abnormality of this sense is rapidly perceived and can overshadow all other sensations. The sensory organ that encodes the sense of balance is the **vestibular apparatus,** which is located within the bony labyrinth. This apparatus has two functions. The dynamic function encodes the rotation of the head in space and is best activated by acceleration. The static function encodes the position of the head. These

functions are encoded by anatomically distinct entities within the vestibular apparatus.

The vestibular system consists of a complex structure that contains multiple canals. The whole structure is suspended within the bony labyrinth by fibrous filaments (Fig. 9-8). The area between the vestibular apparatus and the bone is filled with perilymph that has an ionic composition similar to cerebrospinal fluid, namely, a high concentration of sodium and chloride and a low concentration of potassium. The canals of the vestibular apparatus are filled with endolymph that resembles intracellular fluid. The endolymph has a very high concentration of potassium (150 mM) and a low concentration of sodium (2 mM). Because of differences in the ionic concentrations of potassium and sodium, there is an 80-mV potential difference across the membrane that separates prelymph and endolymph (the prelymph is positive with respect to the endolymph). The vestibular apparatus contains two components, the **otolith organ** and the **semicircular ducts.**

Otolith Organ

The otolith organ contains two organs, the **utricle** and the **saccule** (see Fig. 9-8). These structures are connected and contain endolymph. Both structures contain sensory epithela, called the **macula,** which are composed of hair cells. The hair cells of the sensory epithelium extend into the gelatinous membrane. The ends of the hair cells are differentiated into **stereocilia** and **kinocilia** (Fig. 9-9).

The utricle is an oval tube that is located medially within the vestibule. When the head is in an upright position, the macula within the utricle is parallel to the ground. The utricle is covered with a gelatinous membrane that contains numerous crystals of calcium carbonate called **otoliths.** The hair cells have a resting membrane potential of –60 mV, and when they are bent, this membrane potential changes.

The stereocilia vary in length and are oriented from the shortest to the tallest; the tallest cells are located next to the kinocilia. The basal portions of hair cells, which are located in the sensory epithelium, are encapsulated by the peripheral branches of neurons from the vestibular ganglia; synaptic contacts exist between these structures. At rest, there is continuous release of neurotransmitter from the hair cell terminals. When a hair cell bends toward the kinocelia, its membrane potential depolarizes, and there is an increase in neurotransmitter release. In contrast, when a hair cell bends away from the kinocelia, its membrane po-

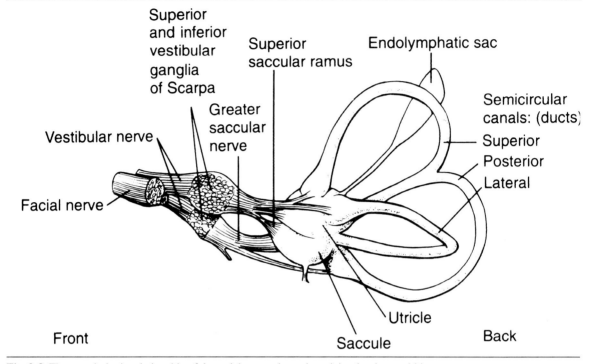

Fig. 9-8. The morphologic relationship of the utricle, saccule, and semicircular ducts within the inner ear.

tential hyperpolarizes, and neurotransmitter release decreases. Stereocilia in the macula of the utricle do not face the same direction. For this reason, linear acceleration in any direction can be encoded by these hair cells.

The **saccule** is located in the medial part of the vestibule just under the utricle. It contains a sensory epithelium called the **saccular macula** that is functionally identical to the utricle macula. Similar to the utricle macula, the hair cells in the saccule macula encode the position of the head. The saccule macula is innervated by a separate branch of the vestibular nerve.

The Semicircular Ducts

Each labyrinth contains three semicircular ducts. These ducts are oriented in planes that are approximately perpendicular to each other. The lumina of the semicircular canals and utricles are connected. Near the junction of one arm of the semicircular canal with the utricle there is a structure called **ampullae** (Fig. 9-10). Within the ampullae of each semicircular canal there is a sensory epithelium called the **crista ampullae.** The ampullae are oriented at

the right angles to the semicircular ducts. The ampulla of each semicircular canal contains hair cells that are all oriented in the same direction. The hair cells extend into a structure called a **cupula.**

The function of the semicircular canals is to detect acceleration of the head. Rotation of the head produces a relative movement of the endolymph in the direction opposite to the direction of the movement. Movement of the endolymph bends the hair cells in the direction of head movement. If the rotation continues, the endolymph moves at the same rate and in the same direction of movement due to friction between the endolymph and the walls of the duct. Because of this property, acceleration of the movement, not its velocity, is encoded by the semicircular canals. When the movement stops, the inertia of the endolymph causes it to bend the hair cell in the opposite direction. The hair cells regain their original state several seconds after the movement has stopped.

The hair cells in each semicircular canal are innervated by a different branch of the vestibular nerve. The afferent fibers from each semicircular canal are most sensitive to the movement in the plane of the duct. For example, fibers

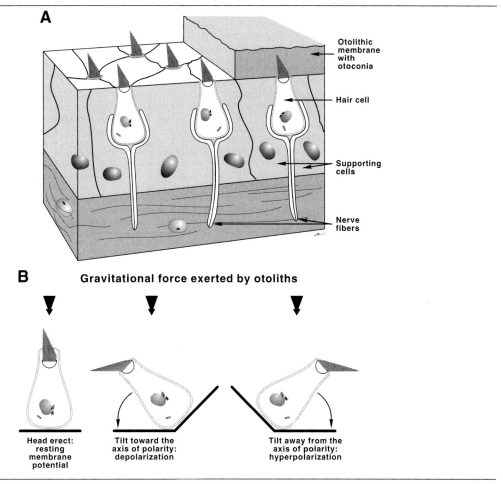

Fig. 9-9. (A) The location of the hair cell and the otolithic membrane. (B) The effect of direction of bending of a hair cell on its resting membrane potential. (Redrawn from: Kandel, E. R., Schwartz, J. H. and Jessell, T. *Principles of Neural Science,* 3rd ed. Norwalk, Conn.: Appleton & Lange, 1991.)

that innervate the horizontal duct respond best to movement of the head in a horizontal plane.

Central Connection of the Vestibular System

The cell bodies of the afferent fibers of the vestibular system are located in the vestibular ganglion. These neurons are bipolar cells. The peripheral branches of these biopolar cells innervate the hair cells, and the central branches travel through the eighth cranial nerve and synapse with cells in the **vestibular nucleus complex.** The vestibular nucleus complex is divided into the lateral, medial, superior, and inferior (descending) vestibular nuclei. Outputs of these nuclei project to the spinal cord, the cerebellum, the nuclei of the extrinsic eye muscles, the reticular formation, and the contralateral vestibular nuclei (Fig. 9-11).

The lateral vestibular nucleus is also known as **Deiter's nucleus** and is divided into two regions. The ventral section of the lateral vestibular nucleus receives inputs from the macula of the utricle and the semicircular ducts. The dorsal region of this nucleus receives inputs from cerebellum and spinal cord. Cells in the lateral vestibular nucleus are tonically active and respond to tilting of the head.

A

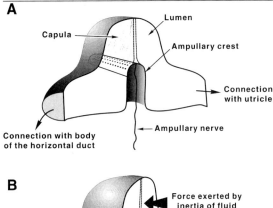

B

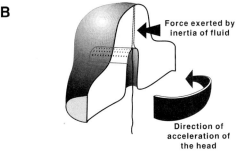

Fig. 9-10. The morphologic characteristics of the ampula of the semicircular duct. The receptor cells are located on the ampullary crest. A gelatinous material (the cupula) stretches from the crest to the roof of the ampula. (Redrawn from: Kandel, E. R., Schwartz, J. H., and Tessell, T., *Principles of Neural Science,* 3rd ed. Norwalk, Conn.: Appleton & Lange, 1991.)

When the head tilts in one direction, the baseline firing of some cells in this nucleus increases. When the head is tilted in the opposite direction, the baseline activities of these cells decrease. The change in the firing frequency depends on the angle of the tilt. The larger the tilt angle, the larger is the change in the firing rate.

Cells in the medial and superior nuclei receive input from the semicircular ducts. These cells are involved in vestibulo-oculomotor reflexes, which coordinate the movement of the eyes with respect to the movement of the head. When the head is tilted in one direction, the eyes move in the opposite direction, which helps in the maintenance of the gaze. The axons of the cells in the medial nucleus project to the cervical spinal cord and innervate motor neurons that control the neck muscles. This pathway is involved in movement of the head with respect to the body.

The inferior vestibular nucleus receives afferents from the semicircular ducts, the utricle, and the saccule. In addi-

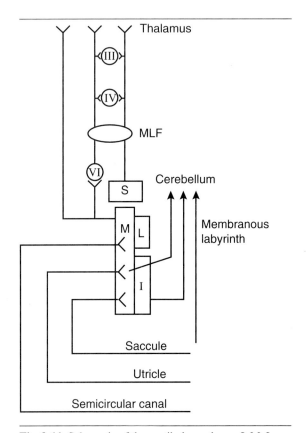

Fig. 9-11. Schematic of the vestibular pathway. I, M, L, and S represent the inferior, medial, lateral, and superior nuclei of the vestibular nuclear complex (MLF, medial longitudinal bundle; III, third nerve [oculomotor] nucleus; IV, fourth nerve [trochlear] nucleus; VI, the sixth nerve [abducens] nucleus).

tion, it receives afferents from the vemis of the cerebellum; the inferior vestibular nucleus sends projections through the vestibulospinal and vestibulo-ocular pathways, innervating motor neurons in these systems.

Summary

The auditory system is designed to change vibration produced by sound into recognizable information. The transduction of sound to changes in the membrane potential takes place at the hair cells. To reach these cells, sound travels through the external auditory meatus and causes vibration of the tympanic membrane. The oscillation of the tympanic membrane causes oscillation of three small bones that transfer vibration to the oval window of the inner ear. Sound is then propagated through the cochlea, an organ with three fluid-filled compartments. Vibration of this fluid causes bending of the hair cells, which leads to the opening of mechanical-sensitive cationic channels. This causes depolarization and hyperpolarization of the hair cell membrane. Changes in the membrane potential of the hair cells alters the firing rate of the auditory nerve. The auditory nerve synapses ipsilaterally with cells in the cochlear nuclei. From the cochlear nuclei the signal is propagated to the superior olivary complex, the inferior colliculi, the medial geniculate nuclei, and finally the auditory cortex. All components of the auditory system show frequency specificity; a tuning curve can be constructed for cells in each component. The sound localization is processed by cells in the superior olivary complex and the higher centers. Cells in the medial geniculate and auditory cortex are tonotropically organized. The auditory cortex is organized in columns, and cells in one column are tuned to the same frequency. Deafness can be produced by damage to the conducting or neural pathways. The conducting pathway can be evaluated by Weber and Rinne tests. Exposure to loud noises also can produce damage that can be permanent.

The vestibular system is involved in the maintenance of posture and reflex movements of the eye. There are two major components in this system. One system, the otolith and saccule, encodes the position of the head. This system responds to movement and tilting of the head. It contributes to those reflex movements of the eye which are very important in maintenance of the field of vision during angular isolation. The second component consists of the semicircular ducts. This system encodes acceleration. The sensory afferents from the vestibular system project to the vestibular nuclei, which in turn have both ascending and descending projections. Vestibular nuclei interact with the cerebellum, the motor nuclei of the eye muscle, and the spinal cord and participate in reflexes that maintain posture and eye movement.

Bibliography

Hudspeth, A. J. The cellular basis of hearing: The biophysics of hair cells. *Science* 230:745, 1985.

Imig, T. J., and Morel, A. Organization of the thalamocortical auditory system in the cat. *Annu. Rev. Neurosci.* 6:95, 1983.

Kornhuber, H. H., ed., Vestibular system: I. Basic mechanisms. In Bullock, T. H., ed., *Handbook of Sensory Physiology,* Vol. VI/1. Heidelberg: Springer-Verlag, 1974.

10 The Chemical Senses: Olfaction and Gustation

Michael M. Behbehani

Objectives

After reading this chapter, you should be able to

Describe the anatomic locations of the neuronal elements involved in processing of smell and taste

Describe how the olfactory receptors transduce the sense of smell

Describe how the sense of smell is encoded by the olfactory bulb and piriform cortex

Explain abnormalities of the sense of smell

Describe the anatomic properties of taste receptors

Describe the four types of taste modality and how they are encoded by taste receptors

Describe how taste is encoded by the nucleus of the solitary tract, ventral posteromedial thalamic nuclei, and gustatory cortex

The chemical senses include the senses of smell and taste. The systems are extremely sensitive. For example, humans can smell some compounds at a concentration of a few parts in 1 trillion. Although both systems respond to chemicals in the environment, the processing of sense of smell is very different from the processing of the sense of taste.

Olfaction

The sense of smell begins by activation of olfactory receptors. In humans, these receptors are located in a 5-cm^2 region of the dorsal posterior recess of the nasal cavity called the **olfactory epithelium** (Fig. 10-1). The olfactory receptors are bipolar cells. Their proximal branches are located in the nasal cavity, and their central branches project to the olfactory bulb. The olfactory epithelium contains the receptors, basal cells, and supporting cells. The proximal branch of each receptor is located in the olfactory epithelium and terminates in a structure called the **olfactory knob** (Fig. 10-2). The olfactory knob contains several cilia that do not move and form a dense mat within the mucosa.

Odorants penetrate the mucosal surface and interact with the membranes of the cilia. The cilia contain a family of binding proteins that act as carriers for lipophilic substances and facilitate the binding of odorants to the receptor sites. The olfactory receptors regenerate, and new receptors are produced from the basal cells every 60 days.

The olfactory receptors are part of a multigene family. These genes encode a series of proteins that are members of a large superfamily of receptor proteins involved in the transduction process in the olfactory receptors. In the mouse, the olfactory multigene family contains more than 900 members. It is not totally clear how these large numbers of receptors are organized within the olfactory epithelium. One possibility is that all receptors that encode one type of odorant are located in a specific region of the olfactory epithelium and their axons project to a specific location in the olfactory bulb and from there to the rest of the CNS sites that process olfactory signals. This type of topographic organization would be similar to signal processing by other sensory modalities such as touch or vision. The second possibility is that odorant receptors are randomly

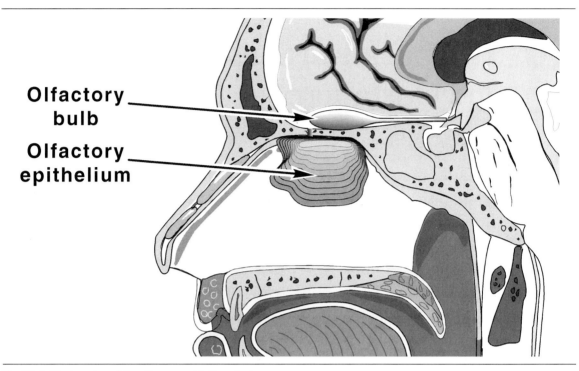

Olfactory bulb

Olfactory epithelium

Fig. 10-1. The location of the olfactory epithelium in the nose.

distributed throughout the olfactory sensory epithelium and there is no topographic organization. Recent experiments using in situ hybridization suggest that odorant receptor genes are expressed in topographically distinct patterns within the epithelium. Each epithelium zone contains several different receptors; however, each odorant receptor gene is expressed in only one zone in the epithelium. These results suggest that similar to the retina, there is a significant signal processing within the olfactory epithelium.

Transduction Processes

The transduction of odors involves the binding of odorant to the olfactory receptor. This binding activates a G protein (G_{olf}). Binding of GTP to this G protein releases its alpha subunit, which stimulates adenylcyclase type III. This causes a transient increase in the cAMP level within the receptor and causes opening of cyclic nucleotide-activated cation channels. Opening of these gates increases both sodium and potassium conductances and leads to depolarization of the receptors. The process is terminated by a

methylxanthine-sensitive phosphodiestrase that rapidly degrades cAMP and lowers its concentration (Fig. 10-3).

In addition to this second-messenger system, there is evidence that inositol-1,4,5-triphosphate (IP_3) is also involved in olfactory transduction. Increased IP_3 level causes opening of calcium channels that allows the entry of calcium into the cell. Calcium binds to calmodulin and activates adenylate cyclase, which can lead to opening of cationic channels. This system is also involved in adaptation of olfactory receptors.

Each olfactory receptor is sensitive to a variety of odorants. Analysis of the structure and types of odor they produce does not show structural specificity. At the receptor level, the specificity of odorants is encoded by their action on a large number of receptors. For this reason, it is believed that the pattern of the activity of the receptors encodes olfactory stimuli.

Absorption of odorants to the receptors produces depolarization that, if large enough, causes the generation of action potentials in the olfactory receptors. The central branches of these receptors synapse with neurons in the olfactory bulb. The olfactory bulb (Fig. 10-4) contains tufted mitral and granule cells. The dendretic branches of tufted

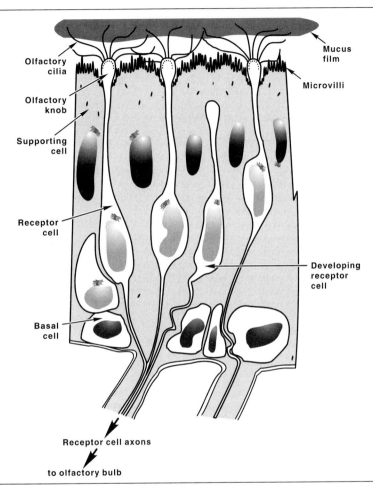

Fig. 10-2. The cellular organization of the olfactory epithelium. The peripheral branch of the cell bodies of the olfactory receptors terminate in the olfactory knob. The olfactory knob contains olfactory cilia that project through the mucous film and contain olfactory receptors. The proximal branches of the olfactory receptor cells form the olfactory nerve and synapse with cells in the olfactory bulb. In addition to the mature olfactory receptors, the olfactory epithelium also contains supporting cells and developing or immature receptor cells. (Redrawn from: Kandel, E. R., Schwartz, J. H., and Jessell, T. M. *Principles of Neural Science,* 3rd ed. New York: Elsevier, 1991.)

and mitral cells form structures called **glomeruli,** and it is within these structures that the receptor terminals interact with mitral and tufted cells. The mitral and tufted cells are the output cells of the olfactory bulb. The granule cells are inhibitory interneurons that form inhibitory feedback loops, which in turn lead to an increase in the signal-to-noise ratio within the olfactory bulb.

The axons of the mitral and tufted cells form the olfac-

tory tract and project to the secondary olfactory area of the cortex. This area consists of five parts: the anterior olfactory nucleus, the olfactory tubercle, the piriform cortex, the cortical nucleus of the amygdala, and the entorhinal cortex. Unlike other sensory systems, such as the somatic sensory system, there is no relation between the topographic area of the olfactory epithelium and the area of the cortex; in other words, the olfactory cortical areas are not

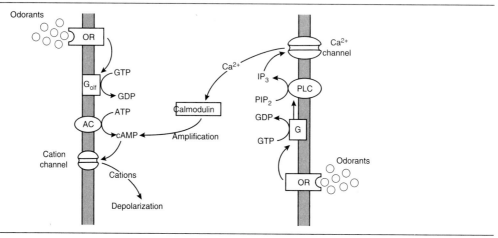

Fig. 10-3. The transduction process in the olfactory receptor. Binding of odorants to their receptors activates a G protein (G_{olf}) that changes GTP to GDP and ATP to cAMP. Increased cAMP level causes opening of cAMP Na^+ and Ca^{2+} channels and depolarizes the membrane. GDP acts on phospholipase C, which transforms phosphatidylinositol-4,5-biphosphate (IP_2) to inositol-1,4,5-triphosphate (IP_3), which opens Ca^{2+} channels. Calcium binds to calmodulin and leads to opening of cation channels and is also involved in adaptation of the receptor. (From: Anholt, R. H., Signal integration in nervous system: Adenylate cyclases as molecular coincidence detectors. *Trends in Neurosci.* 17:37–41, 1991.)

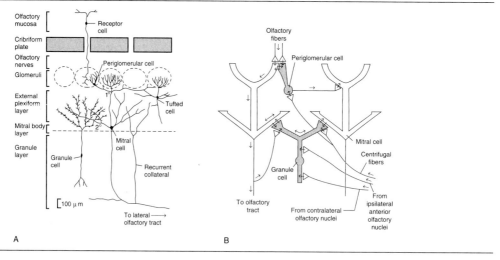

Fig. 10-4. Structure of mammalian olfactory bulb. (A) The cilia of olfactory receptors are located in the olfactory mucosa. The terminals of olfactory receptors synapse with the dendrites of mitral and tufted cells and form glomeruli that are located in the glomeruli layer. The cell bodies of the mitral cells are located in the mitral body layer. The mitral cells have synaptic contact with the granule cells that are located in the granule layer. There is dendrodendritic contact between granule cells and mitral cells. (B) The synaptic interaction between mitral and granule cells. The granule cells are inhibitory interneurons and have contact with many mitral cells. Through activation of the granule cells, excitation of a mitral cell can inhibit the activity of mitral cells that surround it. (From: Shepherd, G. M. Synaptic organization of the olfactory bulb. *Physiology Rev.* 52: 864–917, 1972.)

topographically mapped. The coding of different odorants by the olfactory cortex is not known. However, the intensity of odorant depends on the number of glomeruli that are active at the same time.

Abnormalities of the Sense of Smell

Abnormalities of the sense of smell are divided into three categories. **Hyposmia** is a condition in which the sense of smell is diminished. Hyposmia occurs in a variety of conditions and can be temporary. For example, a head cold produces hyposmia. Hyposmia also occurs in several diseases, such as Parkinson's disease, cystic fibrosis, and adrenal insufficiency. **Specific anosmia** is a condition in which a particular smell is not perceived. **Total anosmia** is a condition in which the sense of smell is not present. This condition occurs when the olfactory epithelium is damaged by chemicals and, on rare occasions, by lesions of the central olfactory systems.

Sense of Taste

The taste receptors are located in structures called **papillae** that are distributed on the tongue, palate, and pharynx. In humans, there are three types of papillae: **circumvallate, foliate,** and **fungiform** (Fig. 10-5). Each papilla contains a cluster of specialized epithelial cells that form the taste buds. Each taste bud contains between 50 and 150 receptors and numerous basal cells and supporting cells. Basal cells are located at the base of the taste buds. They act as immature taste cells and can differentiate into taste cells. The supporting cells behave as glia cells, and they are involved in the maintenance of the other cells by releasing a variety of trophic factors. At the apical portion of each taste cell there are several microvilli that protrude through a pore called the **taste pore** and have contact with the environment of the tongue.

The taste buds are innervated by primary afferents that arise from branches of three separate cranial nerves. Each primary afferent innervates several papillae, and within each papilla, several taste buds are innervated by the same primary afferent. The receptor cells form a synapse-like structure at the site of innervation, and communication between the taste buds and the primary afferent is similar to the chemical synapses.

There is site specificity in the innervation of taste buds (see Fig. 10-5B). The taste buds in the anterior two-thirds of the tongue are innervated by a branch of the seventh cranial nerve, the facial nerve. The cell bodies of these primary afferents are located in the geniculate ganglion, and the axons of these cells form the chorda tympani nerve.

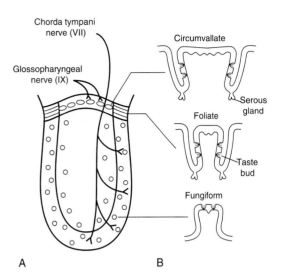

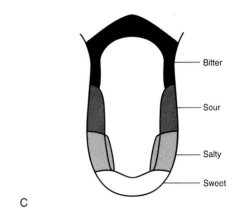

Fig. 10-5. (A) The pattern of innervation of the tongue. The taste buds located in the anterior two-thirds of the tongue are innervated by a branch of the facial nerve (VII) called the *chorda tympani.* The taste buds in the posterior third of the tongue are innervated by a branch of glossopharyngeal nerve (IX). (B) The structure of the three types of taste papillae and their predominant location in the tongue. (C) Regions of the lowest threshold for each type of taste modality on the tongue.

The taste buds in the posterior third of the tongue are innervated by a branch of the lingual branch of the ninth cranial nerve, the glossopharyngeal nerve. The cell bodies of these afferents are located in the petrosal ganglion. The taste buds on the palate are innervated by the greater superficial petrosal branch of the tenth cranial nerve, the vagus. In addition to transmitting taste information, each of these nerves transmits somatosensory information from the areas surrounding the taste buds. The distribution of taste buds in the tongue is not uniform (see Fig. 10-5C). The density of taste buds for sweet is much higher in the anterior of the tongue, the salty and sour taste buds are in the lateral intermediate tongue, and the taste buds for bitter are mostly located in the posterior of the tongue.

Sensory Transduction

There are four modalities of taste: sweetness, sourness, bitterness, and saltiness. For each of these modalities, there are specific receptors that are best tuned for that modality. The transduction of tastant is not the same for these receptors (Fig. 10-6). Sourness is transduced by direct interaction of hydrogen ion with ion channels that cause closure of voltage-dependent potassium channels and thereby produce depolarization. Sodium salts also penetrate the salt receptors and lead to depolarization. The transduction of sweetness involves specific receptor proteins and the cAMP messenger system. Sweet tastants bind to the sweet receptors and activate a G protein. The alpha subunit of this G protein is released by cGMP and activates an adenylcyclase that increases the level of cAMP. Increased cAMP level causes closure of potassium channels and depolarization of the membrane. In addition to these mechanisms, there is evidence that sweet tastants directly open sodium-selective voltage-independent channels that allow movement of sodium into the cell and cause depolarization. The coding of the bitter taste also involves a second-messenger

Fig. 10-6. Transduction of taste by taste receptors. Binding of bitter tastant to its receptor activates IP$_3$, which increases intracellular free calcium and cause depolarization. Binding of sweet tastant activates G proteins that cause formation of cAMP and opening of cationic channels and depolarization. Binding of sour tastants to their receptors directly activates voltage-dependent K$^+$ channels. Salt tastants directly enter actionic channels in the taste bud and cause depolarization. (From Kinnamon, S. C. Taste transduction: A diversity of mechanisms. *Trends in Neurosci.* II:491–496, 1988.)

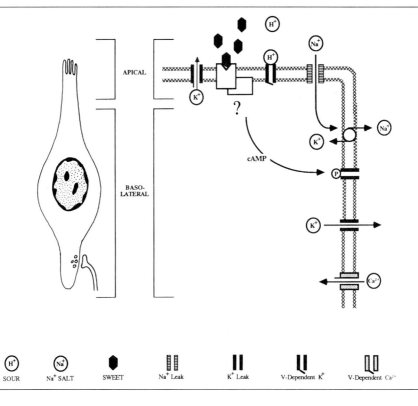

system, the inositol-1,4,5-triphosphate (IP_3) system. In this case, binding of a bitter tastant to a bitter receptor increases the IP_3 level inside the cell. IP_3 causes the release of calcium from intracellular compartments and an increase in the intracellular calcium concentration. This increase causes the release of transmitters from the terminals of the receptors.

Central Pathways for Taste

The first synapse in the central pathway for taste is at the level of the receptor–primary afferent connection. The primary afferents project to the medulla and synapse with neurons in the rostral portion of the **solitary tract nucleus** (STN). Neurons in the STN project in the central tegmental tract and synapse with cells in the gustatory region of the ventral posteromedial nucleus of the thalamus. From this thalamic area, taste-related information is transmitted to the gustatory region of the postcentral gyrus and the inner face of the insular cortex.

The cells in all regions of the central taste pathway respond to all four modalities of tastants (sweet, sour, bitter, and salt) but have a lower threshold for only one particular tastant. In this respect, the response characteristics of taste cells in the STN, thalamus, and cortex resemble the characteristics of auditory cells. That is, each taste cell has a tuning curve and can be described as a salt, sweet, bitter, or sour best cell. The coding of taste by the central neurons is not known. However, there is a likelihood that the pattern of activity of many cells with different tuning characteristics encodes the sense of taste.

Summary

The chemical senses consist of the senses of smell and taste. The sense of smell is encoded by olfactory receptors that are distributed in the olfactory epithelium within the nose. The olfactory receptors are not specific, and each receptor responds to many odorants. The olfactory receptors respond to odorants by depolarization produced by activation of a second-messenger system involving G proteins and cAMP. The olfactory receptors synapse with neurons in the olfactory bulb, which then project to the piriform cortex and cortical areas of the amygdala. Lesions of the olfactory system can produce hyposmia and anosmia. The sense of taste is encoded by taste receptors located in the tongue, palate, and pharynx. There are four specific taste receptors, each encoding the sensation of saltiness, bitterness, sweetness, and sourness. Saltiness and sourness are encoded by direct action of sodium and hydrogen ions on specific receptors. The other two sensations involve activation of second-messenger systems. Taste receptors form synaptic contact with primary afferents that are branches of the seventh, ninth, and tenth cranial nerves. These primary afferents project to the rostral STN, and neurons in this region project ipsilaterally to the ventral posteromedial nucleus of the thalamus. Neurons from this thalamic nucleus project to precentral and insular cortical areas. Neurons in the STN, ventral posterior medial, and cortical areas are responsive to all tastants but have a low threshold for only one tastant. The sense of taste is therefore encoded by the pattern of activities in many neurons within the gustatory regions of the CNS.

Bibliography

Brand, J. G., Teeter, J. H., Cagan, R. H. et al. eds., *Chemical Senses,* Vol. 1: *Receptor Events and Transduction in Taste and Olfaction.* New York: Marcel Dekker, 1989.

Roper, S. D. The cell biology of vertebrate taste receptors. *Annu. Rev. Neurosci.* 12:329, 1989.

Shepherd, G. M. Synaptic organization of the mammalian olfactory bulb. *Physiol. Rev.* 52:864, 1972.

11 Motor Functions of the Spinal Cord

Janusz B. Suszkiw

Objectives

After reading this chapter, you should be able to

Describe the organization of motor neurons in the spinal cord

Explain the function of myotatic and inverse myotatic reflexes

Explain the role of alpha-gamma coactivation in voluntary movement

Describe the flexion-crossed extension reflex

Explain the effect of spinal cord injury on the spinal reflexes

The spinal cord is the seat of all the motor neurons supplying the skeletal muscles of the body. These skeletomotor or alpha motor neurons provide "the final common pathway" (Sherrington) through which the CNS effects muscular activity and thus movement. The supraspinal control of the motor neurons is exerted via the corticospinal tracts from the cerebral cortex and the rubrospinal, reticulospinal, vestibulospinal, and tectospinal tracts from the brainstem. The signals conveyed by these pathways are for the most part relayed to the motor neuron via spinal interneurons, but direct monosynaptic connections are also present. The main features of spinal motor organization are considered in this chapter, and the role of supraspinal motor systems in control of movement is discussed in the following chapter.

Motor Outflow of the Spinal Cord

An alpha motor neuron together with the muscle fibers it innervates is termed a physiologic **motor unit** because an action potential in that motor neuron will cause essentially a synchronous contraction of all the muscle fibers supplied by it. The motor units supplying the same muscle(s) form columns of motor neuronal pools located within the anterior horns of the spinal cord. There is a mediolateral distribution of motor units, with the most medial supplying the axial muscles and the most lateral supplying the distal muscles (Fig. 11-1).

Force of Muscle Contraction Is Graded by Recruitment of Motor Units and Rate of Firing

In general, motor neurons are appropriately matched with the types of muscles they innervate (Fig. 11-2). Fast muscles used for high-intensity, short-duration activity are innervated by motor neurons that can fire phasically at high frequencies and have fast conduction velocities and are thus characterized as **phasic motor units.** Fast muscles are characterized by rapid contraction and relaxation, can develop large tension, but fatigue easily. Conversely, slow muscles, used for long-term, sustained contraction necessary in maintenance of posture, are innervated by the smaller motor neurons that fire at lower frequencies and have slower conduction velocities. These are referred to as **tonic motor units.** Slow muscles contract and relax slowly,

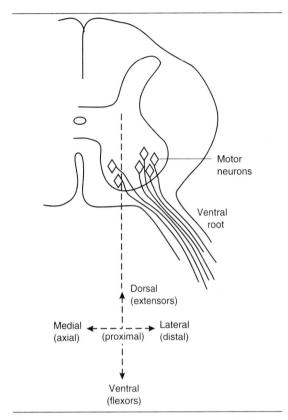

Motor neurons

Ventral root

Dorsal
(extensors)

Medial ←————→ Lateral
(axial)   (proximal)   (distal)

Ventral
(flexors)

Fig. 11-1. Motor neurons in the spinal cord are distributed according to the various muscle groups they innervate.

develop tension over a narrow range, and are relatively resistant to fatigue. Note, however, that there are many intermediate categories of muscles that share to various extents the properties of both "pure" phasic and tonic muscles.

The force of muscle contraction can be graded by recruitment of motor neurons as well as by changes in the rate of motor neuron firing (**rate coding**). Motor neurons are recruited in an orderly fashion according to their size. Small motor neurons have the lowest threshold for excitation and are recruited by even weak synaptic inputs. As the strength of synaptic signal increases, larger motor neurons (larger motor units) are progressively activated; the activation of large motor units results in a progressively greater increment of force added. Increased rate of firing will produce greater muscle force because activation of muscles by successive action potentials whose interval is less than the twitch contraction time leads to summation of the forces generated by each impulse, producing a state of sustained contraction, or **tetanus.**

Role of Muscle Stretch Receptors in Regulation of Muscle Length and Tension

In order that the CNS may generate the desired force or displacement, it must be continuously appraised about the length and tension in the muscle. This is accomplished by two distinct kinds of muscle stretch receptors, the **muscle spindle** and the **Golgi tendon organ.** Muscle spindles respond to changes in muscle length and the rate of change of length, whereas Golgi tendon organs signal muscle tension (Fig. 11-3).

The spindles are composed of small, 3- to 4-mm-long specialized muscle fibers enclosed within spindle-shaped (fusiform) capsules that are attached to and lie in parallel with the large muscle fibers. These small specialized fibers are called the **intrafusal** muscle fibers (within the fusiform capsule) to distinguish them from the bulk of force-producing, large **extrafusal** muscle fibers. Muscle spindles are innervated by group Ia and group II sensory fibers, which respond to deformation of the intrafusal fibers with an increase in the rate of action potential discharge during muscle lengthening (stretch) and a decrease in the action potential discharge during muscle shortening (contraction). The group Ia fibers form the so-called primary endings, and the group II fibers form the so-called secondary endings. The primary endings sense both the change in length of the muscle and the velocity of stretching. The secondary endings sense mainly the change in length of the muscle. The increase in afferent discharge during actual (rapid) stretching is called a **dynamic** spindle response. This response is mediated by the nuclear bag fibers and is recorded in the primary afferent (Ia). Afferent discharge during maintained stretch is called a **static** response. This response is transduced by the nuclear chain intrafusal muscle fibers and is recorded from both group Ia and group II afferents (note both group Ia and group II fibers innervate the nuclear chain fibers, but only group Ia fibers innervate the bag fibers). Intrafusal muscles are also innervated by small motor neurons called **gamma motor neurons,** which maintain the sensitivity of the spindle to changes in extrafusal muscle length.

The Golgi tendon organ (GTO) informs the CNS about muscle tension. The receptor is located near the muscle-tendon junction and consists of the end ramifications of the group Ib sensory fibers around several tendon fascicles. When a muscle is stretched or contracts, the developed tension is sensed by the GTO, and this results in the discharge of action potentials in the afferent fiber.

In summary, muscle spindles are situated "in parallel" with the contractile elements of the extrafusal muscle so

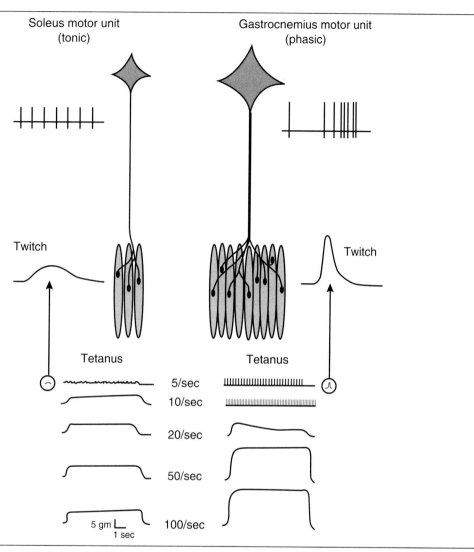

Fig. 11-2. Characteristics of phasic and tonic motor units. Note the differences in (1) size of motor neuron, (2) number of muscle fibers innervated by a single motor neuron, (3) size of muscle fibers, (4) frequency and amplitude of action potentials, (5) time course and amplitude of the motor unit twitch, and (6) tetanic fusion frequencies. (Modified from: Eyzaguirre, C., and Fidone, S. J. *Physiology of the Nervous System,* 2nd ed. St. Louis: Mosby–Year Book, 1975.)

that the degree of spindle stretch is a measure of the change in the muscle length. The Golgi tendon organs sense tension because they are arranged "in series" with the muscle and tendon; i.e., forces that act on the muscle are transmitted directly to the tendon and GTO. The discharge of spindles and Golgi tendon organs generally has a reciprocal relationship. Contraction of extrafusal muscle

tends to decrease muscle length ("unload" the spindle) and increase the tension in the tendons (i.e., "load" the Golgi tendon organ). During passive muscle stretch, muscle lengthening stretches, i.e., loads, the spindles but has less or no effect on GTO firing.

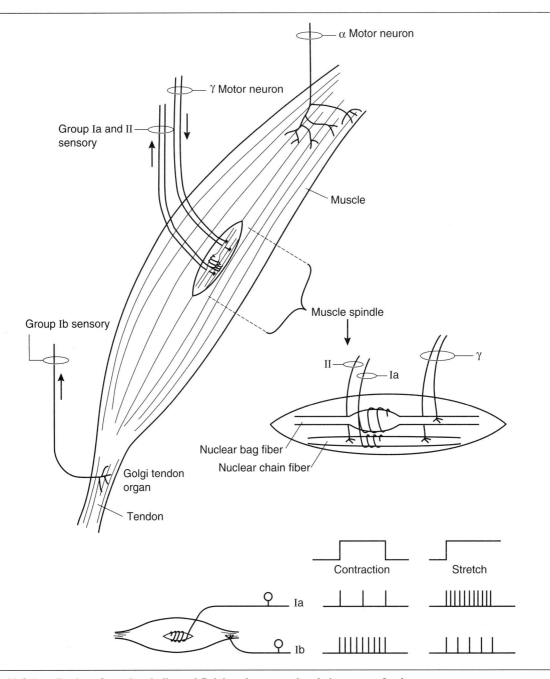

Fig. 11-3. Localization of muscle spindles and Golgi tendon organs in relation to extrafusal muscles. Enlarged view of the muscle spindle illustrates the two types of intrafusal muscle fibers and their innervation. Responses of muscle spindle and Golgi tendon organ to muscle stretch and contraction are illustrated at the lower right part of the figure.

Spinal Reflexes

There are a number of relatively simple neuronal networks in the spinal cord the activation of which produces simple, stereotyped motor responses. These automatic responses to certain stimuli are called **reflexes.**

The components of circuitry mediating a reflex are termed a **reflex arc.** A reflex arc consists of a peripheral receptor (e.g., in skin, muscle, or joint), an afferent sensory fiber that carries information from the receptor to the spinal cord, and a motor neuron and its efferent axon to the muscle.

In most instances, a reflex involves several interneurons between the afferent sensory and efferent motor neurons. A reflex arc involving a single interneuron (therefore, with two synapses in the arc) is called **disynaptic.** Those involving more than one interneuron are called **polysynaptic.** The only **monosynaptic** reflex, involving a direct connection between the afferent sensory and efferent motor neuron (i.e., no interneurons), is the muscle stretch reflex.

The Stretch (Myotatic) Reflexes

The **monosynaptic stretch reflex** arc consists of (1) a muscle spindle, (2) group Ia afferent fibers from the spindle to the spinal cord, and (3) the skeletomotor neuron innervating the same (homonymous) muscle from which the group Ia fibers originate (Fig. 11-4). As explained above, stretching a muscle activates the muscle spindles and increases the frequency of action potentials in group Ia afferents. The group Ia afferents monosynaptically excite motor neurons to the homonymous muscle, causing the muscle to reflexly contract. A classic example of a monosynaptic stretch reflex is the knee jerk produced by tapping the patellar tendon, which stretches and causes reflex contraction of the quadriceps muscle. Group Ia fibers also make direct excitatory connections with inhibitory interneurons, which in turn inhibit alpha motor neurons to antagonist muscles. Thus group Ia fibers monosynaptically excite the homonymous and synergist muscles (agonist muscles with the same action on the joint) and disynaptically inhibit motor neurons, which excite the antagonist muscles, thus causing their relaxation. The inhibition of antagonist motor neurons at the same time that homonymous and synergist neurons are excited is called **reciprocal inhibition.**

The stretch reflex is the basic mechanism for maintaining muscle tone. Stretch reflexes are more pronounced in the physiologic extensor muscles (muscles that oppose

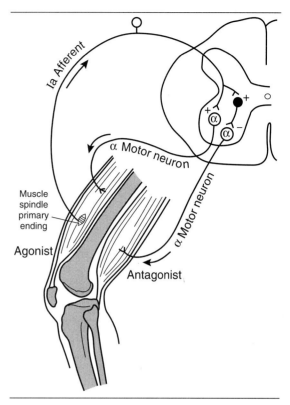

Fig. 11-4. The elements of the monosynaptic stretch reflex, including reciprocal inhibition.

gravity) than in flexors. Also, the reflex tension developed in an extensor is better maintained over time than in a flexor. The purpose of this is that in the human the weight of the body tends to flex the supporting limbs. Since the sensitivity of the extensor reflex is very high, a slight stretch causes development of tension that assists in the maintenance of postural muscle tone. The role of the reflex in the maintenance of muscle tone is illustrated following the section of dorsal root fibers, a condition that interrupts the afferent limb of the arc. In this case, the affected muscles become hypotonic.

Alpha-Gamma Coactivation

During active movement, contraction of the extrafusal muscle causes the spindle to become flaccid, a condition in which the spindle cannot adequately monitor the length of the muscle. Activation of gamma motor neurons causes the intrafusal muscle to contract (to shorten) and restores their sensitivity to any stretch of the extrafusal muscles (Fig. 11-5).

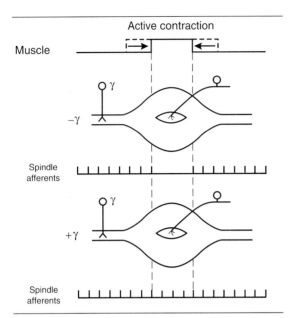

Active contraction

Muscle

γ

−γ

Spindle
afferents

γ

+γ

Spindle
afferents

Fig. 11-5. Response of muscle afferents to muscle contraction without and with activation of gamma motor neurons. During active contraction, discharge in afferent fibers ceases in the absence of gamma activation because the spindle becomes unloaded as extrafusal muscles shorten. Activation of gamma motor neurons prevents unloading of the spindle, and the discharge in the afferents from the spindle is maintained.

Thus an important function of the gamma motor neuron system is to reload the spindle during active contractions, thereby preserving a high sensitivity over a wide range of muscle lengths when muscle is shortening during reflex and voluntary contraction. During voluntary muscle movement, the skeletomotor and fusimotor neurons to a given muscle are activated simultaneously by descending pathways from higher motor centers. The simultaneous activation of skeletomotor and fusimotor neurons is called **alpha-gamma coactivation.** Coactivation of alpha and gamma motor neurons allows continuous flow of sensory information from the spindle to the CNS, informing it about changes in muscle length during ongoing activity.

Activation of gamma neurons alone can produce a reflex contraction of the muscle. Since gamma motor neurons are smaller than alpha motor neurons, they have a lower threshold for excitability than the alpha motor neurons, are more easily excited, and have higher tonic discharge rates. Therefore, tonic discharge of the gamma motor neurons may be responsible in large part for maintenance of muscle tone. Overactivity of the gamma system may lead to hypertonia.

Inverse Myotatic Reflex

Activation of group Ib afferent fibers from the Golgi tendon organ causes inhibition of the homonymous motor neurons returning to the same muscle (Fig. 11-6). The reflex inhibition is disynaptic, i.e., via an inhibitory interneuron. The inhibition is also exerted on the synergistic muscles. The antagonist muscles are facilitated disynaptically via an excitatory interneuron (this is another example of the principle of reciprocal innervation).

The inverse myotatic reflex serves to regulate muscle tension. An increase in muscle tension beyond a desired point would produce negative feedback from the Golgi tendon organ and inhibit further development of tension. A decrease in muscle tension (e.g., during muscle fatigue) would have an opposite effect, since less activation of the Golgi tendon organ would reduce the inhibition onto the homonymous and synergistic muscles.

In pathologic situations, a reflex called the **clasp-knife reflex** can be elicited and is attributed to the Golgi tendon organs. The best way to demonstrate this reflex is in the decerebrate animal. In this type of preparation, there is extensor rigidity due to overfacilitation of the stretch reflex.

Fig. 11-6. Elements of the inverse myotatic reflex arc.

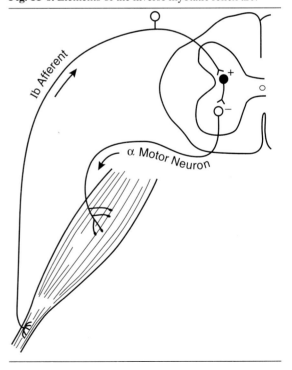

Ib Afferent

α Motor Neuron

If one attempts to flex the rigid limb, it offers a great deal of resistance. As the force exerted to flex the limb is increased, the limb begins to flex, but then it offers more resistance and a greater force must be exerted to flex it further. At one point, suddenly, the extensor tone disappears, the limb no longer offers resistance, and it collapses. This sudden disappearance of the extensor tone has been attributed to activation of group Ib afferent fibers from the Golgi tendon organ that reflexly inhibits the homonymous stretched muscle. However, this explanation has been questioned, and it has been suggested that clasp-knife reflex is mediated by group II, III, and IV afferents via polysynaptic pathways.

Flexion Reflex

Flexion reflexes are important in a number of behavioral patterns; e.g., flexion of limbs is part of the activity involved in walking. One of the most obvious functions of the flexion reflex is withdrawal of a limb from painful, noxious stimuli. Hence the flexion reflex is frequently called the **withdrawal reflex.** Also, since flexion of the limb ipsilateral to the stimulus is usually accompanied by an extension of the contralateral limb(s), this reflex is also referred to as the **flexion-crossed extension reflex.**

The flexion reflex is polysynaptic (Fig. 11-7). The afferent fibers enter the spinal cord and excite interneurons of the dorsal horn. The interneurons then act on alpha motor neurons through relay pathways involving other interneurons. The response is an excitation of alpha motor neurons to the flexor muscles and inhibition of alpha motor neurons to the extensor muscle of the stimulated limb (ipsilateral). In addition, this is frequently accompanied by excitation of alpha motor neurons to extensor muscles and inhibition of flexors to the contralateral muscle. This be-

Fig. 11-7. Schematic of the organization of the flexion–crossed extension reflex.

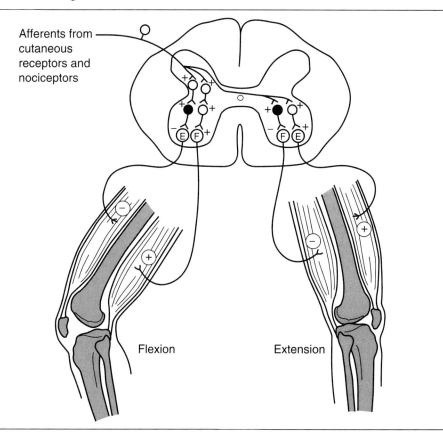

Afferents from cutaneous receptors and nociceptors

Flexion   Extension

havior is the appropriate response to painful stimuli; for example, if a person steps on a sharp object, the injured foot is withdrawn (flexion), while the other limb of the pair is extended, thereby providing support for the body and preventing the person from toppling.

The flexion reflex can be initiated by activity in afferent fibers from a variety of sensory receptor organs. These sensory receptors may be in the skin, in muscle, and in joints and involve afferent fibers II, III, and IV; collectively, these are called **flexor reflex afferents** (FRA). The degree of flexion response can vary from a flexor twitch in response to relatively innocuous stimulation to a complete withdrawal of the limb from a noxious stimulus. A very strong stimulus to the FRA fibers results in activity of all four limbs. This response is mediated via intersegmental connections and is sometimes referred to as **irradiation of the stimulus;** the stronger the stimulus, the more extensive is the reflex reaction.

Motor reactions are directed to the afferent source of the reflex; i.e., reaction is localized to the site of afferent stimulation. The variation in the pattern of a reflex according to the source of afferent input is referred to as the **local sign.** Local sign can override the type of skeletomotor neurons that are excited and inhibited. For example, nociceptive stimulation of the skin overlying an extensor facilitates that extensor and inhibits its antagonist, i.e., the opposite of a flexion reflex. This is very useful because if limbs always flexed in response to painful stimuli, in some situations flexion could drive a limb toward the stimulus rather than away from it.

Pathologic Reflexes

Changes in reflex activity may be noted in certain pathologic conditions. For example, a reduction in stretch reflexes **(hyporeflexia)** is observed when there is peripheral loss of muscle spindle afferent fibers or motor axons in a peripheral neuropathy. Reduced stretch reflexes occur also with diseases affecting the dorsal root or motor neurons, such as poliomyelitis and amyotrophic lateral sclerosis. Certain diseases of the brain also may cause a reduction in stretch reflexes. Conversely, **hyperreflexia,** or excessive reflex activity, is associated with either increased excitability of alpha motor neurons or an increased activity of gamma motor neurons. This may result in an increase in the number of motor neurons that will discharge in response to muscle stretch, e.g., hyperactive tendon jerk response. The tone of muscles supplied by overactive motor neurons also may be increased **(hypertonia)**. In the latter condition, the patient is said to be **spastic.** Spasticity typi-

cally results from damage to the motor cortex involving its extrapyramidal system.

In sufficiently marked hyperreflexia, the phenomenon called **clonus** can be observed. Clonus is a series of spasmodic contractions following sudden stretch of the hyperreflexic muscle. For example, rapid dorsiflection of the foot in hyperreflexia will elicit ankle clonus. Stretch of the triceps surae muscles causes a reflex contraction of these muscles and plantar flexion of the foot. As the triceps surae muscles relax from their contraction, the spindle is stretched. Since the fusimotor tone is heightened in a spastic state and spindle sensitivity is increased, the spindle stretch triggers a new barrage of powerful excitation in group Ia afferents with repeated reflexive muscle contraction. This cycle of contraction and relaxation may continue for some time, depending on the level of hyperexcitability of the stretch reflex. One reason why clonus does not develop under normal physiologic conditions is that normally the skeletomotor neurons discharge with considerable asynchrony during reflex contraction. However, in a spastic condition, with increased fusimotor tones, all skeletomotor neurons are "ready to go," so that muscle stretch produces powerful synchronous cycles of contraction and relaxation.

Spinal Shock Following Damage to the Spinal Cord

Complete transection of the spinal cord results in immediate paralysis and loss of sensation in all body regions innervated by the cord segments below the section. After spinal cord section, all segmental reflexes below the site of the lesion are depressed. This depression of the segmental reflex is called **spinal shock.** The duration of the spinal shock increases with ascent on the phylogenetic scale. For example, in the frog spinal shock lasts a few minutes, whereas in primates and in humans it may last several weeks. The hyporeflexia is due to discontinuation of the descending impulses from the brain. One can show this by making a second section in the cord after recovery from the shock has occurred. The second section will not result in spinal shock. The earliest reflex to reappear after spinal shock is the plantar reflex. In a normal person, stimulation of the sole of the foot results in the plantar flexion of the toe. If stimulation is sufficiently strong, the plantar reflex may be accompanied by a generalized flexion and withdrawal of the entire limb. In humans with a transected spinal cord, the plantar reflex is characterized by dorsiflexion and fanning of the toes. This reflex is called the **Babinski sign** and is due to discontinuation of the influence of the pyramidal tract on the spinal motorneuron. With time, the threshold for flexor reflexes continues to fall, and the person eventually may enter a state of hyperreflexia. In this state, a moderate stimulation leads to massive flexion reflex accompanied by autonomic reactions, such as emptying of the bladder and bowels, sweating, etc.

Summary

The final motor output from the CNS to the muscles of the body is via the skeletomotor neurons localized in the ventral horn of the spinal cord. The activity of the skeletomotor neurons is regulated by descending pathways from higher motor centers in the brain and locally through spinal reflexes. The muscle spindle is a component of the monosynaptic stretch reflex arc that plays an important role in regulation of muscle tone. Muscle spindle senses and informs the CNS about the change and rate of change in muscle length. Its ability to respond to changes in muscle length during active contraction is regulated by gamma motor neurons. The Golgi tendon organ is a component of the disynaptic, inverse myotatic reflex arc. The Golgi tendon organ responds to and informs the CNS about the change in muscle tension. The flexion-crossed extension reflex is a polysynaptic reflex that mediates the flexion and withdrawal of a limb in response to painful stimulus and is accompanied by extension of the contralateral limb. Reflex activity may change in various pathologic conditions, resulting in hyporeflexia or hyperreflexia. Following transection of the spinal cord, all muscles below the site of section are paralyzed, and all reflexes are depressed due to the interruption of descending impulses from brain.

Bibliography

Carew, T. J. Spinal cord: II. Reflex action. In Kandel, E. R. and Schwartz, J. H., eds. *Principles of Neural Science.* New York: Elsevier, 1981. Chap. 26.

Eyzaquirre, E., and Fidone, S. J. *Physiology of the Nervous System,* 2nd ed. Chicago: Year Book Medical Publishers, 1975. Chaps. 15 and 17.

Henneman, E. Organization of the spinal cord and its reflexes. In: Mountcastle, V. B., ed. *Medical Physiology,* 14th ed., Vol. 1. St. Louis: Mosby, 1980. Pp. 762–786.

12 Motor Functions of the Brain

Janusz B. Suszkiw

Objectives

After reading this chapter, you should be able to

Describe the principles of motor organization of the brain

State the function of the brainstem in regulation of postural muscle tone

Describe the role of the cerebral cortex in voluntary movement

Explain the effects of cortical lesions on motor function

Describe the functional organization and motor connections of the cerebellum

Explain the effects of cerebellar lesions on movement

Describe the functional organization of the basal ganglia, including input-output relationships

Explain movement disorders resulting from damage to the basal ganglia

Overview

The activity of motor neurons and reflexes in the spinal cord is under the control of supraspinal motor centers in the brainstem, basal ganglia, cerebellum, and the cerebral cortex. A simplified overview of the descending motor control pathways is provided in Fig. 12-1. The pathways that convey signals from the higher centers directly to the spinal cord are the corticospinal tract from the cerebral motor cortex and the rubrospinal, reticulospinal, vestibulospinal, and tectospinal tracts originating in the brainstem. Brainstem motor areas are modulated by in-puts from the cortex, basal ganglia, and cerebellum. The cerebellum and basal ganglia influence movement by modulating the motor output from the cerebral cortex and via brainstem mechanisms but have no direct outputs to the spinal cord.

Traditionally, the supraspinal motor pathways have been classified into the **pyramidal** and **extrapyramidal systems.** Strictly speaking, the pyramidal system denotes the corticospinal tract fibers that pass through the medullary pyramids, and the extrapyramidal system comprises all other motor pathways. A more useful classification considers descending pathways with respect to their functional influences on the spinal motor neurons and the associated interneurons. The **lateral system** comprises pathways that act primarily on the dorsolaterally situated motor neurons. The principal lateral system pathways are the lateral corticospinal and rubrospinal tracts. The main function of the lateral system is the control of spatially organized movements involving the distal extremities (manipulatory, skilled movements). The main **medial system** pathways are the reticulospinal and vestibulospinal tracts, which originate in the brainstem. Their influences are largely on the ventromedial motor neurons, which act on the proximal and axial muscle groups involved in controlling body and limb movement. Therefore, the main function of these pathways is the control of posture, equilibrium, and locomotion.

Brainstem

The **brainstem** comprises three distinct anatomic structures: medulla oblongata, pons, and mesencephalon (mid-

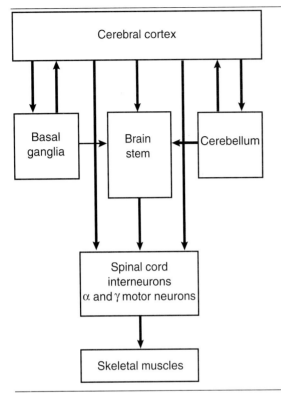

Fig. 12-1. A simplified flow diagram of the major motor centers and their connections.

tory and **extensor inhibitory zones.** The facilitatory zone extends from about middle of the medulla rostrally through the mesencephalic tegmentum and central gray matter into the subthalamus. The inhibitory zone comprises the caudal portion of the medulla. Stimulation in the facilitatory area results in contraction of physiologic extensors, whereas stimulation in the inhibitory area tends to facilitate flexors and inhibit extensors. The neurons in the facilitatory reticular formation are tonically active, and their activity is controlled by descending influences from

Fig. 12-2. Schematic diagram showing the subdivisions and motor pathways of the brainstem. The brainstem receives inputs from ascending sensory fibers from the periphery and descending inputs from the higher motor centers (RTS = reticulospinal tract; RuST = rubrospinal tract; TST = tectospinal tract; VST = vestibulospinal tract).

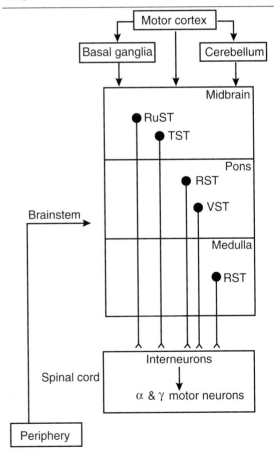

brain). The major lateral motor pathway from the brainstem to the spinal cord is the rubrospinal tract. The fibers of the rubrospinal tract terminate primarily on spinal interneurons. The major medial motor pathways are the reticulospinal and vestibulospinal tracts. These terminate mostly on spinal interneurons. The tectospinal tract originates from nerve cells in the superior colliculus and predominantly terminates on the interneurons at the cervical level of the spinal cord (Fig. 12-2).

The brainstem acts as the major integrating center for regulation of postural muscle tone, equilibrium reactions, and basic orientation reflexes.

Postural Mechanisms

Throughout the extent of the brainstem runs a core comprised of a conglomerate of neurons intermixed with ascending and descending fibers that is known as the **reticular formation.** With respect to its motor functions, the reticular formation can be divided into **extensor facilita-**

the motor cortex, basal ganglia, and cerebellum. The neurons in the inhibitory reticular formation generally are not tonically active but must be activated by descending commands from higher centers. The output from the facilitatory reticular formation to the spinal cord is via the pontine reticulospinal tract, and the output from the inhibitory reticular formation is via the medullary reticulospinal tract. Both tracts influence primarily the ventromedial groups of motor neurons that innervate the axial and proximal muscles; however, the pontine reticular formation is mainly excitatory to the physiologic extensor muscles, whereas the medullary reticular formation is primarily inhibitory to extensors and facilitates flexor muscles.

The pontine reticular formation functions in close association with the vestibular nuclei, which project both to the reticular formation and directly to the spinal cord as the vestibulospinal tract. Like the pontine reticulospinal fibers, the vestibulospinal tract influences the motor neuronal pools in the medial portion of the ventral horn. The activity of the vestibulospinal tract is driven by powerful excitatory inputs from the vestibular apparatus via the vestibular nerve and is modulated by the cerebellum.

In the normal state there is a balance between the facilitatory and inhibitory descending influences, ensuring an appropriate activation of antigravity muscles and regulation of postural tone. The release of brainstem mechanisms from control by the higher centers results in excessive contraction of antigravity muscles, producing various forms of extensor rigidity and spasticity, a condition that can be experimentally demonstrated in the decerebrate animal.

Decerebrate Rigidity

Experimental decerebrate rigidity is produced by transection of the brainstem above the vestibular nuclei at the boundary between the midbrain and pons. In the decerebrate animal, the inhibitory reticulospinal tract in the medulla, the vestibulospinal tract originating in the middle pontine level, the pontine portions of the facilitatory reticular formation, and all the ascending afferents to the medulla and the pons are preserved, but the descending influences from basal ganglia and the cerebral cortex that normally keep the intrinsic activity of reticular and vestibulospinal pathways in check are interrupted (Fig. 12-3). The release from inhibitory control by higher centers results in overactivity of the facilitatory reticular formation, causing overfacilitation and contraction of all postural, antigravity muscles, a condition referred to as **decerebrate rigidity.** The effect is further enhanced by removal of the cerebellum, which keeps in check the activity

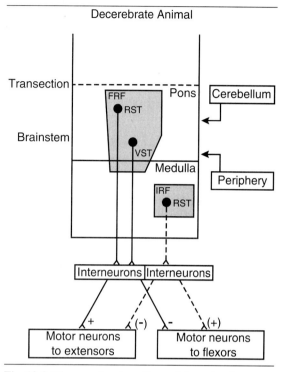

Fig. 12-3. Diagram showing effects of decerebration. Shaded areas indicate the facilitatory reticular formation (FRF) and inhibitory reticular formation (IRF) (RST = reticulospinal tract; VST = vestibulospinal tract). The dashed connections from the medullary reticulospinal tract are used to indicate that this pathway is normally not intrinsically active and is further disfacilitated by interruption of descending inputs that normally activate neurons in the IRF. The major effect of decerebration is overfacilitation of motoneurons to physiologic extensors (antigravity muscles) and reciprocal inhibition of antagonistic flexors.

of the vestibulospinal pathway. Conversely, transection of the vestibular nerve, which provides excitation to the vestibular neurons, or unilateral destruction of vestibular nuclei (Deiter's nucleus) attenuates the rigidity.

With the cerebellum left intact, extensor rigidity in the decerebrate animal is largely reflex in origin. Cutting the dorsal spinal root to a particular limb reduces or abolishes the rigidity in that limb. This indicates that rigidity involves overfacilitation of the gamma motor neurons (myotatic, stretch reflex). This form of rigidity has been termed **gamma rigidity.** On the other hand, when the cerebellum is removed, the rigidity no longer can be abolished by dorsal root transection, indicating that in this condition the rigidity is due mainly to overactivation of alpha motor neurons. Accordingly, this type of rigidity has been termed **alpha rigidity.**

After experimental transection of the neuraxis at a higher level, producing a disconnection of the brainstem from cerebral cortex but leaving other descending influences relatively intact, a **decorticate** condition is produced. In this condition, destruction of vestibular nuclei has relatively little effect, and the rigidity is mainly due to overactivity in the facilitatory reticular formation. Thus the main effect of decortication is overfacilitation of gamma motor neurons and extensor spasticity.

In summary, the reticulospinal and vestibulospinal tracts have important function in regulating the antigravity tone. Release of these pathways from higher controls leads to exaggerated antigravity tone (rigidity). The gamma rigidity resulting from hyperactivity of myotatic reflexes is mainly mediated through the upper (pontine) reticulospinal system. The alpha rigidity is mediated largely by the vestibulospinal system and results from direct overexcitation of the alpha motor neurons.

Clinical Syndromes of Spasticity and Rigidity

The terms **rigidity** and **spasticity** are used frequently in the diagnosis of neurologic disorders. Although manifested in somewhat different ways, both spasticity and rigidity are fundamentally the same phenomenon, in that they reflect **release** of the brainstem mechanisms from descending controls, resulting in an imbalance between the facilitatory and inhibitory influences on the spinal motor circuits.

Spasticity is a hypertonic, hyperreflexive condition characterized by increased resistance of spastic muscle to passive movement that is usually greater in the antigravity muscles **(unidirectional)**. Resistance of spastic muscle depends on velocity of movement. In addition, spastic patients show hyperactive tendon reflexes and **clonus** (repetitive contractions in response to sudden, sustained stretch of a muscle). A clasp-knife reflex is observed.

In humans, spasticity is classically exemplified by the state of arm and leg in hemiplegia resulting from severe injury of certain portions of the frontal lobe or, more commonly, interruption of its extrapyramidal motor projections at the level of the internal capsule. In this condition, limbs contralateral to the site of injury are affected. The leg is stiffly extended and resists passive flexing; the arm is held flexed and resists passive extension. Tendon reflexes are hyperactive, and clonus is evoked if the stretch is prolonged. This is sometimes referred to as **decorticate rigidity.** Actual decerebration, produced, for example, by a

hemorrhage at the mesencephalic level, produces exaggerated extensor rigidity of all four limbs.

The clinical term **rigidity** is one of the major signs of Parkinson's disease, which affects the function of the basal ganglia. In contrast to spasticity, this type of rigidity has the following characteristics: (1) increased resistance to passive movement is bidirectional (i.e., both flexors and extensors are affected); (2) resistance to passive movement of the affected limb is relatively independent of velocity of movement; and (3) patients with Parkinson's disease do not have a hyperactive tendon jerk reflex.

Attitudinal and Postural Reflexes

One of the functions of the brainstem is to control body equilibrium and orientation in space. The ability to stay right-side up is a universal property of animal organisms and depends on a group of specific **righting reflexes** that are integrated at the brainstem level.

Labyrinthine righting reactions are set up by stimulation of the otolithic apparatus. The responding muscles are those of the neck and serve to maintain the normal position of the head. **Body-righting-reflex-acting-on-the head** is a response to asymmetrical stimulation of the body surface. For example, when a decorticate animal without labyrinths is held in air, its head takes a passive position imposed by gravity; however, when it is placed on its side on the ground, the head is righted into normal position. **Body-righting-reflex-acting-on-the body** is elicited by asymmetrical stimulation of the body surface and causes the body to right itself. When the head is righted by either labyrinthine or body-on-head reflexes, the resulting twisting of the neck excites proprioceptively the **neck-righting reflex** that first causes the thoracic, then the lumbar, and finally the pelvic regions to follow the head into the normal, upright position.

The centers for the nonvisual righting reflexes lie chiefly in the medulla and mesencephalon. Additionally, the optical righting reflexes also result in orientation of the head even in the absence of labyrinthine or body stimulation. The visual reflexes depend on the cerebral cortex.

Cerebral Cortex

The motor areas of the cerebral cortex include the primary motor, premotor, and supplementary motor areas. These areas contain somatotopic maps of the body musculature. The primary motor area (Brodmann's area 4) includes the representation of the extremities and the face. The premotor area (Brodmann's area 6) includes mainly the representation of the axial musculature. The supplementary motor cortex is located on the medial surface of the precentral cortex and includes full representation of the body muscles (Fig. 12-4).

Role of Cerebral Cortex in Voluntary Movement

The cerebral motor cortical areas are concerned with organizing and issuing commands for the execution of phasic, goal-oriented movements. Voluntary movement may be considered to involve three main phases: (1) conception and formulation of the goal, (2) defining the plan of action in terms of movement of muscles and joints necessary to achieve the intended goal, and (3) implementation and control of the execution of the plan. According to current concepts, movements appear to be formulated and programmed by the association and sensorimotor cortical areas with the cooperation of the lateral cerebellar hemispheres and the basal ganglia. The plan for movement is then transmitted to the motor cortex, which issues the commands for its execution. Recordings from the scalp of conscious subjects indicate that a buildup of cortical activity commences about 0.8 second before execution of the volitional movement. This activity may be recorded from

widespread areas of precentral cortex in the form of negative surface potential, i.e., the so-called **readiness potential.** About 50 to 100 milliseconds before the onset of muscular activity (i.e., EMG of muscles involved), the readiness potential gives rise to **premotor positivity,** probably reflecting the discharge of pyramidal commands for movement (Fig. 12-5). The readiness potential can be regarded as the neuronal correlate of a "design for voluntary movement." The spatial extent and slow development of this potential suggest that development of voluntary action requires the collaboration of large parts of the cerebral cortex.

Descending commands from the cortical motor areas are conveyed to motor neurons and the associated interneurons in the spinal cord via the corticospinal (pyramidal) tract and through the brainstem pathways (extrapyramidal system). The corticospinal tract has both ventromedial (uncrossed fibers) and dorsolateral (crossed fibers) subdivisions that influence proximal and distal muscles, respectively (Fig. 12-6). Direct connections between cortical pyramidal neurons in the primary motor cortex and motor neurons in the spinal cord appear only in primates and are most extensive in humans, in whom about 10% of corticospinal neurons form direct monosynaptic connections onto motor neurons in the lateral and medial motorneuronal pools. This endows us with the ability to control individual muscles independently from one another, enabling the execution of fine, manipulatory movements.

The patterns of corticospinal influences on the forelimb and hindlimb musculature depend on the degree of antigravity work performed by the muscle and on the degree to

Fig. 12-4. Motor areas of the cerebral cortex.

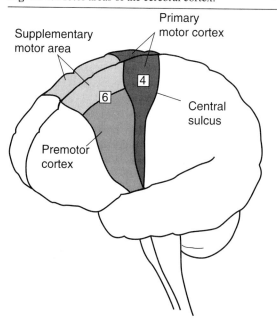

Fig. 12-5. Recordings from the scalp in the left precentral area show the appearance of "readiness potential" in response to voluntary movement of a finger. Zero time is at the onset of movement. (Modified from: Schmitt, F. O., and Worden, F. C., eds. *The Neurosciences: Third Study Program.* Cambridge, Mass.: MIT Press, 1974. Chap. 23.)

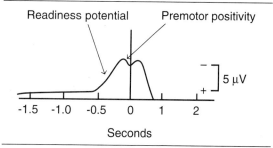

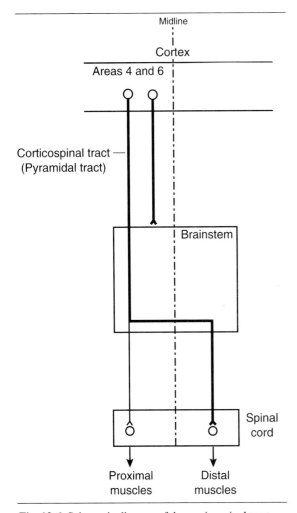

Fig. 12-6. Schematic diagram of the corticospinal tract.

which the muscle participates in phasic, complex motor actions. The greater the postural (antigravity) role of the muscle, the more pronounced is pyramidal inhibition of that muscle. For example, for proximal muscles of a limb, the extensors will be inhibited and the flexors excited. In contrast, if the muscle is involved primarily in manipulatory activity, its motor neurons will be facilitated by the corticospinal tract. For example, in the case of intrinsic muscles of the digits, both flexors and extensors are usually excited by the corticospinal tract. As indicated before, since tonic contraction of antigravity muscles is required for maintenance of normal, upright posture, the dominant effect of the ventromedial brainstem motor centers is the facilitation of proximal extensors (antigravity muscles) and inhibition of antagonist flexors. In contrast, the func-

tion of the pyramidal tract is to effect volitional control of phasic movement, in part, by overcoming the postural set of the animal, i.e., by reducing the excitation of postural muscles that might interfere with execution of the desired phasic movement.

The pyramidal neurons that give rise to the corticospinal tract are organized into columnar **efferent zones.** Pyramidal cells comprising a given efferent zone all have the same action, and their activation causes a contraction of the same muscle or muscle groups. Some neurons increase their activity with flexing, others with extension. As indicated earlier, these neurons typically discharge action potentials shortly before the onset of voluntary muscle contraction.

Cortical columns receive afferent inputs polysynaptically from cutaneous receptors in the path of the movement and from muscle and joint receptors activated during movement of a limb or group of muscles. The general rule is that these sensory stimuli influence the motor cortex in a manner that facilitates movement. For example, stimulation of cutaneous receptors on the ventral surface of a digit will reflexly excite the neurons in the efferent zone to the flexors of that digit. The spindle receptors of the digit flexor are activated when the flexor muscle relaxes (lengthens); slowing of flexing will thus reflexly excite the cortical neurons that drive the flexor (Fig. 12-7). This is one example of corticomotor reflexes, which in all likelihood assist the motor cortex in execution of serial movements. Stereotyped reactions involving cortical motor reflexes include grasping and tactile placing reactions.

Effects of Lesions

Motor deficits produced by lesions of the motor cortex or its outflow depend on the extent to which the pyramidal and extrapyramidal influences are affected. Interruption of the corticospinal tract by unilateral section of the pyramid results in hypotonia and paresis of the distal musculature on the contralateral side. These effects are consistent with a loss of descending facilitatory influences on spinal fusimotor and skeletomotor neurons. With time, the hypotonia gradually abates, and deep tendon reflexes in the affected region approach normal values. The permanent deficit that follows pyramidotomy is a loss of agility and dexterity compared with the unaffected side. In general, the effects of pyramidotomy reflect the role of the corticospinal tract in the execution of fine, manipulative motor tasks involving distal muscles of the extremities.

Experimentally produced localized lesions of cortical primary motor area (area 4) resemble the effects of pyramidotomy, i.e., distal paralysis and hypotonia. When the

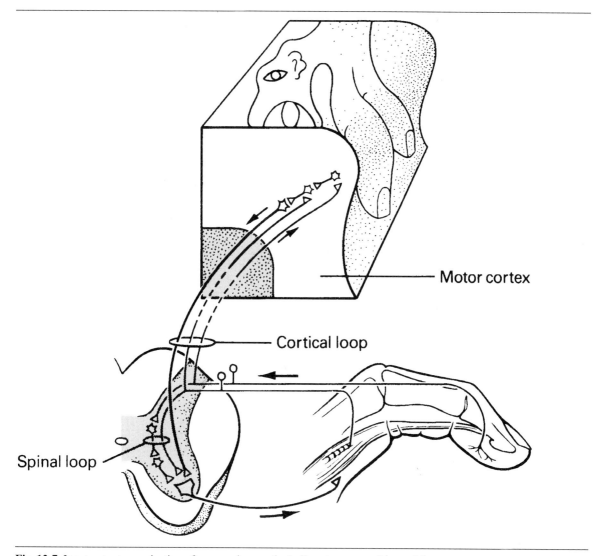

Fig. 12-7. Input-output organization of neurons in a cortical efferent zone to a flexor of the digit. The neurons are activated by either stretch of the muscle or stimulation of the skin. (Modified from: Kandel, E. R., Schwartz, J. H., and Jessell, T. M., eds. *Principles of Neural Science,* 3rd ed. Norwalk, Conn.: Appleton & Lange, 1991.)

sphere of the lesion is increased to include premotor area 6 (in which proximal muscles are represented), the loss of control over brainstem centers generates a state of spasticity that overshadows the concomitant pyramidal loss due to area 4 lesions. Lesions at the level of internal capsule result in the interruption of corticospinal tract fibers as well as projections to the brainstem (extrapyramidal system).

The "extrapyramidal" effects overshadow the "pyramidal" effects. The predominant sign of such a lesion is spasticity.

Basal Ganglia

The basal ganglia participate in the initiation and control of movement involving the axial and proximal muscles and in setting the "postural background" for phasic limb movements.

Functional Organization of the Basal Ganglia

The basal ganglia exert their motor actions largely via reciprocal connections with the cerebral cortex. Nearly all areas of the cerebral cortex project to the striatum (caudate nucleus and putamen). The cortical inputs to the striatum are excitatory and mediated by glutamate. The output from the basal ganglia is via inhibitory (gamma-aminobutyric acid, GABA) neurons from the internal segment of the globus pallidus to the thalamus and then via excitatory pathways to motor and premotor cortices. The flow and processing of cortical signals within the basal ganglia involve two major pathways (Fig. 12-8). The **direct** pathway involves inhibitory GABAergic projection from the striatum to the internal segment of globus pallidus. Activation of this pathway results in inhibition of the inhibitory, pallidal output neurons and hence **disinhibition** of the thalamic relay neurons. This is thought to facilitate movement by exciting premotor and supplementary motor cortical areas. The **indirect** pathway involves a distinct subset of striatal GABAergic neurons that project to the external segment of globus pallidus and inhibit the inhibitory GABAergic projection to the subthalamic nucleus, from which excitatory (glutamatergic) neurons project to the internal segment of globus pallidus, providing excitation to the inhibitory GABAergic pallidothalamic output neurons. The net effect of activation of this pathway is the suppression of thalamic relay neuron activity, disfacilitation of the motor cortical neurons, and inhibition of movement. The activity of the two pathways appears to be modulated by the internal dopaminergic loop between the neostriatum and substantia nigra, probably with the assistance of cholinergic (acetylcholine) interneurons in the striatum. The net effect of dopamine in the striatum appears to be facilitation of the direct pathway and inhibition of the indirect pathway. While the precise circuitry and motor behavioral correlates still have to be worked out in detail, neuropharmacologic studies emphasize the importance of acetylcholine, gamma-aminobutyric acid, and dopamine in basal ganglia function. An imbalance in these transmitters appears to be involved in various motor abnormalities seen in parkinsonism and in Huntington's chorea.

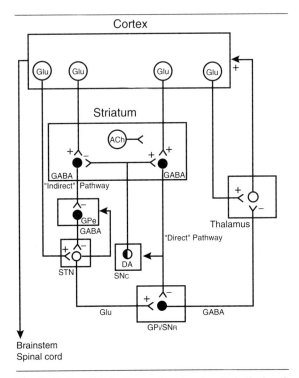

Fig. 12-8. Simplified scheme of motor circuits in the basal ganglia (GPe = external segment of globus pallidus; GPi = internal segment of globus pallidus; SNc = substantia nigra pars compacta; SNr = substantia nigra pars reticulata; STN = subthalamic nucleus; Glu = glutamic acid; GABA = gamma-aminobutyric acid; DA = dopamine; ACh = acetylcholine).

Motor Deficits Associated with Basal Ganglia Dysfunction

Lesions of the basal ganglia induce a spectrum of motor abnormalities ranging from the rigidity and hypokinesia of Parkinson's disease to the hyperkinetic phenomena associated with Huntington's disease and hemiballismus.

Parkinson's disease is associated with degeneration of nigrostriatal dopaminergic neurons and a deficiency in dopamine in the striatum. The disease is characterized by slowness in the initiation and execution of movement (bradykinesia), rigidity, and tremor at rest, usually affecting the extremities. Reduced levels of dopamine in the striatum may be expected to result in reduced inhibition of the striatopallidal component of the indirect pathway and reduced excitation of the striatopallidal component of the direct pathway. Both effects would result in reinforcement of the inhibitory pallidothalamic output and disfacilitation of cortical areas, an effect that has been suggested to underlie the hypokinetic disorders of the basal ganglia. In addition, disinhibition and overactivity of the subthalamic nucleus could play a role in rigidity and tremor. Parkinsonian symptoms can be ameliorated by intravenous administration of L-3,4-dihydroxyphenylalanine (L-DOPA), a precursor of dopamine. Unlike dopamine, L-DOPA penetrates through the blood-brain barrier and is presumably taken up by surviving neurons and perhaps glial cells in the striatum and converted to dopamine. It is then released apparently in amounts large enough to act on appropriate target cells and bring about an amelioration of the parkinsonian symptoms. The treatment does not halt progression of the disease.

Choreas are a group of disorders characterized by rapid (dancelike) involuntary movements (**diskinesia**) largely restricted to muscles of the distal extremities. **Huntington's chorea** is an inherited disease with progressive diskinesia and dementia and death 15 to 20 years after onset (usually in the fourth decade of life). The loss of cognitive functions and dementia in Huntington's disease probably results from the degeneration of cortical neurons. The motor deficits appear to be associated with loss of striatal cholinergic and the GABAergic neurons that project to the external segment of the globus pallidus (indirect pathway). This releases the inhibition of the external pallidum, resulting in suppression of the subthalamic activity, reduced inhibition of the thalamic relay neurons, and greater facilitation of the cortical areas, which has been suggested to account for hyperkinetic disorders of the basal ganglia.

Lesions of the subthalamic nucleus result in **hemiballismus,** a condition referring to involuntary movements, characterized by violent flailing and swinging of extremities due to activity in proximal muscles on the opposite side of the body.

In summary, the spectrum of basal ganglia motor dysfunctions ranging from hypokinesia and hypertonia in Parkinson's disease to hyperkinesia and hypotonia in Huntington's disease seem to reflect opposite alterations in the basal ganglia output, i.e., increased inhibitory output to the thalamus in parkinsonism and a decreased output in Huntington's disease. Involvement of the subthalamic nuclei is implicated in both diseases. The functional disinhibition of subthalamic neurons due to a deficiency of dopamine in Parkinson's disease may be contrasted with suppression of the activity of the subthalamic nucleus due to loss of the inhibitory striatopallidal GABAergic neurons in Huntington's disease. Both functional reduction in the activity of subthalamic neurons in Huntington's disease and loss of subthalamic neurons following lesions of the subthalamic nucleus are manifested in abnormal, uncontrolled movements. The emergence of such abnormal movements is thought to represent a "release phenomenon" from normal control of movement by the basal ganglia.

The Cerebellum

The **cerebellum** acts in coordinating and regulating contractions of muscles and muscle groups so as to provide proper force, direction, and rate of movement.

Functional Organization of the Cerebellum

The cerebellum receives inputs from the peripheral receptors and all levels of the CNS. The two sources of input to the cerebellum are the **mossy** and **climbing fibers.** The climbing fibers comes from the inferior olive, which receives its input from the cerebral cortex, the spino-olivary tract, the red nucleus, and perhaps the caudate. The mossy fibers originate in the spinocerebellar tracts, lateral reticular nucleus, and pontine nuclei. The output from the cerebellum is via neurons in the deep cerebellar nuclei.

The cerebellar afferents carry excitatory signals to neurons in the cerebellar cortex and en route provide excitation to the cerebellar output neurons in the deep nuclei (Fig. 12-9). The cerebellar cortex contains **Purkinje cells,** which project to the deep cerebellar nuclei, and four types of interneurons, the **granule, stellate, basket,** and **Golgi cells.** With the exception of the excitatory (glutamatergic) granule cells, all cerebellar cortical neurons are inhibitory and utilize GABA as the transmitter. Each Purkinje cell receives input from only a single climbing fiber, and each climbing fiber contacts no more than 1 to 10 Purkinje neurons. A single discharge in a climbing fiber initiates a burst of action potentials (**complex spike**) in the Purkinje cell at a frequency of about 1 per second. The mossy fibers activate the granule cells. Through their axons forming the parallel fiber system, the granule cells excite a population of Purkinje cells. Activation of Purkinje cells via mossy fibers results in firing of single action potentials at a rate of about 50 to 100 per second. These fibers thus control the rate of Purkinje neuron firing. The parallel fibers also activate the stellate and basket cells, which feed forward to inhibit Purkinje cells lateral to the main "beam" of Purkinje cells. The granule cells also activate Golgi cells, which synapse back onto the granule cells and inhibit their firing,

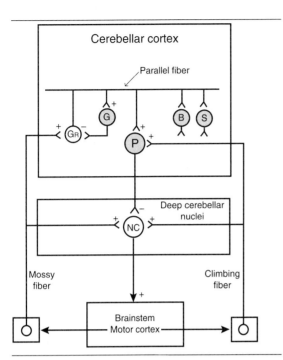

Fig. 12-9. Simplified diagram of cerebellar input-output connections (P = Purkinje neuron; Gr = granule cell; G = Golgi cell; B = basket cell; S = stellate cell; NC = nuclear cell). All shaded neurons are inhibitory.

thus shutting off the activating input. In short, mossy fiber activation of granule cells produces a spatially focused beam of Purkinje cell excitation for a brief period of time. With continuous, incoming stimuli, many such beams are activated in a highly organized spatial and temporal pattern. As indicated, the deep cerebellar nuclei receive excitation from the cerebellar afferents and maintain a high level of tonic activity. This ongoing activity is inhibited by the discharges of Purkinje neurons in precise spatial and temporal fashion. Thus the tonic excitatory influences of the deep cerebellar nuclei on the various targets of the cerebellum are up- or down-modulated by the output from the cerebellar cortex, with spatial and temporal precision appropriate for regulation of rate, range, direction, and force of evolving/ongoing movements. Precisely how such regulation is effected is at present not known; however, it is interesting to note that neurons in the interposed nuclei (spinocerebellum) tend to show altered discharge during and after a movement, implying response to proprioceptive feedback. By contrast, neurons in the dentate nucleus frequently discharge before the movement, supporting the notion that the lateral cerebellum participates in the initiation of movement.

The cerebellum has three functionally divisions (Fig. 12-10). The flocculonodular lobe, or **vestibulocerebellum,** receives information from vestibular labyrinths and sends efferent signals to the lateral vestibular nuclei. The principal destination of the output from the vestibulocerebellum is to the medial systems, and its function is in the control of axial muscles and equilibrium reactions. The **spinocerebellum** is comprised of the vermis and pars intermedia. The vermis receives input from the neck and trunk as well as from the labyrinths and the eyes. Its efferent signals act on the medial system, i.e., via reticulospinal, vestibulospinal, and corticospinal fibers that regulate axial and proximal musculature. The pars intermedia receives information from the limbs and controls the lateral systems, i.e., rubrospinal and lateral corticospinal tracts that act on the distal limb musculature. The function of the spinocerebellum is the regulation of axial, proximal, and distal musculature during evolving and ongoing movement. It performs this function by comparing the efferent cortical motor commands with the sensory feedback it receives from the periphery and then sending "correcting" signals to adjust muscle activity as necessary. The **cerebrocerebellum** comprises the lateral hemispheres (pars lateralis). The cerebrocerebellum receives cortical input via the pontine nuclei and sends signals via the thalamus (ventrolateral nucleus) back to the motor and premotor cortices. It does not receive direct sensory input from the periphery; thus its function is thought to involve planning, initiation, and timing of movements. In particular, it may be important in controlling skilled movements that are performed too rapidly to be adequately regulated by the sensory feedback from peripheral receptors.

Cerebellar Motor Deficits

The deficits associated with lesions of the cerebellum can be grouped into three main classes: disturbances of synergy, equilibrium, or tone. **Asynergia,** or impaired coordination, results from errors in rate, force, range, and direction of movements. Asynergia can manifest itself in a number of ways. **Dysmetria,** or errors in direction and force of movement, results in limb overshooting **(hypermetria)** or undershooting **(hypometria)** the desired position. In the case of lower limbs, it produces **ataxic,** or unsteady, broadly based gait (sailor's walk). Asynergia involving complex movements is often expressed as **decomposition of movement,** where a sequence of movements cannot be performed smoothly, but rather, movements are

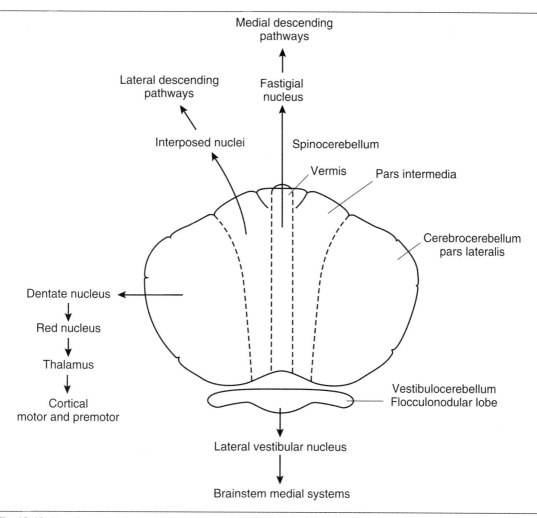

Fig. 12-10. Functional divisions of the cerebellum and their major destinations. Output is via deep cerebellar nuclei: lateral vestibular (vestibulocerebellum), fastigial (spinocerebellum, vermis), interposed (spinocerebellum, pars intermedia), dentate (cerebrocerebellum).

executed in discrete steps. The **intention tremor** is a form of asynergia involving temporal relationship between the contractions of agonistic and antagonistic muscles. Asynergia of the extrinsic eye muscles produces **nystagmus;** if muscles of speech are affected, **dysarthria** is manifested.

Disturbances of equilibrium, i.e., impairment of the ability to maintain an upright posture, occur as a consequence of the lesions involving the vestibulocerebellum. Disturbances of muscle tone associated with cerebellar lesion in humans and other primates result in **hypotonia.** Pendular limb can be observed. For example, after elicita-

tion of a patellar tendon reflex, the limb will swing back and forth in a pendular fashion.

The distribution of motor deficits may be predicted in terms of functional subdivisions of the cerebellum. As indicated, lesions of the vestibulocerebellum (flocculonodular lobe) will affect equilibrium. Lesions involving the medial (vermal) zone will produce primarily ipsilateral truncal deficits. Lesions confined to the intermediate zone affect principally the ipsilateral proximal limbs, muscles involved in postural adjustments. Lesions of the lateral hemispheres compromise spatially organized movements of the limbs but have little effect on posture. The effects are ipsilateral. As might be expected, lesions involving deep nuclei produce more profound impairment than those of the cerebral cortex.

Summary

The supraspinal motor systems are organized hierarchically as well as in parallel. With the exception of the corticospinal tract, which provides a direct connection from the cerebral cortex to the spinal cord, all other descending signals to the spinal cord are funneled through the brainstem. The brainstem is an important component of the medial system responsible for the maintenance of appropriate posture through regulation of contractions in the musculature of the neck and trunk and proximal portions of the limbs. The cerebral cortex is responsible for the formulation, organization, and execution of skilled, voluntary movements. The principal output from the motor cortical areas involved in execution of movement is through the corticospinal tracts, which together with the rubrospinal tract of the brainstem constitute the lateral system controlling the distal muscles. The basal ganglia and cerebellum are responsible for modulation of the cortical and brainstem motor centers. Diseases of the basal ganglia result in a spectrum of motor abnormalities ranging from the hypokinesia and hypertonia of Parkinson's disease to the hyperkinesia and hypotonia of Huntington's disease. The cerebellum is essential for organization and coordination of muscle groups during purposeful, particularly highly skilled movements and for the moment-to-moment corrections during ongoing motor activity.

Bibliography

Henneman, E. Motor functions of the brain stem and basal ganglia. In: Mountcastle, V. B., ed. *Medical Physiology,* St. Louis: Vol. 1. C. V. Mosby, 1981. Chap. 29.

Henneman, E. Motor functions of the cerebral cortex. In: V. B. Mountcastle ed., *Medical Physiology,* Vol. 1. St. Louis: C. V. Mosby, 1981. Chap. 32.

Kandel, E. R., Schwartz, J. H., and Jessell, T. M., eds. *Principles of Neural Science,* 3rd ed. New York: Elsevier, 1991.

Thatch, W. T. The cerebellum. In: V. B. Mountcastle, ed. *Medical Physiology,* Vol. 1. St. Louis: C. V. Mosby, 1981.

13 The Limbic System: Feeding, Thirst, and Regulation of Temperature

Michael M. Behbehani and Ernest C. Foulkes

Objectives

After reading this chapter, you should be able to

Describe the components of the limbic system

Describe the brainstem nuclei that are involved in feeding

Explain the hypothalamic areas that are involved in feeding behavior, and describe how these areas interact with the limbic and the brainstem

Explain what neurotransmitters are involved in feeding behavior

Describe the components and mechanisms of thirst

Discuss temperature regulation in terms of energy balance, resulting from the input of food energy and output of external work, in addition to heat exchange

Define body temperature

Describe heat gain and loss by the body through conduction, convection, and radiation

Explain the importance of evaporative heat loss

Define the basal metabolic rate

Explain the principle of indirect calorimetry

Describe the compensatory mechanisms by which the body responds to heat and cold

Explain the importance of circulation in temperature control

Define fever and distinguish it from physiologic hyperthermia

---

The **limbic system** includes the limbic lobe, a portion of the hypothalamus, the septum, and the nucleus accombens. The **limbic lobe** consists of three layered structures sandwiched between the midbrain and neocortex and includes the amygdala, hippocampus, cinglum, septum, fornix, mammillary bodies, and olfactory bulb. The limbic system is involved in emotional drive and affective behavior such as fear, rage, and maintenance of homeostasis of the body. In this chapter we will consider the regulation of feeding, thirst, and temperature by the limbic system.

Regulation of Feeding

The function of all body organs requires an expenditure of energy that must be gained by eating. The process of feeding involves both **reflex** and **motivational** aspects. The reflex aspect of feeding regulates the events that occur during feeding. These include swallowing, rejection of unpleasant food, and termination of eating when appropriate amounts of food have been consumed. The neuronal elements underlying this reflex activity include the sensory receptors in the tongue, esophagus, and digestive tracts, the nucleus of the solitary tract (NST), the vagal nucleus complex, and the vagus nerve. This reflex activity requires only the brainstem. Decerebrate animals in which the brainstem has been isolated from the rest of the brain chew and swallow food if it is placed in their mouth and also reject unpleasant food. However, these animals do not seek food and will die unless force fed.

The drive to seek food is mediated through the limbic system. Early studies of feeding behavior indicated that lesions of the **ventromedial nucleus of hypothalamus** (VMH) cause overeating. Animals with this type of lesion consume more food, feed more often, and gain weight. In contrast, lesions of the **lateral hypothalamus** (LH) will render animals aphagic. These animals do not eat even when they are deprived of food. Stimulation of these hypothalamic areas produces an effect opposite to that observed with their lesions. Stimulation of the VMH causes termination of eating even when the animal is deprived of food; stimulation of the LH causes an animal to eat even if it has been fed to satiety.

Because of these properties, it was believed that the VMH is the satiety center and the LH is the feeding center and that they negatively interact. A problem with lesion studies is that the procedures (electric lesioning or knife cuts) not only destroy cell bodies but also destroy fibers that pass through the lesion site. Since numerous pathways sends fibers through the VMH and the LH, it is not clear whether the effect of lesions is related to a destruction of the cell bodies in the nuclei or destruction of the tracts that pass through them. Another problem with the satiety and feeding center hypothesis is that if an animal with an LH lesion is kept alive by force feeding, eventually it will feed itself and will maintain normal weight. More recent studies using injection of toxins that destroy cell bodies but do not damage fibers of passage have shown that both the LH and the VMH are involved in feeding and satiety but that they are not the only feeding centers within the brain.

Additional studies of feeding behavior indicate that other hypothalamic areas in addition to the VMH and LH as well as brainstem areas function in concert to produce both short- and long-term regulation of feeding. In this system, the cortical structures modify the functions of the brainstem structures that modulate short-term feeding. Activation of feeding behavior requires signals from both the peripheral and central gustatory systems. Some of these signals have been well characterized. For example, a decrease in **blood glucose concentration** of an animal activates glucose-sensitive hypothalamic neurons, and activation of these neurons increases the drive for food such that the animal will eat if presented with food. Other signals are more complex and are not well understood. For example, all animals including humans adjust their caloric intake such that the ratio of caloric intake (in kCal) to body weight, raised to 0.75, is equal to 70, that is, kCal/body weight$^{0.75}$ = 70. If an animal is maintained on a restrictive diet and loses weight, the caloric intake declines to maintain the ratio at 70. Similarly, if an animal is force fed or allowed to eat more palatable food, it will gain weight and then will eat more to maintain its new weight. These properties indicate that there is a weight set-point and that this set-point is maintained. However, a new set-point can be established by long-term changes in feeding behavior. The mechanisms and signals that modulate the set-point for weight are not known.

Feeding Behavior Signals

Numerous factors produce signals that cause modification of feeding behavior. Animals including humans and monkeys will eat after satiety if they are presented with a food other than the one just consumed. An implication of this behavior is that a person will eat more when offered a variety rather than a single type of food. In addition, the lack of certain types of food increases the hunger for that food. For example, if an animal is fed a diet that lacks salt, it will seek salt. Similar drives exist for carbohydrate, protein, and fat.

To determine the neuronal basis of this behavior, one group of investigators has recorded electrical activity from a large number of cells in the gustatory-related areas of the brain. These studies have shown that a distinct number of neurons in the lateral hypothalamus and substantia innominata respond to the taste or sight of food. However, the responses of these cells depend on the type and concentration of the substance in the food. For example, some cells responded to glucose but not to water or salt, and these responses increase if the concentration of glucose is increased. More important, these cells only respond when the animal is hungry.

The fact that hunger changes the response of hypothalamic cells indicates that these cells are influenced by the motivational state of the animal. A signal for this motivational behavior is gastric distension. If a monkey is fed to satiety and then the contents of the stomach are removed artificially, it will immediately begin feeding. A similar situation occurs if food is removed from the duodenum soon after eating. Since there is insufficient time for digestion to have occurred, the signal from the gastric system must be relayed through a neuronal sensory system. Data indicate that signals related to distension of the digestive tract is relayed by branches of the vagus nerve that innervates these structures.

The motivational aspect of feeding involves cortical and limbic structures. In the hypothalamus, there are neurons that respond to sight or taste of food. These hypothalamic regions have direct projection to the prefrontal cortex and to the supplementary and principal motor cortexes. In addition, these areas project to the NST and to the motor nucleus of the vagus. Therefore, these hypothalamic areas form a neuronal structure that is involved in motivational aspects of feeding.

Neurotransmitters Involved in Feeding Behavior

The earliest transmitter that was shown to have a direct effect on feeding was **norepinephrine** (NE). Injection of NE into the **paraventricular nucleus** of the hypothalamus (PVN) causes a satiated animal to begin feeding. The effect of NE on feeding is now well established. It has been suggested that NE inhibits PVN neurons via alpha$_2$ receptors, signaling a negative energy balance. The PVN receives afferents from the locus ceruleus, and the activity of this system is modulated by vagal afferents. In addition, the number of alpha$_2$ receptors is modulated by adrenal **corticosterone,** a process that modulates the effect of NE.

In addition to NE, **dopamine, epinephrine,** and **serotonin** are also involved in feeding. Injection of these neurotransmitters into the hypothalamus produces anorexia. The effect of dopamine can be blocked by specific dopamine antagonists, and the effect of epinephrine can be blocked by beta-adrenergic blockers. Activation of the dopaminergic system has been used for weight reduction. For example, drugs such as amphetamine that cause release of dopamine suppress eating and are used for control of obesity and overeating. Another classical transmitter, 5-hydroxy-tryptamine (5HT) (serotonin), acts on $5HT_{1B}$ receptors and decreases the food drive. Similar to dopamine and epinephrine, injection of 5HT into the hypothalamus reduces food intake. Drugs that increase serotonin content, such as L-tryptophan, reduce appetite and body weight.

In addition to the preceding classical neurotransmitters, several peptides, including **cholecystokinin** (CCK), **neuropeptide Y** (NPY), **opioid peptides,** and **galanin,** play a role in food intake. CCK is released from the gastrointestinal tract following ingestion of food. This peptide activates vagal sensory afferents and therefore is a major transmitter that signals the presence of food in the gut to the brain. In the human, CCK administration reduces food intake. Injection of NPY into the paraventricular nucleus of the hypothalamus causes feeding in satiated animals. This peptide acts on Y_1 receptors and increases the appetite for carbohydrate. Galanin and opioid peptides act on the medial hypothalamus and increase intake of fat.

Sensation of Thirst

Thirst is the desire to ingest water. The quantity of water that humans ingest is highly variable, and only about half the water intake is the result of water drinking. The remaining water needs of the body are met by water that is the by-product of metabolism or water from solid food. Solid foods have at least 50% water, and 90% of the weight of vegetables is water. Metabolism of carbohydrate and fat produce 60 and 100 ml of water per 100 g weight, respectively. Ingestion of 100 g protein produces 45 ml water as a by-product.

Several factors produce thirst. **Dryness of the mouth** and **reduced salivary secretions** are the most common signals. For example, eating a very dry food produces the desire to drink water because the salivary secretion is not adequate to keep the mouth moist. Increase in the osmolarity of the blood produced by dehydration or increased salt intake is another signal that drives water intake. Finally, **decrease in blood volume** that can occur during hemorrhage is another factor that produces thirst.

Brain Regulation of Thirst

The major site regulating water intake is the hypothalamus. Injection of hyperosmotic saline in the **lateral hypothalamic** nucleus in awake animals causes drinking. In addition, lesions in this area produces adipsia (absence of thirst or abnormal avoidance of drinking). These responses indicate that the lateral hypothalamus is an essential component of the thirst network and that cells in this area can detect changes in osmolarity. Studies of the lateral hypothalamic nucleus have shown that it contains neurons that act as mechanoreceptors and that these cells increase their firing rate when the osmolarity of the extracellular fluid is elevated.

Hypothalamic neurons are also activated by a decrease in blood volume. The volume of blood is detected by receptors located in the right atrium and in the large veins. The mechanisms by which low blood volume increases the drive to drink involve the **renin-angiotensin** system. Low blood volume increases renin secretion from the kidney. Renin cleaves plasma angiotensin I to angiotensin II. Angiotensin II penetrates the walls of capillaries of the subfornical organ. This organ is a collection of neurons that extends into the third ventricle. These cells are supplied by capillaries that have relatively large, tight junctions, and angiotensin II can pass through these structures. Cells in the **subfornical organ** contain angiotensin II receptors and are excited by this peptide. These cells project to the **preoptic and lateral nuclei** of the hypothalamus and excite these neurons, which causes the animal to drink water.

Temperature Regulation

Temperature reflects the heat content of a system, and heat is a form of energy. Maintenance of a constant body temperature therefore represents a special aspect of the wider topic of energy balance.

The commonly used unit of heat energy is the **calorie,** which is the energy required to raise one gram of water 1°C. (Strictly speaking, the 1°C increment refers to a rise of from 14.5 to 15.5°C, which is approximately the point of highest density of water.) For physiologic purposes, the large calorie, or **kilocalorie** (Calorie), where 1 Calorie equals 1000 calories, is usually employed. Because units of energy and work are freely interchangeable, the energy content of food and work output also may be expressed in Calories. Work also can be measured in units that are based on a standard force acting over a standard distance. The equivalence of work and heat was first appreciated by Rumford 200 years ago, when he realized that the heat produced during the boring of gun barrels is proportional to the number of revolutions of the drill. Subsequently, the **work equivalent of heat** (Joule's equivalent) was determined to be 4.18 joules per calorie, where the joule or newton-meter is the work done when a **force** of one newton acts over a **distance** of one meter. Finally, **power** is calculated as work/time and measures the rate at which work can be performed; for instance, one watt (power) equals one joule (work) per second.

Heat Transfer

Direct transfer of heat energy involves three processes: **conduction, convection,** and **radiation.** Heat also can be transferred indirectly, for instance, as a result of physicochemical changes such as evaporation of water. Evaporation of water at body temperature requires 0.58 Cal per milliliter, as will be further discussed in relation to insensible heat loss from the body and sweating.

Heat transfer through a medium depends on its **conductivity.** Conductivity is measured as heat flow (Cal/min) across a unit area (m^2), all divided by the temperature gra-

dient (°C), i.e., in Cal/min/m^2/°C. Metals are better heat conductors than is water, which in turn conducts heat more efficiently than does air. Some representative values for the heat conductivity of different materials are listed in Table 13-1.

The **conductivity of air** varies with its water content and with density and pressure. Thus severe heat loss through conduction may be encountered in the humid and high-pressure atmosphere of a diving bell or an underwater habitation. Because of its high air content, snow is a poorer heat conductor than water. The relatively high conductivity of water also accounts for the fact that an unprotected person can survive for only a very brief time in water that is near the freezing point.

The inverse of heat conductance is **insulation or resistance to heat flow.** The insulating properties of clothing, for instance, are expressed as 1/conductivity, i.e., as the temperature gradient/heat flow, divided by the area, or °C/min/m^2/Cal. In other words, this measures the temperature gradient that the material can maintain for a given rate of heat flow.

Convection in the physiologic context is defined as the transfer of heat to moving air or water. Thus heat loss from the body to the air is increased when air warmed at the skin is replaced by cold air. The chilling effects of cold air are accentuated by wind, creating the wind chill factor. Conversely, a wet diving suit restricts the movement of water in contact with the skin and in this manner helps conserve heat.

Heat transfer by **radiation** describes an electromagnetic process that is independent of the intervening medium. When the skin temperature is less than the temperature of a distant source, such as a radiator or the sun, heat is gained by radiation. Inversely, heat may be lost to a distant sink, such as a cold window or the night sky.

Heat transfer by conduction, convection, or radiation can be modified by protective clothing that insulates (reduces conductance), minimizes convection, or reflects ra-

Table 13-1. Heat Conductivities

Substance	Cal/min/ °C × m^2
Silver	600.00
Water	0.90
Snow (compacted)	0.30
Wood	0.18
Dry air at sea level	0.03

diation. In the desert, heat gain by radiation from sun and sand can best be minimized by covering the skin with thin white clothing. At the other temperature extreme, the Eskimo in the Arctic wears highly insulating clothing to reduce conductive heat loss. The amount of added clothing that can be worn to resist extreme cold is limited, however, by its weight and bulk. In addition, the insensible perspiration from the skin, if trapped in the clothing, will increase heat conductance. Together with respiratory heat loss, this fixes at about –70°C, the maximum cold exposure humans can survive without help from outside sources of heat.

Body Temperature

The **heat content** of the body is reflected by its temperature. Although the mean body temperature is normally considered to be 37°C, there are actually significant variations not only among different parts of the body but also in any given region at different times. Because the skin is the main heat exchange organ of the human body, its temperature is determined by both the temperature and humidity of the environment and by the needs of the body to conserve or dissipate heat. The temperature of the hands and feet may be several degrees lower than that in the core. Venous blood draining actively metabolizing tissues is likely to be warmer than pulmonary venous blood after it has undergone evaporative cooling in the lungs. The right heart is therefore likely to be warmer than the left heart. Similarly, rectal temperature exceeds oral temperature and, in fact, provides the most convenient approximation to mean core temperature. More accurate values, if required, can be obtained with a probe in the esophagus or by measurement of urine temperature during voiding.

The **core temperature** in warm-blooded animals (homeotherms) is also influenced by intrinsic factors such as the menstrual cycle or by diurnal and seasonal cycles. Both metabolic rate and body temperature tend to fall somewhat during sleep and then rise again during the day. Major physiologic temperature shifts occur in some mammals during hibernation. Even reptiles and other normally cold-blooded animals (poikilotherms) can raise and maintain their body temperature above ambient levels in response to physiologic demands; certain snakes, for instance, incubate their eggs. The differences between homeotherms and poikilotherms are therefore only relative.

Energy Balance

The body gains or loses energy primarily by conduction or radiation and by evaporation from the skin or from the respiratory passages. Even in the absence of sweat, some water is lost through so-called **insensible perspiration.** Of particular importance is the heat lost from the respiratory passages. This is a necessary process because relatively cool and dry inspired air must be warmed and saturated with water at 37°C. Although some of the respiratory heat loss may be recovered upon exhalation by heat exchange at the external nares, the net respiratory heat loss may be very significant. This is especially true at high altitudes, where low atmospheric oxygen pressure leads to the need to hyperventilate with cold and dry air.

Food consumption is the major pathway of energy gain. Table 13-2 summarizes the heat content of different classes of food. For several reasons, the total heat content that is physiologically available is less than that liberated by the combustion of these foods in a calorimeter. For instance, one of the end-products of protein metabolism is urea, whose chemical energy is lost to the body. The net energy gained by food intake also may be reduced if the food stimulates metabolism; the classic instance is the so-called **specific dynamic action** of proteins or amino acids.

The **minimal energy input** required to maintain steady-state is the **basal level.** To maintain this basal level in a patient on parenteral feeding may therefore require infusion of around 1600 Cal per day. This corresponds to the heat

Table 13-2. Heat Content of Various Types of Food

Food	Physiologically Available (Cal/g)	O_2 Consumed (liters/g)	CO_2 Produced (liters/g)	RQ	Cal/liter O_2
Fat	9.0	1.96	1.39	0.71	4.6
Protein	4.0	0.94	0.75	0.80	4.2
Carbohydrate	4.0	0.81	0.81	1.00	4.9
Standard average				0.82	4.8

RQ = respiratory quotient, i.e., CO_2 produced/O_2 consumed.

content of 400 g of glucose or of a fifth of 80-proof alcohol, neither of which can be infused without overloading the kidneys and other organs. Procedures have been worked out, however, that not only maintain patients at steady-state but also permit normal growth of children. Such intravenous alimentation is based on administration of fat suspensions in concentrated glucose and amino acid solutions into a central vein.

Energy is lost from the body through work on the environment. Walking 3 miles per hour consumes 140 Cal per hour. The performance of 100 Cal of external work is associated with the production of approximately 400 Cal of heat. In other words, the mechanical efficiency of the body only amounts to around 20%; the remaining 80% of the metabolic energy consumed is liberated as body heat. **Heat dissipation** during exercise can therefore limit the maximum work output. This is especially true of humans who, unlike the camel and some other species, cannot tolerate much of a rise in body temperature and thus cannot store appreciable amounts of heat. The camel, in contrast, accumulates heat during the day, readily tolerating a rise in its core temperature of 5°C. This heat is then dissipated by conduction during the cool of the night, without necessitating loss of water for evaporative cooling.

Indirect Calorimetry

The major source of heat is the **metabolic breakdown of food;** this also furnishes the energy needed for doing work. The physiologic combustion of one gram of each type of food consumes a characteristic number of liters of O_2, as shown in Table 13-2. At the same time, it liberates the stated volume of CO_2, and the ratio of CO_2 produced to O_2 consumed defines the respiratory quotient. A diabetic patient, because of the preferential utilization of fatty acids rather than glucose, is likely to exhibit a lower respiratory quotient than normal.

As shown in Table 13-2, a subject primarily using glucose as a source of energy will have a respiratory quotient of close to 1.00 and will accordingly liberate 4.8 Cal for each liter of O_2 consumed. This observation provides the basis for **indirect calorimetry.** The total heat output of the body is most accurately measured in a whole-body calorimeter, but this is not a convenient procedure and is not easily applicable in a work or exercise setting. In indirect calorimetry, expired air is collected in a bag for subsequent analysis, and the estimated number of liters of O_2 consumed is multiplied by 4.8. If the respiratory quotient is also determined and is well below 1.00, then a value

somewhat lower than 4.8 must be used in order to calculate the caloric yield per liter of O_2.

Indirect calorimetry also can be used to determine the heat output of a single organ. For instance, calories produced by the brain can be calculated, based on the fact that the metabolic substrate is primarily glucose. If O_2 consumption is determined as the product of blood flow and the arteriovenous difference in O_2 concentration, caloric consumption is yielded by the formula: $4.8 \times$ blood flow $\times O_2$ concentration difference.

One disadvantage of indirect calorimetry is that it ignores the **O_2 debt,** which is the transient accumulation of lactic acid and other incomplete combustion products during exercise when glucose breakdown exceeds its oxidation to CO_2 and water. During hard and prolonged exercise, the O_2 debt will reach a steady-state value, at which time measurement of O_2 consumption will yield the correct value of caloric output. Indirect calorimetry performed on subjects engaged in short and violent exercise, such as a 100-yard dash, must be adjusted for the O_2 debt by continuing gas collection until respiration returns to normal. However, return to normal may be delayed if metabolism is stimulated postexercise, independently of O_2 debt.

Basal Metabolic Rate

Even at rest, the body requires a significant expenditure of energy for the maintenance of homeostasis: Blood pressure and muscle tone must be maintained, respiration continued, and ionic gradients restored. In addition, the body temperature must not fall much below 37°C. This basal requirement defines the **basal metabolic rate** (BMR).

To ensure basal conditions for the **measurement of BMR,** the subject must be awake, fasting, and resting horizontally so that the need to pump blood against gravity is minimized. The ambient temperature must be that at which basal heat production is counterbalanced by passive heat loss (see Chap. 63). This temperature is defined as the neutral temperature. It is the temperature at which compensatory activity is minimal.

Under all these conditions, the BMR of a 70-kg male is around 80 Cal per hour, corresponding approximately to the heat output of a 100-watt bulb. The surface area of this average male is 1.73 m^2. Because heat exchange primarily involves the skin, the BMR is often expressed as 50 Cal/m^2 of body surface/hour, referred to as **1 MET.** During sleep, caloric requirements fall below basal levels, so the daily basal requirement is 1600 Cal, or somewhat less than that yielded strictly by multiplying 80 Cal per hour by 24 hours. Homeostasis, even under basal conditions, cannot be maintained on less than 1600 Cal/day, as is made dramatically obvious in pictures of famine victims.

A variety of factors determine the BMR. For instance, the value for females generally is somewhat less than that for males, because females have a smaller muscle mass relative to their body surface area, and because of better insulation. Reduced muscle tone, as occurs in the absence of gravity or in advanced age, also lowers the BMR. Finally, changes in hormonal activity, especially of the thyroid gland, alter the BMR.

Heat Sensors and Integration

Sensors that detect changes in body temperature are located in both peripheral areas and in the CNS. The chief sensory activity, however, and the integration of all the various **feedback loops** involved in the maintenance of a constant body temperature take place in the **preoptic hypothalamus.** This conclusion is based on the type of evidence illustrated in Fig. 13-1. Among other findings, the suggested role of the hypothalamus in temperature control

is supported by the existence of both heat-sensitive and cold-sensitive neurons in this area.

The data depicted in Fig. 13-1 were obtained in a dog. The animal's initial rectal temperature was 37.8°C, and while resting in a room at 32°C, its metabolic rate as measured by O_2 consumption was close to basal. At **point A,** the temperature of the hypothalamus was raised, which can be achieved by perfusing the frontal sinuses or ears with warm water. The rectal temperature began to fall even though the room temperature was not lowered, and body temperature fell further when the ambient temperature was allowed to drop at **point B.** The continued warming of the hypothalamus in this situation is the equivalent of holding a candle under the thermostat in an otherwise cold room: No compensatory heat production or adequate heat conservation takes place. It was only at **point C,** when the hypothalamic or ear perfusion was stopped, that the dog's hypothalamus could sense the core body temperature and the signal went out to the compensating mechanisms. Metabolic heat production rose sharply, and body temperature began to return to normal. Clearly, it was the hypo-

Fig. 13-1. Body temperature and heat production in a resting dog. The hypothalmic temperature was raised between points A and C; at B the room temperature was lowered. (Temperatures are T-air = ambient; T-hypo = hypothalamic; T-rect = rectal, as a measure of core temperature.) (Based on: Hensel, H. Symposium on temperature acclimation: Thermoreceptors. *Fed. Proc.* 22:1156, 1963.)

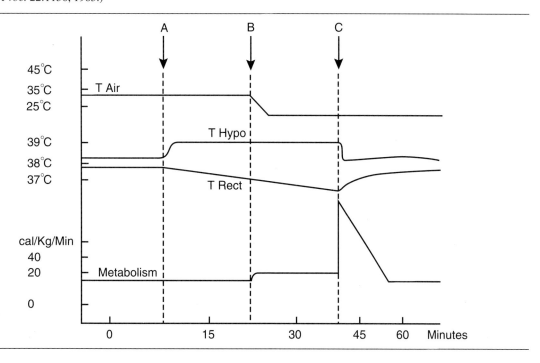

thalamic cooling that triggered this response. Even though central heat control resides in the hypothalamus, this does not exclude cortical influences from contributing to temperature homeostasis. For instance, the subjective feeling of cold may provide the motivation for warm-up exercises.

Spinal and peripheral sensors also participate in temperature control. A good example of the action of a peripheral mechanism is the reduced sweating rate observed when the forearm of a hot individual is cooled, even though the central heat drive from the hypothalamus has not been altered.

Response to Heat

Sweating

Secretion of sweat to reduce body temperature is the function of the two to three million eccrine sweat glands located over most of the body surface. Under extreme heat stress, they can produce sweat at a rate as high as 2 liters per hour. In composition, sweat resembles a dilute ultrafiltrate of plasma. Unless salt and water loss are therefore replenished, high sweating rates may lead to circulatory failure. The evaporation of 1 ml of sweat requires the expenditure of 0.58 Cal (the heat of evaporation of water). When this evaporation is diminished in a highly humid environment, a major source of heat dissipation is lost, so humans cannot maintain a normal body temperature at an environmental temperature of 37°C at 100% relative humidity.

Sweat is first secreted as an isosmotic fluid into the proximal portion of the sweat duct, and salt reabsorption in the diluting segment of the duct produces the final form of sweat. The systemic administration of **cholinergic drugs** provokes sweating, and thermoregulatory sweating is abolished by **atropine,** showing that the postganglionic fibers innervating the sweat glands are cholinergic. However, sweating also can be stimulated by adrenergic agonists.

Vasodilatation and Cardiac Output

The evaporation of sweat provides only local cooling, and it is the **peripheral blood flow** that determines how much heat can be carried from the core to be dissipated on the body surface. If sweating has cooled the skin to 32°C, each liter of blood from a core temperature of 37°C can lose 5 Cal upon equilibration with skin temperature. In other words, the amount of heat lost depends on the evaporative cooling of the skin and the blood flow to the skin. A piece of steak, which has the same composition as human tissue, can evaporate as much water from its surface as can human skin, but in the absence of circulation, it will be cooked at a temperature that humans can survive for some time.

An early response to heat exposure is therefore **decreased peripheral** (skin) **resistance** to blood flow. This **vasodilatation** permits increased peripheral blood flow, especially as cardiac output also begins to rise. This is illustrated in Table 13-3 for heat production at rest, as well as during strenuous or maximal exercise. For the purposes here, it will be assumed that the core temperature is 37°C and the skin temperature is cooled by heat conduction and sweat evaporation down to 32°C. The core-to-skin temperature gradient would therefore equal 5°C, such that each liter of blood from the core loses 5 Cal at the periphery. During strenuous exercise, peripheral blood flow can thus carry $1.9 \times 5 \times 60$, or 570 Cal per hour, to the skin for dissipation. This more than compensates for the heat production of 360 Cal per hour. If, however, work output is raised to maximal levels, with a caloric output of 600 Cal per

Table 13-3. Role of Circulation in Heat Control During Exercise

Variables	Rest	Strenuous Exercise	Maximal Exercise
O$_2$ consumption (liters/min)	0.14	1.20	2.00
Heat production (Cal/min)	0.7	4.8	8.0
Cardiac output (liters/min)	5.8	17.5	25.0
Skeletal muscle			
Blood flow (liters/min)	1.2	12.5	22.0
Vascular resistance (% of normal)	100.0	12.0	8.0
Skin			
Blood flow (liters/min)	0.5	1.9	0.6
Vascular resistance (% of normal)	100.0	40.0	115.0

hour, the blood flow to skeletal (and cardiac) muscle must take precedence over that to some other areas of the body, including the skin. The blood flow to the brain remains constant, but that to mesentery and kidneys is greatly decreased. These conditions initiate peripheral vasoconstriction, such that the peripheral resistance to blood flow increases. The total peripheral blood flow in this example can now dissipate only $0.6 \times 5 \times 60$, or 180 Cal per hour, in the face of a caloric output of 600 Cal, and body temperature will rise rapidly to the point of exhaustion. These calculations ignore the contribution of respiratory heat loss to total heat dissipation, which is an important factor, especially at high rates of ventilation. Nevertheless, this example does illustrate how the ability to dissipate heat may limit the maximal work output.

Response to Cold

Humans possess three main physiologic mechanisms for responding to cold: **shivering, nonmyogenic heat production,** and **vasoconstriction.** If the core body temperature in the cold declines by more than about 2°C, despite the maximal activity of these three compensators, hypothermia eventuates, with loss of coordination, inappropriate responses such as vasodilation, and inability to prevent further heat loss.

Shivering

The muscular (or myogenic) response to cold in humans is the shivering reflex. It is a noncoordinated activity of skeletal muscle that achieves no outside work and therefore represents a 100% efficient source of metabolic heat. However, when violent, it can interfere with normal motor movement, and it may actually increase heat loss by convection because it agitates the surrounding medium.

Nonmyogenic Heat Production

In response to cold, the body also can reflexly increase heat production in nonmuscular tissues, particularly in adipose tissue. This is triggered by catecholamine secretion; this response is perhaps less important in humans than, for example, in rodents, which maintain relatively large brown fat deposits into adult life.

Vasoconstriction

The third major reflex response to cold in humans is peripheral vasoconstriction. This lowers skin temperature and therefore the conductive heat loss that is determined by the temperature gradient from the skin to environment. The heat conductance of fully vasoconstricted skin approximates 0.12 Cal/m^2/°C/min, similar to that of cork. Such extreme vasoconstriction is not uniform over the en-

tire body. For instance, circulation to the hands and feet is little depressed in the cold, which helps minimize the pain of excessive cooling of the extremities, but at the price of greater heat loss.

Obviously, vasodilating drugs such as alcohol also elevate heat loss. While the monks at the St. Bernard Pass may have transiently restored the morale of travelers lost in the snow by providing brandy in flasks tied around the necks of their dogs, they also may have caused the victims to lose heat at a faster rate. Alcohol consumption in someone who is hypothermic is absolutely contraindicated until the victim has been returned to warm surroundings.

Fever

Fever occurs when hypothalamic control permits the steady-state core temperature of the body to rise above normal levels. Fever implies hyperthermia, but not all cases of hyperthermia constitute fever. This important distinction is predicated on the fact that the heat-producing or -conserving mechanisms in fever are promoting an increased body temperature, whereas during exercise-induced hyperthermia, for instance, the cooling mechanisms are striving to return the body temperature to its normal steady-state. This is illustrated in Table 13-4, which compares theoretical data from two hyperthermic individuals, one who has just completed a 440-yard sprint and the other who suffers from fever. Both are now resting at a normal neutral environment of 31°C. This is cooler than the neutral temperature for the fever patient, so this

Table 13-4. Thermal Response During Fever and Physiologic Hyperthermia*

Variables	Exercise Hyperthermia	Fever
Body temperature		
Actual	39	39
Steady-state	37	39
Environmental temperature		
Actual	31	31
Neutral	31	33
Responses		
Sweating	+	0
Vasoconstriction	0	+
Reflex heat production	0	+

*The two individuals were resting at 31°C. All temperatures are given in degrees Celsius. + = increased; 0 = no response.

person reflexly produces heat by shivering. This reduces heat loss by vasoconstriction, and the sweat response is also stopped. In the other person with exercise-induced hyperthermia, heat loss is increased through evaporation and vasodilatation. When the fever "breaks," the patient begins to sweat in order to lower the body temperature to normal.

The fever response can be observed in quite primitive animals, but its pathologic significance and survival value remain unclear. Fever usually results from the action of **endogenous pyrogens** (interleukins) on the hypothalamic heat control center. They are produced by a variety of cells in the body, under the influence of bacterial products and other compounds (the exogenous pyrogens). Antipyretic drugs such as aspirin interfere with the hypothalamic response to pyrogens by inhibiting cyclooxygenase activity.

Summary

The limbic system consists of several structures that communicate with both the brainstem and cortical structures. The limbic system is involved in motivational aspects of feeding and drinking. The major components of the CNS network that regulate feeding are located in the lateral and ventromedial nuclei of the hypothalamus. Cells in these regions respond to the sight and taste of food only when the animal is hungry. The activation of cells in the lateral hypothalamus causes a satiated animal to eat; stimulation of ventromedial hypothalamus causes a hungry animal to refuse food. These hypothalamic areas have reciprocal connections with the amygdala, prefrontal cortex, and brainstem. The major brainstem nuclei involved in feeding are the vagal nucleus and the nucleus of the solitary tract. These brainstem nuclei are involved in reflexes that occur during a meal, such as cessation of food intake when the stomach is distended.

Water intake depends on the moistness of the mouth and the osmolarity of the blood. The major brain area involved in thirst is the paraventricular nucleus of the hypothalamus. Cells in this nucleus are responsive to changes in the osmolarity of the blood. A major signal for thirst is the renin-angiotensin system. Activation of this system causes formation of angiotensin II, which acts on hypothalamic neurons and increases the drive for water intake.

The exchange of heat energy between the body and the environment is regulated in such a way that a stable core temperature can be maintained with the aid of well-defined compensatory mechanisms. The discussion therefore centers on heat gain yielded by metabolism or by energy uptake from the environment, as well as on heat loss to the environment. The mechanisms that permit the body to increase net heat production in the cold and minimize it in the heat are also considered. Neutral temperature is defined as the ambient temperature at which compensatory activity is minimal, and the resting metabolism at that temperature defines the BMR. The steady-state value of the deep body (core) temperature is controlled primarily by a heat loss center in the hypothalamus. When the setting is raised, a higher steady-state body temperature is achieved, as in fever. Fever must be clearly distinguished from physiologic hyperthermia, which is an increase in body temperature resulting from an imbalance between heat loss and heat gain, not a change in the set-point or gain of the system.

Bibliography

Benzinger, T. H. The human thermostat. *Sci. Am.* 204:134–147, 1961.

Dinarello, C. A., and Wolff, S. M. Pathogenesis of fever in man. *N. Engl. J. Med.* 298:607–612, 1978.

Dudrick, S. J., and Rhoads, J. E. New horizons for intravenous feeding. *J.A.M.A.* 215:939–949, 1971.

Epstein, A. N., Fitzsimons, J. T., and Rolls, B. J., et al. Drinking induced by injection of angiotensin into the brain of the rat. *J. Physiol. (Lond.)* 210:457–475, 1970.

Keesey, R. E. Physiological regulation of body weight and the tissue of obesity. *Med. Clin. North Am.* 73:15–27, 1989.

Quinton, P. M. Physiology of sweat secretion. *Kidney Int.* 32(Suppl.21):S102–S108, 1987.

Rolls, E. T. Neuronal activity related to control of feeding. In: Ritter, R. C., Ritter, S., and Barnes, C. D., et al., eds., *Feeding behavior: Neuronal and Hormonal Controls.* New York: Academic Press, Inc., 1986.

14 Higher Cortical Functions: Learning, Memory, and Sleep

Michael M. Behbehani

Objectives

After reading this chapter, you should be able to

Describe habituation and sensitization forms of learning, and explain a possible cellular mechanism for each type

Describe associative or conditioned learning and a possible cellular mechanism to account for this process

Explain the phenomenon of long-term potentiation, explain its role in short-term memory, and describe a cellular mechanism for this phenomenon

Describe the mechanisms that lead to long-term memory, and explain some of the mechanisms that have been proposed to account for long-term memory

Describe the neural mechanisms of sleep

Explain the neural mechanism that accounts for the electroencephalogram (EEG)

Describe the stages of sleep and EEG patterns that are associated with each stage

Explain what is the circadian rhythm, and describe its major neuronal components

Explain and describe the major disorders of sleep

Learning

Learning is essential for survival, and all animal species have the capability to learn. There are several types of learning, some requiring only a few neurons and others involving nearly all the cortex. Two simple forms of learning are **habituation** and **desensitization.** Habituation is the decrease in response that occurs when a novel stimulus is applied repeatedly. For example, an unusual sound, when first heard, produces a response such as visual localization of the origin of the sound or startle. However, if the same sound is heard repeatedly, it will not produce any response. Habituation involves modification of synapses in the affected pathway. The cellular mechanisms of habituation have been studied in detail by examining simple reflexes in a variety of species. In particular, the analysis of the gill-withdrawal reflex in *Aplysia* has been very fruitful. *Aplysia*

is a sea snail that has a simple nervous system containing 20,000 neurons. The cells are very large and are highly suitable for electrophysiologic and chemical studies. In response to stimulation, *Aplysia* shows several protective reflexes. It withdraws its gill if its tail or siphon is stimulated. The pathway for this reflex is shown in Fig. 14-1. The gill-withdrawal reflex habituates, and after several siphon stimulations, the magnitude of the reflex decreases. The habituation effect is temporary, and after a period of rest, the reflex returns. Modification of the synaptic interaction depends on training. For example, in a training series, the tail is stimulated several times during a short period of time. Initially, stimulation of the tail causes gill withdrawal. When this stimulation is repeated several times, its effect decreases, and eventually, stimulation of the tail will not produce gill withdrawal. If no stimulation is applied for several minutes and the tail is again stimu-

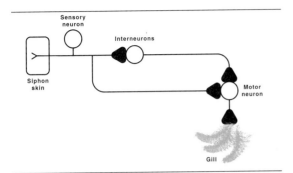

Fig. 14-1. The pathway for gill withdrawal reflex in *Aplysia* and elements of this pathway that are involved in habituation. (Redrawn from: Kandel, E. R., Schwartz, J. H., and Jessell, T. M., eds. *Principles of Neural Science*, 3rd ed. Norwalk, Conn.: Appleton & Lange, 1991.)

lated, it will cause gill withdrawal. However, several series of training periods can cause a decrease in the magnitude of reflex that will last for as long as several weeks.

Habituation is due to a decrease in the **efficacy of synaptic transmission** between the sensory neurons and the motor neuron. This decrease is in part due to inactivation of one type of **calcium channel** (N type) that is present in the presynaptic terminal. This inactivation decreases the amount of calcium that enters the presynaptic terminal per action potential and causes a reduction in the amount of transmission released. Thus there is a decrease in the effectiveness of the sensory stimulus to activate the motor neuron that causes withdrawal.

The second type of simple learning is **sensitization.** The network involved in sensitization is shown in Fig. 14-2. In this network, noxious stimulation of the tail activates facilitory interneurons that have synaptic contact with neurons involved in the gill-withdrawal reflex. The facilitory interneurons release several neurotransmitters, but in particular, serotonin. The biochemical mechanism of sensitization has been studied, and the following mechanism for this process has been proposed: The release of serotonin from the presynaptic terminals of the facilitory interneurons produces several effects. First, it activates a **G protein,** G_s, which in turn causes an increase in the activity of **adenyl cyclase** and causes conversion of ATP to cyclic AMP (cAMP). The cAMP attaches to the regulatory subunit of the **cAMP-dependent protein kinase** and releases its active catalytic subunit. The catalytic subunit then **phosphorylates** potassium **channels** and causes their closure, thereby decreasing the potassium current. This increases the duration of the action potential and allows more calcium to enter the presynaptic terminal (through

N-type calcium channels) per action potential and therefore increases transmitter release per action potential. Serotonin-mediated activation of the catalytic subunit of the cAMP protein kinase also causes mobilization of the reserve synaptic vesicle pool. The latter increases the number of vesicles in the releasable pool and thereby increases the efficiency of synaptic release. In addition, serotonin also activates a second type of G protein, G_o, that activates a **phospholipase.** The latter stimulates diacylglycerol, which in turn increases the number of releasable vesicles by mobilization of the reserve vesicle pool.

A more complex form of learning is a process that is referred to as **classic conditioning.** In this type of learning, the subject must learn the relationship between two stimuli and associate one stimulus with the other. In this type of learning, a stimulus that normally does not produce a response, called the **conditioned stimulus** (CS), is paired with another stimulus that produces a response, called the **unconditioned stimulus** (US). Following repeated pairings of these stimuli, presentation of the CS produces a response. The classic experiments by Pavlov demonstrated the nature of this learning procedure. Pavlov showed that by pairing the ringing of a bell with feeding, a dog can be trained to salivate when it hears the sound of the bell. A requirement of conditioning learning is that the conditioned stimulus must precede the unconditioned stimulus (feeding must precede ringing the bell). This type of conditioning occurs in invertebrates and has been studied in detail in *Aplysia.* In *Aplysia,* the gill-withdrawal reflex can be elicited by stimulating either the siphon or another structure called the **mantel.** Each of these structures has its own reflex arc, and each pathway can be conditioned independently by pairing it with an unconditioned stimulus (a shock to the tail). If one pathway, e.g., the siphon-gill pathway, is coupled with the unconditioned stimulus but the mantel-gill is not coupled, the synaptic efficacy of the coupled pathway will be increased significantly as compared with the uncoupled system. The mechanism of this type of classic conditioning can be explained as follows (Fig. 14-3): In the unpaired pathway, application of the unconditioned stimulus (the electric shock) releases **serotonin** from the facilitory interneurons, and through the mechanism that was described earlier, binding of serotonin will cause an **increase in cAMP** and ultimately an increase in **transmitter release.** In the paired pathway, the system is first activated by application of the conditioned stimulus, which causes opening of **calcium channels** and entry of calcium. While this process is underway, the unconditioned stimulus is presented. Consequently, an increased calcium concentration (due to entry of calcium through

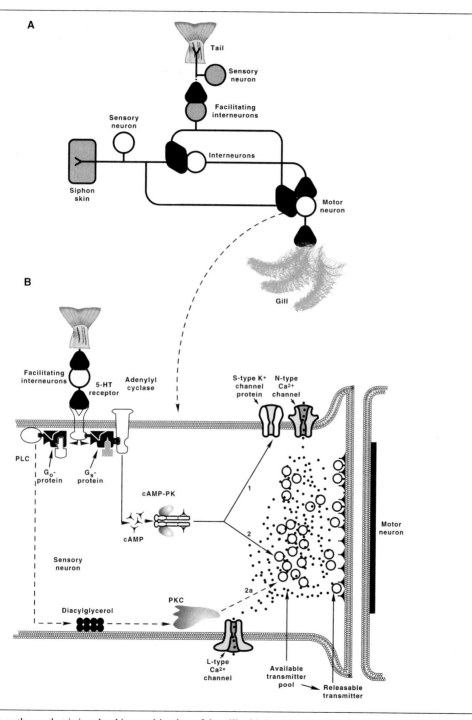

Fig. 14-2. The pathway that is involved in sensitization of the gill withdrawal reflex. (Redrawn from: Kandel, E. R., Schwartz, J. H., and Jessell, T. M., eds. *Principles of Neural Science,* 3rd ed. Norwalk, Conn.: Appleton & Lange, 1991.)

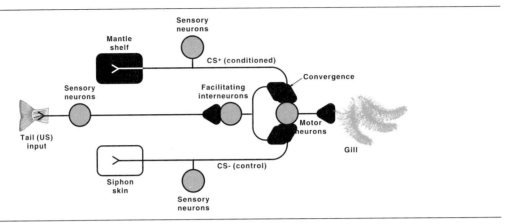

Fig. 14-3. The pathway that is involved in classical conditioning of the gill withdrawal in *Aplysia*. (Redrawn from: Kandel, E. R., Schwartz, J. H., and Jessell, T. M., eds. *Principles of Neural Science,* 3rd ed. Norwalk, Conn.: Appleton & Lange, 1991.)

channels opened by the CS) allows binding of calcium to **calmodulin,** which potentiates formation of **adenyl cyclase** and leads to substantially more adenyl cyclase. This increased adenyl cyclase level leads to formation of a larger amount of cAMP and ultimately an enhanced response to the CS. As can be deduced from this series of events, in order for conditioning to occur, the US must be applied during a short interval after the CS. If this period is too long, then the calcium channels opened by the CS will be closed before the US is applied, and potentiation of the response will not take place.

As mentioned earlier, the modification of synapses during habituation and sensitization are temporary. For learning procedures to produce more permanent changes in the neuronal network, a separate mechanism has been proposed. According to this hypothesis, long-term facilitation requires the **synthesis of proteins.** This synthesis occurs by activation of **protein kinase A** that translocates to the nucleus. Inside the nucleus, protein kinase A phosphorylates one or more **transcriptional activators.** These transcriptional activators are proteins that are members of a family of proteins called **cyclic AMP response element binding proteins.** These activators bind to cyclic AMP regulatory elements that are located in the upstream region of cAMP-inducible genes. Activation of these genes leads to synthesis of two classes of proteins. One set of proteins is a specific protease and causes down-regulation of the regulatory subunit of cAMP protein kinase and allows phosphorylation of calcium channels and activation of **diacylglycerol.** The second set of proteins leads to the growth of new synaptic connections.

Memory

There are at least two types of memory, **short-term memory** and **long-term memory.** Short-term memory is very labile and can last for only a few seconds. In the human, short-term memory has a very limited storage capacity. For example, the average person can store between seven and nine digits in their short-term memory. The storage of short-term memory relies on repetition, and any distraction can abolish it. Long-term memory is very persistent and is not affected by distraction. To store information in long-term memory, the learning process must be rehearsed many times.

Anatomic Pathways of Memory

The hypothesis that specific regions of the brain are involved in different aspects of memory storage has been proposed by numerous investigators, and many experiments have been conducted to test this hypothesis. Nonetheless, since these experiments have relied on ablation of one or more brain structures, the validity of this approach has been questioned because nearly all structures in the brain are interconnected, and a loss of function due to ablation of one structure does not prove that a particular structure is the site of memory storage. On the other hand, some areas of the brain do play a more significant role in memory than other areas. Among the areas that have been implicated in memory, parts of the **limbic areas,** the **amygdala,** the **hippocampus,** and the **prefrontal cortex** have received most attention. In this group of structures, the hippocampus is the most crucial for storage of short-term memory. In humans, bilateral ablation of the hippocampi totally abolishes short-term memory. In addition, diseases of the nervous system that damage the hippocampus produce profound short-term memory loss.

Short-Term Memory

Evidence suggests that short-term memory involves a procedure that is similar or identical to the sensitization process described earlier and involves changes in synaptic efficacy. A mechanism proposed for short-term memory is the **long-term potentiation** (LTP) that occurs in many areas of the CNS, including the hippocamus. Long-term potentiation can be demonstrated by the following experiment: If a recording is made from a hippocampal neuron and the input to that cell is recorded, single-pulse stimulation of the afferent pathway produces a response. If the afferent pathway is stimulated with a several-second train of stimuli and then a single stimulus is applied, the response to the single shock is significantly larger than the original response to the single shock. It is believed that LTP is a major mechanism for short-term memory. There are several mechanisms that can lead to the production of LTP. One mechanism is the sensitization that was described earlier and involves a presynaptic mechanism; i.e., repeated stimulation causes an increase in the efficacy of the presynaptic release. Another mechanism for LTP is postsynaptic and involves **glutaminergic synapses.** Glutamic acid is a major excitatory neurotransmitter in the brain. It acts on three types of receptors, the alpha-amino-3-hydroxy-5-methyl-4-isoxazolepropionate (**AMPA**), the **kianate,** and the methyl-D-aspartate (**NMDA**) receptors. The NMDA receptor has a Mg^{2+} **binding site** that is normally occupied by Mg^{2+} at the resting membrane potential and at a hyperpolarized state of the cell. When the cell is depolarized, Mg^{2+} is removed from its binding site, and the receptor can be activated by the glutamic acid released from the presynaptic terminal. Because of this property, activation of a glutaminergic system by a single shock does not produce any response or only a very small response. However, when the same pathway is activated by a train of stimuli, the cell depolarizes and Mg^{2+} is removed from its binding site. In this condition, a single shock can then produce depolarization through activation of the NMDA receptor. The involvement of the NMDA receptor in LTP and learning has been documented by experiments that use NMDA antagonists. Application of these antagonists to hippocampal tissue blocks

LTP, and in animals, these antagonists abolish short-term memory.

Long-Term Memory

The cellular mechanisms of long-term memory are not totally known. One mechanism is activation of genes that lead to synthesis of specific proteins that remain in the cell nucleus and permanently enhance synaptic transmission; this mechanism was described earlier. In addition, several lines of evidence indicate that **synthesis of new synapses** and the formation of new connections in the CNS are involved in long-term memory. For many years it has been known that if animals are raised in a sensory-rich environment, the number of synaptic terminals and the number of dendrite branches in that sensory system increase. These morphologic changes are specific to the sensory system that is being stimulated. For example, if an animal is raised in a visually rich environment, the visual system shows synaptic and connectivity changes, whereas other systems, such as the auditory or somatic sensory system, do not. The opposite situation occurs if an animal is raised in a poorly stimulating environment. For example, animals raised in total darkness show much fewer synaptic buttons and dendrite trees with a smaller number of branches than animals raised under a normal visual environment. At this time it is not known what signals produce these morphologic changes.

Physiology of Sleep

Our understanding of sleep has been derived from studies using electroencephalographic (EEG) techniques that permit the monitoring of brain waves noninvasively. The **EEG** is a record of the electrical activity of the brain and can be recorded by placing electrodes on the surface of the skull. The EEG is due to the summation of all **excitatory and inhibitory synaptic potentials** that arise from afferent inputs on the dendrites of cortical neurons. Since the EEG is due to minute currents produced by these synaptic activities, only cortical activities can be monitored by the EEG; subcortical currents are too small, and they decimate rapidly. For these reasons, the activities of subcortical structures such as the thalamus or hippocampus cannot be recorded by EEG electrodes placed on the skull.

EEG patterns are not uniform. The most dominant EEG pattern is the **alpha rhythm,** which has a frequency between 8 and 12 Hz. This pattern is recorded when a subject is awake and relaxed. During mental activity or sensory stimulation, the frequency of the EEG pattern increases and the amplitude of the waves decreases. The EEG pattern recorded during this state is called the **beta rhythm, or a desynchronized pattern.** When the subject becomes drowsy, the frequency of the EEG pattern decreases and the amplitude increases. This pattern is referred to as a **delta wave.** During deep sleep, the EEG pattern is dominated by a large-amplitude, low-frequency waveform called the **theta wave.**

Sleep is characterized by the absence of response to most sensory and environmental stimuli and voluntary movement. Originally, it was taught that sleep is the result of an absence of sensory stimuli. This hypothesis was suggested because animals in which the sensory inputs to the cortical areas were abolished (by cutting the connection between the cortical areas within the pons and medulla) remained in a state that resembled deep sleep. However, lack of sensory stimulation does not produce sleep in normal subjects and indicates that this hypothesis is not correct. The current view is that sleep is induced by activation of several regions of the brain rather than an inactivity or lack of stimulation.

By recording the EEG pattern of normal subjects as they fall asleep, five sleep cycles have been identified. These stages fall into two general categories, a **synchronized** (S) and a **desynchronized** (D) stage. During sleep, humans spend 30 to 45 minutes in the four S stages and 5 to 10 minutes in the D stage. As a subject falls asleep, the EEG progresses through all four S stages fairly rapidly (Fig. 14-4). Stage 1 is dominated by small-amplitude, relatively low frequency waves. With each subsequent stage, the frequency of the waves declines and the amplitude increases. Stage 4 is dominated by large-amplitude, low-frequency patterns of activity. After spending some time in stage 4, the EEG pattern changes and returns to stage 1. At this time, EEG patterns become desynchronized and resemble the patterns normally seen when a subject is highly excited. During this stage there are rapid eye movements, and for this reason, this stage of sleep is referred to as **rapid eye movement** (REM) **sleep.** This stage of sleep is associated with dreaming. However, dreaming also occurs at other stages of sleep, but recall is better if the subject is awakened while in REM sleep.

During the REM stage, skeletal muscle tone is nearly absent, and all muscles (except those muscles which control breathing, eye movement, and ear ossicles) are paralyzed. Muscle paralysis during this stage is due to activation of descending systems that originate in the pons. The predominantly noradrenergic-containing region called the **locus ceruleus** plays a significant role in this process. In cats, lesioning of this nucleus releases the inhibitory effects of the brain on the motor neurons, and the cat shows predatory behavior, rage, and grooming during the REM sleep. During the REM phase of sleep, temperature regulation is absent, and the core body temperature moves toward the ambient temperature. The threshold for arousal by environmental stimuli is increased; therefore, it is harder for these types of stimuli to awaken the subject. However, the likelihood of spontaneous arousal is actually increased during this stage of sleep. In addition, during

Fig. 14-4. The patterns of EEG waveforms at different stages of arousal.

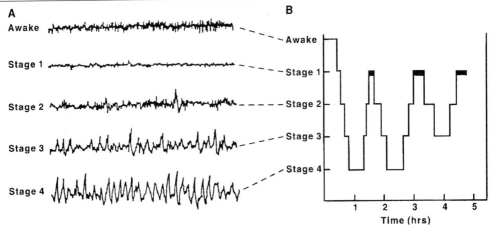

each REM period, males have **penile erection.** This phenomenon is of significant importance, since penile erection during sleep can be used to distinguish physical abnormalities of sexual dysfunction from emotional problems.

The common belief that every individual requires 8 hours of sleep per night is not correct. The required number of sleep hours varies from individual to individual and even for a given individual is not a constant value. Some individuals require as little as 2 hours of sleep, whereas other individuals may require 12 hours of sleep per 24 hours. Sleep requirement is age-dependent (Fig. 14-5) and decreases with age.

Disorders of Sleep

Disorders of sleep are divided into two major categories, **narcolepsy** and **insomnia.**

Narcolepsy

Narcolepsy is defined as an inappropriate attack of sleep. Individuals with this disorder suddenly fall asleep without regard for the time of day, location, or the activity in which they are engaged. Narcolepsy can have any of the following four characteristics: sleep attacks, cataplexy, sleep paralysis, and hypnagogic and hypnopompic hallucinations. **Sleep attacks** are brief, lasting between 15 and 20 minutes, and can occur at any time without any warning. **Cataplexy** is a complete loss of muscle tone that frequently occurs following emotional excitement. During a cataplexy attack, the knees buckle and the subject falls, but the subject is awake. **Sleep paralysis** occurs when a person is in bed and is ready to fall asleep. Sleep paralysis is similar to cataplexy. However, during sleep paralysis, the subject can be aroused by external stimuli such as touch or sound. **Hypnagogic and hypnopompic hallucinations** occur during sleep paralysis as the subject experiences auditory or visual hallucinations. When the hallucination occurs as the subject is falling asleep, it is called **hypnagogic,** and when it occurs while the subject is waking up, it is called **hypnopompic.** The hallucinations are normally unpleasant and often frightening.

Insomnia

Insomnia is defined as the inability to obtain the amount and quality of sleep required to maintain normal function. The emphasis in this case is on the **quality** of the sleep. Since most insomniacs have a normal sleep onset time (approximately 15 minutes) and sleep 7 to 8 hours, these individuals have an abnormal sleep pattern. In particular, their stages 3 and 4 sleep are interrupted many times during the

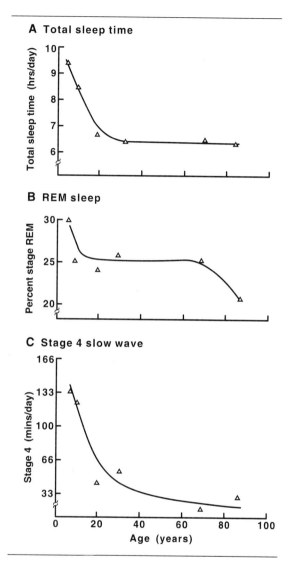

Fig. 14-5. Sleep pattern during one night of sleep. Stages 1–4 are synchronized sleep and the wavefom of the EEG patterns during these stages show progressively lower frequency and larger amplitude. Stage 1 is the light sleep and stage 4 is the deep sleep. The synchronized sleep is interrupted by a period of desynchronized sleep during which EEG patterns resemble those in awake individuals performing mentally demanding activities. During these periods there are many rapid eye movements. This stage (denoted by black lines in the figure) is called the rapid eye movement or REM sleep. (Redrawn from: Kandel, E. R., Schwartz, J. H., and Jessell, T. M., eds. *Principles of Neural Science,* 3rd ed. Norwalk, Conn.: Appleton & Lange, 1991.)

night. Stage 4 is normally deep sleep, but insomniacs are easily awakened in this stage by sounds that would not cause awakening in normal individuals. There are four major causes of insomnia: (1) **disturbances in the circadian rhythm,** (2) **emotional disturbances,** (3) **anticipation of not being able to sleep,** and (4) **restless leg syndrome.** All animals have a circadian rhythm that is dependent on the day-night cycle. Two important hypothalamic nuclei are essential for circadian rhythm, the **suprachiasmic** and the **preoptic nuclei.** Neurons in these areas have a significant dendrodendretic interconnection, and because of this, their firing is synchronized. These areas receive direct afferents from the retina, and their firing activities are related to light. Lesions of the suprachiasmic nucleus block circadian rhythm. Circadian rhythm can be entrained by the day-night cycle, and once a rhythm has been established, any change in this rhythm causes insomnia. Restless leg syndrome is a condition in which patients have the urge to keep their leg in motion before falling asleep.

Pharmacologic Treatment of Insomnia

Barbiturates were used frequently for the treatment of insomnia. However, studies of their effects on sleep indicate that they reduce the duration of stage 3 and 4 sleep and in most patients can totally eliminate these stages. In addition, they reduce the time that is spent in REM sleep. Therefore, treatment with barbiturates increases the amount of time the patient sleeps but reduces the quality of sleep. Moreover, barbiturates are metabolized by several liver enzymes, and chronic barbiturate treatment upregulates these enzymes, resulting in a tolerance to barbiturates and other related drugs. For these reasons, the use of barbiturates for the treatment of insomnia is not recommended.

Benzodiazepines are a group of drugs that act on benzodiazepine receptors that are coupled to gamma-aminobutyric acid receptors. Benzodiazepines decrease the sleep onset time and increase the duration of sleep. However, they reduce the duration of stage 4 sleep. In addition, all diazepams are addictive. Since these agents decrease stage 4 sleep, they are used in behavioral disturbances that are associated with sleep.

Behavioral Disorders Associated with Sleep

There are four major disorders associated with sleep. **Nocturnal enuresis,** or **bed wetting,** is common among young children, and its incidence declines with age. The incidence of bed wetting is much higher in boys than in girls. **Somnambulism,** or **sleep walking,** is a disorder in which patients get up and get out of the bed and move around as if they were awake. During sleep walking episodes, these patients can perform complex tasks such as operating appliances. **Night terror** affects children, and its incidence declines with age. Very few adults are affected by night terrors. **Nightmare** affects adults and is not age-dependent. **Sleep apnea** is a condition in which breathing stops for 1 or 2 minutes. There are two types of sleep apnea, **central** and **obstructive.** Central sleep apnea occurs when the medullary respiratory centers do not drive the respiratory muscles. Patients afflicted with this type of apnea stop breathing for a period of 1 or 2 minutes. During this period, the blood CO_2 concentration increases, and when its concentration reaches a very high level, it activates the respiratory center and the patient breathes. After several minutes of normal breathing, the process is repeated again. A patient can have as many as 500 episodes of sleep apnea per night. This type of disorder may be a cause of **sudden infant death syndrome** (SIDS). Obstructive apnea is caused by the collapse of the upper respiratory pathways. The collapse of these airways is due to total relaxation of these muscles during stage 4 of sleep. Once the airways are blocked, the CO_2 level in the blood increases, and the patient emerges to stages 2 and 1, and muscle tone is regained. This allows opening of the airways, and breathing takes place. Obstructive sleep apnea can be treated by weight loss or by maintenance of positive pressure to keep the airway passages from collapsing.

Summary

Learning and memory are interrelated processes that are essential for survival. There are several types of learning, including habituation, sensitization, associative learning or conditioning, and complex learning behavior. Both habituation and sensitization are temporary and involve changes in the efficacy of synaptic interaction in a specific neuronal network. Conditioning involves modification of one network in association with a separate neuronal network. Conditioning also involves modification of synaptic interactions. Memory is the ability to store information that has been learned. There are at least two types of memory, short- and long-term memory. Short-term memory involves modification of both presynaptic and postsynaptic processes. The hippocampus is an essential component of the brain pathway involved in short-term memory. A mechanism of short-term memory is the process of long-term potentiation. This process involves modification of presynaptic terminals through activation of protein kinase that causes phosphorylation of several proteins in the presynaptic terminals of afferent pathways in the hippocampus and enhancement of the entry of calcium into the presynaptic terminals and an increase in synaptic release. In addition to these presynaptic processes, changes in the postsynaptic processes also contribute to long term potentiation. A postsynaptic mechanism for long-term potentiation is related to the magnesium-binding properties of NMDA receptors for glutamic acid. Long-term memory involves synthesis of new proteins and formation of new synaptic contacts.

Sleep is essential for normal living. Induction of sleep is due to activation of regions within the reticular activating system. Sleep can be monitored by recording the electrical activity of the brain by placing electrodes on the surface of the skull. The records of these activities is the electroencephalogram (EEG). Sleep can be classified by the EEG patterns. Five stages of sleep have been defined. Stages 1 through 4 show synchronized EEG patterns, and with progressive stages, the EEG patterns show progressively lower frequency and higher amplitude. Stage 4, which is the deepest stage of sleep, is dominated by low-frequency, large-amplitude EEG patterns referred to as delta waves. Synchronized sleep is interrupted periodically by desynchronized periods that last 15 to 30 minutes. In this stage, EEG patterns show high-frequency, small-amplitude waveforms that resemble the waking EEG patterns. In this phase there are rapid eye movements, and therefore, this stage is referred to as REM sleep. The amount of sleep and the period of stage 4 sleep decline with age.

A serious disorder of sleep is narcolepsy. In this condition, patients fall asleep at inappropriate times. They lose all muscle tone and fall. Another sleep disorder is insomnia. Insomnia is a condition in which the quality of sleep is not sufficient for normal living. Although there are many causes of insomnia, emotional disturbances are the most significant. Sleep cycles are due to a circadian rhythm. An essential component of circadian rhythm is the supraoptic and preoptic thalamic nuclei that receive direct input from the retina. Circadian rhythm can be trained by the dark-light cycle. A disturbance of the circadian rhythm can cause insomnia.

There are several behavioral disorders that are associated with sleep. These include nocturnal enuresis, somnambulance, night terrors, and sleep apnea. Most of these disorders occur in stage 4 of sleep and can be treated by drugs that reduce the time spent in stage 4.

Bibliography

Baghdoyan, H. A., Spotts, J. L., Snider, S. G. Simultaneous pontine and basal forebrain microinjection of carbachol supress REM sleep. *J. Neurosci.* 13:227–240, 1993.

Hawkins, R. D., Kandel, E. R., and Siegelbaum, S. A. Learning to modulate transmitter release: themes and variation in synaptic plasticity. *Ann. Rev. Neurosci.* 16:625–665, 1993.

Kandel, E. R. and Schwartz, J. H. Molecular biology of learning: Modulation of transmitter release. *Science* 218:433–443, 1992.

Steriade, M., and McCarley, R. W. *Brainstem Control of Wakefulness and Sleep.* London: Plenum Press, 1990.

15 Autonomic Nervous System

Edward S. Redgate

Objectives

After reading this chapter, you should be able to

Compare the structural features distinguishing the somatic and autonomic nervous systems

Describe how an autonomic reflex pathway is organized at cranial levels and at the thoracolumbar and sacral levels of the spinal cord

Explain how integration of signals may occur at synapses in the ganglia and at neuroeffector junctions

Describe the distinguishing characteristics of the enteric nervous system

Identify the neurosecretory functions of the hypothalamic output to the pituitary gland

Identify the different forms of synergism and antagonism that occur in interactions between the sympathetic and parasympathetic outflows

Compare the classic and modern views of neurotransmission and receptor activation

Describe the operation of the baroreceptor reflex pathways controlling the activity of the sinoatrial and atrioventricular nodes and the atria and ventricles of the heart

Describe the autonomic outflow to vascular smooth muscle

Describe the innervation of pelvic organs by somatic, thoracolumbar, and sacral nerves

Explain how visceral innervation plays a role in controlling genital functions, micturition, and defecation, and compare their salient features

Peripheral Autonomic Nervous System

When an action potential is generated in a motor nerve to skeletal muscle, the ensuing events are very predictable. Depolarization of the nerve terminals of a skeletal muscle motor unit results in a release of acetylcholine, which binds to nicotinic cholinergic receptors in the motor end-plate region. The resulting motor end-plate potentials of the skeletal muscle fibers induce action potentials in the skeletal muscle fibers of the motor unit, and these muscle cells shorten. When one considers a comparable sequence of events in the **peripheral autonomic nervous system** (ANS), although the action potential conduction in the nerve fibers is similar, there are significant differences in

each of the other events in the motor pathway that render the outcome less certain. Inasmuch as the ANS plays an important role in the control of body functions, it is important to understand the differences in the output pathways of the somatic and ANS (Table 15-1).

The peripheral ANS possesses several distinctive features:

1. It consists of craniosacral (hypothalamus, the brainstem, and sacral spinal cord) and thoracolumbar outputs.
2. It innervates smooth muscle, the heart, and glands, as well as the enteric nervous system (ENS), which innervates the gastrointestinal tract.
3. The efferent pathway consists of two neurons in series, so there is a neuron cell body located along the efferent

Table 15-1. Comparison of Somatic and Autonomic Nervous System

Somatic Nervous System	Autonomic Nervous System
OUTPUT NEURONS	
Brainstem	Hypothalamus
Spinal cord	Brainstem
	Thoracolumbar spinal cord
	Sacral spinal cord
	Enteric system
TYPE OF OUTPUT	
Cranial somatic or ventral horn cells of spinal cord to slow or fast skeletal muscle fibers	Hypothalamic secretory neuron
	Postganglionic neuron
	Enteric system motor neuron
	Andrenal medullary chromaffin cell
SECRETIONS FOR TARGET ORGANS	
Acetylcholine	Hypothalamic releasing factors
	Pituitary hormones
	Acetylcholine
	Norepinephrine
	Nonadrenergic, noncholinergic
POSTSYNAPTIC RECEPTORS	
Skeletal muscle nicotinic cholinergic	Ganglionic nicotinic cholinergic
	Muscarinic cholinergic
	Alpha and beta adrenergic
	Nonadrenergic, noncholinergic
TARGET ORGAN RESPONSE	
Skeletal muscle shortens	Smooth muscle contracts or relaxes
	Cardiac performance increases or decreases
	Gland secretion increases or decreases

pathway to the visceral target organs. The efferent pathway to the gastrointestinal system includes additional neurons in the ENS.

4. The nerve cell bodies in these efferent pathways are located in ganglionated chains lying alongside the vertebral column or in ganglia and plexuses in the abdomen or close to and even in the walls of the target organ innervated.

5. It plays a major role in homeostasis but also controls nonhomeostatic organs, such as the reproductive system.

6. Unlike the somatic nervous system, whose output to skeletal muscle is phasic and undergoes periods of repose, the ANS output to many visceral organs is continuous (tonic).

7. ANS activity changes in anticipation of demands.

8. The output of the ANS is coordinated with somatic activity to provide supportive visceral function (e.g., blood flow).

Brief History of Our Knowledge of Visceral Innervation

In dissections performed by early anatomists, the highly visible white fibers linking the visceral organs were named **nerves** (from *nervus,* meaning "sinew"). Galen (about A.D. 130–200) proposed that these sinewy fibers contained channels through which animal spirits flowed from one organ to another, thereby establishing a "sympathy" of interaction among visceral organs. Winslow (1669–1760) thought that these visceral "sympathies" were regulated by the chains of ganglia located anterolateral to the bodies of the vertebrae, which he called "the great sympathetics."

Gaskell (1847–1919) demonstrated three separate outflows to the viscera: (1) a **cranial outflow** that included cranial nerves III, VII, IX, and X, (2) a **thoracolumbar outflow** that connected the spinal cord with the paravertebral ganglionic chain, and (3) a **sacral outflow** that innervated the pelvic viscera and was separate from the thoracolumbar outflow.

Langley (1852–1925) gave the name **autonomic** to the visceral innervation and divided it into thoracolumbar or sympathetic, craniosacral or parasympathetic, and the enteric system of the gastrointestinal tract. The true status of the ENS is only now becoming widely accepted. It is now recognized that the size of the population of neurons in the ENS rivals that of the spinal cord. Immunohistochemical techniques have revealed an ENS extremely rich in transmitters and modulators, and from these investigations, it has been reaffirmed that many gastrointestinal reflex pathways lie entirely within the ENS and may function independently of the CNS.

Efferent Neurons

In the most restricted point of view, the ANS is a system of peripheral nerves that extends from the CNS to the viscera and consists entirely of **efferent neurons** (Fig. 15-1). There are separate outflows from the CNS at the cranial, thoracolumbar, and sacral levels. The outflows consist of preganglionic and postganglionic neurons in series, and the various outflows innervate not only smooth muscles, glands, and the heart but also the enteric system.

In a broader context, the ANS is comparable to the somatic nervous system and includes afferent pathways and integrating mechanisms at all levels of the CNS. For example, visceral reflex pathways are similar to somatic reflex pathways in that they include visceral receptors, afferent

Fig. 15-1. The principles of the origins and distributions of the sympathetic and parasympathetic divisions of the autonomic nervous system. Only one side of the cranial (cranial nerves III, VII, IX, and X) and spinal outflows is shown.

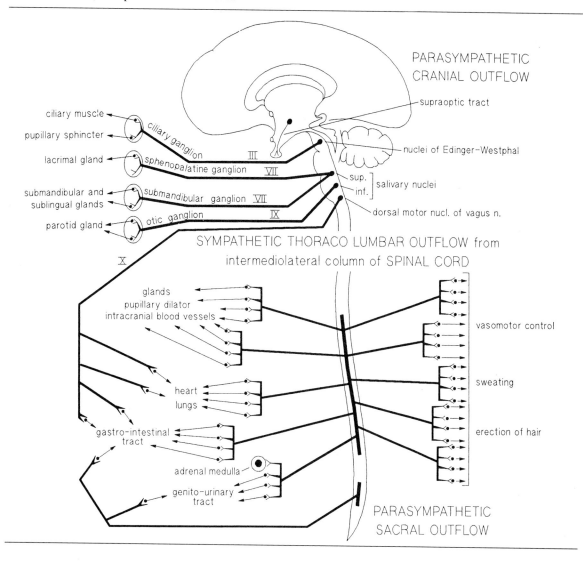

neurons, integrating centers in the CNS, and efferent neurons to effectors.

Visceral Afferent Nerves

Afferent fibers from visceral structures are of great practical significance, since they are responsible for evoking appropriate reflex responses to changes in the internal environment, so it is unfortunate that our knowledge of visceral afferent nerves is less complete than our knowledge of somatic afferent nerves (Table 15-2). Little is known about **visceral receptors,** but many of them appear to be mechanoreceptors, chemoreceptors, or osmoreceptors. The reflex pathways appear to be **multisynaptic,** traveling by way of interneurons in the dorsal horn and connections to preganglionic neurons in the intermediolateral column of the thoracolumbar spinal cord or by ascending spinal pathways to the brainstem and connections via interneurons with preganglionic vagal neurons. Many of these afferent pathways are concerned with the mediation of visceral sensation, such as pain, or with vasomotor, respiratory, gastrointestinal, or other visceral reflexes (see Table 15-2). Some of these visceral afferents play a role in the various reflexes involved in **homeostasis,** but visceral reflexes are not initiated only by visceral afferent fibers, since somatic inputs also may elicit visceral responses, such as vomiting after vestibular stimulation. The **neurotransmitters** released at the synapses of these visceral afferent fibers are not clearly established, but a leading candidate for the mediation of pain is substance P. Somatostatin, vasoactive intestinal peptide, and cholecystokinin are present but are not known to be associated with a particular sensory modality.

Visceral afferent pathways differ from somatic afferent pathways (Fig. 15-2). Afferent nerve fibers from the viscera and blood vessels may be myelinated or unmyelinated and may enter the cerebrospinal axis by different pathways:

1. Afferent fibers from **inner organs** or arising from **large blood vessels,** such as the aorta and its major branches, travel along visceral nerves into the sympathetic trunk and then reach the dorsal root ganglia by way of white or gray rami communicantes.
2. Other visceral afferent neurons from **inner organs** may join somatic spinal nerves and travel to the dorsal root ganglia without traversing sympathetic nerves.
3. Afferent nerves originating from **blood vessels in the extremities** can join peripheral nerves, pass through the rami communicantes into the sympathetic trunks, and enter the dorsal root ganglia.
4. Visceral afferent fibers in the **pelvic nerves** also have their cell bodies in the dorsal root ganglia.
5. Visceral afferents from **taste receptors** (special visceral afferent) and general impulses from the **viscera** (general visceral afferent) enter the brainstem in cranial nerves VII, IX, and X. Visceral afferent fibers in the vagus nerves (cranial nerve X) have their cell bodies in the ganglion nodosum and enter the brainstem.

The sensory column receiving these visceral afferent fibers in the cranial nerves is the **tractus solitarius,** and this is concerned chiefly with visceral afferent input from the mouth, pharynx, lungs, heart, esophagus, and upper part of the gastrointestinal tract. Unlike the afferent projections in the sympathetic system, these afferents do not seem to be involved in pain sensation. Pain sensation from the viscera of the head project via the trigeminal nerve (cranial nerve V) to the sensory nuclei of the trigeminal nerve, such as pain from tooth pulp or the nasal sinuses.

Autonomic Ganglia

In the past, synaptic transmission in the autonomic ganglia was regarded as largely a relay process, with obligatory transmission occurring as at the neuromuscular junction. However, this was an oversimplification. The ganglion cells are **multipolar** with long dendrites. Preganglionic axons branch extensively and synapse in several ganglia with a number of ganglion cells. Fiber counts in preganglionic versus postganglionic nerves have shown that the number of postganglionic nerves exceeds that of the preganglionic nerves, so stimulation of a single preganglionic neuron activates many postganglionic nerves. This is

Table 15-2. Comparison of Inputs to Somatic and Autonomic Nervous System

Somatic	Visceral
RECEPTORS	
Mechanoreceptors of skin	Mechanoreceptors
Thermoreceptors of skin	Chemoreceptors
Cutaneous pain	Osmoreceptors
Proprioceptors	Pain
PERCEPTION	
Usually conscious	Usually not conscious (exceptions: taste, pain)

Afferent Nerves

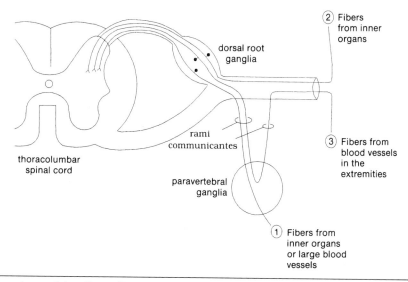

Fig. 15-2. The pathway of the afferent fibers innervating the large blood vessels, the inner organs. and the blood vessels in the extremities.

termed **divergence.** The degree of divergence differs in the two subsystems. In the sympathetic ganglia divergence may be as large as 1:200, while in the parasympathetic it may be as small as 1:2.

On the other hand, there is **convergence** of preganglionic fibers on postganglionic neurons, which is about 50:1 in the human superior cervical ganglia. The preganglionic inputs elicit a variety of fast and slow synaptic potentials in the postganglionic neuron. Summation of both these potentials, especially the fast excitatory synaptic potentials resulting from the action of acetylcholine (ACh) on nicotinic cholinergic receptors, is usually sufficient to produce transmission.

Anatomy of the Sympathetic System

The sympathetic system (thoracolumbar outflow) originates in the preganglionic neurons lying in the **intermediolateral cell column** of the spinal cord, which extends from the first thoracic segment to the second or third lumbar segment. In these segments, this cell column is prominent, and the total number of preganglionic neurons in it exceeds the total number of somatic motor neurons in the ventral horn. The preganglionic nerves are thin, myelinated fibers. They leave the spinal ventral roots in the

white rami communicantes to terminate on postganglionic cells. There are four patterns exhibited by the sympathetic preganglionic fibers (Fig. 15-3):

1. The preganglionic fibers exit from the spinal cord in the ventral roots, traverse the white rami communicantes, and synapse in the first sympathetic chain ganglion they enter.
2. The preganglionic fibers pass through the first chain ganglion they enter and travel upward or downward in the sympathetic trunk before synapsing in other sympathetic chain ganglia.
3. The preganglionic fibers pass through the sympathetic chain without synapsing and travel in a visceral nerve, such as one of the splanchnic nerves, to synapse in a prevertebral ganglion.
4. The preganglionic neurons travel as in the third pattern but, instead of synapsing in a prevertebral ganglion, innervate adrenal medullary chromaffin cells, which secrete catecholamines.

Sympathetic fibers that innervate **peripheral structures,** such as sweat glands and blood vessels, exhibit the first pattern. Postganglionic fibers rejoin the same spinal

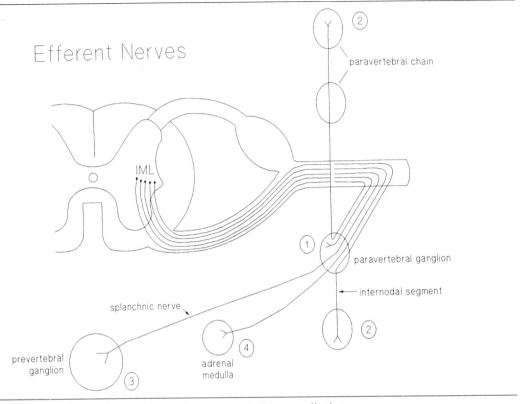

Fig. 15-3. The principles of the outflow and distribution of sympathetic preganglionic nerve fibers from the intermediolateral column of the spinal cord.

nerves from which the preganglionic fibers arose and travel with spinal nerves to the periphery. Sympathetic fibers that innervate structures in the **head** or **pelvic region** demonstrate the second pattern. Preganglionic fibers pass up the sympathetic chain from the thoracic region to the cervical ganglia, where they synapse with postganglionic neurons to supply structures in the head, or the preganglionic fibers descend in the sympathetic chain to innervate the pelvic ganglia. Sympathetic fibers that innervate the **abdominal viscera** display the third pattern. The three prevertebral ganglia (celiac, superior, and inferior mesenteric) are supplied with preganglionic fibers, primarily through the splanchnic nerves, and postganglionic fibers arise from them to innervate the abdominal viscera and the ENS.

Anatomy of the Parasympathetic System

The **parasympathetic system** differs from the sympathetic system not only in its site of origin (craniosacral) but also in the location of its ganglia. Parasympathetic ganglia tend to be near the organ innervated. For example, the cell bodies of cardiac postganglionic parasympathetic fibers are beneath the epicardium in the wall of the heart itself. Similarly, postganglionic fibers innervating the urinary bladder muscle lie within the detrusor muscle of the bladder.

Even when the postganglionic cells are not actually within the walls of the innervated structure, they are in nearby ganglia. For example, the ciliary ganglion contains cell bodies of parasympathetic postganglionic fibers innervating the ciliary muscles and circular muscle of the iris. Other examples are the submandibular, otic, and sphenopalatine ganglia, which innervate the salivary glands and the nasal and pharyngeal mucosa. This arrangement requires that the parasympathetic preganglionic fibers are much longer than the parasympathetic postganglionic fibers, which is the opposite of the arrangement generally found in the sympathetic system.

The **parasympathetic** (craniosacral) **outflow** originates in neurons located in cranial nerves III, VII, IX, and X of the brainstem and in the lateral columns of the spinal cord at sacral segments 2 and 3 (see Fig. 15-1). The divergence along the parasympathetic output is much less than that of the sympathetic output, so the response to stimulation in this system is much more localized than the response in the sympathetic system.

The Enteric Nervous System

The ENS is that system of neurons lying within the walls of the gastrointestinal tract, including neurons in the pancreas and gallbladder. It is an intricate system of neuronal circuits that controls gastrointestinal motility, secretion, and blood flow. There are both internal and external connections of enteric neurons. **Internal connections** are among sensory, associative, and interneurons within the ENS. The **external connections** extend from the ENS to the sympathetic ganglia, the dorsal roots, and the vagal sensory ganglia.

Neuroendocrine Hypothalamus

The **hypothalamus** exerts its influence on both the autonomic nervous and endocrine systems and is the major crossroads of these two regulatory systems. The neural and endocrine systems are intimately interconnected in the hypothalamus. In this section, the ways in which the hypothalamus contributes to endocrine secretion will be considered.

There are numerous examples in the body of how ANS pathways control **exocrine** and **endocrine secretions.** One example is the cranial output to the parasympathetic system that travels over cranial nerves III, VII (intermediate nerve), IX, and X. Many of the nerve fibers included in these cranial nerves synapse with ganglion cells that innervate the glandular epithelium of the salivary, lacrimal, and gastric glands and control their secretion by the release of ACh and a neuropeptide (e.g., vasoactive intestinal peptide) at their nerve terminals. Another example is the major endocrine output of the sympathetic nervous system. Secretion from the chromaffin cells of the adrenal medulla is controlled by preganglionic sympathetic fibers. In addition to the preceding examples, certain neurons that originate in the hypothalamic nuclei secrete hormones directly into the blood and for this reason are called **neurosecretory neurons.**

One group of these hypothalamic neurons, referred to as **magnocellular neurons,** has its nerve terminals in the posterior pituitary. These hypothalamic neurons secrete either vasopressin (antidiuretic hormone) or oxytocin. The nerve terminals of these neurons end at capillaries in the posterior pituitary. The hormones are then released by exocytosis into the blood and act on target organs located at some distance from the pituitary.

Another group of hypothalamic neurons, called **parvocellular neurons,** originates in various nuclei of the hypothalamus, and these neurons terminate on the capillaries of a highly vascular structure at the base of the hypothalamus called the **median eminence.** Most of the blood supply of the anterior pituitary originates in these capillaries and flows through the **hypothalamohypophysial portal system** to supply the various types of secretory epithelium in this structure. This arrangement enables hypothalamic neurons to integrate input from a number of different sources and then send an endocrine signal, called a **releasing** or **inhibiting hormone,** to the anterior pituitary that stimulates or inhibits secretion of a specific pituitary hormone. The names of several of these hypothalamic hormones are listed in Table 15-3. In each case, the primary action of the hormone is included in its name, but most of them have more than one effect.

Actions and Interactions of the Sympathetic and Parasympathetic Systems

Some visceral organs receive innervation from both the sympathetic and parasympathetic systems, and in some of these organs, the impulse discharge from this dual innervation exerts **antagonistic effects** so that the amount of activity depends on the balance between the discharges over the two autonomic outflows. The innervation of the **pacemaker of the heart** exhibits this antagonistic pattern. The heart receives excitatory innervation from the sympathetic outflow of the upper four or five thoracic segments, which acts on the sinoatrial pacemaker node, the atrioventricular conduction system, the atrial and ventricular myocardium, and the coronary vessels. Excitation of this outflow accelerates the heart rate and increases the force of contraction. The parasympathetic innervation originates in the **medulla oblongata** in the vicinity of the dorsal motor nucleus of the vagus and the nucleus ambiguus, and this influence is exerted on the sinoatrial and atrioventricular nodes and the atrial myocardium. Excitation of this output decelerates the heart rate. When the impulse discharge of the sympathetic system dominates, the heart rate accelerates, but when the parasympathetic system is dominant, the heart rate slows. The impulse discharge of these two systems to the heart pacemaker is tonic. In the absence of innervation,

Table 15-3. Hypothalamic Releasing and Inhibiting Hormones

Hypothalamic Hormone	Origin*	Pituitary Anterior Hormones
Corticotropin-releasing factor (CRF)	PVN	ACTH
Growth hormone–releasing hormone (GHRH)	ARC	GH
Growth hormone–inhibiting hormone (or somatostatin) (GHIH)	AHA	GH, TSH
Thyrotropin-releasing hormone (TRH)	PVN	TSH, PRL
Gonadotropin-releasing hormone (GnRH)	POA	LH, FSH
Prolactin-inhibiting hormone (or dopamine) (PIH)	ARC	PRL

*Hypothalamic nuclei.
ACTH = adrenocorticotropic hormone; AHA = anterior hypothalamic arcuate; ARC = arcuate; FSH = follicle-stimulating hormone; GH = growth hormone; LH = luteinizing hormone; POA = preoptic area; PRL = prolactin; PVN = paraventricular; TSH = thyroid-stimulating hormone.

the intrinsic heart rate is about 100 beats per minute, but in the innervated heart in a resting individual, vagal tone is dominant, and it decreases heart rate to about 70 beats per minute. When a reflex adjustment of heart rate occurs in response to a decrease in arterial blood pressure, there is a reciprocal change in the discharge frequency in the sympathetic and parasympathetic systems: The sympathetic discharge frequency increases, while the parasympathetic discharge frequency decreases. In view of the reciprocal changes in discharge frequencies, the functional characteristics of the two subdivisions of the ANS are regarded as **synergistic** and not antagonistic.

A second example is found in the innervation of the smooth muscle of the **gastrointestinal tract,** but it is unlike the innervation of the pacemaker of the heart in that the pathways of the two subsystems terminate on different target tissues. The circular layer of smooth muscle in the nonsphincter regions of the gastrointestinal tract is innervated by a parasympathetic outflow that consists of vagal preganglionic fibers synapsing with enteric neurons. Excitation of this pathway increases the force of contraction of circular smooth muscle during peristalsis. Sympathetic postganglionic fibers from the prevertebral ganglia mainly terminate on the excitatory parasympathetic pathway in the enteric system, instead of circular smooth muscle. Excitation of the sympathetic fibers inhibits the excitatory parasympathetic outflow to the circular layer of smooth muscle and decreases the force of its contraction. In this instance, the opposing actions of the parasympathetic and sympathetic systems are exerted at different points along the pathway to the smooth muscle target organ, and the roles of the sympathetic and parasympathetic systems are reversed, in that the parasympa-

thetic system is excitatory and the sympathetic system is inhibitory.

In the **pupil of the eye,** another form of interaction occurs between the sympathetic and parasympathetic innervation. In this instance, separate but antagonistic muscles are innervated by the autonomic outflows, and both outflows are excitatory. Contraction of the constrictor muscle of the iris is controlled by parasympathetic preganglionic nerve cells in the oculomotor nucleus of the midbrain. These axons synapse with postganglionic neurons in the ciliary ganglion. Excitation of this pathway contracts the constrictor muscle, constricting the pupil and restricting the amount of light admitted. Contraction of the radial muscles of the iris is controlled by sympathetic preganglionic nerve cells in the upper thoracic intermediolateral cell column. These axons synapse with postganglionic neurons in the superior cervical ganglion of the sympathetic trunk. Excitation of this pathway contracts the radial muscle of the iris, dilating the pupil and increasing the amount of light admitted. When the impulse frequency in the sympathetic pathway increases, the pupil dilates, but when the discharge frequency of the parasympathetic pathway increases, the pupil constricts.

The **salivary glands** are innervated by both sympathetic and parasympathetic fibers. Both cause secretion but activate different subcellular processes. However, the sympathetic innervation plays only a minor functional role.

These examples illustrate that the antagonism between the sympathetic and parasympathetic systems is far less absolute than originally proposed, and they show that the structures that receive autonomic innervation exhibit different forms of antagonistic and synergistic actions. In certain other structures, neither antagonism nor synergism can occur, since the autonomic effector receives innervation from only one division of the ANS. The effectors that receive only excitatory sympathetic innervation are sweat glands, vascular smooth muscle, and the pilomotor muscles of hair follicles. The absence of a common pattern of autonomic innervation of target organs suggests that different adaptive arrangements have occurred in the various tissues and organs of the body.

Probably no example of synergism between the sympathetic and parasympathetic systems has been so often portrayed to illustrate this concept as the **fight-or-flight response** so well described by Cannon. This response is elicited in an emergency situation. In the fight-or-flight response, the sympathetic innervation of many visceral structures becomes dominant, so there is

1. Increase in the rate and force of heart contraction
2. Redistribution of blood from the viscera to active skeletal muscles brought about by selective vasoconstriction in the visceral vascular bed and preferential vasodilation in active skeletal muscle
3. Inhibition of gastrointestinal activity
4. Glycogenolysis and lipolysis
5. Adrenal medullary and adrenocorticotropin (ACTH) secretion
6. Dilation of respiratory airways

A CNS neuropeptide may play a role in integrating this assortment of responses because they are elicited by administration of a single peptide (corticotropin-releasing factor) in the brain. This suggests that ACTH release and sympathetic activity in an emergency may be promoted by release of corticotropin-releasing factor into the pituitary portal systems and at various synapses in the brain.

Neurotransmitters

Our understanding of the events that occur during transmission of a signal at a synapse between the preganglionic and postganglionic neurons and at the neuroeffector junction is undergoing rapid development, so we will refer to a **classic** as well as a **modern** view of neurotransmitters of the ANS. In the classic view, **acetylcholine** (ACh) is the transmitter released onto the ganglionic neurons at the synapse between preganglionic and postganglionic neurons and is responsible for evoking action potentials in these neurons in both the parasympathetic and sympathetic systems. According to the classic view, ACh is the transmitter at neuroeffector junctions in the parasympathetic

system, and its action at these sites may be excitatory (e.g., constrictor muscle of the iris, salivary gland secretion) or inhibitory (e.g., cardiac pacemaker). The transmitter at neuroeffector junctions in the sympathetic system is **norepinephrine** (NE), and its action on effectors may be either excitatory (e.g., vascular smooth muscle, cardiac pacemaker) or inhibitory (e.g., bronchial smooth muscle, detrusor muscle). The visceral target organs are integrative and may summate excitatory and inhibitory signals.

A prominent feature of the classic view is **Dale's law,** which states that each neuron contains only one neurotransmitter. In the modern view, Dale's law has been found to be invalid because two or more chemical messengers have been found to coexist at most ganglionic synapses and neuroeffector junctions. These chemical messengers may modulate synaptic excitability in either an excitatory or inhibitory way and may elicit action potentials. Consequently, a number of these substances are regarded as putative neurotransmitters. Many of these putative neurotransmitters are peptides — enkephalin, neuropeptide Y, vasoactive intestinal peptide, luteinizing hormone–releasing hormone, and neurotensin — and they may coexist with the classic neurotransmitters — ACh, NE, serotonin, dopamine — in nerve terminals.

Recently, an entirely different type of molecule has been found to exhibit neurotransmitter activity. Nitric oxide (NO) is a simple gas with free radical chemical properties that is formed by the enzyme NO synthase (NOS). NO is a physiologic mediator of blood vessel relaxation. It binds to the iron in the heme of guanylyl cyclase, stimulates formation of cyclic GMP (cGMP) and phosphorylation of myosin, and causes smooth muscle relaxation. Unlike the classic neurotransmitter, NO is not stored in synaptic vesicles but instead is generated on demand and diffuses out of the neurons of origin. It is very labile, with a half-life of about 5 seconds. In the enteric nervous system it is found in association with another smooth muscle–relaxing substance, vasoactive intestinal peptide (VIP). NOS occurs in inhibitory neurons of the myenteric plexus along with VIP. NOS also occurs in neurons surrounding the deep cavernous artery and the sinusoids of the erectile corpora cavernosa of the penis.

The neurotransmitters involved in the innervation of blood vessels and sweat glands include both the classic neurotransmitters and the neuropeptides. In the classic view, control of vascular smooth muscle regulating blood flow to tissues is regarded as arising through alterations in vasoconstrictor neural activity mediated by NE and the local concentration of vasodilator metabolites. In the modern view, besides the classic adrenergic nerves, vasodilator nerves containing neither NE nor ACh (called **nonadrenergic, noncholinergic nerves**) supply a wide variety of vascular beds and can produce local hyperemia. According to this modern view, two of the most active are NO and VIP. Other putative neurotransmitters include dopamine, ACh, serotonin, purines (adenosine and purine nucleotides), substance P, neuropeptide Y, calcitonin gene–related peptide, neurotensin, and dynorphin.

Receptors for Autonomic Transmitters

The concept of **cellular receptors for neurotransmitters** in the ANS was originally suggested by Langley in 1913 and states that a specific "receptive substance" mediates the actions of neurohumors or related drugs. As this concept evolved, a **receptor** came to be regarded as a specific component of a cell whose interaction with a neurohumor, a hormone, or a drug (agonists) produces a biologic response. The specificity of receptors is remarkable, since even minor differences in configuration (e.g., stereoisomers) of an agonist can lead to marked quantitative differences in the biologic response. Other molecules (**antagonists**) may interact with the receptor and block the biologic response to an agonist. The action of an agonist and of many antagonists may be completely reversible.

Two of the best understood responses to receptor activation are activation of a **second-messenger system** and change in **ion channel permeability.** In the second-messenger type of system, an extracellular chemical (first messenger) interacts with a receptor in the plasma membrane and, by changing the intracellular levels of second messengers (e.g., cyclic adenosine and guanine 5'-monophosphate, Ca^{2+} and calmodulin, inositol triphosphate, diacylglycerol), causes phosphorylation of specific proteins that may be effectors of the biologic response. The nerve impulse also may stimulate an influx of Ca^{2+}, which may regulate phosphorylation of specific proteins. In the channel-forming type of system, the neurotransmitter binds with receptors directly coupled to ion channels, and this interaction produces a change in ion permeability. The second-messenger system includes the receptors to NE (alpha and beta) as well as the smooth muscle muscarinic receptor. The channel-forming system includes the nicotinic cholinergic receptors present in ANS ganglia. Receptors differ in their response to drugs, chemical structure, molecular configuration, actions, and location in a cell (e.g., plasma membrane, nucleus). Most receptors were first identified on the basis of their different responses to certain drugs.

Cholinergic Receptors

The effect of ACh released by preganglionic fibers of either the sympathetic or parasympathetic systems can be simulated by **nicotine.** Conversely, the action of ACh released by postganglionic parasympathetic terminals at target organs can be simulated by **muscarine.** The selective action of nicotine and muscarine is convincing evidence for the presence of two types of receptors for ACh — the nicotinic type at ganglia and the muscarinic type at target organs. There are drugs that are specific antagonists of nicotinic receptors (hexamethonium) and muscarinic receptors (atropine). Activation of nicotinic receptors in the autonomic ganglia produces fast excitatory postsynaptic potentials of the ganglionic neurons that elicit nerve impulses in the postganglionic neuron. Activation of muscarinic receptors at neuroeffector junctions may be either excitatory or inhibitory, depending on the effector. At the neuroeffector junctions in smooth muscle, subthreshold excitatory (excitatory junction potentials) or inhibitory (inhibitory junction potentials) effects may be observed that can summate to produce a greater or lesser effect. Summation of junction potentials of like sign increases the excitatory or inhibitory effects, while summation of junction potentials of unlike sign decreases the effect.

The nicotinic cholinergic receptor is a large protein consisting of five subunits (alpha$_1$, alpha$_2$, beta, gamma, delta) that span the cell membrane. The two alpha subunits are the primary recognition sites for ACh. When each alpha subunit is occupied by an ACh molecule, a rapid conformational change of the receptor occurs, so an aqueous channel is formed which permits fluxes of both Na^+ and K^+ (inward Na^+, outward K^+). Initially, inward Na^+ flux exceeds outward K^+ flux, and the membrane depolarizes. The duration of the channel opening is about 1 millisecond. In the presence of an agonist, the frequency of opening of the channels increases, while the frequency decreases in the presence of a competitive antagonist. With each channel opening, a square-wave pulse of current carried by the cations crosses the cell membrane.

The sites of action and effects of the cholinergic receptors are summarized in Table 15-4.

Adrenergic Receptors

As with the innervation of target organs by the parasympathetic system, the innervation of target organs by the sympathetic system may exert either excitatory or inhibitory actions. An early explanation of this dual response to adrenergic stimulation, popular in the 1930s and 1940s, was that there were two substances — sympathin E and sympathin I — that mediated these excitatory or inhibitory

Table 15-4. Cholinergic Stimulation

Tissue	Receptors	Action	Response
Sinoatrial node of the heart	Muscarinic	↓ Depolarization	↓ Heart rate
Postganglionic parasympathetic neurons of the enteric system	Nicotinic	↑ Discharge	↑ Motility ↑ Secretion
Smooth muscle of bronchi	Muscarinic	↑ Constriction	↑ Air flow resistance

actions through a single receptor. Contradicting this explanation were findings from experiments that showed the pressor response to intravenous epinephrine could be reversed by certain types of adrenergic antagonists. In 1948, Ahlquist proposed that adrenergic receptors could be divided into two types, alpha and beta, which could be distinguished by their relative sensitivity to adrenergic agents and by the actions of pharmacologic blocking agents. Each of these receptor types has subsequently been divided into two subtypes: alpha$_1$, alpha$_2$, beta$_1$, and beta$_2$.

Alpha receptors are responsible for the contractile responses of the spleen, vascular smooth muscle, sphincter muscles of the gastrointestinal tract and bladder, and radial iris muscle. Antagonists for alpha receptors are phentolamine (alpha nonselective), prazosin (alpha$_1$ selective), and rauwolscine (alpha$_2$ selective).

Beta receptors are responsible for adrenergic mediation of increased heart rate and force (beta$_1$), relaxation of bronchiolar smooth muscle (beta$_2$), and inhibition of the parasympathetic excitatory input to the ENS innervating gastrointestinal smooth muscle (beta$_2$). Examples of beta-receptor blockers are propranolol (beta nonselective), metoprolol (beta$_1$ selective), and butoxamine (beta$_2$ selective).

The sites of action and effects of the adrenergic receptors are summarized in Table 15-5.

Central Autonomic Nervous System

Neural Control of Cardiac Function and Vasomotion

Autonomic Pathways to the Heart and Neural Control of Cardiac Function

The heart has an autogenic rate that is modulated by tonic discharge of both divisions of the autonomic nervous system. When this tonic discharge of the vagal innervation is removed, the heart rate increases to a rate greater than the resting rate. On the other hand, when the tonic discharge of the sympathetic innervation is removed, the heart rate slows to less than the resting rate. The **autogenic rhythm** of the heart is greater than the resting rate. Under resting conditions, there is a dominant vagal tone that causes the heart to beat slower than its intrinsic rhythm.

Sympathetic Innervation

The preganglionic sympathetic outflow to the heart originates in the upper eight thoracic segments of the spinal cord (Fig. 15-4A). The preganglionic fibers emerge in the **white rami communicantes** of the upper thoracic segments and enter the sympathetic trunk. Synaptic terminations of preganglionic cardiac sympathetic fibers may exist in the upper thoracic ganglia, including the stellate ganglia (a fusion of the first thoracic ganglion and the inferior cervical ganglion; rarely the second thoracic ganglion is also fused) and the superior, middle, intermediate (also called **vertebral**), and inferior cervical ganglia. The postganglionic fibers enter a complicated **cardiac plexus** at the base of the heart beneath the arch of the aorta.

Parasympathetic Innervation

The preganglionic parasympathetic fibers are located in the **dorsal motor nucleus** of the vagus or the **nucleus ambiguus,** or both. The preganglionic parasympathetic fibers travel in the vagus nerves and join the cardiac plexus containing the synapses between vagal preganglionic and postganglionic neurons.

Innervation of the Sinoatrial and Atrioventricular Nodes

The sinoatrial and atrioventricular nodes are innervated by both sympathetic and vagal fibers from the cardiac plexus, but although the left and right sympathetic innervations of these structures are relatively uniform, the left and right vagal fibers are not distributed equally to these two nodes. The **sinoatrial node** is primarily innervated by fibers in the right vagus, and the **atrioventricular node** is primarily

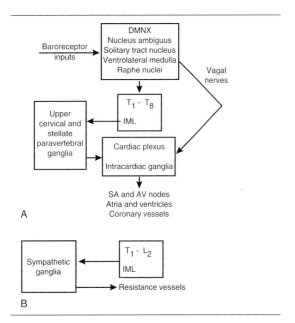

Fig. 15-4. (A) The major anatomic structures of the carotid sinus baroreceptor reflex pathway involved in innervation of the heart. The output from the integrating centers in the brainstem is divided into a parasympathetic pathway of vagal preganglionic fibers and a descending spinal pathway to the thoracic sympathetic preganglionic cells in the intermediolateral column (IML) of spinal segments T1 to T8. The postganglionic fibers of the sympathetic and parasympathetic outputs innervate the sinoatrial (SA) and atrioventricular (AV) nodes of the heart (DMN X = dorsal motor nucleus; N. ambig. = nucleus ambiguus). (B) The sympathetic fiber innervation of the vascular smooth muscle of the resistance vessels. This outflow originates in the intermediolateral column of spinal segments T1 to L2 and projects to ganglion cells in paravertebral and prevertebral ganglia.

innervated by fibers in the left vagus, so the dominant effect of right vagal stimulation is cardiac deceleration and the dominant effect of left vagal stimulation retards atrioventricular conduction.

Innervation of the Cardiac Atria and Ventricles

The atria and ventricles are innervated by both sympathetic and vagal fibers from the cardiac plexus, but the vagal innervation is distributed unevenly. Sympathetic activity strongly affects the atria and ventricles. It increases atrial and ventricular contractility, coronary blood flow, and cardiac output. The vagal fibers are much more densely distributed in the atria than in the ventricles. Vagal stimulation causes a small reduction in ventricular contractility and a large reduction in atrial contractility. Because the postganglionic sympathetic and vagal nerve terminals lie very close to one another within the walls of the heart, complex interactions occur between them. There is cholinergically mediated inhibition of norepinephrine (NE) release from the sympathetic nerve terminals and interactions between second-messenger systems of the myocardial cells.

Neural Control of Systemic Blood Vessels

Perfusion of individual tissues and organs as they perform their diverse tasks requires continuous adjustment of the **resistance to flow** of each vascular bed so that the desired flow is obtained. The cardiovascular system maintains a constant systemic arterial pressure despite alterations in resistance of various vascular regions by adjusting the resistance in other vascular beds and the cardiac output in a compensatory direction. These changes in resistance are primarily due to adjustments in the caliber of the arteri-

Table 15-5. Adrenergic Stimulation

Tissue	Receptors	Action	Response
Heart	Beta$_1$	↑ Heart rate ↑ Force	↑ Cardiac output
Arteries	Alpha$_1$	↑ Constriction in skin, kidney, mesentery	↑ Resistance
	Beta$_2$	↑ Dilation	↓ Resistance
Veins	Alpha$_1$	↓ Compliance	↑ Venous return
Bronchi	Beta$_2$	↑ Dilation	↓ Air flow resistance
Liver	Beta	↑ Glycogenolysis	↑ Blood sugar
Fat	Beta	↑ Lipolysis	↑ Blood free fatty acids

oles. This is accomplished by the CNS, which integrates information from both the **baroreceptors** and the CNS so that the autonomic output to the cardiovascular system may be apprised of current and anticipated requirements. Noradrenergic nerves play a key role in reflex regulation of the resistance vessels. In the classic view, an increase in adrenergic sympathetic activity results in vasoconstriction, and a decrease results in vasodilation. Recently, it has been found that an endothelium-dependent relaxing factor (EDRF) shown to be NO and the neuropeptide VIP are involved in producing vasodilation. NO is also released by nerves in the cerebral vasculature, the myenteric plexus, the posterior pituitary, the adrenal medulla, and erectile tissue of the penis.

Central Baroreceptor Input to the Intermediolateral Cell Column

Baroreceptor input from the carotid and aortic regions projects to neurons in the vicinity of the **solitary tract nucleus** (see Fig. 15-4A). Solitary tract nucleus outflow is involved in controlling several descending bulbospinal pathways that converge on preganglionic sympathetic neurons in the **intermediolateral cell column.** There is evidence that the activity of a descending excitatory bulbospinal path to this cell column arises in neurons in the **rostral ventrolateral medulla** (RVLM). The excitatory activity of these RVLM neurons is held in check by GABAergic inhibitory neurons in the caudal mediolateral medulla (MLM), which are driven by the baroreceptor input. The neurotransmitters at the excitatory synapses in this pathway appear to be excitatory amino acids. Other descending bulbospinal pathways appear to be serotonergic; they arise from the raphe nuclei and either excite the sympathetic preganglionic outflow or inhibit it at the spinal cord by means of interneurons. In addition, there is evidence of suprabulbar components in the baroreceptor reflex pathway and these include structures in the midbrain and hypothalamus.

Autonomic Nerves to Blood Vessels

Adrenergic Innervation

The sympathetic nervous system innervates all blood vessels, including arterioles and veins (see Fig. 15-4B). Postganglionic sympathetic nerve terminals form a network of **unmyelinated varicose fibers** that are in close apposition to the smooth muscle of the blood vessels. NE is released from the varicosities as they are depolarized during the passage of action potentials. The NE binds to vascular smooth muscle cell alpha-adrenergic receptors which initiate contraction. In many vascular beds, the arterioles are endowed with both alpha- and beta-adrenergic receptors. Stimulation of the beta-adrenergic receptors causes vasodilation, but these receptors are not close to sympathetic nerve endings, and thus the vasoconstrictor effect of the NE released from sympathetic nerve fibers predominates.

Cholinergic Innervation

The vascular smooth muscle in skeletal muscle appears to be innervated by postganglionic sympathetic fibers that release ACh instead of NE. This innervation does not possess the tonic activity of the adrenergic innervation but is activated during emotional states such as rage or fear (defense reaction or fight-or-flight reaction). There is parasympathetic cholinergic innervation of salivary and sweat glands and release of ACh is accompanied by vasodilation, but this vasodilation may be due to release of NO from NANC nerve fibers, and NANC fibers also appear to be responsible for the expansion of venous sinuses in the erectile tissue of the penis.

Nonadrenergic, Noncholinergic Innervation

The view that vasodilation that is not mediated by adrenergic nerves is mediated by cholinergic nerves is now being challenged by evidence indicating that many of these responses are mediated by substances such as NO, peptides, purines, and indolamines (i.e., the **nonadrenergic, noncholinergic system**). These substances are found in nerves supplying blood vessels, including the cerebral arteries, salivary gland vessels, cutaneous blood vessels, and penile vessels. It appears that innervation by classic transmitters cannot account for all the vascular responses that follow stimulation or denervation of sympathetic innervation. In addition, there is evidence that the role of ACh in vasodilation may be indirect, in that it acts on endothelial cells to produce a relaxing factor called **endothelium-dependent relaxing factor,** which has been found to be NO.

Innervation of the Pelvic Organs

Motor Innervation

Pelvic organ function depends on innervation by the sympathetic (T10–L2), parasympathetic (S1–S4), and somatic (ventral horn cells) outflows (Fig. 15-5). This innervation controls smooth muscle, striated muscle, and glandular secretions involved in genital function, micturition, and defecation. The **sympathetic preganglionic outflow** emerges from the lumbar spinal cord, passes through the sympathetic chain ganglia, and then synapses with gan-

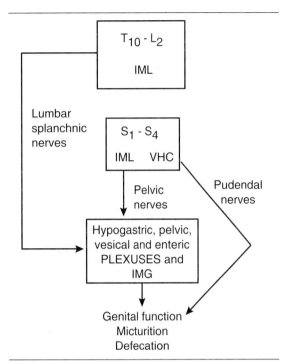

Fig. 15-5. The autonomic innervation of the pelvic organs. The sympathetic preganglionic outflow originates in the intermediolateral column (IML) cells of spinal segments T10 to L2. The parasympathetic preganglionic outflow originates in the lateral column cells of spinal segments S1 to S4 and passes in the pelvic nerves to ganglion cells in the pelvic organs. The pudendal nerves carry the somatic innervation (VHC = ventral horn cell [somatic motor]; IMG = inferior mesenteric ganglion).

glion cells in the pelvic plexuses. The outputs from the ganglion cells travel in the hypogastric, pelvic, vesicular, and enteric plexuses to innervate the smooth muscle and glands of the urogenital organs, the rectum, and the internal anal sphincters. **Parasympathetic preganglionic axons** from the intermediolateral region of the sacral spinal cord pass through the pelvic nerves to ganglion cells in the pelvic plexuses, which innervate the urogenital and anorectal structures. **Sacral somatic pathways** from sacral ventral horn cells travel in the pudendal nerves to innervate the bulbocavernosus, ischiocavernosus, and the external urethral and external anal sphincter muscles.

Afferent Innervation

Afferent axons from the pelvic organs travel in the **pelvic, hypogastric,** and **pudendal nerves.** These afferent fibers pass through the dorsal roots and enter the dorsal horn,

where they terminate primarily on the lateral side in the intermediolateral region. A number of neuropeptides, including vasoactive intestinal peptide, substance P, cholecystokinin, calcitonin gene–related peptide, and dynorphins, are present in these afferent fibers.

Genital Function

The sexual response of the male consists of several successive phases: erection of the penis, emission of semen from the cauda epididymidis into the posterior urethra, and ejaculation of semen from the penile urethra. Similar vascular and secretory responses are present in both sexes. The genital reflex pathways mediating these responses include the sympathetic, parasympathetic, and pudendal innervations.

Erection

Inputs evoking erection arise at both spinal and forebrain levels. At the **forebrain level,** erections induced by psychogenic stimuli involve descending pathways from an integrating center in the anterior hypothalamus. At the **spinal level,** afferent pathways from the penis and other genital regions that excite erection travel in the pudendal nerves to make reflex connections in the sacral spinal cord. Excitation of the parasympathetic output to the erectile tissue induces vasodilation and engorgement of the genital erectile tissue. Since blockers of NOS completely abolish penile erection in the rat, it appears that NO may be the major, if not sole, mediator of penile erection.

Emission and Ejaculation

Reflex activity in the sympathetic outflow from an integrating center in the thoracolumbar spinal cord (1) elicits contractions of the smooth muscles of the epididymis, vas deferens, seminal vesicles, and prostate, (2) propels semen into the posterior urethra, and at the same time (3) causes contraction of the internal sphincter of the bladder to prevent reflux of secretions into the bladder. After emission, rhythmic contractions of the bulbocavernosus and ischiocavernosus striated muscles that compress the urethra provide the propulsive force of ejaculation. The afferent and efferent pathways controlling ejaculation travel in the **pudendal nerves.**

Micturition

Bladder function is divided into two relatively discrete phases: bladder filling and urine storage, and bladder voiding. **Bladder filling** and **urine storage** require accommodation of increasing volumes of urine at low pressure and closure of bladder sphincters during the increased filling.

Bladder voiding requires contraction of bladder smooth muscle (detrusor muscle) and opening of the internal smooth and external striated muscle sphincters.

The neural mechanisms regulating micturition are operating in either the storage or voiding mode. In each mode there is reciprocal activity of the bladder and sphincters. During storage, the bladder is relaxed and the sphincters are contracting tonically. During voiding, the bladder contracts and the sphincters relax. Tension receptors in the bladder wall signal filling of the bladder. At low filling, there is low-frequency afferent activity in the pelvic nerves and bladder reflexes are in the storage mode.

During storage (Table 15-6), sacral ventral horn cells **(Onuf's nucleus)** are tonically active and cause contraction of the external striated muscle sphincter by means of axons in the pudendal nerve. The sympathetic output from intermediolateral column cells in the lumbosacral spinal cord travel in the **hypogastric nerve** and tonically excite the smooth muscle of the internal sphincter (alpha receptors) and tonically inhibit detrusor smooth muscle (beta receptors). The micturition center in the **dorsomedial pons** permits passive distension of the bladder during filling. When urine accumulation is 250 to 500 ml, afferent activity in the pelvic nerves increases to a high level, and bladder reflexes, if unopposed by forebrain influence, operate in the voiding mode. In the voiding mode (see Table 15-6), the high-frequency afferent activity in the pelvic nerves

excites a **spinobulbospinal reflex** pathway to the micturition center in the dorsomedial pons. The dorsomedial pontine neurons project directly to the sacral spinal cord. Excitation of this pathway elicits detrusor muscle contraction and relaxation of the sphincter muscles.

Defecation

The external anal sphincter is under voluntary control and consists of striated muscle that is tonically contracted. The rectum is usually empty, but distension of the rectum initially increases the tone of the external anal sphincter and produces subjective rectal sensations. The internal anal sphincter is made up of smooth muscle, which is part of the circular layer of muscle of the rectum. This internal sphincter is not under voluntary control and relaxes when the rectum is distended. The mechanism of reflex relaxation is believed to depend on the enteric system of the rectum.

Distension of the rectum initiates reflex activity in the sacral spinal cord and sends impulses in **ascending sensory pathways** to the forebrain that reach consciousness and permit voluntary control over the spinal reflexes. If inhibitory signals are not sent by the forebrain mechanisms, distension of the rectum is followed by relaxation of the internal and external anal sphincters.

The **pattern of reflex activity** controlling defecation

Table 15-6. Micturition

Operating Mode	Level of Integration	Efferent Nerve	Effector Organ	Muscle Receptor	Response of Muscle
Storing	Sacral VHC	Pudendal	External sphincter	N	Tonically excited
	IML T10–L2	Hypogastric (symp.)	Internal sphincter	α	Tonically excited
	IML T10–L2	Hypogastric (symp.)	Detrusor	β	Tonically inhibited
	Sacral IML	Pelvic (parasymp.)	Detrusor	M	Inactive
Voiding	Sacral VHC	Pudendal sphincter	External	N	Relaxes
	IML T10–L2	Hypogastric (symp.)	Internal sphincter	α	Relaxes
	IML T10–L2	Hypogastric (symp.)	Detrusor	β	Inactive
	Sacral IML	Pelvic (parasymp.)	Detrusor	M	Phasically excited

VHC = ventral horn cells; IML = intermediolateral column cells; N = nicotinic cholinergic receptor; M = muscarinic; α = alpha-adrenergic receptor; β = beta-adrenergic receptor.

appears to be similar to that controlling micturition. The reflex pathway responsible for tonic innervation of the external anal sphincter consists of (1) afferent fibers to receptors in the anal and perianal skin region, (2) integration in Onuf's nucleus in the ventral horn of the sacral spinal cord of sensory input and descending signals from the forebrain, and (3) somatic output in the pudendal nerves to the striated muscle of the external sphincter. The tonic reflex activity in this pathway may be overruled by a descending signal from brain structures regulating voluntary defecation.

The **enteric neurons** controlling the internal anal sphincter are influenced by sympathetic and parasympathetic outputs. The sympathetic outflow is from the lumbar spinal cord. After synapsing in the inferior mesenteric ganglion, it travels in the hypogastric nerves to the enteric plexus. This sympathetic pathway activates noradrenergic neurons in the enteric plexus that excite tonic contraction of the internal anal sphincter by acting on alpha receptors of the sphincter smooth muscle. The parasympathetic outflow from the intermediolateral region of the sacral spinal cord synapses in the enteric plexus with the NANC neurons that inhibit internal anal sphincter tone but are not active tonically.

Defecation involves (1) the coordinated inhibition of the somatic motor output in the pudendal nerves to the external sphincter, (2) excitation of parasympathetic output to the enteric plexus neurons activating rectal and colonic smooth muscle, (3) inhibition of tonic sympathetic tone to the internal sphincter, and (4) excitation of the parasympathetic outflow to the NANC neurons that relax internal sphincter tone.

Summary

The activity of smooth muscle, cardiac muscle, and glands is controlled by a distinctive outflow from the CNS called the autonomic nervous system (ANS). This outflow to viscera arises from several levels of the CNS — the hypothalamus, the brainstem, and the thoracolumbar and sacral spinal cord — and is divided into two subdivisions, the sympathetic and the parasympathetic. A distinctive characteristic of these autonomic outflows to the viscera is that there are synaptic connections to neurons that lie outside the CNS in various types of ganglia. Major formations of these ganglia, collectively called the enteric nervous system (ENS), reside in the walls of the gastrointestinal tract where they exert control over the vasomotor and secretomotor neurons and external muscle layer motility. Sympa-

thetic and parasympathetic outflows innervate the ENS, but the system is to a large degree independent of the CNS. Within the CNS, there is a multitude of reflex pathways controlling other visceral functions. These reflex pathways consist of afferent neurons from visceral receptors that make synaptic contact through interneurons with autonomic outflows from the craniosacral (parasympathetic) and thoracolumbar (sympathetic) levels of the CNS. The terminations of these outflows overlap in many of the target organs and, as a result, interact in a variety of ways but usually synergistically. Each part of the afferent and efferent pathways is characterized by the presence of specific neurotransmitters. While the major classic neurotransmitters of the ANS are ACh and NE, the modern view includes a number of monoamines (dopamine, serotonin, histamine) and a growing list of neuropeptides, as well as NO, which all together are referred to as the nonadrenergic, noncholinergic system (NANC). This variety of neurotransmitters is coupled with different receptors, each of which is characterized by the presence of distinct subtypes, such as $alpha_1$, $alpha_2$, $beta_1$, $beta_2$ adrenergic or nicotinic, and muscarinic cholinergic. As a result, the ability to selectively influence autonomic outflows by treating subjects with selective agonists or antagonists of the various receptors has become a highly specialized science.

The autonomic outflows to the cardiovascular system, the gastrointestinal tract (Chap. 46), and the pelvic organs are among the most significant in the body. Autonomic nerve discharges control heart rate and contractility as well as vasoconstriction of arteriolar smooth muscle. The sympathetic and parasympathetic outflows control heart rate by releasing NE and ACh at the sinoatrial and atrioventricular nodes of the heart, and they control myocardial contractility by releasing these neurotransmitters at the myocardial cells. In contrast, the sympathetic outflow alone innervates the vascular smooth muscle of resistance vessels controlling systemic arterial pressure. There are additional autonomic innervations controlling blood flow in specialized regions where diverse neurotransmitters are released by sympathetic or parasympathetic nerve terminals. While many parts of the CNS play a role in regulating systemic blood pressure as well as blood flow in specialized regions, a major integrating center for reflex control lies in the medulla and receives multiple inputs, including inputs from baroreceptors. The synaptic connections of this integrating center are found in the solitary tract and ambiguus nuclei and in the ventrolateral medulla. These structures give rise to the vagal outflow to the heart and to the descending bulbospinal pathways controlling sympathetic innervation of the heart and blood vessels. In the lower abdomen, the smooth muscle and glandular tissues of the pelvic organs are innervated by sympathetic and parasympathetic outflows, while the striated muscle of the anal and urethral sphincters and the striated muscles involved in ejaculation are innervated by somatic nerves. There are spinal and spinobulbospinal reflex pathways involving both subdivisions of the autonomic nervous system, and these control genital function, micturition, and defecation. These reflex pathways are highly regulated by descending pathways from the forebrain.

Bibliography

Brodal, A. *Neurological Anatomy,* 3rd ed. New York: Oxford University Press, 1981.

Burnstock, G. The changing face of autonomic neurotransmission. *Acta Physiol. Scand.* 126:67, 1986.

Cooper, J. A., Bloom, F. E., and Roth, R. H. *The Biochemical Basis of Neuropharmacology,* 5th ed. New York: Oxford University Press, 1986.

de Groat, W. C., and Booth, A. M. Autonomic systems to bladder and sex organs. In: Dyck, P. J., Thomas, P. K., Lambert, E., and Bunge, R., eds., *Peripheral Neuropathy,* 2nd ed. Philadelphia: W. B. Saunders, 1984.

Gabella, G. *Structure of the Autonomic Nervous System.* London: Chapman and Hall, 1976.

Gershon, M. D. The enteric nervous system. *Annu. Rev. Neurosci.* 4:227, 1981.

Janig, W. The autonomic nervous system. In: Schmidt, R. F., ed., *Fundamentals of Neurophysiology,* 2nd ed. New York: Springer-Verlag, 1978.

Johnson, R. H., and Spalding, J. M. K. *Disorders of the Autonomic Nervous System.* Oxford: Blackwell Scientific Publications, 1974.

Nishi, S. Cellular pharmacology of ganglionic transmission. In: Narahashi, T., and Bianchi, C. P., eds. *Advances in General and Cellular Pharmacology.* New York: Plenum Press, 1976. Pp. 179–245.

Pick, J. *The Autonomic Nervous System: Morphological, Comparative, Clinical and Surgical Aspects.* Philadelphia: J. B. Lippincott, 1970.

Schuster, M. M., and Mendeloff, A. I. Motor action of rectum and anal sphincters in continence and defecation. In: Code, C. F., and Heidel, W., eds., *Handbook of Physiology* (Section 6: Alimentary Canal), Vol. IV: *Motility.* Washington, D.C.: American Physiological Society, 1968. Pp. 2121–2145.

Part II Questions: Neurophysiology

1. An excitatory postsynaptic potential (EPSP)
   A. is a hyperpolarizing potential.
   B. is always of sufficient amplitude to trigger an action potential in the postsynaptic neuron.
   C. has an equilibrium potential at about –80 mV.
   D. causes depolarization of the postsynaptic membrane.
   E. is associated with an outward current through the synaptic channels.
2. The stretch reflex
   A. is absent in flexors.
   B. is activated only during voluntary muscle contraction.
   C. is activated by an increase in muscle tension.
   D. is the basic mechanism for maintaining muscle tone.
   E. is inoperative during voluntary muscle activity.
3. Bradykinesia would be most likely associated with lesions of the
   A. flocculonodular lobe.
   B. brainstem facilitatory reticular formation.
   C. basal ganglia.
   D. cerebellum.
   E. cerebral motor cortex.
4. Decerebrate rigidity is
   A. produced by disconnecting the cerebellum from the brainstem.
   B. characterized by hyperreflexia and hypertonia of the flexor muscles.
   C. characterized by hyperreflexia and hypertonia of the extensor muscles.
   D. exacerbated by transection of the brainstem at the intercollicular level.
   E. similar to the muscle rigidity observed in Parkinson's disease.
5. In the somatosensory system,
   A. each neuron in the dorsal column nuclei responds to all modalities of somatic sensation such as touch and vibration.
   B. the receptive field of cells decreases as higher cortical centers are reached.
   C. the areas of the cortex devoted to analysis of input from different regions of the body are equal.
   D. the majority of the neurons in somatosensory area I respond only to painful stimuli.
   E. pain can be blocked by chemicals that cause the release of enkephalin in the dorsal horn.
6. In the visual system,
   A. light causes the production of action potentials in the photoreceptors.
   B. cells in the visual cortex are arranged in columns, and each column contains cells that have identical positional and directional receptive field properties.
   C. all neurons in the visual cortex respond to a line that has a specific orientation and moves in a specific direction.
   D. neurons in the visual cortex can encode the magnitude of the intensity of light (number of photons/cm^2).
   E. the synaptic organization is present when the animal is born and is not subject to modification.
7. In the auditory system,
   A. the amplification of sound through mechanical processes occurs because the surface area of the tympanic membrane is much larger than that of the oval window.
   B. the critical frequency is the frequency at which an auditory nerve fiber has the most sensitivity (lowest threshold).
   C. there is a significant lateral inhibition process.
   D. the sensory receptors are directly influenced by the activity of higher brain centers, whereas similar processes seldom occur in other sensory systems.
   E. All of the above.
8. In the chemical senses systems,
   A. there is a specialized receptor for each type of odor that is perceived.

B. the olfactory cortex is organized such that each region of the cortex analyzes a particular type of odorant.

C. the cells in the gustatory region of the solitary tract nucleus respond to only one type of tastant.

D. the cells in the gustatory region of the insular cortex respond to only one type of tastant.

E. None of the above.

9. In the limbic system,

A. The sense of hunger is mediated by activation of cells in the lateral hypothalamus only.

B. The medial hypothalamic areas interact with brainstem regions and modulate short-term feeding behavior.

C. The feeding behavior can be fully explained by assuming that there are two hypothalamic areas, the hunger and satiety centers.

D. The only signal for activation of thirst sensation is an increase in the osmolarity of the blood.

E. All of the above.

10. Which statement regarding learning and memory is *not* correct?

A. Habituation occurs when synaptic activity in a particular sensory system becomes more efficient.

B. Long-term memory is produced when a particular learning process is repeated and causes synthesis of new proteins.

C. Short-term memory involves long-term potentiation that occurs primarily in the hippocampus.

D. Protein kinase A is an important intracellular message that causes modification of synaptic transmission.

E. All of the above.

III Muscle Physiology

Part Editor

Richard J. Paul

16 Muscle: Overview of Structure and Function at the Cellular Level

Richard J. Paul and Judith A. Heiny

Objectives

After reading this chapter, you should be able to

Describe the sequence of events that occur at the cellular level and the relevant cellular structures involved in muscle contraction, from excitation through excitation-contraction coupling, the production of force by filament interaction, and the mobilization of energy metabolism

Draw a diagram of a skeletal muscle, showing the repeating subunits

Explain the difference between a muscle fiber and a myofibril

Define and draw a sarcomere, showing the arrangement of the thick and thin filaments

Describe the relationship between muscle length, sarcomere length, and isometric force

Cite the evidence for constant filament length and relative sliding of interdigitating filaments in contraction, known as the *sliding-filament model*

Describe the relationship of the force versus muscle length curve to the sliding-filament model

Explain how a muscle is stimulated to contract

Identify the initial membrane stimulus that triggers contraction in a striated muscle

Describe how the membrane stimulus is conveyed to the filament system and converted to mechanical force

Describe the intermediate steps and the chemical second messengers involved in the process of excitation-contraction coupling

Explain the role of the sarcolemma, the transverse tubule system, the sarcoplasmic reticulum, and the regulatory proteins of the filament system in excitation-contraction coupling

List the features common to all muscle systems, and explain the role of Ca^{2+} and ATP in these systems

---

Muscle physiology has long fascinated both the scientist and the lay person for a variety of reasons, the most obvious of which is that we are mostly muscle. Approximately 40% of our body weight is skeletal muscle; if one includes cardiac and smooth muscle, the total is closer to 50%. Consequently, muscle plays an important role in the metabolism of the whole organism: at rest, approximately 30% of basal metabolism is devoted to muscle, and up to 90% during strenuous exercise. Muscle also plays a major role in temperature regulation. Because approximately

50% of the energy mobilized for muscle contraction is degraded to heat, muscle heat production can be a significant load on the temperature regulation system. Finally, muscle is a major site for storage and mobilization of glucose and such important body electrolytes as H^+, K^+, and Mg^{2+}.

The major focus of this part will be on the primary function of muscle, that of serving as the engine for the direct conversion of chemical energy to mechanical work. As a chemicomechanical energy converter, muscle is one of the most efficient systems known. Due to its highly organized and repeating substructure, striated muscle is one of the best biologic systems for understanding the relation between structure and function at the molecular level.

In this part we will focus on the following key questions: (1) What are the mechanisms that underlie the generation of force and the ability to shorten? (2) What are the mechanisms that underlie the control of contractile activity? (3) How is chemical energy, in the form of ATP, provided by metabolism and transduced to mechanical work, and how is metabolism coordinated with the energetic requirements of muscle activity?

This chapter will examine muscle structure and function at the cellular level and serve as a general overview. In Chap. 17, there will be further discussion of structure-function relationships that exist at the molecular level. Chapter 18 will focus on the variety and plasticity of different muscle types to meet a variety of necessary mechanical tasks. Chapter 19 will go into further depth on the special features of excitation-contraction coupling in cardiac and smooth muscle.

Muscle Structure

The description throughout this chapter will pertain to generalized striated or striped muscle, which includes cardiac and skeletal muscle. There are many aspects shared by different skeletal muscles as well as cardiac and smooth muscle. The differences in muscles with regard to their physiologic function will be considered in Chapter 18.

Muscle structure can be divided into two important systems: (1) a **filament system,** which underlies the mechanochemical energy conversion, and (2) an interrelated **membrane control system,** consisting of the sarcolemma (cell membrane), transverse-tubule network, and the sarcoplasmic reticulum, which together control contractile activity. The filament system gives muscle its most obvious structural characteristic, that of **banding** or **striations.** Figure 16-1 illustrates muscle structure at various levels of resolution. The structure consists of both longitudinal and transverse repeating units of the filament system. Though most of the nomenclature arose from observations made by optical microscopy, the structure is probably most easily understood at the electron micrograph level. The longitudinal repeating unit of muscle, called the **sarcomere,** consists of two intersecting filament lattices. The thick (14 nm in diameter) filaments contain **myosin,** and the thin (7 nm in diameter) filaments contain **actin.** The sarcomere is defined as the region between repeating structures, called **z-bands,** to which the thin filament lattices are an-

chored. When a muscle is at its in vivo resting length, the sarcomere is about 2.2 µm long.

The terms **A-band** and **I-band** arose from studies at the light microscope level. One of the bands is optically **anisotropic,** or nonhomogeneous with respect to its light-refracting properties, and the other is **isotropic,** or homogeneous. These optical properties arise because the I-band contains only thin filaments, while the A-band contains the overlap region of both thin and thick filaments. The A-band is 1.6 µm long and, as seen in Fig. 16-1, is equal to the length of the thick filament. A less dense central region of the A-band can be distinguished at higher resolution. This is known as the **H-zone** and corresponds to a region in which the thick filaments are not overlapped by thin filaments. The I-band varies in length because of variable degrees of interdigitation of the filaments. The thin filaments are 1 µm long on each side of the z-band.

Sarcomeres are organized into **myofibrils** (1 µm in cross-sectional diameter), which in turn form the repeating unit of the muscle cell, also known as a **muscle fiber.** Muscle fiber diameters range from 20 to 100 µm, and fiber length can be as long as the length of the entire muscle. Single muscle fibers can thus be centimeters long, and this accounts for their characteristic multinucleate structure. Muscle cells are organized into fiber bundles. A **motor unit** consists of a motor neuron and all its innervated muscle fibers.

Muscle Mechanics

Our next step toward understanding muscle function will be to describe the mechanical characteristics of muscle fibers, i.e., muscle mechanics. The two most common types of contraction are **isometric,** whereby the total length of the muscle is held constant, and **isotonic,** in which the load on the muscle is constant. Most in vivo muscle contractions occur under mixed isotonic-isometric conditions.

The time course of the force generated by a muscle fiber under isometric conditions following stimulation is depicted in Fig. 16-2. A single electric stimulation, sufficient to elicit a propagated action potential, provides a response known as a **twitch.** As seen in Fig. 16-2, increasing the stimulus frequency leads to summation of the force responses until, at a certain frequency, a smooth fused response is obtained. This response is known as an isometric **tetanus,** because isometric conditions exist. From our own experience of muscle contraction, we know that smooth contractions occur at submaximal levels of force. As

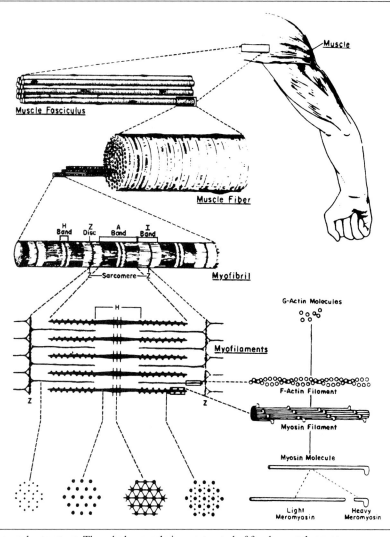

Fig. 16-1. Skeletal muscle structure. The whole muscle is constructed of fundamental repeating units. A muscle cell or fiber is composed of myofibrils, and its fundamental repeating unit is the sarcomere. All views are longitudinal except the cross-sections of the sarcomere shown in the bottom left drawings. (From: Bloom W., and Fawcett, D. W. *A Textbook of Histology.* Philadelphia: W. B. Saunders, 1968. Drawn by Sylvia Colard Keene.)

shown in Fig. 16-2, this does not occur at the single fiber level. We will return to this topic in Chap. 18, where behavior of muscle at the tissue level is discussed.

The next stage in correlating muscle function with structure involves understanding the link between the force generated under isometric tetanic conditions and the length of the muscle fiber. The experimental apparatus for determining the isometric force-length relationship shown

in Fig. 16-3 is similar to that in Fig. 16-2, but the apparatus permits the length of the muscle to be adjusted. Increasing the length of the muscle at rest causes an exponential increase in force. This behavior is similar to that of a rubber band, and the relationship between isometric force and muscle length under these conditions is known as the **passive force-length curve.**

This protocol can be repeated so that the muscle is stim-

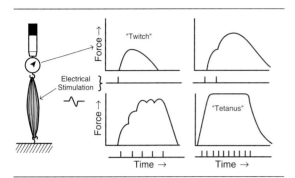

Fig. 16-2. Effects of stimulus frequency on isometric force in a single muscle fiber cell. The additive nature of the force response is called *temporal summation*.

ulated tetanically at each length. Activation of the muscle produces a force that adds to the passive force at each length. This relationship between the total force and length is known as the **total force-length curve.** Subtracting the passive force from the total isometric force yields the **active force-length relationship,** or that force attributable to the activation of the muscle. This relationship is central to understanding muscle structure and function and is unusual in that active force decreases at both long and short lengths. For most materials, such as rubber bands or springs, force simply increases with lengthening. This active force-length relation would not be expected for a contraction mechanism that involved folding of continuous filaments.

Fig. 16-3. The relationship between isometric force and muscle length. (For details of the experimental methodology, see text.)

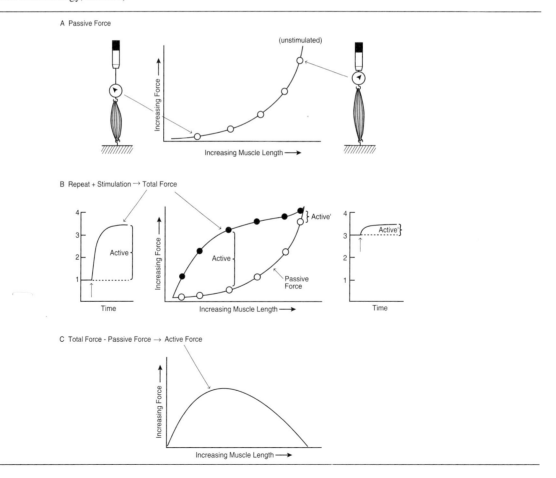

The Sliding-Filament Theory of Contractility

The most widely accepted theory of muscle contraction is the **sliding-filament model.** This theory states that muscle force is generated by the interaction between thick and thin filaments of fixed length, which are free to interdigitate or slide past one another. The isometric force generated is proportional to an active region that corresponds to the overlap area between the thick and thin filaments. Figure 16-4 summarizes the structural and functional evidence supporting this mechanism. The relationship between force and muscle length is best illustrated by the descending limb of the active force-length curve, in which both the overlap between thick and thin filaments and the

Fig. 16-4. Structural basis for the active isometric force-length relationship. (From: Gordon, A. M., Huxley, A. F., and Julian F. J. The variation in isometric tension with sarcomere length in vertebrate muscle fibers. *J. Physiol. (Lond.)* 184:170, 1966.)

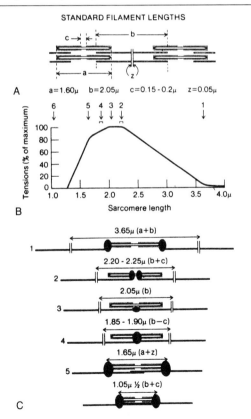

active isometric force decrease with increasing muscle (and hence sarcomere) length. For example, no overlap and thus no force would be expected to occur at a muscle length corresponding to a sarcomere length equal to the length of the thick filament plus that of two thin filaments, or 3.6 μm. The decline in force at short muscle lengths is attributable to double-filament overlap or filament compression at the z-bands.

The constancy of filament length is a critical component of this theory and is supported by x-ray diffraction and electron microscopy findings. In addition, optical measurements of contraction in living muscle indicated that the A-band (and hence thick-filament length) remained constant over a wide range of total muscle lengths. (Fig. 16-5).

Muscle Energetics

The study of the energy requirements for contraction is known as **muscle energetics.** The immediate source of energy for contraction is the free energy furnished by the hydrolysis of ATP. The protein myosin, the major component of the thick filament, is an ATPase that catalyzes the hydrolysis of ATP. The ATPase activity of myosin is enhanced by interaction with actin, the major component of the thin filament. Production of heat by muscle is a consequence of this hydrolysis. Thus, in studies of muscle energetics, muscle heat production is often used to characterize the mechanochemical energy conversion transduced by the actin-myosin interaction. The nature of myosin ATPase and its role in muscle energetics will be considered in detail in Chap. 17. However, for our present purposes, the critical fact is that both ATP hydrolysis and its concomitant heat production exhibit a similar dependence on the length of muscle, as does active force. Thus both force generation and the required energy transduction are dependent on the degree of interaction between thick and thin filaments, which in turn is governed by the degree of interdigitation of the filaments. How this interaction is regulated in muscle will be considered in subsequent sections.

Excitation-Contraction Coupling in Striated Muscle

Skeletal muscle is optimized to contract rapidly and forcefully in response to neural input, in keeping with its primary physiologic role in movement. For example, to twitch the little toe, a signal is sent from the brain, via the spinal cord, to the motor neurons that innervate the toe muscles. In response, the toe muscle contracts once and then relaxes and remains relaxed until the next signal from

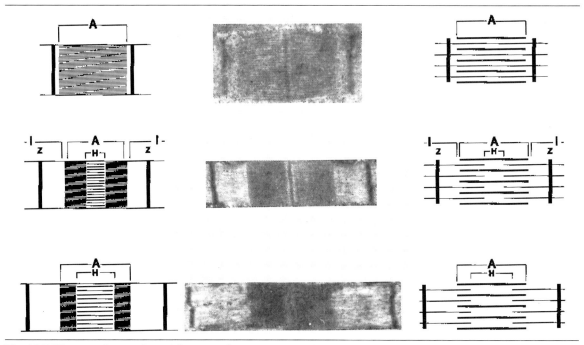

Fig. 16-5. Electron micrographs and diagrams of sarcomeres at various muscle lengths. The sliding-filament theory is based on the constancy of the thick and thin filaments (A = A-bands; I = I-bands; Z = Z-bands; H = H-zone.)

the neuron arrives. At the muscle cell level, a sequence of control processes, collectively referred to as **excitation-contraction coupling,** receives the electric signal and activates mechanical force.

To understand these processes, remember that muscle consists of two major structural systems — a filament system and a **membrane control system,** which surrounds the filament system and triggers activation. This control system is illustrated in Fig. 16-6 and consists of three interrelated membrane compartments — the **sarcolemma,** the **transverse (T) tubules,** and the **sarcoplasmic reticulum** (SR). The sarcolemma, or outer cell membrane, is an electrically excitable membrane that propagates action potentials in a manner analogous to that of nerve fibers. At regular intervals, the outer cell membrane invaginates and forms narrow transversely (T)-oriented tubules that remain open to the extracellular fluid (ECF). For fast-twitch skeletal muscle, these tubules occur at the junction where the A-and I-bands intersect (thus two intersections per sarcomere); for other striated muscles, tubules are found at the z-band level (thus one per sarcomere). These tubules branch and interconnect with other tubules. This network of T-tubules is referred to as the **T-system.** The T-tubules are also electrically excitable and serve as the electric pathway

for propagation of the action potential into the fiber. Thus, both structurally and functionally, the T-tubules are an extension of the outer cell membrane. The T-tubules link the external cell membranes and the internal SR.

Along most of their length, the T-tubules associate with the SR at specialized junctions called **triads,** so named because each T-tubule is flanked on two sides by SR. A narrow 10-nm gap, spanned by connecting "feet" proteins, termed the **ryanodine receptor,** separates the T-tubule and the SR membranes at the triadic junctions.

The SR is an internal membrane system that is specialized to store and rapidly release Ca^{2+} during activity. It has three anatomically and functionally distinct regions. Over most of the sarcomere, the SR consists of narrow, longitudinally oriented saclike structures called the **longitudinal SR.** The SR membrane in these regions contains a high density of Ca^{2+}-ATPase transport proteins, which actively accumulate Ca^{2+} in the SR and maintain resting cytosolic free Ca^{2+} levels very low (100-nM range). Near the regions of junctional contact with the T-tubules, the SR widens into larger saclike regions, termed **terminal cisternae,** or junctional SR. Most of the Ca^{2+} that is accumulated by the SR is stored in these cisternae in bound form, complexed to the Ca^{2+}-binding protein **calsequestrin.**

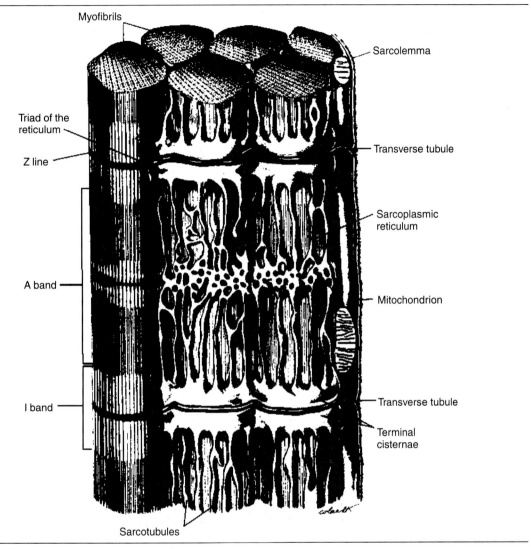

Fig. 16-6. Membrane systems controlling contractile activity in striated muscle. (Modified after L. Peachey; from: Fawcett, D. W., and McNutt, S. The ultrastructure of the cat myocardium. I: Ventricular papillary muscle. *J. Cell Biol.* 42:1, 1969. Drawn by Sylvia Colard Keene.)

Those regions of the terminal cisternae that lie immediately across from the T-system are called the **junctional SR.** Figure 16-7 schematically summarizes the control sequence that initiates contraction. It begins when the motor neuron releases the neurotransmitter acetylcholine (ACh) into the neuromuscular junction and activates channels concentrated at the muscle end-plate. These nonselective cation channels produce local depolarization of the end-plate region to open and initiate a propagating action potential (see Chap. 6). The action potential propagates longitudinally along the outer membrane and radially inward along the T-tubule membranes. This signal is somehow transmitted across the triad junctions to the SR. The SR responds to the T-tubule depolarization by releasing stored Ca^{2+} into the cytosol. Within a few milliseconds, the intracellular Ca^{2+} concentration increases more than a hundredfold, to micromolar levels.

The increased Ca^{2+} concentration is translated into increased actin-myosin interaction by the regulatory proteins troponin and tropomyosin, which are located on the thin

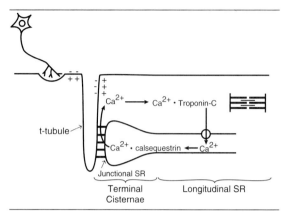

Fig. 16-7. Diagram of the membrane systems important for excitation-contraction coupling in skeletal muscle and the control sequence that initiates contraction. A T-tubule invaginates from the sarcolemma, forming a triad junction with the terminal cisternae (TC) of the SR (one-half triad drawn). "Foot" proteins span the gap between the T-tubule and TC-SR.

filament. A subunit of troponin, troponin-C, is the intracellular receptor protein for Ca^{2+}. (The intracellular receptor for Ca^{2+} in smooth muscles differs from that in striated muscle, as described in Chapter 18.) The Ca^{2+} released from the SR rapidly diffuses and binds to troponin-C. The conformational change elicited by this binding is propagated along the thin filament by tropomyosin and releases the inhibition on the interaction between actin and myosin. When Ca^{2+} is bound to troponin-C, actin and myosin inter-

act, sliding past one another and generating force. Contraction stops when Ca^{2+} is reaccumulated in the SR by the Ca^{2+}-ATPase transport proteins on the SR membrane, and the intracellular free Ca^{2+} concentration returns to resting levels.

Summary

This chapter focuses on the mechanisms responsible for the generation of mechanical force and shortening and the regulation of contractile activity at the cellular level. The sliding-filament theory of muscle contraction and its structural and functional bases are presented. The systems underlying regulation of contractility, termed excitation-contraction coupling, are also described. A flowchart of the events associated with muscle contraction is given in Table 16-1.

Bibliography

Rüegg, J. C. *Calcium in Muscle Activation.* Heidelberg: Springer-Verlag, 1986.

Squire, J. *The Structural Basis of Muscular Contraction.* London: Plenum Press, 1981.

Woledge, R. C., Curtin, N. A., and Homsher, E. *Energetic Aspects of Muscle Contraction.* London: Academic Press, 1985.

Table 16-1. Summary of Muscle Contraction at the Cellular Level

Excitation
1. Propagation of an AP and depolarization of the muscle cell membrane.
2. Inward spread of the AP along the tubule system.
3. Interaction of the tubule system and SR at the triad junction, leading to release of Ca^{2+} from TC-SR.
4. Diffusion of Ca^{2+} to the contractile filaments.

Contraction
5. Binding of Ca^{2+} to troponin on the thin filament.
6. Removal of troponin-tropomyosin inhibition of myosin interaction with actin.
7. Myosin heads on the thick filaments interact cyclically with actin sites on the thin filaments, producing force.
8. Force production is proportional to the overlap between thick and thin filaments and hence the number of potential myosin head-actin interaction sites.
9. ATP provides the energy for this process, with one ATP molecule consumed in each crossbridge cycle.

Relaxation
10. Uptake of Ca^{2+} by the SR, lowering the cytosolic concentration.
11. Release of Ca^{2+} from the contractile protein complex and restoration of the inhibition by troponin-tropomyosin of the actin-myosin interaction.
12. Decay of the tension-developing state as actin-myosin crossbridge links are broken.

17 Muscle Physiology: Molecular Mechanisms

Richard J. Paul, Donald G. Ferguson, and Judith A. Heiny

Objectives

After reading this chapter, you should be able to

Describe the sequence of events that occur at the molecular level and the relevant subcellular structures involved in muscle contraction, from excitation through excitation-contraction coupling, filament interaction, and mobilization of energy metabolism

Describe the relationships that exist between muscle length, tension, and velocity of contraction and relate these to molecular structure

Discuss the molecular mechanisms involved in the conversion of chemical free energy into force and shortening

Describe the structure and protein composition of the thick and thin filaments

Describe the initial membrane stimulus that triggers contraction in striated muscle

Describe how this membrane event is conveyed to the filament system and transduced to mechanical force

Describe the intermediate steps and the chemical second messengers involved in excitation-contraction coupling

Describe the role of the sarcolemma, the transverse tubule system, the sarcoplasmic reticulum, and the regulatory proteins of the filament system in the regulation of contractility

Describe the biochemical interactions between the isolated muscle proteins actin and myosin

Explain the effects of adding ATP to a mixture of purified actin and myosin

Describe the interactions between tropomyosin, troponin, actin, and calcium

Describe the effects of ATP added to myosin plus "regulated" actin filaments (i.e., actin filaments with troponin and tropomyosin)

Explain the effects of adding 10^{-6} M Ca^{2+} to the components described in the preceding objective

Describe the structural considerations that lead to the concept of crossbridge cycling

Describe the molecular structure of thick and thin filaments and integrate this with the biochemical data on isolated proteins to explain potential mechanisms for sliding filaments

Give an order of magnitude for the number of crossbridge cycles per second and the consequent ATP use by muscle

Discuss the energy sources and stores in skeletal muscle

Describe how contractile ATP requirements are coordinated with metabolic energy sources

---

This chapter continues our study of the mechanisms underlying force production and shortening, their mechanical and energetic consequences, and the regulation of contractility. This will be described from the molecular perspective, and the approach will be similar to that used in Chap. 16, where the cellular aspect was considered. We will investigate structure and function and then integrate the two in terms of the mechanisms involved.

Muscle Proteins

Approximately 12% of muscle by weight is protein, not counting collagen and other connective tissue. The major proteins are listed in Table 17-1. Their assembly into the major filaments and the highly organized structure of muscle make them amenable to x-ray diffraction. As such, they serve as models for non-muscle motile systems.

Proteins of the Contractile Machine

Thick Filaments

Myosin, the major component of the thick filament, is a dimer of approximately 500 kDa. Each monomer consists of a heavy chain (approximately 200 kDa) and two light chains (20 kDa) (Fig. 17-1). The **light chains** are thought to be involved in the modulation of contractility. The **heavy chain** consists of a long tail region (120 nm) and a globular head. The **globular head** contains the enzymic site for the catalysis of ATP hydrolysis and an actin-binding site. The long tail region is important in the self-assembly of myosin into thick filaments.

The assembly of myosin molecules into a thick filament

Table 17-1. Relative Proportions of Myofibrillar Proteins in Rabbit Skeletal Muscle

Protein	Total Structural Protein (%)
Myosin	43
Actin	22
Titin	10
Nebulin	5
Tropomyosin	5
Troponin	5
C-protein	2
M-protein	<2
Alpha-actinin	2
Beta-actinin	2

Fig. 17-1. The myosin molecule is a dimer containing two heavy chains and two pairs of light chains. Proteolytic fragments are shown as S_1 (subfragment 1), HMM (heavy meromyosin), and LMM (light meromyosin).

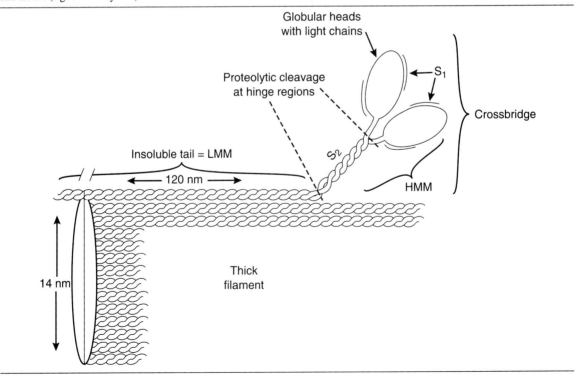

is depicted in Fig. 17-2. Because the myosin molecules assemble with opposite polarity from the center of the filament, there is a central region, known as the **bare zone,** which is devoid of the **globular** (or S_1) **heads.** This structure underlies the plateau region in the **force-length relationship** (See Fig. 17-4).

Knowledge of the geometry of filament organization is crucial to an understanding of the molecular mechanisms of force generation. Based on x-ray diffraction evidence, sites for myosin head projections exist every 14.3 nm along the thick filament. In vertebrate striated muscle, the thick filament has three strands, yielding three myosin molecules arranged symmetrically at 120 degrees at each site (like a three-bladed propeller). Each consecutive site is rotated 40 degrees so that an identical site occurs at 43-nm intervals. Because each myosin molecule contains two S_1 heads, there are six heads per site. Looking endwise at a

thick filament, one would thus see nine projected myosin molecules, each containing two heads. Because the length of a thick filament is 1.6 μm, one filament has approximately a hundred sites (1.6 μm/0.014 μm). There are thus approximately 300 myosin molecules and 600 S_1 heads on each thick filament. Minor thick-filament proteins include C-protein, which may be involved in the self-assembly of the thick filament.

Thin Filaments

Actin is the major protein component of the thin filament (Fig. 17-3) and is a ubiquitous protein found in many types of cells. It has a globular form, known as **g-actin,** with a molecular weight of 42 kDa and a diameter of about 5.5 nm. Actin in muscle has a filamentous form known as **f-actin.** Actin filaments are often depicted as a double string

Fig. 17-2. Thick filament. (A) A rendition of the thick-filament structure based on current evidence. (B) The initiation of filament self-assembly in a tail-to-tail fashion. (C) The filament viewed on end. (Adapted from: Murray, J. M., and Weber, A. The cooperative action of muscle proteins. *Sci. Am.* 230:58, 1974.)

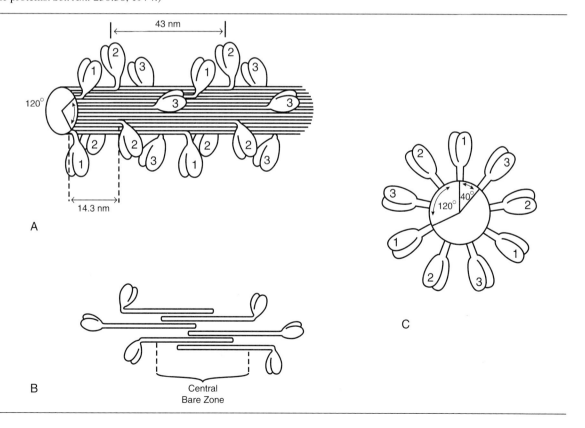

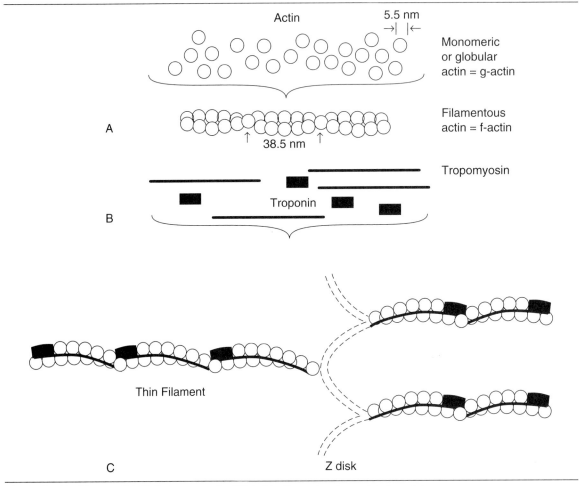

Fig. 17-3. Thin filament. (A) Globular or g-actin. (B) A thin filament and associated regulatory proteins, troponin, and tropomyosin. (C) The attachment of thin filaments to the z-disk (z-band) characteristic of striated muscle. (See text for further description.) (Adapted from: Murray, J. M., and Weber, A. The cooperative action of muscle proteins. *Sci. Am.* 230:58, 1974.)

of pearls, with a twist or repeat unit occurring every 7 g-actin units, or every 38.5 nm, though g-actin is not symmetrical. This is one of the characteristics that underlie the unidirectional nature of muscle contraction. Muscle can only shorten; it cannot actively lengthen.

The native thin filament contains two accessory proteins, tropomyosin and troponin, which are involved in the regulation of contraction. Tropomyosin is a long molecule that is situated near the groove of the double strands of actin. Each tropomyosin molecule interacts with seven actin molecules and forms the regulated unit. Troponin is a more globular molecule and is composed of three subunits:

Troponin-C is the Ca^{2+} binding subunit, troponin-T is the subunit that interacts with tropomyosin, and troponin-I binds to actin and underlies the inhibition of the actin-myosin interaction.

Minor protein components include alpha- and beta-actinin, which are z-band components, and very large-molecular-weight proteins, titin and nebulin, which may serve as templates for the sarcomere superstructure.

A high-resolution electron micrograph of a single sarcomere, which forms the basis for much of our structural knowledge, and a schematic summary are presented in Fig. 17-4.

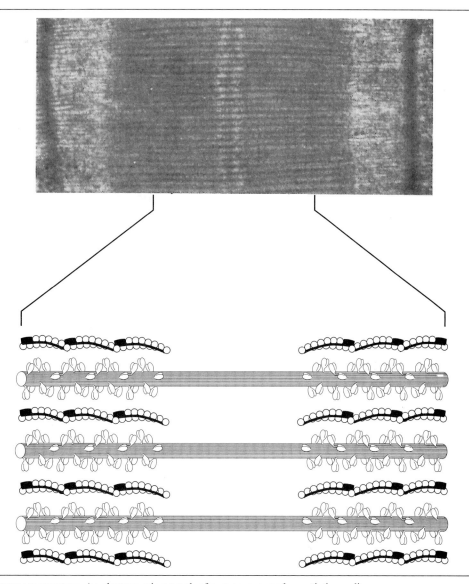

Fig. 17-4. Sarcomere structure. An electron micrograph of a sarcomere and an artistic rendition of the structure based on current knowledge. (Adapted from: Murray, J. M., and Weber, A. The cooperative action of muscle proteins. *Sci. Am.* 230:58, 1974.)

Molecular Mechanics and Biochemical Function

In parallel with our structure and function considerations at the cellular level (see Chap. 16), it is important to consider the biochemical function of isolated actin and myosin filaments, as shown in the experiments depicted in Fig. 17-5. Using purified muscle proteins, we can obtain an index of the actin-myosin interaction, based on the turbidity or cloudiness of the solution measured with a spectrometer. In addition, we can measure the ATPase activity by measuring the hydrolysis products ADP or inorganic phosphate (P_i), or, alternatively, by the disappearance of

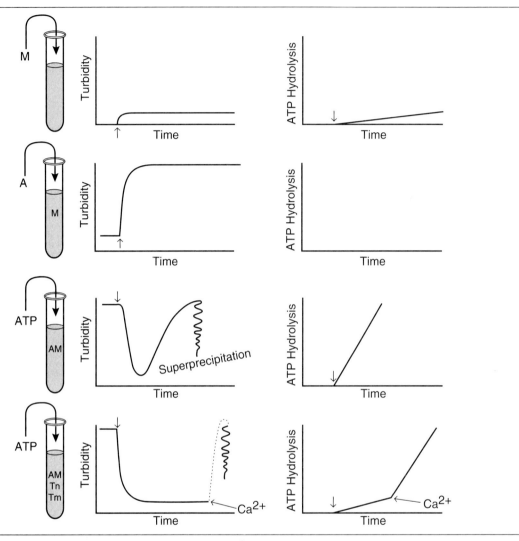

Fig. 17-5. Actin-myosin interactions. The effects of ATP and Ca^{2+} on solutions of actin (A) and myosin (M) and in combination with regulatory proteins troponin (Tn) and tropomyosin (Tm).

ATP. When ATP is added to a solution of myosin, the solution remains relatively clear, and a low level of ATPase activity is recorded. The addition of actin to a solution of myosin, on the other hand, causes a rapid increase of turbidity, indicating a strong interaction between actin and myosin. The actin-myosin complex formed in the absence of ATP is known as a **rigor complex** because of the very stiff state of an intact muscle when ATP is depleted. The addition of ATP initially leads to rapid clearing of the solution, followed by increased turbidity to the point where

actin-myosin complexes precipitate out of solution, due to contraction of the actin-myosin gel and **superprecipitation.** A large increase in ATPase activity is seen shortly following the clearing. If troponin and tropomyosin are present, the addition of ATP produces only the rapid-clearing response without an increase in ATPase activity. Finally, the addition of Ca^{2+} initiates superprecipitation, with a concomitant increase in ATPase activity.

Several salient points can be made from these observations:

1. Myosin alone possesses only weak ATPase activity. Actin and myosin spontaneously form a complex, which can be dissociated by ATP.
2. The ATPase activity of myosin is greatly enhanced (200-fold) by actin.
3. Superprecipitation and the enhanced ATPase activity are inhibited by troponin and tropomyosin.
4. Ca^{2+}, in micromolar quantities, can remove this inhibition.

Crossbridge Cycling

Now we combine the structural and functional evidence to advance a molecular mechanism of muscle contraction. How does the interaction between actin and myosin, which is proportional to filament overlap, generate force and shortening? Figure 17-4 depicts the structural constraints in the overlap region. A very important consideration here is that muscle can operate over a wide range of lengths, roughly corresponding to sarcomere lengths of 1.6 to 3.6 μm. A site for force generation on the thick filament can

operate over a distance of about 1 μm, relative to a thin filament. Given that myosin heads exist every 14.3 nm (0.0143 μm) along the thick filament, a myosin head cannot remain attached to a thin-filament actin site over the entire range of filament motion during shortening. Many attachment-detachment cycles of myosin to actin must occur during muscle contraction. This structural information, plus the fact that ATP breaks the actin-myosin rigor complex and actin activates the myosin ATPase, has led to the **crossbridge cycling theory** of muscle contraction, namely, that there are multiple cycles of myosin-head attachment and detachment to actin during a contraction. Several biochemical steps in the crossbridge cycle have been proposed based on observations made during kinetic analysis of the actin-activated, myosin-catalyzed hydrolysis of ATP, and a number of hypothetical crossbridge states have been postulated, based on findings from mechanical studies of muscle. Some of the major features of the crossbridge cycle consist of the stages shown in Fig. 17-6. It is assumed that the muscle is activated; i.e., Ca^{2+} is present.

In the resting state, in which the actin-myosin interac-

Fig. 17-6. The crossbridge cycle. This depiction represents the combined information gleaned from muscle mechanics and the biochemical kinetics of the actin-activated myosin ATPase (P_i = inorganic phosphate; A = actin; M = myosin).

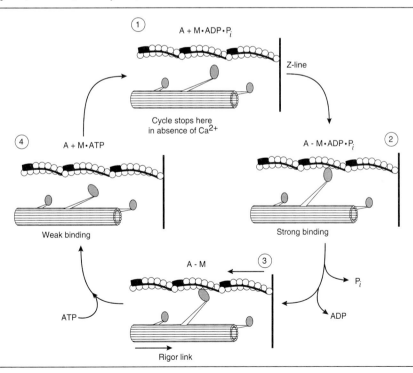

tion is inhibited by the regulatory proteins and ATP is present, the myosin heads have ADP and P_i bound. The orientation of the heads is almost perpendicular to the filament axes. Stimulation increases the intracellular Ca^{2+} concentration, which removes the inhibition, and myosin now exhibits a high affinity for actin. The S_2 region of the myosin molecule appears to serve as a flexible hinge, permitting movement of the head region (S_1) toward the thin filament (see Fig. 17-1). The binding of a myosin head to actin accelerates the removal of ADP and P_i, and the attached myosin head changes conformation by about 45 degrees with respect to the thin filament. This conformational change causes a relative filament movement of about 10 nm and underlies the generation of force. In the absence of ATP, the crossbridge cycle stops here, forming a **rigor link,** analogous to the strong binding of actin to myosin seen in studies of isolated proteins (discussed previously). The next stage in the crossbridge cycle is the binding of ATP to the myosin head, leading to a low affinity for actin and dissociation of the rigor complex. ATP is then hydrolyzed on the myosin head, and the energy from this is stored in the myosin molecule by restoring the perpendicular conformation with a renewed high affinity for

actin. A new cycle can be initiated at this point, or, if Ca^{2+} is absent and regulatory protein inhibition is restored, the cycle is terminated here. This is equivalent to the state of the myosin head under resting conditions.

Only one ATP molecule is hydrolyzed per cycle, and the free energy from this hydrolysis is transduced into mechanical energy by changing the conformation of the myosin head. One can get a rough estimate of the rate of crossbridge cycling by measuring ATP hydrolysis in active muscle. Though widely varying, a typical number for skeletal muscle ATP utilization is about 20 μmol/sec·g (Table 17-2). The myosin content of muscle is about 0.2 μmol/g, so the crossbridges cycle about a hundred times per second. Current evidence favors an independent action of the two S_1 myosin heads, but some form of cooperative interaction cannot be ruled out.

From this estimate of the crossbridge cycling rate, at 100 cycles per second and a potential movement of 10 nm per cycle, each half of the sarcomere could shorten at a rate of 1 μm per second. Thus maximal shortening velocity would be about one muscle length per second such that if a muscle is 3 cm long, the speed would be 3 cm/sec. The ways in which the speed of muscle contraction and energy

Table 17-2. Skeletal Muscle Chemical Energy Utilization and Stores

Rate of ATP Utilization (μmol/sec·g)	$ATP \xrightarrow{Ca2+\text{-pump, myosin}} ADP + Pi = 5\text{–}30 \, \mu mol/g$			
	ENERGY STORE (μMOL/G)	**ENERGY SOURCE**	**ATP EQUIVALENT (μMOL/G)**	**REACTION TIME SCALE**
ATP	3–5		3–5	Immediate energy source
PCr	15–30	Lochmann reaction: PCr + ADP → Cr + ATP ATP → ADP + P_i Net: PCr → Cr + P_i	15–30	Extremely rapid Only measurable chemical changes during contraction
Endogenous glycogen	75	Glycolysis	225	Rapid but limited energy store
		Oxidative phosphorylation	2925	Slowest and most efficient source
Exogenous (plasma) free fatty acids, triglycerides, glucose, and amino acids (in apparent order of preference)		Oxidative phosphorylation	Very large	

PCr = phosphocreatine; Cr = creatine; P_i = inorganic phosphate.

utilization depend on the load on the muscle will be considered in the next section.

Correlates of Crossbridge Cycling: Force-Velocity Relationship and Energetics

With a clearer picture of the crossbridge cycle and its regulation, it is possible to consider other important mechanical and energetic characteristics of muscle. The mechanical constraints can alter the crossbridge cycle and the consequent energy turnover. The terms used to describe the relationship between muscle load (or force developed) and the speed of shortening reflect the early experimental apparatus used but are important to know because this terminology persists.

Force-Velocity Relationship

Figure 17-7 depicts the experimental apparatus used for measuring the **force-velocity relationship.** Using the lever system, a **preload** is placed on the unstimulated muscle. The muscle stretches to the length at which the preload matches the force on the passive force-length relationship. A mechanical stop is then placed so that no further lengthening can occur. Thus the preload determines the initial length of the muscle and consequently the **maximum force** possible, in keeping with the active force-length relationship. Additional loads, known as the **afterload,** can be placed on the apparatus. The name *afterload* derives

Fig. 17-7. Relationship between velocity of shortening, power output, and load. (A) The experimental apparatus used to simulate afterloaded, isotonic conditions. (B) The experimental results yielded by various loads. (C and D) The derived relationships between velocity and load and power and load, respectively (L = length; V = velocity; dl = change in length; dt = change in time; F × V= force × velocity = power).

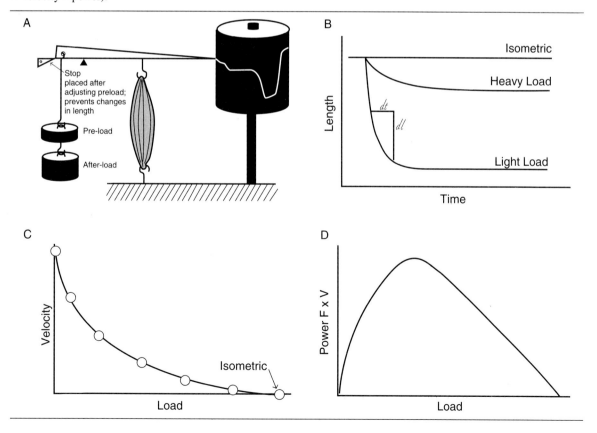

from the fact that the muscle is not influenced by this load, since it is borne by the mechanical stop until "after" the muscle is stimulated. When the muscle is stimulated and generates an isometric force that just exceeds the afterload, the muscle begins to shorten, as shown in Fig. 17-7B. During the initial moments after shortening begins, there is a steady rate of shortening, which subsequently declines and ceases as the muscle reaches its final shortened length. This length corresponds to that point in the active force-length curve matching the afterload. Both the distance shortened and the velocity are dependent on the afterload. The relationship between shortening velocity and afterload (Fig. 17-7C) is hyperbolic, indicating that the velocity decreases rapidly as the afterload is increased. The power output of muscle can be calculated from the relationship between afterload and velocity. Maximal power occurs at a load of about one-third the maximal isometric force for skeletal muscle (Fig. 17-7D).

From the force-velocity relationship, it appears that the potential for actin-myosin interaction is reduced as the relative filament velocity increases.

Muscle Energetics

A fixed amount of energy is liberated for each ATP hydrolyzed. This energy could be recovered as work or dissipated as heat. However, it has been shown that the total energy released (heat plus work) during contraction is not constant but depends on the mechanical conditions. During an isotonic contraction, when work is produced by the muscle, the total energy liberated is up to threefold greater than that for a similar contraction occurring under isometric conditions. This phenomenon, known as the **Fenneffect,** indicates that there is feedback between the mechanical constraints and the rate of crossbridge cycling.

Muscle Metabolism and Mechanisms for Coordination with Contractility

Energy Utilization

Muscle contraction is accompanied by a large increase in energy transduction. The turnover of ATP during maximal contractile activity may be over one thousand times greater than the basal rate (amphibian skeletal muscle at 0°C). As indicated previously, crossbridge cycling at a rate of 100 cycles/sec leads to an ATP hydrolysis of about 20 μm/sec·g. Other energy-dependent processes accompany muscle ac-

tivity, predominantly Ca^{2+} translocation, which can use up to 25% of the energy for crossbridge interaction.

Muscle mass represents about 40% of total body weight in humans, which amounts to 28 kg in a 70-kg person. Thus an ATP hydrolysis of 0.56 mol/sec would be necessary to achieve maximal levels of contractile activity. The heat production from this chemical reaction would heat a 70-kg person at a rate of 0.08°C/sec, or 1°C every 12.5 sec. Thus muscle activity has a number of consequences for the organism. The mechanisms available to the whole organism for dealing with this substantial heat load will be discussed in Chap. 63.

Energy Sources and Stores

Table 17-2 presents the major metabolic sources of ATP and the size of these chemical energy stores. These vary considerably with muscle type and function; however, some generalizations can be made. Skeletal muscle is often characterized by short bursts of intense activity. To meet these energy demands, skeletal muscle has adopted a "buy now, pay later" strategy. A store of a high-energy compound, **phosphocreatine,** is used to meet the energy required for these short bursts of activity. The reaction involved in re-forming ATP from ADP, driven by the conversion of phosphocreatine to creatine, is known as the **Lohmann** or **creatine kinase reaction.** Although the size of the phosphocreatine pool is relatively small, ATP can be provided rapidly. This reaction is very efficient, and for most muscle activity, little change in ATP can be measured, with a breakdown of phosphocreatine the only consequence of muscle activity. The phosphocreatine broken down during muscle activity is restored following activity, a process referred to as **repayment of the oxygen debt.**

Skeletal muscle also stores energy in the form of **glycogen,** a glucose polymer. Glycolysis, with lactate as the end-product, also can produce ATP relatively rapidly, but compared with complete oxidation, it is relatively inefficient. Glycolysis is important in supporting moderate to heavy muscle activity, characterized by increasing levels of lactate.

The ultimate source of ATP for contraction is oxidative phosphorylation. As shown in Table 17-2, the stores of substrate for the oxidative production of ATP are large. This is the most efficient source but, as a multistep process, the slowest of the pathways for meeting contractile energy needs.

The optimal performance of muscle is limited by these energy sources and rate of ATP production. Figure 17-8 shows the rate of running, as an index of muscle power output, and the time over which a given level of power output can be maintained, reflecting these distinct metabolic pathways.

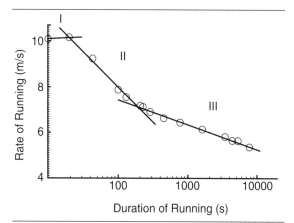

Fig. 17-8. The maximal power output of muscle estimated from the rate of running derived from world track records as a function of the duration of time for which it can be sustained. The data suggest a dependence on distinct energy sources, paralleling those listed in Table 17-2 and described in text (I = Lohmann reaction; II = glycolysis; III = oxidative phosphorylation).

Coordination of ATP Production with Contractile ATP Utilization

Large and rapid changes in energy demand are characteristic of muscle, making the control mechanisms for metabolism critical for normal muscle function. There are a wide variety of regulatory mechanisms, and the major systems will be reviewed.

The products of ATP hydrolysis, ADP and P_i, represent an important feedback mechanism. An increase in ADP levels resulting from contractile activity is a signal for increased mitochondrial oxidative phosphorylation. This is a key mechanism for skeletal muscle, but its role in cardiac and smooth muscle is less certain. ADP production is also a key control for glycolysis, since an increase in ADP or decrease in ATP levels activates phosphofructokinase, an enzyme controlling a rate-limiting step in the glycolytic pathway. An increase in the P_i content also enhances the rate of glycolysis.

The mobilization of substrate plays a role in the coordination of metabolism with contractility. Increases in the intracellular Ca^{2+} concentration, besides activating muscle contraction, are involved in activating the phosphorylase cascade that catalyzes the production of glucose from glycogen.

There are also several mechanisms involved in increasing blood flow to working muscles. This increased flow is important to tissue oxygenation and the removal of metabolic products, notably lactate.

Molecular Mechanisms of Excitation-Contraction Coupling

Membrane Excitation and Intracellular Signaling at the Triad Junctions

As discussed in Chap. 16, the triggering event for muscle contraction is the electrical excitation of the sarcolemma and T-tubule membranes during the action potential. At the triad junctions, this depolarization is transduced into a signal for the SR to release Ca^{2+}. The specialized junctional surfaces of both the **T-tubule** and the **terminal cisternae** contain proteins that play a major role in this signal transduction. The structural organization of the triad is depicted in Fig. 17-9.

The junctional surface of the terminal cisternae contains rows of specialized proteins, spaced at periodic intervals, that bridge the gap between the terminal cisternae and the T-tubule. These proteins, variously termed **"feet,"** **bridg-**

Fig. 17-9. Three-dimensional reconstruction of a half-triad, showing the relative positions of foot proteins, transverse (T)-tubule system proteins, Ca^{2+}-ATPase, and calsequestrin. The junctional surface of the terminal cisternae of the SR bears two rows of feet. The nonjunctional SR contains densely packed Ca^{2+}-ATPase molecules, which are abundant on the longitudinal or free SR, which is continuous with the terminal cisternae. The lumen of the terminal cisternae of the SR contains calsequestrin, a high-capacity Ca^{2+}-binding protein. (Modified from: Block, B. A., et al. Structural evidence for direct interaction between molecular components of the transverse tubule/sarcoplasmic reticulum junction in skeletal muscle. *J. Cell Biol.* 107:2587, 1988.)

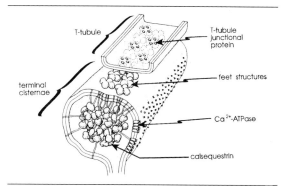

ing, or **spanning proteins,** are aligned in two rows in a skewed pattern (see Fig. 17-9), with a center-to-center spacing of approximately 30 nm. A "foot" protein is composed of four identical subunits, each containing a membrane-spanning domain and a large cytosolic domain. The membrane-spanning domain inserts into the junctional SR bilayer, and the cytosolic domain extends across the junctional gap. The "foot" protein is a large-molecular-weight protein termed the **ryanodine receptor** because of its high-binding affinity to the plant alkaloid ryanodine. This ryanodine receptor functions as a type of Ca^{2+} channel and can release Ca^{2+} from the SR at high rates.

The junctional face surfaces of the T-tubules also have been found to contain specialized proteins aligned with a regular periodicity. The T-tubule network of mammalian skeletal muscle cells is one of the richest sources of a voltage-activated Ca^{2+} channel, which is termed the **dihydropyridine** (DHP) **receptor** because of its high sensitivity to this class of Ca^{2+} channel-blocking drugs. The DHP receptors are localized in the junctional regions of the T-tubule membrane that directly face the junctional surfaces of the terminal cisternae of the SR. Electron microscopy suggests that the DHP receptors are clustered in groups of four, termed **tetrads,** and these tetrads are aligned in parallel rows with a regular periodicity. Figure 17-9 illustrates this pattern for a fish skeletal muscle fiber, in which the tetrads line up opposite every *other* ryanodine receptor in a 1:2 ration. In fast-twitch mammalian skeletal muscle, the tetrads may line up opposite every ryanodine receptor in a 1:1 ratio.

The complementary periodicity and symmetrical fourfold molecular structure of these two major junctional proteins imply that they interact directly in the coupling mechanism between the T-tubules and SR. Thus, during excitation-contraction coupling, a Ca^{2+} channel on the outer cell membrane controls the opening of a second type of Ca^{2+} channel on an internal membrane. The triad junctions are the specialized membrane structures that bring these two kinds of Ca^{2+} channels together in a unique macromolecular complex that permits their interaction.

The exact mechanism by which the Ca^{2+} channels of the T-tubules communicate with the Ca^{2+}-release channels of the SR is not completely understood. However, it is known that junctional coupling in skeletal muscle is tightly controlled by the T-system membrane potential. If the ion channels mediating the action potential (i.e., the Na^+, K^+, and Cl^- channels of the surface and the T-system membranes) are blocked experimentally and the T-system membrane is depolarized to the same potential using electronic feedback, the SR will continue to release Ca^{2+}. In

other words, it is the absolute value of the electrical potential difference across the T-system membrane, not the inflow of ions during the action potential, that controls junctional coupling. (This contrasts with cardiac muscle, in which an influx of extracellular Ca^{2+} occurs during the cardiac action potential and is absolutely required for contraction; see Chap. 19.)

Therefore, the junctional DHP receptors of the T-system membranes are thought to function as voltage-sensor molecules that respond to the depolarization during the action potential, and somehow these receptors communicate the depolarization to the Ca^{2+}-release channels of the SR. The DHP receptor contains mobile, charged regions (dipoles), termed **gating** or **voltage-sensing domains,** within its intramembrane domains. These charged regions move rapidly in response to a change in the transmembrane potential. This early fast movement of the gating domains controls a slower conformational change that leads to channel opening and an influx of Ca^{2+} current. Thus the early rapid conformational changes associated with the gating movement of the protein, and not the Ca^{2+} current that follows after a delay, appear to control the opening of the SR Ca^{2+}-release channels during excitation-contraction coupling.

Failure at the level of excitation-contraction coupling underlies some skeletal muscle disease states, most notably malignant hyperthermia. This disorder is characterized by a hereditary predisposition to sustained Ca^{2+} release in response to certain general anesthetic agents. If not treated rapidly, the hyperthermia is lethal. The genetic locus has been identified as an alteration of the gene coding for the ryanodine receptor. Many commonly used muscle relaxants, such as dantrolene sodium, also alter coupling at the triad junction.

Ca^{2+} and Regulation of Actin-Myosin Filament Interaction

Ca^{2+} removes the inhibition of the actin-myosin interaction. In striated muscle, troponin-C is the intracellular receptor protein for Ca^{2+}. The binding of Ca^{2+} initiates a conformational change in the troponin protein complex, which is transmitted to tropomyosin. Tropomyosin lies in the groove of the double-stranded helix of the actin filament. X-ray diffraction indicates that the position of the tropomyosin molecule relative to the axis of the actin filament is altered by Ca^{2+}, as mediated by the Ca^{2+}-troponin interaction depicted in Fig. 17-10. In the **steric hindrance model,** this movement of tropomyosin elicited by Ca^{2+} removes a steric constraint or blockage of the site for the actin-myosin interaction.

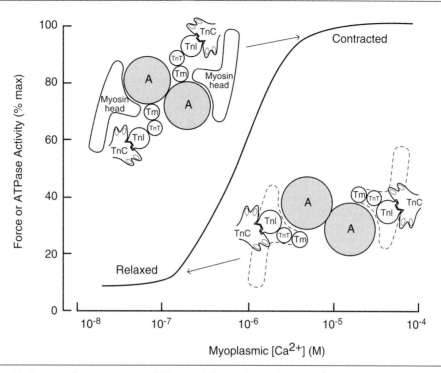

Fig. 17-10. Relationship between force (or myosin ATPase activity) and myoplasmic Ca^{2+} concentration. The insets indicate the relative positions of the myosin heads (M), actin (A), tropomyosin (Tm), and the troponin subunits (TnI, TnC, and TnT).

Because the mode of actin-myosin interaction in striated muscle involves thin-filament proteins, regulation of striated muscle is sometimes termed **thin-filament regulated.** Regulation in some invertebrate muscle as well as in smooth muscle involves mechanisms on the myosin molecule, and this type of regulation, described further in Chap. 18, is called **thick-filament regulation.**

Relaxation

Relaxation involves a lowering of the intracellular free Ca^{2+} concentration. The **Ca^{2+}-transport proteins of the SR** constitute the major Ca^{2+}-removal system in the muscle cell. These are highly concentrated in the longitudinal regions of the SR and use energy stored in ATP to transport Ca^{2+} back into the SR. There, Ca^{2+} is bound again to calsequestrin, a low-affinity high-capacity Ca^{2+}-binding protein. The pumped Ca^{2+} moves back to the terminal cisternae regions, where it is available for the next twitch. Thus Ca^{2+} is continuously recycled within the muscle cell, following the pathways outlined in Fig. 16-7. Additional

Ca^{2+} removal systems operate during sustained muscle activity. Following a single twitch, the transport capacity of the SR Ca^{2+}-ATPase proteins is sufficient to rapidly restore the cytosolic Ca^{2+} concentration to resting levels. However, during sustained activity, as occurs in a tetanus, the cytosolic Ca^{2+} level may exceed the total capacity of the SR ATPase Ca^{2+}-transport system. In this event, a number of cytosolic proteins, such as parvalbumin, serve as Ca^{2+} buffers that temporarily hold and then release Ca^{2+} to the SR Ca^{2+}-ATPase.

Besides the Ca^{2+} transport systems of the SR and cytosolic Ca^{2+}-buffering proteins, several other mechanisms operate in parallel to lower the cytosolic Ca^{2+} concentration. The coupling between the T-system and SR is turned off when the T-system transmembrane potential returns to the resting potential. There is also evidence that the Ca^{2+}-release channel of the SR has a Ca^{2+}-dependent inactivating mechanism that automatically closes the channel. In other words, this channel has a bimodal response to Ca^{2+}: Micromolar levels of Ca^{2+} activate it, and higher levels inactivate it.

Summary

This chapter focuses on the mechanisms needed in the generation of mechanical force and shortening and the regulation of contractile activity at the molecular level. Muscle contractile proteins and their assembly into the sarcomeric structure are discussed. The crossbridge cycle is examined, and the mechanical and biochemical correlates presented. The behavior of intact muscle is then related to the crossbridge cycle and its regulation. This includes the force-velocity relationship, energetics, metabolism, and the coordination of metabolism with muscle function. Muscle regulatory proteins at the membrane system and filament levels are also considered. The mechanisms of excitation-contraction coupling at the molecular level are elaborated on, and extrapolated to the whole tissue level.

Bibliography

Rüegg, J. C. *Calcium in Muscle Activation.* Heidelberg: Springer-Verlag, 1986.

Squire, J. *The Structural Basis of Muscular Contraction.* London: Plenum Press, 1981.

Woledge, R. C., Curtin, N.A., and Homsher, E. *Energetic Aspects of Muscle Contraction.* London: Academic Press, 1985.

18 Diversity of Muscle

Richard J. Paul, Judith A. Heiny, Donald G. Ferguson, and R. John Solaro

Objectives

After reading this chapter, you should be able to

Describe the structural and functional differences at the cellular level of the major skeletal muscle fiber types

Describe the potential physiologic significance of isoform differences among the major muscle proteins

List the major factors influencing the development of a smooth, graded contractile force in a whole muscle

Compare and contrast the major structural and functional differences between cardiac and skeletal muscle

Compare and contrast the major structural and functional differences between smooth and skeletal muscle

Compare and contrast the major modes of activation of striated and smooth muscle

Explain how the Ca^{2+} sensitivity of smooth muscle may be altered

---

Motile systems in biology show great diversity that allows adaptation to specific functions. Two major and quite different protein systems underlie most motile cells. Muscle cells use **myosin** and **actin**, whereas the flagella and cilia of bacteria use **dynein** and **tubulin.** Within muscle cells, the diversity is equally as great; for example, contractile velocities for smooth and skeletal muscle differ by a factor of 500. Another striking characteristic of muscle is its **plasticity**, or ability to adapt to different conditions by changing its structure. How both the diversity and adaptation of muscle can arise using the same component proteins myosin and actin is a central question in the study of muscle physiology at the tissue level.

Skeletal Muscle

Differences between skeletal muscle cells (fibers) are quite striking and obvious, as illustrated by the clear difference between red and white meat. Table 18-1 lists some of the characteristics of the different muscle fiber types and their

nomenclature. The different systems of names have evolved from the various functional or histologic techniques used to differentiate the muscle cells. From both a histologic and functional perspective, there are basically three fiber types, as depicted in Fig. 18-1. For our purposes here, we will use the fiber-type nomenclature that is based on function, namely, **fast glycolytic (FG)**, **fast oxidative-glycolytic (FOG)**, and **slow oxidative (SO)**. Most muscles are a mixture of these three types of fibers, although the proportions vary considerably in different muscles. All such heterogeneous muscles appear pale compared with red muscle, which is mainly composed of SO fibers. The red color is imparted by the presence of myoglobin, a protein that facilitates the diffusion of oxygen through the cell. In primates, the prevalence of FOG fibers is relatively low.

The differences in fiber types are perhaps most easily understood in terms of their adaptation to the different power outputs required and the corresponding difference in the fuels used. Many activities require large forces that are developed rapidly but are not necessarily sustained. The FG fibers are large, and their well-developed sar-

Table 18-1. Morphologic and Histochemical Types of Twitch Fibers in Mammalian Skeletal Muscle

Classification	Fast Glycolytic (FG)	Slow Oxidative (SO)	Fast Oxidative-Glycolytic (FOG)
Other nomenclature	Fast, fatigable	Slow, fatigue-resistant	Fast, fatigue-resistant
	Fast-twitch white	Slow-twitch intermediate	Fast-twitch red
	White	Medium	Red
	A	B	C
	IIB	I	IIA
	I	III	II
	White	Intermediate	Red
Morphologic properties			
Mitochondrial content	Small	Intermediate	Large
Sarcoplasmic reticulum	Dense	Intermediate	Dense
Fiber diameter	Large	Intermediate	Small
Histochemical properties			
Oxidative enzyme activities	Low	High or intermediate	Intermediate or high
Mitochondrial ATPase	Low	Intermediate	High
Glycolytic activities	High	Low or variable	Intermediate or low
Myoglobin content	Low	High	High
Glycogen content	Intermediate	Low	High

coplasmic reticulum (SR) facilitates rapid control of contraction and relaxation. Their metabolism is highly glycolytic, and ATP synthesis can respond rapidly to demand, though with limited capacity.

Other tasks, such as those required of postural muscles, involve a more continuous level of activity. The fatigue-resistant SO fibers are designed for this. Highly oxidative, their metabolism can efficiently support moderate levels of ATP use. Their relatively high capillary density and the presence of myoglobin are directed toward eliminating oxygen diffusion as a possible rate-limiting process. From the utilization aspect, the economical maintenance of force is facilitated by the lower actin-activated myosin ATPase of SO fibers relative to FG. The tradeoff, however, is that the speed of shortening is also slower.

FOG fibers are a less common component, and it is difficult to identify a muscle composed of predominantly FOG fibers, unlike other fiber types. Some ocular muscles appear to pose the best example. Their contractile speed and twitch duration are intermediate between those of SO and FOG fibers, and they are characterized by a high level of both oxidative and glycolytic metabolism. They appear to be specialized for fine, fast movements and for near-continuous activity.

FG, FOG, and SO fiber types also differ significantly in their speed of activation, which is about threefold faster in FG than in SO fibers. In FG fibers, each step of the excitation-contraction coupling is enhanced, including the action potential, the amount of charge movement in the transverse tubule system (T-system), and the rate of Ca^{2+}-release from the SR. These differences in the speed of excitation-contraction coupling correlate well with differences in the junctional surface area of the T-system and SR, as well as with the size of the junctional contact area. The different fiber types and their respective metabolism are summarized in Table 18-2.

Diversity of Contractile and Regulatory Proteins

An interesting feature of the structure-function relationship of mammalian striated muscle is that most of the myofilament proteins are now known to exist as populations of isoforms. This raises important questions concerning the functional significance of a particular isotype population as well as the regulation of the expression of the various isoforms.

Isoforms of Myosin Heavy and Light Chains

Myosin is the most well studied of the **isoforms** of myofilament proteins. Among various muscle types there is diversity in the expression of both the heavy and light chains. It is clear that one way nature has chosen to regulate muscle function for long-term adaptation to loading conditions is to alter the expression of myosin heavy- and light-chain isoforms.

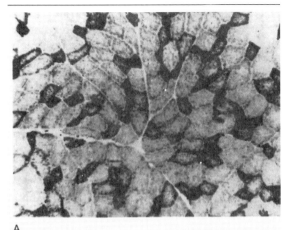

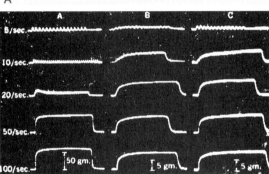

Fig. 18-1. Skeletal muscle fiber type: histology and function. (A) Cross-section of cat gastrocnemius muscle stained for mitochondrial ATPase activity. Large fibers are fast glycolytic; small dark fibers are fast oxidative-glycolytic; and fibers of intermediate size and density are slow oxidative. (From: Henneman, E., and Olson, C. B., Relations between structure and function in the design of skeletal muscles. *J. Neurophysiol.* 28:581, 1965.) (B) Isometric force as a function of stimulus frequency for different fiber types. (A = fast glycolytic; B = slow oxidative, both from cat gastrocnemius; C = fast oxidative-gycolytic from the soleus.) (From McPhedran, A. M., et al. Properties of motor units in a homogeneous red muscle (soleus) of the cat. *J. Neurophysiol.* 28:71, 1965.)

There are three types of light chains in fast skeletal muscle: LC1, LC2, and LC3. There are two types of light chains in heart and slow skeletal muscle: LC1 and LC2. LC2 is the substrate for myosin light-chain kinase and is also known as the **regulatory light chain** or the **P-light chain.** The other forms of the light chain are essential to the activity of myosin. They are referred to as the **A1** and **A2 light chains** or the **essential light chains.** The compo-

sition of the particular light chain affects the rate of ATPase activity of myosin.

The heavy chain of myosin also exists in several isoforms that are products of a multigene family. In the case of heart muscle, which serves as a prototype, two heavy-chain isomers are known as **alpha** and **beta monomer.** Three isoforms are known; two are homodimers and one is a heterodimer. The ATPase activity and velocity of shortening are highly correlated with the relative proportions of isoforms.

Isoforms of Actin and Tropomyosin

There are also several isoforms of actin that have subtle but potentially significant differences. Isoform populations vary with development and with longterm adaptation. There is no convincing evidence showing that shifts in the actin isoforms have significant functional consequences.

Actin exists in many parts of the cell besides the myofilaments and may have activity unassociated with contraction. For example, both cardiac and skeletal alphaactins are expressed in the fetal rat heart, whereas only the alpha-cardiac form is expressed in the adult. There is no strong evidence indicating that these two forms of actin affect thin-filament function.

Tropomyosin (Tm) also exists as alpha and beta isomers, the populations of which appear to be developmentally regulated. Alpha-Tm is predominant in the adult heart of small animal species, but in the neonate there is a relative abundance of striated muscle beta-Tm and both smooth and nonmuscle beta-Tm. As with actin, the structural changes are subtle, and the functional significance is not clear.

Isoforms of Troponin-C, Troponin-T, and Troponin-I

The thin-filament Ca^{2+}-receptor protein **troponin** (Tn-C) exists as two tissue-specific isoforms: fast skeletal Tn-C and slow cardiac Tn-C. Only one isotype exists within a particular mammalian muscle type. Fast Tn-C has four Ca^{2+}-binding sites, two of which are regulatory. Slow Tn-C, which is the same gene product as cardiac Tn-C, has three Ca^{2+}-binding sites, one of which is regulatory. The nonregulatory metal-binding sites of Tn-C bind Mg^{2+} with high affinity and may be important in thin-filament structure.

The presence of multiple isoforms of cardiac **troponin-T** (Tn-T) has been demonstrated in several species and muscle types. Five isoforms of Tn-T have been identified in rabbit heart. The proportion of each isoform varies with postnatal age, and there is some evidence that adaptational responses of muscle may involve shifts in the Tn-T isoform population. Isoform populations of Tn-T and Tm

Table 18-2. Summary of the Major Modes of Activation of Smooth, Cardiac, and Skeletal Muscle

Muscle Protein Type	Membrane Stimulus	Ca^{2+} Source	Ca^{2+}-Binding Regulatory Protein
Skeletal	Depolarization, largely CNS controlled	Intracellular Ca2+ release from SR	Skeletal troponin-C
Cardiac	Depolarization, largely ANS-controlled or hormones	Ca^{2+} influx through voltage-activated Ca^{2+} channels; intracellular Ca^{2+} release mediated by Ca^{2+}; reverse Na^+-Ca^{2+} exchange	Cardiac troponin-C
Smooth	Depolarization, largely ANS-controlled or hormones	Intracellular Ca^{2+} release from SR mediated by IP_3; Ca^{2+} influx through voltage-activated and/or receptor-activated Ca^{2+} channels; reverse Na^+-Ca^{2+} exchange	Calmodulin

CNS = central nervous system; ANS = autonomic nervous system; SR = sarcoplasmic reticulum; IP_3 = inositoltris-phosphate.

may be the major determinants of the different responses to Ca^{2+} observed in fast skeletal muscle fibers.

Three variants of **troponin-I** (Tn-I) are known: fast, slow, and cardiac. Slow Tn-I is expressed as an embryonic isoform in heart muscle. Shifts in the Tn-I isotype may be related to differential effects of acidic pH on Ca^{2+}-activation of myofilaments.

Modification of Myofilament Proteins

Activation of second-messenger cascades alters the state of phosphorylation of myofilament proteins. The Ca^{2+}-calmodulin–dependent pathway is associated with phosphorylation of myosin LC2 by activation of myosin light chain kinase. In striated muscle, this phosphorylation is not responsible for activation. The state of phosphorylation of myosin does, however, modify the level of force achieved at submaximal levels of Ca^{2+}. The combined beta-adrenergic receptor–cyclic adenosine-3′, 5′ monophosphate (cAMP) pathway is associated with the phosphorylation of Tn-I in heart muscle, which reduces the affinity of Tn-C for Ca^{2+} and thus may act as a negative feedback signal. Tn-T, which is an elongated molecule, is phosphorylated at one end by a Tn-T kinase. Tn-T is also phosphorylated by phosphorylase kinase and protein kinase C at the other end of the molecule, which might be involved in Ca^{2+} signaling and in thin-filament cooperativity. There are also sites of phosphorylation in Tm that are strategically located at the region of overlap between adjacent molecules. The functional significance of Tn-T and Tm phosphorylation remains unclear.

Plasticity of Muscle

While the physiologic significance of these isoforms is not completely understood, it is clear that muscle is very plastic, and depending on conditions, fiber type can be modified. For example, denervation of an SO fiber elicits a change toward the mechanical characteristics of an FG fiber. Cross-innervating an SO fiber with a nerve originally from an FG fiber also elicits a change in the SO fiber toward FG characteristics. Whether a trophic factor from the nerve or the stimulus frequency is the major stimulus for the transition is not certain.

Factors Influencing Total Force Developed During Contraction

Let us return to the question originally posed in Chap. 16. If submaximal stimuli result in nonfused tetani (see Fig. 18-1), how do muscles produce smooth submaximal contractions? The functional unit of muscle at the whole tissue level is the **motor unit.** It consists of one motor neuron, its axon, and all the muscle cells innervated by that motor neuron. Individual motor units are composed of the same fiber types, but the individual fibers are not necessarily localized in the same area. Smooth submaximal contractions in whole muscle can result from the asynchronous firing of a large number of motor neurons. This type of force summation is different from the smooth contraction in a single fiber resulting from a tetanus. Smooth contractions in whole muscle are sometimes referred to as **spatial summation** and involve the interplay of various factors, including (1) twitch duration of individual fibers, (2) frequency of firing, (3) number of motor units recruited, and (4) size of the motor units, i.e., the number of fibers per motor neuron. In graded smooth contractions of whole muscle in the lower ranges, force is increased through the addition of motor units, which are recruited in order of their size. At the highest forces, with most motor units involved, increases in force are achieved by increased frequency of firing.

Cardiac Muscle

Cardiac Muscle Structure

Cardiac muscle cells are rod-shaped and intermediate in size between skeletal and smooth muscle. Typically, the working ventricular cell is 15 to 20 μm in width and 150 μm long. The basic elements are similar to those in skeletal muscle, but the relative amounts differ. The sarcolemma contains transverse (T) tubules as in other striated muscle, but their diameters are bigger in the heart. The T-tubules also snake along the length of the cell in ventricular heart muscle. The SR content of heart muscle cells is about half that of skeletal muscle. Overall, the role of the membrane systems in excitation-contraction coupling is similar to that described for skeletal muscle in Chap.17. A major exception is that the regulated influx of extracellular Ca^{2+} is an important factor both in the mechanism of the action potential and for activation of the contractile apparatus. Details of these mechanisms are described in Chap. 19. Cardiac muscle has about one-half the number of myofilaments of skeletal muscle. Moreover, the relative amount of mitochondria is large in heart. These specialized features of cardiac muscle are related to its relatively slow but constant active contraction and relaxation cycles.

Cardiac Muscle Function

The force per unit cross-sectional area generated by cardiac muscle cells is about half that of skeletal muscle. The basic mechanism for force generation is the same as that described for skeletal muscle, but there are about half as many myofilaments acting in parallel to generate force. The energy cost of force generation is about one-fifth that

for fast skeletal muscle, owing to a slower crossbridge cycling rate and unloaded velocity of shortening.

The force-velocity and length-tension relationships of cardiac muscle are essentially the same as those for fast and slow skeletal muscle. The fundamental operation of the sliding-filament mechanism does not differ for these muscle types. An interesting feature of the length-tension relationship in heart muscle is that force falls off much more steeply than it does in skeletal muscle, when the muscle shortens beyond lengths associated with optimal overlap. The shape of the length-tension relationship is important because it is the basis of the Frank-Starling relationship, which underlies the pump characteristics of the heart (see Chap. 23). The mechanism for this difference between heart and skeletal muscle appears to stem from the length dependence of excitation-contraction coupling, involving either Ca^{2+}-release from the SR or the process by which Ca^{2+} activates the myofilaments.

Normally cardiac muscle contraction relies on aerobic metabolism, although there is a capability for anaerobic glycolysis. As expected for a system in which energy demand is normally matched by aerobic energy supply, heart muscle cells have a higher density of mitochondria and a lower amount of phosphocreatine than is found in fast skeletal muscle. When the oxygen supply is limited in heart muscle, force is inhibited by the accumulation of metabolites, especially protons and inorganic phosphate. This is important to the protection of heart cells under pathophysiologic conditions, since this automatically reduces energy demand. This permits preservation of the cells until oxygen can be restored. (Additional protective mechanisms are discussed in Chaps. 19 and 21.)

Smooth Muscle

Smooth muscle, so-called because it lacks the sarcomeric banding characteristic of striated muscle, is an important tissue that typically lines the hollow organs of, for example, the vasculature and gastrointestinal tract. Its structure is less organized than that of skeletal muscle, making it less amenable to biophysical experimentation. However, for health professionals it is of major importance, since many diseases, such as hypertension, coronary artery disease, stroke, asthma, and gastrointestinal disorders, are related to smooth muscle pathology. Many theories of smooth muscle contraction have been extrapolated from those of skeletal muscle. While there are many similarities, striking differences have been shown between striated and smooth muscle, particularly in terms of the regulation of contraction.

One characteristic of smooth muscle is its ability to maintain large forces at relatively low energy cost. It is superbly adapted to this function. How is this accomplished using a basically similar actin-myosin–based contractile system? Our presentation of smooth muscle will follow the structure-function analysis used for skeletal muscle.

Smooth Muscle Structure

Smooth muscle cells are spindle-shaped and very small compared with skeletal muscle. They are about 5 to 10 μm in diameter (one-tenth that of skeletal muscle) and up to several hundred micrometers long. Like striated muscle, smooth muscle cells contain thick, myosin-containing and thin, actin-containing filaments. However, in smooth muscle, the thick and thin filaments are not organized into myofibrils or regular sarcomeres. A cell cytoskeleton serves as attachment points for thin filaments and allows force transmission to the ends of cells. There are no z-bands per se, but specialized cytoskeleton regions, known as **dense bodies** or **patches,** appear to serve as comparable structures for the attachment of thin filaments. These areas contain alpha-actinin, a protein also found in the z-bands of skeletal muscle. Intermediate filaments with 10-nm diameters (intermediate between thin, 7-nm and thick, 15-nm filament diameters) link the dense bodies to form a cytoskeleton network. The ratio of thin to thick filaments in smooth muscle (approximately 15 : 1) is considerably higher than that of striated muscle (2 : 1), and the myosin content is approximately one-fifth that of skeletal muscle. Electron micrographs of smooth muscle and a drawing of the filament structure are shown in Fig 18-2.

Smooth muscle also contains a reticular membrane system which, in terms of its ability to store and release Ca^{2+}, is analogous to the SR of skeletal muscle. The volume of the SR in smooth muscle ranges from about 2% in phasic spike-generating smooth muscles, like the taenia coli, to 5% to 7.5% in tonic smooth muscle, such as that found in the large elastic arteries. The time required for diffusion of intracellular Ca^{2+} is not a limiting factor because of the small diameters of smooth muscle cells.

Smooth Muscle Function

The isometric force per cross-sectional area generated by smooth muscle can be as large as or larger than that of skeletal muscle, which is surprising in light of its smaller myosin content. As was previously indicated, the energy cost of tension maintenance (the rate of ATP hydrolysis per force/cross-section area) can be up to 500-fold lower than that of skeletal muscle. Again, the tradeoff is in con-

traction speed, with smooth muscle velocities being one to two orders of magnitude lower.

The force-length relationships for smooth muscle are qualitatively similar to those for skeletal muscle, providing evidence for an analogous sliding-filament mechanism. How such a mechanism is visualized for the less organized filament structure of smooth muscle is shown in Fig 18-2.

The force-velocity relationship is also qualitatively similar to that of skeletal muscle, albeit with much slower velocities. This suggests a similar crossbridge cycle for smooth muscle contractility. The actin-activated myosin ATPase activity of smooth muscle is substantially less than that of skeletal muscle. This and the lower crossbridge cycle rate can account for the slower shortening speeds and lower energy cost.

In addition, smooth muscle appears to possess mechanisms for regulating the rate of crossbridge cycling as well as the number of activated bridges. Following stimulation, contraction velocities decrease, while the ability to maintain isometric force remains constant. This state of maintaining force at reduced velocities is known as the **latch state.** As many smooth muscles are always tonically activated, e.g., those in blood vessels, the latch state may be dominant under certain physiologic conditions. The regulatory mechanisms involved will be discussed below.

Smooth muscle metabolism is primarily oxidative. The density of mitochondria is generally similar to that of FG skeletal fibers. Because the contractile energy requirements are low, oxidative ATP synthesis generally matches energy demand. Thus, in spite of low phosphocreatine (PCr) pools compared with skeletal muscle, little change in either the PCr or ATP concentration can be measured during contraction, because increases in oxidative phosphorylation provide the ATP as needed. Thus the oxygen debt phenomenon observed in skeletal muscle (oxidative resynthesis of PCr after cessation of contraction) in general does not exist for smooth muscle. An unusual aspect of smooth muscle metabolism is its production of substantial amounts of lactate when it is fully oxygenated. In some smooth muscles, notably vascular smooth muscle, this lactate production may be related to the energy requirements of membrane processes, such as ion pumps. Presumably the ATP-synthesizing, glycolytic enzyme cascades are colocalized in the plasma membrane.

Excitation-Contraction Coupling in Smooth Muscle

As in our treatment of skeletal muscle (Chaps. 16 and 17), regulation in smooth muscle can be conveniently divided into mechanisms for (1) controlling $[Ca]_i$, (2) transduction

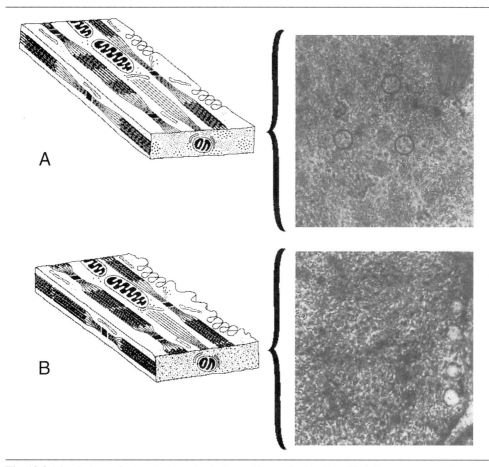

Fig. 18-2. Morphology of relaxed and contracted smooth muscle. (A) Simplified diagram representing a portion of a relaxed smooth muscle cell, highlighting the arrangement of the actin-containing thin filaments and the myosin-containing thick filaments. Thin filaments arise at dense bodies and project to interact with thick filaments, forming the contractile apparatus. The filaments are distributed in a nonuniform manner, with thick filaments forming clusters surrounded by groups of thin filaments. This arrangement is shown in the electron micrograph *(circled),* which is a cross-section of a relaxed visceral smooth muscle cell. (B) A contracted smooth muscle cell. The notable differences are that the thin filaments overlap considerably more of the thick filaments. drawing the dense bodies closer together and shortening the cell. The thin and thick filaments are randomly distributed to form a uniform pattern. The electron micrograph is a cross-section of a contracted visceral smooth muscle cell, which shows more uniform distribution of the thin and thick filaments. (Diagrams are modified from: Heumann, H. G. Smooth muscle: Contraction hypothesis based on the arrangements of actin and myosin filaments in different states of contraction. *Philos. Trans. R. Soc. Lond. (Biol.)* 265:213, 1973.)

of the Ca^{2+} signal at the level of the contractile proteins, and (3) modulation of the Ca^{2+} sensitivity.

Control of Intracellular Ca^{2+} Concentration

The control of intracellular Ca^{2+} concentration ($[Ca]_i$) in smooth muscle is complex, involving both extracellular and intracellular sources, Ca^{2+} uptake by the SR, and ex-

trusion by pumps and exchangers on the plasma membrane. These will be considered in detail in Chap. 19.

Ca^{2+} Control of Contractile Filaments

Until the mid-1970s, the mechanism for the regulation of contractile activity in smooth muscle was postulated, by analogy to skeletal muscle, to be a thin-filament–linked

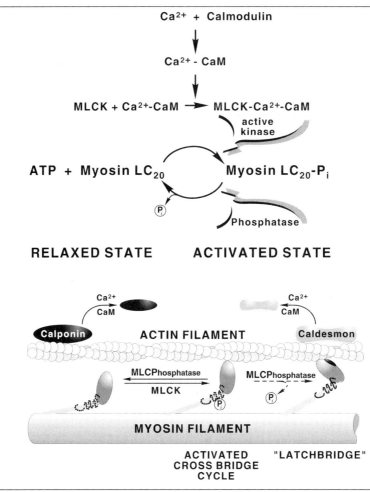

Fig. 18-3. The molecular basis of regulation of smooth muscle contraction. Stimulation of muscarinic receptors increases the $[Ca]_i$ due to entry of external Ca^{2+} and release of Ca^{2+} from internal stores. Ca^{2+} binds to calmodulin (CaM); and the Ca^{2+}-CaM complex then binds to and activates myosin light-chain kinase (MLCK). Phosphorylation of myosin by MLCK stimulates actin-activated myosin-ATP hydrolysis, which produces contraction. Relaxation begins with cessation of agonist stimulation. This results in decreased $[Ca]_i$, dissociation of Ca^{2+} from CaM, inactivation of MLCK due to dissociation of CaM, dephosphorylation of myosin by phosphoprotein phosphatases (P'tase) and relaxation.

mechanism involving Tn and Tm. However, smooth muscle does not contain the Ca^{2+} receptor protein Tn.

It is instructive to compare the biochemical behavior of purified actin and myosin from skeletal and smooth muscles. In skeletal muscle (see Fig. 17-5), when ATP is added to actin and myosin, the myosin ATPase is activated and actin and myosin interact. The presence of the thin-filament proteins Tn and Tm inhibits this interaction, and Ca^{2+} removes this inhibition. In smooth muscle, on the other hand, actin and myosin are inactive and myosin ATPase activity is low. Therefore, a Ca^{2+}-linked activator, rather than a deinhibitor, is required for activity.

The activating factor for the smooth muscle actin-myosin interaction was found to be a covalent modification of the myosin itself, specifically the phosphorylation of the 20-kDa light chain. Ca^{2+}-sensitivity for this phosphorylation resides in the Ca^{2+} dependence of the enzyme **myosin light-chain kinase,** which catalyzes the phosphorylation of the myosin light chain. The Ca^{2+}-receptor protein involved is the ubiquitous Ca^{2+}-binding protein **calmodulin.** The activation sequence involves the binding of Ca^{2+} to calmodulin. In turn, this complex binds to myosin light-chain kinase and activates its ATP-dependent phosphorylation of myosin, allowing actin-myosin interaction.

In contrast to skeletal muscle, relaxation in smooth muscle does not simply involve reversal of the activation process. The dephosphorylation of myosin necessary to inactivate the actin-myosin interaction is catalyzed by a separate enzyme **myosin light-chain phosphatase.** Current evidence suggests that this phosphatase also may be a control point of contractility.

This basic scheme of Ca^{2+} control of smooth muscle contractility is depicted in Fig. 18-3. It is generally accepted that phosphorylation of myosin plays an obligatory role in the regulation of smooth muscle contraction. Other thin-filament–linked, Ca^{2+}-dependent modulators have been postulated, particularly for control of the latch state. The basic scheme has a large number of potential regulatory sites.

Modulation of Ca^{2+}-Sensitivity

It is important to note that while alteration of $[Ca]_i$ is a major mechanism for regulating smooth muscle tone, it is not the sole mechanism. Many previous efforts toward a therapeutic intervention in diseases in which smooth muscle is the final effector system (e.g., hypertension or asthma) involved manipulation of $[Ca]_i$. Calcium-entry blockers are an example of this type of drug development.

Much recent attention has focused on alteration of Ca^{2+}-sensitivity — i.e., the alteration of the response to a given level of $[Ca]_i$. Since activation of smooth muscle depends on the level of phosphorylation of the myosin regulatory light chains (MLC-P_i), there are many avenues for alteration of a response to a given level of $[Ca]_i$. For example, drugs that inhibit the binding of Ca^{2+}-calmodulin to MLCK would reduce the activity of this enzyme, resulting in less MLC-P_i and fewer activated crossbridges for a given $[Ca]_i$. Similarly, stimulation of MLC phosphatase activity also would lead to less force for a given Ca^{2+} level. This approach may enable one to specifically relax smooth muscle. By targeting $[Ca]_i$, one might, however, also involve other muscles unsuitably, for example, if one treated coronary artery disease to improve blood flow with a drug that dilated the coronary arteries but also reduced cardiac contractility.

Summary

The diversity of muscle is described at the cellular level for different types of skeletal muscle fibers. This is further developed at the molecular level in terms of the isoforms of the major muscle proteins. Our consideration of skeletal muscle concludes with a discussion of the factors influencing the generation of total force in a whole muscle. Next, cardiac and smooth muscle are considered in the context of the structure-function paradigm, paralleling that of skeletal muscle. The major differences in the contractile proteins and the regulation of contractility are also considered. Table 18-2 summarizes the major modes of activation of skeletal, cardiac, and smooth muscle.

Bibliography

Paul R. J. Smooth muscle: Mechanochemical energy conversion, relations between metabolism and contractility. In: Johnson, L. R., et al., eds. *Physiology of the Gastrointestinal Tract,* vol. 1, 2nd ed. New York: Raven Press, 1987. Pp. 483–506.

Rüegg, J. C. *Calcium in Muscle Activation.* Heidelberg: Springer-Verlag, 1986.

Solaro, R. J. *Protein Phosphorylation in Heart Muscle.* Boca Raton, Fla.: CRC Press, 1986.

19 Regulation of Intracellular Ca²⁺ in Cardiac Muscle and Smooth Muscle

Nicholas Sperelakis

Objectives

After reading this chapter, you should be able to

Describe the differences in excitation-contraction coupling between cardiac muscle and smooth muscle and how these differ from that for skeletal muscle

List the various routes by which Ca^{2+} enters the cell to initiate contraction and the various mechanisms by which free Ca^{2+} concentration in the myoplasm is reduced to the resting level to bring about relaxation

Discuss the properties of the voltage-dependent Ca^{2+} channels and their regulation

Describe how vasodilators and vasoconstrictors act to alter the tone of arterioles

Discuss the concept of receptor-operated ion channels

As discussed in previous chapters, Ca^{2+} is the key intracellular messenger for the regulation of contraction in all types of muscles. In addition, Ca^{2+} serves as a second messenger for activation of some enzymes and several types of ion channels. Therefore, it is important to examine how the intracellular Ca^{2+} concentration ($[Ca]_i$) is regulated. $[Ca]_i$ can be regulated by (1) controlling Ca^{2+} *influx* into the cell through several types of ion channels and exchangers in the sarcolemma, (2) controlling Ca^{2+} *efflux* from the cell through pumps and exchangers, (3) controlling Ca^{2+} release from the sarcoplasmic reticulum (SR), and (4) controlling Ca^{2+} uptake back into the SR. $[Ca]_i$ is also regulated indirectly by controlling the duration of the action potential (AP) and hence the period that the Ca^{2+} conductance remains elevated. Relaxation is produced by the lowering of $[Ca]_i$ back to the resting level.

The relationship between contractile force and $[Ca]_i$ is sigmoid on a logarithmic scale. The $[Ca]_i$ level of a myocardial cell at rest is about 1×10^{-7} M; elevation to 1×10^{-6}

M produces about half-maximal force generation. The curve plateaus (saturates), so elevation beyond 1×10^{-5} M does not further increase contraction. This **force versus Ca^{2+} sensitivity curve** can be shifted to the left or right under certain conditions, such as acidosis or alkalosis and the action of some drugs, thereby affecting how much force can be developed for a given rise in $[Ca]_i$.

Cardiac Muscle

In cardiac muscle, the force of contraction depends on the extracellular Ca^{2+} concentration ($[Ca]_o$). When $[Ca]_o$ goes below the normal level of about 1.8 mM, the contractile force is diminished and ultimately abolished when the $[Ca]_o$ becomes zero. Conversely, when $[Ca]_o$ is elevated, the contractile force is augmented up to a maximum level. This close dependence on $[Ca]_o$ in cardiac muscle is qualitatively and quantitatively different from that for skeletal muscle, which has much less immediate dependence on $[Ca]_o$. In isolated hearts perfused through the coronary arteries, the time constant for a change in contractile force following a step change in the $[Ca]_o$ of the perfusate is very short, namely, about 5 to 10 sec. Most of this time for equilibration is occupied by diffusion from the vascular compartment to the interstitial compartment. The effect of change in Ca^{2+} concentration at the outer surface of the membrane is virtually instantaneous.

Elevation of $[Ca]_i$ to Initiate Contraction

Slow Ca^{2+} Channels

The reason for the strong dependence of contraction on $[Ca]_o$ is that Ca^{2+} influx into the myocardial cell during excitation is greater when $[Ca]_o$ is greater (Fig. 19-1). This Ca^{2+} influx mainly passes through the voltage-gated slow

Fig. 19-1. Summary of Ca^{2+} influx pathways in myocardial cells and smooth muscle cells. There is Ca^{2+} influx through the sarcolemma via two types of voltage-dependent Ca^{2+} channels: a slow (L-type) channel and a fast (T-type) channel. There is some Ca^{2+} influx via the Ca^{2+}-Na^+ exchange reaction operating in the reverse mode because of the prolonged depolarization during the AP. The entering Ca^{2+} also triggers release of considerable additional Ca^{2+} stored in the sarcoplasmic reticulum (SR) by activating the Ca^{2+}-release channels in the SR membrane. Thus there are two pools of Ca^{2+} for contraction: the extracellular (interstitial) pool and the SR pool ($I_{Ca(T)}$ = inward fast Ca^{2+} current; G-Prot = GTP-binding protein; PK-C, PK-A = protein kinase C and A; DAG = diacylglycerol; IP_3 = inositol-tris-phosphate; PL-C = phospholipase C; ROC = receptor-operated channel; Ag = agonist).

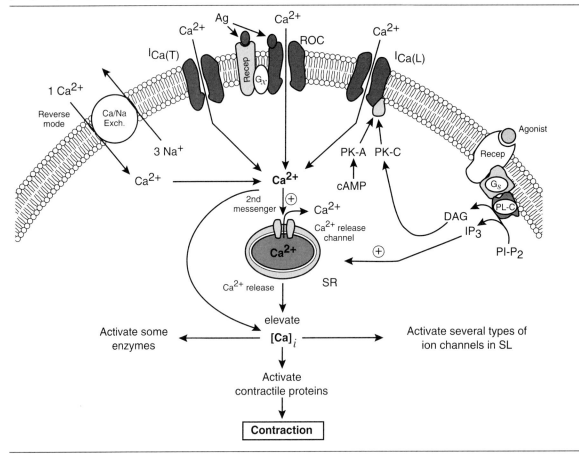

Ca²⁺ channels (also known as the L-type Ca²⁺ channels) in the sarcolemma and can be recorded as the **inward slow current or slow Ca²⁺ current.** Some of the major properties of the slow Ca²⁺ channels are summarized in Table 19-1. As the name *slow channel* implies, these channels (on a population basis) are **kinetically slower** than fast channels, in that they turn on (activate) more slowly, turn off (inactivate) much more slowly, and recover more slowly. In addition, slow channels operate over a different voltage range, namely, less negative (more depolarized); in other words, the slow channels activate and inactivate at more depolarized voltages. Tetrodotoxin (TTX), a specific blocker of fast Na⁺ channels, has no effect on slow channels. The conductance of each slow Ca²⁺ channel is about 25 pS (25 x 10^{-12} siemens or ohm⁻¹). These slow Ca²⁺ channels are opened (made conducting) during the membrane depolarization produced during the cardiac AP. The slow Ca²⁺ current flows during the entire period of the plateau component of the cardiac AP, and this inward Ca²⁺ current actually contributes to the plateau component. (see Chap. 21).

Ca²⁺ Release from the SR

The Ca²⁺ influx into the myocardial cell during the cardiac AP plateau acts on the SR to release additional Ca²⁺ into the myoplasm. Thus the Ca²⁺ required for contraction comes from two sources: (1) the extracellular Ca²⁺ pool, as a Ca²⁺ influx through voltage-gated slow Ca²⁺ channels, and (2) the Ca²⁺ pool in the SR lumen (see Fig. 19-1). Ca²⁺ entry from the extracellular pool triggers release of Ca²⁺ from the intracellular pool (SR). It is estimated that of the Ca²⁺ required to elevate the myoplasmic Ca²⁺ level ([Ca]ᵢ) to that required for maximum force development (about 10^{-5} M, about 10% is derived from the Ca²⁺ influx across the sarcolemma, and the remaining 90% is derived from Ca²⁺ release from the SR. However, the Ca²⁺ influx is the key controlling factor for determining the force of contraction, because it provokes further Ca²⁺ release in a proportional manner. Thus the greater the Ca²⁺ influx (the inward slow Ca²⁺ current), the greater is the force of contraction.

The Ca²⁺ release from the SR, triggered by the Ca²⁺ influx in a proportional manner, occurs through the **Ca²⁺-release channels** embedded in the SR membrane. These channels appear not to be voltage-gated but are gated by Ca²⁺ and inositol-tris-phosphate (IP₃); ATP is also required for release. Hence Ca²⁺ acts on the outer (myoplasmic) surface of the Ca²⁺-release channel to open the channel and allow Ca²⁺ to pass into the myoplasm down a large concentration gradient. The Ca²⁺ concentration in the SR lumen is much higher (e.g., >1.0 mM) than that in the myoplasm (e.g. 1 x 10^{-7} M in a cell at rest), and so there is a large concentration gradient for the movement of Ca²⁺ from the SR lumen into the myoplasm. (It is not known whether a membrane potential normally exists across the SR membrane.)

IP₃ also can activate the Ca²⁺-release channels of the SR to release Ca²⁺. IP₃ is a second messenger that is produced by the activation of several types of sarcolemmal receptors for neurotransmitters and hormones. IP₃ is one end-product of phosphatidyl inositol (PI) metabolism in the cell membrane (alone with diacylglycerol [DAG], which activates protein kinase C). The IP₃ so produced diffuses to the SR membrane, where it acts to bring about Ca²⁺ release. This mechanism is especially important in pharmacomechanical coupling in smooth muscles but also may be

Table 19-1. Summary of Major Differences Between the Slow (L-Type) and Fast (T-Type) Ca²⁺ Channels

Properties	Ca²⁺ Channels	
	Slow (L-Type)	Fast (T-Type)
Duration of current	Long-lasting (sustained)	Transient
Inactivation kinetics	Slower	Faster
Activation kinetics	Slower	Faster
Threshold	High *ca.* −20mV	Low *ca.* −50mV
Single-channel conductance	High	Low
Regulated by cAMP and cGMP and phosphorylation	Yes	No
Blocked by Ca²⁺ antagonist drugs	Yes	No

cAMP = cyclic adenosine-3′,5′-monophosphate; cGMP = cyclic guanosine-3′,5′-monophosphate.

involved in cardiac muscle and skeletal muscle excitation-contraction coupling. The drug **ryanodine** has been shown to activate the Ca^{2+}-release channels in the SR of cardiac muscle and skeletal muscle. Therefore, as anticipated, this drug initially produces contracture by emptying the SR of its Ca^{2+} store.

Fast Ca^{2+} Channels

Myocardial cells possess a second type of voltage-gated Ca^{2+} channel, namely, a **fast Ca^{2+} channel,** also known as the **T-type Ca^{2+} channel,** which is responsible for the fast Ca^{2+} current (see Fig. 19-1). As the name implies, this channel behaves much like a fast Na^+ channel, except that it is selective for Ca^{2+} (and not Na^+) and is not

blocked by TTX. Table 19-1 summarizes the differences between the slow and fast Ca^{2+} channels. As shown, the fast Ca^{2+} channels have a low threshold, activate quickly, inactivate quickly (hence are transient [T-type]), are not blocked by the calcium antagonist drugs, are not regulated by cyclic nucleotides and phosphorylation, and have a lower single-channel conductance (about half that of the slow Ca^{2+} channels, e.g., 10–12 pS). The number (per cell) of fast channels is usually much less than that of the slow channels. The function of the fast Ca^{2+} channels is not known, but some investigators believe that they provide a rapid change in $[Ca]_i$ that gives a more effective release of Ca^{2+} from the SR (see preceding section).

Fig. 19-2. Summary diagram to illustrate the mechanisms by which $[Ca]_i$ is lowered to the resting level to produce relaxation of cardiac muscle and smooth muscle. (A) Ca^{2+} is pumped back into the SR by the SR Ca^{2+}-ATPase pump. (B) Ca^{2+} is pumped out of the cell by the sarcolemmal (SL) Ca^{2+}-ATPase pump. (C) Ca^{2+} is exchanged across the SL for extracellular Na^+ by the Na_o-Ca_i exchanger (forward mode). (D) The influx of Ca^{2+} through the Ca^{2+} channels is shut off by repolarization of the AP.

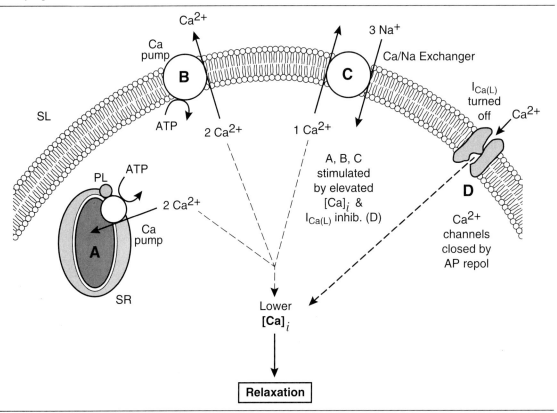

Ca²⁺-Na⁺ Exchange Reversal

The Ca²⁺-Na⁺ exchange reaction contributes to the removal of Ca²⁺ from the cell, in that it helps the sarcolemmal Ca²⁺-ATPase pump in this job (Fig. 19-2). In a cell at rest, the Ca²⁺-Na⁺ exchange helps maintain the ion distributions, namely, a very low free $[Ca]_i$. The exchange in a resting cell is directed to trade one intracellular Ca²⁺ ion for three extracellular Na⁺ ions (see Chap. 3). The energy for the uphill transport (movement) of Ca²⁺ comes from the downhill transport of Na⁺ (down its large electrochemical gradient), and the energetics are such that the outward movement of 1.0 mol Ca²⁺ from the cell requires the inward movement of 3.0 mol Na⁺. Therefore, this exchange reaction contributes to the relaxation of cardiac muscle (immediately after the AP), which requires the rapid lowering of the elevated $[Ca]_i$ (see the following section).

In addition, the Ca²⁺-Na⁺ exchange probably contributes to excitation-contraction coupling by bringing extracellular Ca²⁺ into the cell via this pathway by running in the reverse direction during excitation (see Fig. 19-1). In the reverse mode, the Ca²⁺-Na⁺ reaction exchanges three intracellular Na⁺ ions for one extracellular Ca²⁺ ion. The exchange reverses because the cell membrane is depolarized during the long-duration cardiac AP, and the energetics are now more favorable for the reverse reaction. In some hearts, such as frog atrial myocardial cells, a significant fraction of the Ca²⁺ influx during the AP that initiates contraction occurs by means of this reversed exchange pathway.

Because of this Ca²⁺-Na⁺ exchange, anything that causes $[Na]_i$ to rise will secondarily cause $[Ca]_i$ to rise, thereby leading to a more forceful contraction, known as a **positive inotropic effect** in cardiac muscle. For example, cardiac glycoside drugs, such as digitalis and ouabain, which inhibit the sarcolemmal Na⁺,K⁺-ATPase pump and thereby cause $[Na]_i$ to rise, have a potent positive inotropic effect. Such drugs are often used in patients with failing hearts, such as congestive heart failure.

Lowering of the Elevated $[Ca]_i$ to Produce Relaxation

For the heart to relax and refill after contraction, the elevated $[Ca]_i$ must be reduced to the resting level of about 1 x 10^{-7} M. This is accomplished by the operation of three pathways stimulated by the higher $[Ca]_i$ during the AP: (1) the exchange of intracellular Ca²⁺ for extracellular Na⁺ across the sarcolemma, (2) the sarcolemmal Ca²⁺-ATPase pump, and (3) the SR Ca²⁺-ATPase pump (see Fig. 19-2). As with Na⁺,K⁺-ATPase, in which intracellular Na⁺ and extracellular K⁺ stimulate this enzyme pump, a rise in $[Ca]_i$ stimulates the two Ca²⁺-ATPases (sarcolemmal and SR). These two pumps thereby act to lower $[Ca]_i$ to the resting level. The SR Ca²⁺ pump is probably the more important because it is present at a very high density in the SR membrane.

In addition, the high $[Ca]_i$ during the AP stimulates the Ca²⁺-Na⁺ exchange to operate in the *forward* direction: internal Ca²⁺ for external Na⁺. When the membrane potential reverts to the original resting level following the AP, this makes the energetics favorable again for the exchanger to operate in the forward direction. A combination of these three factors (two pumps and one exchanger), coupled with the shutting off of the enhanced Ca²⁺ entry into the cell because the AP has terminated (and therefore the depolarization-gated slow Ca²⁺ channels have reclosed), lowers $[Ca]_i$ to the resting level and relaxes the muscle (see Fig. 19-2).

Regulation of Force of Contraction

The force of heart contraction can be quickly increased or decreased. This fast regulation is primarily enabled by the special properties of the slow Ca²⁺ channels of the heart. Most of the Ca²⁺ influx into the myocardial cell during excitation is by means of the slow Ca²⁺ channels because (1) there are more slow Ca²⁺ channels than fast Ca²⁺ channels, (2) the conductance of the slow channels is about double that of the fast channels, and (3) the slow-channel conductance remains activated for a much longer time. The activity of these slow Ca²⁺ channels is stimulated by phosphorylation with cyclic adenosine-3′,5′-monophosphate (cAMP)–dependent protein kinase (PK-A) and inhibited by phosphorylation with cyclic guanosine-3′, 5′-monophosphate (cGMP)–dependent protein kinase (PK-G) (Fig. 19-3). Therefore, any intervention that elevates the cAMP level increases the force of contraction, and any intervention that elevates the cGMP level decreases the force of contraction. Thus cAMP and cGMP act in an antagonistic manner.

The cAMP is elevated by the action of a number of agents, including the sympathetic nerve neurotransmitter norepinephrine and circulating epinephrine, both of which bind to and activate the beta-adrenergic receptors. Other agents that elevate cAMP include histamine (via the H_2 receptor) and phosphodiesterase inhibitors such as theophylline and caffeine. Drugs such as forskolin directly stimulate adenylate cyclase to elevate the cAMP level. Therefore, all these agents, as well as isoproterenol (a more selective beta-adrenergic activator), are positive in-

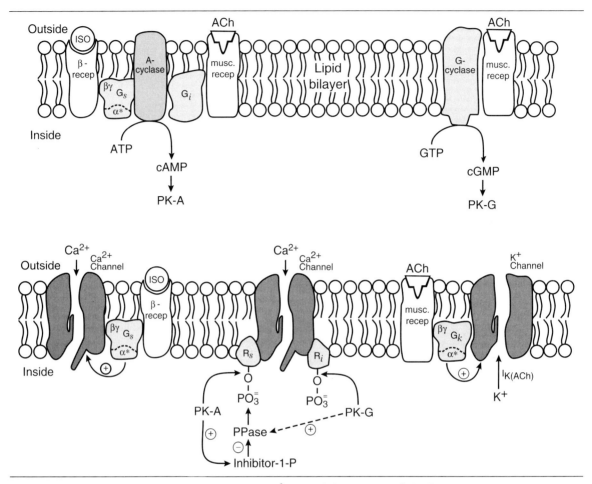

Fig. 19-3. Diagram summarizing the regulation of slow Ca^{2+} channels in the myocardial cell membrane. Included are the mechanism of action of beta-adrenergic agonists (neurotransmitter and hormones), e.g., isoproterenol (ISO), on stimulating the Ca^{2+} channel *(lower middle)* and several methods of antagonism by the muscarinic cholinergic agonist acetylcholine (ACh). The latter includes the activation of a K^+ channel by ACh ($I_{K(ACh)}$), one type of receptor-operated channel *(lower right)*, which shortens the AP. This type of channel is not present in ventricular cells. Also depicted *(lower left)* is the direct stimulation of the Ca^{2+} channel by the activated alpha subunit of the G_s coupling protein (*$G_{s\alpha}$) (SA = sinoatrial; AV = atrioventricular; ISO = isoproterenol; ACh = acetylcholine; ß-rec = beta-adrenergic receptor; Musc rec = muscarinic cholinergic receptor; A-cycl = adenylate cyclase; G-cycl = guanylate cyclase; PK = protein kinase).

otropic agents, in that they make the heart contract more forcefully. The GTP-binding proteins (G-proteins) serve to couple membrane receptors to membrane enzymes (or to ion channels). G_s-protein stimulates adenylate cyclase, whereas G_i-protein inhibits this enzyme.

The parasympathetic nerve neurotransmitter acetylcholine (ACh), which activates the muscarinic cholinergic receptors, is a negative inotropic agent, in that it makes the

heart contract less forcefully. It acts by a number of mechanisms, several of which are depicted in Fig. 19-3. As one mechanism, the G_i coupling protein reverses the stimulation of adenylate cyclase produced by the beta-adrenergic receptor (via G_s coupling protein), thus lowering the elevated cAMP level. As a second mechanism, the activation of guanylate cyclase raises the cGMP level. cGMP activates PK-G and, as described above, phosphorylates the

Ca^{2+} channel to inhibit it. PK-G also may phosphorylate and stimulate a phosphatase that dephosphorylates the site phosphorylated by PK-A and thereby inhibits the Ca^{2+} channel. Another mechanism involves activation (gating) of a special type of K^+ channel by means of a G_k coupling protein that increases the outward (repolarizing) K^+ current, resulting in the early termination of the cardiac AP that deactivates the slow Ca^{2+} channels. These G-protein–gated K^+ channels, which are responsible for the ACh-activated K^+ current, exist in atrial myocardial cells and nodal cells but not in ventricular myocardial cells of mammals. Thus the cardiac sympathetic and parasympathetic innervations act in an antagonistic manner on the force of contraction of the heart. The sympathetic nerves stimulate the heart to contract more forcefully, whereas the parasympathetic nerves cause the heart to contract less forcefully.

Special Properties of the Ca²⁺ Slow Channels

The slow Ca^{2+} channels in cardiac muscle possess some special properties that are different from other types of ion channels. These features are summarized in Table 19-2. One special property is that the activity of the slow Ca^{2+} channels **depends on metabolic energy** in the form of ATP. Thus, under conditions of hypoxia or ischemia, which are known to inhibit metabolism and lower ATP level, the slow Ca^{2+} channels are selectively inhibited. The other types of ion channels continue to function, at least initially, and so almost normal APs continue to be generated. Only the plateau of the AP becomes slightly more triangular because the Ca^{2+} current contribution to the plateau is missing (see Chap. 21). However, contraction is greatly depressed or abolished because of the loss of the

Table 19-2. Special Properties of Slow Ca^{2+} Channels in Myocardial Cells

1. Activity dependent on metabolic energy (ATP)
2. Activity inhibited (quickly and reversibly) by acidosis (half-inhibition at pH 6.6)
3. Activity stimulated by cAMP and phosphorylation by cAMP-PK
4. Activity inhibited by cGMP and phosphorylation by cGMP-PK
5. Activity inhibited by calcium antagonist drugs and stimulated by calcium agonist drugs

cAMP=cyclic adenosine monophosphate; cGMP=cyclic guanosine monophosphate; PK=protein kinase.

Ca^{2+} influx through the slow Ca^{2+} channels; i.e., there is uncoupling of contraction from excitation.

A second important special property is that the slow Ca^{2+} channel activity is **selectively inhibited by acidosis** (see Table 19-2), e.g., during ischemia. This allows almost normal APs to continue to be generated, although the contractions are greatly depressed. Therefore, ATP is conserved by the ischemic myocardial cells, and this protects them. Half-inhibition occurs at a pH of about 6.6 and almost complete inhibition at pH 6.1. The effect of acidosis is quick in onset and in offset (i.e., rapidly reversible).

The third and fourth important properties are that slow Ca^{2+} channel activity is **stimulated by cyclic AMP** and **inhibited by cyclic GMP** (see Table 19-2 and Fig. 19-3). cAMP activates PK-A, and cGMP activates PK-G. As discussed in the preceding section, this antagonistic relationship allows the two sets of autonomic nerve innervation to the heart to exert antagonistic effects on the force of contraction and heart rate by regulating Ca^{2+} entry into the cells, in accordance with the physiologic needs. The two cyclic nucleotides exert their regulatory effects on the slow Ca^{2+} channels by **phosphorylation of the channel protein** itself or of **associated regulatory proteins** (see Fig. 19-3). The PK-A site stimulates channel activity, whereas the PK-G site inhibits channel activity. Phosphorylation by PK-A increases both the probability that the Ca^{2+} channel will be opened (at a given voltage) and the mean open time. Some silent (inactive) channels also are recruited into activity by phosphorylation. Phosphorylation by PK-G decreases the probability of channel opening and the mean open time.

A fifth special property of slow Ca^{2+} channels is that they are preferentially blocked by a class of drugs known as **calcium antagonists** or **slow-channel blockers** (see Table 19-2). Four major chemical types of such drugs are represented by verapamil, bepridil, diltiazem, and nifedipine. A small chemical change in the dihydropyridine molecule (e.g., nifedipine) causes the drug to act as a Ca^{2+} channel opener or so-called **calcium agonist** (e.g., Bay-K-8644). Thus the activity of slow Ca^{2+} channels is inhibited by Ca^{2+} antagonist drugs and stimulated by Ca^{2+} agonist drugs.

The special properties of the slow Ca^{2+} channels of the heart protect the heart under ischemic conditions. For example, if vasospasm develops in one of the major coronary arteries supplying the heart muscle, the resulting acidosis quickly shuts off the slow Ca^{2+} channels but allows the other types of ion channels to function normally. Therefore, the myocardial cells in the ischemic zone stop contracting because most of the Ca^{2+} influx into the cells has ceased. Therefore, these myocardial cells have become excitation-contraction *un*coupled.

In addition to direct regulation of slow Ca^{2+} channels, Ca^{2+} influx is indirectly controlled by regulating the activity of one type of K^+ channel that is inhibited by ATP. Therefore, in normal hearts, with normal ATP level, the activity of this K^+ channel is continuously suppressed. This channel becomes unmasked (available to be voltage activated) when the ATP level is lowered in ischemic myocardial cells. Thus, during the AP, a large outward repolarizing K^+ current is increased earlier, thereby terminating the AP prematurely and causing brief APs. Hence the Ca^{2+} channels are turned back off prematurely by the AP repolarization, causing considerably less contraction.

Inhibition of contraction allows the ischemic cells to conserve their ATP content, because most of the ATP use is associated with contraction. Thus, when the blood flow returns to normal (vasospasm relieved), the cells can fully recover and resume contracting. Therefore, the slow Ca^{2+} channels and ATP-sensitive K^+ channels serve to protect ischemic myocardial cells.

Smooth Muscle

In smooth muscle, the force of contraction or state of tone depends on $[Ca]_o$, but some agents can trigger the release of intracellular Ca^{2+} from the SR (e.g., via IP_3 production) and so produce contraction even at very low $[Ca]_o$ (Figs. 19-1 and 19-4). As in cardiac muscle, the relationship between contractile force and $[Ca]_i$ is sigmoid on a logarithmic scale. In smooth muscle, Ca^{2+} acts as a **second messenger** to activate the myosin light-chain kinase for the phosphorylation of the myosin light chains and production of force (see Chap. 18).

Examples are the smooth muscles of the gastrointestinal tract, uterus, and blood vessels. The visceral smooth muscles generally fire APs that propagate at a velocity of about 5 cm/sec. Some vascular smooth muscles fire APs in response to graded excitatory postsynaptic potentials — or excitatory junction potentials (EJPs) — that depolarize to a threshold potential (Fig. 19-5). Other smooth muscles normally do not discharge APs, but contraction is controlled by graded changes in the membrane potential (graded depolarization) produced by neurotransmitters, hormones, and autocoids (local "hormones").

Resting Potential and Action Potentials

The resting potential of smooth muscle cells is generally about –55 mV, although this may range from –40 to –70 mV depending on the location of the smooth muscle. There is an electrogenic Na^+-K^+ pump contribution to the resting potential of about 8 mV. The resting potential in smooth muscle cells is considerably lower than that in cardiac muscle or skeletal muscle because of a higher ratio of Na^+ to K^+ permeability (see Chap. 3).

In those smooth muscle cells which normally fire APs, the AP overshoots to about +10 mV. Thus the AP amplitude is about 65 mV (from –55 to +10 mV). The maximum rate of rise of the AP is about 10 V/sec, which is much slower than that in myocardial cells (approximately 200 V/sec) and skeletal muscle fibers (about 600 V/sec). The AP duration at 50% amplitude (APD_{50}) is about 30 msec, compared with about 3 msec in skeletal muscle fibers and 100 to 200 msec in myocardial cells. However, some vascular smooth muscles (e.g., aorta of rat) exhibit a prolonged plateau component that follows the spike, thus giving long APD_{50} values of about 100 msec. In some smooth muscles, the rate of repolarization of the AP is even faster than the rate of depolarization, suggesting a large, fast turn-on of the delayed-rectifier K^+ conductance and current (see Fig. 19-5). If activation of the K^+ conductance occurs earlier, this prevents the AP spike from attaining its normal overshoot potential (+10 mV), thus causing undershooting APs (e.g., peak voltage reached of about –10 mV) and even inexcitability. The rising phase of the AP in most smooth muscles is produced by an inward Ca^{2+} current carried through slow Ca^{2+} channels (see Fig. 19-5). Most smooth muscle cells do not normally possess functional Na^+ fast channels.

Following the AP spike, there is often an **afterpotential** (see Chap. 4) of the hyperpolarizing type, produced by the increase in the delayed-rectifier K^+ conductance persisting beyond the spike and causing hyperpolarization toward the K^+ equilibrium potential (E_K).

Many smooth muscles have spontaneous contractions and electrical activity; i.e., they possess **automaticity.** Automaticity is produced by pacemaker potentials that depolarize the cell to its threshold potential (see Chaps. 3 and 21). Some smooth muscles, such as the longitudinal layer of small intestine, have a peculiar type of pacemaker potential known as **slow waves,** which are slow oscillations in the membrane potential with a periodicity of several seconds. During their depolarizing phase, a train of APs is elicited, the frequency of the burst gradually diminishes, and the APs stop when the repolarizing phase of the slow wave is underway. Thus the APs occur in bursts during successive **slow-wave oscillations.** The peak-to-peak amplitude of the slow wave is about 15 to 30 mV. One hypothesis for generation of the slow waves is based on **oscillations in the electrogenic Na^+-K^+ pump.** Some smooth muscles behave like **stretch receptors,** in that

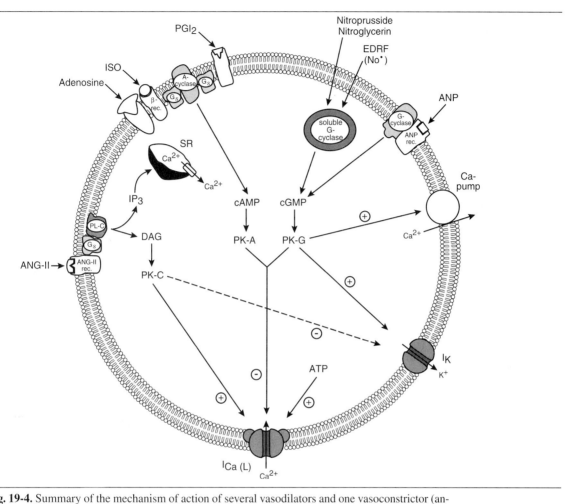

Fig. 19-4. Summary of the mechanism of action of several vasodilators and one vasoconstrictor (angiotensin-II) in vascular smooth muscle. The nitrovasodilators (nitroprusside and nitroglycerin) and endothelial-derived relaxing factor (EDRF) act directly on the soluble (cytosolic) guanylate cyclase (G-cyclase) to stimulate its activity and elevate the cGMP level. Atrial natriuretic peptide (ANP) stimulates the sarcolemmal G-cyclase via its membrane receptor. The beta-adrenergic agonist isoproterenol (ISO) and the prostaglandin (PGI₂) prostacyclin act on their respective receptors, thus stimulating the adenylate cyclase (A-cyclase) (via the G_s coupling protein) and elevating cAMP level. cAMP and cGMP activate their respective protein kinases (PKs), resulting in phosphorylation of the slow Ca²⁺ channel protein (or associated regulatory protein) and inhibiting their activity. cAMP and cGMP also stimulate the delayed-rectifier K⁺ channels, which depresses excitability and AP generation, therefore indirectly inhibiting Ca²⁺ influx. Thus such vasodilators inhibit Ca²⁺ influx and stimulate K⁺ efflux. In addition, cGMP may stimulate Ca²⁺ efflux via the sarcolemmal Ca²⁺ pump and thereby also act to lower $[Ca]_i$ and produce relaxation and vasodilation. Angiotensin stimulates phosphoinositol turnover; and thereby inositol-tris-phosphate (IP₃) and diacylglycerol (DAG) production. IP₃ activates the Ca²⁺-release channels of the SR, resulting in Ca²⁺ release, $[Ca]_i$ increase, and hence contraction. DAG activates PK-C, which phosphorylates the slow Ca²⁺ channel, stimulating channel activity and hence Ca²⁺ influx. Angiotensin also inhibits the delayed-rectifier K⁺ channel, prolonging the AP and the Ca²⁺ influx through the slow Ca²⁺ channels (I_K= K⁺ current, $I_{Ca(s)}$ = slow Ca²⁺ current; NO• = nitric oxide).

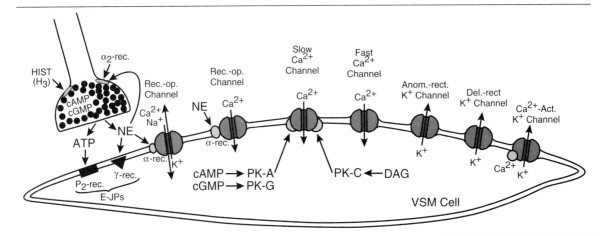

Fig. 19-5. Various types of ion channels in a vascular smooth muscle (VSM) cell. Depicted are three different types of Ca^{2+} channels (fast, slow, and receptor-operated) and a nonselective ion channel (receptor-operated), which allows Ca^{2+}, Na^+, and K^+ to pass through. Also depicted are three different types of K^+ channels (anomalous-rectifier, delayed-rectifier, and Ca^{2+}-activated). Also shown is an adrenergic nerve terminal from which norepinephrine (NE) and ATP are released to activate alpha and gamma receptors and purinergic (P_2) receptors, respectively, on the postsynaptic membrane. Release of neurotransmitters may be modulated by substances such as NE, histamine, and cyclic nucleotides (E-JP = excitatory junction potential).

stretch of the muscle leads to partial depolarization and initiation of AP bursts and contractions.

Nerve Control

As stated earlier, some smooth muscles are closely controlled by the autonomic nervous system. In these cases, most of the smooth muscle cells are not very far from a nerve terminal and so can be influenced by the diffusion of neurotransmitter (see Fig.19-5). Depending on the type of neuron (sympathetic or parasympathetic) and neurotransmitters released, the smooth muscle can be either stimulated to contract or be inhibited to relax. Because of cell-to-cell propagation of APs, the effect of the neurons can be quickly reflected over greater distances than the diffusion of the neurotransmitter alone would predict. In some smooth muscles (e.g., intestinal and uterine), excitation can be propagated over relatively long distances with little decrement (fall-off or dying-out) of activity.

Control of Contraction and Relaxation by $[Ca]_i$

Contraction

As discussed for cardiac muscle, elevation of $[Ca]_i$ initiates contraction (see Fig. 19-1), and lowering $[Ca]_i$ pro-

duces relaxation (see Fig. 19-2). Elevation of $[Ca]_i$ is produced by three events: (1) **Ca^{2+} influx** through the voltage-dependent slow Ca^{2+} channels and fast Ca^{2+} channels, (2) **Ca^{2+} release** from the SR stores through activation of the Ca^{2+}-release channels in the SR membrane by Ca^{2+} ("trigger" Ca^{2+}) or by IP_3 or both, and (3) reversed **Ca^{2+}-Na^+ exchange** (see Fig. 19-1). In addition, Ca^{2+} influx can occur by means of the **receptor-operated ion channels** (not voltage-gated) that are selective for Ca^{2+} (see Figs 19-1 and 19-5). In most smooth muscles examined, the number of **fast Ca^{2+} channels** is relatively small compared with the number of **slow Ca^{2+} channels,** as is true of myocardial cells.

Thus the Ca^{2+} current that is responsible for the **rising phase of the propagated AP** also serves as one **second messenger** involved in initiating contraction. The Ca^{2+} influx not only contributes to the elevation of $[Ca]_i$ but also **triggers the release** of more Ca^{2+} from the SR (see Fig. 19-1). As discussed in Chap. 18, the Ca^{2+}-calmodulin complex activates the myosin light-chain kinase, which phosphorylates the myosin light chains to bring about contraction.

Relaxation

Relaxation of smooth muscle, as in cardiac muscle, is produced by lowering of $[Ca]_i$ back to the resting level of about 1×10^{-7} M (see Fig. 19-2). This is accomplished by turning off Ca^{2+} influx and Ca^{2+} release, coupled with stimulation of the Ca^{2+} pumps. The Ca^{2+} pumps of both the sarcolemma and SR are stimulated by the elevated $[Ca]_i$. Stimulation of Ca^{2+} sequestering into the SR speeds relaxation, as would an increase in the rate of the Ca_i-Na_o exchange (in the forward direction, ie., Ca^{2+} transported out). Inhibition of the Ca^{2+} APs and excitability causes relaxation. The high $[Ca]_i$ stimulates the Ca^{2+}-Na^+ exchanger to exchange in the *forward* direction: internal Ca^{2+} for external Na^+. When the membrane potential reverts to the original resting level following the AP, this makes the energetics again favorable for the exchanger to run in the forward direction.

In summary, a combination of these factors (two pumps and one exchanger), coupled with the shutting off of the enhanced Ca^{2+} entry into the cell because the AP has terminated (and therefore the voltage-gated slow Ca^{2+} channels have reclosed), allows $[Ca]_i$ to be lowered to the resting level and the muscle to relax (see Fig. 19-2).

Modulation of Contraction

In myocardial cells we learned that cAMP stimulated the activity of the slow Ca^{2+} channels, whereas cGMP inhibited their activity. In contrast, in vascular smooth muscle, both cyclic nucleotides act in the same direction, namely, to inhibit the activity of the slow Ca^{2+} channels (see Figs. 19-4 and 19-5). Therefore, any agent that elevates cAMP or cGMP in vascular muscle would tend to cause vasodilation by relaxing the vascular smooth muscle. For example, atrial natriuretic peptide and endothelial cell nitric oxide (which stimulate guanylate cyclase and raise cGMP) and beta-adrenergic agonists (which stimulate adenylate cyclase and raise cAMP) are vasodilators. Drugs such as nitroprusside, which directly activate the soluble (cytosolic) guanylate cyclase to elevate cGMP, also act as vasodilators (see Fig. 19-4). The effects of the cyclic nucleotides are mediated by their respective protein kinases and phosphorylation of the slow Ca^{2+} channel protein (or associated regulatory protein).

ATP has been shown to be required for activity of the slow Ca^{2+} channels in vascular smooth muscle. Lowering the cellular ATP level inhibits (half-inhibition value of 0.3 mM) the slow Ca^{2+} channels and Ca^{2+} influx and hence would tend to cause vasodilation in response to metabolic inhibition.

Because the slow Ca^{2+} channels are preferentially blocked by the calcium antagonist drugs (see section on cardiac muscle), and because the binding of these drugs is sensitive to the membrane potential, and thus their blocking effect is greater at lower (i.e., less negative) resting po-

tentials, their effect is more pronounced on smooth muscles than on cardiac muscle. Therefore, they can exert substantial vasodilating effects (and thus be a therapeutic treatment for angina pectoris and hypertension) without significantly depressing the heart's pumping action. A new class of antihypertensive vasodilator drugs (e.g., pinacidil) has been developed recently that act by opening K^+ channels, thereby hyperpolarizing and relaxing the vascular smooth muscle.

Another mechanism proposed for the inhibition of the tonic contraction of some smooth muscles by cyclic nucleotides is stimulation of the sarcolemmal Ca^{2+}-ATPase pump (see Fig. 19-4) to lower $[Ca]_i$ and so inhibit contraction. Thus agents that elevate cAMP or cGMP levels in vascular smooth muscle produce vasodilation by at least three mechanisms: (1) inhibition of the slow Ca^{2+} channels, (2) stimulation of the delayed-rectifier K^+ channels, and (3) stimulation of the sarcolemmal Ca^{2+} pump.

Some vasoconstrictor agents, such as angiotensin-II, stimulate phosphatidylinositol turnover and production of IP_3 and diacylglycerol (see Fig. 19-4). As stated previously, diacylglycerol activates PK-C, and IP_3 acts as a second messenger on the SR membrane. IP_3 activates the Ca^{2+}-release channels, which release Ca^{2+} from the SR stores. Elevation of $[Ca]_i$ by this mechanism stimulates contraction. Thus angiotensin-II stimulates contraction through the operation of at least three mechanisms: (1) production of diacylglycerol and activation of PK-C for phosphorylation of the slow Ca^{2+} channels, (2) production of IP_3 and release of Ca^{2+} from the SR, and (3) inhibition of the delayed-rectifier K^+ channel, thereby prolonging the APs and augmenting Ca^{2+} influx.

Summary

In myocardial cells, the activity of the slow Ca^{2+} channels is regulated by a number of mechanisms, including cyclic nucleotide levels, the ATP level, and pH. These Ca^{2+} channels can be opened or stimulated by some drugs (e.g., dihydropyridine Ca^{2+} agonists) and blocked or inhibited by others (e.g., dihydropyridine Ca^{2+} antagonists). cAMP, through phosphorylation of the slow Ca^{2+} channel protein (or of an associated regulatory protein) by PK-A, stimulates the channels. cGMP, through phosphorylation by PK-G, inhibits the channels. Therefore, cAMP and cGMP have antagonistic effects. Thus the heart has a number of extrinsic ways for the Ca^{2+} influx to be regulated, ensuring that the force of contraction and frequency of contraction can be controlled and adjusted to meet the physiologic demands.

The myocardial cells also have a number of intrinsic ways to regulate the Ca^{2+} influx under adverse conditions and so can protect themselves from irreversible damage. One type of K^+ channel is constantly suppressed by the normal ATP level, but this repression is reversed when the ATP level falls (e.g., during ischemia). This shortens the AP plateau and depresses Ca^{2+} influx and contraction and hence conserves ATP and protects the cells. The ACh-activated K^+ channel ($I_{K(ACh)}$), which is directly gated by the alpha subunit of the G_k-coupling protein, is activated when the muscarinic receptor is activated, thus shortening the AP plateau and depressing contraction.

The regulation of $[Ca]_i$ and excitation-contraction coupling in smooth muscle is similar in some ways to that in cardiac muscle. The ion channels and membrane receptors allow the force and frequency of contraction of the smooth muscle, as well as its state of tone (sustained contraction), to accommodate to the physiologic demands. The inward current during the rising phase of the AP in smooth muscle cells is carried through the slow Ca^{2+} channels. This Ca^{2+} influx during the AP also acts as a second messenger to alter the state of contraction.

In vascular smooth muscle, for example, the activity of the slow Ca^{2+} channels is regulated by a number of mechanisms, including the cyclic nucleotides (cAMP and cGMP), the ATP level, and the protein kinase C activity (see Fig. 19-4). Phosphorylation of the channel protein by PK-A and PK-G inhibits channel activity, whereas phosphorylation by PK-C stimulates channel activity. Therefore, agents that elevate the cAMP or cGMP level act as vasodilators (inhibit contraction), whereas agents (such as angiotensin-II) that stimulate IP_3 and diacylglycerol production (thereby activating PK-C) act as vasoconstrictors (see Fig. 19-4).

Contraction of smooth muscle is inhibited not only by direct inhibition of the slow Ca^{2+} channels but also by indirect inhibition exerted through stimulation of the K^+ channels. cAMP and cGMP stimulate the activity of K^+ channels (delayed-rectifier type) and thereby increase K^+ efflux, hyperpolarize, and depress excitability (see Fig. 19-4). This prevents the turn-on of the voltage-dependent slow Ca^{2+} channels, thereby inhibiting Ca^{2+} influx. Activation of the Ca^{2+}-sensitive K^+ channels or the ATP-regulated K^+ channels would have the same effect, namely, vasodilation.

One major difference between smooth muscles and cardiac muscle is the presence of receptor-operated Ca^{2+} channels in smooth muscles (see Figs. 19-1 and 19-5). The presence of such non-voltage-gated Ca^{2+} channels underlies the concept of **pharmacomechanical coupling,** such that some agents are able to produce contraction without producing a change in the resting potential or initiation of APs.

Bibliography

Fabiato, A. Calcium release in skinned cardiac cells: Variations with species, tissues, and development. *Fed. Proc.* 41:2238–2244, 1982.

Sperelakis, N. Regulation of calcium slow channels of heart by cyclic nucleotides and effects of ischemia. In: Bosnjak, Z. J., and Kampine, J. P., eds. *Proceedings of 1993 Symposium on Anesthesia and Cardiovascular Disease: Advances in Pharmacology,* Vol. 31. London: Academic Press, 1994. Pp. 1–24.

Sperelakis, N., and Kuriyama, H., eds. *Ion Channels of Vascular Smooth Muscle Cells and Endothelial Cells.* Amsterdam: Elsevier, 1991.

Sperelakis, N., and Ohya, Y. Electrophysiology of vascular smooth muscle. In: Sperelakis, N., ed. *Physiology and Pathophysiology of the Heart,* 3rd ed. Amsterdam: Kluwer Academic Publishers, 1994. Pp. 859–893.

Part III Questions: Muscle Physiology

1. An increase in the total isometric force with increases in length seen at long muscle lengths (sarcomere lengths greater than 3.6 μm) can best be attributed to
   A. the passive elastic behavior of muscle.
   B. an increase in overlap between thick and thin filaments.
   C. an increase in thin-filament length.
   D. stimulation of ATP synthesis.
   E. increased release of Ca^{2+} from the SR.
2. Relaxation of skeletal muscle is associated with
   A. rapid dissociation of thick filaments into myosin dimers.
   B. uncoupling of the T-tubules from the surface membrane.
   C. reduction of intracellular Ca^{2+} by uptake into the SR.
   D. inhibition of creatine kinase.
   E. formation of "rigor" links.
3. During a single crossbridge cycle,
   A. troponin is cleaved from tropomyosin.
   B. Ca^{2+} dissociates from myosin, eliciting a change in conformation to that of a rigor link.
   C. the hydrolysis of ATP on the myosin crossbridge is the force-generating step.
   D. one ATP molecule is hydrolyzed.
   E. one molecule of lactate is produced.
4. If a muscular disorder is characterized by low-level activity of glycogen phosphorylase, an enzyme which is rate limiting for glycolysis, which of the following symptoms would be characteristic of this condition?
   A. Moderate muscle activity would be normal, but intensive muscle activity would be disabling.
   B. Muscles would contract spontaneously and irregularly.
   C. Contraction would be normal but relaxation would be impaired.

   D. There would be pronounced atrophy in all muscle fibers.
   E. There would be insenstivity to normal Ca^{2+} levels.
5. Relaxation of smooth muscle is associated with
   A. dephosphorylation of myosin light chains.
   B. activation of myosin light-chain kinase.
   C. increases in the concentration of inositol-tris-phosphate.
   D. increased oxidative metabolism.
   E. formation of the latch state of the crossbridges.
6. In comparison to fast-twitch (type IIB, FG) fibers, slow-twitch (type I, SO) fibers have
   A. a higher myoglobin content.
   B. a higher glycolytic capacity.
   C. more T-tubule–sarcoplasmic reticulum junctional surface area.
   D. similar myosin isoforms.
   E. different force-length relationship.
7. Ca^{2+} release from the SR is brought about physiologically by at least two mechanisms, one of which is?
   A. Long-range forces
   B. IP_3 production
   C. Caffeine
   D. Ryanodine
   E. Mechanical squeezing
8. Which one of the following statements is *correct* for the Ca^{2+}-Na^+ exchanger working in the *reverse* direction?
   A. Exchanges intracellular Ca^{2+} with extracellular Na^+
   B. Exchange stoichiometry is one extracellular Ca^{2+} to three intracellular Na^+
   C. Exchange stoichiometry is three Ca^{2+} to one Na^+
   D. Exchange is nonelectrogenic
   E. None of the above

IV Cardiovascular Physiology

Part Editor
Richard A. Walsh

20 Basic Principles of Cardiovascular Physiology

Richard A. Walsh

Objectives

After reading this chapter, you should be able to

Describe the functional anatomy of the heart and valves

Explain the normal sequence of blood flow through the heart and cardiovascular system

Identify the principal determinants of blood flow through the cardiovascular system

---

> A man is as old as his arteries.
> Thomas Sydenham

The principal function of the heart and circulatory system is to provide oxygen and nutrients and to remove metabolic waste products from tissues and organs of the body. This is accomplished by a closed-loop system in which large blood vessels provide the conduits for delivering and receiving these materials. The heart is a muscular pump that provides the energy for transporting the blood through this system to facilitate the exchange of oxygen, carbon dioxide, and other metabolites through the tiny thin-walled capillaries. An appreciation of normal cardiocirculatory physiology provides an essential foundation for understanding disease states that affect the heart and blood vessels and the actions of various cardioactive drugs.

Heart and vascular disease is the most common cause of morbidity and mortality in adults in the Western world. For example, over one-half million people die each year from heart attacks and over sixty million people in the United States have some form of cardiocirculatory disease. Cardiovascular disease is also the principal cause of all deaths in men between the ages of 35 and 70 years. These statistics emphasize the importance of medical students having a firm understanding of basic cardiocirculatory phenom-

ena. The major elements of the heart and vascular system will be described in this chapter. More detailed considerations of the various aspects of normal cardiovascular physiology will be covered in subsequent chapters.

Overview of the Heart

The heart is a four-chambered pump that is largely composed of a special type of striated muscle, called **myocardium.** Two major pumps operate in the heart, and they are the **right ventricle,** which pumps blood into the pulmonary circulation, and the **left ventricle,** which pumps blood into the systemic circulation. Each of these pumps is connected to a special booster pump, called the **right** and **left atrium.** The heart possesses a specialized electrical system that ensures the overall timing of ventricular and atrial pumping is optimal for producing the **cardiac output,** or the amount of blood pumped by the heart per minute.

Functional Anatomy of the Cardiac Conduction System

The normal pacemaker of the heart is a self-firing unit located in the right atrium and called the **sinoatrial node.**

The electric impulse generated by this tiny structure activates the two atria and stimulates atrial contraction. The electric impulse then reaches the main specialized conduction system by means of conducting pathways within and between the atria. The impulse is delayed at the level of the **atrioventricular node** and is then transmitted down a rapid conduction system, composed of the **right** and **left bundle branches,** to stimulate the two ventricles and cause them to contract. The normal pacemaker and specialized conduction system are influenced by **intrinsic automatic activity** and by the **autonomic nervous system,** which modulates heart rate and the speed with which electrical impulses are conducted through the specialized system, as will be discussed in detail in Chap. 21.

There are many diseases that interfere with the specialized electrical system of the heart and may result in abnormally fast, slow, or irregular heart rhythms.

Functional Anatomy of the Cardiac Chambers

The two atrial chambers are thin-walled structures possessing conduit reservoir and booster pump functions. They passively transmit blood during ventricular filling, store blood during ventricular contraction, and augment ventricular filling by contraction toward the end of ventricular relaxation. The **right atrium** receives unoxygenated venous blood from the **superior** and **inferior venae cavae,** and the **left atrium** receives oxygenated blood from the **pulmonary veins** (Fig. 20-1). The right and left ventricles provide the major energy for displacement of blood from the heart into the vascular system. The **right ventricle** pumps blood into the low-pressure pulmonary circulation. Consequently, the right ventricular wall is relatively thin (approximately 3 mm). By contrast, the **left ventricle** pumps blood into the high-pressure systemic circulation, and although the cavity size of the right and left ventricle is similar, the left ventricle has much thicker walls (approximately 6 to 10 mm).

The force and rate of contraction of the heart are highly variable and dependent on many factors (Chap. 23). These factors include heart rate, the amount of ventricular filling, the resistance to ejection of blood, and the intrinsic ability of the heart muscle to generate force and eject blood (Fig. 20-2). The autonomic nervous system may greatly modify the contractility of heart muscle in response to changing physiologic or pathologic conditions. For example, the sympathetic nerve terminals in the heart release norepinephrine, which is a powerful stimulant for heart muscle

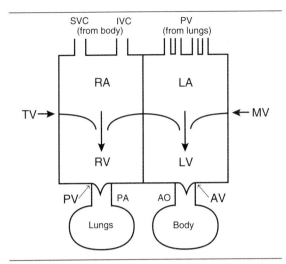

Fig. 20-1. The relationship among the four cardiac chambers, their valves, and the great vessels. Blood flows from the superior vena cava (SVC) and inferior vena cava (IVC) to the right atrium (RA) through the tricuspid valve (TV) and into the right ventricle (RV). Right ventricular contraction propels blood through the pulmonic valve (PV) into the pulmonary artery (PA). After oxygenation of blood and elimination of carbon dioxide in the pulmonary capillaries, oxygenated blood returns to the left atrium (LA) through the pulmonary veins (PV). Left atrial blood traverses the mitral valve (MV) into the left ventricle (LV). During ventricular contraction, the aortic valve (AV) opens and blood is propelled into the aorta (AO). In diastole, the atrioventricular valves (TV, MV) are open, while the semilunar valves (PA, AO) are closed.

contraction during exercise or other stressful conditions (see Fig. 20-2).

A number of diseases impair or destroy a variable amount of heart muscle and lead to **heart failure,** defined as a cardiac output that is inadequate for the metabolic needs of the peripheral tissues. These diseases include those caused by destruction of a region of the heart muscle by an inadequate blood supply, such as occurs during a heart attack, viral infections, and other pathologic processes.

Functional Anatomy of the Cardiac Valves

There are four **intracardiac valves** (see Fig. 20-1). Two of these valves are called the **atrioventricular valves** because they prevent leakage of blood backward from the ventricles into the atria when the right and left ventricles contract to eject blood into the pulmonary artery and aorta,

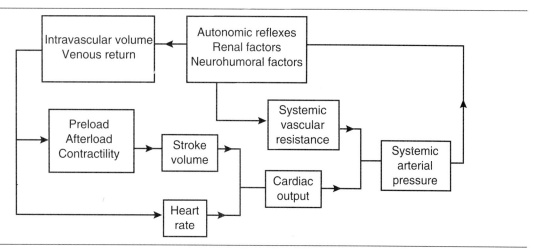

Fig. 20-2. The major determinants of blood flow in the cardiovascular system. Stroke volume (the amount of blood pumped per cardiac contraction [systole]) is determined by the preload (amount of cardiac filling during relaxation [diastole]), afterload (amount of resistance to ventricular ejection), and contractility (ability of heart muscle to develop tension and eject blood independent of preload and afterload). The product of stroke volume and heart rate is the cardiac output. The product of cardiac output and systemic vascular resistance is the systemic arterial pressure. These intrinsic circulatory factors are modulated by reflex, neurohormonal, and renal variables as well as intravascular volume.

respectively. The two-leaflet **mitral valve** serves this function between the left ventricle and left atrium, and the three-leaflet **tricuspid valve** is the barrier to retrograde flow of blood from the right ventricle to the right atrium. The other two valves are situated between the ventricles and the great arteries and are called **semilunar valves.** The **aortic valve** is interposed between the left ventricle and aorta and prevents retrograde flow from this great vessel into the left ventricle; the **pulmonic valve** serves a similar function between the pulmonary artery and the right ventricle. During the contraction phase of the heart, called **systole,** when the ventricles develop pressure and eject blood, the mitral and tricuspid atrioventricular valves close, while the semilunar aortic and pulmonary valves open. During the relaxation phase of the cardiac cycle, called **diastole,** the atrioventricular tricuspid and mitral valves open and allow the ventricles to fill from the atria, while the semilunar valves are closed (see Fig. 20-1).

The timing of normal atrioventricular and semilunar valve closure is important in understanding the generation of normal and abnormal heart sounds as they are heard over the chest using a stethoscope (Chap. 23). The four cardiac valves may be affected by congenital or acquired disease, and this may result in leakage of blood through the valve or obstruction to blood flow.

Functional Anatomy of the Coronary Circulation

The **coronary arteries** are the first arterial branches to arise from the aorta just above the aortic valve. These vessels provide oxygen and nutrients to the heart muscle of all four cardiac chambers (Chap. 24). **Atherosclerosis** (variable obstruction of the coronary vessels by plaques composed of lipid fibrous tissue and calcium) may variably obstruct or completely occlude one or more of the coronary arteries, producing electrical instability of the heart, death of heart muscle (myocardial infarction), or death of the patient.

Functional Anatomy of the Pericardium

The **pericardium** is an extremely thin-walled membranous sack that surrounds the heart. There is a small amount of fluid in the space between the surface of he heart and the pericardium that serves as lubrication. The pericardium anchors the heart within the chest cavity, prevents overfilling of the cardiac chambers, and protects the heart from infectious diseases that may affect the lungs.

Overview of the Circulatory System

Major Circulations

The two principal circulations of the body are linked in sequence so that blood flows through the organs and tissues of the body, returns to the lungs, and recycles throughout the body after oxygen is acquired and carbon dioxide is eliminated through pulmonary respiration (see Fig. 20-1). Unoxygenated venous blood returns by means of the **superior and inferior venae cavae** to the right atrium and subsequently to the right ventricle. The right ventricle pumps blood through the **pulmonary artery** to the lungs, where **pulmonary gas exchange,** defined as uptake of oxygen and release of carbon dioxide, occurs at the level of the capillaries. The oxygenated blood then flows through the pulmonary veins into the left atrium and subsequently to the left ventricle, where it is pumped to the arteries and capillaries of the rest of the body (Chap. 25).

The primary function of the **pulmonary circulation,** also called the **central** or **lesser circulation,** is to transport deoxygenated blood at low pressure through the lungs. The pulmonary circulation contains about 10% of the total blood volume at any given time.

The principal function of the **systemic circulation,** also called the **peripheral circulation,** is to provide a high-pressure source of oxygenated blood for tissue and organ perfusion and to drain venous blood back to the right side of the heart. The phasicity and level of intravascular pressures progressively drop within the components of the systemic circulation as blood flows from the arteries to the veins (Chap. 25). There is high pressure in the systemic arteries and low pressure in the veins. The major cause of reduced pulsatile pressure is the relatively high distensibility of the large arteries as compared with the smaller arteries and arterioles. The progressive decline in pressure from the aorta to the capillary level is mainly brought about by the progressive increase in the total cross-sectional area of the circulation as it branches throughout the body.

The **lymphatic circulation** is composed of tiny thin-walled channels that parallel the blood vessels of the body (Chap. 26). This circulation serves as an additional transport and drainage system. The branching network of these vessels throughout the tissues and the fluid contained within them, called **lymph,** is eventually channeled into the systemic venous circulation. Capillary filtration predominates slightly over capillary reabsorption and this produces tissue lymph flow. About 90% of net filtration is reabsorbed directly into the capillaries and 10% into the lymphatic system.

Hemodynamics and Regional Circulation

The circulation of blood in the pulmonary and systemic circulations largely depends on the interrelationships among **pressure** (force per unit area), **flow** (volume of blood transmitted per unit time), and **resistance** (the resistance to blood flow produced by structural or functional changes at the level of the arterioles). Multiple regional circulations exist in parallel off the systemic circulation. Examples of specialized regional circulations include the **coronary,** the **cerebral, skeletal muscle,** and, during pregnancy, the **placental circulation** (Chap. 25). The determinants of blood flow and tissue perfusion in these specialized circulations may vary considerably but involve a relative predominance of local, neural, or hormonal factors (Chap. 27). These factors ultimately affect resistance and hence perfusion of the relevant regional circulation. The major determinants of resistance can be understood by analogy to **Ohm's law of electrical circuits:** current flow = voltage/resistance. In circulatory physiology, this is rendered as:

$$\text{Flow} = \frac{\text{pressure difference}}{\text{vascular resistance}}$$

The systemic arterial pressure is in turn a product of flow and peripheral vascular resistance. The level of systemic arterial pressure is held relatively constant by means of reflexes elicited from the autonomic nervous system. The prevailing level of systemic arterial pressure is ultimately determined by the interplay among intravascular volume, cardiac pump performance, and neural and endocrine factors (see Chap. 27 and Fig. 20-2). Alterations in any or all of these determinants of arterial pressure may provoke abnormally elevated blood pressure or systemic arterial hypertension.

21 Initiation and Propagation of the Cardiac Action Potential

Ira R. Josephson

Objectives

After reading this chapter, you should be able to

Describe the anatomic pathways for the spread of excitation through the heart

Compare the characteristics of the action potentials generated in different regions of the heart

Explain the ionic basis for the generation of cardiac action potentials

Describe the central role of the Ca^{2+} current in excitation-contraction coupling, and understand how it is regulated

Explain the electrophysiologic basis of cardiac arrhythmias

The normal heartbeat is initiated by a complex flow of electric signals that provide the rhythm of the heart. The properties of the electric signals, or **action potentials** (APs), that are generated in the different regions of the heart are diverse, but they all have a characteristic long duration (100 to 300 msec) as compared with nerve or skeletal muscle APs. The APs generated in cells residing in the **sinoatrial** (SA) **node** display **automaticity;** that is, they undergo spontaneous and rhythmic depolarization in the absence of external stimuli. The SA node is the primary pacemaker of the heart, and impulses originating in this region propagate over the heart and drive the quiescent tissues. The electrogenesis of the cardiac AP is similar to, but somewhat more complex than, that of nerve (Chap. 4). Besides contributions from Na^+ and K^+ currents, a third current, carried by Ca^{2+}, plays a central role in coupling cardiac excitation with contraction. External influences, including the autonomic nervous system, hormones, and autacoids, modulate the force and rate of cardiac contraction through their action on the Ca^{2+} current and other currents.

In this chapter we will first examine the pathways and mechanisms for the overall spread of electrical excitation in the heart. We will then focus on the properties of the APs in different regions of the heart and the ionic currents that generate them.

Functional Anatomy of the Heart and Spread of Excitation

For the heart to act as an efficient pump for the circulation of blood, it is essential that there is precise and sequential activation of the contraction of the atria and ventricles during each heartbeat. If the atria and ventricles were depolarized simultaneously, this would cause incomplete filling of the ventricles and reduced cardiac output. The pattern of electrical activation of the heart can be recorded at the body surface and is called the **electrocardiogram** (see Chap. 22).

The primary pacemaker for the normal heartbeat is the SA node, which is located near the junction of the superior vena cava and the right atrium. It is composed of a small group of muscle cells that spontaneously and rhythmically fire APs. The SA nodal APs **propagate** (i.e., they elicit APs) in neighboring right and left atrial muscle, leading to contraction of the atria. There are three bundles of muscle fibers — the internodal tracts of **Bachmann, Wenckebach,** and **Thorel** — which ensure that the atrial musculature is rapidly and nearly simultaneously activated and that the depolarization reaches the **atrioventricular** (AV) **node.** The atria are electrically isolated from the ventricles by nonconductile connective tissue, and the spread of excitation in the ventricles can only occur by way of the AV node and the **bundle of His,** which are fine-muscle fiber tracts linking the two regions. Once excited, the AV node conducts the impulse slowly (e.g., about 3 cm/sec), permitting ample time for ventricular filling prior to contraction.

The rate of firing of the SA (and AV) node is modulated by the **sympathetic** and **parasympathetic** divisions of the **autonomic nervous system.** Sympathetic stimulation speeds up the SA node (sinus tachycardia), and parasympathetic activation slows the SA node firing (sinus bradycardia). In addition to the effects on heart rate, the autonomic neurotransmitters increase (sympathetic) or decrease (parasympathetic) the velocity of propagation of excitation through the AV nodal region. Further, the force of contraction of the heart is augmented by sympathetic stimulation and diminished by parasympathetic stimulation. The autonomic nerves innervate the atrial and ventricular myocardium.

After passing through the AV node and the bundle of His, the excitation reaches a specialized conduction system, which serves to rapidly and nearly synchronously activate the ventricular myocardium. The propagation velocity in this **Purkinje system** is the fastest in the heart, or about 1.0 m/sec. The Purkinje fibers, which comprise this system, are large-diameter muscle fibers that, at their terminals, ramify and form junctions with the ventricular myocardial cells. The Purkinje system terminates in the inner surface of the ventricular myocardium (the endocardium). Thus the excitation is transferred from the Purkinje network to the myocardial cells, thus effecting rapid and nearly simultaneous activation of the two ventricles. Propagation velocity in the ventricular myocardium is about 0.4 m/sec.

Conduction of the Cardiac AP

To understand the process by which excitation is propagated from cell to cell, it is necessary to appreciate the microscopic anatomy of the heart tissue. Cardiac muscle consists of a tight "bricklike" packing of cells, with dimensions of approximately 100 by 15 µm. The ends of neighboring cells are joined at interdigitation regions called **intercalated disks.** Within the disks, the membranes of the two cells are occasionally in close apposition and form a **nexus** or **gap junction.** Within the nexus there may be one or many **gap junction channels** that form a low-resistance pathway for the spread of current from one cell to another. The cardiac AP propagates along the myocardial fiber in a manner similar to that described for the propagation along a cable in elongated nerve and skeletal muscle cells (Chap. 5). **Local-circuit currents,** which precede the AP wavefront, depolarize the adjacent membrane, bring it to the threshold potential, and activate the inward Na^+ current. With depolarization, the local-circuit currents can flow through the gap junction channels and thereby depolarize the neighboring cell membrane to generate an AP. It is also possible that the close apposition of the neighboring cell membranes and the associated electrical field generated by the AP causes transfer of excitation in the absence of gap junction channels.

The **velocity of conduction** of the cardiac AP through each region of the heart depends on several factors. The **amplitude** and the **rate of rise of the AP** are the major determinants of propagation velocity (see Chap. 5). The amplitude represents the potential difference between the polarized (resting) and depolarized regions of the cell. Because the magnitude of the local circuit currents is directly proportional to this potential difference, the larger the amplitude of the AP, the larger and more extensive are the local-circuit currents. The result is faster conduction of the AP. The rate of rise of the AP is directly related to the density of the (net) inward current. The greater the inward current, the more extensive are the local-circuit currents, and hence faster excitation of adjacent membrane. For the normal, fast-rising AP, the inward current is supplied by the large, fast Na^+ current. For slowly rising APs in the SA and AV nodes, as well as the slow AP in the myocardium, the inward current is relatively small and is carried by the Ca^{2+} current. The difference in the density of the inward current produces a corresponding difference in the propagation velocity of these tissues.

The **size** of the fiber is directly proportional to the velocity of propagation. For example, Purkinje fibers are among the largest cells in the heart and have the largest conduction velocity. A decrease in **temperature** decreases the conduction velocity, mainly by slowing the activation of the fast Na^+ currents.

General Characteristics of Heart Action Potentials

The transmembrane potential can be recorded from individual myocardial cells by means of a microelectrode. When the microelectrode tip is outside the cell membrane, there is a potential difference of 0 mV between the microelectrode and the reference (ground) electrode. As the microelectrode tip is advanced and punctures the cell membrane, the potential difference abruptly shifts to a negative value. This negative potential is referred to as the **resting potential.**

If a myocardial cell is electrically stimulated to depolarize beyond a critical value, called the **threshold potential,** then an AP is generated that is characteristic for that cell type. The cardiac AP can be divided into several phases: **Phase 0** represents the rapid upstroke or depolarization phase of the AP, **phase 1** is the initial rapid repolarization, **phase 2** is the long-duration plateau, **phase 3** is the terminal repolarization, and **phase 4** is the resting potential (or pacemaker potential). This general description applies to a ventricular AP and should be slightly modified for the other cell types in the heart. The different properties of APs from each part of the heart will be reviewed in the following sections.

SA and AV Nodal APs

As mentioned previously, the SA node is the **primary pacemaker** of the heart, and APs recorded from these cells do not possess stable resting potentials but display a slow diastolic depolarization called the **pacemaker potential** (Fig. 21-1). The most negative potential reached (approximately –60 mV) is called the **maximum diastolic potential.** The membrane potential continues to depolarize until the threshold for firing an AP is reached (at about –40 mV). The upstroke of the SA node AP is quite slow (about

1 to 5 V/sec), as compared with the working myocardium (200 to 300 V/sec). The maximum overshoot is usually 20 to 30 mV. The plateau phase also may be briefer than that in ventricular cells. Finally, phase 3 repolarization causes the membrane potential to return to the maximum diastolic potential.

The AV node AP is similar in waveform to the SA node AP, as shown in Fig. 21-1.

Atrial AP

The atrial AP (Fig. 21-1) displays a fast rate of rise (100 to 200 V/sec) from a stable resting potential of –80 mV. The overshoot ranges from 20 to 30 mV. In most species there is a prominent phase 1; this may abbreviate the plateau and give the AP its characteristic triangular appearance.

Ventricular AP

The ventricular AP (Fig. 21-1) has a stable resting potential of –80 to –85 mV. The upstroke velocity is about 200 V/sec, and the overshoot ranges from 20 to 30 mV. The duration of the ventricular AP is intermediate between atrial and Purkinje APs, ranging from 200 to 250 msec.

Purkinje AP

Although normally large and stable (–95 mV), under pathologic conditions, the resting potential of the Purkinje fiber may depolarize spontaneously, giving rise to **automaticity.** Normally the SA node drives the heart at a rate that is faster than the intrinsic rate of discharge of the Purkinje system. The upstroke velocity of Purkinje fibers (200 to 500 V/sec) is the greatest of all the different myocardial tissues and accounts for the rapid conduction of these fibers. A long plateau and terminal repolarization are seen following a **prominent phase 1** "notch" (see Fig.

Fig. 21-1. Typical action potentials recorded from a sinoatrial (SA) node cell, atrial cell, atrioventricular (AV) node cell, ventricular cell, and a Purkinje fiber.

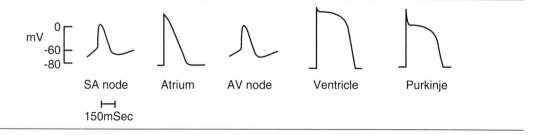

21-1). The plateau phase of the Purkinje AP is longer than that for other cardiac tissues and may help prevent reexcitation of the ventricles between beats.

Refractory Periods

In nerve cells, APs can be elicited at rates approaching 1000 per second, but this is not the case for cardiac muscle. The long duration of the AP plateau in the heart limits its ability to be driven at a high frequency. This long plateau provides ample time for ventricular filling so that the heart can serve as an effective pump.

Based on their operation, it is possible to identify at least two types of refractory periods (Fig. 21-2). The **functional** (or effective) **refractory period** is the shortest interval after the initiation of the first AP when another normal AP can be initiated. The **absolute refractory period** is the interval during which no AP can be elicited, regardless of the stimulus intensity. The **relative refractory period** is the interval during which a second AP can be elicited, but at a higher stimulus intensity. The functional refractory period lasts for the entire absolute refractory period and over half the relative refractory period. As can be seen in Fig. 21-2, the absolute refractory period lasts the entire upstroke and plateau of the AP and ends when the

Fig. 21-2. Refractor periods during the cardiac action potential. The absolute refractory period (ARP) extends from the upstroke to approximately the middle of the repolarization phase; during this time, a second action potential cannot be elicited, regardless of the stimulus intensity. The interval between the ARP and the relative refractory period (RRP) is that time when a second action potential may be elicited, but usually with a slow upstroke velocity and slower propagation. The functional refractory period (FRP) is the shortest time interval after the first action potential when another action potential can be elicited.

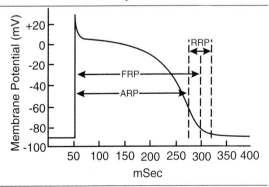

terminal repolarization of the AP reaches about –60 mV. The relative refractory period begins at the end of the absolute refractory period and continues until membrane excitability returns to normal (usually when the membrane potential returns to the resting potential). Because the current for stimulation of a not-yet-activated region is limited by the propagating AP, this defines the maximal current intensity available for stimulation, and thus defines the functional refractory period.

Effect of Resting Potential on the AP

Elevation of the extracellular K^+ concentration ($[K]_o$) reduces the K^+ equilibrium potential (E_K) and thereby depolarizes the membrane potential. Membrane **depolarization reduces the rate of rise** of the AP and eventually **decreases the overshoot.** At membrane potentials positive to –55 to 60 mV, APs (in ventricular, atrial, and Purkinje cells) may not be elicited, even by supranormal currents. Conversely, if the membrane potential were **hyperpolarized** beyond the normal resting potential (e.g., by lowering $[K]_o$ or by injecting negative current into the cell), this would **increase the rate of rise** and **overshoot.**

Basis of the Resting Potential

As described in Chap. 3, the resting potential that develops across the membrane of heart cells results from the difference in concentration of certain ions (mainly K^+ and Na^+) inside and outside the cell and from the selective permeability of the membrane to these ions. In cardiac muscle, as in nerve and skeletal muscle, K^+ plays a major role in determining the magnitude of the resting potential.

Microelectrode measurements of the membrane potential at varying $[K]_o$ show that the membrane potential does parallel E_K closely at high $[K]_o$ (exceeding 10 mM) but that the membrane potential deviates increasingly from E_K as $[K]_o$ goes below 10 mM to the physiologic level. This implies that at lower $[K]_o$, the membrane potential is not determined solely by the membrane conductance to K^+. This occurs because, as $[K]_o$ is reduced, the membrane permeability for K^+ itself is also reduced. At low $[K]_o$, Na^+ makes a proportionately larger contribution to the resting potential. Because Na^+ has a positive equilibrium potential (+60 mV), it exerts a depolarizing influence on the membrane potential, which becomes more important at low $[K]_o$. This behavior at low $[K]_o$ can be accounted for by the **Goldman constant-field equation** (see Chap. 3).

Because the resting potential is generally more positive than E_K, there is a small efflux of K+ from the cell, even at rest. As mentioned previously, the offset of the membrane potential from E_K is caused by the small influx of Na+ into the cell at rest. Over time, the loss of K+ and gain of Na+ would lead to depolarization of the membrane. The rundown of the K+ and Na+ gradients is prevented by the **Na+-K+ pumps,** which are protein transport mechanisms residing in the cell membrane that translocate Na+ out of and K+ into the cell. In both cases, the replenishing action must work against the existing concentration and electric gradients (electrochemical) for Na+ and K+, and therefore requires chemical energy from the hydrolysis of ATP.

Ion Channel Types

The diversity of the waveforms of APs recorded from cells in different regions of the heart reflects the number and type of **voltage-dependent ionic channels** residing in their cell membranes. Channels are **transmembrane proteins** that allow ions such as Na+, K+, and Ca2+ to cross the impermeable (lipid) bilayer. Membrane channels are **gated** to open or close as the result of changes in the transmembrane potential. Following a voltage change, some channels open or close. as a function of time. The major types of ionic channels that are known to exist in certain heart cell membranes are listed in Table 21-1. Ionic channels can be identified on the basis of their **ionic specificity,** their **conductance,** their **voltage dependence,** and their **kinetics** (i.e., how long it takes for them to turn on or off).

Ionic Basis of Cardiac AP

Rising Phase

The rapidly rising APs generated by ventricular, atrial, and Purkinje cells have in common that their **phase 0** is caused by the rapid influx of Na+ across the cell membrane. Depolarization leads to Na+ influx, which leads to further depolarization, and so on. The upstroke is therefore a regenerative process, as in nerve. Early evidence that supported this conclusion was obtained from experiments in which the Na+ concentration in the solutions bathing the heart cells was varied, and the effects on the rate of rise and overshoot of the AP were analyzed. It was found that both the overshoot and rate of rise of the AP were directly proportional to the external Na+ concentration.

More recent experimentation, employing the voltage-clamp method to measure the membrane currents directly (see Chap. 4), has left little doubt that a **fast Na+ current** is responsible for the upstroke of ventricular, atrial, and

Table 21-1. Types of Ion Channels in the Heart

Type	Heart Tissue
Na+ fast channels	Atrial myocardial cells
	Ventricular myocardial cells
	Purkinje fibers
	AV nodal cells (low-density)
Ca2+ slow channels	Atrial myocardial cells
	Ventricular myocardial cells
	Purkinje fibers
	SA nodal cells
	AV nodal cells
K+ channels	
Inwardly rectifying K+ channels	Atrial myocardial cells
	Ventricular myocardial cells
	Purkinje fibers
Delayed K+ channels	Atrial myocardial cells
	Ventricular myocardial cells
	Purkinje myocardial cells
	AV nodal cells
	SA nodal cells
Transient outward K+ channels	Atrial myocardial cells
	Purkinje fibers
Pacemaker channels	
"Funny" currents	Purkinje fibers
Hyperpolarizing currents	SA nodal cells
	AV nodal cells
Ligand-operated channels	
Ca2+-activated nonspecific channels	Ventricular myocardial cells
	Purkinje fibers
ATP-sensitive K+ current	Ventricular and atrial myocardial cells
ACh-sensitive K+ current	Atrial myocardial cells
	SA nodal cells
	AV nodal cells

AV = atrioventricular; SA = sinoatrial; ACh = acetylcholine.

Purkinje APs. The term *fast* refers to the short time it takes for the current to turn on (activate) and turn off (inactivate). During a voltage-clamp step (from an initial, or holding, potential of −80 mV), the fast Na+ current **activates** and reaches a peak in 0.1 to 1.0 msec (depending on the potential at which it is measured). It then spontaneously declines, or inactivates, in 1 to 10 msec. A rapid activation of a fast Na+ current of large magnitude (usually

10 to 100 times larger than the other ionic currents) is required to produce the rapid rates of depolarization measured for these cells.

We may think of the **fast Na+ channel** as existing in one of three **states** (Chap. 4). It may be in the **resting, active,** or **inactivated state.** What determines the particular state of the channel is the membrane potential and the amount of time that the channel has "experienced" that potential. We say, therefore, that fast Na+ channels are **voltage-dependent and time-dependent.** Each Na+ channel has two gates in series that govern the movement of Na+ through the pore. One gate is called the **activation (A) gate,** and the other is the **inactivation (I) gate.** If both gates are open, Na+ is permitted to flow through the channel and into the cell. If one or both gates are closed, the channel does not conduct Na+.

If the membrane is depolarized (e.g., by a voltage-clamp circuit) above a critical level from the resting potential, the A-gates of individual Na+ channels open rapidly and Na+ flows into the cell (see Chap. 4). At the same time, the I-gate, which was originally open at rest, begins to close. The channel must then experience repolarization of the membrane potential for a certain time before it can conduct Na+ again. This process is called **recovery.** As mentioned, all the transitions between the three states of the Na+ channel are both voltage-dependent and time-dependent. Because activation is faster than inactivation, it is possible for the channels to activate briefly and then return to the resting state, without incurring inactivation. Such a procedure gives rise to **tail currents** that display the time course for channel deactivation, and these may be used to determine the voltage dependence of the conductance.

Direct measurements of single-channel currents in isolated heart cells can now be obtained experimentally using the **patch voltage-clamp method** (see Chap. 4). For example, single Na+-channel currents can be recorded from a membrane patch. The amplitude of the single Na+-channel currents is 1 to 2 picoamps (10^{-12} amps), and their average duration is several milliseconds. Although the individual openings of the channel appear to occur **randomly** in time, an average of many samples shows the characteristic activation and inactivation time courses described for the total Na+ current. During a voltage step, the channel may open and close more than once, before becoming inactivated. Individual cardiac cells have thousands of Na+ channels.

Plateau

The long-duration plateau is a **unique characteristic** of the cardiac AP, and its electrogenesis has been the subject

of continuing study for over three decades. The most obvious features of the plateau are that the membrane potential is maintained at a positive value and that it is relatively constant for hundreds of milliseconds. Because the membrane potential is always the result of the sum of all the inward and outward membrane currents, the plateau must represent a fine balance of inward and outward currents. Experiments in which the membrane resistance was measured during the phases of the AP by the injection of current pulses have shown that the membrane resistance is highest during the plateau. These results have led to the conclusion that both the inward and outward currents flowing during the plateau must be of small magnitude. This has been supported directly by the voltage-clamp experiments in which the inward and outward currents have been examined separately.

Repolarization: Outward K+ Currents

We have already learned that the plateau results from a balance of inward (Ca^{2+}) and outward (K^+) currents. The final repolarization of the AP must then be caused by inactivation of the Ca^{2+} current and an increase in the outward current, which then repolarizes the membrane back to the resting potential. Several **K+ currents** contribute to the plateau and repolarization, and these will be discussed briefly.

The **inwardly rectifying K+ current** (I_{K1}) is that K+ conductance which is turned on at rest and generates the resting potential. The channels allow current to flow inward more easily than outward, hence inwardly rectifying. During depolarization of the AP upstroke, I_{K1} **turns off** and remains so until the membrane potential begins to repolarize. Late in the repolarization, I_{K1} generates a small outward current, which further aids in repolarization.

The **transient outward K+ current** is mainly present in Purkinje and atrial cells and is responsible for producing the **initial phase 1 repolarization** (or "notch") of the AP. It turns on rapidly with depolarization and inactivates during the AP.

The **delayed outward K+ current** (I_K) is the main current responsible for initiating the **final repolarization** of the AP. As the name suggests, I_K turns on very slowly, and its contribution occurs at the final phase of the AP. Recent evidence has shown that I_K is regulated by the autonomic nervous system, thereby controlling the AP duration. Norepinephrine (which increases cyclic adenosine-3′,5′-monophosphate [cAMP] levels) increases the magnitude of the outward K+ current, thereby tending to shorten the AP duration.

A diagram of the ionic currents that contribute to the ventricular AP is given in Fig. 21-3.

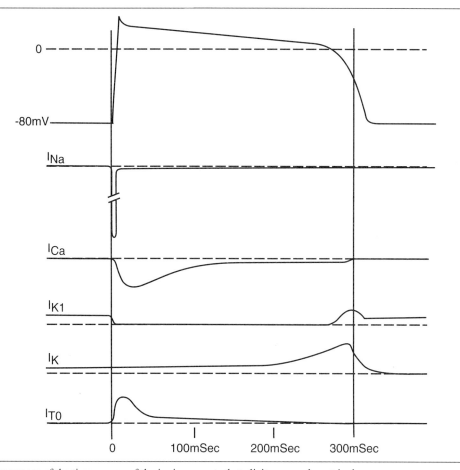

Fig. 21-3. A summary of the time course of the ionic currents that elicit a normal ventricular cardiac action potential. All of the currents, except the inwardly rectifying current (I_{K1}), are off at rest and turned on during depolarization, as indicated. I_{K1} is turned on at rest and turns off with depolarization. The fast Na$^+$ current (I_{Na}) is interrupted, since it is much larger than the other currents and would be off the scale in this diagram (I_{Ca} = inward Ca^{2+} current; I_K = delayed outward K$^+$ current; I_{TO} = transient outward K$^+$ current).

Properties of the Ca^{2+} Currents

In the absence of the fast Na$^+$ current (by voltage inactivation or by the addition of tetrodotoxin), a small second inward current, carried by Ca^{2+}, is recorded when there is depolarization under voltage-clamp conditions. The **Ca^{2+} current** (sometimes called the **slow inward Ca^{2+} current** to differentiate it from the fast Na$^+$ current) activates at membrane potentials above –50 mV, is maximal around 0 to +10 mV, and has a positive reversal potential (above +100 mV). The Ca^{2+} current peaks within a few millisec-

onds but inactivates very slowly over several hundred milliseconds.

There are **two types of Ca^{2+} channels** in certain cardiac cells. One type, called **low-threshold,** is activated over a more negative potential range, and these channels inactivate relatively rapidly. The other type, called **high-threshold,** is activated at less negative potentials, and the channels inactivate very slowly. At the single-channel level, these two types of Ca^{2+} channels also may be differentiated by their differing conductances and kinetics. (Some of their other properties will be discussed in the following sections on the regulation of Ca^{2+} currents.) Ca^{2+} channels are about 10 times less numerous than Na^+ channels in the cell membrane, which partly accounts for the smaller magnitude of the total Ca^{2+} current.

Regulation of Ca^{2+} Currents

The influx of Ca^{2+} serves as the **trigger** and **modulator** of the force of contraction of the myocardial cell (see Chap. 19). In light of this central role of the Ca^{2+} current, it is not surprising that several levels of regulation exist to control the activity of the voltage-dependent Ca^{2+} channels and hence Ca^{2+} influx.

The first and most direct regulation of Ca^{2+} influx occurs as a result of Ca^{2+} flowing through the Ca^{2+} channel itself. Studies have demonstrated that inactivation of the Ca^{2+} channel is at least partially dependent on the **accumulation of Ca^{2+} ions at a binding site** at, or near, the inner surface of the channel. Thus Ca^{2+} influx through the Ca^{2+} channel provides a negative feedback signal that inhibits subsequent Ca^{2+} influx during depolarization. Such a mechanism serves to limit Ca^{2+} influx and help maintain $[Ca]_i$ at very low levels at rest.

Another level of regulation over the Ca^{2+} current is mediated by the **autonomic nervous system.** We are all familiar with the increased heart rate and force of cardiac contraction when fear or anger is provoked or upon exertion. This primitive fight-or-flight response is triggered by the increased activity of the sympathetic nervous system. The neurotransmitter **norepinephrine** is released from nerve terminals located throughout the heart in response to sympathetic activation. Norepinephrine molecules diffuse from the nerve terminals to the myocardial cells, where they bind to specific receptor proteins on the outer surface of the membrane. By binding to the receptor, a stimulatory signal is transmitted to an associated enzyme (located on the inner surface of the membrane), called **adenylate cyclase.** The adenylate cyclase catalyzes the reaction that converts ATP to **cAMP.** cAMP is regarded as a second (intracellular) messenger, whereas norepinephrine is considered a first (extracellular) messenger. The importance of cAMP is that it activates a **protein kinase** that, among many other functions, **phosphorylates the Ca^{2+}-channel protein,** thereby increasing its activity. It is clear that norepinephrine elevates intracellular cAMP levels, and this is tightly correlated with an increase in the magnitude of the Ca^{2+} current and the force of contraction. At the single-channel level, norepinephrine increases the probability of the high-threshold Ca^{2+} channel being open during depolarization. Because the channel is more often open, more current can flow through it, thus increasing the total current.

The restorative branch of the autonomic nervous system, the **parasympathetics,** counteracts the sympathetics by slowing the heart rate and decreasing the force of contraction. Activation of parasympathetic nerve fibers leads to release of acetylcholine from nerve terminals, which can occupy and activate another set of specific receptors located on the heart cell membrane. **Acetylcholine** reduces the portion of the Ca^{2+} current that was increased by norepinephrine. Thus acetylcholine restores the Ca^{2+} current to its original or basal magnitude. The reduction of the Ca^{2+} current by acetylcholine is thought to be related to a reduction in the cAMP levels and dephosphorylation of the Ca^{2+} channels. Alternatively, acetylcholine may increase in the **cyclic guanosine-3',5'-monophosphate level,** which itself acts to reduce the Ca^{2+} current.

Another level of regulation of the Ca^{2+} current is imposed by agents carried in the systemic circulation. An example of these agents is the peptide **angiotensin-II,** which has been shown to increase the Ca^{2+} current.

Ca^{2+}-Dependent Slow AP

Normally, the fast Na^+ current is responsible for the rapid depolarization of the upstroke of the cardiac AP. Experimentally, however, it is possible to block the fast Na^+ current with **tetrodotoxin,** which binds specifically to and **blocks fast Na^+ channels** at low concentrations. Another method takes advantage of the fact that the Na^+ current is **voltage inactivated** (blocked) if the membrane potential is held at a depolarized level, less than -50 mV. Depolarization may be induced either by injection of a constant positive current into the cell or by elevation of the external K concentration to about 25 mM, thereby decreasing E_K and consequently depolarizing the membrane (Fig. 21-4).

If the partially depolarized membrane is stimulated by applying current pulses, it will not respond and will appear unexcitable. If the cardiac cell is exposed to a positive inotropic agent (which increases the force of contraction), such as norepinephrine, electric stimulation causes a **regenerative, slowly rising** (10 to 20 V/sec) **overshooting AP** (the slow response) and associated contractions (see Fig. 21-4). The rising phase of the slow AP is caused by the influx of Ca^{2+}. The Ca^{2+} influx, and therefore the slow AP, is blocked by the addition of certain known Ca^{2+}-blocking (or antagonistic) agents. These include manganese, cobalt, cadmium, nickel, and lanthanum (inorganic blockers), as well as verapamil, nifedipine, and other **dihydropyridines** (organic blockers).

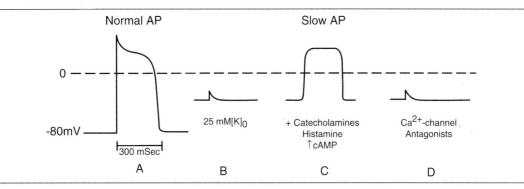

Fig. 21-4. The slow, Ca^{2+}-dependent action potential (AP). (A) The normal action potential. (B) The external K^+ concentration ($[K]_o$) is raised to 25 mM, causing partial depolarization of the membrane potential and loss of excitability. (C) The addition of certain positive inotropic agents (such as catecholamines, histamine, or cyclic adenosine-3′,5′-monophosphate [cAMP]) induces a slowly rising, overshooting, slow-response action potential. (D) The slow Ca^{2+}-dependent action potential is abolished by Ca^{2+}-channel antagonists, such as cobalt, cadmium, nickel, lanthanum, verapamil, and nifedipine.

Many positive inotropic agents increase the Ca^{2+} current and thereby induce the slow AP. Elevation of the intracellular cAMP levels is a common mechanism for many of these agents. In addition, the slow AP may be induced simply by elevating the $[Ca]_o$, thereby increasing the current flowing through the "basal" Ca^{2+} channels. The slow AP also may be induced by reducing the amount of outward K^+ current by the addition of a K^+-channel blocker, such as tetraethylammonium ion.

The slow AP is important in that it may replace the normal fast AP in a region of the heart tissue during pathologic states, such as **ischemia.** During ischemic damage, there may be an elevated $[K]_o$, leading to depolarization and partial block of the fast Na^+ current, and increased concentrations of norepinephrine, brought about by the sympathetic discharge. These conditions will lead to slow AP formation. Because the slow AP propagates more slowly than does the fast AP (the propagation velocity is proportional to the density of inward current during the upstroke), propagation of excitation through the ischemic depolarized region may be disrupted, leading to **arrhythmia.**

Ionic Basis of Automaticity

The unceasing rhythmic contraction of the heart is normally driven by the spontaneous electrical activity of a small group of cells — the SA node. Other heart tissues (e.g., the AV node and Purkinje fibers) are also capable of displaying **automaticity** but are usually suppressed by the faster rate of firing of the SA node. The rate of firing is determined by several factors (Fig. 21-5), including the **slope of the pacemaker potential.** A more **positive slope** means that the membrane potential is depolarizing more rapidly and will therefore more rapidly reach the threshold for firing an AP. The rate is also determined by the **maximum diastolic potential,** in that, given the same slope, the AP arising from a more negative potential will take longer to reach threshold. A third factor is the **threshold potential** itself, which may change and also affect the time it takes to reach threshold.

The rate of firing of the SA node AP is modulated by the **autonomic neurotransmitters.** Sympathetic stimulation (releasing norepinephrine) accelerates the rate of firing by increasing the slope of the pacemaker potential, and parasympathetic stimulation (releasing acetylcholine) reduces the rate of firing by decreasing the slope and hyperpolarizing the pacemaker potential.

In contrast to the stable resting potential of ventricular and atrial cells (net inward and outward currents are balanced, i.e., equal zero), cells of the SA and AV nodes and the Purkinje fibers have **imbalanced inward and outward currents** and hence display automaticity. The slow depolarization of the pacemaker potential implies that there is either a time-dependent increase in the net inward current or a time-dependent decrease in the net outward current or both.

The ionic mechanisms that generate automaticity can be examined using the voltage-clamp method (Fig. 21-6). Several ionic currents may be involved in generating the

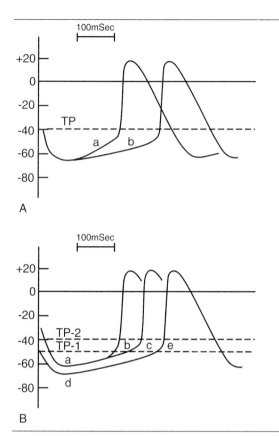

Fig. 21-5. The mechanisms for changing the firing rate of a pacemaking cell. (A) A decrease in the slope of the pacemaker potential (b) lengthens the time to reach the threshold potential (TP) and hence causes a greater cycle length. (B) A less-negative TP (compare a to b [TP-1] and a to c [TP-2]) lengthens the cycle. In addition, hyperpolarization of the maximum diastolic potential (d to e) also increases the time to TP and the cycle length.

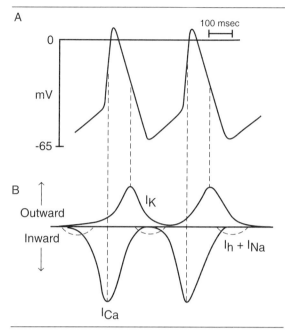

Fig. 21-6. The ionic currents responsible for the generation of pacemaker action potentials in the SA node. (A) The spontaneous APs of the SA node. (B) The inward and outward ionic currents (I_{Ca}, I_K, I_h, and I_{Na}) that contribute to the generation of the APs.

pacemaker potential, and the specific currents in the SA node may differ from those in the Purkinje fibers. In the SA node, a low-threshold Ca^{2+} current is responsible for contributing inward current to the pacemaker potential. This current is increased by norepinephrine and reduced by acetylcholine. An outward delayed K^+ current that is activated during the plateau and turned off (or deactivated) during the pacemaker potential also contributes to depolarization. Nodal cells do not have a large conductance for K^+ at rest because they lack inwardly rectifying K^+ channels. This condition also promotes automaticity, because the resulting high membrane resistance allows entry of only a small inward current to promote depolarization. In Purkinje fibers, a background Na^+ current, which may result from

the slow component of inactivation of the fast Na^+ current, contributes inward current to the pacemaker potential, along with a low-threshold Ca^{2+} current. Deactivation of the delayed outward K^+ current also promotes depolarization. The inwardly rectifying K^+ current is present in Purkinje fibers but tends to turn off with depolarization from the maximum diastolic potential (about –90 to –95 mV).

Another current, called the I_f **("funny" current),** is turned on by repolarization of the AP and contributes inward, depolarizing current. This "funny" current is carried by Na^+ and K^+; it is increased by norepinephrine and reduced by acetylcholine. A similar current exists in the SA node, where it is called the **hyperpolarizing current,** but it may not play a major role in pacemaking in those cells, since the membrane potential does not reach the negative values necessary for full activation.

Cardiac Arrhythmias

Any disturbance in the normal rate or rhythm of cardiac electrical activation may lead to **cardiac arrhythmias.** Because, as already emphasized, the electrical activity of cardiac muscle triggers and modulates the force of contraction, the inherent danger from arrhythmia is that the heart may not perform as an efficient pump of blood. Clinically, the electrocardiogram is a useful tool for detecting cardiac arrhythmia and discerning its origin within the heart (see Chap. 22).

Arrhythmia may arise from an alteration in the normal sequence of excitation. Normally, the SA node is the fastest pacemaker of the heart, and it determines the heart rate. Other cardiac tissues, including the AV node, Purkinje fibers, and even the atrial and ventricular muscle, may, under pathologic conditions, display automaticity. If the rate of firing of these ectopic pacemakers is greater than that from the SA node, or if the signal from the SA node is blocked, they will supersede in the job of driving ventricular depolarization. The latter behavior is demonstrated when conduction between the atria and ventricles is slowed or blocked by an alteration in the properties of the AV node. Then the AV node itself or the Purkinje system may take over as the pacemaker, usually driving the ventricles at a slower than normal rate.

Another type of arrhythmia, termed **reentrant arrhythmia,** arises when cardiac excitation reenters tissues of an **abnormal anatomic circuit** that would normally be refractory to excitation. The continued abnormal excitation is called **circus movement,** since it may travel around the path without cessation.

Reentrant arrhythmia results from several causes. One of these was mentioned previously and is the slow, Ca^{2+}-dependent AP that forms in a region of depolarization caused by ischemia or hypoxia, with consequential slow propagation through that region of the ventricle. Because the excitation travels slower through the damaged region, it may reach and reexcite normal tissue, which, because of the delay, is no longer refractory. If the timing is "right" and a nonrefractory pathway is available, the ectopic impulse may be continuously reflected around the abnormal circuit, with dire effects on cardiac pumping.

Arrhythmias may result from **early** and **delayed afterdepolarizations.** An early afterdepolarization occurs when a second premature AP is generated during the plateau or repolarization phase of a preceding AP. A delayed afterdepolarization occurs after the repolarization of the preceding AP is completed and may give rise to a premature AP. In either event, the premature AP may display abnormally slow conduction, leading to reentry.

The most serious form of arrhythmia is **ventricular fibrillation,** in which multiple circus movements cause totally uncoordinated ventricular excitation. During fibrillation, the pumping ability of the heart is lost, so this condition must be terminated within minutes for patient survival. Ventricular fibrillation can be converted to nor-

mal sinus rhythm by the application of a large electric shock to the heart.

Alterations in the cellular electrophysiology of cardiac cells can be studied to provide insight into the mechanism of the generation of certain arrhythmias. For example, arrhythmia may be brought about by high doses of the cardiac glycoside **digitalis,** which is used to treat cardiac failure. This agent produces depolarizing APs, which may lead to the formation of premature APs and arrhythmia. Recently it has been shown that elevation of $[Ca_i]$, produced by digitalis, activates a **transient inward current,** which is responsible for the depolarization.

Summary

The heart rate is determined by the firing of spontaneous APs in the SA node. Excitation is propagated throughout the myocardium by means of specialized conduction pathways. APs from the different heart tissues have different waveforms and properties. These different waveforms are a consequence of the type and amount of specific ionic currents that generate the APs. The upstroke of APs in rapidly conducting tissues and the myocardial cells is caused by the fast Na^+ current. The slowly rising APs of SA and AV nodes are caused by an inward Ca^{2+} current through voltage-dependent slow channels. The Ca^{2+} current is a major component of the AP plateau; it also initiates and modulates contraction of the myocardial cell. Outward K^+ currents repolarize the AP back to the resting potential. Cardiac arrhythmias are disturbances in the rate or rhythm, or both, of excitation, and arise from alterations in the generation or conduction of the AP.

Bibliography

Cranefield, P. F. *The Conduction of the Cardiac Impulse.* Mount Kisco, N.Y.: Futura, 1975.

Hoffman, B. F., and Cranefield, P. F. *Electrophysiology of the Heart.* Mount Kisco, N.Y.: Futura, 1976.

Noble, D. *Initiation of the Heartbeat.* Oxford: Clarendon, 1979.

Sperelakis, N. Electrogenesis of the cardiac resting potential. In: Berne, R. M., and Sperelakis, N., eds. *Handbook of Physiology,* Vol 1: *The Cardiovascular System.* New York: Oxford University Press, 1979. Pp. 187–267.

Sperelakis, N., ed. *Physiology and Pathophysiology of the Heart.* 2nd ed. Boston: Kluwer Academic Publishers, 1989.

22 Physiologic Basis of the Electrocardiogram

Gunter Grupp, Ingrid L. Grupp, and William C. Farr

Objectives

After reading this chapter, you should be able to

Identify the sequence of electrical events of the heart by obtaining a body surface electrogram — the electrocardiogram

Describe the normal conduction pathways from the sinoatrial node through the atria, atrioventricular conduction system, His-Purkinje system, to and through the ventricles

Explain the importance of the anatomic and electrophysiologic sequence of depolarization in an efficiently coordinated cardiac contraction

Describe the difference between the conduction pathways of depolarization and the process of repolarization

Name each component of the electrocardiographic complex and describe the underlying physiologic reasons for each component

Use the concept of a cardiac dipole to explain why the different electrocardiographic leads record different-appearing QRS complexes, although they are produced by the same electrical forces

Determine the mean electrical axis of the QRS complex of an electrocardiogram, using any two bipolar limb leads, and explain why any two limb leads yield the same finding

Suggest reasons for the different appearance of a QRS complex initiated by an ectopic ventricular pacemaker, as compared with a normally conducted impulse

---

The electrocardiogram (ECG) provides clinically useful information about the electrical orientation of the heart, the relative size of the heart chambers, conduction defects in the heart, consequences of changes in coronary blood flow (ischemia), and others. It does *not* reflect the state of the mechanical performance of the heart.

A great deal of our current knowledge of the equipment, recording techniques, and the theoretical basis of the ECG was gained from the work of Willem Einthoven. In 1903 he began a systematic study of the potential differences between different parts of the heart recorded on the body surface. The ECG is a composite picture of the changing potential differences during cardiac excitation, depolariza-

tion, and repolarization recorded between electrodes on the skin surface and plotted on moving paper (Fig. 22-1).

Many theories have been proposed to explain the ECG tracing based on cellular events. Stated simply, depolarization of one sector of the heart causes a difference in the potential between the depolarized and polarized regions that produces an electric current. Because electrolytes contained in the tissues and fluids of the body surrounding the heart are good conductors, these electric currents reach the skin surface. Two ECG electrodes placed on the skin detect these changing potential differences. These continuously changing potentials are greatly amplified and recorded on calibrated moving paper.

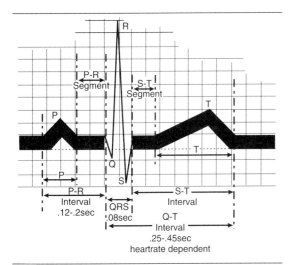

Fig. 22-1. Nomenclature of the deflections, intervals, and segments of the normal electrocardiogram.

The source of the electrical force, the heart, can be considered as a single electrochemical generator located in the center of a sphere, and this "generator" is made up of positive and negative charges — a **dipole.** A dipole is best described mathematically using a vector. A **vector** can describe brief instants during the excitation process (instantaneous vector), or it can be used to summate a large number of instantaneous vectors (a mean vector). Over the 0.4- to 0.7-second (400- to 700-msec) duration of one heartbeat, a multitude of dipoles can be described by an equal number of vectors, giving insight into the electrical activity of the heart. The algebraic mean of all ventricular vectors is represented by the **mean electric axis.**

Terminology of the ECG

As described in the preceding chapter, the heartbeat is initiated by a spontaneous depolarization in the **sinoatrial (SA) node,** which is located at the junction of the superior vena cava and the right atrium. The impulses travel rapidly (1.0 to 1.5 msec) through all right and left atrial fibers, depolarizing them. This atrial depolarization wave is recorded on the skin surface as the **P wave** of the ECG (see Fig. 22-1). This wave is normally a small, smooth wave without obvious notching, about 2 mm in height and 0.08 second in duration. The depolarization then traverses slowly (0.02 to 0.05 msec) through the **atrioventricular**

(AV) **node** to the bundle of His and its branches and emerges again in the very fast-conducting Purkinje system (2.0 to 4.0 msec) to enter both ventricles, thereby initiating the **QRS complex.** The conduction velocity through the ventricular myocardium is very fast (1.0 to 2.0 msec). As a result, the duration of ventricular depolarization (QRS) is only 0.05 to 0.10 second. In general, the first downward deflection after the P wave is called the **Q wave** (see Fig. 22-1). The first upward component after the Q wave is the **R wave,** and the downward deflection after an R wave is the **S wave** (see Fig. 22-1). If there is a second upward deflection (caused by ventricular depolarization) after the S wave, it is labeled an **R′ wave,** and so on. Independent of the sequence of depolarization waves, the complex is always called the **QRS complex.** Ventricular repolarization occurs during the **T wave.** This wave is generally upright and about 0.15 to 0.25 second in duration.

The **PR interval,** which is the period between the beginning of the atrial depolarization and the beginning of the ventricular depolarization, is normally 0.12 to 0.2 second in duration. Shorter PR intervals may indicate AV conduction shortcuts, and longer intervals may indicate partial or complete AV block.

The **QT interval** encompasses the time from the beginning of the QRS complex to the end of the T wave, or that period from the beginning of ventricular depolarization to the end of repolarization. The duration of the QT interval therefore somewhat mimics the total of all ventricular action potential durations (see Chap. 21). Heart rate has a profound effect on the duration of the action potential and consequently on QT interval duration; increases in the heart rate shorten the QT interval and decreases lengthen it. Table 22-1 lists the average QT intervals at different heart rates for men. The PR, ST, and TP segments are electrically quiet and therefore **isoelectric.**

Table 22-1. Heart Rate Dependence of QT Intervals of Normal Male Subjects

Heart Rate (beats/min)	Normal
50	0.41
60	0.39
80	0.34
100	0.31
120	0.28
150	0.25

The Basis of the ECG Recording

The following generalizations can be made about the recording of the ECG and the mechanisms that underlie it.

1. Currents flow only during **depolarization** and **repolarization.**
2. Depolarization of the heart causes **potential differences** to form between polarized and depolarized regions. The same is true during repolarization.
3. Current flows from **polarized to depolarized areas,** from plus to minus, causing potential differences.
4. Arrows (force vectors) point in the direction of the **propagation of the wave of depolarization.**
5. The **polarity** of the recording voltmeter (ECG machine) is arranged so that, in bipolar recordings, the direction of the wave of propagation toward the positive pole produces an upright deflection; conversely, if the wave of propagation is toward the negative pole, it produces a downward deflection.
6. In unipolar recordings, upright deflection indicates movement of the propagation wave toward the positive (exploring) electrode, and downward deflection, movement away from it.
7. The flow of electric currents generates **electrical fields.**
8. The field always travels in the direction the charge wants to move, from **positive to negative.**
9. Because **depolarization** runs from cell to cell until the whole heart is depolarized, current changes also run in this direction.
10. Current changes are picked up on the body surface in the form of the **changes in potentials surrounding the currents.**
11. The body is a nearly uniform **volume conductor** (a bag of saline), and the skin is a good conductor; therefore, potential differences in the heart can be measured and recorded from the surface of the body.

In brief, there are currents flowing during depolarization and repolarization; there are potential differences when currents flow; there are no potential differences when there is *no* current flow; and there are no potential differences when the heart is completely polarized (at rest) or completely depolarized (after activation and before reactivation).

Equipment and Lead System

The **electrocardiograph** is an elaborate **voltmeter** that measures the potential differences between the electrodes and records them. The arrangement of a pair of electrodes on the body surface constitutes a **lead.** In clinical practice, two lead systems are used: **bipolar** and **unipolar.**

There are **three bipolar leads,** and these are placed on the **frontal plane** of the body (Fig. 22-2IA). **Lead I** records the potential difference between the right and left arms (or shoulders); **lead II,** between the right arm and left leg; and **lead III,** between the left arm and left leg. The right leg is used to ground the patient. The three bipolar leads form the **Einthoven triangle** (dashed-line triangle in Fig. 22-2IA), with the heart at its center. An imaginary line between two electrodes of a lead is called the **lead axis** (denoted by dashed lines in Fig. 22-2).

Unipolar leads are used to add additional lead axes in the frontal plane and to obtain the V leads in the **horizontal plane.** In clinical practice, no truly unipolar lead system exists, but it can be approximated by use of **Wilson's central terminal** (denoted as *CT* in Figure 22-2IB and II). A unipolar system assumes that **one electrode** is an indifferent electrode, and the central terminal (CT) assumes this function. This "indifferent" electrode is considered to be close to zero potential (denoted as a minus in Fig. 22-2IB and II). The **second,** or exploring, **electrode** constitutes the actual recording electrode, and this detects the potential changes relative to zero from its various locations on the body surface (denoted as plus in Figure 22-2IB and II). On the frontal plane, **Goldberger's augmented unipolar limb leads** are unipolar (shown as aVF, aVL, and aVR in Fig. 22-2IB). The term **augmented** has an historical origin, in that Wilson's earlier unipolar leads recorded 50% less voltage than did the bipolar leads. Goldberger's arrangement "augmented" the sensitivity of Wilson's bipolar leads by 50% to 87%. The exploring electrodes of these three leads record potential changes manifested at the right arm, left arm, and left leg, respectively. The lead axes (dashed lines in Fig. 22-2) fit reasonably well between the lead axes of the bipolar frontal leads I, II, and III. These six frontal leads provide the so-called **hexaxial arrangement,** which constitutes a nearly all-encompassing frontal view of the electrical activity of the heart. The six chest leads (shown as V leads in Fig. 22-2, part II) are also unipolar and record the local potentials at six points along the **horizontal axis** (plane) of the thorax (V_1 to V_6).

In clinical practice, one records all twelve leads. By doing so, the distribution of the potentials on the frontal and horizontal planes of the body can be studied. This pro-

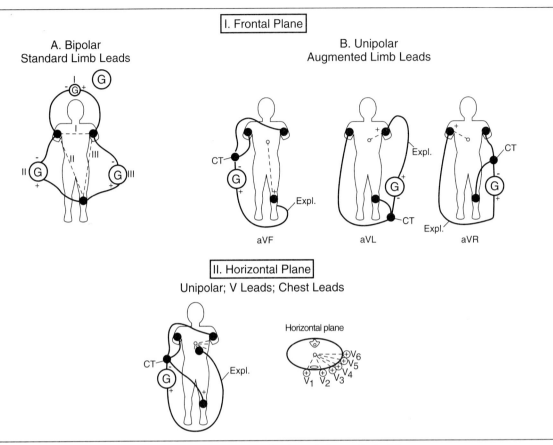

Fig. 22-2. Bipolar and unipolar lead systems of the frontal and horizontal planes (*dashed lines = lead axes*; G = galvanometer showing the potential differences on the electrodes; CT = Wilson's central terminal; Expl. = exploring electrode).

vides a reasonable amount of information about the three-dimensional distribution of the heart's potential field. The potentials recorded from various areas of the body differ because of variations in the distance of the electrodes from the heart, the amount of intervening tissue, the tissue resistance, and the arrangement of the recording leads. Because of this, the shapes and directions of the P, QRS, and T waves **are different at the various leads, although they all result from the same heartbeat.**

The Heart's Electrical Field in a Volume Conductor

When the cells of one area of the heart depolarize, their outside becomes electrically negative with respect to the quiescent positive areas. **Current flows from the positive to the negative area.** In contrast, the direction of the propagation wave of the impulse goes from outside negative (depolarized) to outside positive (polarized) areas, leaving depolarization in its wake. The **body** is not a homogeneous conducting medium. It does, however, permit currents to reach the skin surface, and therefore, it can be considered a **volume conductor.** There are areas of equal potential called **isopotential lines** (see PR and ST segments in Fig. 22-1). If two electrodes are placed in this electrical field, a potential difference is recorded, provided the electrodes are at different potentials. The potential recorded depends on how far the two electrodes are from the source and on the resistance of the conducting medium. Different potentials are recorded when the electrodes are moved relative to the source. Likewise, if the electrode position is held in a fixed site (as is the case with a given ECG lead) and the electrical field changes over time (the fields in the heart change during electrical activity), a change in the potential difference over time is recorded, and **this is what the electrocardiograph does.**

The Rotating Dipole

The ever-changing depolarization pathways in the heart and the changing cardiac mass contributing to the potentials form a very complex relationship. At any instant, there are thousands of cardiac cells depolarizing in different locations in the heart and depolarizing in various directions at different distances from the electrodes. In addition, each cell has its own characteristic action potential and conduction velocity. Therefore, there is a **multiplicity of conductive resistances** between the cells of the heart and the skin surface. To better understand this complexity, the ECG theoreticians have represented the total excitation process as a single positive and negative charge — a **dipole** (Fig. 22-3A). If one regards the cardiac dipole as the center of the chest, one can describe its magnitude and direction three dimensionally by using **vectors.** The complex excitation process of the heart can then be described with an infinite number of vectors. In reality, only a few instants in time are used; these are called **instantaneous vectors.**

By convention, a vector has a positive and negative end (see Fig. 22-3A, B). The magnitude of the arrow representing the vector is determined by the magnitude of the potential difference recorded. The potential difference recorded by an ECG can be estimated using the simple rules of **vectorial projection.** To project a vector onto a lead axis (see

Fig. 22-3B), perpendicular lines are dropped from the ends of the vector to the axis. If the vector projects onto the positive half of the lead axis, the voltage registered by the lead is positive, and the ECG records an upward deflection (see Fig. 22-3C). The magnitude of the deflection indicates the potential difference measured. The projected length of the vector in Fig. 22-3B is equal to the length of the actual vector, because both vector direction and the lead axis are parallel. In most cases, the projected length is smaller because the in situ vectors diverge from the lead axis. Consequently, if the vector projects onto the negative portion of the lead axis, the lead voltage is negative and a downward deflection is recorded. If the vector parallels or coincides with the lead axis, it projects maximal voltage onto the lead. A vector directed perpendicular to a lead axis does not project onto the lead axis, and so the ECG shows zero voltage. Rotation of the dipole vector between these two extremes yields a continuum of intermediate values. **Thus the magnitude of the potential recorded is proportional to the length of a line projected onto the lead axis.** The polarity of the recorded event is upward when a positive-recording electrode is in the heart's positive field and downward or negative when in the negative field of the heart.

The **changing electrical forces of the heart** in three-dimensional space can be described with a rotating dipole and a series of instantaneous vectors.

Mean Instantaneous Vectors

The development of several mean instantaneous vectors is depicted in Fig. 22-4. During the first part of ventricular depolarization, the left endocardial surface of the interven-

Fig. 22-3. (A) Dipole vector recorded in leads A(–) and B(+). (B) Vector projected onto lead axis. (C) Strength of vector recorded on moving paper.

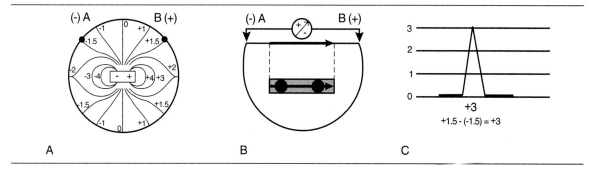

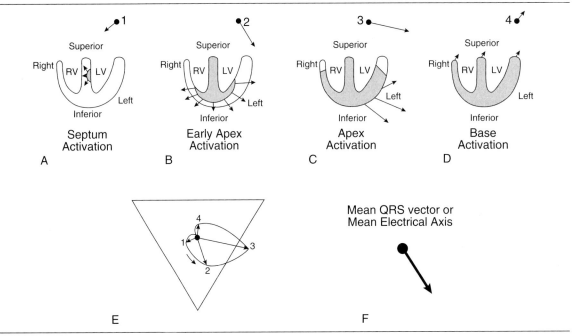

Fig. 22-4. (A–D) Time sequence and instantaneous vectors 1 to 4 during ventricular depolarization (RV = right ventricular; LV = left ventricular). (E) Vector cardiogram from vectors 1 to 4. (F) Summation of all vectors, i.e., mean QRS vector of mean electrical axis.

tricular septum is activated (see Fig. 22-4A). This takes about 5 to 10 msec. If, at that instant, all these electrical forces are averaged, a **mean instantaneous vector** can be obtained (labeled 1 in Fig. 22-4A). This vector is small and points to the right ventricle. During the subsequent phases of ventricular excitation, the forces occurring at other instants also can be averaged and represented by their respective vectors: **early apex activation** can be summarized by vector 2 (see Fig. 22-4B); **late apex activation** by vector 3 (see Fig. 22-4C); and the final **base activation** by vector 4 (see Fig. 22-4D). It follows from the example developed in this figure that a whole continuum of vectors can describe ventricular depolarization. These vectors can be used to produce a **continuous vectorial analysis** (see Fig. 22-4E). A loop can be inscribed within the Einthoven triangle, originating from the midpoint and going from there to the tips of vectors 1, 2, 3, and 4 and back to the midpoint. This is a **vector cardiogram.** Such a loop can be constructed for P, QRS, and T wave activity for any of the ECG leads. Using the method of **vector summation** in the frontal plane (see Fig. 22-4F), a total **mean QRS vector,** also called the **mean electrical axis,** can be computed.

Quantitation of a QRS Complex

Figure 22-5 (*left panel*) shows two frontal plane projections, lead I and lead III, of the four instantaneous vectors elaborated in Fig. 22-4. These projections describe the electrical forces of the ventricles at four different instants during one ventricular depolarization. In the top part of the left panel of Fig. 22-5, the vectors are projected onto lead I. Using the method described previously (see Fig. 22-3B), one can project these vectors onto the axis of lead I and quantitatively calculate the ECG deflections shown at the right of the figure. Vector 1 reflects onto the lead I axis with –2, vector 2 with +1, vector 3 with +6, and vector 4 with +1. These deflections can be plotted against time. The resulting QRS complex is shown to the right. If the exact same four electrical vectors are projected onto lead III (see lower part), a very different ECG complex is derived. Similarly, if lead II is used, or an augmented unipolar aVR, or even one of the V leads, the same electrical forces would produce **different** ECG complexes, depending on the spatial arrangement of the vectors in the respective leads. These observations explain why it is important to record all twelve leads in clinical practice.

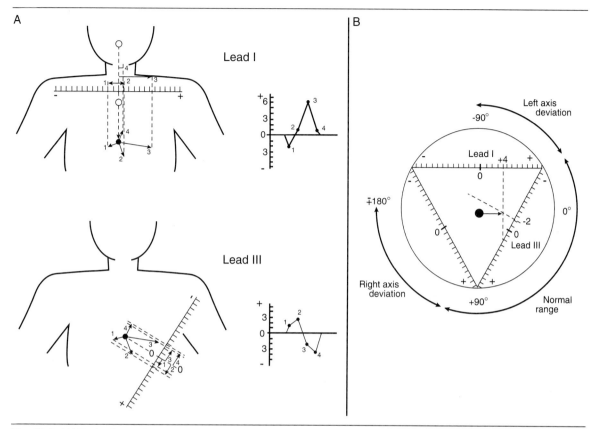

Fig. 22-5. (A) Projection and recording of instantaneous vectors 1 to 4 in leads I and III. (B) Construction of the mean electrical axis from two of the three bipolar limb leads: leads I and III.

Mean Electrical Axis

Because vectors can be used to calculate precisely the type of the ECG deflection recorded (see Fig. 22-5), the reverse is also true. In clinical practice, an ECG tracing is obtained and then used to calculate mean vectors for the P, QRS, and T waves. Most often, the inscription of the QRS complex is used to provide general insight into the direction and distribution of the electrical forces of the ventricular myocardium. This is called the **mean QRS vector,** or **mean electrical axis.**

The **mean electrical axis** is an important descriptor of the ECG, since it can be abnormal in a variety of cardiac disorders. It is determined by the anatomic position of the heart (vertical or horizontal, with the former more likely in young people and the latter more likely in obese individuals) and by the direction of electrical depolarization of the ventricles. The **mean QRS axis** is determined from the

mean QRS vector and is reported in degrees. The normal mean QRS axis in the frontal plane lies between –30 and +100 degrees. If the mean QRS axis is –30 degrees or more negative, there is **left-axis deviation,** indicating left ventricular preponderance (e.g., hypertrophy). If the mean QRS axis lies to the right of +100 degrees, there is **right-axis deviation,** indicating right ventricular preponderance.

Computation of the Mean Electrical Axis from the Three Standard Limb Leads

The mean electrical axis can be computed from any two of the three standard limb leads. In the example given in Fig. 22-5B, this was determined from leads I and III. The sum of the downward deflections of the QRS complex is subtracted from the sum of the upward deflections. In this example, the R wave of lead I has a vertical height above baseline of +6 mm with a downward deflection of –2 mm. These values are added algebraically, giving a net value of +4. At a point 4 units toward the plus sign on the lead I axis of the triangle (Fig. 22-5, *right panel*), a perpendicular line is erected. Similar measurement of lead III yields a net amplitude of upward and downward deflections of –2 (+3 –5). A perpendicular line erected 2 units toward the minus sign on lead III is extended to intersect the perpendicular line from lead I. An arrow drawn from the center of the triangle to the intersection of these two perpendicular lines indicates the **mean electrical axis,** pointing in the example to 0 degrees. Any combination of any two of the three standard limb leads will give the same result.

Ventricular Repolarization: The T Wave

Whereas the activation or **depolarization** of the ventricles occurs rapidly in the form of a progressive wave that passes from cell to cell, which is generally directed from the endocardium to the epicardium and from the apex to the base of the heart, the recovery or **repolarization** is an independent, prolonged, and complicated process that seems to be an innate property of each cell. Consequently, repolarization *does not* occur as a propagated wave. Instead, there are **multiple areas of potential difference** that are oriented in many directions, and these relationships change frequently as the recovery is completed. Although the recovery process may be depicted by a single vector, recovery actually represents the summation of the effects of the very complicated process of repolarization. Another difference between depolarization and repolarization can be gleaned from the time courses of the two events. Based on the duration of the single action potential, it is obvious that depolarization, which is associated with phase 0, is a rapid process. It requires less than 1 msec to depolarize a single cell and only 60 to 80 msec to depolarize both entire ventricles. On the other hand, repolarization, which occurs during phases 2 and 3 of the action potential, is a much longer process, requiring 150 to 300 msec to repolarize each cell and 300 to 400 msec to repolarize both ventricles.

Intuitively one might expect the T wave to be of opposite polarity from the QRS complex, because repolarization is the reverse of depolarization at the cellular level. However, because of the considerations described, this assumption is not supported by the facts: QRS and T waves in leads I and II are both upright (positive) in most normal ECGs.

The Isoelectric Line

Several segments of the ECG tracing are flat: the PR, ST, and TP segments. These segments, from which all deflections "take off," form the **isoelectric line.** The **PR segment** is not influenced by heart forces, since the mass of tissue activated during this period is too small (depolarization of the AV node, common-bundle branches). The **ST segment** probably represents that interval when most ventricular muscle cells are already completely depolarized and not yet repolarized. Because "all" cells are equally depolarized during the ST segment, no current flows and no potentials are recorded. During the **TP segment,** the ventricles are repolarized, and therefore no current flows until the next heartbeat.

Some Clinical Applications of the ECG

Heart rate and rhythm can be monitored with the ECG. **Tachycardia,** a heart rate of more than 100 beats per minute, and **bradycardia,** a heart rate of less than 60 beats per minute, can be calculated from the R-R interval and the known paper speed of the ECG. The occurrence and frequency of extra beats originating from **premature atrial depolarization** or from **premature ventricular depolarization** also can be observed. When these events originate outside the normal pacemaker area, a compensatory pause ensues until the normal rate takes over again.

The PR interval of the ECG is an important indicator of **AV conduction.** Its normal duration is 0.12 to 0.2 second. A PR interval shorter than 0.12 second may indicate a ventricular preexcitation syndrome. A PR interval longer than 0.2 second indicates **first-degree AV block** if each P wave is followed by an R wave. Intermittent failure of the conduction of the supraventricular impulse implies **second-degree AV block** with varying conduction ratios of 2:1 or 3:1 or other P waves per QRS complex. If the atrial and ventricular activities are completely independent, **third-degree** or **complete AV block** exists.

The ECG is very helpful in indicating the orientation of the heart within the body. The mean electrical axis gives an estimate of the orientation and preponderance of the heart. The normal mean electrical axis lies between about –30 and +100 degrees. Figure 22-6A is an example of an ECG in the normal range. In this instance, the QRS complexes of leads I and II are both positive overall. Figure 22-6B shows the recording from leads I, II, and III from a patient with left ventricular hypertrophy. In this instance, lead I

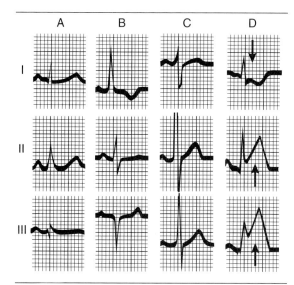

Fig. 22-6. (A–C) Mean electrical axis from leads I, II, and III. (A) Normal axis, +18 degrees; leads I and II positive. (B) Left-axis deviation, –50 degrees; lead I positive, lead II negative. (C) Right-axis deviation, +120 degrees; lead III negative, lead II positive. (D) Acute anterior myocardial infarction in which the ST segments are elevated in leads II and III. (Adapted from: Winsor, T. The electrocardiogram in myocardial infarction. *Clin. Symp.* 29:16–17, 1977. CIBA-GEIGY Pharmaceutical Co.)

Summary

When depolarization proceeds in an orderly and predictable fashion over the atria and ventricles of the heart, this generates current flows. Because the human body behaves as a volume conductor, the potential differences created by these current flows can be measured and recorded on the surface of the body, producing the ECG. Depending on the placement of the recording electrodes, the sequence of the current flows (depolarization) in the heart can be observed from many different aspects. Ordinarily, the frontal and horizontal planes of the heart are recorded, each in six different aspects; these consist of the hexaxial limb leads and the precordial V leads. The original three limb leads, introduced by Willem Einthoven in 1903, are bipolar; the augmented limb leads and V leads are unipolar. In contrast to the cell-to-cell conduction that occurs during depolarization, the process of repolarization is not conducted. Instead, it is produced by the innate properties of each cell and is therefore prolonged and complicated. The ECG is a major tool in the diagnosis of conduction defects of the heart; these include first-, second-, and third-degree heart block, arrhythmias, ectopic beats, and myocardial infarction. The recording from the different leads allows a quick assessment of the mean electrical axis of the heart, showing whether it is normal or has left- or right-axis deviation. The ECG does not, however, appraise the quality of the contractile function of the heart.

Bibliography

Chou, T. *Electrocardiography in Clinical Practice,* 3rd ed. Philadelphia: W. B. Saunders, 1991.

Cooksey, J. D., Dunn, M., and Massie, E. *Clinical Vector-cardiography and Electrocardiography,* 2nd ed. Chicago: Year Book Medical Publishers, 1977. Part I.

Einthoven, W. *Pflugers Arch.* 99:472, 1903.

Pozzi, L. *Basic Principles in Vector Electrocardiography.* Springfield, Ill.: Charles C Thomas, 1961.

Scher, A. M., and Spach, M. S. *Handbook of Physiology,* Sec. 2. Vol. I. New York: Oxford University Press, 1979. Pp. 357–392.

Snellen, H. A. Contribution of Willem Einthoven to physiology. *News in Physiol. Sci.* 4:162–165, 1989.

shows an overall positive reading and lead III a negative value: this translates into a mean axis of –50 degrees, according to the text discussion for Fig. 22-5B. This indicates a left-axis deviation. Figure 22-6C shows a right-axis deviation of +120 degrees, representing right ventricular hypertrophy; in this example, lead I had an overall negative value, and lead III, a positive one.

A **normal QRS duration** is between 0.06 and 0.1 second. About one-half the adult population exhibits a QRS value of 0.08 second. Any ventricular conduction disturbance is reflected in the QRS complex. In particular, myocardial ischemia and infarction alter the QRS complex dramatically. Figure 22-6D shows the ECG recording from leads I, II, and III of a patient with acute anterior myocardial infarction. Typical changes consist of the substantial elevation of the normally isoelectric ST segments in leads II and III. Similar radical changes in the QRS configuration can occur in a healthy ventricle that is depolarized outside its normal site (ectopic beat).

23 Determinants of Left Ventricular Performance and Cardiac Output

Brian D. Hoit and Richard A. Walsh

Objectives

After reading this chapter, you should be able to

Describe the determinants of contraction in isolated cardiac muscle and in the intact left ventricle

Describe pressure, volume, and flow phenomena during the cardiac cycle and graphically depict these events using the pressure-volume loop

Explain the significance of ventricular-vascular coupling

Left ventricular performance may be assessed by evaluating the mechanics of constituent muscle fibers; these are the **development of force** and **the velocity and extent of muscle shortening** (see Chap. 18). However, a more integrated analysis considers the left ventricle as a **muscle pump** coupled to the vascular (arterial and venous) system. The principal determinants of left ventricular function include the loading conditions (preload and afterload), the inotropic (contractile) state, and the heart rate. In this chapter, principles derived from studies in isolated cardiac muscle will be used to explain how performance is modulated in the intact left ventricle. The cardiac cycle will be described in terms of its temporal relationship with left ventricular pressure, volume, and flow and in the context of the ventricular pressure-volume relationship. Finally, coupling of the left ventricle to the vascular system will be discussed briefly.

Determinants of Myocardial Performance

Isometric Contraction

When a strip of heart muscle (such as cat papillary muscle) is attached at both ends so that the length is fixed and then electrically stimulated, the muscle develops force without shortening. A fundamental property of striated muscle is that the strength of this **isometric twitch** is dependent on the initial resting muscle length, or **preload** (see Chap. 17). As cardiac muscle is stretched passively (increased preload), the resting tension rapidly rises and prevents overstretching of the **sarcomeres.** If additional load is applied before contraction (preload), stimulation causes contraction with an increased **peak tension** and rate of **tension development** (dT/dt) (Fig. 23-1A, B). Thus total tension includes both active and passive tension. The **length-tension relationship,** derived from variably preloaded fibers, is depicted in Fig. 23-1C. The length-tension relationship forms the basis for the Frank-Starling relationship in the intact heart, which will be discussed later.

The **inotropic state** is often defined operationally as a change in the rate or extent of force development that occurs independently of the loading conditions. The inotropic state is determined directly by subcellular processes that regulate myocyte cytosolic calcium and actin–myosin crossbridge cycling (Chap. 18). In isolated cardiac muscle, changes in the inotropic state are measured by changes in the peak isometric tension and dT/dt at a fixed preload. Thus positive inotropic agents, such as **catecholamines** or **digoxin,** increase the peak tension and dT/dt of an isometric contraction at a given preload. The

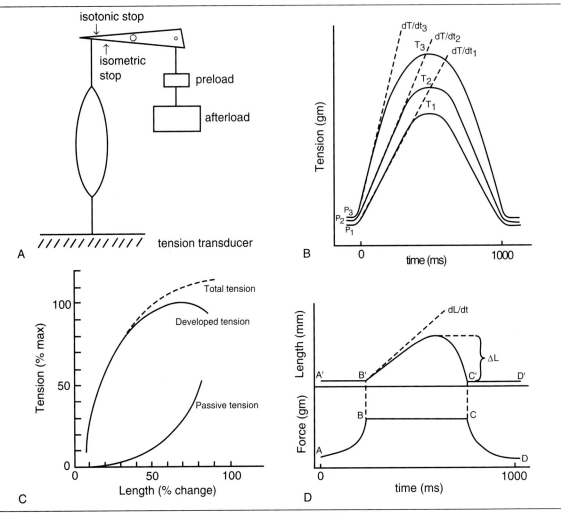

Fig. 23-1. Contractions in isolated muscle. (A) Isolated muscle preparation. Muscle is attached to a lever arm at one end and fixed to a tension transducer at the other. The muscle is stretched by applying a weight (preload) at one end of the lever arm. A stop prevents muscle shortening. (B) Tension-time curves of isometric twitches at three levels of preload. With increased preload peak tension (T_1, T_2, and T_3) and the maximum rate of tension development (dT/dt_1, dT/dt_2, and dT/dt_3) are increased. The time to peak tension is unchanged. (C) Length–total tension relationship and its components, passive and active tension. As muscle is stretched, the absolute passive tension increases, along with its contribution to total tension. (D) Superimposed tension-time and length-time recordings from afterloaded isotonic contractions. After preload is applied, a stop is placed to prevent further stretching. Afterload is added and the muscle is stimulated. Muscle shortens when generated tension equals total load (preload and afterload). Measures of shortening in the isotonic contraction include total shortening (ΔL) and the initial velocity of contraction (dL/dt). (Redrawn with permission from: Ross, J., Jr. In: *Best and Taylor's Physiological Basis of Medical Practice,* 12th ed. Baltimore: Williams & Wilkins, 1990. P. 213.)

opposite occurs when negative inotropic interventions, such as hypoxia and beta blockers, are used.

Isotonic Contraction

If isolated cardiac muscle is allowed to shorten, the contraction (Fig. 23-1D) is termed **isotonic.** Initial muscle length is determined by applying a preload; an additional load, known as the **afterload,** affects muscle behavior after stimulation. Muscle shortening occurs when tension development equals the total load (preload plus afterload). During shortening, tension remains constant (hence the term **isotonic**). With dissipation of the active state, the muscle returns to its initial preloaded length, and finally tension declines.

If preload is altered while the afterload is kept constant, **length-shortening** and **length-velocity curves** are obtained; these are analogous to the **length-tension curve** seen in isometric muscle (Fig. 23-2).

An inverse hyperbolic curve relating afterload and the initial velocity of shortening, the **force-velocity curve,** can be obtained from a series of variably **afterloaded contractions.** As shown in Fig. 23-3, when the afterload is so great that the muscle cannot shorten (the X intercept, P_O), the contraction becomes isometric. Because preload always

exists, the velocity of an unloaded contraction (the Y intercept, V_{max}) must be extrapolated from the force-velocity curve. V_{max} is determined by physiochemical properties unique to cardiac muscle and is therefore considered a measure of the inotropic state. Although changes in pre-

Fig. 23-3. Force-velocity relationship from variably afterloaded contractions. Increased preload causes an increase in the maximum isometric tension (P_{O_1} to P_{O_2}) without a change in the extrapolated velocity of an unloaded contraction (V_{max}). An increase in the inotropic state increases P_o and V_{max} (dL/dt = velocity of contraction).

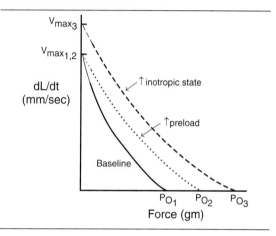

Fig. 23-2. Length-shortening and length-velocity relationships from isotonic contractions at a constant afterload. As muscle length (preload) increases, shortening (ΔL) and velocity of shortening (dL/dt) increase. An increased inotropic state shifts the curve upward and to the left; conversely, a decreased inotropic state shifts the curve downward and to the right.

Fig. 23-4. Length-tension curves from variably loaded isotonic contractions. Beats 1 and 2 are isotonic and contract from the same preload but a variable afterload (beat 2 is greater than beat 1). Beats 3 and 4 are isometric and contract at a preload matched to the end-contraction length of beats 1 and 2, respectively. Isotonic beats 1 and 2 contract to the same point on the isometric length-tension curve as isometric beats 3 and 4.

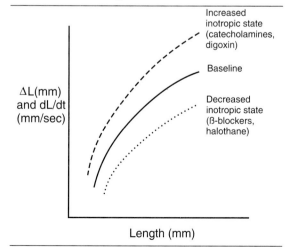

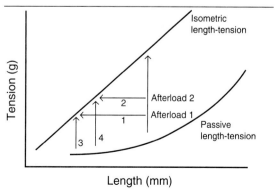

load shift P_O without changing V_{max}, a positive inotropic agent increases V_{max} and P_O by means of a parallel upward shift of the force-velocity curve; a negative inotropic agent causes the opposite (see Fig. 23-3). Similar operational definitions of the inotropic state may be applied to the **preloaded isotonic contraction,** in that a positive inotropic agent produces an upward shift of the length–shortening and length–velocity curves (see Fig. 23-2).

An important property of cardiac muscle is that the isometric passive length-tension curve establishes the limits of tension for an isotonic contraction. In other words, the tension at the end of an isotonic contraction is the same as the tension developed for an isometric contraction **at the same resting muscle length** (Fig. 23-4).

Besides load and the contractile state, cardiac muscle performance is influenced by the frequency of stimulation (heart rate). An increase in stimulation frequently causes an increase in tension in isolated cardiac muscle, known as **Bowditch's phenomenon.**

Cardiac Cycle

The cardiac cycle describes **pressure, volume,** and **flow phenomena** in the ventricles as a function of time. This cycle is similar for both the left and right ventricles, although there are differences in timing stemming from differences in the depolarization sequence and the levels of pressure in the pulmonary and systemic circulations. For simplicity, the cardiac cycle for the left heart during one beat will be described (Fig. 23-5).

The **QRS complex** on the surface ECG reflects ventricular depolarization (Chap. 22). Contraction begins after a 50-msec delay and results in closure of the mitral valve. The left ventricle contracts isovolumetrically until the ventricular pressure exceeds the systemic pressure; the aortic valve opens and ventricular ejection occurs. Bulging of the mitral valve into the left atrium during isovolumetric systole causes a slight increase in left atrial pressure (C wave). Shortly after ejection begins, the active state declines, and ventricular pressure begins to decrease. The aortic valve closes when left ventricular pressure falls below aortic pressure. In late systole, momentum briefly maintains forward flow despite greater aortic than left ventricular pressure. Ventricular pressure then declines exponentially during isovolumic relaxation, when both the aortic and mitral valves are closed. Left atrial pressure rises during ventricular systole (V wave) as blood returns to the left atrium by means of the pulmonary veins. When ventricular pressure declines below left atrial pressure, the mitral valve opens, and ventricular filling begins. Initially, ventricular

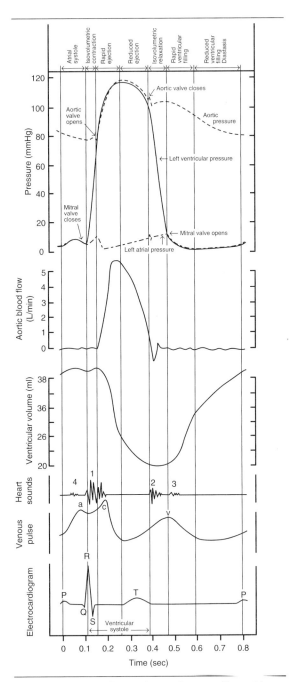

Fig. 23-5. Pressure, flow, volume, electrocardiographic and phonocardiographic events constituting the cardiac cycle (see text for elaboration). (Reproduced with permission from: Berne, R. M. and Levy, M. N. *Physiology,* 2nd ed. St Louis: Mosby, 1988, P. 444.)

filling is very rapid, because of the relatively large pressure gradient between the atrium and ventricle. Ventricular pressure continues to fall after mitral valve opening because of continued ventricular relaxation; its subsequent rise (and the fall in atrial pressure) slows ventricular filling. Especially at low end-systolic volumes, ventricular **early rapid filling** may be facilitated by ventricular suction produced by elastic recoil. Ventricular filling slows during **diastasis,** when atrial and ventricular pressures and volumes rise very gradually. Atrial depolarization inscribes a P wave on the ECG and is followed by atrial contraction, increased atrial pressure, and a second, late rapid-filling phase. A subsequent ventricular depolarization completes the cycle.

Valve closure and **rapid-filling phases** are audible with a **stethoscope** placed on the chest and may be recorded by a phonocardiograph after electronic amplification (see Fig. 23-5). The **first heart sound,** resulting from cardiohemic vibrations with closure of the atrioventricular (mitral, tricuspid) valves, heralds **ventricular systole.** The **second heart sound,** shorter and composed of higher frequencies than the first, is associated with **closure of the semilunar valves** (aorta and pulmonic) at the end of ventricular ejection. **Third** and **fourth heart sounds,** low-frequency vibrations caused by early, rapid filling and rapid filling due to atrial contraction, respectively, may be heard in normal children but in adults usually indicate disease.

The Pressure-Volume Loop

An alternative time-independent representation of the cardiac cycle is obtained by plotting instantaneous ventricular pressure and volume. During **ventricular filling,** pressure and volume increase nonlinearly (see Fig. 23-6A, phase 1). The instantaneous slope of the diastolic pressure-volume curve (dP/dV) is chamber stiffness and its inverse (dV/dP) is compliance. As chamber volume increases, the ventricle becomes stiffer (less compliant). In a normal ventricle, operative compliance is high, in that the ventricle operates on the flat portion of its diastolic pressure-volume curve.

During **isovolumetric contraction** (see Fig. 23-6A, phase 2), pressure increases and volume remains constant. During **ejection** (see Fig. 23-6A, phase 3), pressure rises and falls until the minimum ventricular size is attained. The maximum ratio of pressure to volume (maximal active chamber stiffness or elastance) usually occurs at the end of ejection. **Isovolumetric relaxation** follows (see Fig. 23-6A, phase 4), and when left ventricular pressure falls below left atrial pressure, ventricular filling begins. Left ventricular pressure-volume diagrams can illustrate the ef-

fects of changing preload, afterload, and inotropic state in the intact left ventricle, and this will be discussed.

The Atrial Cycle

A pressure-volume loop can also be described for atrial events. During ventricular ejection, descent of the ventricular base lowers atrial pressure and thus assists in atrial filling. Filling of the atria from the veins results in a **V wave** on the atrial and venous pressure tracing (see Fig. 23-6). (The **C wave** is inscribed on the atrial pressure tracing during ventricular isovolumetric contraction.) When the **mitral** and **tricuspid valves** open, blood stored in the atria empties into the ventricles. The atria also act as conduits for blood flow from the veins into the atria during passive atrial **emptying** and atrial **diastasis.** Atrial **contraction,** denoted by an **A wave** on the atrial pressure tracing, actively assists ventricular filling. Thus, the atria function as reservoirs, conduits, and booster pumps. In the normal ventricle, atrial systole contributes approximately 15 percent of the ventricular filling; when ventricular filling is impaired, such as occurs in hypertensive heart disease, the active atrial contribution may rise significantly.

Determinants of Performance and Cardiac Output in the Left Ventricle

Measures of Ventricular Performance

Measures of overall ventricular performance include cardiac output, stroke volume, and stroke work. **Cardiac output** is defined as the quantity of blood delivered to the circulation (usually expressed in liters per minute). Cardiac output is the product of stroke volume and heart rate. **Stroke volume** is the quantity of blood ejected by the heart in each beat and equals the ventricular end-diastolic volume minus the end-systolic volume. **Stroke work** is the product of pressure and stroke volume and equals the area bounded by the ventricular pressure-volume loop. In the clinical setting, stroke work may be approximated as (LVSP – LVDP) × stroke volume × 0.0136, where LVSP and LVDP are the mean left ventricular systolic and diastolic pressures, respectively, and 0.0136 converts mmHg·ml to g·m.

Cardiac output responds to changes in the oxygen requirements of tissues, as provoked, for example, by exercise. The extraction of nutrients by tissue can be expressed as the **arteriovenous difference** across the tissue. Accord-

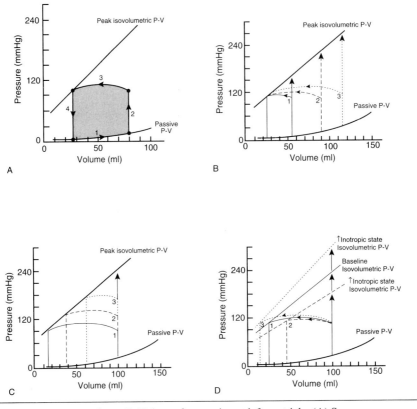

Fig. 23-6. Left ventricular pressure-volume (P-V) loops from an intact left ventricle. (A) Segments of the P-V loop correspond to events of the cardiac cycle: diastolic ventricular filling along the passive P-V curve (phase 1), isovolumetric contraction (phase 2), ventricular ejection (phase 3), and isovolumetric relaxation (phase 4). The ventricle ejects to an end-systolic volume determined by the peak isovolumetric P-V line. An isovolumetric contraction (*dashed line*) from the end-diastolic volume falls on the same isovolumetric P-V line. (B) A series of beats contracting from increasing preload to the same peak isovolumetric P-V line. Note the progressive increase in stroke volume with increasing preload. Pressure-volume curves from variably afterloaded beats (C) and beats after different inotropic interventions (D). (C) As afterload increases (3 > 2 > 1), stroke volume decreases, although end-ejection points fall on the same isovolumetric pressure–volume (P-V) line. (D) End-ejection points from beats with different inotropic states (3 > 1 > 2) fall on different isovolumetric P-V lines. Beat 1 is from baseline, beat 2 is after administration of a negative inotropic drug, and beat 3 is after application of a positive inotropic drug.

ing to the **Fick principle,** the consumption of a particular nutrient (e.g., oxygen) by a tissue equals the rate of delivery of that nutrient, i.e., the cardiac output times the arteriovenous difference (see App. 2). Changes in cardiac output necessary to meet the metabolic needs of the tissues can be produced by changes in the stroke volume or heart rate or both. Changes in stroke volume are mediated by altered loading conditions, inotropic state, and heart rate.

Thus those factors which influence the strength of contraction in isolated muscle are the same factors that determine cardiac output.

Attempts to extrapolate experimental results from isolated muscle to the intact left ventricle have been hampered by the complexity of chamber geometry and myocardial fiber orientation, which make it difficult to estimate initial fiber length (preload) and the force opposing left ventricular ejection (afterload). In contrast to isolated cardiac muscle, contraction of the intact left ventricle is **auxotonic,** in that force rises and falls during ejection of viscous blood into a viscoelastic arterial system. As with isolated cardiac muscle, performance of the intact left ventricle depends on the interplay among preload, afterload, the inotropic state, and heart rate. However, unlike isolated cardiac muscle, ventricular performance is modulated by neurohumoral influences, central and local autonomic reflex pathways, right and left ventricular interaction, the restraining effects of the pericardium, and atrial function (Chap. 27).

Preload and the Frank-Starling Relationship

The influence of preload on measures of ventricular performance defines the left ventricular function curve, known as the **Frank-Starling relationship:** Increasing left ventricular end-diastolic volume increases stroke volume in ejecting beats and increases peak left-ventricular pressure in isovolumetric beats (see Fig. 23-6B). The modulation of ventricular performance by changes in preload, termed **heterometric regulation,** operates on a beat-by-beat basis and is responsible for matching outputs of the right and left ventricles (e.g., after standing or with respiration). The Frank-Starling relationship also represents an important compensatory mechanism that maintains left ventricular stroke volume (by increasing left ventricular end-diastolic volume) when left ventricular shortening is impaired, owing either to myocardial contractile dysfunction or to excessive afterload. The atria also exhibit a Frank-Starling relationship that becomes clinically important during exercise and when there is resistance to early diastolic left ventricular filling (e.g., caused by mitral stenosis, left ventricular hypertrophy, or impaired left ventricular relaxation).

Because a representative fiber length (preload) is difficult to determine in the left ventricle, changes in the myocardial fiber length are estimated from changes in the left ventricular end-diastolic volume. In the clinical setting, end-diastolic pressure or pulmonary capillary wedge pressure are used frequently as measures of preload. However, the passive pressure-volume relationship (analogous to the passive length-tension curve in isolated muscle) is not linear, but exponential. Thus the ratio of change in left ventricular pressure and volume is greater at higher than at lower left ventricular volumes. Not surprisingly, under certain circumstances, ventricular pressure may inaccurately reflect the ventricular volume (preload). Moreover, changes in ventricular volume may erroneously be inferred

from changes in cardiac pressures, which, in fact, result only from alterations in ventricular compliance. Compliance of the left ventricle is affected by pericardial pressure, right ventricular pressure and volume, and coronary artery perfusion (turgor), besides changes in the elastic properties of the left ventricle.

Afterload

Afterload in the intact heart may be considered as either the **tension** (stress) in the left ventricular wall during ejection or as the **arterial input impedance** (a function of arterial pressures, elasticity, vessel dimension, and blood viscosity). Although force within the ventricular wall is difficult to measure and varies throughout its thickness, initial estimates of systolic wall stress can be derived from application of the **Laplace relationship,** in which tension = P × r/2h, where P refers to the pressure, r to the ventricular radius, and h to the wall thickness. This relationship assumes spherical ventricular geometry, however. Complex derivations, based on more realistic geometric assumptions, are used in laboratory investigations. Measurement of aortic input impedance requires instantaneous measurement of pressure and flow and is therefore impractical in a clinical setting. Accordingly, peak left ventricular pressure and systemic vascular resistance are used clinically as measures of afterload.

An increase in afterload (stress) causes a decrease in stroke volume (see Fig. 23-6C) and the velocity of left ventricular shortening. The resulting stress-shortening and stress-velocity curves are analogous to those obtained from variably afterloaded isotonic contractions in isolated muscle.

The Inotropic State

The ideal method of measuring the inotropic state in the intact left ventricle should incorporate the variables of **force, length, velocity,** and **time,** be **independent of external loading conditions,** and relate to **physicochemical processes** at the **sarcomeric level.** Because of these constraints, changes in the inotropic state are usually defined operationally by shifts of the various ventricular function curves. For example, a drug with positive inotropic activity (e.g., digoxin) shifts the Frank-Starling relationship (analogous to the length-tension curve) upward and to the left, and changes the stress-shortening relationship (analogous to the force-velocity curve) upward and to the right (see Figs. 23-2 and 23-3).

The intact left ventricle can be made to contract isovolumetrically over a range of left ventricular end-diastolic volumes to produce an isovolumetric pressure-volume line, analogous to the isometric length-tension curves in isolated muscle. Moreover, end-systolic pressure-volume plot points from ejecting beats (obtained from variably preloaded and afterloaded contractions) fall reasonably close to the isovolumetric pressure-volume line for a given inotropic state (see Fig. 23-6B). Thus changes in the inotropic state, **independent of the loading conditions,** can be identified by changes in the slope of the end-systolic pressure-volume relationship (see Fig. 23-6D). **End systole** may be defined as end ejection or as that time of maximal elastance (the maximal pressure-volume ratio) during systole. In the normal heart, these two points are closely related in time.

The **rate of pressure development** in the left ventricle during isovolumic systole (dP/dt) has been used as an index of the inotropic state. However, because of the direct influence of preload on dP/dt, dP/dt at a common developed pressure and the slope of the dP/dt–end-diastolic volume curve have been proposed as preload-independent indices of the inotropic state.

Heart Rate

Increasing heart rate causes a small, but measurable, increase in the inotropic state through the force-frequency (Bowditch) relationship. Heart rate is an important determinant of left ventricular performance under certain circumstances, by virtue of the relationship between cardiac output and heart rate: **cardiac output = stroke volume × heart rate.** In a normal left ventricle, pacing between heart rates of 60 and 160 beats per minute has little effect on cardiac output, because the diminished diastolic filling time (and hence the stroke volume determined by the Frank-Starling relationship) offsets the modest increase in the inotropic state. Heart rate is normally determined by the interplay between the intrinsic automaticity of the sinoatrial node and the activity of the autonomic nervous system. Sympathetic stimulation increases and parasympathetic stimulation decreases the heart rate (see Chap. 27).

Ventricular-Vascular Coupling

In isolated muscle, loading conditions represent the force applied to muscle before (preload) and after (afterload) the onset of contraction. In the intact left ventricle, preload and afterload are also determined by the characteristics of the arterial and venous circulations. Thus loading conditions are not only important direct determinants of left ventricular performance; they also function indirectly, by coupling the left ventricle to the vascular system.

The **venous return curve** describes the inverse relationship between venous pressure and cardiac output. This relationship is a function of arterial and venous capacitance (the change in volume per change in pressure [dV/dP]) and the peripheral resistance provided by the microcirculation (resistance = pressure gradient for flow divided by the cardiac output).

Ventricular contraction transfers blood from the venous to the arterial side of the circulation, and arterial and venous capacitances determine the respective pressures that result from the shift in blood volume. These pressures determine the **driving force** (pressure gradient) across the peripheral resistance and are primarily responsible for venous return to the heart. In contrast to convention, the venous return curve plots the independent variable (cardiac output) on the vertical axis and the dependent variable (venous pressure) on the horizontal axis. The X intercept is the mean circulatory pressure, or that pressure in the vascular system in the absence of cardiac pumping. The **mean circulatory pressure** is a function of the capacitance of the vascular system and the total blood volume. The plateau of the venous return curve and the Y intercept represent the **maximal obtainable cardiac output** as venous pressure is reduced. In the normal heart, cardiac output is limited by venous return, and the operating venous pressure is near the plateau of the venous return curve.

Coupling of the venous system to the heart is graphically represented in Fig. 23-7. In this analysis, developed by Guyton and coworkers, the intersection of the ventricular function (Frank-Starling) curve and the venous return curve represents the steady-state operating values of cardiac output and venous pressure. At this **equilibrium point,** the ability of the venous system to provide venous return at a given pressure is matched with the ability of the ventricle to pump that venous return when distended to the same pressure. For example, an increase in venous pressure causes an increase in cardiac output (Frank-Starling) but a decrease in cardiac output, according to the venous return curve; the resultant cardiac output is determined by the dynamic equilibrium of these forces.

Increased blood volume and venoconstriction shift the venous function curve upward and to the right, increasing the mean circulatory pressure and the maximal cardiac output (see Fig. 23-7A). The venous system contains the major fraction of blood in the vascular system, because of the greater capacitance of veins than of arteries. As a re-

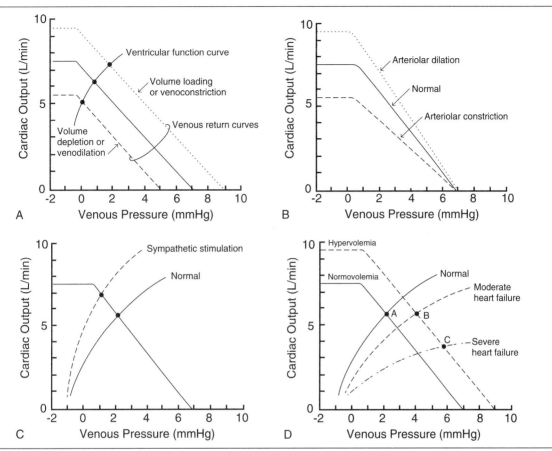

Fig. 23-7. Venous pressure–cardiac output curves. The equilibrium point is defined by the intersection of the ventricular function curve with the venous return curve. (A) Volume loading and venoconstriction shift the venous return curve to the right, resulting in an equilibrium point with a higher cardiac output and higher mean circulatory pressure (P_v). Volume depletion and venodilation shift the curve to the left, resulting in an equilibrium point with a lower cardiac output and a smaller P_v. (B) The effects of arteriolar constriction and dilation on the venous return curves are more complex. (C) Sympathetic nerve stimulation (a positive inotropic intervention) causes a leftward shift of the ventricular function curve, resulting in an equilibrium point with a lower venous pressure and higher cardiac output. (D) Chronic heart failure causes rightward shifts of both the ventricular function and venous return curves. At B (moderate heart failure), cardiac output is preserved at the expense of venous pressure. At C (severe heart failure), cardiac output is decreased and venous pressure further increased. (Redrawn with permission from: Berne, R. M., and Levy, M. N. *Physiology,* 2nd ed. St Louis: Mosby, 1988, Pp. 529, 530, 532, 533.)

sult, venoconstriction shifts significant quantities of blood from the peripheral to central circulation. Because arteries contain only a small percentage of the total blood volume, their contractile state does not affect the mean circulatory pressure. Moreover, because venous pressure varies inversely with systemic vascular resistance, arteriolar

constriction (increased afterload) shifts the curve downward and to the left without changing the mean circulatory pressure; conversely, arteriolar dilation (decreased afterload) shifts the curve upward and to the right (see Fig. 23-7B). An increased inotropic state (e.g., that arising from sympathetic nervous stimulation; see Fig. 23-7C) shifts the ventricular function curve to the left without significantly altering the venous return curve. Conversely, in chronic heart failure (see Fig. 23-7D) there is a rightward shift of the ventricular function curve and, because of renal salt and water retention, a parallel rightward shift of the vascular function curve. In this way, cardiac output is initially maintained at the expense of increased venous pressure and congestion. If the compensatory mechanisms fail, venous pressure rises further and cardiac output falls.

Summary

Although the complexities of the intact left ventricle are considerable, the Frank-Starling and force-shortening relationships, which are analogous to the length-tension and force-velocity curves, respectively, in isolated cardiac muscle are useful for characterizing left ventricular performance. The Frank-Starling curve relates preload, and the force-shortening curve relates afterload, to measures of ventricular performance. The inotropic or contractile state is recognized by shifts in the ventricular function curves, such as the end-systolic pressure-volume relationship. The sequence of events in each cardiac cycle and changes in left ventricular performance can be represented graphically by the pressure-volume loop. Cardiac output is a measure of ventricular performance that, in turn, is linked to the metabolic needs of the tissues. The concept of ventricular-vascular coupling accounts for the interplay between the ventricular pump and the arterial and venous circulations that regulate cardiac output.

Bibliography

Braunwald, E. Assessment of cardiac performance. In: *Heart Disease. A Textbook of Cardiovascular Medicine.* Philadelphia: W. B. Saunders, 1980. Pp. 472–492.

Guyton, A. C., Jones, C. E., and Coleman, T. G. *Circulatory Physiology: Cardiac Output and Its Regulation.* Philadelphia: W. B. Saunders, 1973. Pp. 146–233.

Ross, J., Jr., and Sobel, B. E. Regulation of cardiac contraction. *Annu. Rev. Physiol.* 34:47, 1972.

Sagawa, K. The ventricular pressure-volume diagram revisited. *Circ. Res.* 43:677, 1978.

Sonnenblick, E. H. Force-velocity relations in mammalian heart muscle. *Am. J. Physiol.* 202:931–939, 1962.

24 Coronary Circulation, Myocardial Oxygen Consumption, and Energetics

Laura F. Wexler and Richard A. Walsh

Objectives

After reading this chapter, you should be able to

Describe the anatomy of the coronary circulation

Describe at least four factors that determine coronary blood flow

List four major determinants of myocardial oxygen consumption

Describe how coronary blood flow is regulated to match myocardial oxygen requirements

Characterize and compare the metabolic pathways used by the heart to obtain energy under normal conditions and under conditions of limited blood flow

Under normal conditions, cardiac muscle metabolism is almost exclusively aerobic, depending on oxidative phosphorylation to resynthesize the ATP continuously utilized for repetitive excitation-contraction-relaxation. Myocardial oxygen requirements are therefore high and unremitting, even under resting conditions. During stress or exercise, oxygen requirements may increase abruptly by three- to fourfold. Unlike skeletal muscle, cardiac muscle cannot obtain significantly more oxygen by extracting a greater percentage of the oxygen delivered to it, since myocardial oxygen extraction is near maximal at rest. The major mechanism by which oxygen delivery to the myocardium can be augmented is by an increase in the amount of coronary artery blood flow. This chapter describes the anatomy of the coronary circulation and the means by which coronary flow is regulated to continuously meet the demands of a variable level of myocardial work.

Anatomy of the Coronary Circulation
Arterial Supply

Two main **coronary arteries** arise from the **aortic sinuses** just above the **aortic valve leaflets** and give rise to a series of branches that run along the outer (epicardial) surface of the heart (Fig. 24-1).

The main epicardial vessels and their branches subdivide several times on the surface of the heart before giving off small penetrating branches that give rise to an extensively branching network of small **intramural arteries, arterioles,** and **capillaries,** which traverse the myocardial wall from epicardium to endocardium. Capillary density is very high in heart muscle, commensurate with the high oxygen requirements of myocardial cells. Capillaries are situated close to each myocardial cell, providing a conduit for rapidly diffusible oxygen for ATP production in the cell and for removal of metabolic waste products. Considered

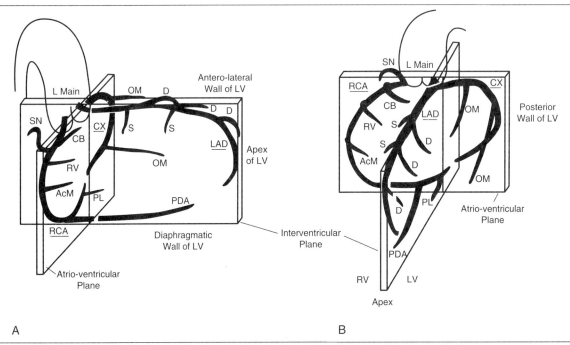

A   B

Fig. 24-1. The coronary anatomy relative to the atrioventricular groove and the interventricular groove, as seen in a right anterior oblique (A) and left anterior oblique (B) orientation. Coronary branches: L main = left main; LAD = left anterior descending; D = diagonal; S = septal perforator; CX = circumflex; OM = obtuse marginal; RCA = right coronary artery; CB = conus branch; SN = sinus node artery; AcM = acute marginal; PDA = posterior descending artery; PL = posterior left ventricular (LV = left ventricle; RV = right ventricle).

collectively, the coronary vasculature and the blood it contains account for approximately 15% of the total mass of the heart (Fig. 24-2).

Venous Drainage

As in other parts of the systemic circulation, **myocardial capillaries** feed into a network of **intramural venules** that eventually drain into large **epicardial collecting veins.** Right ventricular venous blood drains into several anterior cardiac veins that empty into the right atrium. Most of the left ventricular venous blood drains into the **coronary sinus,** a large venous channel that runs along the atrioventricular groove and empties into the right atrium.

Coronary Artery Collaterals

Coronary collaterals constitute direct arterial connections between one coronary artery and another. If a coronary

artery is occluded, collateral vessels may provide some degree of arterial blood supply beyond the obstruction, thus protecting the myocardium distal to the obstruction. Certain species (e.g., dogs) normally possess an extensive network of large preformed arterial collaterals. Abrupt occlusion of a proximal coronary artery will cause only limited myocardial damage, since there is an alternative source of arterial flow provided by preexisting collaterals. In contrast, other species (e.g., humans, nonhuman primates, pigs) have a minimal collateral network under normal circumstances. After acute coronary occlusion of a proximal coronary artery, small intramural collaterals can supply less than 10% of the normal flow, and a more extensive and predictable amount of myocardial damage results. However, in the event of gradual chronic coronary obstruction, as may occur with atherosclerotic coronary artery disease, these small collaterals may greatly enlarge over time. Even after complete occlusion of the diseased coronary artery, well-developed coronary collaterals may provide normal or near-normal flow to the distal segment of the

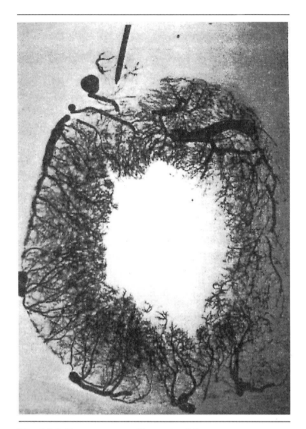

Fig. 24-2. Postmortem radiograph of the coronary vascular tree in a cross-section of the left ventricle. Note the extensive arborization of the intramural vessels.

diseased artery. However, although the flow rate may be normal at rest, the capacity to augment myocardial blood flow during exercise or stress (coronary reserve) is usually limited in collateral vessels.

Regulation of Coronary Blood Flow

Resting coronary blood flow is normally between 60 and 90 ml/min/100 g of myocardium and may rapidly increase by four- to fivefold during exercise or other conditions requiring augmented flow. The coronary **flow rate** is determined by the **coronary artery perfusion pressure** and by the **resistance to flow** exerted by forces generated within and outside the coronary vascular bed.

The pattern of blood flow to the **left ventricle** (which receives the greatest proportion of coronary flow) is unique

in that arterial flow is markedly decreased during **systole,** since the intramyocardial pressure generated by contracting myocardial fibers effectively shuts off flow from the epicardial to the intramural arteries. Most of the coronary flow to the left ventricle occurs during **diastole,** and coronary perfusion pressure is largely determined by aortic diastolic pressure. Blood flow to the right ventricular myocardium is also phasic, but because the systolic pressure transmitted to the right ventricular myocardium is much lower, the difference between systolic and diastolic flow is less marked (Fig. 24-3).

Coronary Autoregulation

If there is a sudden change in aortic pressure (within certain limits), coronary vascular resistance will adjust itself proportionally within 8 to 12 seconds so that a constant blood flow is maintained. This phenomenon is called **autoregulation** (Fig. 24-4), and it protects the myocardium from inadequate blood flow if there is a decline in coronary perfusion pressure. During periods of abnormally high aortic pressure, the role of autoregulation is less clear. It may attenuate endothelial wall stress and protect the vasculature from damage resulting from elevated coronary distending pressures.

Autoregulation also occurs in **localized areas** of the coronary vasculature when partial obstruction of an artery

Fig. 24-3. Comparison of epicardial coronary blood flow to the left and right ventricles. Flow to the left ventricle is abolished in early systole because of high intraventricular pressures. Most flow takes place during early to mid-diastole. Coronary flow to the right ventricle is also cyclic, but is less affected during systole because of the lower pressure generated within the right ventricular myocardium.

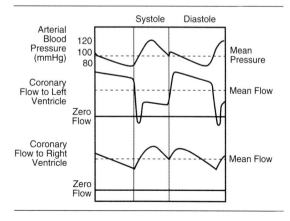

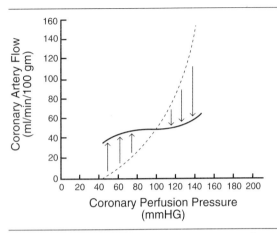

Fig. 24-4. Autoregulation of coronary artery flow during alterations in coronary perfusion pressure. The *dashed line* represents the instantaneous (nonautoregulated) coronary artery flow that would be observed immediately after altering coronary perfusion pressure between 20 and 160 mmHg. The *solid line* depicts the effects of autoregulation: appropriate adjustments in coronary vascular resistance (*arrows*), occurring within 8 to 12 seconds, compensate for the acute changes in coronary perfusion pressure and return flow to a level that is maintained fairly constant between pressures of about 60 and 140 mmHg. The level to which coronary flow is autoregulated at any given time is determined by the instantaneous oxygen requirements of the heart.

causes a decrease in the coronary perfusion pressure. The vessel distal to the obstruction will dilate, thus normalizing flow by decreasing coronary vascular resistance. The normal coronary vascular bed can autoregulate over a range of systemic arterial pressures, usually 60 to 140 mmHg. Above or below these limits, autoregulation fails, and coronary flow increases or decreases in a linear fashion, with corresponding increases or decreases in aortic pressure.

Autoregulatory reserve refers to the maximal degree of vasodilation possible in the coronary vascular bed and determines the range of decreased perfusion pressures over which myocardial flow can be maintained. Autoregulatory reserve will depend on the level of chronic vasodilation in the coronary vasculature as a whole or in any specific region of the heart. If a region of the vascular bed is already vasodilated to compensate for a localized decrease in coronary perfusion pressure, the capacity to autoregulate during further declines in aortic diastolic pressure will be impaired. In other words, autoregulatory reserve will be impaired, and the affected area of myocardium will be more vulnerable to transient decreases in aortic pressure.

Several mechanisms have been proposed to explain au-

toregulation, but the most compelling evidence points to the existence of a chemical mediator. **Adenosine,** a breakdown product of ATP, is a likely candidate. Adenosine is a potent vasodilator that is generated continuously in myocardial cells from AMP by the action of an enzyme (5'-nucleotidase) that is located at the inner surface of the cell membrane (Fig. 24-5). Adenosine freely diffuses across the cell membrane; any decrease in perfusion pressure, by causing an initial decrease in coronary artery flow, leads to a diminished rate of adenosine washout and an increase in local tissue concentration. This, in turn, results in vasodilation and increase in coronary flow. An increase in perfusion pressure precipitates an initial increase in flow and more rapid washout of adenosine. This results in diminished vasodilation and subsequent decrease in the coronary flow rate. It is also possible that tissue PO_2 or the level of other metabolic products in tissue, by changing

Fig. 24-5. Proposed mechanism of coronary autoregulation. As ATP is hydrolyzed during excitation, contraction, and relaxation, some is broken down to AMP and then to adenosine (which is freely diffusible across the cell membrane) by an enzyme (5'-nucleotidase) at the inner myocardial cell membrane, so that adenosine promptly diffuses out of the myocardial cell at a rate proportional to its rate of production. The degree of vasodilation it induces in surrounding arterioles would be determined by its rate of production and also by its rate of washout after diffusing into the intramural vessels. If the rate of washout decreases because coronary flow rate decreases, the local tissue concentration of adenosine would increase, leading to more vasodilation and increased flow rate. As the flow rate increases, washout would be accelerated, the local tissue concentration of adenosine would lower (assuming its rate of production has been stable), and vasodilation would diminish, thus readjusting flow (CPP = coronary perfusion pressure; IMP = inosine 5'-monophosphate).

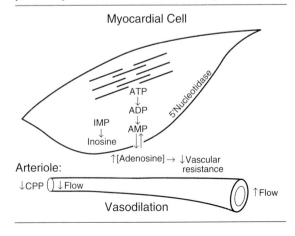

slightly as perfusion pressure rises and falls, may directly affect coronary artery tone.

Metabolic Regulation of Coronary Artery Blood Flow

Coronary blood flow must be modulated continuously so that a sufficient supply of oxygen is delivered to the myocardium to support **oxidative energy production** at a rate that matches energy utilization. The means by which coronary flow is so precisely regulated is still debated, but the mechanism clearly involves some signal that induces rapid changes in coronary vascular resistance. The most likely mediator is again **adenosine.** As the rate of ATP use increases with increased cardiac work, there is a relative accumulation of its breakdown products, including adenosine. This adenosine induces coronary vasodilation, and blood flow increases, which then furnishes the additional oxygen required for accelerated ATP resynthesis (Fig. 24-6).

Several other factors have been hypothesized to be involved in metabolic regulation of coronary blood flow, including PO_2, partial pressure of carbon dioxide (PCO_2), K^+ concentration, and pH. However, adenosine remains the most likely mediator in that its concentration is directly proportional to the rate of ATP turnover, it diffuses readily across the myocardial cell membrane, and it is a potent coronary artery vasodilator.

Fig. 24-6. Elements of a metabolic blood flow control system in which the cellular energy state (ATP potential) determines the rate of production of vasoregulatory metabolites, and thereby the rate of substrate delivery. The symbol (–) indicates that a change in one variable causes a reciprocal change in another. Thus, an increased rate of ATP hydrolysis leads to a decrease in the ratio of ATP to ADP + inorganic phosphate (P_i) and an increase in the rate of production of adenosine. This leads to a decrease in smooth muscle tone and an increase in the rate of oxygen delivery as coronary flow increases. (Adapted from: Olsson, R. A. and Bunger, R., Metabolic control of coronary blood flow. *Prog. Cardiovasc. Dis.* 29:369–387, 1987.)

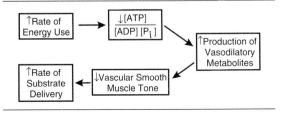

Epicardial versus Endocardial Blood Flow

Several factors affecting blood flow are markedly different in the inner (subendocardial) and outer (subepicardial) layers of the myocardium. Systolic compression is much higher in the **subendocardial layers** than in the **subepicardial layers** of the heart such that subendocardial blood flow is virtually absent in systole. There also may be some degree of mechanical interference with flow in the subendocardial vessels in late diastole as pressure is exerted on the inner layers of the heart by the blood filling and distending the ventricular chamber. This may account for the fact that flow in the subendocardial layers rises rapidly in early diastole but falls off in late diastole. In contrast, flow to the midwall of the heart is approximately equal in systole and diastole; in the outer layers of the subepicardium, flow is slightly higher in systole than in diastole.

The arrangement of intramural vessels partially compensates for the almost complete absence of blood flow to the subendocardium during systole, in that vascular density is increased in the subendocardium so that net flow is augmented. In addition, despite the greater external forces exerted on the subendocardial arteries, their intrinsic coronary vascular resistance is lower, such that blood flow per gram of myocardium is normally higher in the subendocardium than in the subepicardium. The ratio of subendocardial to subepicardial flow is about 1.1:1. This is consistent with the fact that oxygen requirements are higher in the subendocardium because it develops higher wall stress and shortens more than the subepicardial layers. However, because of the lower resting coronary resistance of the subendocardial vessels. the capacity to **further augment flow** in response to increased metabolic demands (i.e., the **coronary reserve** of the subendocardial vessels) is inherently less than in the midwall and epicardial vessels. This makes the subendocardium more vulnerable to injury if coronary perfusion pressure drops or coronary flow is impeded. Some oxygen does diffuse directly into the subendocardium from the arterial blood that fills the left ventricular chamber, but it reaches only the most superficial layers.

Neurohumoral Modulation of Coronary Blood Flow

The **autonomic nervous system** influences the smooth muscle tone of the **coronary arteries,** and this modulates coronary flow to some extent, although its role is overshadowed by metabolic and mechanical influences under normal conditions. The larger epicardial coronary arteries have both alpha-adrenergic receptors, which mediate vasoconstriction, and beta-adrenergic receptors, which mediate vasodilation. The smaller intramural arteries contain a larger percentage of beta-adrenergic receptors.

Release of **norepinephrine** during sympathetic stimulation can cause coronary artery vasoconstriction, but this response is normally overridden by metabolic factors because sympathetic stimulation also increases heart rate and contractility, thereby augmenting myocardial oxygen consumption and ATP turnover and resulting in vasodilation by autoregulatory and metabolic mechanisms. There does, however, appear to be a small degree of resting coronary vasoconstrictor "tone," since coronary denervation or pharmacologic alpha-adrenergic blockade will result in a small increase in coronary blood flow at rest and during exercise, suggesting loss or withdrawal of a vasoconstrictor substance. The significance of sympathetic innervation of the normal coronary arteries is not clear. Abnormal increases in vasoconstrictor tone have been suggested as a mechanism underlying certain types of coronary artery disease states, but there is little evidence to support this.

Stimulation of **beta₂ receptors** in the smaller coronary arteries by endogenous circulating catecholamines or by pharmacologic beta agonists results in coronary vasodilation. The extent to which coronary beta receptors contribute to coronary blood flow regulation is difficult to assess, since beta stimulation of the myocardium increases oxygen consumption by increasing heart rate and contractility, which lead to metabolically mediated vasodilation. However, autonomically mediated vasodilation can be demonstrated when sympathetic nerves are stimulated in a fibrillating (nonbeating) heart.

Endothelial Regulation of Coronary Blood Flow

Endothelium-derived relaxation factor (EDRF) is a potent vasodilator that is elaborated by vascular endothelial cells in response to a number of "stress" signals, including hypoxia, ADP accumulation, and serotonin secretion. EDRF release is also stimulated by distending forces in the vascular wall; i.e., it is released when coronary perfusion pressure or flow increases. This may serve to amplify the coronary flow response to conditions such as exercise when it may be appropriate for both coronary perfusion pressure and flow to increase (in contrast to the autoregulatory response, which keeps flow constant during inappropriate changes in coronary perfusion pressure).

Determinants of Myocardial Oxygen Consumption

Under normal conditions, the rate of coronary blood flow is regulated so that oxygen delivery will match oxygen consumption. **Myocardial oxygen consumption** is relatively high, even under resting conditions in the beating heart (approximately 8.0 ml/min/100 g of myocardium). The oxygen requirements of the heart are largely related to the energy requirements of cardiac contraction and relaxation, i.e., the oxygen consumed in the resynthesis of ATP expended during crossbridge cycling and Ca^{2+} reuptake by the sarcoplasmic reticulum. Oxygen consumption will markedly increase when the contractile work of the heart increases.

Left ventricular myocardium is responsible for the largest proportion of oxygen consumed by the heart, since it does the most contractile work. The **right ventricle** pumps the same volume of blood as the left ventricle during each cardiac cycle but has to generate much less pressure because the resistance of the pulmonary arterial system is much lower than that of the systemic arterial system. The three most important determinants of left ventricular work (and therefore of myocardial oxygen consumption) are the **number of beats per minute** (heart rate), the **tension** or **pressure** developed during systole, and the **inotropic state** (the ability of the left ventricle to generate pressure and eject blood independent of loading conditions; see Chap. 23). To a lesser extent, the volume of **blood ejected** (i.e., the extent of shortening of ventricular muscle) is also a factor.

Mycardial oxygen consumption increases with heart rate in an almost **linear fashion.** The energy cost of each heartbeat is actually slightly higher at rapid rates than at slow rates by virtue of a small increase in contractility that occurs at higher heart rates, a phenomenon termed the **positive staircase,** or **Bowditch, effect** (see Chap. 23).

Mycardial oxygen consumption also increases in a near-linear fashion with the development of **systolic tension.** In experimental studies of isolated hearts in which the inotropic state can be held constant, there is a close positive correlation between oxygen consumption and the product of systolic pressure and heart rate. This product is usually derived as the **tension-time index,** which is calculated as the integrated area under the left ventricular pressure curve per beat or per minute.

Systolic tension, or wall stress, which is the force exerted per unit area of myocardium (see Chap. 23), is determined by the level of the systolic pressure generated but also by the radius of curvature of the ventricle at the onset of contraction, which is determined by the end-diastolic volume. The components determining systolic wall stress or tension are expressed in the **Laplace relationship:** Wall stress = P × r/2h, where P is the systolic pressure, r is the radius of the ventricle, and h is the wall thickness. For any degree of pressure development, the wall stress will be higher, and thus more oxygen consumed per beat, during contraction of a large dilated ventricle than during contraction of a small ventricle. Elevated wall stress is diminished or normalized for any given pressure or chamber size by thickening or hypertrophy of the myocardial walls.

The **energy cost** of developing tension (pressure work) can be considered separately from the cost of actual shortening (volume work) and is substantially greater. Ejection of blood only accounts for about 15% of oxygen consumption. An increase in systemic vascular resistance requiring an increase in systolic tension is far more energy costly than an increase in the volume of blood ejected.

Contractility, or the inotropic state of the heart, is also a major determinant of oxygen consumption. In clinical situations, an increase in contractility enables the heart to do more work, i.e., to pump a greater volume of blood or to develop more tension and pump against a greater resistance. However, the enhanced inotropic state in itself affects energy use. In an experimental preparation in which heart rate, stroke volume, and systolic pressure are held constant, a positive inotropic drug such as digitalis increases the velocity of contraction or the rate at which pressure develops and oxygen consumption increases even though the actual mechanical work performed by the heart has not increased. It is not clear why myocardial oxygen consumption increases when there is an increase in the inotropic state. The intracellular event that appears to be a common factor in the mechanism of action of many positive inotropic drugs or interventions is that more calcium is made available to the contractile proteins. Thus the increase in oxygen consumption is most likely related to the energy cost of the calcium pumps. Whether they cycle faster when presented with more calcium or whether additional pumps are recruited is not known.

In clinical situations, contractility and the other determinants of myocardial oxygen consumption are interrelated and usually cannot be analyzed separately. Drugs that increase contractility usually accelerate ventricular emptying (shortening), which, in turn, affects myocardial oxygen consumption. The resulting increase in cardiac output causes reflex changes in the heart rate and systemic resistance that also affect the myocardial oxygen consumption.

Energy is also required (but to a much lesser extent) for **noncontractile processes.** Even if there is no external work, the heart still consumes oxygen. A small component of oxygen consumption is related to **electrical excitation,** which utilizes membrane pumps and is consequently an energy-requiring process. There is also a **"basal" oxygen requirement** that is unrelated to contractile or electric activity; it can be measured when the heart is arrested with potassium chloride. It accounts for approximately 15% to 20% of the total cardiac oxygen consumption and is associated with intracellular chemical reactions unrelated to excitation or contraction.

Myocardial Energy Metabolism

ATP is the immediate source of energy for all energy-requiring processes in the heart — for electrical excitation, for contraction itself, and for relaxation and restoration of resting electrochemical gradients across the membranes of the heart. Compared with other tissues, the myocardium contains a low concentration of **high-energy phosphates,** given the continuous energy requirements of excitation, contraction, and relaxation. Furthermore, the heart can abruptly increase its work output at least sixfold and thus requires a substantial energy reserve.

ATP levels are buffered in the heart by the much larger concentration of **phosphocreatine** (PCr), which regenerates ATP by the reaction ADP + PCr = ATP + Cr, catalyzed by the enzyme creatine kinase. Regeneration of ATP from phosphocreatine can protect the heart from ATP depletion during a mild or brief increase in energy demand, but the heart is fundamentally dependent on continuous resynthesis of mitochondrial ATP.

The metabolic pathways by which ATP is synthesized in the myocardium utilize a variety of substrates but are almost exclusively aerobic. Unlike skeletal muscle, the heart cannot function anaerobically for extended periods of high demand, building up an "oxygen debt" to be repaid during subsequent periods of rest. Because the heart is continuously active, oxidative ATP synthesis must continuously match ATP utilization.

Under normal resting conditions, the heart generates 60% to 70% of its ATP from **beta oxidation** of free fatty acids and 30% from metabolism of **carbohydrates,** including exogenous glucose and lactate (Fig. 24-7A). Amino acids and ketones are also used as substrates, but to a much lesser extent. During exercise, the large amounts of lactate produced by skeletal muscle become a major substrate for meeting the energy requirements of cardiac muscle, entering the Krebs cycle after conversion to pyruvate.

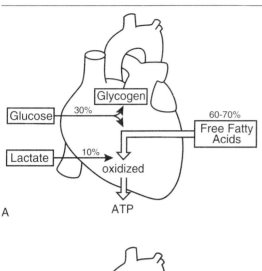

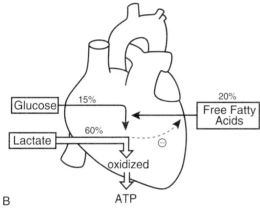

Fig. 24-7. (A) Preferred substrate use by the heart under normal resting conditions. Oxidation of free fatty acids is the source of most of the ATP produced by the heart. (B) During acute exercise, the blood lactate level rises, and lactate becomes the major fuel of the heart. Lactate inhibits the uptake of free fatty acids. Carbohydrate metabolism can account for 70% to 75% of the ATP generated.

Oxidation of free fatty acids is inhibited, and carbohydrates become the predominant substrate for energy metabolism (see Fig. 24-7B).

Coronary Artery Disease and the Consequences of Impaired Coronary Artery Flow

The most common cardiovascular disease in the Western world is **atherosclerosis,** a process of progressive thickening and calcification of the inner arterial walls that charac-

teristically affects the lower abdominal aorta and the large arteries of the heart, brain, lower extremities, and kidneys. Atherosclerotic coronary artery disease remains a leading cause of death in the United States and in other industrialized nations. The disease may be diffuse but most commonly is manifested as focal narrowings (plaques) in one or more of the **epicardial coronary arteries.** The diseased coronary artery segment may become gradually narrowed by progressive plaque enlargement, or it may be abruptly occluded by thrombus (clot) formation or vascular spasm, both of which can be triggered by vascular injury caused by the atherosclerotic process.

The functional and metabolic consequences of fixed focal narrowing of a coronary artery depend on the severity of the stenosis, whether collateral vessels have developed distal to the stenosis, and the extent of the myocardium supplied by the involved vessel. Resting flow does not decrease until there has been a very marked reduction in the arterial lumen, at least a 70% reduction in inner diameter (which corresponds to a 90% reduction in lumen size). This is so because the coronary artery (and branches) distal to a stenosis can vasodilate so as to restore resting flow. However, even though resting flow is not impaired until a very tight stenosis has developed, **coronary reserve,** which is the residual capacity of the coronary vascular bed to autoregulate and augment flow in response to an increase in myocardial oxygen consumption or further decrease in coronary perfusion pressure, becomes impaired once the luminal area is reduced by more than 50%. Furthermore, neurogenic and endothelial modulation of coronary flow may become markedly abnormal in atherosclerotic vessels, leading to an impaired vasodilatory response or even inappropriate vasoconstriction (coronary spasm).

Once coronary flow cannot adequately meet the oxygen requirements of the contracting muscle, the muscle is said to be ischemic. **Ischemia** can result from reduced coronary perfusion pressure below that to which autoregulation can restore flow (below the level of coronary reserve) or from an increase in myocardial oxygen demand beyond the capacity of the vascular bed to augment flow through metabolic regulation. Myocardial ischemia has almost immediate functional consequences, including electric instability leading to abnormal cardiac impulse formation (arrhythmias), diminished force of contraction, diminished rate and extent of shortening, and impaired relaxation, presumably because of inadequate ATP for Ca^{2+} resequestration by the sarcoplasmic reticulum. In addition, myocardial ischemia often causes a very distressing type of chest pain, known as **angina pectoris.**

The combination of inadequate mitochondrial ATP synthesis due to lack of oxygen and the toxic metabolic waste products (particularly H$^+$) that accumulate at low flow rates because of impaired washout produces impaired cardiac function during myocardial ischemia.

When there is a lack of oxygen, myocardial cells can produce only limited amounts of ATP by anaerobic glycolysis of endogenous glycogen stores, and the heart is very limited in its ability to subsist on ATP generated anaerobically. Although the rate of glycolysis is accelerated in ischemia, the net yield of ATP from the initial nonoxidative steps of the glycolytic pathway (2 mol of ATP per mole of glucose; 3 mol of ATP per mole of glycogen) is meager compared with the yield from complete cycling of glucose or glycogen during oxidative phosphorylation (Fig. 24-8). Furthermore, myocardial glycogen stores are soon depleted. The accumulation of lactate and NADH, which cannot be metabolized in the absence of oxygen, has a negative feedback effect on several key enzymes of the

glycolytic pathway, thus effectively halting anaerobic glycolysis. Lactate accumulation produces intracellular acidosis. This further impairs cardiac function, since a high concentration of H$^+$ has a direct negative inotropic effect in that it diminishes the sensitivity of the contractile proteins to Ca^{2+}.

As long as there is a **small residual blood flow** through a narrowed coronary artery to provide some oxygen and substrate for oxidative phosphorylation and to wash out lactate produced by accelerated anaerobic glycolysis, the heart can function for extended periods during mild to moderate low-flow ischemia. However, the heart will be exceedingly vulnerable to any increase in myocardial oxygen demand (stress, exercise) or any further impairment of coronary flow.

The consequences of **total occlusion** of a coronary artery depend on whether the occlusion is permanent or transient (as might occur with spontaneous resolution of a clot or reversal of spasm) and whether there are collateral vessels supplying an alternative source of blood flow distal to the obstruction. **Complete cessation** of coronary flow within seconds causes profound malfunction of the myocardium supplied by that vessel and within 20 to 40 minutes leads to myocardial cell necrosis or **myocardial infarction.**

Transient obstruction of a coronary artery, if relieved before the onset of irreversible cell damage, leads to a variable degree of cardiac dysfunction (diminished contractility and impaired relaxation) that may persist for hours, days, or weeks after flow has been restored and is known as **myocardial stunning.** Patients with coronary artery disease often present with evidence of a "stuttering" coronary obstruction, in that the artery appears to be repetitively occluding and reperfusing, causing repeated episodes of chest pain at rest. This is called **unstable angina.** Many of these patients go on to suffer myocardial infarction when the artery occludes permanently or remains occluded long enough to cause irreversible damage.

Fig. 24-8. ATP balance during anaerobic and aerobic glycolysis in the heart. Anaerobic glycolysis produces 4 moles of ATP during the conversion of 1 mol of glucose to 2 mol of lactate. However, 2 mol of ATP are consumed during the initial conversion of 1 mol of glucose to 2 mol of glyceraldehyde-3-phosphate and 1 mol of ATP is consumed during the initial metabolism of 1 mol of glycogen. Thus the net yield of ATP from anaerobic glycolysis is 2 mol of ATP per mole of glucose and 3 mol of ATP per mole of glycogen. In contrast, complete oxidative metabolism of 1 mol of glucose, including aerobic glycolysis to 2 mol of pyruvate, oxidation of pyruvate to acetylcoenzyme A, and then oxidation of acetylcoenzyme A through the Krebs tricarboxylic acid (TCA) cycle, yields 36 mol of ATP.

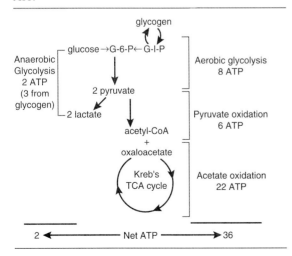

Summary

Metabolism in cardiac muscle is predominantly aerobic and synthesizes the large amounts of ATP it requires for contraction and relaxation by oxidative phosphorylation in the mitochondria, with only a small contribution from anaerobic glycolysis. The oxygen requirements of the myocardium are therefore very high, even under resting conditions, and markedly increase under conditions of stress or exercise. The major factor that determines the amount of oxygen supplied to the myocardium is coronary blood flow, since oxygen extraction by myocardial cells is near maximal at rest and can be augmented only slightly in response to the oxygen requirements of increased cardiac work. The determinants of coronary flow are the aortic perfusion pressure (mainly diastolic pressure, since flow to the intramyocardial vessels is largely shut off during systole) and coronary vascular resistance, which is the key factor in the regulation of coronary flow. Three mechanisms regulate coronary vascular resistance: (1) metabolic regulation by adenosine, a vasodilatory breakdown product of ATP that accumulates when ATP use is heightened (increased work) or ATP synthesis is decreased (ischemia or hypoxia), (2) neurogenic regulation by means of the autonomic nervous system, and (3) regulation by endothelial-derived factors, the best defined being EDRF, which is elaborated in response to a variety of stress signals.

Bibliography

Berne, R. M. The role of adenosine in the regulation of coronary blood flow. *Circ. Res.* 47:807–813, 1980.

Katz, A. M. *Physiology of the Heart.* New York: Raven Press. 1977.

Klocke, F. J. Measurement of coronary blood flow and degree of stenosis: current clinical implications and continuing uncertainties. *Am. J. Coll. Cardiol.* 1:31–41, 1983.

McAlpine, W. A. *Heart and Coronary Arteries: Anatomic Atlas for Radiologic Diagnosis and Surgical Therapy.* New York: Springer-Verlag, 1975.

Neely, J. R., Morgan, H. E. Myocardial utilization of carbohydrate and lipids. *Prog. Cardiovasc. Dis.* 15:289–329, 1972.

Olsson, R. A., and Bunger, R. Metabolic control of coronary blood flow. *Prog. Cardiovasc. Dis.* 29:369–387, 1987.

Opie, L. H. *The Heart: Physiology and Metabolism.* New York: Raven Press, 1991.

25 Hemodynamics and Regional Circulation

Harriet S. Iwamoto and Richard A. Walsh

Objectives

After reading this chapter, you should be able to

Describe in a general way how each of the following characteristics vary among the aorta, arterioles, capillaries, venules, and veins: compliance, resistance, pressure, capacitance, volume, and vessel diameter

Explain how total peripheral resistance is affected by amputation of a limb

List the major determinants of vascular resistance, and identify which is the most important one under normal conditions

Describe the relationship among blood flow, resistance, and driving pressure

Define *compliance,* and describe why it is important in the peripheral circulation

---

The adult cardiovascular system is a closed loop made up of two separate circulations arranged in series: the **systemic** and **pulmonary circulations** (Fig. 25-1). At rest, **cardiac output** is 5 to 6 liters/min. A major portion of the systemic blood flow is distributed to the renal and splanchnic circulations. During strenuous exercise, cardiac output increases to as much as 25 liters/min. The relative distribution of systemic blood flow changes dramatically, such that blood flow to the skin and skeletal muscle increases to constitute as much as 85% of cardiac output. Note that the heart receives about 5% of cardiac output at rest and during strenuous exercise. This represents a fivefold increase in blood flow during exercise over baseline values (1250 versus 250 ml/min). The brain receives about the same amount of blood flow in each situation (750 ml/min), whereas the kidneys receive less during strenuous exercise than at rest (500 versus 1000 ml/min). Regulation of blood flow to the different regions of the systemic circulation balances the needs of the body as a whole against the needs of the individual tissues for oxygen and nutrient uptake and waste removal. The factors that regulate the distribution of cardiac output under various conditions are the topics for this and the next two chapters.

An important principle that governs the distribution of cardiac output is based on a physiologic analogy of **Ohm's law of electrical resistance.** Ohm's law states that the amount of current (I) that flows is related directly to the voltage gradient across the system $(V_1 - V_2)$ and inversely to the resistance in the circuit (R): $I = (V_1 - V_2)/R$. The heart and peripheral circulations (systemic and pulmonary) are analogous circuits in which the voltage generator is the heart pump that generates a pressure gradient $(P_1 - P_2)$, current is blood flow (Q), and the systemic and pulmonary circulations are resistance elements (R). Blood flow increases with an increase in the pressure gradient $(P_1 - P_2)$ or a decrease in resistance according to the relationship $Q = (P_1 - P_2)/R$.

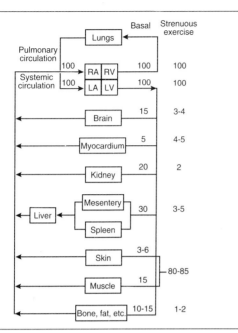

Fig. 25-1. Distribution of blood flow in the adult circulation. Blood flow that returns from the systemic circulation to the right atrium (RA) is ejected by the right ventricle (RV) and perfuses the pulmonary circulation. Blood returns to the left atrium (LA) and is ejected by the left ventricle (LV) and perfuses the systemic circulation. Cardiac output is the amount of blood ejected by each ventricle per minute and is indicated as 100%. Major components of the systemic circulation are depicted. The two columns of numbers represent the approximate percentage of cardiac output each organ receives under basal conditions (*left column*) and during strenuous exercise (*right column*). Cardiac output under basal conditions is 5 to 6 liters/min; cardiac output during strenuous exercise can reach 25 liters/min.

Pressure

Definitions

Vascular pressures are **absolute pressures,** i.e., the difference between total and atmospheric pressures, and are expressed in mmHg or the SI unit kilopascals (where 1 kPa = 7.50 mmHg). **Transmural pressure** (P_{TM}) is the difference between the pressure inside and the pressure outside a structure. P_{TM} is the net pressure that distends structures, such as the cardiac chambers or blood vessels. **Driving pressure** represents the difference between absolute pressure upstream and the absolute pressure downstream, e.g.,

$P_1 - P_2$. For blood to flow from one point to another, P_1 must exceed P_2.

Pressure Changes Through the Circulation

The **absolute pressures** that exist in the circulation are depicted in Fig. 25-2. The pumping action of the left ventricle generates the energy that propels blood flow through the systemic circulation. Absolute pressure in the normal left ventricle oscillates between 3 and 120 mmHg. In the aorta, blood pressure oscillates between 80 and 120 mmHg. The lowest pressure (80 mmHg) is the **diastolic pressure,** and the highest pressure (120 mmHg) is the **systolic pressure.** The difference between these two values (systolic pressure – diastolic pressure = 40 mmHg) is the **pulse pressure.** The **mean arterial pressure** is the average arterial blood pressure during the entire cardiac cycle (see Chap. 22) and can be approximated from these two values. Mean arterial pressure is not simply the arithmetic mean of these values, because systole normally lasts only about half as long as diastole. Mean arterial pressure can be estimated to be a weighted average: mean arterial pressure = one-third the systolic pressure + two-thirds the diastolic pressure. Thus mean arterial pressure in this example is 93 mmHg.

As blood courses through the large arteries, systolic pressure increases slightly and diastolic pressure decreases. The decrease in diastolic pressure is greater than the increase in systolic pressure, so pulse pressure increases gradually and mean arterial blood pressure decreases in the systemic arteries as a direct function of the distance from the heart. The arterioles provide the greatest resistance to blood flow in the circulation. Consequently, absolute blood pressure decreases by the greatest amount in the arterioles. In addition, the oscillations of blood pressure are abolished in the arteriolar portion of the systemic circulation.

Blood enters the capillaries of the **systemic circulation** with pressures that range from 30 to 38 mmHg. As blood flows through the capillaries, the blood pressure decreases to 20 mmHg, and in the venules, it decreases to 5 mmHg. Blood pressure decreases further in the large veins and vena cava, so blood returns to the right atrium with an absolute pressure nearly equal to the atmospheric pressure.

The right ventricle is another pump with the same cavity size but smaller mass than the left ventricle. The right ventricle generates pressure pulses that oscillate between 0 and 25 mmHg. Pressure in the pulmonary artery oscillates between 8 and 25 mmHg, and the mean pulmonary arterial blood pressure is about 15 mmHg. As with the systemic

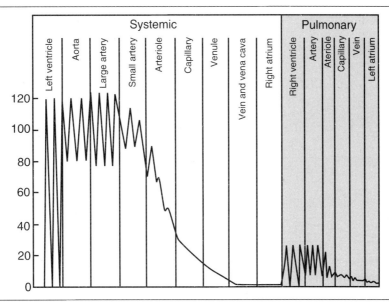

Fig. 25-2. Absolute pressures in major portions of the systemic and pulmonary (*shaded portion*) circulations. In the systemic circulation, blood flows from the left ventricle, through arteries, capillaries, venules, and veins, to the right atrium. The driving pressure for the systemic circulation is the difference between aortic and right atrial pressures. In the pulmonary circulation, blood flows from the right ventricle, through pulmonary vessels, to the left atrium. The driving pressure for the pulmonary circulation is the difference between right ventricular and left atrial pressures.

circulation, the pulmonary arterioles exert the greatest resistance to blood flow in the **pulmonary circulation,** and therefore, the greatest pressure decrease occurs in the arteriolar portion. Unlike the systemic arterioles, the pulmonary arterioles do not completely dampen the pressure pulses. The mean pressure in the pulmonary capillaries is about 7 mmHg. A further decrease in blood pressure occurs in the remainder of the pulmonary circulation, such that the mean pressure in the left atrium is about 2 to 3 mmHg.

Relationship Between Pressure and Volume

Changes in blood volume have very important effects on blood pressure and blood flow. One of the major variables affected by changes in blood volume is the **mean circulatory pressure,** which is defined as the equilibrium pressure of the circulation. Mean circulatory pressure is the absolute pressure measurable when blood flow is zero. It is an index of the "fullness" of the circulation. Under normal circumstances, mean circulatory pressure is 7 mmHg. When blood volume is increased above normal, mean cir-

culatory pressure increases. As a result, venous return, ventricular filling, and cardiac output increase. The increase in cardiac output increases arterial blood pressure in accordance with Ohm's law. The increase in arterial blood pressure tends to be buffered by baroreceptor-activated mechanisms, as discussed in Chap. 26.

Another relationship between blood volume and blood pressure is defined as **compliance.** When a distensible structure such as a balloon is inflated, the volume it attains depends on the distending or transmural (P_{TM}) pressure and the elastic properties of the balloon material. A change in volume is accompanied by a corresponding change in the P_{TM}, the magnitude of which depends on its compliance. Compliance (C) represents the ease with which a structure can be stretched and is expressed mathematically as $C = \Delta V/\Delta P_{TM}$. Note that differences (Δ) rather than absolute values are used in this expression and that compliance is the **change** in pressure required to produce a **change** in volume. For a very compliant structure, a large change in volume will produce a relatively small change in P_{TM}; for a stiff structure, a small change in volume will produce a large change in P_{TM}.

Figure 25-3 depicts the **relationship between volume**

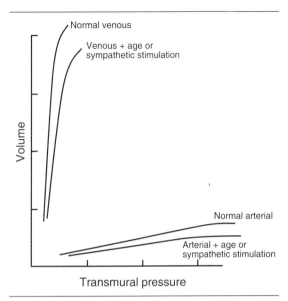

Fig. 25-3. Relationship between transmural pressure (P_{TM}) and volume in an artery and vein. Note that the slope of the relationship ($\Delta vol/\Delta P_{TM}$) is equal to compliance. Veins are more compliant than arteries. Aging and sympathetic stimulation (indicated by *thin lines*) render both arteries and veins less compliant.

and P_{TM} for the arterial and venous portions of the circulation. The slope of the relationship is equal to compliance. The slope of the arterial curve is less than the slope of the venous curve; arteries are much less compliant than veins. That is, a small amount of volume added to an artery produces a large increase in P_{TM}, whereas a large amount of volume added to a vein produces only a small increase in P_{TM}. Normal aging or an increase in sympathetic stimulation decreases the slopes of the curves and thus compliance of both arteries and veins. Aging decreases arterial compliance gradually primarily because there are gradual increases in arterial blood pressure and abundance of relatively nondistensible structural proteins such as collagen in the arterial vessel wall. Sympathetic stimulation decreases vessel compliance by constricting vessels and increasing vascular tone.

Because of differences in compliance in the arterial and venous portions of the circulation, more blood volume resides in the venous than in the arterial component at any given time (Table 25-1). The greatest proportion of total blood volume exists in the accommodating, compliant venous part of the circulation, which is an important blood reservoir. When necessary, an increase in sympathetic stimulation constricts venous vessels and increases venous

Table 25-1. Distribution of Blood Volume in the Circulation

	% Total Volume*
Heart	8–11
Systemic arteries	10–12
Capillaries	4–5
Systemic veins	60–70
Lungs	10–12

*This represents the fraction of total blood volume in residence in each area of the circulation at any given time.

pressure. Because only a small increase in venous pressure can markedly reduce venous blood volume, blood can be effectively returned to the heart to maintain cardiac output and arterial blood pressure. This is an important adaptive mechanism that operates in normal day-to-day activities as well as in pathologic situations.

Arterial Blood Pressure

Transformation of the Ventricular Pressure Pulse

The output of blood from the ventricles is intermittent, whereas blood flow in the capillaries is continuous. Intermittent blood flow ejected from the ventricles is converted to a more continuous flow in the aorta and large arteries. The example shown in Fig. 25-4 explains how this is accomplished. A rigid tube is connected to a piston pump on one end and a resistance unit on the other end. A reservoir and a one-way valve are placed between the pump and the resistance unit. Pressure is measured between the valve and the resistance unit (Fig. 25-4A). Initially, the reservoir is filled, the valve is closed, and the pressure measured is equal to the atmospheric pressure. The pump is activated, and the piston moves to the right, fluid flows out of the reservoir as the valve opens, and a positive deflection of pressure is recorded. Then the piston is pulled back. The pressure in the reservoir becomes less than that in the tube, the valve closes, and the pressure returns to the atmospheric pressure. A pump connected to a rigid tube then delivers intermittent flow, and pressure oscillates between atmospheric and a positive value (Fig. 25-4B).

Such wide oscillations in intraluminal pressure would damage those vessels of the systemic circulation which are thin-walled. By contrast, the circulation is similar to the system shown in Fig. 25-4C, in which a distensible tube has replaced the rigid tube. As fluid is ejected from the

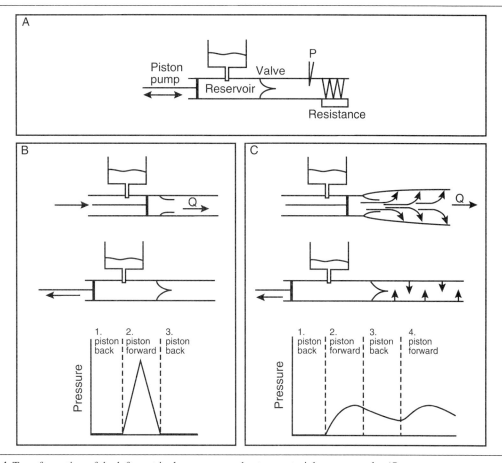

Fig. 25-4. Transformation of the left ventricular pressure pulse to an arterial pressure pulse (Q = fluid flow; P = pressure; see text for details).

reservoir, the tube stretches and expands. Some of the energy imparted by the pump is converted into kinetic energy in the form of moving fluid, and some of the energy is stored as potential energy in the tube wall. As the piston draws back, the one-way valve closes, and pressure decreases in the reservoir and tube. However, the pressure in the tube decreases more slowly than in the reservoir. During this phase, the stored potential energy in the distensible tube is converted to the kinetic energy of fluid flow as the wall of the tube recoils. If the frequency of piston movement is relatively high, the pressure is maintained at a level above atmospheric pressure. In this way, driving pressure throughout the cardiac cycle is maintained at a level greater than atmospheric pressure. Intermittent flow and large pressure changes in the reservoir (ventricle) are transformed into continuous flow and

smaller pressure changes in the distensible tube (peripheral circulation).

Factors That Alter the Arterial Pressure Waveform

Normal Arterial Pressure Waveform.   During the ejection phase of the cardiac cycle, the aortic valve is open, and pressures in the left ventricle and aorta are approximately equal (see Chap. 22). When the left ventricle begins to relax during ventricular diastole, pressure in the ventricle falls, and the aortic valve closes. This causes the aortic valve leaflets to pull in slightly, bringing about a brief backflow of blood followed by cessation of backflow. A corresponding fall and rise in arterial pressure occurs, and this is inscribed as a **dicrotic notch** on the arterial pressure pulse. When the aortic valve is closed, ventricular and aortic pressures differ (see Chap. 23). During the remainder of ventricular diastole, absolute pressure in the aorta decreases gradually until the aortic valve opens at the beginning of the next ejection phase.

Effect of Heart Rate.   Changes in heart rate largely affect the diastolic pressure. For example, let us say that diastolic pressure in the aorta is 80 mmHg when heart rate is 60 beats per minute. When heart rate increases to 120 beats per minute, the duration of ventricular systole is not affected. However, the duration of ventricular diastole is reduced so that the aortic valve opens much sooner than previously. As a result, aortic pressure does not have time to decrease to 80 mmHg before the aortic valve reopens. The net effect is to increase diastolic pressure and decrease pulse pressure. Systolic pressure is not affected if there is *only* a change in the heart rate. However, an increase in heart rate is often initiated by heightened sympathetic stimulation, which increases ventricular contractility. If this occurs, systolic arterial pressure also would increase.

Effect of Altered Stroke Volume.   Pulse pressure is related directly to stroke volume and inversely to arterial compliance. During ventricular systole, which lasts about 0.25 second, the stroke volume ejected by the ventricle, about 70 ml, enters the aorta during the first 0.1 second. This quick increase in aortic volume produces an increase in aortic pressure that is proportional to the increase in volume, as dictated by aortic compliance. An increase in stroke volume increases pulse pressure because the aorta is relatively noncompliant, and a small increase in volume produces a relatively large increase in pressure, i.e., systolic pressure. Diastolic pressure is altered to a much smaller extent.

Effect of Altered Aortic Valve Function.   **Aortic regurgitation** or **aortic valve insufficiency** occurs when the aortic valve does not close normally. In the extreme, the aortic valve does not close completely, and ventricular and aortic pressures are equal throughout the cardiac cycle. However, in this syndrome, the aortic valve usually closes, but later than normal. As a result, diastolic pressure in the aorta decreases and pulse pressure increases. Ventricular filling is altered because the ventricle relaxes when the aortic valve is still open. This allows backflow of blood from the aorta to the ventricle and results in increased ventricular volume. Because of **Starling's law,** increased stretch of the myofibers results in more forceful con-

traction and increased stroke volume. The net effect of aortic valve insufficiency is an increase in the force of contraction, ultimately an increase ventricle size and wall tension (the work of the heart) and a decrease in diastolic pressure. The end result of these effects is an increase in aortic pulse pressure.

Aortic stenosis is the inability of the aortic valve to open fully during systole. Aortic stenosis decreases the radius of the outflow tract and increases resistance to ventricular ejection (increased afterload). Consequently, a pressure gradient develops between the left ventricle and aorta, in accordance with **Ohm's law.** To maintain normal aortic pressures, the left ventricle must generate pressures higher than normal. Thus myocardial work is increased, and left ventricular hypertrophy results.

Decrease in Arterial Compliance.   Arterial compliance decreases with increased sympathetic stimulation and normal aging and in certain diseases such as atherosclerosis. Decreased compliance renders the arteries stiffer and less able to accommodate the stroke volume ejected by the ventricle with each heartbeat. The arteries become more like rigid tubes, as shown in Fig. 25-4. As a result, pulse pressure increases, and the arterial pressure wave becomes more peaked and angular.

Pressure Wave Transmission Throughout the Arterial Circulation.   As shown in Fig. 25-2, the blood pressure contour in large arteries differs from that in the aorta. In large arteries, systolic pressure is greater, diastolic pressure is less, and pulse pressure is greater than in the aorta. The mean arterial blood pressure is slightly less than that in the aorta because the **decrease in diastolic pressure** is proportionately greater than the rise in systolic pressure. The explanation for the latter is related to the fact that an arterial pressure wave is composed of a number of different waves with different amplitudes and frequencies. High-frequency pressure waves are transmitted faster than low-frequency waves, and these transmitted frequencies summate to form a different pressure profile at points distant from the heart. A second factor that alters the arterial pressure waveform is related to **arterial compliance.** As each segment of the arterial tree is stretched and recoils, the intraluminal pressure is altered, as previously described. Third, as the pressure wave hits major branch points, there is a **reflection** of the wave. These reflected waves summate with oncoming waves from subsequent beats. The net effect of these factors is that the arterial pressure waveform is continually altered as it is transmitted from the heart to the periphery.

Capillary Dynamics

For an in-depth discussion on capillary dynamics, the reader is referred to Chap. 26.

Venous Blood Pressure

Central venous blood pressure is that pressure measured at the level of the heart and normally is close to atmospheric pressure. It is the downstream pressure that influences **cardiac output,** according to the relationship cardiac output = (aortic pressure – central venous pressure)/systemic vascular resistance. The pressure in the venous circulation is expressed by the relationship, venous return = (capillary pressure – central venous pressure)/venous resistance. Variations in venous pressure alter venous capacitance and the amount of blood stored in the venous reservoir; they also affect ventricular filling and cardiac function.

Venous Pressure Waves

In the systemic circulation, the pressure pulse waves generated by the left ventricle are dampened in the arterioles and capillaries, and venous pressures are low. However, pulses can still be observed in the systemic veins near the heart. These pressure waves are quite unlike the arterial pressure pulse, though they are cyclic in nature. They reflect the pressure changes in the right atrium.

There are **three pressure waves** in the right atrial pulse. The **a wave** occurs during atrial contraction. During late diastole, the right ventricle is filled with nearly all of its end-diastolic volume. The right atrium contracts, right atrial pressure increases, and additional blood is transmitted to the right ventricle. The increase in right atrial pressure is reflected retrograde into the large veins near the heart. As the atrium relaxes, pressure in the right atrium and large veins falls. This rise and fall in pressure inscribes the a wave. The next wave is the **c wave,** and this coincides with ventricular contraction. Right ventricular contraction increases ventricular pressure, which is transmitted retrograde into the right atrium, producing a second increase in pressure in the atrium and large veins. When the pressure in the right ventricle exceeds that in the pulmonary artery, the pulmonic valve opens. Pressures in the ventricle, pulmonary artery, atrium, and large veins rise and then fall. This pressure wave generated in the atrium and veins is the c wave. During ventricular systole and isovolumetric relaxation, the tricuspid valve is closed (see Chap. 22). Toward the end of these phases, the systemic veins and right atrium are stretched, and intraluminal pressure rises. This pressure buildup is relieved only when the tricuspid valve opens at the beginning of diastole. This rise and fall in pressure is called the **v wave.** These three pressure waves can be seen in the cardiac cycle diagram in Chap. 22. In the normal person, these pressure waves are evident only when the person is quietly recumbent. They can become prominent in certain disease states such as atrioventricular nodal block.

Normal Variations in Venous Pressure

Hydrostatic Effects.   In a recumbent person, the absolute pressures as defined in Fig. 25-2 are fairly accurate. However, for a person standing upright, the values are much different. Absolute blood pressure is a function of the energy imparted by the pumping action of the heart plus the hydrostatic pressure imposed by a column of fluid. Blood in the hand, which is about 2 ft (60 cm) below the heart, has a 2-ft column of blood resting on it compared with blood in the heart. Gravity and the specific density of blood produce a **hydrostatic pressure** of about 35 mmHg. The arterial blood pressure in the hand, relative to atmospheric pressure at the level of the heart, is 95 + 35 mmHg, or 130 mmHg. Venous blood pressure in the hand is about 40 mmHg. Because of the effects of gravity, arterial blood pressure is 185 mmHg and venous pressure is about 95 mmHg in the foot. For this reason, absolute blood pressures are measured at the same level as the heart, by convention.

Skeletal Muscle Pump.   Gravitational effects on blood can reduce venous return. After only 15 minutes of quiet standing, as much as 15% to 20% of the blood volume is retained in the lower extremities. The resulting increase in capillary hydrostatic and filtration pressures promotes capillary filtration and loss of fluid from the vascular compartment. In this situation, **skeletal muscle activity** can increase venous return. Skeletal muscle contraction increases the pressure surrounding the veins. Blood is prevented from flowing backward by one-way valves in the lumina of peripheral veins, so blood is propelled back to the heart. Regular cycles of muscle contraction and relaxation thus pump blood and assist venous return.

Skeletal muscle activity is not the only mechanism that enhances venous return in the peripheral veins. As will be discussed in detail in Chap. 26, a decrease in venous return is perceived by sensory nerve endings located in the large veins and atria. The **sympathetic nervous system** and **endocrine mechanisms** are activated. Vasoactive factors, thus stimulated, constrict peripheral vessels. Venous pressure increases, venous compliance decreases, and additional blood is returned to the heart.

Thoracoabdominal Pump. The thoracoabdominal pump is another pumping mechanism that promotes venous return to the heart. The inferior vena cava returns blood from the abdomen to the heart in the thoracic cavity. Relative to atmospheric pressure, intra-abdominal pressure is a few millimeters of mercury positive and intrathoracic pressure is a few millimeters of mercury negative. During inspiration, the diaphragm contracts, the abdominal pressure increases, and intrathoracic pressure decreases. This pressure gradient favors venous return. On expiration, abdominal pressure decreases and intrathoracic pressure increases yet remains negative. Rhythmic breathing thus produces a rhythmic oscillation of intra-abdominal and intrathoracic pressures that alternately results in a more and less favorable pressure gradient for venous return.

Blood Flow and Blood Flow Velocity

Blood flow refers to the bulk flow of fluid in the circulation. This flow of blood from the heart, through the aorta, through the total arteriolar system, through the capillaries, and through the venous system is equal to cardiac output. **Blood flow velocity** is the speed with which blood moves along the circulation in any particular segment and is expressed in units of distance per time. Blood flow velocity is related directly to blood flow and inversely to cross-sectional area, according to the relationship average blood flow velocity = blood flow/cross-sectional area. Thus blood flow velocity is greatest in the aorta and least in the capillary bed.

In the circulation, blood flows predominantly in a streamline or laminar pattern. There is friction between the blood vessel wall and that blood flowing close to the vessel wall, causing blood flow velocity to be almost zero next to the wall. Shear stresses between adjacent layers of blood cause blood to flow in a laminar pattern in much of the circulation. When blood flows in this fashion, it appears to move in concentric cylinders of ever-faster-moving blood, with the blood cells moving with their long axes parallel to the long axis of the vessel. The laminar pattern of blood flow is interrupted and converted to a turbulent flow pattern in the ventricles and, to a certain extent, in the atria. Turbulence in these portions of the circulation ensures

mixing of the blood. Turbulence also occurs at branch points in the circulatory tree, where blood flow increases above a critical value when there is an abrupt change in vessel diameter, such as one secondary to atherosclerotic plaque development, and in the aorta, where turbulence is greater than expected, probably because flow in the aorta is pulsatile. When blood travels in a laminar pattern, it makes little or no discernible noise. Turbulent blood flow in a region where wall resonance is prominent, such as the cardiac chambers and large vessels, produces a sound or murmur that can be discerned by auscultation with a stethoscope.

Resistance

As stated previously, blood flow and blood pressure are directly proportional and equal to vascular resistance. Several factors influence resistance to blood flow. **Viscosity** refers to the thickness of a fluid. The more viscous a fluid is, the more energy is required to overcome frictional forces to initiate and maintain fluid movement. For a homogeneous fluid such as water or plasma at a given temperature, viscosity is constant. The viscosity of plasma at 37°C is about 1.7 times that of water. For suspension solutions such as blood, viscosity is not constant. In vitro, the viscosity of blood is about three to four times greater than that of water. In vivo, however, the viscosity of blood is only one to two times greater than that of water. Several factors are responsible for this. In large blood vessels, **laminar blood flow** and the alignment of red blood cells parallel to the axis of motion greatly reduce viscosity. When blood flow falls below a critical level, the cells fall out of alignment and tumble end over end. This increases the apparent viscosity. In small blood vessels, red blood cells flow in the center of the vessel, away from the no-flow zone next to the vessel wall. This reduces viscosity.

Temperature is another factor that affects viscosity. Viscosity increases approximately 2% for each 1°C decrease in temperature. Another factor that affects viscosity is **red blood cell mass** and **protein concentration.** As the red blood cell mass (hematocrit) or protein concentration increases, viscosity increases. Viscosity is often expressed as η and directly affects resistance (R). Thus $R \propto \eta$. As the length (l) of the resistance pathway, the blood vessel, increases, the greater is the resistance. Thus: $R \propto l$.

The most important factor that influences resistance to blood flow is the vessel radius (r). The relationship between radius and resistance is rendered as $R \propto 1/r^4$. Thus the vessel radius has a very important effect on resistance, such that when the radius is halved, resistance increases by a factor of 16. The relationship between viscosity, length, and vessel radius is quantified in Poiseuille's law:

$$R = \frac{8\eta l}{\Pi r^4}$$

and

$$Q = \frac{(P_1 - P_2)\Pi r^4}{8\eta l}$$

Although this relationship was originally developed to describe the flow of a homogeneous fluid through a rigid tube, it approximates the flow of the circulation.

The **circulation** is not a single circuit but is composed of a number of circuits arranged in series as well as in parallel. Each circuit provides resistance to blood flow, and the type of circuit determines its contribution to total peripheral resistance. For a circuit that has resistances arranged in series, the total resistance is equal to the sum of component resistances. For resistances connected in parallel, the reciprocal of the total resistance is equal to the sum of the reciprocals of the component resistances.

Resistances connected in parallel are more efficient than resistances connected in series because the heart pump does not have to generate a large driving pressure. A parallel system has the advantage not only of efficiency but also of continuity. This means that when the resistance of one circuit changes markedly, blood flows to other circuits change only slightly. This is so because driving pressure, more specifically arterial blood pressure, is maintained within narrow limits (see Chap. 27). When one circuit is eliminated (e.g., by tying a tight tourniquet around one's leg), total resistance and arterial blood pressure increase immediately. The increase in arterial blood pressure is sensed by the baroreceptors (see Chap. 27) that mediate changes which cause arterial blood pressure to return to its original value. This mechanism serves to keep blood flow to other areas of the circulation relatively constant. Even though less efficient, series resistance units are sometimes necessary, e.g., the portal venous connection between the gastrointestinal tract and liver.

The total peripheral vascular resistance is the sum of all resistances in the systemic circulation that the left ventricle must overcome to eject blood. For the systemic circulation, if the driving pressure is 90 mmHg (aortic –

right atrial pressures) and cardiac output is 5 liter/min, the total peripheral vascular resistance is 18 mmHg·min/liter. Total vascular resistance across the pulmonary circuit is much less; driving pressure [16 – 2 mmHg (pulmonary arterial – pulmonary venous)] divided by cardiac output (5 liters/min, or 2.4 mmHg·min/liter). This difference in systemic and pulmonary resistances accounts for why the left and right ventricles differ in wall thickness and mass.

Peripheral Blood Flow

Distribution

The proportion of cardiac output that various areas of the peripheral circulation receive is shown in Fig. 25-1, and the blood flow each organ receives is given in Table 25-2. In this section the factors that regulate blood flow to the brain, muscle, and skin are discussed. Blood flow regulation in other organs is discussed in detail elsewhere in this text.

Brain

Preserving blood flow to the brain is the most important function of the circulation, because cerebral tissue cannot survive on anaerobic metabolism and begins to die if blood flow is arrested for more than a few minutes. Several mechanisms maintain **cerebral blood flow,** one of which is dependent on **arterial blood gases.** There is a positive curvilinear relationship between cerebral blood flow and arterial carbon dioxide tension. Small increases in arterial blood carbon dioxide tension above normal values produce large increases in cerebral blood flow. Decreases in carbon dioxide decrease blood flow. It is generally believed that this response is mediated in part through changes in extracellular pH. The increase in cerebral blood flow, when carbon dioxide tension or hydrogen ion concentrations increase, maintains the concentration of these substances in the cerebrospinal fluid (CSF) within narrow limits. This is an important feature because pH changes alter membrane potentials and function of nerve cells. Oxygen also alters cerebral blood flow. When arterial oxygen content decreases, cerebral blood flow increases exponentially. This is an important relationship, because cerebral oxygen delivery (the product of cerebral blood flow and arterial oxygen content) stays constant. This response appears to be locally regulated because it is observed in animals in which innervation of blood vessels has been interrupted surgically or pharmacologically or hormonal responses have been inhibited.

Cerebral blood flow is also controlled by autoregulation

Table 25-2. Blood Flow to Individual Organs

| Organ | Mass (kg) | Basal Blood Flow | | Maximum Blood Flow (liters/min) |
		Liters/min	Ml/min/100 g	
Brain	1.5	0.75	50	2.1
White	0.9	0.23	25	0.9
Gray	0.6	0.60	100	2.0
Heart	0.3	0.24	80	1.2
Muscle	30.0	1.0	3–5	18.0
Skin	2.0	0.2	3–5	3–4.0
GI tract	2.5	1.0	40	5.0
Liver*	1.4	0.5	40	3.0
Kidney	0.3	1.2	400	1.4
Bone	27.0	0.8	3	4.0

*These values denote hepatic arterial contribution only.

of blood flow in the face of widely varying perfusion pressures of from 60 to 150 mmHg (see Chap. 23). When arterial blood pressure decreases below 60 mmHg and cerebral blood flow falls, the brain tissue begins to become ischemic. This response, particularly in the portions of the brain that regulate cardiovascular function, can elicit powerful stimulation of the peripheral sympathetic nervous system, which produces generalized vasoconstriction and an increase in arterial blood pressure (see Chap. 27). This response is effective down to arterial blood pressures of 15 to 20 mmHg and is so powerful that blood flow to other areas can drop to zero in an effort to preserve cerebral blood flow. This reflex response is called the **central nervous system ischemic response.** Coronary blood flow is maintained (see Chap. 22) because the sympathetic activation simultaneously increases myocardial work by increasing heart rate and contractility. Since the myocardial blood flow is regulated predominantly by metabolic factors, intense sympathetic nervous system activation tends to increase myocardial blood flow.

Cerebral blood vessels are innervated, but these neural mechanisms modify cerebral blood flow only weakly. Any effect nerve stimulation has on cerebral blood flow can be overpowered by other factors that regulate cerebral blood flow.

Skeletal Muscle

The blood flow to resting skeletal muscle is relatively low, normally only 3 to 4 ml/min/100 g of muscle, and only 10% of the capillary beds are perfused. This is sufficient to meet the basal metabolic needs of resting muscle. Blood vessels in skeletal muscle are innervated; they constrict in

response to alpha-adrenergic stimulation and dilate in response to beta-adrenergic or cholinergic stimulation. When skeletal muscle is not working and blood flow is needed elsewhere, neural mechanisms constrict muscle vessels to divert blood to the needed areas. When skeletal muscle is active, however, neural influences on blood flow are overridden by powerful local metabolic and vascular control mechanisms. Strenuous exercise can increase blood flow to muscle by as much as 25-fold, to a maximum of about 80 ml/min/100 g, in which *all* capillary beds are perfused. The primary regulators of skeletal muscle blood flow during exercise are **metabolic factors.** When muscle contracts, it necessarily consumes oxygen and nutrients (primarily glucose) and produces carbon dioxide and other metabolic waste products. These resulting changes — a decrease in oxygen tension and increases in the concentrations of carbon dioxide, lactic acid, hydrogen ions, and potassium ions — directly increase muscle blood flow. The predominant effector has not been clearly identified, and it is probable that endothelial-derived substances are involved (see Chap. 27) and all factors make some contribution to the change in blood flow. As the increase in blood flow reverses these changes (i.e., the increased perfusion washes out these substances), tissue concentrations return to normal. With aerobic exercise, blood flow is maintained at a steady level, albeit one higher than normal, in pace with the increase in metabolic rate. On average, blood flow is matched to metabolic rate, although this may vary from moment to moment because the muscle can depend on anaerobic metabolism for only short periods of time. Under anaerobic conditions, muscle blood flow remains elevated until the concentrations of all effector substances return to normal. Thus, for a given period of exercise, the increase in metabolic rate is matched by an increase in blood flow, even if the exercise is maximal for a time and blood flow remains elevated into the period of recovery from exercise.

Skin

Blood flows to the skin to nourish the epidermis and to help regulate body temperature. A brief description of the **anatomy of cutaneous circulation** is important to an understanding of the physiology of cutaneous blood flow. Blood enters the skin in the dermis in arterioles. The arterioles branch into metarterioles, and these give rise to capillary loops that radiate out toward the epidermal layer. The capillary loops then drain into venules that drain into a venous plexus located in the dermal layer. In certain areas of the body (soles of feet, palms, ears, lips, and nose), blood that enters a cutaneous artery can either flow through the capillary loops via the arterioles or bypass the capillaries by flowing through short communications between the venous plexus and artery, the arteriovenous anastomosis. These vessels are richly innervated with sympathetic nerve fibers. Sympathetic nerve stimulation constricts arterioles and arteriovenous anastomoses; intense stimulation can reduce cutaneous blood flow to nearly zero.

Blood flows through the capillaries much more slowly than through the arteriovenous anastomoses. This is an important feature of cutaneous blood flow and its role in temperature regulation. When the body is cold, the sympathetic nervous system is activated, and arterioles and arteriovenous anastomoses constrict. Blood flow then bypasses the cutaneous circulation and returns quickly to the body's core. The heat in the blood is thus retained, and body temperature is maintained. When the body is warm, the sympathetic activation of the skin is inhibited, and the arterioles dilate. A major portion of blood flows through the capillaries, and heat is dissipated in venous plexus in the dermis and epidermal skin layers and is ultimately lost to the atmosphere.

Regional Circulation in the Fetus and the Transition at Birth

The Fetal Circulation

Course of Blood Flow
The placenta is the site of nutrient, oxygen, and waste exchange between the mother and fetus such that the placenta functions as the gastrointestinal tract, lungs, and

kidneys for the fetus. **Placental exchange** poses a unique problem of blood flow distribution for the fetus, in that maintenance of blood flow to the placenta is essential for survival.

Blood rich in oxygen and nutrients returns to the fetal body from the placenta in the umbilical veins (Fig. 25-5). Blood flows from the umbilical veins to the portal sinus to enter, in approximately equal portions, either the hepatic microvasculature or the **ductus venosus,** a conduit vessel that connects the umbilical vein and inferior vena cava. Well-saturated blood derived from the umbilical vein joins poorly saturated blood derived from venous drainage of lower-body organs in the inferior vena cava. These bloodstreams do not mix but streamline alongside each other, with the well-saturated stream medial to the poorly saturated stream. About half the inferior vena caval return

Fig. 25-5. Course of the circulation in the fetus (* = ductus venosus; ** = foramen ovale; *** = ductus arteriosus; LA = left atrium; LV = left ventricle; RA = right atrium; RV = right ventricle).

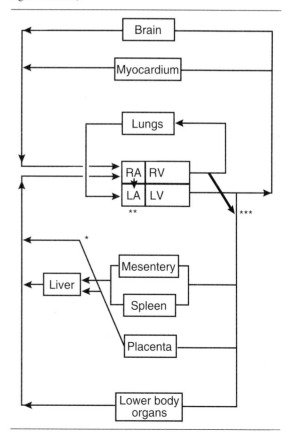

flows through the right atrium to the right ventricle. The remaining half, composed primarily of well-saturated blood, flows through the communication between the right and left atria, the **foramen ovale,** to the left ventricle. Thus shunting of umbilical venous blood across the ductus venosus and foramen ovale delivers high concentrations of oxygen and nutrients primarily to upper-body organs, which include the brain and heart of the fetus.

Venous drainage from upper-body organs returns to the heart in the superior vena cava. This blood, along with half the return from the inferior vena cava, is ejected by the right ventricle. Because pulmonary vascular resistance is quite high in the fetus, most of right ventricular output bypasses the pulmonary circulation and flows through the **ductus arteriosus,** a large communication between the main pulmonary trunk and descending aorta. A major portion of blood flow in the descending aorta is directed toward the placenta. In this way, venous drainage from upper- and lower-body organs is shunted toward the placenta, where wastes are eliminated and oxygen and nutrients are acquired.

There are important differences between the fetal and postnatal circulations. The **fetal circulation** is a parallel circuit, and the **postnatal circulation** is a series circuit. In the fetus, left and right ventricular outputs are not equal; the right ventricular output exceeds the left ventricular output by a factor of 2, and they perfuse different portions of the peripheral circulation. By virtue of the large vascular shunts in the fetal circulation, pressures in the left and right ventricles are roughly equivalent, as are pressures in the aorta and pulmonary artery. Right atrial pressure is greater than left atrial pressure, so blood flows through the foramen ovale from the right to left atrium.

The Transition at Birth

Immediately after birth, several events occur. Pulmonary ventilation and gas exchange are initiated, and the placenta is removed from the circulation. The environmental temperature decreases as the newborn leaves the warm, humid amniotic cavity for a drier, cooler environment. These events produce marked cardiovascular changes. With the initiation of pulmonary ventilation, pulmonary vascular resistance decreases dramatically. Factors responsible for this include the establishment of an air-liquid interface that reduces surface tension and an increase in oxygen content of the blood, which is a vasodilator in the pulmonary circulation. These factors appear to be mediated by local activation of arachidonic acid metabolism and increased prostacyclin production and increased production of nitric oxide by endothelial cells (see Chap. 27). When pul-

monary vascular resistance decreases, pulmonary blood flow increases and pulmonary arterial pressure decreases. As a consequence, the quantity of blood flowing through the ductus arteriosus decreases, and pulmonary venous return to the heart increases. Left atrial pressure increases, and the foramen ovale closes functionally soon after birth. These changes reverse the blood pressure gradient across the foramen ovale so that left atrial pressure exceeds right atrial pressure. Elimination of the placental circulation increases the systemic vascular resistance. The decrease in pulmonary vascular resistance and increase in systemic vascular resistance cause a separation of blood pressures in the aorta and pulmonary artery. With these changes, the parallel fetal circulation is transformed into a series circulation in the newborn. The foramen ovale and ductus venosus close within a few days after birth, and the ductus arteriosus closes within 7 to 10 days.

At birth, oxygen consumption increases by a factor of 2 to 3 because of the necessity of maintaining body temperature in a colder environment. In addition, heart rate and cardiac output increase. Normal thyroid function before birth and sympathetic stimulation at birth are necessary for these changes to occur.

Summary

From the time organogenesis is complete until death, blood flow is propelled by the heart to peripheral organs and maintained at a level that is appropriate for the physiologic situation and function. Each portion of the peripheral circulation serves a function that is important for maintaining cardiovascular homeostasis. The heart generates all the energy required to maintain blood flow to the pulmonary and systemic circulations. The left ventricle ejects blood intermittently and generates pressures that oscillate between 0 and 120 mmHg. The arteries are relatively stiff structures that conduct blood flow from the heart to peripheral organs. The physical properties of the arteries convert the intermittent flow and large pressure changes in the left ventricle to more continuous flow and smaller pressure changes in more peripheral portions of the circulation. The arterioles are the site of the majority of resistance in the circulation. Regulation of their diameters inversely alters vascular resistance. Capillaries are the site where the "work" of the peripheral circulation is carried out. Ten billion capillaries carry nutrients to and waste products from every cell in the body; each cell is only 20 to 30 μm away from a capillary. The venous side of the peripheral circulation is the collection portion of the circulation. Blood drains from capillaries into venules, venules empty into veins, and the entire venous return enters the right atrium via the superior or inferior vena cava. Most of the blood resides in the venous side of the circulation. At times of need, the blood can be squeezed out and returned to the arterial side of the circulation.

Physical principles that describe the hydraulic behavior of a fluid and current flow through an electric circuit apply in large part to the behavior of the circulation. Thus the relationship among blood flow, perfusion pressure, and vascular resistance is analogous to the relationship among current flow through a circuit, voltage gradient, and resistance such that blood flow is directly proportional to the blood pressure gradient and inversely proportional to vascular resistance. Vascular resistance is directly related to the length of the circuit and viscosity of the blood and indirectly related to the fourth power of the radius. Vascular resistance is thus exquisitely regulated by changes in arteriolar diameter. Compliance is the relationship between a change in transmural pressure and volume. High compliance of the venous side of the circulation is important for the reservoir function of the venous circulation. Changes in compliance on the venous side of the circulation alter the quantity of blood that can be stored in the venous reservoir. Changes in compliance on the arterial side of the circulation directly affect the arterial pressure waveform.

Individual vascular beds are affected by a number of vascular regulators. Of note is the inverse relationship between carbon dioxide tension and cerebral blood flow, the direct relationship between skeletal muscle work and blood flow, and the direct relationship between body temperature and skin blood flow. Superimposed on hemodynamic regulators of the peripheral circulation are local, neural, and hormonal mechanisms that ensure adequate blood flow to every area of the body throughout the lifetime of an individual.

Bibliography

Berne, R. M., and Levy, M. N. *Cardiovascular Physiology.* St. Louis: Mosby Year Book, 1992.

Heller, L. J., and Mohrman, D. E. *Cardiovascular Physiology.* New York: McGraw-Hill, 1991.

Rudolph, A. M., Iwamoto, H. S., and Teitel, D. F. Circulatory changes at birth. *J. Perinat. Med.* 16:9–21, 1988.

26 Microcirculation and Lymphatic Circulation

Patrick D. Harris and Gary L. Anderson

Objectives

After reading this chapter, you should be able to

Describe vasomotion

List the factors important in determining diffusion

Explain the meaning of *reflection coefficient* and *permeability*

Explain the Starling hypothesis in terms of water movement from the capillaries

List the normal values for arteriole, capillary, and venule hydrostatic and colloid osmotic pressures

Explain how capillary pressure is regulated by arteriole and venule pressures and resistances

Describe lymphatic drainage

Explain the problems associated with tissue edema

Various organs and issues have a microcirculation made up of small blood vessels (arterioles, capillaries, and venules) that can be seen clearly only under a microscope. Blood travels into a tissue through the muscular arterioles and then into the capillaries, which have a single layer of endothelial cells through which oxygen and nutrients diffuse to the nearby tissues. Arterioles, which range from 10 to 150 μm in diameter, regulate the distribution of blood flow to various groups of capillaries. Some of the smallest arterioles (called **metarterioles**) can serve as thoroughfare channels that bypass the capillary beds by shunting blood directly into the venules.

Because different sizes of arterioles can dilate or constrict somewhat independently of each other, flow patterns throughout the microcirculation can vary in speed and direction and from continuous to intermittent. There are cross connections between arterioles that permit flow to change directions, but most often, flow through the arterioles is rapid, continuous, and in one direction. In contrast, capillary flow can be highly variable, with long periods (up to 30 minutes) when flow ceases in small groups of adjacent capillaries.

Microvascular Function

Blood flow from the capillaries (which are 0.5 to 1 mm long) collects in venules. The smaller venules (10 to 40 μm in diameter) have an endothelial cell layer surrounded by minimal adventitia and occasional contractile cells, called **pericytes.** These venules are involved in **transvascular exchange,** which is the transport of fluid and large molecules (macromolecules) across the vascular wall. The larger venules and veins are principally collecting and storage vessels for the return of blood to the heart. The large venules have smooth muscle, and some (primarily in the skin) exhibit a regular rhythmic vasomotion of 12 to 20 contractions per minute.

The microvasculature accomplishes two major things: (1) **delivery** (called nutrient flow) of blood flow containing oxygen and other nutrients to the capillaries; and (2) **exchange** of fluid and solutes **across the capillaries** or venule walls.

Capillary Exchange Function

The number of capillaries with flow (i.e., the amount of capillary wall area available for exchange) is a prime factor in the exchange of water and electrolytes between capillaries and tissues. More metabolically active tissues have a greater number of capillaries per gram of tissue, or a high **capillary density.** For example, heart, muscle, brain, and glandular tissues have many more capillaries per gram of tissue than do bone and cartilage. A large capillary wall area allows increased exchange between the capillary blood and the interstitial space. For example, approximately 300 ml of water diffuses every minute across the capillary walls in each 100 g of skeletal muscle because skeletal muscle has a high capillary density.

A second important factor in transvascular exchange is the **lipid solubility** of the material to be exchanged. Molecules such as water, sodium, chloride, and glucose readily diffuse through holes (pores) in the capillary wall, but these molecules do not diffuse as easily through endothelial cell membranes because they are not very soluble in lipid, which is a major component of the cell membrane. Lipid-soluble substances, especially dissolved gases such as oxygen and carbon dioxide, also diffuse through capillary pores, but there is a much higher exchange of these substances through the endothelial cell membranes because they are very soluble in the lipid of the cell membrane. Thus oxygen and carbon dioxide diffuse very rapidly between the blood and the tissue interstitium, while other materials, such as water, move more slowly.

A third important factor in the transvascular exchange of material is the **free diffusion coefficient** for that material being exchanged between the blood and the interstitium. This coefficient is a measure of how fast material placed at the center of a container will disperse or move throughout water in the container. Material that consists of small molecules and molecules with very little net electric charge have very high free diffusion coefficients and disperse rapidly.

A fourth important factor in the transvascular exchange of material is the **relative concentrations of the material** in the blood and the tissue interstitium. A large difference in concentration between these two sites produces a higher rate of transvascular exchange.

All the preceding factors combine to determine transvascular exchange by a process called **diffusion.** Figure 26-1 illustrates diffusion for a material (Q) that is moving from inside the vessel to the outside (the interstitial space). The rate of material movement (quantity per second) is represented by the expression dQ/dt. The amount of capil-

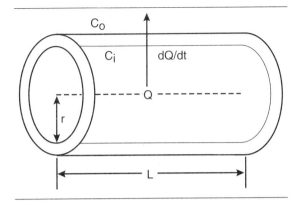

Fig. 26-1. The important components in determining diffusion of substances across the vessel wall. (See text for further explanation.)

lary wall area is defined as the product of circumference and length ($2\pi r l$) of the vessel. The difference between the concentration for Q inside the blood vessel (C_i) and for Q outside the vessel (C_o) represents the **driving force** (ΔC) for the movement of Q across the vessel wall. The ease with which Q can cross the vessel wall is called the **permeability** (P) of the vessel wall to Q. Permeability (expressed as centimeters per second) is determined by the lipid solubility and the free diffusion coefficient for Q. A high lipid solubility and a high free diffusion coefficient yield a high permeability. Overall, the rate of Q movement by diffusion is defined as:

$$\frac{dQ}{dt} = (2\pi r l)(P)(\Delta C)$$

Blood vessel permeability and thus the rate of diffusion is not the same for all blood vessels or for all tissues. For example, liver capillaries have a very high permeability even to large-molecular-weight solutes such as albumin (molecular weight 69,000). Skeletal muscle, on the other hand, has capillaries that are not permeable to albumin. The brain has capillaries that restrict the diffusion of almost all solutes, and the transport of many substances across the endothelial cells of brain capillaries is accomplished only by other processes, called **pinocytosis** and **vesicular transport.** This special barrier property of the brain microcirculation is referred to as the **blood-brain barrier.**

Generally, the venous end of a capillary is more permeable to small lipid-insoluble solutes, primarily because the venous end appears to have more pores than the arteriole end. However, even the most liberal estimates indicate that pores occupy less than 1% of the total capillary surface area. Thus lipid-insoluble materials exchange slowly, even at the venous end of the capillary, and lipid-soluble substances, which can diffuse through the cell membrane as well as through pores in the capillary wall, move readily across the vessel wall at both the arterial and venous ends. Lipid-insoluble materials, such as glucose, albumin, and small charged solutes (e.g., sodium and chloride), are slow to enter the bloodstream from many tissues. In contrast, lipid-insoluble materials, such as carbon dioxide, are essentially not stored in tissues. Other lipid-soluble materials, such as oxygen, can be depleted from the blood quickly when blood flow to tissues is severely reduced.

The arrival of lipid-soluble materials in the tissue interstitium is limited primarily by the amount of these materials that enters the capillary through blood flow and not limited by diffusion of these materials across the blood vessel wall. This means that lipid-soluble materials are **flow-limited** in their entry and exit from the tissue interstitium.

The arrival of lipid-insoluble materials, such as albumin and glucose in the tissue interstitium, is primarily **limited by the diffusion** of these materials across the blood vessel wall and not by the quantity that enters the capillary through blood flow. The interstitial level of these materials is primarily regulated through tissue control of the microvessel wall permeability to these materials. There is one major exception. Water is a lipid-insoluble material, but the interstitial water level is not regulated by tissue control of vessel permeability to water. The mechanism of water exchange is described in the next section.

Transvascular Exchange of Water

The net transfer of water from the capillaries to the interstitial space is only minimally influenced by diffusion, because the driving force for water is almost zero. Instead, the transvascular exchange of water between the blood and the interstitium occurs primarily through the **bulk flow of water.** The pumping action of the heart creates hydrostatic pressure in the blood vessels, and the difference between the hydrostatic pressure in the capillaries and that in the tissue interstitium forces water through pores in the capillary wall. The amount of bulk flow is determined by the magnitude of the hydrostatic pressure difference across the capillary wall and by the pore resistance to bulk flow.

In addition to the hydrostatic pressure, the presence of molecules other than water produce **osmotic** or **oncotic**

pressures that influence the bulk flow of water. Plasma contains dissolved protein (mainly albumin) which, because of its large size (molecular weight 69,000), cannot readily diffuse through the small capillary pores. The presence of protein in blood plasma produces a **capillary oncotic pressure,** also called **plasma colloid osmotic pressure,** which keeps water from leaving the capillaries. In contrast, proteins in the tissue interstitium exert a **tissue colloid osmotic pressure** that draws water out of the capillaries.

The net water movement across the capillary wall is determined by the sum of these four separate forces: the hydrostatic forces within and outside the capillary and the colloid osmotic forces within and outside the capillary. The **net outward force** is a hydrostatic force. The **net inward force** is a colloid osmotic force. The combined effect of these forces on transvascular water movement is described by the following equation, which was developed by Starling in 1896:

$$\dot{Q}(H_2O) = CFC\,[(CHP - THP) - \sigma(COP - TOP)]$$

where $\dot{Q}(H_2O)$ is the transvascular water flow, CFC is the capillary filtration coefficient, CHP is the capillary hydrostatic pressure, THP is the tissue (interstitial) hydrostatic pressure, σ is the reflection coefficient for the movement of proteins (colloids) across the capillary wall, COP is the capillary (colloid) osmotic pressure, and TOP is the tissue (colloid) osmotic pressure.

The **capillary filtration coefficient** is represented by the product of surface area and permeability, because it is determined by the length and diameter of the capillaries (surface area) and the number and size of the pores through which water can exit the blood vessel (water permeability). This coefficient is sometimes expressed as a **hydraulic conductivity factor.**

The **protein reflection coefficient** is the inverse of the permeability of the vessel wall to protein. A molecule in the blood that "reflects" from the capillary wall and does not cross the capillary wall into the interstitium has zero permeability and a maximum reflection coefficient of 1. A molecule that does not reflect from the capillary wall but easily passes through the capillary wall into the interstitium has a high permeability and a reflection coefficient of zero. The normal reflection coefficient for plasma proteins at the capillary wall is almost 1.0, indicating low permeability and a high reflection coefficient, since these plasma proteins are almost totally reflected at the capillary wall.

The **plasma colloid osmotic pressure** is about 20 mmHg. Approximately 12 mmHg of this is provided by the plasma proteins. Because the plasma proteins are negatively charged, they exert an electric attraction on sodium and other positively charged ions. Thus these positive ions are somewhat retained in the vascular space and add 8 mmHg to the plasma protein effect on osmotic pressure. Some protein does leak into the interstitial space, primarily through the venules. With time, this protein is returned to the circulation by the lymphatic system. This protein leakage means that the interstitial space contains a small amount of soluble protein that exerts approximately 4.5 mmHg of **tissue colloid osmotic pressure.**

Capillary hydrostatic pressure varies from tissue to tissue; it is particularly high in kidney glomerular capillaries (45 mmHg) and low in intestinal (10 mmHg) and lung (8 mmHg) capillaries. In skeletal muscle, capillary pressure is nearly 40 mmHg at the arterial end and 12 mmHg at the venous end. The interstitial fluid space has a hydrostatic pressure that may be slightly positive or even slightly negative, depending on factors such as tissue structure, muscle activity, and interstitial fluid volume. Over time, the tissue hydrostatic pressure is normally small and is assumed to be approximately zero.

The combined hydrostatic and oncotic pressures determine a net force for water movement across the capillary wall. If the net force is positive, water moves out of the capillary blood, called **filtration.** If the net force is negative, water moves into the capillary blood, called **reabsorption.** Filtration actually occurs near the arterial end of the capillary and reabsorption occurs near the venule end, because the balance of hydrostatic and osmotic forces is different at various locations along the capillary.

As shown in Fig. 26-2, the **net hydrostatic pressure** (the difference between the capillary and tissue hydrostatic pressure, shown as a solid line) decreases in a linear fashion from 40 to 12 mmHg along the length of capillary. In contrast, the **net colloid osmotic pressure** (the difference between the capillary and tissue osmotic pressures, shown as a dashed line) changes in a curvilinear fashion along the length of the capillary. At the arterial end of the capillary, where the net hydrostatic pressure exceeds the net oncotic pressure, net filtration occurs, and water leaves the capillary. This increases the concentration of protein within the capillary, since the capillary wall is not very permeable to protein. The higher protein concentration near the midpoint along the capillary length produces a higher plasma colloid osmotic pressure at that point. At the venule end of the capillary, where the net hydrostatic pressures is less than the net oncotic pressure, there is net reabsorpion of water, and water enters the capillary to restore the colloid osmotic pressure to normal.

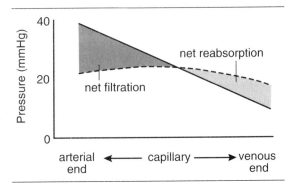

Fig. 26-2. The distribution of pressure and the sites of net filtration and net reabsorption of fluids within capillaries of skeletal muscle.

In skeletal muscle there is slightly more filtration than reabsorption throughout the whole capillary, with the excess filtration becoming lymph drainage from that tissue area. In contrast, glomerular capillaries in the kidney have filtration along most of their length, and the capillaries in the intestine and lung have reabsorption along most of their length. The primary physiologic mechanism underlying the transcapillary exchange of water in all capillaries is the **capillary hydrostatic pressure.**

Determinants of Capillary Pressure

Capillary hydrostatic pressure is controlled by the arterioles, venules, and heart, according to the following formula:

$$CHP = \frac{R_V}{R_A} P_A + P_V$$

where CHP is the pressure at the midpoint in the capillary microvasculature, R_V is the resistance of the venule microvasculature, R_A is the resistance of the arteriole microvasculature, P_A is the pressure at the beginning of the arteriole microvasculature (similar to mean arterial pressure), P_V is the pressure at the end of the venule microvasculature (similar to central venous pressure), and F is the flow through the microvasculature This is diagrammed in Fig. 26-3.

The capillary pressure will increase whenever arterial pressure increases (as in hypertension), venous pressure increases (as in congestive right-sided heart failure), venule

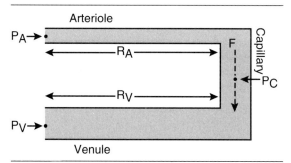

Fig. 26-3. The important factors in determining capillary pressure. (See text for further explanation.)

resistance to flow increases (as in obstructive venous clots), or arteriole resistance to flow decreases (as in arteriole vasodilation).

The most important point is that capillary pressure is much more sensitive to changes in venous pressure than to changes in arterial pressure. The ratio of venule to arteriole resistance (R_V/R_A) is normally about 0.1. Thus arterial pressure (P_A) must increase 10 mmHg to cause a 1-mmHg increase in capillary hydrostatic pressure. In contrast, a 1-mmHg increase in venous pressure will cause about a 1-mmHg increase in capillary hydrostatic pressure. This means that capillary hydrostatic pressure is somewhat protected from changes in arterial pressure but is highly influenced by even small changes in central venous pressure.

Lymphatic Drainage

In many tissues, capillary filtration predominates slightly over capillary reabsorption, and this produces **tissue lymph flow.** About 90% of the net filtration is reabsorbed directly into the blood of capillaries or postcapillary venules. The lymphatics return the remaining 10% of the filtered fluid. Of course, changes in capillary pressure vary this balance between filtration and reabsorption and thus alter lymph flow. When capillary pressure decreases significantly, as in hemorrhagic shock, reabsorption can occur along the entire capillary to stop lymph flow in any tissue. Some tissues, such as skin, have a specialized vascular smooth muscle (called precapillary sphincters) at the entrance to the capillary bed. When the precapillary sphincters in these tissues close completely, capillary pressure decreases to the venous pressure level, which triggers reabsorption along the entire capillary.

The **lymphatics** form a closed, separate fluid-flow system composed of endothelium-lined vessels that closely parallel the larger arterioles and venules. Lymph capillar-

ies originate as blind-ended sacs close to blood capillaries and are anchored by fine filaments to the surrounding tissue. The lymphatic sacs have one-way valves that open when tissue pressure exceeds lymph pressure. Lymph vessels contract to propel the lymph fluid into the larger collecting lymph vessels that eventually connect to the thoracic duct, where the lymph fluid empties into the venous circulation. The total volume of lymph fluid returned to the circulation is approximately 3 to 4 liters/day. This lymph circulation system is especially important for transporting fluid containing chylomicrons absorbed from the intestine and plasma proteins that leak from the microcirculation.

Edema

Edema is the accumulation of excess fluid in the interstitial or extravascular space. Edema is clinically detectable only when considerable excess fluid accumulates in the soft-tissue spaces. One cause of edema is **reduced concentrations of plasma protein,** which reduce colloid osmotic pressure. This oncotic pressure problem can result from liver disease, since the liver normally synthesizes many of the plasma proteins. Another cause of edema is reduced outflow of lymph brought about by blockage of lymph vessels or by increased pressure within the vena cava, which prevents lymph fluid from leaving the thoracic lymph duct to enter the circulation.

Histamine release during inflammation can substantially dilate arterioles and can increase capillary hydrostatic pressure and net filtration. Histamine release also decreases the reflection coefficient for plasma proteins so that protein leak from the vascular space into the interstitium is increased. This leakage happens in the small postcapillary venules (not in capillaries) where histamine causes large gaps (up to 1.0 μm in length and 0.4 μm in width) to form between venule endothelial cells.

Bacterial toxins and **burns** also cause increases in capillary permeability, which results in edema. Edema is particularly serious in the lungs because it widens the distance between the lung capillaries and the alveolar air sacks, and this increases the diffusion distance for the movement of oxygen from the lung air into the red blood cells.

Summary

The microcirculation consists of small arterioles, capillaries, and venules that serve as the exchange sites for water, nutrients, and the waste products from cell metabolism.

Arterioles help control the amount of blood flow to the capillaries by dilating or contracting in response to signals from the CNS or from certain endocrine organs. Arterioles also exhibit vasomotion (rhythmic contractions) that helps regulate capillary blood flow. The exchange of solutes between blood and interstitial fluid occurs when materials move across the vessel wall by diffusion, which partly depends on the permeability of the capillary and venule walls. Small lipid-soluble substances (like oxygen) diffuse rapidly, while large lipid-insoluble substances (like albumin) diffuse very slowly. The balance between hydrostatic and colloid osmotic pressures across the vessel wall regulates the exchange of water. High-pressure capillaries (such as glomerular capillaries in the kidney) filter fluid out of the capillary and low-pressure capillaries (such as intestinal villus capillaries) reabsorb fluid back into the bloodstream. Edema arises when the net filtration of fluid into the interstitium exceeds the capacity of the lymph system to return fluid to the circulation. Agents such as histamine, which increase venule wall permeability to plasma proteins (such as albumin), promote net fluid filtration and can result in edema.

Bibliography

Schmid-Schonbein, G. W., and Chien, S. The microcirculation in hypertension. In: Zanchetti, A. and Tarazi, R. C., eds. *Handbook of Hypertension: Cardiovascular Aspects.* New York: Elsevier Science Publishers, 1986. Pp. 465–489.

Staub, N. C., and Taylor, A. E. *Edema.* New York: Raven Press, 1984.

27 Regulation of the Cardiovascular System

Alvin S. Blaustein and Richard A. Walsh

Objectives

After reading this chapter, you should be able to

Outline the general organization of the systems that control circulation and explain the importance of these systems

Explain the basic properties of control systems, principally feedback and gain

Identify the major sensor, integrating, and effector components involved in reflex control

Explain the regulatory mechanisms involved in postural changes and Valsalva's maneuver

Explain and give examples of the autocrine, paracrine, and endocrine control of arterial pressure and volume

Describe the mechanisms responsible for the distribution of cardiac output during exercise

---

Effective control of cardiac output and arterial pressure requires coordinated interaction between the vasculature and heart. This is accomplished by three major regulatory systems: the nervous system, a system of peptides that affects vascular tone and is important in volume regulation, and local factors in the heart, endothelium, and organ circulations (Table 27-1). These systems adjust the volume and resistance in various circulatory compartments and modify the force and rate of cardiac contraction and relaxation.

Basic Features of Circulatory Control

Blood flow is distributed to many organs with individual requirements that may vary by as much as 25 times over the basal demand. Flow is regulated by local factors that match need to perfusion. These local perfusions form the major determinant of cardiac output through their combined effect on venous return. This local control usually involves physical factors, metabolic products, and peptides that regulate function through either **autocrine** or **paracrine mechanisms.** Autocrine control occurs when a substance elaborated by a cell regulates the function of that cell; paracrine control results when such substances regulate the function of neighboring cells. **Neural control components** consist of widely distributed receptors and neuroeffector junctions in the heart and blood vessels and integrating areas in the brain. Neuroendocrine interactions are responsible for much cardiovascular endocrine regulation, producing effects distant from their site of hormone elaboration.

The primary goal of circulatory control is to maintain an arterial pressure sufficient to provide the energy for perfusion without damaging vital organs or vessels. Regulation of pressure or volume involves a **sensor,** the control system or integrator, and **effector organs** that form a loop to maintain the variable within physiologic limits (Fig. 27-1A). Changes in arterial pressure or volume represent **inputs,** or perturbations, to the control system and initiate **outputs,** or

Table 27-1. Elements of Circulatory Control

Sensors and Integrators	Effectors
Detectors	Vascular smooth muscle
Baroreceptors	Arteries
Chemoreceptors	Arterioles
Cardiac receptors	Venules
Osmoreceptors	Veins
Ergoreceptors	
Thermoreceptors	Microcirculation
	Endothelial junctions
Endothelium	
Relaxing factors(s)	Volume regulators
Endothelins	Kidney
Prostacyclin	Hypothalamus
Prostaglandins	Neurohypophysis
	Adrenal cortex
Vasoactive peptides	
Angiotensins	Specialized tissues
Atrial natriuretic peptide	Adrenal medulla
Vasopressin	
Vasoactive intestinal	Heart
peptide	Sinoatrial or atrioven-
Opioids	tricular nodes
Substance P	His-Purkinje system
Catecholamines	Atrial muscle
Norepinephrine	Ventricular muscle
Epinephrine	
Dopamine	
Specialized substances	
Histamine	
Serotonin	
Kinins	
Autonomic nervous system	
Cortical centers	
Vasomotor areas	
Hypothalamus	
Neurohypophysis	
Sympathetic ganglia	

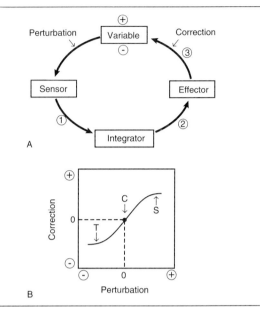

Fig. 27-1. Characteristics of a negative feedback system. (A) The basic elements of a control system (loop) regulating a variable are the *sensor,* which detects a perturbation, the *integrator,* which interprets the sensor's signal and "instructs" an *effector,* which in turn corrects the variable. Site 1 represents a potential opening in the loop commonly used to study integrating systems by controlling the signal to the integrator. A second system may also contribute a signal to the same integrator, modifying the response. Site 2 is used to isolate the effector and study the range and intensity of its responses to putative or known mediators. Here responses may be elicited in other systems as well. At site 3, the specific nature and characteristics of the effector's output can be observed, leading, for example, to the discovery of changes in effector sensitivity. The effector's output may also perturb another system, as when sympathetic renal vasoconstriction reduces renal blood flow and initiates alterations in volume regulation. (B) The behavior of a control system can be expressed as the relationship between the perturbation (i.e., the degree to which the controlled variable is disturbed) and the correction. Most often this relationship is sigmoid. The threshold (T) is the smallest disturbance that will initiate any correction; the equilibrium point (C) is the usual operating point of the system and need not be in the middle as it is on this diagram. However, it generally lies along the steepest portion of the response curve. The *saturation plateau* (S) represents the maximum output of the control system, regardless of the magnitude of the perturbation. In a system with negative feedback, if the perturbation shifts the equilibrium point upward (+), a negative correction (−) will move the system back toward C.

corrections, that restore pressure or volume to normal. When the control system suppresses the perturbation, it exhibits **negative feedback,** and this is characteristic of most control systems in the body. Thus, when systemic pressure or volume falls, adjustments increase resistance and cardiac function and mobilize or retain fluid. The relationship between the input and output characterizes the ability of the control system to maintain homeostasis and is called the **gain.** The gain is defined as the ratio of the **correction** (the degree to which adjustments compensate) to the **error** (the deviation from homeostasis remaining after adjustment). For example, if arterial pressure falls acutely from a mean of 80 mmHg to a mean of 50 mmHg and subsequent compensation returns the pressure to 70 mmHg, the gain would be the ratio of 20 (the correction of 50 to 70) to 10 (the difference between 70 and 80).

For most control systems, the relationship between the magnitudes of the output, or response, and the input is neither constant nor linear. Instead, at one extreme, the system may be relatively insensitive to the input, which must achieve a **threshold** before an output is elicited; at the other extreme, there is a **saturation zone,** whereby the output is maximum regardless of the perturbation. Between these, the system exhibits a steep relationship between input and output such that any displacement from equilibrium quickly activates a brisk corrective response (see Fig. 27-1B). For the regulation of both arterial pressure and volume, either can be affected by a number of inputs that open the simple loop between the sensor and the effector. In addition, the pressure and volume loops interact such that changes in one of the variables may initiate a correction in the other system (see Fig. 27-1A; sites 2 and 3). These systems function as open-loop, negative feedback systems. In experiments, a loop is deliberately opened, usually at the sensor (Fig. 27-1A, site 1), so that the investigator can control the perturbations detected by the receptor and determine the response of the system.

In almost all cases, **positive feedback** in biologic systems is maladaptive and results when control systems are inadequate or ill-suited to overcome perturbations. In this event, the original disturbance is not corrected but accentuated. For example, in chronic congestive heart failure, there is increased intravascular volume and frequently ventricular dysfunction. The sympathetic division of the autonomic nervous system is activated and stimulates the heart to contract more frequently and forcefully. Resistance vessels also constrict, reducing renal blood flow and initiating mechanisms responsible for salt and water retention. The result is further circulatory overload and eventually edema formation.

Overview of Circulatory Function

For the most part, the circulation constitutes a **closed system** of blood vessels whose pressure and volume are tightly regulated. The most important elements of this control system are summarized in Fig. 27-2. The fluid in the vascular system is in **dynamic equilibrium** with interstitial fluid bathing the cells, which leaves and enters the cir-

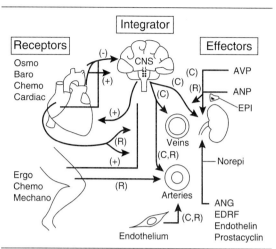

Fig. 27-2. Elements of circulatory control for systemic arterial pressure and volume. On the left are the *receptors,* which sense a variety of variables to which there are circulatory responses. Generally, their outputs are proportional to the perturbation, though for each variable there are some receptor types that are activated only at physiologic extremes. Much of the *integration* and *coordination* takes place in the central nervous system (CNS), where neural and hormonal elements are in direct contact. The response is determined by a balance of *effectors,* listed on the right, which ultimately depend on chemical mediators acting at target organs. These target organs include circulatory elements such as the heart and blood vessels, as well as volume regulators such as the kidney and neurohypophysis (AVP = arginine vasopressin; ANP = atrial natriuretic peptide; EPI = epinephrine; NE = norepinephrine; ANG II = angiotensin-II; EDRF = endothelium-derived relaxing factor; (−) = inhibitory; (+) = excitatory; C = constrict; R = relax).

culation through the capillaries and lymphatics. The heart connects the venous and arterial sides of the circulation and imparts the mechanical energy required for all fluid transfers. The amount of blood leaving the heart during each contraction is called the **stroke volume** and the amount flowing through the arterial tree per unit of time, the **cardiac output,** is equal to the **heart rate** times the stroke volume.

The cardiac output is delivered to the peripheral tissues by the **large arteries** such as the aorta. These conductance vessels have relatively little smooth muscle in their walls and are not significantly affected by vascular control. They do, however, contain mechanoreceptors (the carotid sinus and aortic arch baroreceptors) that initiate circulatory reflexes important in controlling systemic arterial pressure. The elastic tissue of the aorta and its branches converts pulsatile cardiac flow into a continuous, steady-state flow optimal for perfusion of the smaller arteries and arterioles. These smaller vessels are surrounded by layers of smooth muscle cells in direct contact with endothelium on the luminal side and are richly innervated on the adventitial side. Both the endothelium and neural connections provide an important regulatory input that determines the tension in the smooth muscle encircling the vascular lumen. This, in turn, changes the cross-sectional area of these vessels. The **effective cross-sectional area** in the muscular arteries, arterioles, and venules is the most important determinant of steady-state peripheral resistance. By the time blood reaches the microcirculation, the loss of energy across the arterial resistance has caused the mean pressure to decline from between 80 and 100 mmHg to approximately 20 mmHg near the arteriolar end of the capillaries and to between 5 and 10 mmHg in the small veins distal to the venules. The pressure drop that occurs from artery to vein is the most important source of energy for venous return. It is likely that some **tissue metabolites** such as adenosine or locally synthesized **vasoactive substances** such as prostaglandins or kinins exert their effects near the arteriolar and venulocapillary junctions. In this way, tissue factors can "feed back" to regulate local flow.

In contrast to arteries, **veins** are highly distensible and, together with the venules and venous sinuses, contain 60% to 65% of the blood volume, one-third of which is in the splanchnic veins. By regulating the functional cross-sectional area of the venous compartment, the body can control the amount of blood available for translocation from the venous to the arterial side of the circulation (the cardiac output). An increase in the venomotor tone decreases venous capacitance and redistributes blood volume, thus increasing cardiac output; a decrease in venomotor tone has the exact opposite effect. The large veins pass between major body compartments and are affected by local external pressures, such as normal positive pressures exerted by exercising skeletal muscles and the normally negative pressures in the thoracic cavity. Because venous pressures are relatively low and capacitance (volume-pressure relationship) is large, such external forces may variably facilitate or inhibit venous return, with only small changes in venous pressure adding dynamic modifiers to the more static behavior of the vascular system.

Ultimately, the amount of venous return is largely influenced by the **pressure difference** between the venules and right atrium. Because dynamic factors are superimposed on more static behavior, the heart must be able to adjust to momentary changes in venous return arising during altered respiration or posture or the more sustained increases produced by exercise. Intrinsic cardiac mechanisms, such as the **length-tension relationship** (see Chap. 23), allow the heart to vary the **stroke volume** with each beat; **neurohormonal influences,** including catecholamines, mediate changes in the cardiac rate and force of contraction that can be sustained somewhat longer.

Neural Influences on Circulatory Control

Overview of the Autonomic Nervous System

The most pervasive and well-understood integrating regulatory system controlling cardiac output and arterial pressure is the **autonomic nervous system.** This system directly influences vasomotor tone and cardiac function (heart rate and contractility) through its two major divisions, sympathetic and parasympathetic. It also affects systemic volume and peripheral resistance by modulating the release of certain **peptide hormones. Neural control** involves the assimilation of inputs from the cerebral cortex (motor, visual, labyrinthine, and olfactory) and specialized sensors (mechanoreceptors, chemoreceptors, osmoreceptors, and thermoreceptors) and their integration into several regions (hypothalamus, pons, and medullary) to conduct efferent nerve impulses to the periphery over the sympathetic and parasympathetic pathways. The dynamic balance between these two systems determines the **net response.**

Central integrating components of the autonomic nervous system are organized longitudinally so that axons from both the central and peripheral sites converge on the sympathetic and parasympathetic neurons throughout the hypothalamus, pons, and medulla. All these regions contain synapses important to cardiovascular autonomic regulation. It is not possible to organize these into discrete anatomic-functional centers because of the complexity of their interconnections; however, there are some general descriptions that apply to their organization (Fig. 27-3).

The **hypothalamus** is located on the floor of the third cerebral ventricle and connects the endocrine functions of the pituitary, the vasomotor areas in the pons and medulla, and the higher cortical centers. This organization facilitates patterned cardiovascular responses to behavioral states, such as aggression and sex, and provides one of the places where the cardiovascular and volume control systems communicate. The hypothalamus can modify thirst

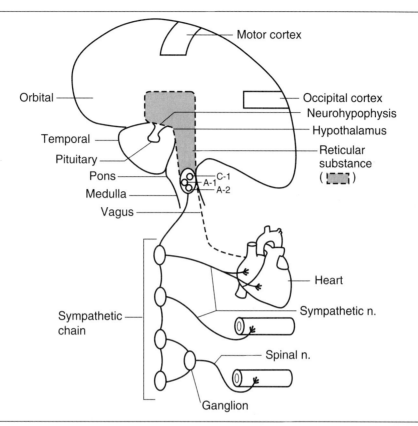

Fig. 27-3. Relationship between vasomotor centers and major target organs. Input from the cortex and peripheral or central sensors converges on the *hypothalamus* and *vasomotor areas* in the pons and medulla, where preganglionic autonomic neurons are concentrated. This figure focuses on inputs arising from other cortical centers, particularly behavioral (*temporal lobe*), motor (*motor cortex*), and visual (*occipital cortex*). There are some connections from these centers to the hypothalamus, which also has osmoreceptors and thermoreceptors. The hypothalamus has outputs to the *pituitary,* as well as to the pons and medulla. Control over the circulation by the vasomotor centers is largely the result of balancing the sympathetic (*sympathetic chain and spinal sympathetic nerves*) and parasympathetic (*vagus*) neural outflow to the heart, resistance vessels; and kidney, where renal renin release is modulated (C1 = vasoconstrictor area; A1 = vasodilator area in the lower anterolateral medulla; A2 = sensory area which integrates C1 and A1).

and modulate serum osmolarity by controlling the secretion of **arginine vasopressin** (a hormone that modifies the renal control of urine osmolarity) from the posterior pituitary. Cardiovascular responses to thermal stress are also likely to originate in the hypothalamus.

The overall organization of the **vasomotor areas** is complex, but there appear to be three functionally overlapping anatomic zones that interact extensively (see Fig. 27-3). These include a **vasoconstrictor** area in the upper anterolateral medulla, a **vasodilator** area in the lower anterolateral medulla, and a **sensory** area that integrates the vasoconstrictor and vasodilator areas and is located bilaterally in the nucleus tractus solitarii of the posterolateral medulla and lower pons. Regions that seem more devoted to modifying heart rate than vasomotor tone are located in the thalamus, posterior and posterolateral regions of the hypothalamus, and dorsal region of the medulla (the traditional cardioaccelerator region). Accelerator regions are located primarily on the right sides of both the hypothalamus and medulla.

The heart and blood vessels are under continuous stimulation by sympathetic and parasympathetic impulses. Changes reflect an altered balance between these two divisions, which generally behave in a roughly reciprocal fashion. This reciprocal behavior represents interaction among the higher centers. The effects of the two divisions are further modified at the effector organ by the distribution and density of the innervation.

Effects of Sympathetic Neural Control

Stimulation and withdrawal of sympathetic nervous activity represent the most potent factors controlling the **peripheral circulation.** Broadly categorized, fibers travel either in specific sympathetic nerves (those innervating the viscera and heart) or join the paravertebral sympathetic chain, synapsing in various secondary ganglia that give rise to spinal nerves (innervating peripheral vessels) (see Fig. 27-3). The **vascular nerves** terminate on small arteries, arterioles, venules, and veins, allowing neural modulation of resistance and vascular volume. **Cardiac nerves,** many of which descend from the stellate ganglia, innervate both the atria and ventricles.

Most often, reflex sympathetic stimulation causes vasoconstriction by releasing norepinephrine (NE) from sympathetic nerve endings and is an example of **paracrine function.** If the sympathetic nerve to a limb is stimulated, local vascular resistance increases, blood flow shows a corresponding decrease, capillary pressure falls (absorbing local interstitial fluid), and blood volume is displaced from the limb. In a metabolically active organ, local influences may override the autonomic ones. The inhibition of sympathetic outflow allows vessels to dilate and respond to local humoral and myogenic stimuli.

Although most reflex sympathetic stimulation produces vascular constriction, a subset of fibers release acetylcholine (ACh) rather than NE. These fibers arise in the motor cortex of the cerebrum and then pass through the hypothalamus and medulla before joining other sympathetic nerves. For the most part, these neurons innervate the vasculature of skeletal muscle and provoke an **anticipatory increase** in local blood flow prior to exercise. Another secondary outcome of the sympathetic stimulation of these fibers is the release of epinephrine from the adrenal medullae. Unlike NE, epinephrine stimulates both alpha and beta receptors. In low quantities, epinephrine causes vasodilation and cardiac stimulation; at higher concentrations, vasoconstriction predominates.

Direct cardiac effects of reflex sympathetic stimulation include increased heart rate, more forceful and rapid cardiac ejection, and faster relaxation and filling. Its effect on the pacemakers and conduction tissue initiate the **increased heart rate.** Beta-adrenergic stimulation of the sinoatrial node causes the pacemaker cells to have faster intrinsic rates of depolarization. The result is an action potential with increased amplitude, faster upstroke, and shorter duration. **Greater contractility** is the consequence of higher cytosolic calcium concentration (enhanced release from the sarcoplasmic reticulum) and enhanced calcium responsiveness of the contractile proteins. Finally, **faster relaxation** is due to enhanced phosphorylation of both troponin I and phospholamban.

Reflex sympathetic stimulation is important in the increase in cardiac output necessary during exercise or other forms of stress. These cardiac stimulating effects of the sympathetic nervous system increase the metabolic requirements of heart muscle, and this forms the basis for using graded exercise stress to evaluate cardiac reserve in disease states. Sympathetically mediated actions are largely responsible for maintaining systemic arterial pressure and vital organ perfusion during hypovolemic states and cardiac dysfunction.

Effects of Parasympathetic Neural Control

The parasympathetic nervous system has a **cranial division,** supplying the blood vessels of the head and viscera, and a **sacral division,** with fibers innervating the vessels of the genitalia, bladder, and large intestine. Because these fibers supply only a small percentage of the resistance vessels, ordinarily the parasympathetic component of the autonomic nervous system has little involvement in the regulation of arterial pressure. It does, however, play an important role in modulating the cardiac rate. Fibers traveling in the **vagus nerve** innervate the sinoatrial and atrioventricular nodes as well as the atrial musculature. Changes in heart rate arise from the shift to P cells, with slower intrinsic rates of depolarization and changes in membrane depolarization secondary to ACh stimulation. When the vagus nerve is stimulated, heart rate and the force of atrial contraction both decline. Because of effects on atrioventricular conduction, the coordination of atria and ventricles is often disrupted. This combination of effects may lower cardiac output by 40% to 50%. The effects of vagal stimulation are evident following external massage of the carotid sinus, which stimulates the glossopharyngeal afferent limb of the baroreceptor reflex and modifies efferent parasympathetic outflow. This slows cardiac rate and atrioventricular conduction.

Other Neurovascular Transmitters

Although most neurovascular communications are transmitted by NE or ACh, other neurotransmitters are involved in cardiovascular reflexes. **Substance P** is a neurotransmitter peptide that is widely distributed in the brain and peripheral nervous system. Its cardiovascular regulatory potential is suggested by its relatively high concentration in the vasomotor areas (particularly the nucleus tractus solitarii and dorsal motor nucleus of the vagus), where it may interact with the opioid peptide system. In addition, it is present in the nerves innervating virtually every vascular bed, where its release triggers vasodilation through a specific receptor. **Opioids** such as the enkephalins and endorphins are also widely distributed in the brain and spinal cord. While infusion of these neurotransmitters produces transient vasodilation, they are thought to cooperate with other neurotransmitters operating in the same synaptic cleft to modulate the responses. They appear to be most involved in the behavioral responses to pain and exercise. **Vasoactive intestinal polypeptide** is found in the brain (in descending order of concentration: cerebral, cerebellar, basilar vertebral, and spinal arteries), gut, salivary glands, uterus, and skeletal muscle. It is a potent vasodilator and also increases heart rate above that obtained with sympathetic stimulation only.

Baroreceptors and Control of Arterial Pressure

A complex set of afferent inputs to the central cardiovascular areas arises from both within and without the brain. Among these are the peripheral sensors such as the baroreceptors, chemoreceptors, and cardiac mechanoreceptors. The **baroreceptor system** consists principally of the carotid sinus and aortic arch mechanoreceptors, central vasomotor integrating areas, and autonomic efferents and exerts short-term control over arterial pressure. In vivo, the baroreceptor system operates as an open loop, with negative feedback and its components buffering potentially large changes in arterial pressure (e.g., those produced by changes in posture). Under resting conditions, the system is static; however, it can be modified by periodic or transient perturbations, such as respiration or exercise, and therefore it also has dynamic characteristics. The neural outflow from the vasomotor centers modulates the smooth muscle tone of resistance vessels, the force of myocardial contraction, and the heart rate, which buffer changes in systemic arterial pressure or blood volume. The sympathetic efferent flow is not uniformly distributed to all resistance beds but exhibits a characteristic pattern.

The **carotid sinus** baroreceptor is located at the bifurcation of the common carotid artery. The receptors are in the adventitia of the sinus wall and are innervated by a branch of the glossopharyngeal nerve, which carries afferent traffic to the nucleus tractus solitarii in the medullary area of the brainstem. **Strain energy density** (the force required to produce an incremental stretch) in the wall of the sinus is linearly related to pressure over a wide range of values from 50 to 250 mmHg. Over much of this range, the physical distortion produced by an increase in pressure also has a direct linear relationship with afferent nerve activity. The rate of afferent nerve discharge is largely influenced by the mean arterial pressure and to a lesser extent by pulse pressure (Fig. 27-4). Therefore, for any given mean pressure, a narrower pulse pressure decreases afferent activity. Because the rate of nerve discharge is closely related to the stretch associated with dimensional changes in the sinus wall, physiologic (catecholamines) and pathologic (hypertension or atherosclerosis) factors that modify the distensibility of the carotid sinus also change the relationship between intraluminal pressure and stretch.

The **aortic arch** baroreflex system is similar to that of the carotid sinus. Nerve endings are concentrated at the junction between the adventitia and media and serve as stretch receptors with their afferent impulses traveling through both myelinated and unmyelinated fibers in the vagus nerve. The threshold of pressure stimulation for aortic receptors is about 90 mmHg, compared with 60 mmHg for the carotid receptors (Fig. 27-5). Therefore, the carotid sinus is still important in modulating blood pressure and heart rate at lower pressures, a feature especially important for maintaining cerebral perfusion in an upright posture. This difference in characteristics of the two systems allows the aortic reflex to buffer the carotid reflex. If the afferent nerves from the aortic arch receptors are transected (i.e., the loop is opened at a sensor) and pressure in the vascularly isolated carotid sinus is lowered from 100 to 50 mmHg, systemic arterial pressure rises from 85 to 150 mmHg. This demonstrates the unopposed action of the carotid sinus reflex at lower pressures. With the aortic nerves intact, arterial pressure rises only to 120 mmHg, illustrating the buffering action of the aortic on the carotid sinus reflex.

As a demonstration of this, if blood pressure increases, the carotid and aortic receptors are activated by the deformation caused by changes in local wall stress. This produces an increase in afferent impulses traveling through the vagus and glossopharyngeal nerves, respectively.

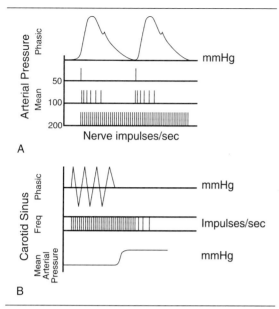

Fig. 27-4. Baroreceptor nerve responses to alterations in mean and phasic pressures. (A) The discharge rate of the baroreceptor nerve increases as mean arterial pressure increases. These discharges generally inhibit central vasomotor centers. At lower pressures, the effects of phasic (pulsatile) variations in arterial pressure are superimposed on the effects of mean pressure, but, at higher systemic pressures, this variation is no longer evident, indicating receptor saturation. (B) The difference between baroreceptor nerve responses to pulsatile and constant pressure stimuli. When the input is phasic, the discharge rate in the nerve remains higher than that when the input is constant, indicating that receptors adapt under these conditions. Thus, phasic stimuli are more effective in maintaining baroreceptor function than are continuous ones. (Modified from: Berne, R. M., and Levy, M. N., eds. *Physiology,* 2nd ed. St. Louis: C. V. Mosby, 1988. Pp. 519–520.)

These impulses reach synapses in the central vasomotor centers of the pons and medulla, inhibiting sympathetic efferent nerve activity to heart and resistance vessels and veins (particularly splanchnic). Parasympathetic outflow to the heart then increases. The net effects are cardiac slowing and a fall in blood pressure, due both to arterial and venous dilation and to the decreased force of cardiac contraction, which correct the increase in blood pressure.

Chemoreceptors

Arterial chemoreceptors are located in the carotid arteries and aortic arch in the same regions as baroreceptors. They

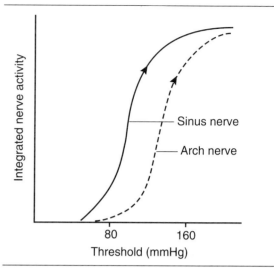

Fig. 27-5. Difference in carotid sinus and aortic arch baroreceptor responses. As pressure sensed by the receptors is increased from 50 to 200 mmHg, the afferent nerve discharges detected from the carotid sinus and aortic arch exhibit differences. The carotid baroreceptor has an almost immediate threshold response, which is steepest up to pressures of 160 mmHg, where there is saturation. In contrast, the threshold of the aortic baroreceptor is between 80 and 90 mmHg, and saturation occurs at 200 mmHg. This allows the two receptor systems to interact, particularly at lower pressures.

are formed by a varying number of specialized type I and type II cells. The **type I cells** form synapses with nerve fibers, and a group of four to six cells is encircled by a type II cell. This array is close to an extensive capillary network. The type I cells are excitable and act as receptors that release neurotransmitters (e.g., NE or substance P) which activate the afferent nerves. **Type II cells** are inexcitable, and though essential for sensor function, their function is not well understood. Hypoxia or decreased pH slows mitochondrial electron transport, and this changes the ratio of ADP to ATP. This leads to mitochondrial calcium release, a rise in the cytosolic calcium level, and a decrease in the frequency of action potential formation in type I cells.

The **carotid bodies** are innervated by a branch of the glossopharyngeal nerve, and the **aortic bodies** are supplied by a branch of the vagus. The fibers from each may be either myelinated or unmyelinated. Nerve discharges are stimulated by decreases in pH or the oxygen tension (Po_2) or by increases in the carbon dioxide tension (Pco_2)

and temperature. Po_2 and Pco_2 interact during afferent nerve activity. For any given arterial Po_2, the number of discharges increases at higher Pco_2; conversely, for any given Pco_2, the number of impulses increases with lower Po_2. No entirely satisfactory overview of the role of chemoreceptors in cardiovascular regulation has been formulated, unlike the prominent role that has been identified for them in ventilatory regulation.

Systemic hypoxia produces profound cardiovascular adjustments, mediated by peripheral chemoreceptors, the direct effects of hypoxia on the CNS, and the effects of increased ventilation on lung inflation and Pco_2. The carotid and aortic body chemoreflexes are responsible for the reflex systemic arterial hypertension, which is mediated by sympathetic outflow from the vasomotor areas. Increases in heart rate, contractility, and cardiac output are most likely due to the combined effects of CNS hypoxia and increased ventilation, since chemoreceptor denervation does not abolish the cardiac responses, while lung denervation largely prevents or reverses them.

Cardiac Mechanoreceptors

Mechanoreceptors in the heart possess both vagal and sympathetic afferents. Sensors on the atria and ventricles receive vagal afferents; sensors on the pulmonary veins and coronary vessels receive sympathetic afferents.

Vagal Afferents
Atrial A and B receptors are distinguished by their location at the **venoatrial junctions,** as well as by their function. Type A receptors seem to react primarily to heart rate, but they adapt (gradually decrease their rate of discharge after an initial increase) to long-term changes in atrial volume. Type B receptors respond to short-term changes in atrial volume, increasing discharges during atrial distension. **C fibers** arise from receptors scattered throughout the atria. These discharge with a low frequency and respond with increased discharge to increases in atrial pressure. The A and B receptors are thought to mediate the increase in heart rate associated with atrial distention, known as the **Bainbridge reflex.** In contrast, activation of the **atrial C fibers** is generally vasodepressor in nature, with cardiac slowing and peripheral vasodilation.

Ventricular mechanoreceptors also have afferents with myelinated and unmyelinated fibers. Discharge in the myelinated fibers decreases periodically with inspiration and increases with a rise in ventricular pressure. Ventricular C fibers are located primarily in the **epicardium** and discharge more rapidly in response to increases in both

systolic and diastolic pressure. They exhibit a sharp threshold, discharging only at high systolic pressures, but progressively increase as diastolic pressures rise from 5 to 20 mmHg. Ventricular distension can produce powerful depressor reflexes during both bradycardia and hypotension, called the **Bezold-Jarisch reflex.** C fibers appear to be more important than myelinated ones in conducting the relevant afferent nerve traffic. The central connections for this reflex are in the nucleus tractus solitarii, which has both sympathetic and parasympathetic synapses. Activation of cardiac C fibers also induces marked relaxation of the stomach by means of vagal noncholinergic fibers and is part of a more generalized activation of the vomiting reflex.

Sympathetic Afferents
The sympathetic afferents are less well understood than the vagal afferents. **Atrial fibers** appear to increase activity with rises in atrial pressure and volume and can respond to phasic changes in atrial volume. **Ventricular fibers** may be either myelinated or unmyelinated and show modest increases in discharge rate when end-diastolic pressure (unmyelinated) or ventricular systole (myelinated) is elevated. Receptors on the coronary vessels discharge more frequently as blood flow or intracoronary pressures fall. The increased discharge rate during interrupted coronary flow may be important during myocardial ischemia. Recently, a class of receptors has been identified that are activated by low pressures in the atria and ventricle.

The importance of **cardiac mechanoreceptors** in the short-term regulation of arterial pressure is unknown, although they are much less involved than the baroreceptors. There is evidence that these atrial and ventricular receptors may affect the release of vasopressin and the renal release of renin by modifying selected efferent sympathetic outflow.

Circulatory Control During Postural Changes

The circulatory changes associated with standing up from a recumbent position illustrate how rapid control by neural mechanisms is integrated. Upon standing, **gravity** initially displaces blood from the thorax and splanchnic beds to the lower extremities and buttocks within a few heartbeats. The **labyrinthine organs** are also stimulated due to the change in position. The magnitude of the displaced blood helps to determine the ultimate response. There is a reduction in cardiac volumes, with atrial pressures falling from 2 or 3 mmHg to −8 to −10 mmHg, and a resulting decline in cardiac filling. **Stroke volume** and **cardiac output** fall rapidly. The reduction in central volume stimulates atrial and ventricular receptors, increasing traffic through the sympathetic afferents and decreasing traffic through the vagal afferents. In addition, the **stretch** on the carotid sinus and aortic arch baroreceptors decreases, reducing the frequency of afferent discharge in the glossopharyngeal and vagus nerves. The result is both disinhibition and direct stimulation of vasoconstrictor and cardiac accelerator regions of the vasomotor areas.

Sympathetic outflow from the nucleus tractus solitarii and vasoconstrictor regions increases to offset the potential decrease in systemic arterial pressure produced by upright posture. The first detectable changes are venous and arterial vasoconstriction that leads to decreased venous caliber and capacitance, particularly in the splanchnic veins, which are nearly maximally constricted in the upright position, and increased peripheral resistance; arterial pressure also increases. Shortly thereafter, heart rate rises, and contractility is enhanced, but despite this, stroke vol-

ume and cardiac output are reduced predominantly by the effects on preload (decreased cardiac volumes) that result from venous pooling.

Circulatory Changes During Valsalva's Maneuver

Valsalva's maneuver, which involves straining to expire against a closed glottis, is often performed during defecation and parturition. Discussing it is a useful way to evaluate the integrated autonomic control of the circulation and demonstrates how neural and intrinsic cardiac control systems compensate for a physical stress (Fig. 27-6). At the onset of the maneuver, intrathoracic pressure increases abruptly, compressing the great vessels, raising the aortic pressure, and displacing blood volume out of the chest (**phase I**). In **phase II,** the increased intrathoracic pressure narrows veins at the thoracic inlet and obstructs systemic venous return. Intracardiac volumes decrease by 25% to 30%, reducing cardiac preload and hence stroke volume;

Fig. 27-6. Hemodynamic responses to Valsalva's manuever. (A) The changes in systemic arterial pressure. (B) The heart rate responses. (C) Representative left ventricular minor axis dimensions during diastole and systole, as measured by reflected ultrasound. During the strain phase (II), arterial pressures and pulse pressures fall, heart rate increases, and cardiac volumes decline. After release of the strain (IV), there is a brief overshoot in arterial pressure which reflects the persistent effects of circulatory adjustments made during phase II (phase I = onset of maneuver; phase III = release of strain).

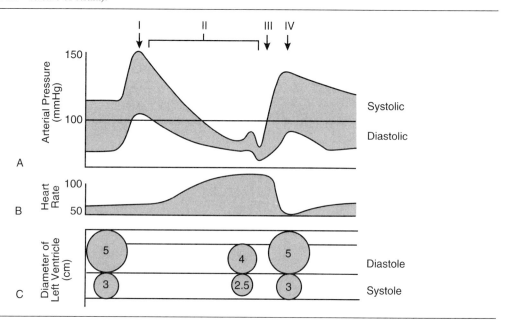

arterial pressure falls and pulse pressure narrows. Low-pressure cardiac receptors are stimulated, and this leads to sympathetic afferent stimulation of vasoconstrictor regions. Baroreceptor impulses originating from the carotid sinus and aortic arch decrease because of lowered mean aortic pressure and pulse pressure. The resulting sympathetic outflow increases heart rate and contractility and constricts peripheral arteries (increasing resistance) and veins (increasing venous pressure outside the chest). As a result, cardiac volume, stroke volume, cardiac output, and arterial pressure stabilize and may even increase. At the moment the strain is released **(phase III),** intrathoracic pressure falls, relieving constraining effects on the thoracic vena cava, heart, and aorta. Immediately, there is a transient fall in systemic pressure. The sympathetically mediated vascular responses initiated and sustained during straining then produce a large venous pressure gradient between the extrathoracic capacitance vessels and the underfilled low-pressure right atrium, driving an explosive venous return. Within a few seconds, intracardiac volumes return to premaneuver levels. This recruitment of the cardiac length-tension mechanisms coupled with sympathetic cardiac support increases stroke volume and translocates the increased venous return into the constricted arterial circulation. The sudden transfer of this additional volume raises arterial and pulse pressures above premaneuver levels **(phase IV).** This increases wall stress in the heart and baroreceptor regions. Afferent nerve traffic from these sensors increases, inhibiting central outflow and leading to recovery.

Local Influences and Circulatory Control

Vascular Smooth Muscle

Vascular smooth muscle can constrict tonically and change its tension in response to both **centrally dispatched signals** and **local factors.** These characteristics permit flexible and precise circulatory control.

Vasodilator Mechanisms

Atrial natriuretic peptide (ANP) is a recently discovered endocrine hormone synthesized in the heart and found predominantly in granules in the atrial appendage. **Release of ANP** is promoted by atrial stretch, beta-adrenergic stimulation, and increased heart rate.

ANP is a direct-acting vasodilator that antagonizes the vasoconstrictor **angiotensin-II** but cannot overcome high doses of NE. ANP stimulates membrane-bound cyclic guanosine-3′,5′-monophosphate (cGMP) as a second messenger to induce its vasodilating effects. In vivo, ANP promotes arterial and venous dilation. When infused systemically, ANP reliably reduces arterial pressure almost immediately in a dose-dependent manner. Because the drug also dilates veins, cardiac output falls and peripheral resistance is therefore unchanged. Renin secretion is suppressed and plasma levels decline, perhaps due to the accelerated sodium delivery to the macula densa. ANP also blocks the effects of angiotensin-II on aldosterone release, as well as lowering angiotensin levels. About 1 hour after the start of the infusion, arterial pressure returns to preinfusion levels, reflecting the influence of other compensatory mechanisms. These effects are most important as part of the short-term regulation of **volume** and **pressure.** Levels of ANP are elevated during heart failure; however, its effects are offset by potent vasoconstrictor mechanisms and stimuli for sodium retention.

The **kinins** are a group of polypeptide vasodilators. As with other vasoactive peptides, they are synthesized and circulate in the form of larger, inactive molecules in the blood and tissue fluid. Bioconversion to active molecules occurs locally, where concentrations may be a good deal higher than systemic levels. The best understood of these is **bradykinin,** which is formed from **kallikrein.** Bradykinin has only local effects on the circulation, because it is quickly inactivated by **carboxypeptidases** or converting enzyme. Bradykinin is an important mediator of the inflammatory response influencing endothelial permeability and plays a regulatory role in the control of local circulations in the skin, kidney, and salivary glands. **Histamine, serotonin,** and **prostaglandins** have highly specific functions but no known systemic role in circulatory control.

The **endothelium** is also an important modulator of smooth muscle activity. Its role in mediating smooth muscle relaxation was first recognized when the vasodilator response to ACh observed in larger arteries was abolished by denuding the endothelium (Fig. 27-7). The search for an **endothelium-derived relaxing factor** (EDRF) that diffused into smooth muscle resulted in the identification of **nitric oxide,** generated from L-arginine by nitric oxide synthase. This represented the first, but not necessarily only, EDRF. Nitric oxide has a half-life of only a few seconds and is quickly inactivated by the superoxide anion. It exerts paracrine control on vasodilation by stimulating the accumulation of cGMP, a breakdown product of guanosine triphosphate.

In the microcirculation, EDRF may mediate the vasodi-

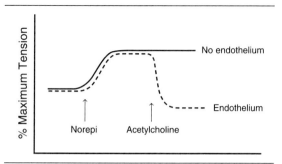

Fig. 27-7. Endothelium-dependent relaxation of vascular smooth muscle. This is a typical example of the effects of endothelial-derived relaxing factor. Two strips or rings of vascular smooth muscle are bathed in a nutrient buffer, one with the endothelium intact and the other with the endothelium gently abraded or digested. The vessel is then preconstricted, in this example with norepinephrine (NOREPI), and then exposed to the test agent. If tension falls in the vessel with intact endothelium but not in the vessel without endothelium, this indicates endothelial-induced relaxation. This is an example of paracrine function which is important in the local control of the circulation. Acetylcholine is the standard against which other substances are compared.

lation associated with **inflammation** and **trauma,** which are local hyperemic responses. EDRF is also released in normal vessels in response to **platelet aggregation** and **shear stress** exerted by flowing blood. When diseases such as atherosclerosis disrupt the endothelium, they may interfere with the synthesis of EDRF or the ability to vasodilate in response to a number of stimuli. Recently, the excessive vasodilation associated with **bacteremic shock** has been linked to uncontrolled production of nitric oxide. **Prostacyclin** is a vasodilator derived from the family of prostaglandins synthesized in endothelial cells. It also inhibits platelet aggregation and works synergistically with EDRF. Their combined effects may wash away platelet plugs formed during physiologic vascular trauma. Because it is not stored and has a short half-life, prostacyclin's effects are only local and promote smooth muscle relaxation.

Vasoconstrictors

The endothelium is also the source of substances that initiate smooth muscle contraction, including **thromboxane A$_2$, prostaglandin H$_2$,** and the **superoxide anion,** all of which are short acting. A group of active peptides, **endothelins,** has recently been isolated. They are formed by enzymatic cleavage from a larger, inactive precursor and

constrict both arterial and venous smooth muscle in all vascular beds, acting through a unique receptor in the media. Endothelins open a voltage-sensitive Ca^{2+} channel that activates inositol-tris-phosphate and diacylglycerol. This further increases intracellular Ca^{2+} concentrations. Pretreatment with Ca^{2+}-channel blockers prevents the vasoconstrictor actions of endothelin, demonstrating its dependence on the extracellular Ca^{2+} level. The constriction produced by endothelin follows a brief vasodilation and is slow in onset and sustained. It is reversed by stimulation of cAMP or by glyceryl trinitrate, which increases cGMP levels much like EDRF does.

Endothelin causes arterial constriction, and thus arterial resistance is augmented. Its venoconstrictor actions decrease capacitance and increase cardiac preload. It is also a potent antinatriuretic. However, its effects on arterial resistance generally predominate, and cardiac output falls during endothelin infusions. In the heart, endothelin has an **inotropic effect,** at least on atrial muscle, and stimulates the secretion of ANP. The role of endothelin in cardiovascular control is currently unknown, as are details about the regulation of its synthesis and release. It is known to be released in response to raised thrombin levels, suggesting that it may be important in the evolution of responses to hemorrhage. Its slow secretion and onset of action, as well as its sustained action, are not consistent with the properties needed for rapid circulatory regulation. Recently, it has been noted to possess the characteristics that mitogen exhibits in smooth muscle cells, fibroblasts, and mesangial cells, suggesting a role in systemic arterial hypertension.

Endothelial cells, as well as cardiac and renal cells, contain intrinsic **renin-angiotensin systems. Angiotensin-II** is a powerful vasoconstrictor peptide. It is formed by the action of the enzyme renin on its precursor, angiotensinogen. The product, angiotensin-I, is not vasoactive but is cleaved to angiotensin-II by a converting enzyme, for which potent pharmacologic inhibitors have been synthesized. Angiotensin-II is also a **salt-retaining hormone** when released into the circulation, stimulating the synthesis and release of aldosterone. It also has cardiac **inotropic properties.** In these capacities, it functions as an endocrine hormone. Its release is modulated by the sympathetic division of the autonomic nervous system, representing another interaction of the pressure and volume control systems. Angiotensin appears to be involved chiefly in the intermediate- and long-term regulation of **systemic pressure** and **volume.** Local angiotensin systems may play a role in the regulation of **organ perfusion** and serve as a **growth factor** for myocytes and fibroblasts. These regulatory functions are examples of **autocrine reg-**

ulation. Regulation of growth may be critical to cardiovascular adaptation in hypertension.

Arginine vasopressin (AVP) and its precursor **neurophysin** are synthesized in the magnicellular neurons of the supraoptic, paraventricular, and suprachiasmatic nuclei of the hypothalamus. Neurosecretory granules are transported axonally to the neurohypophysis, where they are released from nerve endings into the systemic circulation. AVP is also a neurotransmitter found in central regions involved in circulatory control, including the nucleus tractus solitarii and dorsal motor nucleus of the vagus. AVP also projects to the cerebral cortex and spinal cord. Thus AVP exhibits features of both **paracrine** and **endocrine control.**

AVP has **two major circulatory roles:** (1) to maintain arterial pressure in the presence of reduced blood volume and (2) to regulate osmolality in the face of an increased plasma solute concentration. Its actions on arterial pressure reflect its interaction with vasoconstrictor V_1 receptors, and its central action augments the baroreceptor reflex by modifying sympathetic outflow and accentuating the bradycardia. In contrast to its constricting effects in the periphery, AVP induces vasodilation in cerebral vessels, and this depends on EDRF. AVP's role in maintaining volume is mediated through arterial and atrial receptors, which inhibit systemic AVP secretion when activated.

Summary

The circulation maintains local environmental conditions essential for cellular function. Control of the circulation is important for the integration of the local blood flow requirements largely related to metabolic demands. Control of the systemic arterial pressure provides the energy for perfusion of all tissues. Three important systems interact to exert and coordinate control. The first is the autonomic nervous system, consisting of peripheral receptors, central integrating vasomotor centers, and neuroeffector junctions on the heart and blood vessels. The second comprises the local regulators in the tissues. These include intrinsic cardiac mechanisms such as the length-tension relationship, which permit the heart to adjust to momentary changes in venous return, and paracrine regulation of local circulations. The third system consists of the endocrine regulators of systemic vascular volume. These systems overlap (e.g., in the hypothalamus) and interact extensively to permit acute and long-term regulation of arterial pressure and blood volume. At the same time, they preserve the autonomy of organ and tissue blood flow, which is the cornerstone of circulatory flexibility and adaptation. The control systems involved in circulatory regulation exhibit negative feedback, responding with adjustments that oppose the perturbations from equilibrium values.

Bibliography

Laragh, J. H., and Atlas, S. Atrial natriuretic hormone: a regulator of blood pressure and volume homeostasis. *Kidney Int.* 34(Suppl. 25); S64–71, 1988.

Shepherd, J. T. Reflex control of arterial pressure. *Cardiovasc. Res.* 16:357–383, 1982.

Shepherd, J. T., and Abboud, F. M., eds. *Handbook of Physiology,* Vol. III: *The Peripheral Circulation,* Part 2: *Cardiovascular Reflexes and Circulatory Integration.* New York: Oxford University Press, 1984.

Vane, J. R., Anggard, E. E., and Gotting, R. M. Regulatory Functions of vascular endothelium. *N. Engl. J. Med.* 323:27–36, 1990.

Vanhoutte, P. M. Endothelium-derived relaxing and contracting factors. *Adv. Nephrol.* 19:3–16, 1990.

Yanagisawa, M., and Masaki, T. Endothelin: A novel endothelium-derived peptide. *Pharmacology* 38:1877–1883, 1989.

Part IV Questions: Cardiovascular Physiology

1. Major functions of the pericardium include
   A. preventing overdistention of the ventricles.
   B. tethering the heart within the chest cavity.
   C. protecting the heart from inflammation and infection from the lungs.
   D. all of the above.
2. During phase 2 of the ventricular AP, the inward current is carried by the
   A. Na^+ current.
   B. transient outward K^+ current.
   C. Ca^{2+} current.
   D. "funny" current.
3. The AV conduction time is reflected in the
   A. PR interval.
   B. PR segment.
   C. QRS duration.
   D. QT interval.
   E. T-wave duration.
4. A drug with a positive inotropic effect (increased inotropic state) will
   A. lower the blood pressure.
   B. shift the force-velocity relationship upward, increasing P_o and V_{max}.
   C. shift the length-tension relationship downward and to the right.
   D. increase the peak isometric tension but not change dT/dt.
5. The Frank-Starling relationship
   A. relates the influence of changing preload on measures of ventricular performance.
   B. is an inverse hyperbolic curve, relating afterload (wall stress) and cardiac output.
   C. is determined during isovolumetric systole.
   D. is the principal force for ventricular filling.
6. When oxygen use by the myocardium increases, oxygen delivery is augmented to match this by
   A. increased coronary perfusion pressure.

B. a shift in the oxygen-hemoglobin dissociation curve so that more oxygen is released per gram of hemoglobin.
   C. increased extraction of oxygen from the coronary artery blood.
   D. increased coronary artery blood flow.
   E. increased oxygen uptake by the lungs.
7. The most important mechanism by which coronary blood flow is regulated to match myocardial oxygen requirements is
   A. adenosine-mediated vasodilation.
   B. neurogenic reflex control of coronary artery tone.
   C. autonomic reflex control of the heart rate and other determinants of myocardial work.
   D. alterations in the coronary perfusion pressure.
   E. augmentation of the intramyocardial blood flow during diastole by enhanced myocardial relaxation.
8. An agent that increases vascular compliance will
   A. decrease the volume of blood in the arteries.
   B. decrease the volume of blood in the veins.
   C. increase arterial blood pressure.
   D. increase right atrial pressure.
   E. decrease venous return.
9. Edema will most likely result from each of the following conditions *except*
   A. high venous pressure.
   B. lymphatic obstruction.
   C. low plasma protein concentration.
   D. increased mean arterial pressure.
   E. increased capillary hydrostatic pressure.
10. Local regulatory mechanisms are most important in the circulatory control in which scenario?
    A. Change in posture
    B. Systemic hypoxia
    C. Moderate exercise
    D. Valsalva's maneuver
    E. Weightless environment

V Hemostasis and Blood Coagulation

Part Editor
Robert F. Highsmith

28 Platelet Function and Blood Coagulation

Robert F. Highsmith

Objectives

After reading this chapter, you should be able to

Define *hemostasis* and describe conceptually where the hemostatic mechanism is operative in relation to the conditions of thrombosis and hemorrhage

Explain why the hemostatic mechanism is a "potential" one, and describe the adequate stimuli necessary to elicit the response

Illustrate how the hemostatic mechanism may be stimulated by abnormal processes leading to thrombosis

Explain why an inability of the mechanism to respond to a stimulus such as vascular injury may result in fatal hemorrhaging

List the basic components of the normal hemostatic response to vessel injury

Describe the mechanisms by which platelets interact with an injured vessel wall to form a temporary hemostatic plug

Delineate those factors which necessitate the transformation of the temporary hemostatic plug to a definitive mass of fibrin

Describe the production of coagulation factors and the role of vitamin K in coagulation factor synthesis

Describe the major enzymatic pathways of blood coagulation and the mechanisms by which they are initiated

Contrast the kinetics of thrombin evolution via the extrinsic pathway versus the intrinsic pathway

Explain the necessity of having both pathways of coagulation operative for normal coagulation

List the diverse effects of thrombin and explain its pivotal role in the overall hemostatic response to vessel injury

---

All organs and tissues of the body depend on a fluid medium (blood) for oxygen delivery, exchange of gases and nutrients, biologic waste removal, and hormonal communication. This design, in turn, demands the presence of a very competent mechanism to ensure that the circulating blood stays within the vascular compartment (no bleeding) and remains fluid at all times (no clotting). Injury to vessels transporting blood under considerable pressure can lead to life-threatening bleeding, or **hemorrhage.** Fortunately, an elaborate host defense mechanism is normally operative that in most cases, depending on the site and severity of the trauma, can completely halt the extravasation of blood from the vascular compartment. This mechanism, termed **hemostasis,** represents the concert of events responsible for the rapid repair of any break in the vascular endothelium without compromising the fluidity of the blood. These events greatly assist in maintaining the constancy of the internal environment and thus represent a classic example of a homeostatic control system.

The hemostatic mechanism is a **potential system** designed to reseal the endothelial surface in response to injury. However, this potential for rapid localized hemostasis within a fluid medium is not without risk, for essentially the same processes responsible for the arrest of bleeding, if abnormal, may result in hemorrhage or intravascular clotting **(thrombosis).** Since it is a potential system, the hemostatic mechanism must be triggered. If the mechanism fails to respond to the stimulus, or if one or more of its components are not functional, a hemorrhagic condition may develop. Conversely, if the hemostatic mechanism triggers spontaneously or is not regulated properly, a thrombotic condition may develop. Fortunately, a number of checks and balances exist that collectively permit the timely arrest of bleeding after injury without compromising blood fluidity.

Overview and Components of Hemostasis

A competent hemostatic mechanism involves the proper triggering and interplay of (1) blood vessel constriction, (2) platelet aggregation and fusion, (3) activation of blood coagulation factors, and (4) regulation and limitation of coagulation. In response to vessel injury, blood vessels rapidly constrict and platelets aggregate to form a **temporary hemostatic plug.** These events, involving smooth muscle shortening in the vessel wall and alterations in platelet biochemistry, comprise the **primary hemostatic response.** Steps 3 and 4, encompassing the **secondary phase of hemostasis,** are also activated on vessel injury but are temporally sequenced so as to permit localized stoppage of bleeding. Thus activation of coagulation leads to the deposition of a blood clot (insoluble **fibrin**) that serves to anchor the hemostatic plug and provide for definitive hemostasis. In addition, numerous other regulatory factors and/or systems are present that limit the coagulation process and restrict it to the site of vessel injury.

The relative importance of each of these components in the overall hemostatic response is determined by the region of the vasculature in which the injury occurs, the caliber or size of the vessel, and the pressure differential between the inside of the vessel and the outside. For example, vasoconstriction plays a predominant role in halting bleeding in the arterioles and venules due to the relatively high proportion of smooth muscle in these vessels. On the other hand, platelet aggregation and fusion are particularly important elements in the hemostatic response to injury at the capillary level due to lower blood flow and pressure, as well as the lack of smooth muscle. Bleeding from dam-

aged larger arteries can be profuse due to the high pressure; the formation of fibrin is an absolute requirement for effective hemostasis in these vessels. Obviously, none of the components is effective in halting bleeding from laceration or rupture of the major conduit arteries, in which case pressure must be applied and immediate surgical repair of the damaged vessel undertaken. The extent of bleeding is also influenced by the pressure in the perivascular area surrounding the injury. For example, bleeding into joints and skeletal muscle is strongly limited by the elevated tissue pressures in these restricted areas, whereas hemorrhage in the gastrointestinal tract is often difficult to control.

The remainder of this chapter deals with the major events in the normal hemostatic response to vessel injury, namely, the roles of blood vessel constriction, platelet activation, and blood coagulation. The next chapter contains information relating to the regulatory factors that localize and restrict the coagulation process, the most common screening tests for hemostatic abnormalities, and a conceptual approach to bleeding and thrombotic disorders.

Vascular and Platelet Responses to Injury
Blood Vessel Constriction

When small-resistance vessels **(arterioles)** are severed, the immediate control of hemorrhage is accomplished very efficiently by vasoconstriction. The importance of vasoconstriction in effective hemostasis is exemplified by the profuse bleeding that may accompany trauma to vascular tumors **(hemangiomas)** or inflamed vessels **(vasculitis),** conditions in which the blood vessel contractile responses are limited. Although capillaries do not have smooth muscle fibers, some control of bleeding is probably gained by means of precapillary sphincter contraction. The type of injury, whether transecting or crushing in nature, will determine the efficiency of vasoconstriction to halt blood loss. Although larger arteries and veins do contract when injured, the reflexive constriction is usually not sufficient to minimize bleeding in areas of rapid blood flow and elevated pressures.

The vasoconstriction response has two components, a **rapid reflexive** contraction lasting 10 to 30 seconds that depends on sympathetic neural inputs and a **slower** (about 60 minutes) **myogenic** component that may be mediated by the release of local vasoactive substances. Possible chemical mediators are **serotonin** (5-hydroxytryptamine) or **thromboxane A₂,** released from aggregating platelets, or the potent vasoconstrictor **endothelin,** released from damaged endothelial cells.

Role of Platelets in Hemostasis

Normal Platelet Production and Structure

Platelets are anuclear, discoid cells produced from the cytoplasm of megakaryocytes in the bone marrow. Substantial reserves of mature platelets are not available in the marrow; platelet production is regulated to meet circulating demands by means of humoral stimulation by thrombopoietin, analogous to red blood cell (RBC) regulation by erythropoietin. Platelets normally circulate at a concentration of about 200,000 to 400,000 platelets per microliter of blood and have a half-life of about 9 to 10 days. Under normal conditions, about two-thirds of the total platelets are present in the systemic circulation, with the remainder sequestered in the spleen. Enlargement of the spleen **(splenomegaly)** can lead to increased splenic pooling of platelets and to a decrease in the availability of circulating platelets **(thrombocytopenia),** thus increasing the tendency for bleeding to occur. **Platelet turnover,** calculated from the platelet count divided by the platelet survival time, directly estimates the rate of platelet removal from the circulation and, as discussed in Chap. 29, is an important factor in arterial thrombosis. In normal subjects, platelet turnover is about 25,000 to 35,000 platelets per microliter of blood per day. Thus, if circulating platelet levels are suddenly depleted, due to an increase in either platelet consumption or destruction, approximately 5 to 7 days is required to restore the platelet count to normal.

Platelets are the smallest of the circulating formed elements with an average diameter of 3 to 4 μm and a thickness of about 1μm. The plasma membrane has numerous invaginations and is continuous with an open canalicular system that serves as a pathway for both the uptake of extracellular calcium and the release of intracellular material. A dense tubular system is also present, consisting of smooth endoplasmic reticulum that interdigitates with the canalicular system. These two tubular systems are involved in Ca^{2+} regulation. The plasma membrane is rich in phospholipids, cholesterol, and glycolipids. The membrane phospholipids are important because they serve as cofactors in the coagulation process and as a source of arachidonic acid for the production of thromboxane A₂. Just below the plasma membrane is a circumferential band of microtubules that serves as a cytoskeleton in the maintenance of cell shape.

Platelets contain a variety of proteins characteristic of contractile cells, including actin, myosin, tropomyosin, calmodulin, myosin light-chain kinase, filamin, and troponin. Energy for platelet contraction is provided by ATP from both anaerobic glycolysis and mitochondrial oxidative metabolism. The largest organelle is the electron-dense body or granule. Other organelles include the alpha granules, small mitochondria, and glycogen stores. The **alpha granules** contain platelet-specific proteins such as beta-thromboglobulin, platelet-derived growth factor, and platelet factor 4, as well as proteins also present in plasma (fibrinogen, albumin, and fibronectin). The **dense granules** contain ADP, calcium, and serotonin. In response to stimulation (see below), platelet secretion involves activation of the contractile machinery and release of storage granule contents into the open canalicular system and ultimately into the extracellular fluid space.

Platelets and the Response to Vessel Injury

Platelets are essential for normal hemostasis and play several important roles: (1) maintenance of **vessel integrity** by sealing over minor disruptions of the vascular endothelial surface, (2) formation of **hemostatic plugs** following vessel injury and disruption of the endothelium, (3) provision of **procoagulant activity** and phospholipid, which are required for efficient formation of fibrin, the end-product of the coagulation pathway, and (4) provision of **platelet-derived growth factor** (PDGF), which may be an important mitogen in the wound-healing process and in the development of atherosclerosis.

Platelet Adhesion.   Normally, platelets circulate freely and do not adhere to the endothelial surface. This may be due to the basal secretion of **prostacyclin** (PGI₂), a potent inhibitor of platelet aggregation, by endothelial cells. However, on disruption of the endothelial surface, platelets rapidly accumulate at the site of vessel injury in a process termed **platelet adhesion.** This reaction initiates platelet involvement in hemostasis and occurs within seconds; it is characterized by the formation of pseudopodia in the platelets in contact with connective-tissue elements in the subendothelial space. The platelet has high affinity for **collagen** and tends to migrate to this subendothelial protein. The process of platelet adhesion requires a plasma cofactor protein termed **von Willebrand factor** (vWF), named after the individual who first described the inherited bleeding disorder associated with its deficiency. vWF is synthesized by endothelial cells and is adsorbed by circulating platelets and by exposed subendothelial tissue. A specific platelet **membrane glycoprotein** (GP), termed **GP1b** (or **GP1b-IX**), serves as the surface receptor for multimers of vWF (see Fig. 28-2). Hereditary absence of this glycoprotein receptor (**Bernard-Soulier syndrome**) or absence of vWF results in defective platelet adhesion and a severe bleeding tendency. These observations indicate that both vWF and platelet membrane glycoproteins are key elements in the interaction of the platelet membrane with the subendothelium.

Platelet Activation and Aggregation.   Blood vessel disruption and exposure to subendothelial tissue also result in activation and aggregation of platelets. These overlapping events involve (1) platelet shape changes, (2) the release of ADP and serotonin from the dense granules, (3) liberation and oxidation of arachidonic acid from the platelet membrane, (4) formation of thromboxane A_2, and (5) the simultaneous formation of small amounts of thrombin via coagulation with subsequent thrombin-induced changes in platelet function. **Collagen** and the

initial **thrombin** formed after vessel injury are the primary triggers for platelet activation and aggregation. After binding to specific glycoprotein receptors on the platelet membrane, these substances result in activation of membrane phospholipases and the liberation of arachidonic acid (Fig. 28-1). The arachidonate in the platelet is rapidly converted to **thromboxane A_2.** In addition to its potent vasoconstrictor activity, thromboxane A_2 mobilizes calcium from various intracellular storage sites, particularly the dense tubular system. The resulting elevation in cytosolic calcium is most likely the final mediator of platelet aggregation and release; calcium complexes with calmodulin and leads to phosphorylation of myosin, contraction of actomyosin, and release of intracellular granule contents (e.g., ADP and serotonin). The elevated calcium also activates membrane phospholipases that further amplify the process.

As noted in Fig. 28-1, **aspirin** is a potent inhibitor of the

Fig. 28-1. Oxidation of arachidonic acid in the platelet in response to platelet aggregating agents (ADP = adenosine diphosphate; TxA_2 = thromboxane A_2; PGG_2 and PGH_2 = cyclic endoperoxides; PGI_2 = prostacyclin). Metabolism of arachidonate via the lipoxygenase pathway, leading to the formation of leukotrienes is not shown; its potential role in the platelet aggregation response is not clearly known. To the right of the dashed line is depicted the metabolism of endoperoxides by the endothelial cell.

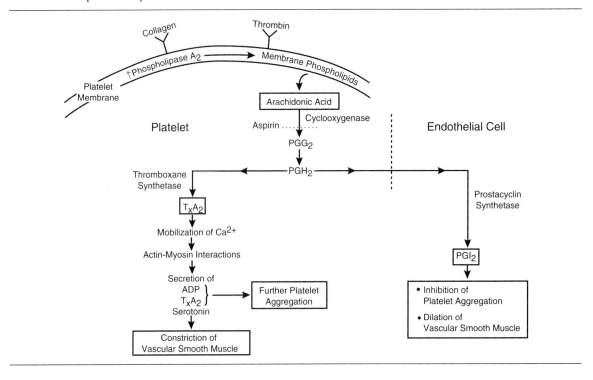

cyclooxygenase enzyme that converts arachidonate to the endoperoxides. A brief exposure to aspirin acetylates and inactivates cyclooxygenase. Furthermore, since the platelet is incapable of de novo synthesis of proteins and enzymes, inactivation of cyclooxygenase by aspirin is irreversible for the life span of the platelet. Although aspirin does prolong the bleeding time test of platelet function, it does not usually cause a bleeding tendency.

The ADP released by platelets in contact with collagen or thrombin induces further platelet aggregation and thereby increases the size of the platelet plug. ADP initiates aggregation by binding to specific receptors on the platelet, thereby mobilizing fibrinogen-binding sites (complex between membrane glycoproteins GPIIb and GPIIIa). Bridging between platelets is mediated by a calcium-dependent binding of fibrinogen molecules at the membrane. Thus normal platelet aggregation requires fibrinogen and calcium and does not occur in conditions in which the glycoproteins GPIIb and GPIIIa are abnormal (Fig. 28-2.)

Endothelin (released from damaged endothelium), as well as serotonin and thromboxane A$_2$ (released by stimulated platelets), causes vasoconstriction in regions containing smooth muscle fibers. The net effect of these reactions is a contracted blood vessel and a propagating platelet

mass that may be sufficient (without fibrin formation via coagulation) to halt bleeding. However, depending on the severity and site of the injury, anchoring of the temporary hemostatic plug with the coagulation product fibrin may be necessary. In addition, the released ADP is slowly metabolized, and the adherent platelets tend to disaggregate.

Mechanisms of Blood Coagulation

The overall purpose of **blood coagulation** is to seal damaged vessels and to anchor platelet plug formation by forming a definitive insoluble fibrous meshwork **(fibrin)** from a soluble precursor in plasma **(fibrinogen).** In simplest terms, the clotting of blood involves the enzymatic activation of several plasma proteins possessing highly specific functions **(coagulation factors).** This process consists of a series of cascading proteolytic reactions in which an inactive precursor is converted to an active proteolytic enzyme **(serine protease),** which then cleaves and activates the next inert precursor. Despite considerable sequence identity in the coagulation factors, they also possess highly specific and unique substrate binding sites. The cascading nature of the activation of coagulation allows for numerous points of control and for **amplification** —

Fig. 28-2. Schematic of the major events involved in platelet adhesion, aggregation, and vasoconstriction in response to vessel injury (VWF = von Willebrand factor; ADP = adenosine diphosphate; TXA$_2$ = thromboxane A$_2$; ET-1 = endothelin-1).

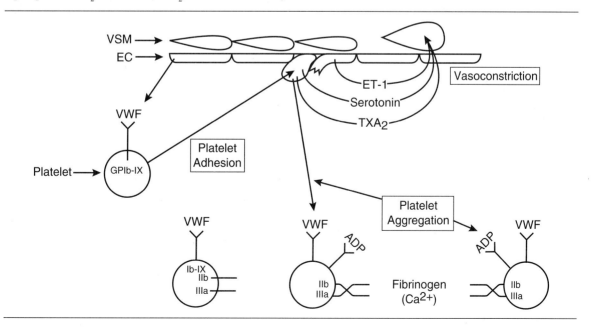

the activation of a few molecules of protease results in the formation of many molecules of product. In many of the reactions, Ca^{2+} is required and phospholipid (derived primarily from platelet membranes) and other substances serve as required cofactors for coagulation. The cofactors are important regulatory elements because they (1) accelerate the reaction rates so that ample product is formed rapidly, (2) provide a "surface" upon which the reactions can occur, protected from inhibition and blood flow dilution, (3) confer specificity to the reactions by aligning the proteases with the correct substrates, and (4) are provided primarily at the site of damaged tissues and thereby localize the coagulation process.

Both Roman numerals and common names are used to identify the factors involved in blood coagulation (Table 28-1). Although an international committee agreed to assign Roman numerals to the various factors, some of the synonyms are still used. For example, fibrinogen, prothrombin, tissue thromboplastin, and calcium ion are rarely referred to as factors. The numerals were assigned in the order of their discovery and do not reflect the reaction sequence. The majority of the coagulation factors exist in plasma as inactive precursors termed **procoagulants.** After activation by the process of **limited proteolysis,** the activated factors are identified by affixing the lowercase letter "a" to the factor number; for example, inactive factor X is converted to factor X_a during the clotting process. Fibrinogen is an exception to this general rule, for it is converted to an insoluble and nonenzymatic fibrin molecule that is the major structural protein of the blood clot.

Table 28-1. Glossary of Coagulation Proteins

Factor	Synonym
I	Fibrinogen
II	Prothrombin
III	Tissue thromboplastin, tissue factor
V	Proaccelerin, labile factor
VII	Proconvertin, stable factor
VIII	Antihemophilic factor
IX	Christmas factor
X	Stuart factor
XI	Plasma thromboplastin antecedent
XII	Hageman factor
XIII	Fibrin-stabilizing factor
Prekallikrein	Fletcher factor
HMWK	Fitzgerald factor

Production of Coagulation Factors and the Role of Vitamin K

All the factors circulate in plasma in concentrations ranging from about 1 to 150 µg/ml, except for fibrinogen, which is about 1000-fold greater at 2.5 mg/ml. Thus, under normal circumstances, there is virtually an inexhaustible supply of fibrinogen as the final substrate for coagulation (and thrombosis). The liver is the source of production of all the factors except factor VIII, the antihemophilic factor, which is most likely produced in endothelial cells and/or megakaryocytes. Therefore, the plasma concentrations of all other clotting proteins fall dramatically in severe liver disease, thereby promoting a hemorrhagic condition.

Vitamin K (Fig. 28-3A) is a fat-soluble vitamin that is required for the synthesis of certain Ca^{2+}-binding domains in factors II (prothrombin) (see Fig. 28-3B), VII, IX, and X and protein C (discussed in Chap. 29). Vitamin K is needed for the hepatic formation of gamma-carboxyglutamic acid residues (GLA), which form a unique negative charge density and a Ca^{2+}-binding site that permits the vitamin K–dependent factors to bind to phospholipid via Ca^{2+} bridges. Deficiencies of vitamin K can lead to severe bleeding tendencies and ineffective coagulation. The vitamin K–dependent proteins lack the unique GLA residues and are therefore ineffective during the coagulation process. Deficiencies in vitamin K can be due to inadequate dietary intake or to fat malabsorption in the intestine. The vitamin is also produced endogenously as the result of gastrointestinal bacterial action. Most of the clotting factors have short intravascular half-times relative to other plasma proteins, ranging from just a few hours (factors VII, VIII, and IX) to up to 7 days (factor XIII).

Enzymatic Pathways of Coagulation

The first clotting protein, discovered by Malpighi in the seventeenth century, was **fibrin** — the insoluble ropelike meshwork of a blood clot that is formed rapidly upon exposure of blood to foreign surfaces. It was quickly recognized that fibrin cannot exist as such in the normal circulation, and a soluble precursor form of the molecule, now known as **fibrinogen,** was correctly predicted. In the late 1800s, some key observations were made by Buchannan and Schmidt, who noted that a substance was evolved during the clotting process (was present in **serum** but absent in **plasma**) that could hasten the conversion of fibrinogen to fibrin. This process was later confirmed to be

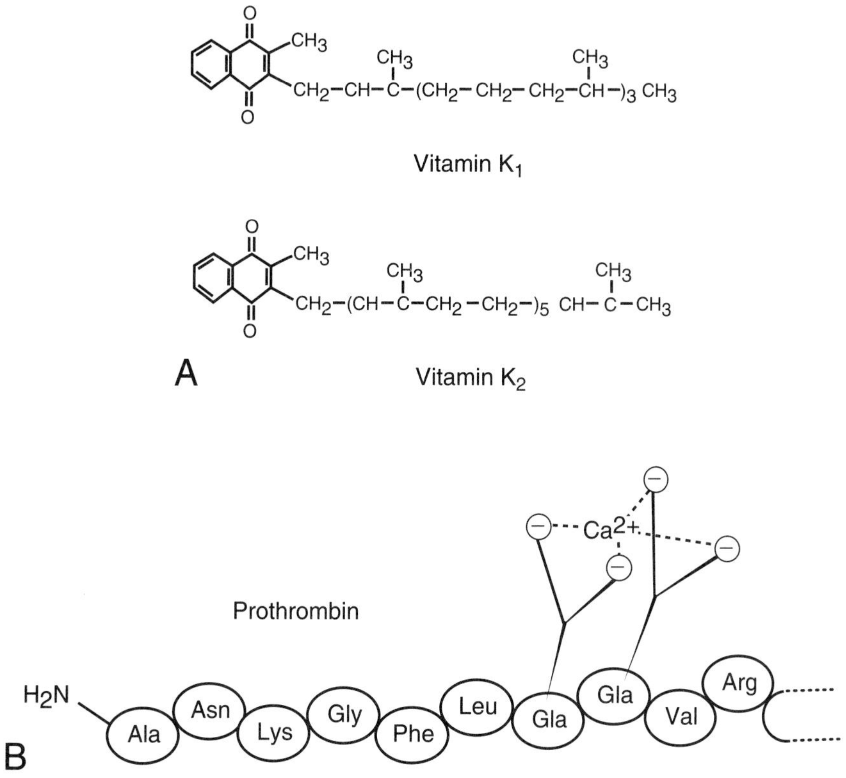

Fig. 28-3. Structure and action of vitamin K. (A) Two forms of vitamin K, one from dietary sources (plant, type K_1) and the other from bacteria (type K_2). Vitamin K is a napthoquinone derivative with a hydrophobic side chain that differs in the two forms. (B) An example of the vitamin K–dependent, posttranslational insertion of gamma-carboxyglutamic acid residues (GLA) into the amino-terminal sequence (Ala, Asn, Lys, etc.) of prothrombin. Several similar insertions are made into each of the vitamin K–dependent clotting factors. The resulting GLA residues form a negatively charged region that serves as a Ca^{2+}-binding domain through which the factors bind to phospholipid surfaces. (Modified from: Ogston, D. *The Physiology of Hemostasis.* Cambridge: Harvard University Press, 1983; and from: Thompson, A. R., and Harker, L. A. *Manual of Hemostasis and Thrombosis,* 3rd ed. Philadelphia: F. A. Davis, 1983. P. 119.)

due to the action of a proteolytic enzyme now known as **thrombin.** This discovery led to the obvious postulation that in circulating blood, thrombin must exist as an inactive precursor termed **prothrombin.** In trying to understand the mechanisms underlying the conversion of prothrombin to thrombin, numerous coagulation factors were discovered as being essential components of the normal hemostatic mechanism. Nearly all the factors were detected by studies on patients who displayed abnormal bleeding due to an inherited deficiency of the factor. Many of the hemorrhagic disease states and the deficient factors

involved were named after the afflicted family or persons involved (e.g., Hageman factor and Hageman trait; Christmas factor and Christmas disease).

Mechanisms of Thrombin Formation

The reactions leading to the formation of thrombin from prothrombin can be simplified and divided into three major enzymatic pathways: **intrinsic, extrinsic,** and **common pathways** (Fig. 28-4). All the components required for the intrinsic pathway are present in circulating blood,

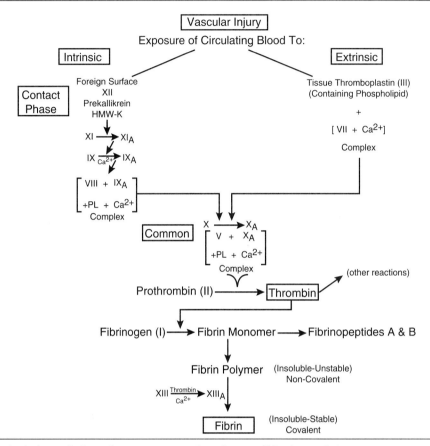

Fig. 28-4. The intrinsic, extrinsic, and common enzymatic pathways of blood coagulation. (See text for detailed description.) (HMW-K = high-molecular-weight kininogen; PL = phospholipid.)

hence the name **intrinsic.** However, the extrinsic pathway is initiated by a factor not normally present in the bloodstream but contributed by damaged tissue, hence the term **extrinsic.** Activation of either of these two reaction chains leads to the activation of factor X, which in turn converts prothrombin to thrombin, followed by conversion of fibrinogen to fibrin. That portion of the overall reaction sequence shared by both the intrinsic and extrinsic pathways, beginning at the factor X step, is referred to as the **common pathway.** Both the intrinsic and extrinsic pathways become operative in vivo in response to vessel injury and must be functional for normal hemostasis.

The Intrinsic Pathway

The intrinsic pathway leading to the activation of factor X

is initiated by contact of blood with a negatively charged foreign surface and involves six clotting proteins: factor XII, plasma prekallikrein (PK), high-molecular-weight kininogen (HMWK), factor XI, factor IX, and factor VIII. The initial stage of this pathway, involving the first four of these factors, is sometimes referred to as the **contact phase** of coagulation (triggered by contact with a foreign surface). The reactions during the contact phase are not dependent on Ca^{2+}. The factors involved in contact activation of blood coagulation also may participate in other host defense mechanisms, including fibrinolysis, kinin generation in the inflammatory response, as well as complement activation. Although the contact phase can be readily demonstrated in vitro, the pathophysiologic significance of these initial reactions remains questionable. In fact, of the contact factors, only severely depressed levels of factor XI are associated with abnormal bleeding.

Experimental studies have revealed that when factors XII, PK, HMWK, and XI are properly assembled on a negatively charged surface, factor XI is rapidly activated to factor XI$_a$ by the enzymic activated factor XII (XII$_a$). Although the activation of factor XII is not fully understood, reciprocal activation reactions most likely occur. For example, a few molecules of factor XII$_a$ activate prekallikrein to kallikrein, which in turn activates additional factor XII. HMWK has no known enzymatic function but serves as a required cofactor in several of these reactions. Both prekallikrein and factor XI exist in plasma complexed with HMWK. Thus HMWK may function to bring PK and factor XI into close proximity to surface-bound factor XII. In this way, HMWK enhances the ability of factor XII$_a$ to activate not only factor XI but also prekallikrein to kallikrein, which in turn generates additional factor XII$_a$.

Factor XI$_a$, in the presence of Ca^{2+}, next activates factor IX by limited proteolysis at two sites. Once activated, factor IX$_a$ converts inactive factor X to its active form (X$_a$) in the presence of factor VIII, phospholipids, and Ca^{2+}. The latter reaction takes place efficiently only when the factors first form a multimolecular complex on the phospholipid surface with factors IX$_a$ and X bound at their GLA residues to the phospholipid via Ca^{2+} bridges. In vivo, the phospholipid is provided by the platelet membrane, and factor VIII serves as a cofactor to this process. The formation of the multimolecular assembly on the phospholipid surface accelerates the reaction by immobilizing the substrates and enzymes.

The Extrinsic Pathway

An alternative mechanism of activation of factor X via the extrinsic pathway is simultaneously initiated when blood is exposed to underlying tissue (see Fig. 28-4). The combination of a ubiquitous tissue lipoprotein, termed **tissue factor** or **tissue thromboplastin (factor III),** with a plasma protein, factor VII, results in the rapid activation of factor X to X$_a$. Factor VII, a vitamin K–dependent clotting factor present in very low levels in plasma, binds to the phospholipid portion of factor III via its GLA residues and Ca^{2+}. The resulting complex then develops an active site in factor VII to form factor VII$_a$, which then converts factor X to X$_a$ by a mechanism identical to that described previously for the factor IX$_a$–factor VIII–Ca^{2+}–phospholipid complex. Recent experimental evidence indicates that **feedback mechanisms** and interactions may occur at several points between the intrinsic and extrinsic pathways. For example, the activation of factor XII, in addition to

triggering the intrinsic pathway, may activate factor VII in the extrinsic pathway.

The Common Pathway

In a fashion similar to the activation of factor X by factor IX$_a$, the activation of prothrombin by factor X$_a$ requires factor V, phospholipid, and Ca^{2+} as cofactors. (As with factor VIII in the activation of factor X, both the availability of phospholipid from platelet membranes and the binding of factor V to the lipid matrix are enhanced by thrombin.) The vitamin K–dependent proteins, prothrombin and factor X$_a$ bind to the phospholipid via GLA residues and Ca^{2+} bridges. Factor V, a very large molecule (250–300 kDa), also binds to the phospholipid and to prothrombin. Formation of this multimolecular complex on the phospholipid surface requires factor V as a nonenzymatic cofactor that efficiently aligns the substrate (prothrombin) and the enzyme (factor X$_a$) for optimal interaction. Factor X$_a$ induces two sequential proteolytic cleavages in prothrombin. First, an amino-terminal fragment and a carboxy-terminal fragment, termed **prethrombin,** are released. Cleavage at a second site on prethrombin yields the final active protease of coagulation, **thrombin.**

Formation and Stabilization of Fibrin

Fibrinogen is a very large glycoprotein (340 kDa) that circulates in plasma at a high concentration (2–4 mg/ml). It is a dimeric molecule with two identical halves each consisting of three polypeptide chains, termed the Aα_2, Bβ_2, and γ_2 chains, respectively (Fig. 28-5A). The conversion of fibrinogen to fibrin occurs in three distinct stages. In the **first stage** (see Fig. 28-5B, C), thrombin cleaves fibrinogen at the amino-terminal end of each α and β chain to yield four small fragments: two fibrinopeptides A and two fibrinopeptides B. The release of the A peptide (16 amino acids) precedes that of the B peptide (14 amino acids). The action of thrombin thus exposes new amino acid residues in the central nodule region that serve as binding sites for subsequent polymerization of the molecule. Once the fibrinopeptides have been cleaved from fibrinogen, the resulting molecule is the **fibrin monomer.**

In the **second stage,** molecules of fibrin monomer polymerize in a nonenzymatic fashion by end-to-end and side-to-side binding to form **fibrin polymer.** The binding of monomers to form polymeric fibrin occurs via weak noncovalent interactions; this results in the formation of fibrin strands that are insoluble in plasma. This type of fibrin polymer (in the absence of factor XIII$_a$) is very susceptible to hydrolysis by the fibrinolytic enzyme **plasmin** (discussed in Chap. 29). The **final stage** of coagulation is sta-

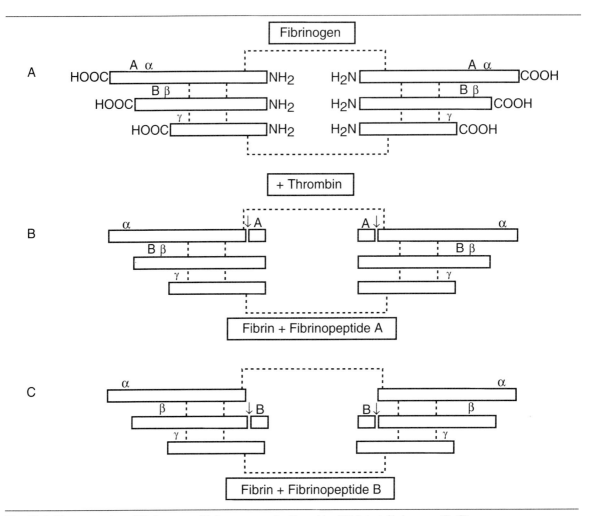

Fig. 28-5. The conversion of fibrinogen to fibrin monomer by thrombin. (A) Intact fibrinogen. (B, C) In the presence of thrombin, two pairs of fibrinopeptides A and B are sequentially removed from fibrinogen to yield monomeric fibrin (broken lines = disulfide bonds). (Modified from: Ogston, D. *The Physiology of Hemostasis.* Cambridge: Harvard University Press, 1983. P. 90.)

bilization of the fibrin molecule by factor XIII, which is activated to its enzymatic form (factor XIII$_a$) by limited proteolysis with thrombin in the presence of Ca^{2+}. Factor XIII$_a$ is a transglutaminase that catalyzes covalent bond formation between adjacent side chains of fibrin polymer (Fig. 28-6). The net effect is an increase in the mechanical rigidity of fibrin and the production of a tightly cross-linked clot that is insoluble in denaturing agents. The stabilized fibrin molecule is highly resistant to the action of the fibrinolytic enzyme plasmin (due to the primary in-

hibitor of plasmin, **alpha$_2$-antiplasmin,** being cross-linked to fibrin by factor XIII$_a$).

Coagulation Kinetics and the Roles of Thrombin

Thrombin plays a central role in the overall process of coagulation. In addition to converting fibrinogen to fibrin and activating factor XIII, it also potentiates the activities of

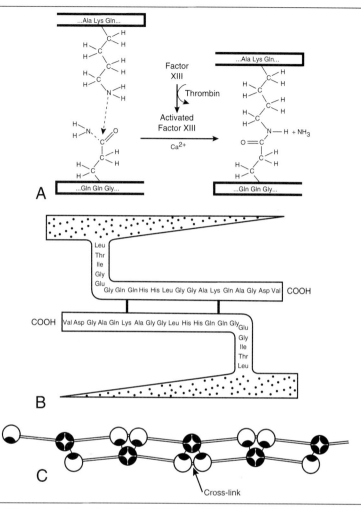

Fig. 28-6. Stabilization of fibrin by activated factor XIII. (A) Factor XIII is activated by thrombin and, in the presence of Ca^{2+}, catalyzes peptide-bond formation between glutamine and lysine residues of adjacent molecules of fibrin. (B) The antiparallel arrangement of adjacent gamma chains and the location of the covalent linkages catalyzed by factor XIIIa. (C) Spatial arrangement of trinodular fibrin molecules after cross-linking with factor XIIIa. (A and B modified from: Doolittle, R. F. Fibrinogen and fibrin. *Sci. Am.* 245: 126–135, 1981; C modified from: Ogston. D. *The Physiology of Hemostasis.* Cambridge: Harvard University Press, 1983. P. 91.)

factors V and VIII in their binding to phospholipid-Ca^{2+} matrices. Another important function of thrombin is its ability to provide phospholipid by virtue of its potent effect on the platelet membrane, providing a surface for coagulation reactions to proceed rapidly and efficiently, most notably those involving factors V and VIII. Thrombin pro-

duction via the extrinsic pathway is initially much faster than that generated by the intrinsic pathway (due to fewer rate-limiting reactions). Efficient operation of the intrinsic pathway has a strong requirement for phospholipid at the factor IX_a–factor VIII–Ca^{2+} stage. However, once phospholipid is made available, the intrinsic pathway becomes fully operative. Furthermore, **amplification** occurs during activation of the intrinsic pathway in that the formation of a few molecules of activated product leads to activation of many more molecules. Thus, in response to vessel injury, a small amount of thrombin is rapidly produced primarily from activation of the extrinsic pathway. By virtue of its action on platelets and factors V and VIII, thrombin, in a positive feedback fashion, then allows unimpeded operation of the intrinsic pathway, explosive generation of more thrombin, and subsequent conversion of fibrinogen to fibrin. Both pathways must be operative in order to achieve the critical thrombin concentration necessary to convert enough fibrinogen to fibrin to bring about effective hemostasis. There is the need to limit the rate of formation of thrombin once effective hemostasis has been achieved. Two important questions that will be addressed in Chap. 29 are (1) How is the coagulation of blood localized to only the site of vessel injury? and (2) How is this explosive system regulated so that coagulation does not occur in the absence of vessel injury (thrombosis)?

Summary

When a vessel is injured, a series of host-defense reactions is initiated at the interface of the blood and vessel wall to arrest bleeding and achieve effective hemostasis. Platelets play a key role in this process by forming a temporary hemostatic plug, which, in addition to smooth muscle contraction, may suffice to halt bleeding from small vessels. The biochemical mechanisms underlying platelet activation and the aggregation response to collagen and thrombin have been largely elucidated. Platelet membranes also contribute phospholipid, which is an important cofactor in the coagulation response. Coagulation is initiated via two pathways when blood is exposed to foreign surfaces and to tissue thromboplastin. A series of cascading reactions, featuring limited proteolysis, amplification, and feedback, produces the insoluble fibrin matrix. Thrombin, platelet phospholipid, and Ca^{2+} play multiple key roles in coagulation. The explosive generation of thrombin, with subsequent formation of fibrin, is a high-risk system that must be carefully regulated to ensure that coagulation is restricted to the site of vessel injury.

Bibliography

Bloom, A. L., Forbes, C. D., Thomas, D. P., and Tuddenham, E. G. D., eds. *Haemostasis and Thrombosis,* 3rd ed., Vols. 1 and 2. Edinburgh: Churchill-Livingstone, 1994.

Ogston, D. *The Physiology of Hemostasis.* Cambridge: Harvard University Press, 1983.

Ratnoff, O. D., and Forbes, C. D., eds. *Disorders of Hemostasis.* Orlando, Fla.: Grune & Stratton, 1984.

Thompson, A. R., and Harker, L. A. *Manual of Hemostasis and Thrombosis,* 3rd ed. Philadelphia: F. A. Davis, 1983.

29 Regulation of Coagulation and Pathophysiology of Hemostasis

Robert F. Highsmith

Objectives

After reading this chapter, you should be able to

List the major regulatory factors that localize and restrict the coagulation process

Explain the role of blood flow dilution and consumption of coagulation factors in the regulation of coagulation

Compare and contrast the counterbalancing effects of arachidonic acid metabolism in the platelet versus the endothelial cell

Describe the role of protease inhibitors in the regulation of coagulation, and predict the consequences of their absence

Describe the components of the fibrinolytic enzyme system, and indicate how it is activated, both physiologically and therapeutically

Explain the mechanism by which fibrin(ogen) degradation products are formed, and define their effects on coagulation

Describe the thrombomodulin–protein C anticoagulant system, and discuss its importance in the regulation of coagulation

Summarize and integrate the reactions of the entire hemostatic mechanism, including how it is initiated and regulated

Conceptually understand hemorrhagic disorders in terms of what components of the hemostatic mechanism are affected

Describe the basic principles underlying the most common tests of platelet and coagulation factor function, and diagnose the specific causes of abnormal bleeding based on the results of these tests

Define thrombosis in terms of what components of the hemostatic mechanism are affected

Understand the pathophysiologic consequences of thrombosis, and define *infarction* and *embolization*

Compare and contrast arterial and venous thrombosis

Understand the concepts of fibrinogen and platelet turnover (and survival times) under normal conditions and during arterial and venous thrombosis

Calculate platelet and fibrinogen turnover and survival time, and understand their relationship in arterial and venous thrombosis

Explain the mechanisms of action of heparin, vitamin K antagonists, and plasminogen activators and their use in the treatment of thrombosis

Regulation of Blood Coagulation

Under normal circumstances, blood remains fluid at all times; platelet fusion and fibrin deposition occur only at sites of vessel injury and only in amounts sufficient to halt bleeding. Because of the virtually unlimited supply of platelets and fibrinogen and the dire consequences of dissemination of the platelet-fibrin mass, it is not surprising that an abundance of mechanisms have evolved to regulate hemostasis. Even more astounding is how effective hemostasis can take place despite such a wealth of inhibitory and regulatory elements.

Stimulus Localization and Blood Flow

The endothelium lines the entire vasculature in a continuous fashion, is nonthrombogenic, and normally does not activate platelets or the coagulation system. This unique property of endothelial cells is in large part due to their basal secretion of **prostacyclin** (PGI_2), a vasodilator and potent inhibitor of platelet aggregation, and production of substances that inhibit or oppose coagulation (activators of fibrinolysis, antithrombin, and protein C; see below). Thus the hemostatic system is a potential one that is only triggered by local perturbations of the endothelium, such as vessel injury. Also, the cofactors necessary for effective hemostasis, such as phospholipid, are provided locally, do not circulate, and serve as sinks for binding certain activated coagulation factors.

One of the most important means by which hemostasis is localized and restricted is by the rapid movement of fresh, "unactivated" blood through the vessels, causing substantial dilution of activated procoagulants generated at the site of injury. In addition, the shear forces and turbulence associated with flowing blood mechanically oppose clot formation. The importance of blood flow in opposing coagulation is clearly illustrated by the increased occurrence of deep venous thrombosis in bed-ridden patients — a situation in which the beneficial effects of blood flow are minimal. Also, the injection of activated coagulation factors into experimental animals does not produce thrombosis unless a vessel segment is occluded shortly after the infusion.

Consumption and Catabolism of Coagulation Factors

During the clotting process, several components in plasma are consumed. For example, **serum,** the cell-free fluid that is obtained from a clot after coagulation has occurred, is depleted of fibrinogen, prothrombin, factors V, VIII, and XIII, and platelets. This consumption constitutes a local means of limiting coagulation, since the levels of these components must be replenished before clotting can proceed. In the case of minor vessel injury, circulating levels of these components are not affected, and replenishment is accomplished by the delivery of fresh plasma to the injury site. However, in conditions in which massive systemic coagulation occurs (e.g., **disseminated intravascular coagulation,** or DIC), circulating levels of these factors may be affected so as to produce a bleeding tendency because of factor depletion. In this instance, replenishment requires de novo synthesis of new protein and platelets or, in severe cases, transfusion of whole blood, plasma, or factor concentrates.

The liver has a major role in both the synthesis and degradation of most coagulation factors. It is not surprising, therefore, that liver disease is frequently accompanied by marked alterations in the coagulation system. In terms of its role in the regulation of coagulation, the liver is capable of removing from the bloodstream activated coagulants but not their unactivated procoagulant forms.

Platelet–Endothelial Cell Interactions

As alluded to earlier, very few platelets normally adhere to the luminal surface of the vessel wall. The nonthrombogenic nature of this surface is in large part attributable to the basal secretion of products of arachidonic acid metabolism from the endothelium. Recall that in both the platelet and endothelial cell, activation of **phospholipase A_2** results in the liberation of arachidonate from membrane phospholipids, which is then rapidly oxidized by cyclooxygenase to form endoperoxides (see Fig. 28-1). In the platelet, the endoperoxide PGH_2 is converted by **thromboxane synthase** to the potent mediator of platelet aggregation and vasoconstriction **thromboxane A_2.** However, in the endothelial cell, oxidation of arachidonic acid generates PGI_2 because of the presence of **PGI_2 synthase** in this cell. In direct contrast to thromboxane A_2, PGI_2 is a potent inhibitor of platelet aggregation and is a vasodilator. Thus, by virtue of its basal secretion of PGI_2, the endothelial cell counterbalances the release of thromboxane A_2 by stimulated platelets. Furthermore, it has been shown in vitro that endoperoxides released from aggregating platelets may be taken up by endothelial cells, metabolized, and released as PGI_2. Therefore, as activated platelets come into contact with an intact endothelial cell capable of producing PGI_2, the transferring of endoperoxide substrates from the platelet to the endothelial cell may represent another means of limiting the growth of platelet hemostatic plugs.

Inhibition of Activated Coagulation Factors

Human plasma contains an abundance of naturally occurring **protease inhibitors** that effectively block the activity of proteolytic enzymes, particularly those possessing serine residues at the active site (Table 29-1). These inhibitors collectively ensure that any "spillover" of serine proteases (e.g., activated coagulant proteases) generated at the site of vessel injury will be rapidly neutralized in the systemic circulation. In vitro, the inhibitors display considerable overlap in their specificity toward different proteases. However, the disease states associated with inherited deficiencies of each inhibitor are very specific, suggesting distinct roles for each inhibitor in vivo.

Antithrombin (sometimes referred to as antithrombin III or heparin cofactor) is of particular importance in the overall regulation of coagulation. This inhibitor forms a stable covalent complex with thrombin (as well as with factors XII_a, XI_a, X_a, IX_a, and kallikrein) so as to

Table 29-1. Plasma Protease Inhibitors

Inhibitor	Deficiency State
Alpha$_1$-anti-trypsin	Pulmonary emphysema
Alpha$_2$-macroglobulin	?
Antithrombin (antithrombin III or heparin cofactor)	Thrombosis
C1 inactivator (C1 esterase inhibitor)	HANE
Alpha$_2$-antiplasmin (alpha$_2$-plasmin inhibitor)	Hemorrhage
Protein C	Thrombosis

HANE = hereditary angioneurotic edema.

completely and irreversibly block the active-site serine residues of these enzymes. In the presence of the anticoagulant **heparin** (and perhaps heparin-like mucopolysaccharides in the vessel wall), the rate of inhibition of thrombin by antithrombin is greatly accelerated. Thus antithrombin serves as a necessary cofactor in the expression of the anticoagulant activity of heparin. (The molecular basis of

Fig. 29-1. The components of the fibrinolytic enzyme system. (See text for elaboration.)

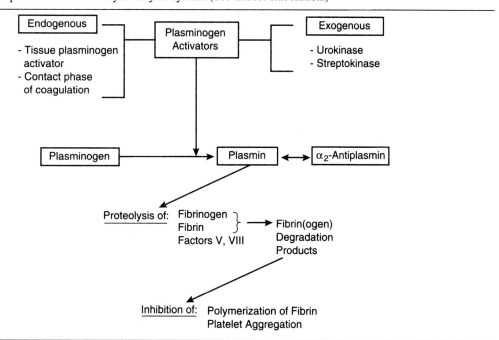

these interactions is discussed later.) The importance of antithrombin in the regulation of coagulation is readily exemplified by the occurrence of severe thrombotic episodes in patients with hereditary deficiencies of this inhibitor.

With the exception of alpha$_2$-macroglobulin, hereditary defects in each of the other antiproteases are also closely associated with specific clinical syndromes. Although the manifestations of these disease states are widely different, a common feature is unopposed proteolysis. Like antithrombin deficiency, the other syndromes illustrate the importance of inhibitors as regulators not only for blood coagulation but also for other proteolytic systems.

Activation of Fibrinolysis

Fibrinolysis is the naturally occurring process by which fibrin clots are dissolved. Like coagulation, the fibrinolytic enzyme system is a potential one that must be activated (Fig. 29-1). In the presence of an endogenous or exogenous activator substance, the single-chain inactive zymogen **plasminogen** is converted by limited proteolysis to a two-chain active serine protease **plasmin.** If plasmin is formed in plasma devoid of clots, it is rapidly and irreversibly inhibited by alpha$_2$-antiplasmin in a fashion analogous to the inhibition of thrombin by antithrombin (a 1 : 1 covalent complex of inhibitor and enzyme). Under unusual circumstances (e.g., alpha$_2$-antiplasmin deficiency or repeated activation of plasminogen by administration of exogenous plasminogen activators), free plasmin can be generated in plasma, in which case widespread proteolysis can occur. Although rare, this event can lead to the breakdown of several proteins necessary for normal coagulation, such as factors V and VIII and fibrinogen, and thereby induce a hemorrhagic condition. However, due to the high affinity of plasminogen activator and plasminogen for fibrin, physiologic activation of plasmin most likely occurs in situ (within the fibrin clot), in an environment protected from inhibition.

When activated on the fibrin surface, plasmin hydrolyzes peptide bonds in fibrin to yield progressively smaller fragments termed **fibrin degradation products** (fdps). If generated in plasma in amounts greater than inhibitor concentrations, plasmin also cleaves fibrinogen in a similar fashion to produce **fibrinogen degradation products** (FDPs). The cleavage of fibrin(ogen) by plasmin occurs in a sequential and asymmetrical fashion, yielding four products: fragments X, Y, D, and finally E (Fig. 29-2). Fibrin that has been cross-linked by factor XIII$_a$ is highly resistant to lysis by plasmin, but degradation products are still formed that contain combinations of the fragments, such as two D fragments and one E fragment.

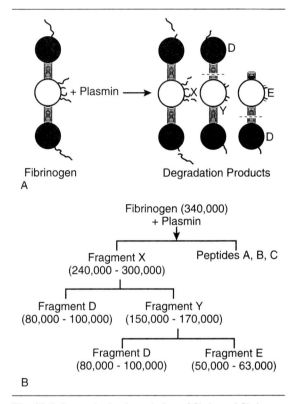

Fibrinogen
A   Degradation Products

Fibrinogen (340,000) + Plasmin

Fragment X (240,000 - 300,000)   Peptides A, B, C

Fragment D (80,000 - 100,000)   Fragment Y (150,000 - 170,000)

Fragment D (80,000 - 100,000)   Fragment E (50,000 - 63,000)

B

Fig. 29-2. Stages in the degradation of fibrin and fibrinogen by plasmin. (A) The trinodular structure of fibrin and fibrinogen and the plasmin cleavage sites. (B) Approximate molecular weights (in daltons) of the major fragments of fibrin and fibrinogen following degradation by plasmin. (See text description.) (A modified from: Rapaport, S. I. Hemostasis. In: West, J. B., ed. *Physiological Basis of Medical Practice,* 11th ed. Baltimore: Williams & Wilkins, 1985. P. 428; B modified from: Ogston, D. *The Physiology of Hemostasis.* Cambridge: Harvard University Press, 1983. P. 148.)

The degradation products of fibrin(ogen) are inhibitory to hemostasis in several ways. For example, the aggregation of platelets is greatly impeded by fragments X, Y, and D. These cleavage products, but not the smaller fragment E, effectively compete with the D-domain of intact fibrinogen for binding to a platelet membrane receptor. The fragments are thus highly inhibitory, since binding of intact fibrinogen to a specific receptor site (GPIIb-IIIa) on the platelet membrane is a prerequisite for the normal platelet aggregation response. In addition, the larger fragments, X and Y, inhibit the polymerization of fibrin by disrupting the interaction of intact monomers.

Plasminogen activators (PAs) play an obvious key role in initiating fibrinolysis, both from a physiologic and a therapeutic viewpoint. The most commonly recognized PAs include the factor XII$_a$–kallikrein–high-molecular-weight kininogen system, urokinase, streptokinase, and tissue-type PA (see Fig. 29-1). **Urokinase,** a urinary protein produced by the renal tubular epithelium, is a potent PA that has been used successfully as a thrombolytic agent. However, since this PA is excreted by the kidney and does not circulate in blood, it most likely plays no role in intravascular fibrinolysis. **Streptokinase,** an exogenous PA, is a product of hemolytic streptococci and, like urokinase, has been used as a therapeutic activator of plasminogen in the treatment of thrombosis.

The most important physiologic PA is termed **tissue-type PA** (t-PA). Since it is produced by vascular endothelial cells, this protein is ideally positioned to interact with circulating plasminogen and to trigger fibrinolysis following clot formation at the vessel wall. t-PA is unique among PAs in that it possesses a very high affinity for fibrin(ogen) as well as plasminogen and is therefore able to elicit plasmin formation within the fibrin matrix — an environment that protects the fibrinolytic enzyme from rapid inhibition by the plasma protease inhibitors. Thus the t-PA molecule can elicit highly specific and localized fibrinolysis. Recombinant t-PA is now available for treating thrombotic complications, and most clinical trials indicate that it is a very effective thrombolytic agent. How the secretion and activity of this important PA are regulated remains uncertain. However, recent research has revealed that endothelial cells also express at least two highly specific inhibitors of t-PA. Although this finding adds yet another level of complexity to the overall regulation of the fibrinolytic system, the t-PA inhibitor molecules are probably very important in coordinating fibrinolysis with coagulation.

The Thrombomodulin–Protein C Anticoagulant System

Protein C is another vitamin K–dependent plasma protein which, when activated, has a profound **anticoagulant** action. When formed during the coagulation process, thrombin is not only bound and inhibited by antithrombin so as to prevent systemic coagulation but also binds locally to **thrombomodulin,** an endothelial cell membrane protein. The resulting thrombin-thrombomodulin complex activates circulating protein C to C$_a$ (Fig. 29-3). Protein C$_a$ has two activities that together promote anticoagulation and stimulate fibrinolysis. First, protein C$_a$ inactivates factor VIII, and in the presence of **protein S,** another vitamin K–dependent protein, protein C$_a$ also hydrolyzes factor V. Inactivation of these two factors effectively blocks further coagulation. In addition, since protein C$_a$ is free to circulate and has a relatively long half-life in plasma, it can limit systemic clotting as well. Second, protein C$_a$ also inactivates the inhibitor of t-PA produced by the endothelium, thereby allowing t-PA to initiate fibrinolysis. The importance of the protein C system as an endogenous anticoagulant is exemplified by the finding of severe recurrent

Fig. 29-3. Thrombin-thrombomodulin activation of protein C. (See text description.) (C$_a$ = activated protein C; t-PA = tissue-type plasminogen activator.)

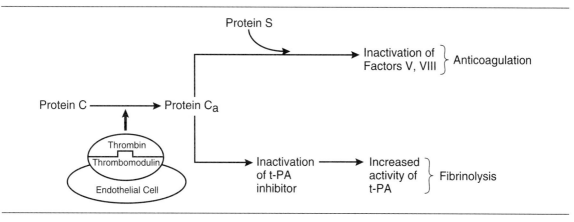

venous thrombosis in patients having genetic deficiencies in this protein.

The Integrated Reactions of Hemostasis

An overall summary of the hemostatic response to vessel injury is given in Fig. 29-4. In response to vessel injury, smooth muscle contraction and platelet aggregation and fusion initiate temporary hemostatic plug formation that, in some cases, may be sufficient to halt bleeding. In most situations, however, fibrin must be deposited at the site in order to accomplish definitive hemostasis. Coagulation is initiated by exposure of blood to tissue thromboplastin (extrinsic) and activation of factor XII by negatively charged foreign surfaces (intrinsic). The subsequent formation of thrombin converts soluble fibrinogen to insoluble fibrin polymer. Thrombin plays a pivotal role in numerous aspects of coagulation and its regulation. For in-

stance, thrombin results in stabilization of the fibrin molecule and further enhances the hemostatic process by virtue of its effect on factors V and VIII and platelets (providing membrane phospholipid upon which reactions occur). Thrombin not only has positive feedback effects causing explosive activation of the coagulation cascade but also initiates negative feedback mechanisms that control its own generation (e.g., the protein C–thrombomodulin anticoagulant system). Finally, numerous regulatory mechanisms, both constant and triggered by the coagulation process itself, ensure that hemostasis is restricted and localized to the site of the vessel injury.

Pathophysiology of Hemostasis

The primary focus of the preceding section has been on the normal physiology of hemostasis. The purpose of the re-

Fig. 29-4. Summary of the integrated hemostatic response to vessel injury. (See text description.)

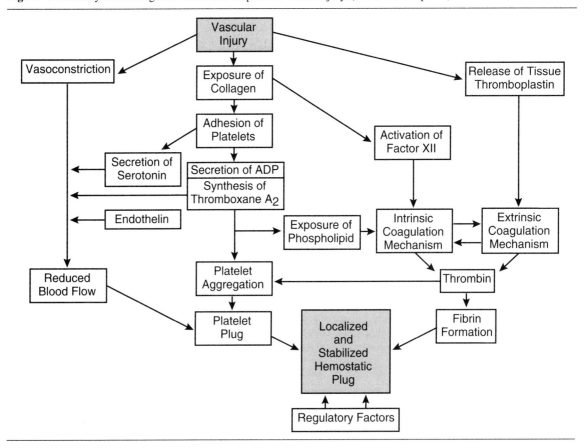

maining two sections is to provide a conceptual approach to the underlying causes and diagnoses of the most commonly used hemorrhagic and thrombotic disorders. The commonly used screening tests of hemostasis are provided as a means of testing your understanding of the underlying mechanisms. The patient with a bleeding or thrombotic disorder can present the clinician with a diagnostic challenge varying in degrees of complexity. Frequently, however, emergency procedures must be initiated in order to properly manage life-threatening hemorrhage or thrombosis. In either case, a thorough knowledge of the basic hemostatic mechanisms and an understanding of the screening tests are required.

Hemorrhagic Disorders

If a stimulus occurs, such as a break in the endothelium, and any of the components of the mechanism do not respond normally (e.g., blood vessel abnormality, platelet or coagulation factor levels below normal in concentration or abnormal in quality, as in genetic defects), a hemorrhagic condition could develop. In fact, if the defect is severe, spontaneous hemorrhage may occur in the apparent absence of trauma. Below are briefly described several commonly used tests to assess abnormalities in platelet number and function, as well as to screen for coagulation factor deficiencies.

Platelet Screening Tests

Platelet Count.   It is customary to evaluate the concentration of platelets in blood as a part of the hemostasis screening profile, particularly since a common cause of defective platelet plug formation is a lowered platelet count (**thrombocytopenia**). The normal ratio of platelets to red blood cells is approximately 1 : 20. The normal platelet count is 250,000 ± 60,000 per microliter of blood. Accurate determination of platelet concentration is done by chamber counting under phase contrast microscopy or by electronic particle counting.

Bleeding Time.   Since the platelet count does not detect abnormalities in platelet function, it is often important to screen for both qualitative and quantitative platelet defects. This is accomplished by the template **bleeding time test,** which screens the overall competence of platelets in forming hemostatic plugs in response to a standardized incision. Bleeding from the wound ceases when sufficient platelets have aggregated and functioned properly to hold against the standardized backpressure. Under usual circumstances, and with platelet counts above

100,000 normal platelets per microliter, the normal bleeding time is about 4.5 ± 1.5 minutes. Borderline prolongation is approximately 8 to 10 minutes, and significant platelet dysfunction and/or thrombocytopenia is suggested with values greater than 10 minutes. It is important to reiterate that the bleeding time can be prolonged due to either a qualitative or quantitative platelet defect and so must be accompanied by a platelet count to differentiate these possibilities.

Coagulation Screening Tests

Partial Thromboplastin Time.   The **partial thromboplastin time** (PTT) measures the overall competency of the intrinsic pathway of coagulation. Partial thromboplastins (such as cephalin or Inosithin) are added to citrated plasma, and the time for coagulation to occur is measured after the addition of phospholipid and Ca^{2+}. A variant of this test, termed the **activated PTT** (aPTT), removes the varying degree of contact activation (a concern with the PTT test), in that the contact factors are maximally activated by first mixing the plasma with particulates. The aPTT and PTT preferentially screen the intrinsic pathway because factor III (tissue thromboplastin) is not available to initiate the extrinsic pathway while the reagents used (a particulate foreign surface, phospholipid, and Ca^{2+}) permit clotting to proceed in the test tube via the intrinsic pathway. Normal values for the aPTT are about 35 to 45 seconds. The aPTT will be prolonged in the presence of a circulating anticoagulant or if any of the factors present in the intrinsic pathway are significantly below normal levels or are defective in quality.

Prothrombin Time.   The **prothrombin time** (PT) assesses the overall competency of the extrinsic pathway of coagulation. The test is performed by adding synthetic tissue thromboplastin (factor III), containing phospholipid, to citrated plasma and measuring the time for coagulation to occur after the addition of Ca^{2+}. The PT preferentially screens the extrinsic pathway because the degree of contact activation of the intrinsic pathway is minimal while the factor III added as a reagent rapidly interacts with factor VII in the plasma sample and clotting proceeds via the extrinsic pathway. The test therefore bypasses the early stages of the intrinsic pathway. Normal values for the PT are approximately 10 to 15 seconds. The PT will be prolonged in the presence of a circulating anticoagulant or if any of the factors present in the extrinsic pathway are significantly below normal levels or are defective in quality.

Thrombin Time.   The **thrombin time** (TT) evaluates the integrity of the final stage of coagulation in which soluble fibrinogen is converted to insoluble fibrin polymer. The test is performed by adding a standard dilute solution of thrombin to citrated plasma and measuring the time for coagulation to occur. The test preferentially screens only the last stage of coagulation because exogenous thrombin is used as a reagent and the patient's ability to generate thrombin via either the intrinsic or extrinsic pathways is therefore bypassed. Normal values for the TT are approximately 18 to 20 seconds. The TT will be prolonged when plasma fibrinogen are significantly low, as well as in the presence of heparin, fibrin(ogen) degradation products, or an abnormal fibrinogen molecule.

Factor XIII Test.   The end point for all the preceding coagulation tests (PTT, PT, and TT) is the appearance of insoluble fibrin polymer in plasma. However, these tests cannot distinguish whether the fibrin formed is a weakly associated or covalently bonded polymer. For this reason, the tests are insensitive to deficiencies of factor XIII. In order to screen for factor XIII defects, the solubility of the patient's clot must be evaluated. If the clot is a covalently linked polymer (i.e., normal factor XIII), it is insoluble in 5 M urea or 1% monochloroacetic acid. In the absence of factor XIII, however, the defective clot is readily soluble in these reagents. Thus clot solubility serves as a means for detecting factor XIII defects.

Differential Diagnosis

Tables 29-2 and 29-3 classify hemostatic disorders based on their screening test profiles. Considerable diagnostic discrimination of hemostatic disorders can be made using just the three classic coagulation screening tests. However, a definitive diagnosis often requires specific immunochemical factor assays.

Examples of Specific Hemorrhagic Disorders

Abnormalities of Platelet Plug Formation

Hemorrhagic disorders can be broadly classified according to which phase of the hemostatic mechanism is affected. For example, abnormalities in the formation of temporary hemostatic plugs can be due to vascular defects, producing an inability of the vessel to constrict properly (inflammation, hemangioma, etc.) or, more likely, due to **quantitative** or **qualitative** platelet defects. These potential causes of bleeding are minimally assessed by the bleeding time

Table 29-2. Evaluation of Hemostatic Deficiencies by the Prothrombin Time and Partial Thromboplastin Time

Deficiency	Partial Thrombo-plastin Time	Prothrombin Time
Prekallikrein	P	N
HMWK	P	N
Factor XII	P	N
Factor XI	P	N
Factor IX	P	N
Factor VIII	P	N
Factor VII	N	P
Factor X	P	P
Factor V	P	P
Prothrombin	P	P
Fibrinogen	P	P
Factor XIII	N	N

HMWK = high-molecular-weight kininogen: P = prolonged; N = normal.

Table 29-3. Classification of Hemostatic Deficiencies Based on Coagulation Screening Tests

Deficiency	Partial Thrombo-plastin Time	Prothrom-bin Time	Thrombin Time
Intrinsic pathway	P	N	N
Extrinsic pathway	N	P	N
Common pathway	P	P	N
Fibrinogen defect	N*	Nª	P

*Prolonged if fibrinogen defect is severe.
P = prolonged; N = normal.

and platelet count. While **hereditary** thrombocytopenia is rare, **acquired** thrombocytopenia is the most common cause of impaired hemostatic function. A decrease in platelet number can be due to a decrease in production (bone marrow disease), an enhanced platelet destruction (autoimmune reactions, such as idiopathic thrombocytopenic purpura, ITP), or increased pooling of platelets by an enlarged spleen (splenomegaly).

Platelet defects can be either hereditary or acquired (e.g., drug-induced or secondary to other diseases). Examples of hereditary platelet abnormalities include a lack of membrane receptors necessary for adherence to collagen (Bernard-Soulier disease) as well as a deficiency in those receptors which normally mediate platelet aggregation

(Glanzmann's thrombasthenia). Von Willebrand's disease is a common heredity hemostatic disorder that is autosomal dominant (nearly all others are autosomal recessive or sex-linked recessive) and is manifest as a qualitative platelet defect coupled with a coagulation factor defect. Platelets from patients with von Willebrand's disease do not adhere normally to injured vessel walls. This abnormality is caused by a decrease in a plasma protein (von Willebrand factor), believed to be a part of the factor VIII complex, that is necessary for normal platelet adhesion. Thus these patients display a prolonged bleeding time. The depression in factor VIII level represents a decrease in both immunologic factor VIII (as measured with an antibody) and functional factor VIII (as measured with a clotting assay). In hemophilia, another hereditary disorder involving factor VIII (see below), immunologic levels of factor VIII are normal, while functional levels are depressed.

Abnormalities of Coagulation

Coagulation defects resulting in a bleeding tendency can be due to a decreased production or an increased destruction of the coagulant proteins, the presence or absence of inhibitory substances, or the production of an abnormal (dysfunctional) coagulant molecule. The prothrombin time, the partial thromboplastin time, the thrombin time, and clot solubility tests are routinely used to screen the competency of the coagulation factors.

The most common congenital bleeding disorder is **factor VIII deficiency,** or **hemophilia** (**hemophilia A,** or **classic hemophilia**). This hereditary defect is a sex-linked recessive disorder affecting only males that accounts for about three-fourths of all congenital defects and has a prevalence of about 1 in 10,000 persons. **Factor IX deficiency (hemophilia B,** or **Christmas disease)** is about one-fourth as frequent as hemophilia A. The coagulant defect in classic hemophilia is a functional deficiency of factor VIII, as measured with clotting assays. The problem is not caused by a deficient rate of production, but by the production of an abnormal factor VIII molecule. Most hemophiliacs have functional factor VIII levels in the 15% to 40% range and do not have spontaneous bleeding. Instead, these patients have hemorrhagic complications in response to trauma, wherein effective hemostasis requires deposition of fibrin, such as surgery, tooth extractions, and injuries. Mild cases of hemophilia can be difficult to distinguish from von Willebrand's disease, another common congenital disorder involving both platelets and an abnormal factor VIII profile. The characteristics of these two disorders are presented in Table 29-4.

Table 29-4. Characteristics of von Willebrand's Disease and Classic Hemophilia

Characteristic	von Wille-brand's Disease	Hemophilia
Common bleeding site	Gastro-intestinal	Joints
Inheritance	Autosomal dominant	X-linked recessive
Prothrombin time	N	N
Partial thromboplastin time	P	P
Platelet count	N	N
Bleeding time	P	N
Factor VIII (antigen)	Low	N
Factor VIII (clotting)	Low	Low

P = prolonged; N = normal.

Thrombosis and Anticoagulants

Thrombosis develops when the hemostatic mechanism is abnormally triggered or when it is not restricted or regulated properly. In comparison with hemorrhagic disease, thrombosis of either the venous or arterial vasculature is very common and, in fact, is a major cause of morbidity and mortality in Western civilizations. In many cases, fatality due to thrombosis is particularly tragic in that it may occur without any apparent clinical warning and frequently at a relatively young age. Thrombosis represents a pathologic occlusion or plugging of a blood vessel due to inappropriate intravascular coagulation. These events may lead to decreased delivery of oxygen and nutrients to the affected area(s), tissue ischemia, and finally, cellular death (**infarction**). The severity of the effect that it may produce is determined by where it is formed or where it may travel to in the event that it is dislodged (**embolization**). For example, small deposits of fibrin often can be tolerated in areas such as skeletal muscle that possess good collateral circulation. Dislodged thrombi in the venous system may embolize to the lung (**pulmonary embolus**), and clots forming in the coronary circulation may produce myocardial infarction, both of which can be life-threatening.

Arterial Thrombosis

Thrombi developing on the arterial side of the circulation are composed primarily of platelets. Relatively little fibrin deposition and trapping of erythrocytes are apparent in the early stages of arterial thrombosis due to the high pressure and rapid flow characteristic of this circulation. The formation of arterial thrombi appears to be dependent on an abnormal vessel wall with damaged or disrupted endothelium. Thus areas of the arterial tree that frequently contain lesions of the vessel wall are particularly susceptible to thrombus formation. For example, atherosclerotic plaque formation, stenotic valves, and chemical or mechanical trauma to the endothelium may represent situations likely to initiate thrombosis.

Atherosclerosis of the coronary arteries, resulting in **ischemic heart disease**, is of particular importance because it is a leading cause of death in the United States. Furthermore, it is now evident that thrombosis (often accompanied by vasospasm) is the most common cause of myocardial infractions in atherosclerotic coronary arteries. The initial event in arterial thrombosis appears to be the development of a platelet mass adhering to the vessel wall lesion or to the damaged endothelium. The platelet mass continues to grow and intrude into the lumen of the vessel. Although occlusion can occur at the site of the lesion, more commonly the platelet mass embolizes, with occlusion taking place downstream at the arteriolar level. After occlusion has occurred, the condition of static blood flow then favors the deposition of fibrin. Myocardial or cerebral infarctions are the most common sequelae.

The platelet is not only the primary component of the arterial thrombus but may be involved in the development of the atherosclerotic lesion as well. During platelet aggregation at the site of damaged endothelium, a substance called **platelet-derived growth factor** (PDGF) is released from the alpha granules, which is a potent mitogen for vascular smooth muscle cell growth in vitro. PDGF may promote growth and proliferation of the underlying smooth muscle cells in vivo, resulting in the invasion of this cell type into the intimal region and plaque formation. Also, in experimental animal models of atherosclerosis, reducing the platelet count markedly retards the development of lesions.

The diagnosis and localization of arterial thrombi can be accomplished by a variety of means, including noninvasive measurements of blood flow and autoradiographic scanning. A cardinal feature is an increase in platelet consumption and platelet turnover (see section below dealing with fibrinogen and platelet turnover). Unfortunately, effective treatment for arterial thrombosis is difficult. Anticoagulant therapies, which are quite effective in treating venous thrombosis, are largely unsuccessful in preventing arterial thrombosis, since the latter involves primarily platelets and not coagulation per se. Platelet suppressive agents, such as aspirin, have met with limited success.

Venous Thrombosis

Thrombi developing on the venous side of the circulation contain primarily fibrin with trapped erythrocytes and some platelets. These thrombi develop in the absence of any apparent lesions of the vessel wall and appear to be dependent on stasis or venous pooling of blood. Since the venous circulation is characterized by low pressures and flow, any events that favor venous pooling of blood and stasis will predispose a person to spontaneous activation of the coagulation process. For this reason, venous thrombosis can be a major problem for bed-ridden patients, older individuals with limited physical activity, or those with occupations restricting movement. Additional conditions associated with an increased risk of venous thrombosis are surgery, pregnancy, congestive heart failure, varicose veins, and obesity. The fact that static blood flow is such a common predisposing feature of venous thrombosis suggests that some degree of coagulation may be occurring continuously and that adequate blood flow accompanying physical activity may be a key factor in preventing its development. These observations also indicate the importance of blood flow dilution as a regulatory factor in localizing and restricting the coagulation process. Another important concern associated with deep venous thrombosis is the potential for embolization, in which case the dislodged fibrin will circulate and be deposited in the lung **(pulmonary embolus).** Widely available methods for detecting venous thrombosis include contrast and isotopic venography, Doppler flow measurements, and radiolabeled fibrinogen uptake. A major feature of venous thrombosis is an increase in fibrinogen turnover (see section below dealing with fibrinogen and platelet turnover). In contrast to arterial thrombosis, venous thrombosis is very amenable to anticoagulant therapy (see below).

Fibrinogen and Platelet Turnover in Thrombosis

The turnover of fibrinogen and platelets in arterial thrombosis and venous thrombosis is a helpful parameter in understanding the major differences between these two conditions. The concentration of any substance ([S]) in whole blood is given by the product of its turnover times the mean survival time:

$$[S]_{blood} = \text{turnover}_s \times \text{survival time}_s \qquad (29\text{-}1)$$

Analysis of this simple equation illustrates why the measurement of static blood concentrations of substances, such as fibrinogen or platelets, is of limited value. For example, during thrombosis, the survival time for platelets and/or fibrinogen is suddenly lowered due to consumption of these substances. In response to this consumption, feedback regulation becomes operative, and more fibrinogen or platelets are produced (i.e., turnover is increased). If the enhanced turnover rate counterbalances the decrease in survival, no change will have occurred in the whole blood concentration. Thus static blood concentrations often do not reflect major changes in the metabolism of substances. A much more useful and dynamic parameter is to estimate the actual turnover of the substances of interest. The turnover of fibrinogen and/or platelets can be calculated from the mean survival times of radiolabeled fibrinogen or platelets following their infusion into patients. Thus, by rearranging Eq. (29-1), the turnover of any substance (T_s) is given by the blood concentration of S ([S]) divided by the mean survival time.

Under normal conditions, platelet turnover (T_p) is approximately 2.5×10^4 platelets/µl/day (2.5×10^5 platelets/µl divided by 10 days), and fibrinogen turnover (T_f) is about 0.5 mg/ml/day (2.5 mg/ml divided by 5 days). The range of normal turnover values and those occurring during a theoretical thrombotic episode in the arterial or venous circulations are shown in Fig. 29-5. In **arterial thrombosis,** there is an increase in platelet consumption and therefore a decrease in survival time as platelet thrombi are formed in the arterial circulation. In an attempt to maintain normal circulating platelet levels, T_p is increased. Since fibrinogen consumption in arterial thrombosis is largely unaffected (unless severe and widespread occlusion has occurred), the T_f value remains unchanged.

In **venous thrombosis,** there is an increase primarily in fibrinogen consumption and therefore a decrease in fibrinogen survival time as fibrin thrombi are formed in the venous circulation. In order to maintain normal circulating fibrinogen levels, T_f is increased. In severe cases in which significant numbers of platelets are trapped within the fibrin thrombi, T_p may increase as well.

Anticoagulants in the Treatment of Venous Thrombosis

Heparin and **warfarin (coumarin** or **Coumadin)** are two widely used anticoagulants that differ markedly in their mechanisms of action. Heparin is a highly sulfonated, negatively charged mucopolysaccharide isolated from animal lungs and intestinal mucosa. It is also present in human

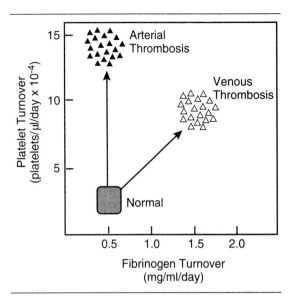

Fig. 29-5. Platelet and fibrinogen turnover under normal conditions and following arterial or venous thrombosis. (See text explanation.)

mast cells and in the extracellular matrix of the endothelium. Heparin alone has little anticoagulant activity. However, in the presence of a plasma cofactor antithrombin, heparin is a potent inhibitor of the coagulation process. Heparin binds to antithrombin and induces a conformational change in the inhibitor molecule so that the reactive site of antithrombin is more favorably positioned for interaction with the active-site serine residue of thrombin. Thus the interaction of heparin and antithrombin produces nearly instantaneous inhibition of thrombin. Nearly all other activated coagulant enzymes are similarly inhibited by antithrombin, with heparin enchancing their rates of interaction as well.

Heparin therapy results in significant prolongation of the clotting times of the three major screening tests (PTT, PT, and TT), with the thrombin time or the partial thromboplastin time being the most sensitive. Although heparin is widely used with success, several factors make it a less than ideal anticoagulant. For example, it is not effective orally and requires injection; repeated infusions may be required, since it is rapidly metabolized with a half-life of about 90 minutes.

Warfarin (coumarin or Coumadin) is an orally effective anticoagulant that is commonly used for the chronic prevention of **venous thrombosis.** It was discovered originally as the active ingredient (bis-hydroxycoumarin) in spoiled sweet clover that induced a hemorrhagic condition after ingestion by cattle. This finding rapidly led to the use of coumarin-like derivatives as rodenticides and, surprisingly, in the prevention of thromboembolism. The coumarin nucleus is chemically similar to vitamin K (see Fig. 28-3); both compounds most likely compete for a common receptor site in the liver. Thus warfarin antagonizes the action of vitamin K in the hepatic synthesis of the vitamin K–dependent clotting factors (prothrombin and factors VII, IX, and X). As discussed earlier, vitamin K allows the posttranslational insertion into these proteins of gamma-carboxyglutamic acid residues that are essential for their clotting function — particularly for their ability to bind Ca^{2+} and phospholipid. The effect of warfarin, then, is to induce an abnormality in the structure of certain key clotting factors. Following warfarin therapy, the levels of the altered vitamin K–dependent factors are simply a reflection of their normal half-life, which ranges from about 5 to 7 hours for factor VII to about 70 to 75 hours for prothrombin (Fig. 29-6).

Fibrinolytic Therapy

As alluded to earlier, activation of the plasminogen-plasmin system by infusing exogenous activator compounds, such as streptokinase and urokinase, has met with some success in acute treatment of patients with ongoing thrombosis. However, both of these compounds have major drawbacks and place the patient at a significant risk of bleeding. Of particular promise is the use of recombinant

Fig. 29-6. Functional levels of prothrombin and factors VII, IX, and X following warfarin administration.

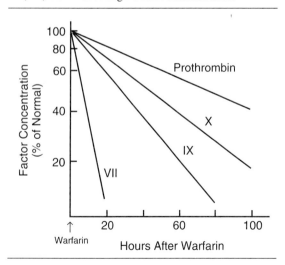

tissue plasminogen activator (t-PA) in fibrinolytic therapy. t-PA appears to mimic the endogenous PA of endothelial cell origin. It binds specifically to the components of the clot matrix, activates plasminogen in situ, and thereby elicits clot dissolution in an environment largely protected from inhibition by alpha$_2$-antiplasmin. Early clinical trials of t-PA indicate that it is a very effective thrombolytic agent in certain conditions and that the secondary risk of bleeding is low.

Summary

An abundance of regulatory factors exist or become operative in order to localize and restrict hemostasis to the site of vessel injury. For example, the endothelium is normally nonthrombogenic and produces substances with antiplatelet and vasodilatory actions. In addition, certain key coagulation factors are consumed during the clotting process, and their activated forms are rapidly diluted by blood flow, cleared by the liver, or effectively inactivated by the plasma protease inhibitors such as antithrombin. Activation of fibrinolysis and the protein C–thrombomodulin proteolytic systems represent two additional major anticoagulant mechanisms.

Although relatively rare, hemorrhagic conditions can develop spontaneously or when the components of the hemostatic mechanism do not respond to the stimulus of vessel injury. As assessed by simple screening tests, hemorrhagic disorders can result from blood vessel dysfunction or from either a qualitative or quantitative defect in the platelets or coagulation proteins. Thrombosis is a common disorder in which the hemostatic mechanism is abnormally triggered or improperly regulated. Arterial and venous thrombosis differ considerably in their etiology and therapy, as well as in the extent of platelet involvement versus activation of coagulation.

Bibliography

Bloom, A. L., Forbes, C. D., Thomas, D. P., and Tuddenham, E. G. D., eds. *Haemostasis and Thrombosis,* 3rd ed., Vols. 1 and 2. Edinburgh: Churchill-Livingston, 1994.

Loscalzo, J., and Schafer, A. I. *Thrombosis and Hemorrhage.* Cambridge, Mass.: Blackwell Scientific, 1994.

Ratnoff, O. D., and Forbes, C. D., eds. *Disorders of Hemostasis.* Orlando, Fla.: Grune & Stratton, 1984.

Thompson, A. R., and Harker, L. A. *Manual of Hemostasis and Thrombosis.* 3rd ed. Philadelphia: F. A. Davis, 1983.

Part V Questions: Hemostasis and Blood Coagulation

1. When platelets contact subendothelial collagen,
   A. the collagen fibrils are rapidly degraded by platelet-derived thrombin.
   B. the platelet-release reaction is initiated, whereby the platelets swell, the cell membrane disintegrates, and the intracellular contents are released.
   C. they are activated by tissue thromboplastin (factor III) and the clotting sequence begins.
   D. ADP is released from the collagen fibrils and causes further platelet aggregation.
   E. antithrombin is released from the platelet, inactivates thrombin, and thereby restricts the coagulation process to the site of vascular injury.

2. Which of the following statements concerning vitamin K is *correct?*
   A. Vitamin K is a fat-soluble vitamin necessary for normal platelet function.
   B. The synthesis of Ca^{2+}-binding GLA residues in factors II (prothrombin), VII, IX, and X requires vitamin K.
   C. Thrombin's action on platelet membranes requires vitamin K.
   D. The only source of vitamin K is from dietary intake.

   E. Although the synthesis of platelets does not require vitamin K, their ability to aggregate in response to collagen strongly depends on vitamin K.

3. A patient with a bleeding disorder had a normal platelet count, normal thrombin time, and normal prothrombin time. Which of the following defects is *not possible* (i.e., can be ruled out as a possible diagnosis)?
   A. Qualitative platelet defect
   B. Classic hemophilia
   C. Factor XIII defect
   D. Vitamin K deficiency
   E. Factor IX defect

4. A person has the following laboratory values: platelet count, 250,000 platelets/μl; mean platelet survival time, 10 days; fibrinogen turnover, 0.4 mg/ml/day; and plasma fibrinogen level, 2.0 mg/ml. Which of the following is *true?*
   A. The bleeding time is significantly prolonged.
   B. The person most likely has ongoing venous thrombosis.
   C. The mean fibrinogen survival time is 50 days.
   D. The platelet turnover is 2.5×10^4 platelets/μl/day.
   E. The person most likely has ongoing arterial thrombosis.

VI Respiratory Physiology

Part Editor

Douglas K. Anderson

30 Introduction to the Pulmonary System

Douglas K. Anderson

Objectives

After reading this chapter, you should be able to

Describe the basic anatomy and functions of the pulmonary system

Define the lung volumes and capacities

Describe the primary functions of the muscles of respiration

The respiratory system is responsible for the exchange of oxygen and carbon dioxide by the body. The gas-exchanging organs are the **lungs.** In addition to gas exchange, the lungs have a variety of other functions, including contributing to the body's acid-base balance, speech, metabolism of certain vasoactive compounds, and defense against infection. In this part, however, discussion will be limited to the gas-exchange function of the pulmonary system.

Metabolizing cells require a continuous supply of oxygen and continuously produce carbon dioxide. To provide adequate oxygen to the cells and remove sufficient amounts of carbon dioxide from them, the lungs must be ventilated and perfused at all times. Gas exchange is limited if the lungs (or a region of the lungs) are ventilated but not receiving adequate blood flow or vice versa. The purpose of this part is to describe the steps required to move oxygen from the air to the mitochondria and carbon dioxide from the cells to the external environment. Discussion will focus on lung mechanics, ventilation, gas exchange and transport, pulmonary blood flow, the regulation or control of ventilation, and the matching of ventilation to blood flow. However, before considering the physiology of respiration, it is necessary to understand the anatomy of the lungs and airways and the remarkable way the structure of the lungs accomplishes their primary function of gas exchange.

Anatomy of the Lungs

Airways and Alveoli

Air passes into the **tracheobronchial tree** (airways) through the nose and mouth. It is warmed to body temperature, humidified, and, if entering through the nose, filtered. The airways bring the inspired air to the gas-exchange region of the lungs; these are the respiratory bronchioles, alveolar ducts, and alveoli. From the trachea to the alveolar sacs, there are approximately 23 generations of sequential branching (Fig. 30-1). The first 16 or so generations constitute the **conducting zone.** The blood flow to this portion of the airways is primarily to provide nutrients to the smooth muscle of the airways that constitute the conducting zone. Because no gas is exchanged in these airways, the conducting zone constitutes the **anatomic dead space.** Each generation of branching increases the collective cross-sectional area of the airways while reducing the radius of each individual airway and the velocity of air flow within that airway. Smooth muscle innervated by autonomic fibers can vary the airway diameter of the conducting zone, but this smooth muscle also responds to certain chemicals and drugs.

Around the sixteenth or seventeenth branching generation (between the terminal and respiratory bronchioles), there is a **transitional zone.** Here, the walls thin out but re-

	Trachea	0
Conducting Airways	Bronchi	1
		2
	Bronchiole	3
		4
	Terminal Bronchioles	5 ↓ 16
Transition Airways	Respiratory Bronchioles	17
		18
		19
Respiratory Airways	Alveolar Ducts	20
		21
		22
	Alveoli	23

Fig. 30-1. Diagram of the airways. The first 16 levels of branching constitute the conducting zone. Branches 17 to 23 are the transition and respiratory zone where gas exchange occurs. (Modified from: West, J. B. *Respiratory Physiology* 4th ed. Baltimore: Willlams &Wilkins, 1990. P. 6.)

tain their smooth muscle coat. Generations 17 to 23 constitute the **respiratory zone,** comprising respiratory bronchioles (with a smooth muscle coat and occasional alveoli), alveolar ducts (with smooth muscle sphincters only), and alveolar sacs. It is in the respiratory zone, principally the alveolar sacs, that gas exchange occurs. There are approximately 300 million alveoli in the lung, each with an average diameter of 0.3 mm.

These multiple generations of branching translate into an enormous area for gas exchange (50 to 100 m², average 70 m²). This large contact area between alveolar gas and pulmonary capillary blood, coupled with a very thin alveolar-capillary barrier (approximately 0.5 μm), highly soluble respiratory gases (oxygen and carbon dioxide), and driving pressures for both oxygen and carbon dioxide between the alveoli and pulmonary capillary blood endow the respiratory system with the ideal characteristics for exchanging gas by passive diffusion.

The movement of air from the nose to the terminal bron-

chioles is accomplished by **bulk flow.** At the level of the terminal bronchioles, where the total cross-sectional area is great, the forward velocity of bulk air flow is negligible, and **gas diffusion** becomes the predominant process. The distance from the terminal bronchiole to alveolar sacs is small (5 mm), so the time required to equilibrate alveolar gas with inspired air is also small (less than 1 second). However, low air velocity in the terminal portions of the conducting zone causes suspended particles such as dust and asbestos to be deposited there.

Gas-Exchange Interface

The pulmonary capillaries are extremely short and heavily interconnected, effectively presenting a sheet of blood to the alveolar wall for gas exchange. There are approximately 250 to 300 billion pulmonary capillaries in the lung, or about a thousand capillaries per alveolus. Each capillary also makes contact with several alveoli (being sandwiched between them), thereby taking maximum advantage of the large available surface area. Alveolar gas must cross **six layers** to enter erythrocytes in pulmonary capillaries. These are (1) a fluid layer containing surfactant (see Chap. 31) on the inner surface of the alveolus, (2) the alveolar epithelium, (3) an interstitial space filled with fluid, (4) the capillary endothelium, (5) plasma in the capillaries, and (6) the erythrocyte membrane. The first four layers (the so-called alveolar-capillary barrier) collectively average 0.5 μm in thickness.

The fluid-filled interstitial space is in contact with **lymphatics,** thereby furnishing a conduit for draining interstitial fluid from the lung. This drainage helps to keep the alveoli dry. Although a general widening of the interstitial space, either by fibrosis (due to such agents as asbestos and coal dust) or interstitial edema, can, theoretically, reduce diffusional gas exchange, thickening of the interstitial space is generally not considered clinically important in reducing gas diffusion across the alveolar-capillary barrier.

Lung Volumes and Capacities

An understanding of the various volumes and capacities (the sum of two or more volumes) that are used to describe lung function is integral to a discussion of pulmonary physiology (Fig. 30-2A). Measurable physiologic lung volumes and capacities can provide an index of pulmonary function but are arbitrarily defined and differ among individuals according to age, body type, conditioning, and gender. Consequently, these volumes are not necessarily of diagnostic value but can aid in differentiating between the two major types of lung disorders — obstructive and restrictive — and in quantifying the extent of the abnormality. All lung volumes, capacities, and ventilations are expressed as BTPS (body temperature, ambient pressure, saturated with water vapor). All gas volumes in blood (e.g., oxygen consumption and carbon dioxide production) are expressed as STPD (standard temperature and pressure, dry gas). Ventilation and gas volumes in blood are covered in Chap. 32.

The **total lung capacity** (TLC) is the total volume of air in the lungs when they are maximally inflated. The **residual volume** (RV) represents the volume of air left in the lungs after a maximal expiration, that is, the lungs do not empty to a completely airless state on exhalation. The RV differs with age and gender. In young adults, the RV accounts for approximately 20% of the TLC, increasing in older individuals to about 30%. These age-related changes stem from alterations in the elastic recoil of the lung and mobility of the chest wall.

The **vital capacity** (VC) is the maximum volume of air that can be exhaled after a maximal inspiration. The VC constitutes 80% of the TLC and has three components. The first is the **tidal volume** (VT), which is that volume of air inspired and expired with each normal breath. VT can increase during exercise to approach the VC. During normal breathing, VT is approximately 500 ml. The second component of VC is the **inspiratory reserve volume** (IRV). This is the quantity of air that can be inhaled into the lungs from a normal end-tidal inspiratory position. The third component is the **expiratory reserve volume** (ERV), which is the amount of air that can be exhaled from the lungs from a normal end-tidal expiratory position. Both the IRV and ERV decrease as the VT increases and approaches the VC; in other words, the VT increases at the expense of the IRV and ERV.

The **functional residual capacity** (FRC) is that volume of air in the lungs at the end of a normal expiration, that is, the FRC is the resting volume of the lung and is the sum of RV and ERV (see Fig. 30-2A). At the FRC, the inward elastic recoil of the lung is in equilibrium with the outward elastic recoil of the chest wall.

The FRC, like some of the other lung volumes and capacities, can differ with age, gender, and body type. However, these lung volumes and capacities also can be considerably affected by mechanical problems that alter the elastic recoil properties of the lung (restrictive lung diseases) or by conditions that block the airways (obstructive lung diseases). Conditions that limit the mobility of the chest wall also can affect the lung volumes and capacities. Asthma is an example of **obstructive disease.** This disorder is caused by a narrowing of the airways due to spasm of the bronchial smooth muscle, bronchial wall edema, or increased mucus production. Air is then trapped

Fig. 30-2. (A) Lung volumes and capacities. (B) Effects of obstructive lung disease (e.g., emphysema) on these lung volumes. (C) Effects of restrictive lung disease (e.g., pulmonary interstitial fibrosis) on these same lung volumes and capacities.

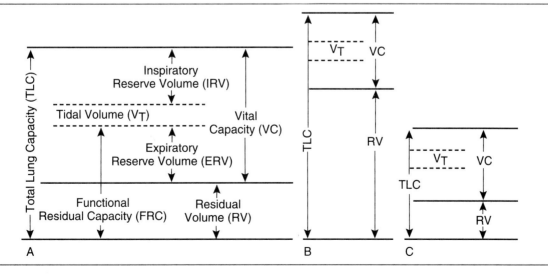

in the lungs distal to the obstruction, resulting in increased FRC, RV, and TLC but decreased VC (see Fig. 30-2B). Other obstructive lung diseases, such as emphysema and chronic bronchitis, also increase the resistance to air flow and can produce similar changes in the FRC, RV, TLC, and VC. Conversely, **restrictive lung disease,** such as pulmonary fibrosis, increase the "stiffness" of the lungs. Because these restrictive disorders augment lung elasticity (i.e., decrease lung compliance and increase lung recoil; see Chap 31), the lungs cannot expand normally and VC, TLC, FRC, and RV all decrease (see Fig. 30-2C).

Respiratory Muscles

The respiratory muscles change the dimensions of the thoracic cavity, causing it to function as a pump. Changing the size of the thoracic cavity alters the dimensions of the lungs. Increasing the volume of the thoracic cavity increases the volume of the lungs, causing air to be inhaled. Reducing the volume of the thoracic cavity decreases the lung volume, causing air to be expelled.

Different muscles accomplish inspiration and expiration. The most important **inspiratory muscle** is the **diaphragm,** which is innervated by the phrenic nerve. Contraction of the diaphragm enlarges the vertical dimension of the thoracic cavity by pushing the abdominal contents down and increases the transverse dimension by pushing the margins of the ribs laterally. Contraction of the **external intercostals** stiffens the chest wall and prevents these muscles from being pulled inward during inspiration, thereby reducing the dimensions of the thoracic cavity. During exercise and hyperventilation, the **accessory muscles of inspiration** are also recruited. These include the **scalene** and **sternomastoid muscles,** both of which enlarge the thoracic cavity by elevating the sternum.

At rest or even during moderate exercise, expiration is a **passive** event, mediated by the return of the diaphragm to its relaxed position and by the elastic recoil of the lungs. With increased levels of ventilation, expiration becomes active and involves the muscles associated with expiration. The **abdominal musculature** (the rectus abdominis, the internal and external obliques, and the transverse abdominal) are the primary expiratory muscles. The **internal intercostals** are also active during forced expiration.

Summary

All metabolizing tissues require oxygen and produce carbon dioxide, and the respiratory system is responsible for their transport. There are a number of steps involved in the movement of oxygen from the air to the tissues and carbon dioxide from the tissues to the external environment. These include the movement of air into and out of the lungs, the matching of the pulmonary blood flow to ventilation, the neural control of ventilation, the movement of oxygen and carbon dioxide between the lungs and the pulmonary circulation, and the transport of respiratory gases between the lungs and tissues.

Bibliography

Cherniack, N. S., Altose, M. D., and Kelsen, S. G. The Respiratory System. In: Berne, R. M., and Levy, M. N., eds. Physiology. Sect. VI, St. Louis: C. V. Mosby, 1983.

Comroe, J. H. *Physiology of Respiration,* 2nd ed. Chicago: Year Book Medical Publishers, 1974.

Levitzky, M. G. *Pulmonary Physiology,* 4th ed. New York: McGraw-Hill, 1995.

Mines, A. H. *Respiratory Physiology,* 2nd ed. New York: Raven Press, 1986.

Taylor, A. E., Rehder, K., Hyatt, R. E., and Parker, J. C. *Clincial Respiratory Physiology.* Philadelphia: W. B. Saunders, 1989.

West, J. B. *Respiratory Physiology,* 5th ed. Baltimore: Williams & Wilkins, 1995.

31 Mechanics of Respiration

Douglas K. Anderson

Objectives

After reading this chapter, you should be able to

Define and discuss the relationships among the pressures responsible for the movement of air into and out of the lungs

Describe the pressure-volume changes in one respiratory cycle

Define the "resistances" to ventilation, that is, those forces that oppose lung expansion and air flow

Define and discuss the factors that affect lung compliance

Define and understand the determinants of air flow resistance

The mechanics of breathing encompass those factors that influence lung elasticity and air flow. They require an understanding of the pressures exerted to overcome the elastic recoil of the lungs and chest wall and the resistance to air flow that together effect volume changes in the lungs. Elastic properties of the lung and chest wall are termed **static** because they are defined during periods of zero air flow. The properties of airway resistance are studied during periods of air flow and are therefore called **dynamic.**

Pressures

For air to move into and out of the lungs, a pressure gradient between the alveoli and the atmosphere must be created. The **atmospheric,** or barometric, **pressure** exists at the nose and mouth and by convention is defined as **0 cmH$_2$O. Alveolar pressure** is the pressure in the alveoli. When there is no air flow, the alveolar pressure equals the atmospheric pressure, or 0 cmH$_2$O. When the aveolar pressure falls below the atmospheric pressure, a **pressure gradient,** extending from the atmosphere to the alveoli, is created, and air moves into the lungs. Conversely, when the alveolar pressure exceeds the atmospheric pressure, the

pressure gradient travels from the alveoli to the atmosphere, and air flows out of the lungs. The pressure that establishes these gradients is the **intrapleural pressure,** which is inside the thoracic cavity but surrounding the lungs in the thin, serous fluid–filled space between the parietal and visceral pleura. The cohesive forces of the fluid molecules cause the two pleural surfaces to adhere to each other. At rest, the lungs are partially inflated and, because of their elastic nature, tend to collapse. The chest wall is drawn inward and, because it also has elastic properties, tends to recoil outward. Because pressure is equal to the force per unit area, these opposing forces act on the pleural surfaces to produce a subatmospheric intrapleural pressure which averages between –3 and – 5 cmH$_2$O at rest. The intrapleural pressure becomes more subatmospheric as the forces trying to pull the two pleural layers apart increase. Because the alveolar pressure always exceeds the pressure in the intrapleural space, the lungs tend to expand into this region of lower pressure. It is this subatmospheric intrapleural pressure that keeps the lungs inflated. Stated differently, the **transpulmonary pressure** (here defined as the transmural pressure across the alveolar wall, which is equal to the difference between the alveolar and intrapleural pressures) is the distending pressure of the alveoli. As long as the intrapleural pressure is less than the alveolar pressure, the alveoli will be partially inflated. When the transpulmonary pressure is increased by making the intrapleural pressure more subatmospheric (or by raising alveolar pressure), the alveoli expand further and their volume increases.

Pressure-Volume Relationships During One Inspiration-Expiration Cycle

Figure 31-1 illustrates the volume, pressure, and air flow changes that take place during a normal quiet breath. The tidal volume (VT), air flow, and intrapleural pressure are all measured directly. Alveolar pressure can only be calculated. The intrapleural pressure can be measured with a pressure-sensitive balloon transducer passed into the esophagus.

At the end of expiration and just before the start of inspiration, air flow is zero because there is no driving pressure (i.e., the atmospheric pressure equals the alveolar pressure, which by definition is 0 cmH$_2$O). Intrapleural pressure is subatmospheric, averaging 5 cmH$_2$O (actually –5 cmH$_2$O) below atmospheric pressure.

Inspiration is initiated when the inspiratory muscles (primarily the diaphragm) contract and thus enlarge the thoracic cavity. With the increasing throacic volume, the intrapleural pressure becomes more subatmospheric, and the lungs expand. With this increased lung volume, alveolar pressure decreases and becomes subatmospheric (–1 to –2 cmH$_2$O), causing air to flow into the lungs down this pressure gradient. Air continues to fill the lungs until the alveolar pressure again equals the atmospheric pressure. At this point, air flow ceases, inspiration ends, and the volume of air that has entered the lungs is the VT.

When inspiration terminates, the diaphragm relaxes and the lungs recoil. As they recoil, the intrapleural pressure becomes less subatmospheric, and lung volume is reduced such that it returns toward the **functional residual capacity** (FRC), or resting volume. This decreased lung volume compresses the alveolar gas, causing alveolar pressure to exceed the atmospheric pressure, which causes air to flow down this gradient from the lungs to the atmosphere. When the alveolar pressure again equals the atmospheric pressure (when the VT has been removed from the lungs), air flow ceases, expiration ends, and the cycle is repeated.

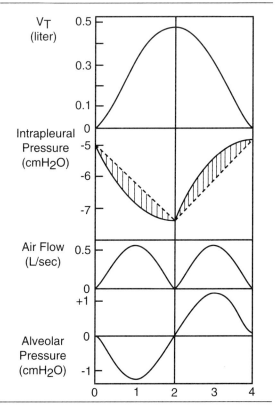

Fig. 31-1. Pressure, volume, and air flow changes in one inspiration-expiration (breathing) cycle (VT = tidal volume). (Modified from: Comroe, J. H. *Physiology of Respiration* 2nd ed. Chicago: Year Book Medical Publishers, 1974. P. 102.)

Resistances to Ventilation

Certain factors oppose lung expansion and air flow. These consist of the **elastic recoil** properties of the lung (which include surface tension forces), the **resistance to air flow** produced when air moves through the airways, and **tissue resistance.** Of the three, tissue resistance (which is caused primarily by the sliding of the lung tissues over each other as the lungs inflate and deflate) is minor and will not be considered in this discussion.

Figure 31-1 describes two pathways by which **intrapleural pressure** is changed during a normal breathing cycle. The dashed line shows the course intrapleural pressure would take if there were no air flow. This is the pressure change necessary for overcoming the elastic recoil forces of the lung only. The solid line describes the changes in intrapleural pressure during air flow. This line diverges from the dashed line because it is the sum of the pressure changes needed to overcome both the lung elastic recoil and the resistance to air flow. Thus the difference between the two lines is the pressure change required to overcome the air flow resistance. The remainder of this chapter concentrates on the factors that produce the elastic properties of the lungs and that contribute to or change the resistance to air flow. These concepts are important because most lung disorders involve changes in lung elasticity or air flow.

Compliance

Compliance is defined as a unit change in the lung volume per the unit change in pressure, expressed as liters per centimeter of water, and is an index of the "expandability" of the lungs. This calculation is termed **static compliance** if the pressure and volume measurements are made when there is no air flow. An increase in the volume change per unit change in pressure indicates **increased lung compliance.** This results from reduced lung elasticity or elastic recoil and means the lungs are easier to inflate. A decrease in the volume change per change in pressure indicates **reduced lung compliance.** This means the lungs are "stiffer," in that they display increased elasticity or elastic recoil and are harder to inflate. Thus compliance is the inverse of elasticity or elastic recoil.

Pressure-Volume (Compliance) Curve of Excised Lungs

The pressure-volume relationship of the lung can be demonstrated in lungs in vitro (Fig. 31-2). By measuring the change in volume that occurs with each change in pressure, compliance curves like those in Fig. 31-2 can be generated. There are several important features of these curves. Even though the lungs have been removed from the body, they are not airless — a small volume of **minimal air** remains. Starting at this point of maximum deflation, increasing the pressure inside the lungs (or decreasing the pressure around the lungs) causes the lung volume to increase. This is not a linear increase but is S-shaped. At a very low lung volume, compliance is low, such that it takes a relatively large change in pressure to achieve a change in volume. This occurs because, at this low volume, most of the alveoli in these excised lungs

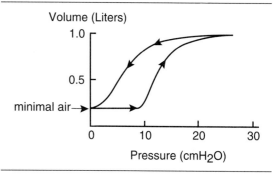

Fig. 31-2. Pressure-volume (compliance) curve of air-inflated excised lungs. Direction of *arrowheads* indicates inflation and deflation curves. (Modified from: West, J. B. *Respiratory Physiology* 5th ed. Baltimore: Williams & Wilkins, 1995. P. 92.)

have collapsed and the cohesive forces at the liquid-liquid interface in these alveoli must be overcome. Thus the initial pressure is expended in opening these closed alveoli, without a substantial change in volume.

Once open, the lungs distend easily. Between 5 and 20 cmH_2O, there is a relatively large change in the volume per unit change in pressure, indicating that the lungs are quite compliant over this pressure range. Above 20 cmH_2O, however, compliance again declines, because at high lung volumes the maximum distensibility of the lung is being reached (the lung is near maximally stretched), and further increases in pressure will produce only small volume increases.

The deflation curve for excised lungs differs from the inflation curve. This **hysteresis loop** results primarily from changes in the surface tension at different lung volumes, which will be discussed later in this chapter.

Anything that changes the lung's elastic properties alters compliance. Figure 31-3 shows how various pathologic states affect compliance. (The curves in this figure correspond to the deflation curve in Fig. 31-2.) **Emphysema** is a condition in which lung tissue is lost. Consequently, the elasticity or elastic recoil of the lung is decreased, and the lungs become more distensible (compliance increases). The curve shifts to the left of normal. In **fibrosis,** connective tissue infiltrates the interstitial space. This makes the lung tissue stiffer, causing increased lung elasticity and decreased compliance. The curve shifts to the right of normal. Compliance is also reduced if the pulmonary vasculature becomes engorged with blood. This can result from increased pulmonary venous pressure due

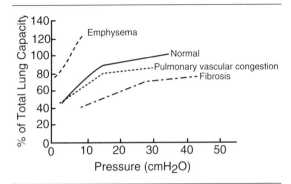

Fig. 31-3. Effects of disease on lung compliance.

to left-sided heart failure. In fact, any condition that decreases the distensibility of the lung, such as alveolar edema or atelectasis (collapsed alveoli), decreases compliance.

Regional Differences in Ventilation

Ventilation (the volume of air inspired and expired per unit time; see Chap. 32 for a more complete discussion) is not uniform throughout the lung. Rather, there is a continuum from the top to the bottom of the lung, with the lowest level of ventilation at the apex and the highest at the base. Thus more air per unit of time is brought into and removed from the lower lung than from the upper lung. This difference in ventilation is illustrated in Fig. 31-4.

Intrapleural pressure is not uniform around the lung because the lungs are suspended in the thoracic cavity, causing their full weight to be supported at the apex. Consequently, the forces tending to separate the parietal and visceral pleura are greater at the lung apex than at its base. As a result, intrapleural pressure increases from the top to the bottom of the lung. In other words, pressure in the intrapleural space is more subatmospheric at the apex of the lung than at its base. Because of this **intrapleural pressure gradient** from the apex to the base of the lung, there is a corresponding transpulmonary pressure gradient. The higher transpulmonary pressure at the apex of the lung causes the alveoli in this region to be more expanded than those at the base. Thus, for a given change in the intrapleural pressure, the alveoli on or near the upper flat portion of the compliance curve (those which are near the top of the lung) will distend less than the alveoli toward the base of the lung, which are on the steep part of the compliance curve. Consequently, over time, more gas is

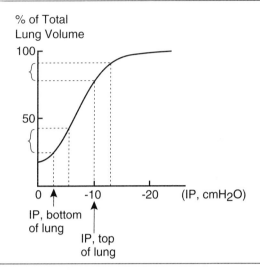

Fig. 31-4. The source of differences in ventilation from the apex to the base of the lung (IP = intrapleural pressure).

moved into and out of the alveoli at the base of the lung than at the apex.

Specific Compliance

To determine if changes in compliance are due to alterations in the elastic properties of the lung and not in the size or volume of the lung, compliance must be normalized to some lung volume that generally approximates the FRC. A person with a normal compliance of 0.2 liter/cmH_2O and FRC of 2.5 liters would have a specific compliance of 0.08 per cmH_2O. **Specific compliance** is relatively consistent across species and normal individuals with widely different lung sizes but changes in disease states that affect the elastic properties of the lungs.

Pressure-Volume (Compliance) Curve of the Lungs and Chest Wall

As mentioned earlier in this chapter, both the lungs and chest wall have elastic properties. Normally, the elastic recoil forces of the lungs and chest wall oppose each other, in that the lungs are inflated and recoil inward toward their equilibrium or resting position while the chest wall is pulled inward and recoils out toward its equilibrium position. Indeed, when the intrapleural space is opened to the atmosphere (pneumothorax) and the intrapleural pressure equals the atmospheric pressure, the lungs collapse and the chest wall springs outward.

The interaction between the lungs and chest wall over a wide range of volumes and pressures is demonstrated in Fig. 31-5. A **relaxation pressure curve** for the entire respiratory system (lungs and chest wall) can be generated if the airway pressure is measured at different lung volumes while the respiratory muscles are relaxed. If the intrapleural pressure is also measured, the individual recoil pressures of the lungs and chest wall can be calculated. Thus the relaxation pressure is the algebraic sum of the recoil pressures of the lung and chest wall.

If no external force is applied to the system (when the respiratory muscles are relaxed), the relaxation pressure is zero at the point when the inward recoil of the lungs is exactly counterbalanced by the outward recoil of the chest wall. This is the **resting respiratory position,** and the volume of air remaining in the lungs is the FRC. With inspiration, the lungs inflate and move away from their equilibrium position, whereas the chest wall moves toward its resting point. Consequently, during this portion of inspiration, the lung elastic forces are the only ones that the respiratory muscles need to overcome. When the chest wall reaches its resting position (at about 70% of vital capacity), the relaxation pressure is entirely due to the lung elastic recoil pressure. Above this point, the chest wall is beyond its equilibrium position, and the inspiratory muscles must then overcome the recoil of both the lungs and the chest wall. Thus **maximum inspiration** (and vital capacity) is determined by the strength of the inspiratory muscles in relation to the recoil forces of the lung and chest wall.

With **maximum expiration,** the lungs approach their resting position, and the relaxation pressure is created almost entirely by the elastic recoil pressure of the chest wall. At this point, there are minimal lung recoil forces, and the expiratory muscles have compressed the chest wall as far as possible from its equilibrium point. This is when the lungs contain minimal air.

If the elastic recoil of either the lungs or chest wall changes without a corresponding change in the other, the FRC is altered, and the relaxation pressure curve is shifted to either the left or right of normal. For example, with the loss of elastic tissue in **emphysema,** there is diminished elastic recoil force in the lungs without an accompanying loss of recoil in the chest wall. Thus the lungs are more compliant and distended (FRC is increased), and the relaxation pressure curve is shifted to the left. Conversely, in **pulmonary fibrosis,** the elastic recoil force of the lungs, but not of the chest wall, is increased. This causes the lung compliance or distensibility to be decreased. Consequently, the FRC is decreased and the relaxation pressure curve is shifted to the right.

Surface Tension

Figure 31-6 depicts the surface tension created when a liquid (such as water) is exposed to air. The open circles represent water molecules, and the solid squares are gas molecules. In liquid, the molecular attracting forces acting on each individual water molecule are equal in all directions (see Fig. 31-6A). At the air-water interface, however, the water molecules beneath the surface exert stronger attracting forces on the surface water molecules than do the gas molecules (see Fig. 31-6B). Thus there are stronger forces pulling the surface water molecules down than there are pulling them up. As a result of this imbalance of attractive forces, the surface shrinks to its smallest possible area. The resulting force between the surface molecules is the **surface tension.**

There is a thin film of fluid that lines the alveoli. Because this alveolar fluid has an air interface, it creates a surface tension. This surface tension of the alveolar fluid–air interface is depicted in Fig. 31-7. Both the elastic recoil forces and the surface tension forces tend to collapse the alveolus. Thus alveolar size is determined by the alveo-

Fig. 31-5. Pressure-volume curves of the lung and chest wall. The relaxation pressure is the algebraic sum of the recoil pressures of the lungs and chest wall. (Modified from: Slonim, N. B., and Hamilton, L. H. *Respiratory Physiology* 2nd ed. St. Louis: Mosby, 1971. P. 52.)

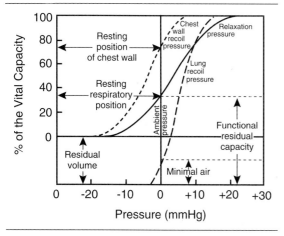

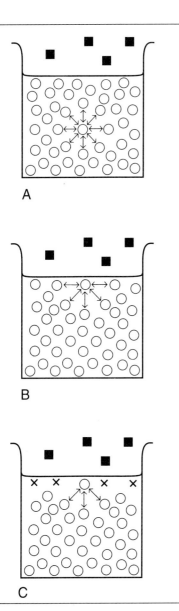

A

B

C

Fig. 31-6. Schematic depiction of the concept of surface tension. The *open circles* represent water molecules; the *closed squares* represent air molecules; and the *x*'s represent surface active or surfactant molecules. (A) The molecular forces acting on each water molecule are equal in all directions. (B) The air-water interface. (C) Action of surfactant molecules. (Modified from: Conroe, J. H. *Physiology of Respiration* 2nd ed. Chicago: Year Book Medical Publishers, 1974. P. 107.)

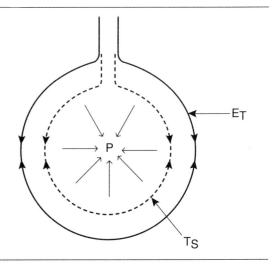

Fig. 31-7. The forces acting at the alveolar liquid–air interface (E_T = tissue tension; T_S = surface tension; and P = intraalveolar pressure). *Arrowheads* indicate the direction of the forces. (Modified from: Levitzky, M. G. *Pulmonary Physiology* 4th ed. New York: McGraw-Hill, 1995. P. 26.)

lar pressure (which expands the alveolus) that balances the sum of the elastic recoil and surface tension forces.

As indicated previously, surface tension plays a major role in the overall **compliance** of the lungs. The contribution of surface tension to lung compliance can be seen when the pressure-volume (compliance) curves in air (see Fig. 31-2) are contrasted with those from the saline-inflated lungs (Fig. 31-8). When filled with air, the lungs' inflation curve differs from their deflation curve (a hysteresis loop) (see Fig. 31-2). When inflated with saline, hysteresis is abolished, and the lungs have much greater compliance than when they are inflated with air (see Fig. 31-8). When the lungs are filled with saline, the air-liquid interface is eliminated, and this abolishes the surface tension forces. This leaves elastic recoil as the only force opposing lung distension and demonstrates that surface tension constitutes a substantial portion of the total recoil force of the lung.

Pulmonary Surfactant

Surfactants are surface-active molecules that reduce surface tension forces in the lung. These molecules accumulate on the surface of the alveolar fluid and interdigitate between the water molecules (see Fig. 31-6C). This separates the surface water molecules and reduces the attractive forces between them, thus decreasing surface tension.

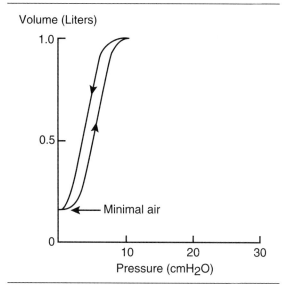

Volume (Liters)

Pressure (cmH2O)

Fig. 31-8. Pressure-volume (compliance) curve for saline-inflated excised lungs. (Compare with Fig. 33-2.) (Modified from: West, J. B. *Respiratory Physiology* 5th ed. Baltimore: Williams & Wilkins, 1995. P. 95.)

Characteristics of Pulmonary Surfactant

Surfactant is a complex phospholipid that is a combination of a dipalmitoyl phosphatidylcholine (DPPC) and other lipids and proteins. It is formed in type II alveolar cells and is rapidly synthesized and turned over. DPPC has two long-chain saturated fatty acids (palmitate) esterified to the first and second carbons of a glycerol molecule. A choline base is located on the third glycerol carbon. The fatty acids are nonpolar and hydrophobic, whereas the charged choline base is polar and hydrophylic. Thus DPPC orients perpendicularly to the air-water interface such that the polar end is dissolved in the water and the nonpolar fatty acids project toward the alveolar lumen (Fig. 31-9).

Physiologic Importance of Pulmonary Surfactant

Surfactant lowers the surface tension in the alveoli, thereby increasing lung compliance. This reduces the effort needed to expand the lungs with each breath.

Surfactant also promotes the stability of alveoli and helps keep them from collapsing. The lung is a collection of 300 million basically spherical alveoli of different sizes, all communicating with each other. There is little variation

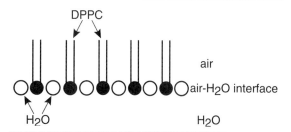

Fig. 31-9. The air-water interface in the presence of molecules of the surfactant dipalmitoyl phosphatidylcholine (DPPC).

in alveolar pressure throughout the lung, meaning that the pressure is essentially the same in all open and functioning alveoli. According to the law of Laplace, the distending pressure in a sphere is equal to 2T/r, where T is the wall tension and r is the radius of the sphere. Thus, if wall tension remains constant, the distending pressure increases if the radius decreases, and vice versa. When this law is applied to alveoli, the wall tension is the tension in the wall of an alveolus (the sum of elastic and surface tension; see Fig. 31-7), and the radius is the alveolar radius. Because the distending pressure is essentially the same in the millions of alveoli of different radii, the wall tension must change commensurate with the change in radius; otherwise, small alveoli will empty into larger alveoli and then collapse. Surfactant is responsible for changing the alveolar wall tension. When the radius is small (during expiration), surfactant molecules are packed tightly together, widely separating the water molecules and reducing the wall tension. When the radius is large, the surfactant molecules are scattered, allowing the water molecules greater access to each other and thereby increasing the alveolar wall tension.

Surfactant helps keep the alveoli dry. Surface tension also tends to draw fluid into the alveoli, causing alveolar edema. Because surfactant reduces the surface tension forces, the affinity for fluid to move into the alveoli is diminished.

Resistance to Air Flow

As discussed previously, two primary factors must be overcome in order to move air into and out of the lungs: the elastic recoil forces of the lungs and chest wall and airway resistance. Of the two, airway resistance is the most important. The factors governing air flow through the airways are the same as those regulating the flow of any fluid through tubes.

Physical Factors Determining the Resistance to Air Flow

As noted in Chap. 25, there are two primary types of air flow in the airways: laminar and turbulent. In **laminar flow,** the stream lines travel parallel to the side of the tubes. Laminar flow occurs in all airways whenever air flow is low, but generally it is limited to the smaller airways because air flow in these regions is usually low. In **turbulent flow,** the flow in the stream lines is agitated. Turbulent flow can develop at the branch points of airways or when there are irregularities in the airways caused by mucus, tumors, or foreign bodies, even at low flow rates. The flow in the larger airways is also turbulent when air flow velocity is elevated.

Laminar flow through straight, smooth tubes is governed by **Poiseuille's law,** as described in Chap. 25. Thus the airway radius is the most important determinant of the resistance to air flow. For example, halving the radius increased resistance 16-fold, but doubling the length of the airway only doubles airway resistance.

Turbulent flow alters the relationship between the driving pressure, resistance, and air flow. When air flow becomes turbulent, the driving pressure has to increase (by the square of the flow) in order to maintain air flow constant. Thus

$$P = V^2R \qquad (31\text{-}1)$$

where P is the pressure difference (the driving pressure), V is the air flow, and R is the resistance.

For much of the tracheobronchial tree, air flow is **transitional,** in that there is a combination of turbulent and laminar flows. Thus, for transitional flow,

$$P = VR_1 + V^2R_2 \qquad (31\text{-}2)$$

For normal individuals, the second (turbulent) component is relatively small during quiet breathing and Eq. 31-2 reduces to

$$P = VR_1 \qquad (31\text{-}3)$$

Principal Sites of Airway Resistance

Total airway resistance is the sum of the resistances from the nose and mouth and from the tracheobronchial tree. The nose and mouth account for a substantial portion of total airway resistance.

For the tracheobronchial tree, the total cross-sectional area of the airways increases from the larger to the smaller airways, even though the individual radii are decreasing (Fig. 31-10). The chief site of airway resistance in the tracheobronchial tree is at the medium-sized segmental bronchi, where the radius of the individual bronchi is decreased but the total cross-sectional area is not yet substantially increased. The least resistance to air flow is in the very small and numerous terminal bronchioles, with their tiny individual radii but enormous cross-sectional area.

Determinants of Airway Resistance

Lung Volume

When lung volumes increase, airway resistance decreases (Fig. 31-11). Lung volume modifies airway resistance in two ways. First, lung tissue is tethered to the airways. With increasing lung volume, the **airways are "pulled open,"** thereby decreasing resistance. Second, increasing the lung volume elevates the **transmural pressure** across the airways, and this increases their radii and decreases resistance. Thus, because lung volume is greater at the apex than at the base of the lung (see Fig. 31-4), airway caliber

Fig. 31-10. Airway resistance (*solid circles*) and total cross-sectional area (*solid line*) plotted as a function of airways branch number. Airway resistance decreases and the total cross-sectional area of the airways increases going from the trachea to the smaller airways. (Modified from: West, J. B. *Respiratory Physiology* 5th ed. Baltimore: Williams & Wilkins, 1995. P. 107.)

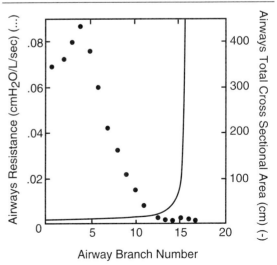

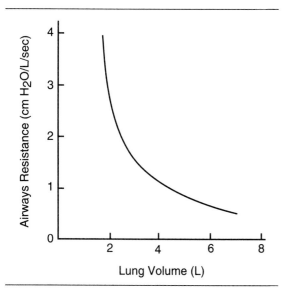

Fig. 31-11. Airway resistance plotted as a function of lung volume. Resistance decreases as lung volume increases. (Modified from: West, J. B. *Respiratory Physiology* 5th ed. Baltimore: Williams & Wilkins, 1995. P. 109.)

is larger at the top than at the bottom of the lung, causing airway resistance to increase progressively from the top to the base of the lung.

Bronchial Smooth Muscle

Airways from the trachea down to the alveolar ducts are supplied with smooth muscle, which is controlled by the autonomic nervous system. **Adrenergic sympathetic** activity or sympathomimetic compounds relax bronchial smooth muscle, whereas **cholinergic parasympathetic** activity or parasympathomimetic agents constrict bronchial smooth muscle. This is the opposite of what takes place in vascular smooth muscle, because beta$_2$ receptors (adrenergic receptors that mediate smooth muscle relaxation) predominate in bronchial smooth muscle.

Irritants such as smoke and dust and certain chemicals such as histamine can cause **reflex constriction** of the airways. These substances may stimulate the **rapidly adapting receptors** in the airways. In addition, emboli that lodge in the pulmonary circulation will cause airways in the poorly perfused areas to constrict. This appears to be a direct effect of decreased alveolar carbon dioxide tension on the smooth muscle of airways and may be one mechanism involved in balancing ventilation and perfusion (see Chap. 35).

Summary

To move air into and out of the lungs, pressures must be generated that overcome the elastic recoil of the lungs and chest wall as well as the resistance to air flow. Atmospheric, alveolar, and intrapleural pressures are the important pressures in creating air flow. The distensibility of the lungs is defined in terms of changes in volume per unit change in pressure and is called compliance. Lung compliance also includes surface tension forces. Surface tension is reduced and varied in the lung through the influence of surfactant, a surface active molecule which is a complex phospholipid. Resistance to air flow is determined by the pressure difference divided by the air flow. The radii of the individual airways decrease going from the larger to the smaller airways, but the total cross-sectional area of the tracheobronchial tree increases. Consequently, the least resistance to air flow is generated in the terminal bronchioles and the greatest air flow resistance in the tracheobronchial tree arises in the medium-sized segmental bronchi. The caliber and, hence, resistance of the airways can be determined passively by changes in lung volume and actively by changes in the autonomic activity to the smooth muscle of the airways.

Bibliography

Cherniack, N. S., Altose, M. D., and Kelsen, S. G. The Respiratory System. In: Berne, R. M., and Levy, M. N., eds. Physiology, Sect. VI. St. Louis: C. V. Mosby, 1983.

Comroe, J. H. *Physiology of Respiration,* 2nd ed. Chicago: Year Book Medical Publishers, 1974.

Levitzky, M. G. *Pulmonary Physiology,* 4th ed. New York: McGraw-Hill, 1995.

Mines, A. H. *Respiratory Physiology,* 2nd ed. New York: Raven Press, 1986.

Taylor, A. E., Rehder, K., Hyatt, R. E., and Parker, J. C. *Clinical Respiratory Physiology.* Philadelphia: W. B. Saunders, 1989.

West, J. B. *Respiratory Physiology,* 5th ed. Baltimore: Williams & Wilkins, 1995.

32 Ventilation, Gas Exchange, and Transport

Douglas K. Anderson

Objectives

After reading this chapter, you should be able to

Describe the basic properties of gases

Define minute ventilation, alveolar ventilation, and dead space

Describe the relationship among alveolar ventilation, alveolar oxygen and carbon dioxide partial pressures, oxygen consumption, and carbon dioxide production

Explain the source of the simplified alveolar gas equation

Describe the factors that govern the diffusion of gases through the alveolar-capillary membrane

Discuss the equilibration times for oxygen and carbon dioxide across the alveolar-capillary membrane

Discuss the factors responsible for the transport of oxygen by the blood

Define oxygen content and capacity and oxyhemoglobin saturation

Define the reasons for the shape of the oxyhemoglobin dissociation curve, and discuss its physiologic significance

Delineate the mechanisms that control carbon dioxide transport by the blood, and describe the carbon dioxide dissociation curves for whole blood

---

The principal function of the lung and chest wall system is the conveyance of air to the alveolar-capillary interface to supply oxygen to and remove carbon dioxide from the pulmonary capillary blood. Ventilation responds to changes in the metabolic demand of the body and the environmental gas composition and pressure. O_2 and CO_2 movement across the alveolar-capillary barrier is accomplished by diffusion and is governed by **Fick's law.** In the blood, O_2 is transported to the tissues attached primarily to hemoglobin, whereas CO_2 is returned to the lungs principally in the form of bicarbonate. The entire process and mechanisms responsible for moving O_2 from the air to the tissues and CO_2 from the tissues to the atmosphere is the topic of this chapter. Preliminary to this, the behavior of individual gases, mixtures of gases, and gases in liquid will be summarized.

Properties of Gases

The factors that determine the pressure of a gas are described by the **general gas law:**

$$P = nRT / V \qquad (32\text{-}1)$$

where P represents pressure, V is volume, n is the number of gas molecules, R is the gas constant, and T is temperature. Thus pressure is directly related to temperature and inversely related to volume. This means that at a constant volume, if temperature is raised, pressure increases. Further, if the volume containing the gas is increased at a constant temperature, the pressure falls.

Dalton's law states that the partial pressure of a single gas (P_g) in a mixture of gases is equal to the product of the total pressure (Pτ) and the mole fraction (f_g) of the single gas (i.e., the fraction of the total number of gas molecules that are molecules of the single gas).

$$P_g = P\tau \times f_g \qquad (32\text{-}2)$$

For example, the pressure of dry air at sea level (P_{ATM}) is 760 mmHg, and O_2 (fo_2) constitutes 20.95 percent of this. Thus the partial pressure of O_2 (Po_2) at sea level is

$$Po_2 = P_{ATM} \times fo_2$$
$$Po_2 = (760)(0.2095)$$
$$Po_2 = 159 \text{ mmHg}$$

In a mixture of gases, the total pressure of the mixture (P_T) is equal to the sum of the partial pressures of the individual gases composing the mixture:

$$P_T = P_1 + P_2 + P_3 + \ldots \qquad (32\text{-}3)$$

Each gas acts as if the others did not exist.

Air is a mixture of gases, including nitrogen, O_2, CO_2, and certain inert (I) gases. Thus, for air,

$$P_{ATM} = PN_2 + PO_2 + PCO_2 + PI \qquad (32\text{-}4)$$

The preceding applies to **dry** gas mixtures. Inspired atmospheric air is warmed and humidified as it passes through the nose and mouth. The water vapor pressure (PH_2O) of a saturated gas varies with temperature. At body temperature, PH_2O is 47 mmHg. Because water vapor is a gas and exerts a partial pressure, the partial pressure of inspired gases in the airways is

$$P_{ATM} = PN_2 + PO_2 + PCO_2 + PH_2O + PI \qquad (32\text{-}5)$$

Thus the Po_2 of inspired air (PIO_2) in the airway is

$$PIO_2 = (P_{ATM} - PH_2O) \times fO_2$$
$$PIO_2 = (760 - 47)(0.2095)$$
$$PIO_2 = (713)(0.2095)$$
$$PIO_2 = 149 \text{ mmHg}$$

Thus the Po_2 has been reduced by approximately 6%, which equals the amount of water vapor added to the inspired air at the nose and mouth. The partial pressures of the other gases are also lessened by the partial pressure of water vapor, so that the sum of the partial pressures of all

the gases that make up the inspired air does not exceed P_{ATM}.

As one ascends to higher altitudes, P_{ATM} declines, but the proportions of the gases that make up air do not change. For example, if P_{ATM} is 349 mmHg at 20,000 ft (6000 m) above sea level, then

$$Po_2 = (349 - 47)(0.2095)$$
$$Po_2 = 63 \text{ mmHg}$$

When a gas (such as O_2 or CO_2) is exposed to a liquid, it will dissolve in that liquid. The amount or concentration of gas (C_g) dissolved is the product of the partial pressure of the gas (P_g) in the gas phase and the solubility of the gas (S) in the liquid such that

$$C_g = P_g \times S \qquad (32\text{-}6)$$

At equilibrium, the partial pressure of a gas in a liquid equals its partial pressure in a gas mixture that is exposed to the liquid. The amount of gas dissolved in a liquid depends not only on its partial pressure but also on its solubility. Thus, if a gas is very soluble, its concentration in a liquid may be high even though its partial pressure is low. For two gases with the same partial pressure, the one with the greatest solubility will be the most concentrated in the liquid. CO_2 is about 24-fold more soluble in water than O_2. Thus, at any given partial pressure, about 24 times more CO_2 than O_2 will be dissolved.

Some **important pressures** (given in millimeters mercury) are alveolar O_2 (PAO_2), 100 to 105; pulmonary vein O_2 (systemic arterial, PaO_2), 95 to 100; alveolar CO_2 ($PACO_2$), 40; pulmonary vein CO_2 (systemic arterial, $PaCO_2$) 40; inspired Po_2, 152; pulmonary artery O_2 (systemic vein), 40; inspired Pco_2, 0.3; pulmonary artery CO_2 (systemic vein), 45; expired Po_2, 120; tissue Po_2, 40 or less; expired Pco_2, 32; and tissue Pco_2, 47 or more.

In the respiratory system, pressure is the driving force, and gases move down the pressure gradients. For O_2, the gradient is directed from the atmosphere to the tissues; for CO_2, the gradient is directed from the tissues to the atmosphere.

In the normal lung, the equilibrium of O_2 and CO_2 between each alveolus and its investing capillaries is very rapid and complete, in that the partial pressures in both the alveoli and capillaries are essentially the same. However, for the lung as a whole and for systemic arterial gas pressures, equilibrium is not complete (PAO_2 exceeds PaO_2 by about 5 to 8 mmHg). This is caused by physiologic ventilation-perfusion mismatching in the lung and arteriovenous shunts (e.g., nutrient circulation to the upper airways). (Ventilation-perfusion inequalities and shunting are discussed in Chap. 35.)

PaO_2 and $PaCO_2$ levels represent a balance between what comes into the lung in inspired air and what is removed (or added) from pulmonary capillary blood. The factors influencing the **levels of inspired gases** include the atmospheric pressure, the percentage of O_2 and CO_2 in the inspired air, and the level of alveolar ventilation ($\dot{V}A$). *(Note that the dot over the letter indicates some volume per unit time — a flow.)* Determinants of what is added or removed by the blood include the Po_2 and Pco_2 in blood (which are functions of the metabolic rate) and the rate or volume of the pulmonary blood flow ($\dot{Q}$). Normally these factors do not change singly but act in concert; for example, if metabolic rate is altered, so is $\dot{V}A$ and $\dot{Q}$. This maintains PaO_2 and $PaCO_2$ as close as possible to optimal values (100 and 40 mmHg, respectively) over a broad range of atmospheric pressures, PIO_2 levels, and degrees of physical activity.

Ventilation

As noted in Chap. 30, all lung volumes, capacities, and ventilation are expressed as BTPS (body temperature, ambient pressure, saturated with water vapor); gas volumes in blood are expressed as STPD (standard temperature and pressure, dry gas). **Ventilation** is the volume of gas that is inspired or expired per unit time. **Minute ventilation** ($\dot{V}E$) is the volume of gas inspired and expired per minute (in liters per minute, BTPS) and is the product of the tidal volume (VT) and the frequency of breathing (n):

$$\dot{V}E = VT \times n \qquad (32\text{-}7)$$

The VT is all the air that enters the lungs with each breath. It includes the volume of air that enters the alveoli (VA) and the air that remains in the conducting zone of the airways (where no gas is exchanged with pulmonary capillary blood), called the **anatomic dead space** (VD). In healthy individuals, VD is estimated to be equal to the body weight in pounds. Thus

$$VT = VD + VA \qquad (32\text{-}8)$$

The **physiologic dead space** is defined as any part of the lung that is ventilated but not perfused. This "wasted ventilation" (as it is more appropriately termed) increases in

certain pathologic conditions, such as pulmonary emboli. In normal individuals, the ratio of VD to VT is approximately 0.3. Like other lung volumes, respiratory dead space is expressed as BTPS.

Alveolar ventilation ($\dot{V}A$) is the volume of fresh gas that reaches the gas exchange zone (alveoli) each minute (liters per minute, BTPS). The $\dot{V}A$ is of key importance because it represents the amount of fresh inspired air that is available for gas exchange. $\dot{V}A$ equals the frequency of breathing times the difference between VT and VD. Thus the magnitude of $\dot{V}A$ depends on the VT, the VD, and the frequency of breathing:

$$\dot{V}A = (VT - VD) \times n \qquad (32\text{-}9)$$

Alveolar Ventilation, Carbon Dioxide, and Oxygen

The purpose of $\dot{V}A$ is to supply the O_2 removed from the blood by the tissues and to remove from the alveoli the CO_2 added to blood by the tissues. Thus $\dot{V}A$ matches O_2 intake with O_2 consumption ($\dot{V}O_2$), and CO_2 elimination with CO_2 production ($\dot{V}CO_2$) and, in the process, maintains alveolar and arterial blood gas levels essentially constant. Consequently, there is a relationship between the PaO_2, $\dot{V}O_2$, and $\dot{V}A$ as well as between $PaCO_2$, $\dot{V}CO_2$, and $\dot{V}A$. In all the following relationships, $\dot{V}O_2$ and $\dot{V}CO_2$ are expressed as STPD and $\dot{V}A$ as BTPS.

Carbon Dioxide

The relationship between $\dot{V}A$ and $PaCO_2$ is given by

$$PaCO_2 = PICO_2 + \dot{V}CO_2 / \dot{V}A \times K \qquad (32\text{-}10)$$

where K is a proportionality constant equal to 0.863 if $\dot{V}CO_2$ is at STPD and $\dot{V}A$ is expressed as BTPS. Because the partial pressure of inspired CO_2 ($PICO_2$) is essentially zero (approximately 0.3 mmHg at sea level), this term can be eliminated, reducing the equation to

$$PaCO_2 = \dot{V}CO_2 / \dot{V}A \times K \qquad (32\text{-}11)$$

At a constant $\dot{V}CO_2$ (200 ml/min), $PaCO_2$, and thus arterial Pco_2 ($PaCO_2$), varies inversely with $\dot{V}A$ (Fig. 32-1). Consequently, if $\dot{V}CO_2$ is unchanged, doubling $\dot{V}A$ will halve $PaCO_2$ and $PaCO_2$, and halving $\dot{V}A$ will double $PaCO_2$ and $PaCO_2$.

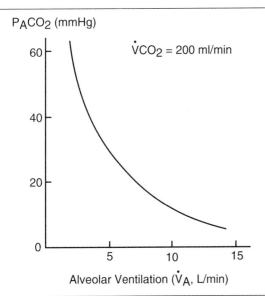

Fig. 32-1. Alveolar CO_2 tension ($PACO_2$) plotted as a function of alveolar ventilation ($\dot{V}A$) at a constant production of $\dot{V}CO_2$. As $\dot{V}A$ increases, $PACO_2$ declines. (Modified from: Cherniack, N. S., Altose, M. D., and Kelsen, S. G. The respiratory system. In: Berne, R. H., and Levy, M. N., eds., *Physiology*. St. Louis: Mosby, 1983. P. 685.)

Generally, $\dot{V}A$ and $\dot{V}CO_2$ do not change independently. Rather, an increase in metabolic rate accelerates $\dot{V}CO_2$. The excess CO_2 produced will stimulate the central and peripheral chemoreceptors (see Chap. 34 for details on respiration regulation). This causes $\dot{V}A$ to increase appropriately, resulting in a relatively constant $PACO_2$ and $PaCO_2$ over a broad range of activity (metabolic) levels.

Oxygen

The relationship for $\dot{V}A$ and PAO_2 is expressed as follows:

$$PAO_2 = PIO_2 - \dot{V}O_2 / \dot{V}A \times K \qquad (32\text{-}12)$$

where K is again 0.863. The PIO_2 is approximately 150 mmHg and, unlike $PICO_2$ cannot be ignored. At constant levels of $\dot{V}O_2$ (approximately 250 ml/min), both PAO_2 and arterial PO_2 (PaO_2) increase with increasing $\dot{V}A$ and approach the PIO_2 (Fig. 32-2). Again, the $\dot{V}A$ does not normally change in the face of a constant $\dot{V}O_2$ but is regulated to meet metabolic demands such that the PAO_2 and PaO_2 remain relatively unaltered over a wide metabolic range.

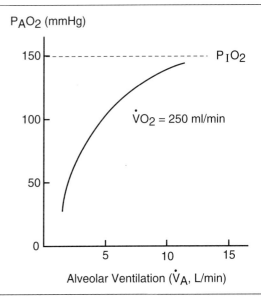

Fig. 32-2. Alveolar O_2 tension (PAO_2) plotted as a function of $\dot{V}A$ at a constant O_2 consumption ($\dot{V}O_2$). As $\dot{V}A$ increases, PAO_2 rises, approaching the level of inspired O_2. (Modified from: Cherniack, N. S., Altose, M. D., and Kelsen, S. G. The respiratory system. In: Berne, R. H., and Levy, M. N., eds., *Physiology*. St. Louis: Mosby, 1983. P. 686.)

Simplified Alveolar Gas Equation

Equations (32-11) and (32-12) can be combined to form the simplified alveolar gas equation:

$$PAO_2 = PIO_2 - PACO_2 / R + F \qquad (32\text{-}13)$$

where R is the respiratory exchange ratio (an index of the metabolic rate), equal to $\dot{V}CO_2/\dot{V}O_2$, and F is a correction factor of approximately 1 to 3 mmHg. In its complete form, the **alveolar gas equation** is expressed as

$$PAO_2 = PIO_2 - PACO_2(FIO_2 + 1 - FIO_2 / R) \qquad (32\text{-}14)$$

where FIO_2 (the fraction of inspired oxygen) is 0.2095. Equation (32-14) indicates that PAO_2 depends on PIO_2 and the respiratory exchange ratio. Also, at a given PIO_2 and a constant respiratory exchange ratio, PAO_2 and $PACO_2$ are inversely related. For example, if $\dot{V}A$ increases, PAO_2 will rise and $PACO_2$ will fall. **Alveolar hypoventilation** occurs when $\dot{V}A$ is less than what the metabolic rate requires. Thus $P_{A}O_2$ and $P_{a}O_2$ will decrease and $P_{A}CO_2$ and $P_{a}CO_2$ will increase. Conversely, **alveolar hyperventilation** arises when $\dot{V}A$ exceeds the metabolic demands. In this event, $P_{A}O_2$ and $P_{a}O_2$ increase and $P_{A}CO_2$ and $P_{a}CO_2$ decrease.

Gas Exchange (Diffusion)

Generally, $P_{a}O_2$ and $P_{a}CO_2$ can be used interchangeably with $P_{A}O_2$ and $P_{A}CO_2$, respectively, in the alveolar gas equation because of the rapid equilibration of O_2 and CO_2 across the alveolar-capillary barrier. These gases move between the alveoli and pulmonary capillary blood through the process of **diffusion.** This transfer of gases is governed by **Fick's law,** which states that the volume of gas ($\dot{V}_g$) transferred across the alveolar-capillary membrane per unit of time is **directly related** to the

1. Driving pressure across the alveolar-capillary membrane, that is, the difference in the partial pressure of the gas between the alveoli and capillary blood (P_A – P_C)
2. Area of the membrane (A)
3. Solubility (S) of the gas

and is **inversely related** to the

4. Length of the diffusion pathway (the thickness of the membrane [T])
5. Square root of the molecular weight (MW) of the gas.

Usually solubility and molecular weight are incorporated into a diffusion constant (D):

$$D \propto S / \sqrt{MW} \qquad (32\text{-}15)$$

The expression for Fick's law is then

$$V_g = A \times D \times (P_A - P_C)/T \qquad (32\text{-}16)$$

The solubility of CO_2 in water and its molecular weight are about 24 and 1.4 times greater than those for O_2, respectively. This combination causes the rate of CO_2 diffusion through both the tissue fluid and into the liquid surface to be about 20-fold higher than that of O_2.

As discussed previously, the lung is well designed to transfer gases between the alveoli and pulmonary capillary blood. There is a large surface area for gas exchange

(about 70 m²) that is primarily due to the subdivision of the lung into approximately 300 million alveoli. In addition, the diffusion pathway is short (averaging 0.5 μm), and there are transmembrane pressure gradients in the correct directions for movement of both O_2 and CO_2.

Transfer of gases across the alveolar-capillary barrier can be either diffusion or perfusion limited. A gas that does not equilibrate across the alveolar-capillary barrier, such that its partial pressure gradient is maintained when the blood is in transit through a pulmonary capillary, is said to be **diffusion limited.** Stated differently, the diffusion-limited transfer of a gas depends on the physical properties of the alveolar-capillary barrier (such as the thickness of the barrier and the area for gas exchange) and not on the blood flow rate in the pulmonary capillary. The movement of carbon monoxide across the alveolar-capillary barrier is diffusion limited.

Conversely, a gas that equilibrates rapidly across the alveolar-capillary barrier is **perfusion limited.** In this case, the partial pressure for the gas in the pulmonary capillary blood becomes virtually equal to that in the alveoli very soon after blood has entered the pulmonary capillary. Once its partial pressure gradient across the alveolar-capillary barrier is eliminated, no additional diffusion of this gas can occur during the remaining time blood is in transit through the pulmonary capillary. Thus the amount of this gas transferred depends on the blood flow and not on the diffusion properties of the alveolar-capillary barrier. Nitrous oxide is a gas that is perfusion limited.

Equilibration of Oxygen

Under normal conditions, O_2 transfer is **perfusion limited.** This is demonstrated in Fig. 32-3, which plots P_{O_2} in blood as a function of the blood transit time in a single pulmonary capillary. It takes blood an average of 0.75 second to traverse one pulmonary capillary. Curve A in Fig. 32-3 shows that under resting conditions, there is essentially complete equilibration between alveolar and capillary P_{O_2} once blood has passed only one-third of the way through the capillary. Thus the rate of blood flow through the capillary can be substantially increased, but essentially complete equilibration between capillary and alveolar P_{O_2} still takes place. For example, during heavy exercise, the increased cardiac output can reduce the capillary transit time by as much as threefold, to 0.25 second. This two-thirds reduction in the transit time does not appreciably alter the alveolar-capillary equilibration of O_2, and the end-capillary P_{O_2} will remain near resting levels. Thus, in normal

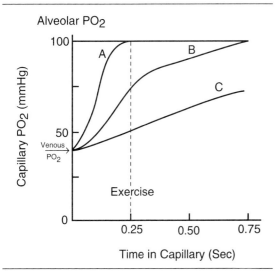

Fig. 32-3. Capillary partial pressure of O_2 (P_{O_2}) plotted as a function of the mean transit time for a red blood cell to pass through a pulmonary capillary. (A) The normal O_2 equilibration curve between the alveolus and the pulmonary capillary. O_2 equilibration is essentially complete by the time the red blood cell is one-third of its way through the capillary. (B) The O_2 equilibration curve if the alveolar-capillary barrier becomes moderately thickened. (C) The O_2 equilibration curve between the alveolus and pulmonary capillary if this thickening becomes severe. (Modified from: West, J. B. *Respiratory Physiology.* 5th ed. Baltimore: Williams & Wilkins, 1995. P. 25.)

individuals, O_2 transfer is perfusion limited even during exercise. In some well-conditioned athletes, the capillary transit time during exercise becomes so short (less than 0.25 second) that O_2 equilibration is incomplete. In this special situation, O_2 transfer becomes diffusion limited.

Theoretically, if the alveolar-capillary barrier thickens because of disease (e.g., interstitial pulmonary fibrosis or edema), O_2 transfer could be impeded and blood may need to traverse almost the entire length of the capillary to achieve equilibrium (see Fig. 32-3, curve B). At rest, the end-capillary P_{O_2} in such a person would be near normal, but the reduced capillary transit time that occurs with exercise would impose a significant diffusion limitation on O_2 transfer, and end-capillary P_{O_2} would fall. If the thickening is extreme, then O_2 equilibration may not occur even at rest (see Fig. 32-3, curve C).

This perfect matching between one alveolus and capillary for O_2 does not occur throughout the whole lung because of the ventilation and perfusion inequalities and shunting that typically exist even in the healthy lung. (This subject is covered in Chap. 35.)

Equilibration of Carbon Dioxide

The equilibration of CO_2 across the alveolar-capillary barrier occurs at about the same rate as oxygen, in that equilibration is complete when blood is slightly over one-third of the way through the capillary (Fig. 32-4, curve A). Thus the transfer of CO_2, like that of O_2, is perfusion limited over a wide range of activity levels. In addition, if thickening of the alveolar-capillary barrier is sufficiently severe, CO_2 transfer could become diffusion limited, and end-capillary P_{CO_2} levels would rise (see Fig. 32-4, curve B). O_2 and CO_2 have essentially the same equilibration times even though CO_2 is 24 times more soluble in water and diffuses 20 times faster through water than does O_2. This is due primarily to two reasons. First, the pressure gradient for CO_2 across the alveolar-capillary barrier is substantially less than that for O_2 (5 versus 60 mmHg, respectively). Second, CO_2 is transported in blood primarily as bicarbonate and carbamino compounds. It takes a finite period to reverse these reactions in the lung to form dissolved

Fig. 32-4. Equilibration of CO_2 across the alveolar-capillary barrier. (A) CO_2 equilibration is essentially complete by the time the red blood cell is a little over one-third of its way through the capillary. (B) With thickening of the alveolar-capillary barrier, CO_2 equilibration may be incomplete (P_{CO_2} = partial pressures of CO_2). (Modified from: West, J. B. *Respiratory Physiology* 5th ed. Baltimore: Williams & Wilkins, 1995. P. 29.)

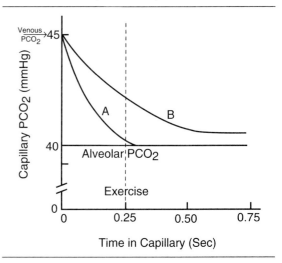

CO_2 so that it can diffuse from blood into the alveoli. Together, these two factors are primarily responsible for the slightly longer Pco_2 equilibration time.

Gas Transport by the Blood

Oxygen

O_2 is transported in the blood in two forms: **physically dissolved** and attached to **hemoglobin.**

At 37°C, each milliliter of plasma takes up 0.00003 ml of O_2 for each 1-mmHg increase in Po_2. Thus there is 0.3 ml of dissolved O_2 in every 100 ml of blood at 37°C with a Po_2 of 100 mmHg. If this were the only way blood could transport O_2, the cardiac output would have to be 83 liters per minute, and every O_2 molecule would have to be extracted from the blood to meet an O_2 consumption in **resting** humans of 250 ml/min. Obviously, O_2 carriage by the blood solely in this form could not meet even the most basic metabolic requirements of the body, and an additional form of O_2 transport is needed. Hemoglobin provides this transport.

Hemoglobin is a remarkable compound made up of four polypeptide chains, each with a **heme** moiety attached. The heme molecule consists of a porphyrin ring with one atom of ferrous iron in the center. Each of these four iron molecules can reversibly combine with one molecule of O_2. The iron molecules stay in the ferrous state when they bind with O_2, so this reaction is more correctly called **oxygenation** than oxidation. Thus the presence of hemoglobin in the blood permits much greater quantities of O_2 to be transported than in the dissolved state alone. O_2 attached to hemoglobin (oxyhemoglobin) accounts for about 98% of O_2 transported by blood. Hemoglobin permits blood to absorb 65 times as much O_2 as plasma at a Po_2 of 100 mmHg.

Definition of Oxygen Content and Capacity and Oxyhemoglobin Saturation

The **O_2 content** of blood is the total amount of O_2 carried in blood; that is, the O_2 content is the sum of the O_2 combined with hemoglobin and the O_2 dissolved in plasma. Thus the O_2 content varies with the total amount of hemoglobin in blood and with the PaO_2.

The **O_2 capacity** of blood is defined as the maximum amount of O_2 that can be carried by hemoglobin. One gram of hemoglobin that is fully loaded with O_2 combines with 1.34 ml of O_2. Whole blood in healthy adults contains approximately 15 g of hemoglobin (Hb) per 100 ml of blood. Thus

$$O_2 \text{ capacity} = 1.34 \text{ ml } O_2 \times g \, Hb / \text{vol. of blood}$$
$$= 1.34 \, ml \, O_2 / g \, Hb \times 15 \, g \, Hb / 100 \text{ ml of blood}$$
$$= 20.1 \, ml \, O_2 / 100 \text{ ml of blood} \quad (32\text{-}17)$$

This calculation reveals that the O_2 capacity varies with the hemoglobin content of blood.

The **percentage saturation of hemoglobin with O_2** is the amount of O_2 actually combined with hemoglobin divided by the O_2 capacity times 100. This quantity (%HbO_2) can be plotted as a function of the PaO_2, yielding the oxyhemoglobin dissociation curve.

The Oxyhemoglobin Dissociation Curve

Plotting the dissolved O_2 content against PaO_2 yields a straight line, but the relationship between PaO_2 and %HbO_2 saturation is not linear but is S-shaped (Fig. 32-5). The slope is steep when PaO_2 is in the lower ranges and is essentially flat at higher PaO_2 values. The S-shaped oxyhemoglobin dissociation curve indicates that the amount of O_2 bound to hemoglobin is relatively constant over a fairly wide range of higher PaO_2 values (flat part of the curve), but at lower PaO_2 levels, there are gradually larger changes in the amount of O_2 bound to hemoglobin for a given change in PaO_2 (steep part of curve). This occurs because

Fig. 32-5. Oxyhemoglobin (HbO_2) dissociation curve (*solid line*) compared with the amount of O_2 in physical solution (*dashed line*). Partial pressure of O_2 in blood, pH, and temperature is held constant at 40 mmHg, pH 7.4, and 37°C, respectively. (Modified from: West, J. B. *Respiratory Physiology* 4th ed. Baltimore: Williams & Wilkins, 1990. P. 70.)

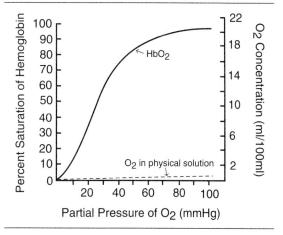

hemoglobin is made up of four subunits that load or unload their attached O_2 molecules with different affinities. As PaO_2 decreases from 100 mmHg, there is little change in the %HbO_2 saturation until PaO_2 reaches about 60 to 70 mmHg. Thus it takes a substantial decline in PaO_2 to off-load the first O_2 molecule, causing the upper portion of the curve to be relatively flat. The unloading of the remaining three O_2 molecules is progressively easier, and this accounts for the steep part of the curve.

Physiologic Significance of the Shape of the Oxyhemoglobin Dissociation Curve

The plateau portion of the oxyhemoglobin dissociation curve provides a "reserve" for the availability of O_2. PAO_2 (and consequently PaO_2) can lower substantially with little change in the %HbO_2 saturation. This means that PaO_2 can vary widely (from 100 to 60 mmHg, or about 40 mmHg), and yet essentially the same amount of O_2 will attach to hemoglobin.

The steep part of the oxyhemoglobin dissociation curve enables tissues to extract relatively large amounts of O_2 from blood with relatively small changes in the PaO_2. Consequently, on the steep part of the curve, almost 60% of the O_2 attached to hemoglobin can be offloaded with a 40-mmHg change in PaO_2 (i.e., from 60 to 20 mmHg). This allows for large quantities of O_2 to be offloaded from hemoglobin when the PaO_2 is low, thereby making it available to metabolically active tissues where it is needed.

Factors Affecting the Oxyhemoglobin Dissociation Curve

The oxyhemoglobin dissociation curve shown in Fig. 32-5 only illustrates PaO_2 as affecting the onloading and offloading of O_2 from hemoglobin. Other factors such as an increase in temperature and Pco_2 and decrease in pH shift the oxyhemoglobin dissociation curve to the right (Fig. 32-6). Conversely, a decrease in temperature and Pco_2 and an increase in pH shift the curve to the left. This effect of Pco_2 and pH on the oxyhemoglobin dissociation curve is called the **Bohr effect.** A rightward shift of the curve means that at a given PaO_2, there is less O_2 bound to hemoglobin (more offloading of O_2); a leftward shift means that at a given PaO_2, there is more O_2 bound to hemoglobin. In metabolizing tissues, Po_2 and pH decline and Pco_2 and temperature increase, facilitating the unloading of O_2 from hemoglobin. Thus additional O_2 is made available to the tissues.

CO_2 and H^+ combine with sites on hemoglobin, changing its configuration and facilitating the offloading of oxygen. Both CO_2 and H^+ bind more avidly to partially

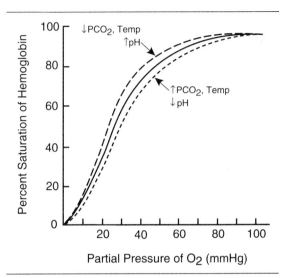

Fig. 32-6. Effects of changing partial pressure of CO_2 (Pco_2), pH, and temperature on the dissociation of O_2 from hemoglobin. Increases in pH and decreases in Pco_2 and temperature shift the oxyhemoglobin dissociation curve to the left. Conversely, a decrease in pH and increases in temperature and Pco_2 shift the curve to the right.

unsaturated hemoglobin. Thus the initial unloading of O_2 from hemoglobin is caused by a decline in PaO_2. However, once partially unsaturated hemoglobin appears, H^+ and CO_2 begin to bind, thereby enhancing the further offloading of O_2 along with the decline in PaO_2.

2,3-Diphosphoglycerate (2,3-DPG) is a metabolite of anaerobic glycolysis and is highly concentrated in red blood cells (15 mol/g of hemoglobin). Like CO_2 and H^+, 2,3-DPG facilitates the unloading of O_2 from hemoglobin. It is generally believed that increases in 2,3-DPG levels can induce a rightward shift of the oxyhemoglobin dissociation curve. However, measurable increases in 2,3-DPG seem to occur only under certain conditions such as at hypoxia (produced by high altitudes) or exercise, and this rise develops only after some delay. For example, 2,3-DPG does not become elevated until after about 1 hour of vigorous exercise, and there may be no increase at all in some well-trained athletes.

The binding of 2,3-DPG to hemoglobin facilitates the release of O_2 by changing the configuration of the hemoglobin molecule. When hemoglobin is essentially completely oxygenated, most of the 2,3-DPG–binding sites are covered. However, when O_2 is released from hemoglobin in the tissues (initiated by decreased PaO_2) and partially reduced hemoglobin appears, binding sites for 2,3-DPG are uncovered. The 2,3-DPG molecules attach to these sites, causing a change in the molecular configuration of hemoglobin and thus enhancing the unloading of O_2. In the lung, hemoglobin is reoxygenated, 2,3-DPG–binding sites are covered, and the 2,3-DPG molecules (along with CO_2 and H^+ from other sites on the hemoglobin molecule) are offloaded from hemoglobin. Thus the loading and unloading of O_2 from hemoglobin is a dynamic process that depends on the PaO_2, the levels of CO_2 and 2,3-DPG, pH, and temperature.

Effects of Anemia and Carbon Monoxide on Oxygen Transport

The curves in Fig. 32-7 are not oxyhemoglobin dissociation curves (%HbO_2 saturation) but represent plots of the **amount** of O_2 bound to hemoglobin (oxyhemoglobin content) as a function of PaO_2. Curve A depicts data from a normal subject, whereas curve C illustrates data from an **anemic** person (a hemoglobin concentration of 6 g/100 ml of blood; normal 15 g/100 ml). Thus the oxyhemoglobin content is reduced in this person, which means the total amount of O_2 carried by hemoglobin is decreased because

Fig. 32-7. Effects of anemia (C) and carbon monoxide poisoning (B) on the oxyhemoglobin (HbO_2) content (the volume of O_2 bound to hemoglobin). (A) The normal curve. Note that both anemia and carbon monoxide poisoning reduce the HbO_2 content but for different reasons (see text). (Modified from: Cherniack, N. S., Altose, M. D., and Kelsen, S. G. The respiratory system. In Berne, R. H., and Levy, M. N., eds. *Physiology.* St. Louis: Mosby, 1983. P. 691.)

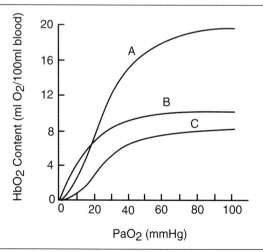

the concentration of hemoglobin is reduced. However, at a PaO_2 of 100 mmHg, the hemoglobin in an anemic individual is still about 97% saturated. Thus, even though the hemoglobin levels are depressed, the remaining hemoglobin is saturable. In anemic blood, as PaO_2 levels are reduced, substantially more O_2 is unloaded from hemoglobin than normal (rightward shift of curve C from curve A). This represents a compensation for the lowered O_2 content in the blood of anemic individuals. This prolonged reduction in O_2 levels is likely to produce lactic acidosis (decreased pH) and to increase 2,3-DPG levels (anaerobic shift in metabolism) in the blood, both of which facilitate the offloading of O_2.

Curve B describes the oxyhemoglobin in a person exposed to **carbon monoxide.** The affinity of carbon monoxide for the O_2-binding sites on hemoglobin is more than 200 times greater than that of O_2. Because carbon monoxide competes with O_2 for binding sites on hemoglobin, exposure to carbon monoxide reduces the oxyhemoglobin content. In this event, the %HbO_2 saturation is reduced, such that the hemoglobin levels are normal but carbon monoxide is bound to about 60% the O_2-binding sites. Carbon monoxide binding causes a leftward shift of the oxyhemoglobin content curve. Because most of the O_2-binding sites are occupied by carbon monoxide molecules that do not respond to declining PaO_2 levels, the O_2 molecules that remain on hemoglobin are more avidly bound and unload slower than normal, resulting in the leftward shift of curve B from curve A.

Carbon Dioxide

Like O_2, the movement of CO_2 between compartments proceeds down its pressure gradient: from tissue PCO_2 to blood plasma to red blood cells to lungs, in descending order. There are three forms of CO_2 transport: (1) physically dissolved, (2) as bicarbonate, and (3) in combination with blood proteins as carbamino compounds. These three mechanisms of CO_2 transport at the tissue are depicted in Chap. 42 (see Fig. 42-2). The reverse process occurs in the lungs.

Because CO_2 is about 24 times more soluble than O_2, **dissolved CO_2** is a more important form of CO_2 transport than is dissolved O_2. Approximately 5% to 10% of the CO_2 is transported in the dissolved form. At 37°C, each milliliter of blood takes up 0.0007 ml of CO_2 for each 1-mmHg increase in PCO_2, which is about 20 times greater than the rate for O_2.

Some of the dissolved CO_2 reacts with water, forming carbonic acid, which immediately breaks down to **bicarbonate** and H^+:

$$CO_2 + H_2O \rightleftarrows H_2CO_3 \rightleftarrows H^+ + HCO_3$$

This reaction is very slow in plasma. However, in the red blood cell it is 13,000 times faster because of the presence of the enzyme **carbonic anhydrase,** which catalyzes the hydration of CO_2 to carbonic acid. The H^+ that is formed is buffered by the partially oxygenated hemoglobin. The bicarbonate that is produced diffuses out of the red blood cells into plasma, and this prevents its accumulation in the red blood cell, which would slow or halt the hydration of CO_2. Thus, even though most of the bicarbonate is formed in red blood cells, much of it diffuses out and is transported in plasma. Between 60% and 65% of the CO_2 in the blood is in the form of bicarbonate.

With the leakage of bicarbonate from erythrocytes into plasma, chloride ions from plasma move into the red blood cell to maintain electric neutrality. This exchange of anions is known as the **Hamburger** or **chloride shift.** Buffering the H^+ reduces the polyvalent anionic charge on hemoglobin. This loss of intracellular negative charge is replaced by the monovalent anions, bicarbonate and chloride. Consequently, the total number of ions in the cell increases, elevating the internal osmotic pressure. Water moves into red blood cells to preserve the **osmotic equilibrium.** This causes a slight swelling of erythrocytes in the venous blood and a consequential increase in the venous hematocrit relative to that of arterial blood.

Carbamino compounds are formed from the reaction of CO_2 with terminal amine groups, **primarily** on hemoglobin (although CO_2 also will form carbamino compounds with plasma proteins, but to a much lesser extent). Carbamino compounds account for about 30% of the CO_2 transported in blood.

Carbon Dioxide Elimination by the Lungs

The pressure gradients for O_2 and CO_2 across the alveolarcapillary barrier initially stimulate the simultaneous movement of these two gases between the alveoli and blood. As CO_2 enters the alveoli from plasma, the **law of mass action** demands that the reaction for the hydration of CO_2 be shifted to the left. This process plus the binding of O_2 with hemoglobin causes both CO_2 and H^+ to dissociate from hemoglobin; the released H^+ then combines with bicarbonate to reform CO_2. Basically, the movement of CO_2 and O_2 at the lungs is the reverse of their movement at the tissues (see Fig. 42-2).

Carbon Dioxide Dissociation Curve

The CO_2 dissociation curve relates changes in the **CO_2 content** of whole blood to changes in the blood Pco_2, not

the changes in binding of CO_2 to some carrier molecule such as hemoglobin (i.e., it is not a percentage saturation curve like the oxyhemoglobin dissociation curve) (Fig. 32-8). Several points distinguish this curve. First, the CO_2 dissociation curve is not S-shaped like the oxyhemoglobin dissociation curve but is essentially linear in the physiologic $PaCO_2$ range (from 40 to 50 mmHg). Second, reducing the O_2 saturation of hemoglobin causes a leftward shift of the CO_2 dissociation curve. Consequently, as O_2 is unloaded from hemoglobin, the CO_2 content of blood is **increased,** primarily because unsaturated or deoxyhemoglobin is a weaker acid than oxyhemoglobin. Thus, as hemoglobin becomes progressively more unsaturated, it more readily binds the H^+ formed by the dissociation of carbonic acid, thereby allowing more CO_2 to be transported as bicarbonate. In addition, as hemoglobin de-

Fig. 32-8. CO_2 (*solid lines*) and O_2 (*dashed line*) plotted as a function of partial pressures of CO_2 (Pco_2) or O_2 (Po_2), respectively. CO_2 content is increased with desaturation of hemoglobin and decreased with increasing saturation of hemoglobin. In the physiologic range, the CO_2 content curve is essentially linear, as compared with the oxyhemoglobin dissociation curve. Note that the CO_2 content of whole blood is approximately twenty times higher than the O_2 content. (Modified from: Mines, A. H. *Respiratory Physiology* 2nd ed. New York: Raven Press, 1986. P. 77.)

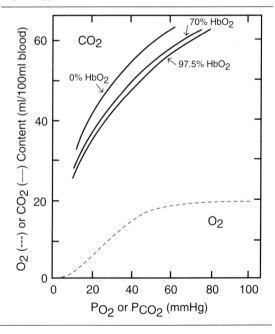

saturates, CO_2 forms carbamino compounds with the deoxyhemoglobin, which also adds to the CO_2 content. Thus just as O_2 dissociation from hemoglobin does not physiologically obey one curve, neither does CO_2 dissociation from whole blood. There is an additional change in CO_2 content resulting from the difference in the oxyhemoglobin concentration between the lungs and the microvasculature of the tissues. Finally, at any partial pressure, the CO_2 content of whole blood is more than twice that for O_2, primarily because of the greater solubility of CO_2 in blood.

Summary

Alveolar ventilation supplies the O_2 needed for metabolism and eliminates the CO_2 produced by the tissues. Consequently, the level of alveolar ventilation is responsive to the metabolic demand. The transfer of O_2 and CO_2 across the alveolar-capillary barrier occurs by means of diffusion down their respective partial pressure gradients. O_2 is primarily transported in the blood from the lungs to the tissues, bound to hemoglobin. The $\%HbO_2$ saturation is predominantly determined by the PaO_2 but is also significantly influenced by CO_2 and 2,3-DPG levels, pH, and temperature.

CO_2 is conveyed from the tissues to the lungs in three forms: physically dissolved, attached to hemoglobin as carbamino compounds, and as bicarbonate. Of the three, bicarbonate is the most important, accounting for up to 65% of the total amount of CO_2 transported. The CO_2 content of the blood is a function of the PCO_2 and the $\%HbO_2$ saturation.

Bibliography

Cherniack, N. S., Altose, M. D., and Kelsen, S. G. The respiratory system. In: Berne, R. M., and Levy, M. N., eds. *Physiology,* Sec. VI. St. Louis: C. V. Mosby, 1983.

Comroe, J. H. *Physiology of Respiration,* 2nd ed. Chicago: Year Book Medical Publishers, 1974.

Levitzky, M. G. *Pulmonary Physiology,* 4th ed. New York: McGraw-Hill, 1995.

Mines, A. H. *Respiratory Physiology,* 2nd ed. New York: Raven Press, 1986.

Taylor, A. E., Rehder, K., Hyatt, R. E., and Parker, J. C. *Clinical Respiratory Physiology,* Philadelphia: W. B. Saunders, 1989.

West, J. B. *Respiratory Physiology,* 5th ed. Baltimore: Williams & Wilkins, 1995.

33 Pulmonary Blood Flow

Douglas K. Anderson

Objectives

After reading this chapter, you should be able to

Define and compare the pressures within the pulmonary vascular system to those in the systemic circulation

Describe the factors affecting pulmonary vascular resistance

Explain the effects of gravity on the distribution of blood flow in the lung

---

The pulmonary circulation is basically a low-pressure, low-resistance, highly compliant system. Its function is to accept the **entire cardiac output** for gas exchange and not to regulate the supply of blood to individual organs to meet metabolic demands, as the systemic circulation does. The walls of the pulmonary vessels are thinner and contain less smooth muscle than the walls of the systemic vessels. In addition, the pulmonary capillary segments are very short, forming a dense meshwork that essentially yields a continuous sheet of blood flow in the alveolar wall.

Pressures in the Pulmonary Vascular System

Pressure in the pulmonary artery is about 25 mmHg systolic and 8 mmHg diastolic, with a mean of about 14 mmHg [calculated as (systolic pressure – diastolic pressure)/3 + diastolic pressure]. Pressure in the left atrium is about 5 mmHg, resulting in a pressure drop across the pulmonary circulation of approximately 9 mmHg. In the systemic circulation, pressure in the aorta averages 93 mmHg, with systolic and diastolic pressures of 120 and 80 mmHg, respectively. If the pressure in the right atrium averages 2 mmHg, then the pressure gradient across the systemic circulation is about 91 mmHg, or 10 times greater than that in the pulmonary circulation.

Pulmonary Vascular Resistance

Pulmonary vascular resistance is 1.8 mmHg/liter/min, and **systemic vascular resistance** is 18 mmHg/liter/min if the cardiac output is 5 liters/min. Thus the pulmonary circulation is a highly distensible system, with a resistance that is only about 10% of the systemic vascular resistance. Although there is some active regulation of the pulmonary circulation, changes in the pulmonary vascular resistance are primarily passive and consist of responses to changes in lung volume and pulmonary arterial and venous pressures.

Passive Changes in the Pulmonary Vascular Resistance
Effects of Lung Volume

The pulmonary circulation is composed principally of two types of vessels: extraalveolar and intraalveolar. The larger arteries and veins constitute the **extraalveolar** vessels. They lie outside the alveoli, are tethered to the elastic tissue of the lung, and are exposed to the intrapleural pressure. The **intraalveolar** vessels (the pulmonary capillaries) lie between the alveoli. These two groups of vessels respond differently to changes in lung volume, with both contributing to the overall pulmonary vascular resistance.

At lower lung (alveolar) volumes, the intraalveolar vessels are near maximally open, and therefore, their resistance to blood flow is minimal (Fig. 33-1, curve B). However, with increasing lung volume, these intraalveolar vessels are compressed by the distended alveoli, and this progressively increases their resistance to blood flow (see Fig. 33-1, curve B). Conversely, at low lung volumes, the caliber of the extraalveolar vessels is small because the transmural pressure gradient across the walls of these vessels is reduced due to the lesser subatmospheric pressure in the intrapleural space. Consequently, vascular resistance in the extraalveolar vessels is high at low lung volumes (see Fig. 33-1, curve C). With increasing lung volume, the intrapleural pressure becomes more subatmospheric, elevating the transmural pressure gradient across the extraalveolar vessels. This increased transmural pressure,

Fig. 33-1. Pulmonary vascular resistance plotted as a function of lung volume. (A) The total pulmonary vascular resistance, which is the sum of the resistance contributed by the intraalveolar vessels (B) and extraalveolar vessels (C). The functional residual capacity (FRC) is that lung volume with the least total vascular resistance. (RV = residual volume; TLC = total lung capacity.) (Modified from: Taylor, A. E., et al. *Clinical Respiratory Physiology*. Philadelphia: W. B. Saunders, 1989. P. 75.)

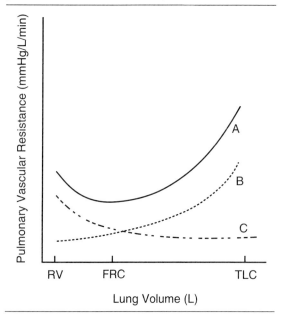

coupled with the added radial traction on the extraalveolar vessels imposed by the surrounding lung tissue as it expands, causes these vessels to distend and thereby decreases their vascular resistance (see Fig. 33-1, curve C).

Because the greatest cross-sectional area exists in the millions of intraalveolar vessels, increasing vascular resistance in these vessels offsets decreased resistance in the extraalveolar vessels. Thus total pulmonary vascular resistance is heightened at higher lung volumes when vascular resistance in the intraalveolar vessels is high (see Fig. 33-1, curve A). Total pulmonary vascular resistance is lowest at the functional residual capacity when there is sufficient lung inflation to open the extraalveolar vessels with minimal closing of the intraalveolar vessels (see Fig. 33-1, curve A).

Recruitment and Distention of Capillaries

As previously indicated, the pulmonary circulation is remarkably compliant. Pulmonary vascular resistance declines as the pressure in the pulmonary circulation rises. This is depicted in Fig. 33-2, which is a plot of the pulmonary vascular resistance as a function of pressure in the pulmonary artery at normal (curve A) and elevated (curve B) left atrial pressures. At normal pressures, approximately half the pulmonary capillaries are closed. With increasing pulmonary arterial pressures, these previously closed capillaries open, in what is known as **recruitment,** and as vascular pressure continues to rise, these patent microvessels become **distended** (see Fig. 33-2, curve A). The net effect is an increase in the total cross-sectional area of the pulmonary capillaries, resulting in decreased pulmonary vascular resistance. If the left atrial pressure is elevated, increasing pulmonary arterial pressure has little effect on the pulmonary vascular resistance because all capillaries are open and fully distended due to the venous back pressure. As a consequence, little further decrease in resistance can occur (see Fig. 33-2, curve B).

Active Regulation of Pulmonary Vascular Resistance

Although changes in pulmonary resistance are achieved mainly by passive factors, resistance can be actively modified by **neural, chemical,** and **humoral** influences. The pulmonary blood vessels are innervated by both sympathetic and parasympathetic fibers but more sparsely than are the systemic vessels. The density of innervation is

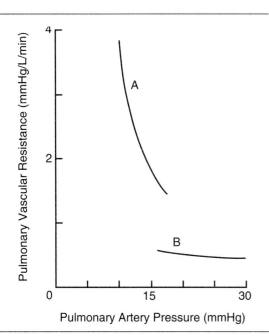

Fig. 33-2. Pulmonary vascular resistance plotted as a function of pressure in the pulmonary artery at normal (A) and elevated (B) left atrial pressures. (Modified from: Taylor, A. E., et al. *Clinical Respiratory Physiology*. Philadelphia: W. B. Saunders, 1989. P. 74.)

greatest in the larger vessels, decreasing with vessel size. **Sympathetic** stimulation constricts the pulmonary blood vessels (or at least increases the tone of the larger blood vessels), whereas **parasympathetic** stimulation causes vasodilation.

There are a variety of **vasoactive compounds** that affect pulmonary vascular resistance. The **vasoconstricting** agents include arachidonic acid, leukotrienes, thromboxane A_2, prostaglandin F_2, angiotensin-II, serotonin, epinephrine, and norepinephrine. The **vasodilating** compounds are: acetylcholine, bradykinin, and prostacyclin.

Alveolar Hypoxia

Local alveolar hypoxia (a decrease in the alveolar oxygen tension in a restricted region of the lung) produces vasoconstriction of the vessels to that portion of the lung. This is an important reaction that shifts blood away from poorly ventilated alveoli to better-ventilated ones, thereby matching perfusion with ventilation (see Chap. 35). It is the re-

duced oxygen tension in the alveoli (and not in the blood) that is thought to cause vasoconstriction of the precapillary small muscular arteries leading to the hypoxic region. This vasoconstriction may be due to the direct effects of oxygen on the vascular smooth muscle or may be mediated by some vasoactive agent or agents.

Effects of Gravity on Pulmonary Blood Flow

As indicated in Fig. 33-3, pulmonary blood flow decreases from the bottom to the top of the lung in upright individuals. This occurs because gravity creates a gradient of vascular pressures from the top to the bottom of the lung such that the pressure is lower at the apex than at the base of the lung. Thus the intravascular pressure in the lung is unlike the alveolar pressure which is essentially constant throughout the lung.

The distance from the apex to the base of the lung is approximately 30 cm. If, for example, the pulmonary artery enters the lung at its midpoint, then the top of the lung is 15 cm above the inlet of the pulmonary artery. If the pulmonary artery has a pressure of 20 cmH_2O, the arterial pressure at the top of the lung is 5 cmH_2O (the arterial pressure at the lung apex equals the pressure at the inlet of the pulmonary artery [20 cmH_2O] less the height of a column of blood extending from the inlet to the top of the lung [15 cm]).

As illustrated in Fig. 33-3, there is a **potential** region (zone A) at the top of the lung where arterial, capillary, and venous pressures are all less than the alveolar pressure. In this situation, the blood vessels would be completely collapsed, and no blood would flow through this region of the lung. If this region continued to be ventilated, it would become **alveolar dead space,** such that it would be ventilated but not perfused. Such a zone does not usually exist; vascular pressure is normally higher than alveolar pressure, so that capillary flow commonly occurs at the top of the lung in standing individuals. However, such a zone can exist if the pulmonary arterial pressure is reduced (e.g., by hemorrhage) or if the alveolar pressure is increased (e.g., by positive-pressure ventilation).

In the erect position, pulmonary arterial pressure increases toward the base of the lung, approaching the pressure in the pulmonary artery near its inlet (see Fig. 33-3, zone B). Below the inlet, arterial pressure in the lung exceeds the pressure in the pulmonary artery (see Fig. 33-3, zone C). Thus, in this example, the arterial pressure would

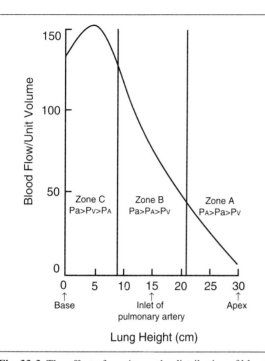

Fig. 33-3. The effect of gravity on the distribution of blood flow in the upright lung. Blood flow is highest at the base of the lung and decreases toward the apex. (See text for detailed description.) (Pa = arterial pressure; Pv = venous pressure; P_A = intraalveolar pressure.) (Modified from: West, J. B. *Respiratory Physiology,* 5th ed. Baltimore: Williams &Wilkins, 1995. P. 40.)

be 20 cmH_2O at the inlet of the pulmonary artery and 35 cmH_2O at the bottom of the lung, 15 cm below the inlet.

In zone B, the arterial pressure is greater than the alveolar pressure, but the alveolar pressure may still slightly exceed the venous pressure. In this case, flow is determined by the difference between the arterial and alveolar pressures and not the difference between the arterial and venous pressures as in most other organs. Thus venules may be partially compressed in the upper portions of zone B, thereby restricting blood flow. However, because the arterial pressure is increasing in zone B, the pressure difference (difference between arterial and alveolar pressure) for flow becomes greater and blood flow increases in the lower regions of this zone. In addition, with the increasing arterial pressure in zone B, capillary recruitment can take place.

In zone C, both the arterial and venous pressures exceed the alveolar pressures, and flow is determined, as in most organs, by the difference between the arterial and venous pressures. In zone C, it is likely that most capillaries are open, and the increases in blood flow are due chiefly to distention of the microvessels.

The gradient in pulmonary blood flow from the top to the bottom of the lung is also caused by the higher lung (alveolar) volumes at the top of the lung. These higher volumes tend to compress the capillaries and increase resistance in the apical region, as compared with the base of the lung, where alveolar volume is less (see Fig. 33-1, curve B). However, as noted previously, at very low lung volumes, resistance in the extraalveolar vessels increases because the transmural pressure is reduced across the wall of these vessels and the radial traction on these vessels is decreased (see Fig. 33-1, curve C). This increased resistance in the extraalveolar vessels is responsible for the decline in blood flow at the base of the lung (the lowest portion of zone C).

When an individual is supine, the pressure differences between the apex and base of the lung are abolished because the lung is not as wide as it is tall. Consequently, pulmonary blood flow is more homogeneous throughout the supine lung than throughout the upright lung.

Summary

The pulmonary circulation represents a low-pressure, low-resistance, highly distensible system. It serves to accept the entire cardiac output for gas exchange. Although there is some active regulation of the pulmonary circulation, pulmonary vascular resistance is determined primarily by passive events, including lung volume and the pulmonary arterial and venous pressures. In addition, gravitational effects on pulmonary arterial pressure cause blood flow to be nonuniform throughout the upright lung, such that blood flow is greatest at the base and progressively decreases toward the apex. These passive changes in blood flow are accomplished primarily by the recruitment and distention of capillaries.

Bibliography

Cherniack, N. S., Altose, M. D., and Kelsen, S. G. The respiratory system. In: Berne, R. M., and Levy, M. N. eds. *Physiology,* Sec. VI. St. Louis: C. V. Mosby, 1983.

Comroe, J. H. *Physiology of Respiration,* 2nd ed. Chicago: Year Book Medical Publishers, 1974.

Levitzky, M. G. *Pulmonary Physiology,* 4th ed. New York: McGraw-Hill, 1995.

Mines, A. H. *Respiratory Physiology,* 2nd ed. New York: Raven Press, 1986.

Taylor, A. E., Rehder, K., Hyatt, R. E., and Parker, J. C. *Clinical Respiratory Physiology.* Philadelphia: W. B. Saunders, 1989.

West, J. B. *Respiratory Physiology,* 5th ed. Baltimore: Williams & Wilkins, 1995.

34 Control of Ventilation During Wakefulness

Shahrokh Javaheri and Douglas K. Anderson

Objectives

After reading this chapter, you should be able to

Give an overview of the control of breathing and distinguish between homeostatic and behavioral functions of the respiratory system

Distinguish various elements of the respiratory system involved in the control of breathing

Describe the role of the brain in the control of breathing

Describe the homeostatic mechanisms that maintain the oxygen and carbon dioxide partial pressures and H^+ concentration

Explain how hypoxemia and hypercapnia differ in their control of breathing

Name and describe the role of the intrathoracic receptors in the control of breathing

Explain the role of upper airway respiratory muscles in regulating upper airway patency

Describe how the control of breathing differs during wakefulness and sleep

---

The major function of the respiratory system is to maintain normal blood partial pressures of the two vital respiratory gases, O_2 and CO_2, along with the H^+ concentration $[H^+]$. This important regulatory function is referred to as the **homeostatic** (chemostatic or metabolic) **function** of the respiratory system and is achieved by adjusting ventilation to the metabolic need (O_2 consumption $[\dot{V}o_2]$ and CO_2 production $[\dot{V}co_2]$) of the organism.

The breathing apparatus, however, is also used for non-homeostatic (behavioral) functions, such as **phonation.** With the ever-occurring variations in metabolic needs and behavioral functions, particularly during wakefulness, the act of breathing becomes complex and must be governed precisely by a hierarchy of control systems.

The metabolic and behavioral functions of the respiratory system are regulated by the CNS, where **respiratory rhythmogenesis** arises. The **central pattern generators** produce the **automatic respiratory rhythm** that underlies the peri-odic cycles of inspiration and expiration. About 70 years ago, it was demonstrated that respiratory rhythm can persist after removal of the entire brain above the brainstem, but automatic breathing ceases after transection of the brainstem at the medullary-spinal level (first cervical level). However, even today, precise histologic localization of the respiratory centers in the pontomedullary area remains ill-defined.

Components of the Respiratory System That Control Breathing

Control of respiration involves three components: sensors, controllers, and effectors (Fig. 34-1). In this complicated system, the **controllers** are "the respiratory centers," and they harbor multiple important functions. These are

1. Respiratory rhythmogenesis — central pattern generation

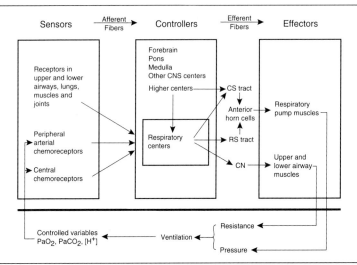

Fig. 34-1. The components of the respiratory system that control breathing. In a broad sense, these include sensors, controllers, and effectors. The respiratory centers receive afferent information from multiple sites (sensors). Axons from the medullary respiratory neurons decussate below the obex of the medulla oblongata and descend in the reticulospinal (RS) tracts in the ventrolateral spinal cord to synapse with spinal motor neurons of the phrenic and intercostal nerves that innervate the thoracic inspiratory and expiratory pump muscles. The voluntary breathing system, which originates in the cerebral cortex, descends via the corticospinal (CS) tract to the spinal motor neurons innervating the respiratory pump muscles and via the corticobulbar tract innervating the upper airway respiratory muscles, by way of the cranial nerves (CN). In this diagram, ventilation is determined by the balance between upper airway resistance (determined by state of activation of muscles of upper airways) and the pressure generated by the pump muscles. Arterial blood partial pressures of O_2 and CO_2 (PaO$_2$ and PaCO$_2$) and the H^+ concentration ([H^+]) are the controlled variables and influence the activity of the chemoreceptors.

2. Neural translation of the central rhythm to the motor output that drives the respiratory muscles
3. Adjustment of the rhythm and motor output to meet the metabolic needs (homeostatic functions)
4. Adjustment of the rhythm and motor output to meet behavioral and voluntary functions (nonhomeostatic functions)
5. Most efficient use of the respiratory system to achieve various functions with minimal energy expenditure

The respiratory centers are the sites of respiratory rhythmogenesis, the basic function underlying the act of automatic breathing. The centers receive multiple inputs from a variety of **sensors** located at various sites (Table 34-1). These sensors perceive changes in a wide variety of variables, such as the partial pressure of CO_2 (Pco$_2$) and O_2 (Po$_2$), [H^+], and lung inflation, and transmit this information (in the form of increased or decreased activity) to the controllers. After processing this information, the con-

Table 34-1. Sensors (Receptors) with Afferent Input to the Respiratory Centers

From within the brain
  Central chemoreceptors
  Hypothalamic (temperature) receptors
  Forebrain centers (voluntary functions)
From outside the brain
  Peripheral arterial chemoreceptors (primarily carotid bodies)
  Upper airway receptors
    Nasal
    Pharyngeal
    Laryngeal
  Pulmonary receptors
    Stretch receptors
    Irritant receptors
    C fibers
  Respiratory muscle receptors
  Costovertebral joint receptors

trollers alter their level of activity, which is conveyed to multiple **effectors** (see Fig. 34-1). The most basic effectors are the respiratory muscles, including the thoracic inspiratory pump muscles and the muscles of the upper airways. As noted in Chap. 30, the main inspiratory muscle is the **diaphragm.** The major respiratory muscles of the upper airways are the so-called **upper airway dilators,** which regulate the cross-sectional area and resistance of the upper airway. These muscles contract in phase with inspiration, increasing the tone in the compliant upper airways and thereby preventing the walls of the upper airways from being drawn inward by the subatmospheric intraluminal pressure generated by the diaphragm.

Although the respiratory centers receive information from various receptors over a variety of neural pathways (see Fig. 34-1), the output information is conveyed to the diaphragm via the phrenic nerves, to the intercostal muscles via the intercostal nerves, and to the muscles of the upper airways via the cranial nerves (see Fig. 34-1). Thus air flows through the upper airway into the lungs, where gas exchange occurs.

This chapter will review the metabolic and behavioral functions of the respiratory system and consider some of the more important reflex arcs involved in the control of breathing. Various sensors, respiratory centers, and muscles of the upper airway will be emphasized. The respiratory thoracic pump muscles were covered in Chap. 30. Control of breathing during sleep and with exercise is beyond the scope of this book and is only briefly considered.

Respiratory Centers and Neurogenesis of Breathing

Over 70 years ago, results of brain transection experiments indicated that the **central automatic respiratory centers** were located in the brainstem and consisted of a **pneumotaxic center** in the rostral pons, an **apneustic center** in the caudal pons, and the **medullary centers** (Fig. 34-2). Transections made above the **upper pons** (level 1) caused no change in the respiration of an anesthetized animal, and this localized the site of respiratory centers to the pons and

Fig. 34-2. Lumsden's experiments with brainstem transections at levels 1 to 4 (see text). The diagram to the left is a dorsal view of the pontomedullary area. The breathing patterns (labeled A to E) represent those which appear following complete transections at each level. These patterns are: normal breathing (A), slow deep breathing (B), apneustic breathing (C), gasping (D), and apnea (E). (SC and IC = the superior and inferior colliculi respectively; (CP) = the cerebellar peduncles.) (Modified from: Comroe, J. H., ed. *Physiology of Respiration.* Chicago: Year Book Medical Publishers, 1974.)

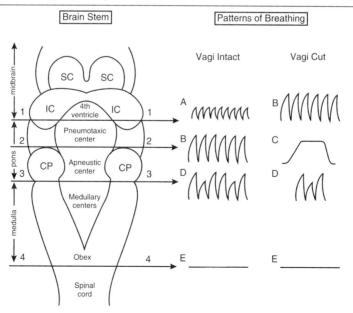

medulla. Sectioning the **vagi** with or without this transection caused slowing and deepening of respiration. This pattern of breathing is due to removal of inhibitory afferent input from pulmonary stretch receptors (to be discussed). A transection made at the **midpons** (level 2) caused some slowing and deepening of respiration with the vagi intact. When the vagi were sectioned, this pontine transection produced a series of prolonged inspirations, punctuated by very brief expirations, termed **apneustic breathing.** This respiratory pattern supposedly arises because a center (called the **apneustic center**) in the lower pons assumes control of the breathing pattern. Because apneustic breathing was unmasked by vagal and upper pontine sections, it was concluded that normal activity in the apneustic center was periodically inhibited by impulses traveling in the vagus and by impulses from the pneumotaxic center in the upper pons.

Removal of the **pontine apneustic center** by transection between the pons and medulla (level 3) produced a gasping, spasmodic respiratory pattern characterized by brief and usually maximal inspiratory efforts that terminated abruptly (see Fig. 34-2). Sectioning between the **medulla** and **spinal cord** (level 4) causes all spontaneous respirations to cease (apnea) in the resting expiratory position (at the functional residual capacity). This indicated that the **medullary centers** were critically important for spontaneous respiration.

Structure and Function of Characteristics of Respiratory Centers

Although these early studies localized the respiratory centers to the pontomedullary areas, detailed anatomic localization had to await the advent of electrophysiologic techniques. Microelectrodes placed in different parts of the brainstem have been used to explore the regions involved in **rhythmogenesis.** These studies revealed the presence of **respiration-related neurons** that link oscillation to respiratory output, such as phrenic nerve motor activity. Although the basic neural mechanism of rhythmogenesis is still unclear, these studies have identified multiple neural aggregates located bilaterally in the various parts of the brainstem (Fig. 34-3). Thus the **pneumotaxic center** corresponds to two rostral pontine nuclei, the **parabrachialis medialis** and the **Kolliker-Fuse nuclear complex.** The **apneustic center** is considered to be a diffuse entity in the pontine reticular formation, and the **medullary centers**

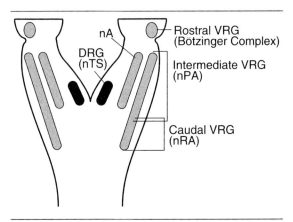

Fig. 34-3. Medulla and part of the spinal cord. showing the two main aggregates of respiration-related neurons, the dorsal (DRG) and ventral (VRG) respiratory groups. These nuclei are spread symmetrically and bilaterally (nTS = nucleus tractus solitarii; nA = nucleus ambiguus; nPA = nucleus paraambigualis; nRA = nucleus retroambigualis). (Modified from: Euler, C. V. Brain stem mechanisms for generation and control of breathing pattern. In: Cherniak, N. S., and Widdicombe, J. G., eds. *Handbook of Physiology: The Respiratory System,* Vol. II. New York: Oxford University Press, 1986.)

consist of at least two separate groups of nuclei, the **dorsal** and **ventral respiratory groups** (see Fig. 34-3).

Dorsal Respiratory Group

The dorsal respiratory group is located in the dorsomedial part of the medulla, corresponding to the ventrolateral nucleus of the tractus solitarii (see Fig. 34-3). This respiratory group contains mainly **inspiratory-related neurons.**

The axonal projections of the neurons of the **nucleus tractus solitarii** terminate in the cervical and thoracic anterior spinal motor neurons of the phrenic and intercostal nerves and exhibit discharge patterns similar to those of the phrenic and intercostal nerves.

Ventral Respiratory Group

The ventral respiratory group is more diffuse than the dorsal one, and consists of multiple neural aggregates extending longitudinally from the rostral to caudal medulla and possibly up to the second cervical segment of the spinal cord. In a broad sense, the ventral respiratory group consists of the **Bötzinger complex,** in the vicinity of the nucleus retrofacialis, the **nucleus ambiguus** and **paraam-**

bigualis, and the **nucleus retroambigualis** (see Fig. 34-3). The ventral respiratory group contains neurons that are active during both inspiration and expiration. The expiration-related neurons project to expiratory intercostal motor neurons.

Pontine Respiratory Group

The respiration-related neurons in the pontine respiratory group include the **parabrachialis medialis** and the **Kolliker-Fuse nuclei** in the dorsolateral rostral pons, which constitute the so-called **pneumotaxic center.** These pontine nuclei transmit information to the **inspiratory-off switch** (IO-S), which has not been fully defined histologically but determines the inspiratory time. This mechanism also receives information from the pulmonary stretch receptors via the vagus nerves. Both vagal stimulation (lung inflation) and input from the pontine respiratory group activate the IO-S neurons, causing termination of inspiration. In contrast, the combination of vagotomy and lesioning of the pontine respiratory group (transection at level 2; see Fig. 34-2) abolishes the IO-S function, resulting in uninterrupted inspiratory activity that lasts for long periods — apneustic breathing. The IO-S mechanism is also stimulated by increased body (or hypothalamic) temperature, and this initiates tachypnea. This mechanism (panting) is used to dissipate heat in some animals when they become hyperthermic.

Simplified Model of Respiratory Rhythmogenesis

Although the respiratory centers of rhythmogenesis have been localized to the brainstem region, it has not been possible to precisely locate the basic rhythm generator, the **central pattern generator,** and the mechanisms underlying respiratory rhythmogenesis remain ill-defined. A simplified working model is presented.

Two important features of this model are the **magnitude** of the central inspiratory activity, which determines the intensity of the desire to inspire and is reflected in the inspiratory flow rate, and the **duration** of the central inspiratory activity, which determines the inspiratory time. Because flow equals the pressure divided by resistance, in the model, **inspiratory air flow** is the function of contractions of the diaphragm (generating pressure) and of the muscles of the upper airway (determining upper airway resistance). The **inspiratory time** is the function of the IO-S mechanism, which, when turned on, stops central inspiratory ac-

tivity, thereby terminating inspiration. **Expiration** begins passively through the elastic recoil of the respiratory system. However, at high levels of ventilation, expiration also can become active, in that the expiratory muscles contract rhythmically to augment expiration. This indicates the presence of central expiratory activity.

Receptors in the Upper Airways and Chest Wall

Aside from the receptors in the tracheobronchial tree and the chemoreceptors, which will be discussed, many other receptors transmit afferent input to the pontomedullary centers. Examples of these receptors include those in the **upper respiratory tract** (including the nose, pharynx, and larynx), the **respiratory muscles** (muscle spindles and tendon organs), and the **costovertebral joints.** The respiratory effects of these reflex arcs are complex and will not be discussed in detail. Some examples are the mammalian diving reflex, induced when water is applied to the nose or face, and the cough reflex or apnea, provoked by stimulation of laryngeal receptors. **Apnea** is of major interest because of the sudden infant death syndrome and sleep apnea syndrome.

Receptors in the Tracheobronchial Tree and the Lung Parenchyma

There are at least three different groups of afferent end organs in the wall of the lower airways and lung parenchyma that may influence the breathing pattern. These are the **pulmonary stretch receptors,** the **rapidly adapting irritant receptors,** and **C fibers.**

Pulmonary Stretch Receptors

The pulmonary stretch receptors are located in the smooth muscle of the trachea and larger bronchi. The afferent nerves originating from these receptors pass primarily in the vagus nerves into the brain (see description of the IO-S mechanism in the section "Pontine Respiratory Group").

Airway distension is the major stimulus of the pulmonary stretch receptors. Many of these receptors discharge spontaneously when functional residual capacity is reached, their activity markedly increasing with airway distension. This increase in activity ebbs slowly with time; hence they are called **slowly adapting receptors.**

In the **Hering-Breuer reflex,** lung inflation inhibits inspiration and prolongs expiration. The pulmonary stretch receptors are stimulated by lung inflation, and this increases their afferent activity in the vagus nerves. This activates the IO-S mechanism, which terminates inspiration, thereby limiting further lung inflation. For this reason, sectioning the vagus nerves in anesthetized, spontaneously breathing animals produces a prolonged inspiratory time. This reflex is active in animals and infants but is not of major importance in adult humans except during deep breathing.

Rapidly Adapting Irritant Receptors

Nerve endings in the epithelium of large airways probably serve as the rapidly adapting irritant receptors. These receptors are stimulated by **intraluminal irritants** such as cigarette smoke and by **inflammatory mediators** such as histamine and prostaglandins. However, they quickly adapt to stimulation and their activity returns to basal levels despite continued stimulation, hence their name. Information from the rapidly adapting irritant receptors travels through the vagal fibers to the brain, where the efferent limb of this reflex (the motor fibers in the vagus) activates contraction of the airway smooth muscle (bronchospasm). This reflex is therefore important in asthma. Rapidly adapting irritant receptors also mediate the cough reflex.

Coughing is an attempt to expel the intraluminal irritants that stimulate the irritant receptors.

C Fibers and Juxtacapillary Receptors

The C fibers and juxtacapillary (J) receptors are present both in bronchi (bronchial C fibers) and in lung parenchyma (pulmonary C fibers or J receptors). The J receptors are located in the interstitium of the alveolar wall juxtaposed to capillaries. J receptors are presumably stimulated by "distension" of the interstitial space, as may occur in pulmonary interstitial edema and fibrosis. The **reflex arc** is otherwise similar to that described for the pulmonary stretch receptors. Stimulation of the J receptors is believed to account for the **rapid breathing** (tachypnea) seen in a variety of cardiopulmonary disorders such as pneumonia, pulmonary edema, embolism, and fibrosis.

Peripheral Arterial Chemoreceptors

The peripheral arterial chemoreceptors include the carotid and aortic bodies. The **carotid bodies** are located in the tissue between the internal and external carotid arteries (Fig. 34-4), and the **aortic bodies** are located at the arch of

Fig. 34-4. (A) The carotid bodies and (B) the related hyperbolic hypoxic ventilatory response. The arterial O_2 tension (PaO_2) must decrease considerably before notable changes in ventilation occur; however, any further decrease in PaO_2 results in progressively increasing ventilation.

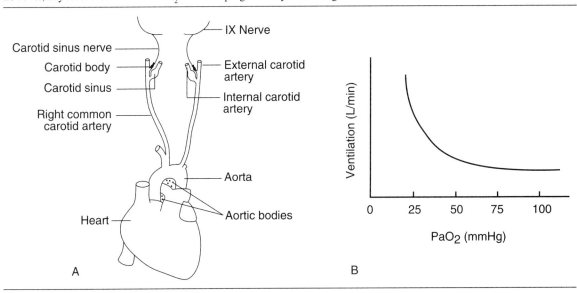

the aorta. The carotid bodies should not be mistaken for the carotid sinuses, which are baroreceptors that detect changes in blood pressure and are located in the wall of the internal carotid arteries. The carotid bodies are highly vascularized with a rich blood flow. Their main nerve supply is provided by the **carotid sinus nerve,** which is a branch of the glossopharyngeal nerve.

In most species, including humans, the carotid bodies are the predominant arterial chemoreceptors mediating the hyperventilatory response to decreased arterial O_2 tension (PaO_2), known as **hypoxemia.** In anesthetized animals, hypoxemia causes ventilatory depression if the carotid bodies are absent. This hypoxic ventilatory depression is probably due to the depressant action of hypoxemia on the brain, mediated by the release of multiple neurotransmitters such as **adenosine. Theophylline,** an adenosine antagonist, partially reverses the hypoxic ventilatory depression.

Ultrastructurally, there are two main cell types in the carotid bodies, the type I and II cells. The **type I** cells are the chief cells involved in **chemotransduction.** The carotid bodies respond to changes in blood PO_2, $[H^+]$, and K^+ concentration ($[K^+]$). Because the systemic circulation furnishes their blood supply, and because of their proximity to the lung and heart, the carotid bodies detect changes in PaO_2, PCO_2, and $[H^+]$ relatively quickly, resulting in the immediate ventilatory response.

This negative feedback loop is illustrated in Fig. 34-5. Hypoxemia, increased plasma $[H^+]$ (acidemia), and heightened $[K^+]$ (hyperkalemia) stimulate the carotid bodies, thus accelerating impulses to the brainstem respiratory centers from these chemoreceptors. Added activity from the respiratory centers to the thoracic and upper airway muscles causes increased ventilation that delivers more O_2 to and removes excess CO_2 from the lungs. The arterial CO_2 tension ($PaCO_2$) therefore decreases (which in turn

reduces the carbonic acid level and $[H^+]$), and PaO_2 increases, partially relieving the initial stimulus — the hypoxemia or acidemia. **Hyperkalemia** also excites these receptors, which may play a role in mediating the hyperpneic response of exercise. **Hypercapnia** also may stimulate the peripheral chemoreceptors independent of associated changes in $[H^+]$.

The importance of the **carotid bodies** in PO_2 homeostasis is demonstrated in people staying at high altitudes, where, despite considerable drops in the atmospheric PO_2, compensatory hyperventilation maintains adequate PO_2 for survival. The hypoxemia associated with pulmonary disease also stimulates the peripheral chemoreceptors in an attempt to increase alveolar ventilation and PaO_2. However, PaO_2 must fall considerably (below approximately 55 mmHg) before the receptors are sufficiently stimulated (see Fig. 34-4). The hyperbolic nature of the changes in the rate of discharge of afferent fibers from the carotid body illustrate this, as do the hyperbolic changes in ventilation when PO_2 is reduced (see Fig. 34-4). It is reemphasized that PaO_2 represents the stimulus to the carotid bodies and not the O_2 content of the arterial blood. This is why anemia and carbon monoxide inhalation are not associated with compensatory hyperventilation.

Central Chemoreceptors

The central chemoreceptors are situated somewhat superficially on the ventrolateral aspect of the medulla. At least **three areas,** designated M, S, and L for the scientists who identified these areas, have been defined (Fig. 34-6). Recent evidence suggests that there also may be some chemoreceptors deeper in the medulla.

The main stimulus to the central chemoreceptors is the

Fig. 34-5. The operation of the negative-feedback system that mediates the compensatory hyperventilation initiated by hypoxemia (PCR) = peripheral arterial chemoreceptors; VA = alveolar ventilation; PaCO₂ and PaO₂ = arterial CO₂ and O₂ tension, respectively). *Arrows* indicate increases or decreases in the level of activity.

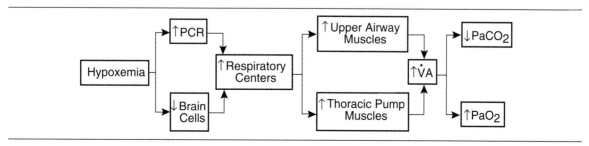

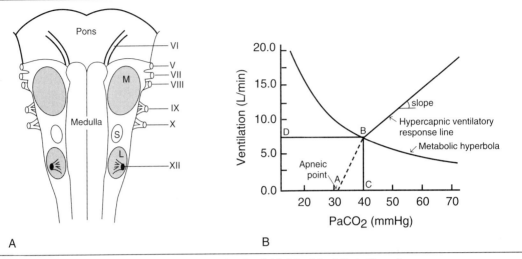

Fig. 34-6. (A) The central chemoreceptors (L = Loeschcke; S = Schlafcke; M = Mitchell) on the ventral aspects of the medulla. (B) The related hypercapnic ventilatory response. Areas M and L are presumably CO_2 sensitive. Note the linear ventilatory response to changes in the arterial CO_2 tension ($PaCO_2$). The slope of the line (reflecting gain in the system) defines the ventilatory response to CO_2. The average slope ranges between 1 and 3 liters/min/1-mmHg rise in the partial pressure of CO_2. Also shown is the metabolic hyperbola. C is the resting $PaCO_2$ (40 mmHg), and D is the resting ventilation. A is the so-called apneic point, or that $PaCO_2$ below which ventilation ceases.

[H^+] of the brain extracellular fluid that bathes these receptors. These receptors are separated from blood by the blood-brain barrier, which is formed by the tight junctions between the endothelial cells of the cerebral capillaries. Because the blood-brain barrier resists ionic diffusion, it takes several minutes for changes in plasma [H^+] to be reflected in the brain extracellular fluid. In metabolic acidosis or alkalosis, the magnitude of steady-state changes in brain extracellular fluid [H^+] is much smaller than the changes in plasma [H^+]. This difference exists because the blood-brain barrier is also equipped with **transport carriers** that can move various ions into and out of the extracellular fluid, thereby regulating its ionic composition. **Central chemoreceptors** are stimulated by increased [H^+] in extracellular fluid during metabolic acidosis; conversely, their activity diminishes when extracellular fluid [H^+] decreases during metabolic alkalosis. This information is signaled to the respiratory centers (see Fig. 34-1) and initiates compensatory changes in ventilation and $PaCO_2$, which in turn mitigate the changes in [H^+] induced initially by the metabolic acid-base perturbation (negative feedback loop of the central chemoreceptors).

Brain extracellular fluid [H^+] rises rapidly with **acute increases in $PaCO_2$** because CO_2 is a lipid-soluble molecule that diffuses quickly across the blood-brain barrier. In the extracellular fluid, CO_2 is hydrated to form carbonic acid, which dissociates to H^+ and HCO_3- (the bicarbonate radical). It is this H^+ that stimulates the central chemoreceptors. However, recent findings have suggested that PCO_2 may exert an independent stimulatory effect on the central chemoreceptors separate from the H^+.

The sensitivity or gain of the central chemoreceptors to changes in [H^+] appears to exceed that of the peripheral chemoreceptors such that most of the steady-state ventilatory response to changes in [H^+] (metabolic or respiratory) is mediated by the central chemoreceptors. Studies in some animal species have revealed that the hyperventilation caused by severe metabolic acidosis is almost equivalent before and after denervation of the peripheral chemoreceptors.

Summary of the Reflex Arcs of the Peripheral and Central Chemoreceptors

Both the peripheral and central chemoreceptors are part of a **negative feedback system** that functions primarily to correct disturbances in P_{O_2} [H^+], and P_{CO_2}. These **reflex arcs** are important elements of the metabolic (homeostatic) function of the respiratory system. The peripheral and central chemoreceptors are stimulated or depressed by altered [H^+] in their chemical environment, initiated by metabolic and respiratory acid-base disturbances. Increases in P_{CO_2} may be independent of [H^+] in activating peripheral and central chemoreceptors. Decreased PaO_2 stimulates the peripheral chemoreceptors and has a central depressant effect. Because of their strategic location, peripheral chemoreceptors respond quickly to changes in the **arterial blood chemistry** (P_{O_2}, [H^+], and $PaCO_2$). The central chemoreceptors are believed to be more sensitive (higher gain) than the peripheral chemoreceptors to changes in [H^+] and $PaCO_2$ and to mediate most of the ventilatory response to changes in [H^+] stemming from either respiratory or metabolic sources.

Voluntary and Behavioral Control of Breathing

During deep anesthesia and slow-wave sleep, breathing primarily accommodates metabolic needs (homeostasis). During wakefulness, however, the breathing apparatus subserves both homeostatic and nonhomeostatic (voluntary) functions (see Fig. 34-1). During **wakefulness,** in keeping with priorities imposed by the prevailing circumstances, the pattern of breathing is adjusted to meet the functional requirements.

During voluntary and behavioral acts, PaO_2 and $PaCO_2$ and [H^+] are disturbed; these represent the controlled variables of the metabolic respiratory control system. Although these disturbances are tolerated to some extent, the metabolic control system soon intercedes. Breathholding is a specific example: If the subject first hyperventilates (lowers P_{CO_2}) or breathes pure O_2, it can be prolonged.

As depicted in Fig. 34-1, the **descending neural signals** that drive the cranial nerves (innervating muscles of upper airways) and the **spinal respiratory motor neurons** (innervating the thoracic pump muscles) consist of those arising from voluntary (e.g., cortical) and involuntary (pontomedullary) sources. The corticospinal (pyramidal) tract may transmit the voluntary information directly from the cortex to the respiratory motor neurons. Alternatively, information from that cortex may pass through pontomedullary respiratory centers before descending to the motor neurons via the reticulospinal tract (extrapyramidal tract).

$PaCO_2$ Homeostasis

The normal resting $PaCO_2$ is determined where the metabolic hyperbola (see Chap. 32, Fig. 32-1) intercepts the curve of the CO_2 response (see Fig. 34-6B). Because of the characteristic linear relationship of P_{CO_2} to ventilation (linear gain), small changes in P_{CO_2} produce immediate compensatory changes in ventilation. This is in contrast to the PaO_2, which can decrease considerably before evoking significant compensatory ventilatory changes (see Fig. 34-4). In addition, because the metabolic rate is tightly linked to alveolar ventilation, as $\dot{V}_{CO_2}$ increases (exercise, ingestion of food high in carbohydrates), alveolar ventilation increases proportionately and $PaCO_2$ remains constant. For these reasons, $PaCO_2$ homeostasis appears to be under tight control.

Respiratory Muscles of Upper Airways

The nose, mouth, pharynx, and larynx that constitute the upper airways serve as the conduit for air flow into the trachea. The upper airways contribute to the **anatomic dead space** because they do not take part in gas exchange. However, **flow-resistive changes** in the upper airways can greatly influence ventilation and hence gas exchange. An example of this is upper airway occlusion, which may occur during sleep and is the underlying cause of **obstructive sleep apnea.** This occlusion occurs because the walls of upper airways are not rigid but contain soft tissues such as muscles and vessels. If the muscle tone is poor and the vascular bed is congested, this can profoundly reduce the cross-sectional area and increase resistance. During inspiration when the inspiratory muscles generate negative suction, a compliant upper airway is prone to collapse.

Of particular importance are those groups of **upper airway muscles** which phasically contract to stiffen the upper airway during each inspiration, preventing its collapse. Activation of these dilator muscles has been shown to precede diaphragmatic activation, which allows the upper airways to withstand the negative intraluminal pressure. These muscles are also stimulated by **hypoxemia** and **hypercapnia,** in a manner similar to that described for the respiratory pump muscles (see Fig. 34-5).

An important dilator muscle is the **genioglossus,** which pulls the tongue ventrally when it contracts. Relaxation of this muscle during sleep, along with gravitational force exerted on the tongue in the supine position, displaces the tongue backward, causing pharyngeal obstruction and sleep apnea.

Summary

The respiratory centers are located in the pontomedullary area of the brain and produce the respiratory rhythmogenesis underlying the act of breathing. The neural signals travel to muscles of the upper airways (via cranial nerves) and to the thoracic pump muscles (via phrenic and intercostal nerves).

The generation of rhythmic neural signals by the respiratory centers depends on afferent inputs from multiple receptors (sensors) located both inside and outside the brain. The carotid bodies constitute the primary peripheral arterial chemoreceptors that mediate the hyperventilatory response to hypoxemia. The increased ventilation caused by hypercapnia is mediated mostly by the central chemoreceptors in the medulla oblongata. These receptors are stimulated by increased $[H^+]$ in the extracellular fluid bathing them. This accounts for most of the compensatory increase in ventilation (and fall in arterial P_{CO_2}) during metabolic acidosis and the compensatory fall in ventilation (and rise in P_{CO_2}) during metabolic alkalosis. Normally, ventilation is maintained proportional to the metabolic rate, such that $PaCO_2$ and PaO_2 remain constant. This is how O_2 and CO_2 levels remain constant during exercise despite several-fold increases in the metabolic rate ($\dot{V}CO_2$). The primary function of the respiratory system is to keep P_{O_2}, P_{CO_2}, and $[H^+]$ as close to normal as possible. This is referred to as metabolic or homeostatic function. Although breathing is chiefly automatic (homeostatic), nonhomeostatic factors (behavioral control) also influence ventilation. The respiratory apparatus is used to achieve important behavioral acts such as speech, swallowing, and control of posture. Normally, there is a complex interaction between the behavioral and homeostatic control of breathing.

Bibliography

Berger, A. J., Mitchell, R. A., and Severinghaus, J. W. Regulation of respiration. *N. Engl. J. Med.* 297:91–97; 138–143; 194–201, 1977.

Comroe, J. H., ed. *Physiology of Respiration.* Chicago: Year Book Medical Publishers, 1974.

Dempsey, J. A., and Forster, H. V. Mediation of ventilatory adaptations. *Physiol. Rev.* 62:262–346, 1982.

Euler, C. V. Brain stem mechanisms for generation and control of breathing pattern. In: Cherniak, N. S., Widdicombe, J. G., eds. *Handbook of Physiology, The Respiratory System,* Vol. II. New York: Oxford University Press, 1986.

Javaheri, S., and Kazemi, H. Metabolic alkalosis and hypoventilation in man. *Am. Rev. Respir. Dis.* 136: 1011–1016, 1987.

35 Matching of Ventilation with Blood Flow

Douglas K. Anderson

Objectives

After reading this chapter, you should be able to

Define the normal alveolar ventilation to perfusion ratio and its extremes

Describe the physiologic and pathologic factors that cause mismatching of ventilation with blood flow

Describe the effects on the blood gases of the alveolar ventilation to perfusion ratio

Low arterial oxygen tension (PaO_2) is frequently seen in patients with cardiopulmonary disease. The most frequent cause of this hypoxemia is uneven matching of ventilation and blood flow (alveolar ventilation/perfusion ratio [$\dot{V}A/\dot{Q}$] inequality). To optimize the efficiency of gas exchange and achieve normal blood gas levels, the alveoli must be **both** adequately ventilated **and** perfused. Thus not only must the alveoli freely inspire O_2 and expire CO_2 (ventilation) but also sufficient blood must perfuse these alveoli to transport O_2 to the tissues and return CO_2 from the tissues to the alveoli for removal.

The Alveolar Ventilation/ Perfusion Ratio

Figure 35-1 illustrates the matching of ventilation and perfusion, the two extremes of $\dot{V}A/\dot{Q}$ mismatching and its effect on alveolar and blood gases. A represents the normal situation in which $\dot{V}A$ and $\dot{Q}$ are matched ($\dot{V}A/\dot{Q}$ = 0.8 to 1.2). B is the extreme circumstance of **venous to arterial shunting of blood,** where $\dot{Q}$ is normal but there is no $\dot{V}A$ ($\dot{V}A/\dot{Q}$ = 0). In this situation, the alveolar and blood partial pressures of O_2 (PO_2) and CO_2 (PCO_2) approach those of

Fig. 35-1. The spectrum of possible alveolar ventilation to perfusion ($\dot{V}A/\dot{Q}$) ratios in the lung. (A) The normal situation, with normal alveolar and blood gas values. (B) The lowest possible $\dot{V}A/\dot{Q}$ ratio — blood flow with no ventilation or a shunt. Alveolar and blood gas values in this situation approach those seen in venous blood. (C) The highest possible $\dot{V}A/\dot{Q}$ ratio, in which there is wasted ventilation or alveolar dead space with alveolar gas values that approach those in inspired air ($P\bar{v}O_2$ = mean venous O_2 tension; PIO_2 = inspiratory O_2 tension; PAO_2 = alveolar O_2 tension; PaO_2 = arteriolar O_2 tension).

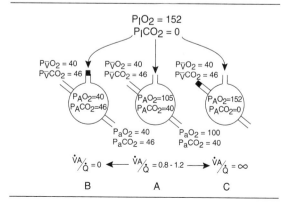

venous blood. C is the extreme condition of **alveolar dead space** in which $\dot{V}A$ is normal but there is no $\dot{Q}$ ($\dot{V}A/\dot{Q} = \infty$). Under these circumstances, alveolar PCO_2 and PO_2 approach the levels in inspired air. Thus B and C represent the extremes of a continuum of possible $\dot{V}A/\dot{Q}$ ratios in the lung.

Factors Responsible for Mismatching of $\dot{V}A/\dot{Q}$

Normal or Physiologic Factors

Figure 35-2 summarizes the normal changes that occur in blood flow, ventilation, and $\dot{V}A/\dot{Q}$ ratios proceeding from the top to the bottom of the lung. As discussed previously, in the normal, healthy, upright lung, ventilation and blood flow decrease from the base to the apex. However, as indicated by the slope of the lines in Fig. 35-2, the rate of the decrease in blood flow exceeds that for ventilation. Consequently, there is a gradient of low to high $\dot{V}A/\dot{Q}$ ratios from the bottom to the top of the lung. In the lower portions of the lung, blood flow exceeds ventilation, causing low $\dot{V}A/\dot{Q}$ ratios. In the upper regions of the lung, ventilation

Fig. 35-2. Plot of ventilation, blood flow, and alveolar ventilation to perfusion ($\dot{V}A/\dot{Q}$) ratios as a function of the height of the lung. Although both ventilation and perfusion decrease progressively from the bottom to the top of the lung, perfusion exceeds ventilation in the lower regions of the lung and vice versa toward the top of the lung. Consequently, $\dot{V}A/\dot{Q}$ ratios increase from the bottom to the top of the lung, in that low $\dot{V}A/\dot{Q}$ ratios are normally found toward the bottom of the lung and high $\dot{V}A/\dot{Q}$ ratios are seen in the upper portion. (Modified from: West, J. B. *Respiratory Physiology,* 5th ed. Baltimore: Williams & Wilkins, 1995. P. 61.)

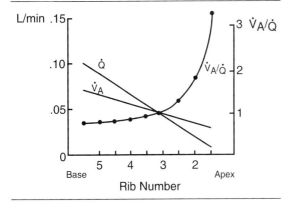

surpasses blood flow, resulting in high $\dot{V}A/\dot{Q}$ ratios. When blood flow and ventilation are essentially equal, $\dot{V}A/\dot{Q}$ ratios are normal. Thus, in the normal upright lung, $\dot{V}A/\dot{Q}$ ratios can range from under 0.5 to over 3.

Regions of the lung with low $\dot{V}A/\dot{Q}$ ratios have low PO_2 and high PCO_2 relative to normal. Areas of the lung with high $\dot{V}A/\dot{Q}$ ratios have relatively high PO_2 levels and low PCO_2 levels. This consequential mismatching of $\dot{V}A/\dot{Q}$ from the bottom to the top of the lung causes a range of values for PO_2 (90 to 130 mmHg) and PCO_2 (35 to 42 mmHg) in the effluent blood from the various regions of the lung. Even though O_2 may essentially be completely equilibrated across the alveolar-capillary barrier for the individual units, the range of $\dot{V}A/\dot{Q}$ ratios (and hence the range of alveolar PO_2 [PAO_2] and arterial PO_2 [PaO_2] values) common in the healthy lung contributes to the difference normally seen between the PO_2 in mixed alveolar gas and the PO_2 in systemic arterial blood — $P(A–a)O_2$ (see Chap. 32 for a description of some of the important pressures).

Another factor that contributes to the overall disparity between the PAO_2 and the PaO_2 is the presence of anatomic venous-to-arterial shunts. Normally a small percentage (2% to 5%) of the venous return is not exposed to the gas exchange surfaces of the lung but instead passes directly into the systemic arterial circulation. This includes nutrient blood flow coming from the upper airways and collected by the bronchial veins and coronary venous blood that drains directly into the left ventricle via the thebesian veins. This "dumping" of unoxygenated blood into the systemic circulation further lowers the PaO_2, causing additional deviation of the PaO_2 from the PAO_2.

Pathologic Factors

There are a number of conditions that can restrict ventilation and blood flow, producing abnormally large mismatching of ventilation with perfusion. This **$\dot{V}A/\dot{Q}$ mismatching** leads to low $\dot{V}A/\dot{Q}$ ratios and to subsequent **hypoxemia.**

Hypoventilation can eventuate from either uneven resistance to air flow within the lung or uneven lung compliance. Examples of **uneven resistance** to air flow include bronchoconstriction (asthma), collapse of airways (emphysema), narrowing of airways (bronchitis), and compression of airways (tumors, edema). Examples of **uneven lung compliance** consist of an increase in elastic recoil (fibrosis), loss of elastic recoil (emphysema), and insufficient surfactant levels (infant respiratory distress syndrome).

Pulmonary blood flow can be restricted by constriction

or compression of blood vessels (tumors, edema), obliteration of vessels (emphysema, fibrosis), or blockage (embolization or thrombosis) of some part of the pulmonary circulation.

When pulmonary arterial blood flows to the systemic circulation without any effective contact with alveolar gas, this creates a **venous-to-arterial shunt.** In the same way that normal venous-to-arterial shunts lower PaO_2, pathologic shunts can cause significant $\dot{V}A/\dot{Q}$ mismatching (low $\dot{V}A/\dot{Q}$ units) and hypoxemia. Interatrial septal defects are examples of pathologic anatomic shunts. Physiologic or functional shunts can arise with any disease process causing atelectasis or a consolidation of alveolar spaces that continue to be perfused. In the respiratory distress syndromes of both adults and children, alveoli either collapse from high surface-tension forces or become filled with edema fluid, hemorrhage, or cellular debris. A physiologic shunt exists for as long as there is perfusion to these areas, and hence hypoxemia develops.

Effects of $\dot{V}A/\dot{Q}$ Inequality on Blood Gases

Figure 35-3 depicts two lung units, one with a low and the other with a high $\dot{V}A/\dot{Q}$ ratio. The levels of PO_2 and PCO_2 in inspired air and in the pulmonary arterial blood supplying these units are normal. If equal volumes of blood are entering and leaving both units, then the low $\dot{V}A/\dot{Q}$ unit is underventilated and the high $\dot{V}A/\dot{Q}$ unit is overventilated.

Oxygen

Capillary blood leaving the low $\dot{V}A/\dot{Q}$ unit will be hypoxemic, in that the PaO_2, percentage of oxyhemoglobin (%HbO_2), and O_2 content will all be reduced. If the PaO_2 from this unit is, for example, 60 mmHg, the O_2 content would be approximately 18.0 ml of O_2 per 100 ml of blood with a %HbO_2 of about 89%. Ventilation in the other unit is increased relative to its blood flow such that the $\dot{V}A/\dot{Q}$ ratio is elevated and blood leaving this unit has an abnormally high PaO_2, %HbO_2, and O_2 content of 125 mmHg, 99%, and 20.2 ml of O_2 per 100 ml of blood, respectively. When the blood from these two units merges, the approximate PaO_2, %HbO_2, and O_2 content of the mixed effluent blood would be 75 mmHg, 94%, and 19.1 ml of O_2 per 100 ml of blood, respectively. Thus, for O_2, the high $\dot{V}A/\dot{Q}$ units only partially compensate for the low $\dot{V}A/\dot{Q}$ units, in that the O_2 values in the mixed-effluent blood are lower

than the normal values of PaO_2, 100 mmHg; %HbO_2, 97.4%; and O_2 content, 19.8 ml of O_2 per 100 ml of blood.

The reason the units with high $\dot{V}A/\dot{Q}$ ratios do not compensate for the low units is that the units with high $\dot{V}A/\dot{Q}$ ratios add relatively little O_2 to the blood compared with the decrement in O_2 caused by the units with low $\dot{V}A/\dot{Q}$ ratios because of the nonlinear shape of the oxyhemoglobin dissociation curve (see Fig. 32-5). Because this curve is almost horizontal when PO_2 exceeds 80 mmHg, raising the PO_2 to 125 mmHg would elevate the saturation of hemoglobin from approximately 97.4% (at a normal PO_2 of about 95 to 100 mmHg) to around 99%. This would increase the volume of O_2 carried by hemoglobin by about 0.32 ml of O_2 per 100 ml of blood. In the low $\dot{V}A/\dot{Q}$ unit (with a PO_2 of 60 mmHg), the volume of O_2 carried by hemoglobin is about 17.8 ml of O_2 per 100 ml of blood. This would represent an O_2 decrement of approximately 1.68 ml of O_2 per 100 ml of blood, rendered as 19.48 ml of O_2 per 100 ml of blood (the volume of O_2 combined with hemoglobin at a PaO_2 of 100 mmHg) minus 17.8 ml of O_2 per 100 ml of blood. Thus the high $\dot{V}A/\dot{Q}$ unit, which adds about 0.32 ml of O_2 per 100 ml of blood, cannot offset the loss of 1.68 ml of O_2 per 100 ml of blood from the low $\dot{V}A/\dot{Q}$ unit. Consequently, the PaO_2, %HbO_2, and O_2 content of the mixed-effluent blood all fall below normal levels.

Carbon Dioxide

In subjects with $\dot{V}A/\dot{Q}$ mismatching, there is often a normal or even subnormal $PaCO_2$. This can arise because the shape of the CO_2 dissociation curve for whole blood, unlike the oxyhemoglobin dissociation curve (compare Figs. 32-5 and 32-9), is essentially linear over a wide range of PCO_2 values. Consequently, the PCO_2 and CO_2 in mixed-effluent blood are essentially the average of their respective contents from high and low $\dot{V}A/\dot{Q}$ units. For the two lung units depicted in Fig. 35-3, blood leaving the low $\dot{V}A/\dot{Q}$ unit has elevated PCO_2 and CO_2 contents (approximately 44 mmHg and 52.1 ml of CO_2 per 100 ml of blood, respectively), but blood from the high $\dot{V}A/\dot{Q}$ unit has low PCO_2 and CO_2 contents (approximately 34 mmHg and 45.3 ml of CO_2 per 100 ml of blood, respectively). Because the CO_2 contents and PCO_2 values from these two units can be averaged (the CO_2 content/PCO_2 relationship is linear; see Fig. 32-8), the mixed-effluent blood has a PCO_2 of 39 mmHg and a CO_2 content of 47.8 ml of CO_2 per 100 ml of blood; both values are essentially normal. Thus, under these circumstances, the decreased PCO_2 and CO_2 content in the high $\dot{V}A/\dot{Q}$ unit compensates for the increase

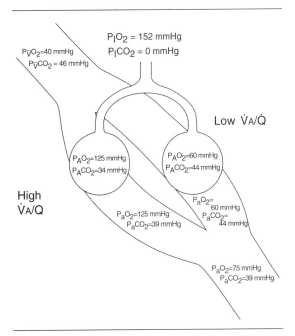

$P_I O_2 = 152$ mmHg
$P_I CO_2 = 0$ mmHg

$P_{\bar{v}} O_2 = 40$ mmHg
$P_{\bar{v}} CO_2 = 46$ mmHg

Low $\dot{V}_A/\dot{Q}$

$P_A O_2 = 125$ mmHg
$P_A CO_2 = 34$ mmHg

$P_A O_2 = 60$ mmHg
$P_A CO_2 = 44$ mmHg

High
$\dot{V}_A/\dot{Q}$

$P_a O_2 = 125$ mmHg
$P_a CO_2 = 39$ mmHg

$P_a O_2 = 60$ mmHg
$P_a CO_2 = 44$ mmHg

$P_a O_2 = 75$ mmHg
$P_a CO_2 = 39$ mmHg

Fig. 35-3. Depiction of two lung units, with equal blood flow to and from both units. One unit has a low $\dot{V}_A/\dot{Q}$ ratio; the other has a high $\dot{V}_A/\dot{Q}$ ratio. Levels of venous blood and inspired gases are normal ($P_{\bar{v}}O_2$ = mean venous O_2 tension; $P_I O_2$ = inspiratory O_2 tension; $P_A O_2$ = alveolar O_2 tension; $P_a O_2$ = arteriolar O_2 tension). (Modified from: Cherniack, N. S., Altose, M. D., and Kelsen, S. G. The respiratory system. In: Berne, R. H., and Levy, M. N., eds., *Physiology.* St. Louis: Mosby, 1983. P. 700.)

in P_{CO_2} and CO_2 content in the blood from the low $\dot{V}_A/\dot{Q}$ unit.

In a disease state, the number of low $\dot{V}_A/\dot{Q}$ units will be increased, causing PaO_2 to fall and $PaCO_2$ to rise. Stimulation of the central and peripheral chemoreceptors by either the elevated $PaCO_2$ or the hypoxic stimulation of the peripheral chemoreceptors augments alveolar ventilation (creating high $\dot{V}_A/\dot{Q}$ ratios) in those regions of the lung which are normal or not yet significantly diseased. In this case, systemic blood is likely to be hypoxemic with a near-normal $PaCO_2$. However, as the disease worsens, the area of the lung with low $\dot{V}_A/\dot{Q}$ ratios will enlarge. Because this occurs at the expense of the normal to high (healthy) $\dot{V}_A/\dot{Q}$ regions, the lung becomes progressively less able to pro-

vide adequate O_2 levels and to expel CO_2, thus intensifying the hypoxemia and CO_2 retention.

Compensatory Mechanisms Matching Ventilation and Perfusion

As mentioned in Chap. 33, alveolar hypoxia, that is, low **alveolar P_{O_2}** in poorly ventilated alveoli, causes **arteriolar constriction,** which increases the resistance to blood flow to these poorly ventilated alveoli. This event, in turn, redistributes blood flow to well-ventilated alveoli. In addition, alveolar hypocapnia, that is, low **alveolar P_{CO_2}** in overventilating alveoli or alveoli receiving a decreased blood flow, **constricts the small airways** leading to these alveoli. This increased airway resistance reduces the ventilation to these alveoli, resulting in a redistribution of gas to other alveoli with adequate blood flow, thereby creating a better match between ventilation and perfusion.

Summary

To achieve maximal gas exchange and normal blood gas levels, alveoli must be both ventilated and perfused. Ventilation with little or no perfusion is called alveolar dead space and results in PaO_2 and $PaCO_2$ levels that approach their respective levels in inspired air. Perfusion without ventilation is termed venous-to-arterial shunt and causes alveolar gas pressures to approximate those in venous blood. Shunts and alveolar dead space represent the extreme limits of low to high $\dot{V}_A/\dot{Q}$ ratios, respectively. Because the progressive decline in blood flow from the bottom to the top of the lung exceeds that for ventilation, there is a normal mismatching of ventilation with perfusion and hence a range of $\dot{V}_A/\dot{Q}$ ratios from the base to the apex of the lung. This $\dot{V}_A/\dot{Q}$ mismatching plus normal shunting causes aortic P_{O_2} levels that are slightly lower than alveolar values. For O_2, units with high $\dot{V}_A/\dot{Q}$ ratios cannot compensate for units with low $\dot{V}_A/\dot{Q}$ ratios because the shape of the oxyhemoglobin dissociation curve is not linear. Thus high $\dot{V}_A/\dot{Q}$ units cannot replace the O_2 lost by the low $\dot{V}_A/\dot{Q}$ units. Conversely, CO_2 retained by units with low $\dot{V}_A/\dot{Q}$ ratios can be eliminated by the units with high $\dot{V}_A/\dot{Q}$ ratios because the CO_2 dissociation curve for whole blood is essentially linear in the physiologic range. Thus, as long as sufficient healthy lung tissue remains, high $\dot{V}_A/\dot{Q}$ units can compensate for low $\dot{V}_A/\dot{Q}$ units and thereby maintain normal or near-normal blood levels of CO_2. However, as increasing areas of the lung become diseased, the ratio of high $\dot{V}A/\dot{Q}$ units to low $\dot{V}A/\dot{Q}$ units decreases, and CO_2 is retained.

Bibliography

Cherniak, N. S., Altose, M. D., Kelsen, S. G. The respiratory system. In: Berne, R. M., and Levy, M. N., eds. *Physiology,* Sect. VI. St. Louis: C. V. Mosby, 1983.

Comroe, J. H. *Physiology of Respiration,* 2nd ed. Chicago: Year Book Medical Publishers, 1974.

Levitzky, M. G. *Pulmonary Physiology,* 4th ed. New York: McGraw-Hill, 1995.

Mines, A. H. *Respiratory Physiology,* 2nd ed. New York: Raven Press, 1986.

Taylor, A. E., Rehder, K., Hyatt, R. E., and Parker, J. C. *Clinical Respiratory Physiology.* Philadelphia: W. B. Saunders, 1989.

West, J. B. *Respiratory Physiology,* 5th ed. Baltimore: Williams & Wilkins, 1995.

Part VI Questions: Respiratory Physiology

1. The vital capacity (VC) is the
   A. volume of air remaining in the lungs after a maximum expiration.
   B. total volume of air in the lungs when they are maximally inflated.
   C. volume of air inspired and expired with each normal breath.
   D. amount of air that can be inspired from the end-tidal expiratory position.
   E. maximum volume of air that can be exhaled after a maximum inspiration.

2. During normal tidal breathing (0.6 liter), a person shows an intrapleural pressure change of 3 cmH_2O. If his FRC is 2.5 liters, his specific compliance (in cmH_2O^{-1}) is
   A. 0.83.
   B. 0.2.
   C. 0.033.
   D. 0.33.
   E. 0.08.

3. Lung compliance is increased
   A. when surfactant levels decrease.
   B. in patients with emphysema.
   C. by pulmonary congestion.
   D. in patients with pulmonary interstitial fibrosis.
   E. when airway resistance is increased.

4. A normal individual is flying in an open-cockpit airplane at 6000 ft (1800 m). At this altitude, his PiO_2 is 120 mmHg and his $\dot{V}A$ is increased. Assuming his respiratory exchange ratio stays at 0.8, what would his $PaCO_2$ be (in mmHg) if his PaO_2 is restored to 100 mmHg by the increased $\dot{V}A$ (ignore the correction factor)?
   A. 32
   B. 16
   C. 25
   D. 42
   E. 56

5. Most CO_2 in the blood is transported in the form of

   A. carbamino compounds combined with plasma proteins.
   B. carbamino compounds combined with hemoglobin.
   C. physically dissolved in plasma and the cytosol of red blood cells.
   D. carbonic acid in plasma.
   E. bicarbonate in plasma.

6. Which of the following produces vasodilation of the pulmonary vasculature?
   A. Epinephrine
   B. Alveolar hypoxia
   C. Arachidonic acid
   D. Angiotensin-II
   E. Acetylcholine

7. Vascular resistance in the pulmonary circulation is highest in the
   A. extraalveolar vessels at low lung volumes.
   B. extraalveolar vessels at the functional residual capacity.
   C. extraalveolar vessels at high lung volumes.
   D. intraalveolar vessels at high lung volumes.
   E. intraalveolar vessels at low lung volumes.

8. Which of the following receptors mediate the hyperventilatory response to hypoxemia?
   A. Central chemoreceptors
   B. Pulmonary stretch receptors
   C. Carotid bodies
   D. Irritant receptors

9. In the normal lung,
   A. low $\dot{V}A/\dot{Q}$ ratios are found primarily at the apex.
   B. low $\dot{V}A/\dot{Q}$ are found primarily at the base.
   C. both $\dot{V}A$ and $\dot{Q}$ are higher at the apex than at the base.
   D. normal $\dot{V}A/\dot{Q}$ mismatching occurs because $\dot{V}A$ is higher at the base than at the apex, whereas $\dot{Q}$ is higher at the apex than at the base.
   E. at the apex, $\dot{Q}$ normally exceeds $\dot{V}A$.

10. With respect to a normal PaO_2 of 100 mmHg and $PaCO_2$ of 40 mmHg, which of the following changes would be exhibited by blood coming from a low $\dot{V}A/\dot{Q}$ unit?

   A. Low PaO_2 and high $PaCO_2$
   B. High PaO_2 and low $PaCO_2$
   C. Low PaO_2 and low $PaCO_2$
   D. High PaO_2 and high $PaCO_2$
   E. No change

VII Renal and Acid-Base Physiology

Part Editor

Robert O. Banks

36 Elements of Renal Function

Robert O. Banks

Objectives

After reading this chapter, you should be able to

List the functions of the kidneys

List the major anatomic structures in the kidney, and describe their functional organization

List and define the three major mechanisms at work in the formation of urine

Cite the formula for renal clearance

Explain why the clearance of a substance that is freely filtered and not reabsorbed or secreted equals the glomerular filtration rate

Describe the application of the Fick principle to the kidney, and explain why the clearance of a substance that is totally cleared by the kidney equals the renal plasma flow

Define the filtration fraction and give normal values

Distinguish between total renal plasma flow and effective renal plasma flow

Explain renal extraction

Define filtered load and fractional excretion, and calculate the filtered Na^+ load per day and the fractional Na^+ excretion

---

The kidney represents the primary organ of homeostasis in its regulation of both the volume and composition of many constituents of the extracellular fluid space. Although this part on renal physiology primarily focuses on the homeostatic role of the kidney, the excretion of metabolic waste products and the regulation of **red blood cell synthesis** through the **production of erythropoietin** represent two other important renal functions.

Anatomy of the Kidney

The anatomy of the kidney is summarized in Figs. 36-1 and 36-2. There are two clearly defined zones in the kidney — an outer region, referred to as the **cortex,** and an inner region, called the **medulla.** In the human kidney, the medulla is divided into a number of conical areas called the **renal pyramids.** Within each pyramid, the medulla can be further partitioned into an **outer medulla,** containing an **outer** and an **inner stripe,** and an **inner medulla.**

The apex of the inner medulla is often referred to as the **papilla** and protrudes into the pelvic space.

As is illustrated in Figs. 36-1 and 36-2, the kidney is highly vascular. Even though the combined kidney weight constitutes a relatively small percentage (0.5%) of the total body weight, approximately 20% of the entire cardiac output perfuses the kidney under resting conditions. Because the normal cardiac output is about 5 liters/min, the combined renal blood flow (RBF) to the right plus left kidney is close to 1 liter/min.

The major sites of **resistance to blood flow** in the kidney are located in the afferent and efferent arterioles. Of the total renal vascular resistance (defined by the ratio of the mean arterial pressure minus the mean renal venous pressure divided by the RBF), most (greater than 90%) is due to the combined resistance of the afferent and efferent arteriole. This **portal system** allows for very efficient regulation of the pressure in the glomerular capillaries, which are interposed between the two arteriolar segments of the renal vasculature.

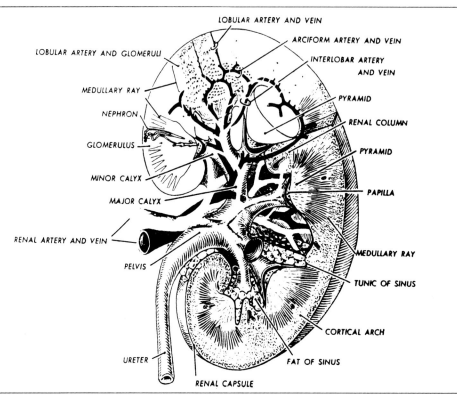

Fig. 36-1. The vascular and tubular networks in the human kidney. Lobular arteries and veins are also referred to as *interlobular vessels; arciform* and *arcuate* are also synonymous. (Reproduced with the permission of Oxford University Press from: Smith, H. W. *Principles of Renal Physiology.* New York: Oxford University Press, 1956.)

The functional unit of the kidney is the **nephron,** and there are approximately 800,000 of these tubular structures in each kidney. Within the closed end of each tubule is the filtering unit of the nephron, the **renal corpuscle.** The renal corpuscle is composed of the glomerular capillaries, generally referred to as the **glomerulus,** and the surrounding tubular element, known as **Bowman's capsule.**

Glomeruli are located only in the cortex. There are, however, three general types of nephrons: those with glomeruli originating in the superficial regions of the cortex, referred to as **superficial** or **outer cortical nephrons;** those with glomeruli originating in the **midcortical regions;** and those with glomeruli in the **juxtamedullary region** (see Fig. 36-2). In the human kidney, approximately 15% of the total nephron population is of the juxtamedullary variety.

There are four major tubular segments of the nephron, the **proximal tubule,** the intermediate tubule or **loop of Henle,** the **distal tubule,** and the **collecting duct** (see Fig.

36-2). Each of these can be further divided. The proximal tubule has a convoluted portion, or the **proximal convoluted tubule,** and a straight segment, also known as the **pars recta.** Three cell types form the epithelial lining of these proximal structures. The **S_1 segment,** composed of S_1-type cells, makes up the beginning and middle portions of the convoluted proximal tubule. S_1 cells are characterized by numerous microvilli and mitochondria. The **S_2 segment** forms the remaining portion of the convoluted tubule and the initial portion of the straight segment. S_2 cells have fewer microvilli and mitochondria than do S_1 cells. Finally, the remaining portion of the pars recta is called the **S_3 segment;** S_3 cells have few microvilli and mitochondria.

The **loop of Henle** is divided into the descending and ascending limbs. These loops descend to varying depths into the medulla of the kidney. In general, those which originate from glomeruli in superficial regions of the kid-

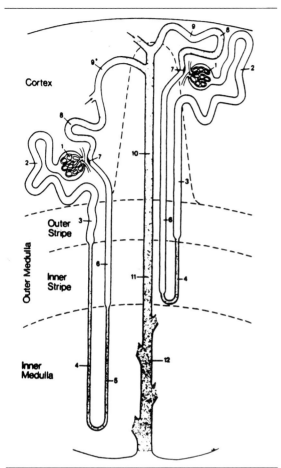

Cortex

Outer Medulla

Outer Stripe

Inner Stripe

Inner Medulla

Fig. 36-2. An illustration, not drawn to scale, of the long-looped and short-looped nephrons (1 = The renal corpuscle; 2 = the proximal convoluted tubule; 3 = the proximal straight tubule; 4 = the descending limb of Henle's loop; 5 = the thin ascending limb; 6 = the thick ascending limb; 7 = the macula densa; 8 = the distal convoluted tubule; 9 = the connecting tubule; 9* = the connecting tubule of the juxtamedullary nephron that forms an arcade; 10 = the cortical collecting duct; 11 = the outer medullary collecting duct; 12 = the inner medullary collecting duct). A medullary ray in the cortex is delineated by a *dashed line.* (Reproduced with permission of: Kritz, W., and Bankir, L. A standard nomenclature for structures of the kidney. *Am. J. Physiol.* 254:Fl–F8, 1988.)

ney descend only to the outer medulla, the so-called **short-looped nephrons;** those of the juxtamedullary variety descend into the inner medulla, often to the tip of the papilla, the so-called **long-looped nephrons.** The lumina of both

the descending and ascending limbs of Henle's loop are lined with relatively thin epithelial cells and are therefore referred to as the **thin descending** and **thin ascending limbs.** These epithelial cells contain very few mitochondria and microvilli.

The initial segment of the distal tubule is the thick ascending limb of the outer medulla, referred to as the **medullary thick ascending limb.** In the cortex, the thick ascending limb is referred to as the **cortical thick ascending limb,** each of which comes into contact with the afferent arteriole of its parent glomerulus, forming a complex known as the **juxtaglomerular apparatus.** This unit is composed of differentiated epithelial cells of the tubule (macula densa cells) and afferent arteriole (juxtaglomerular cells) plus interposed lacis cells.

The terminal segment of the distal tubule (beyond the macula densa) is the **distal convoluted tubule.** The distal convoluted tubules of superficial nephrons return to the surface of the kidney and represent, in addition to the proximal convoluted tubules of these nephrons, one of the tubular regions accessible to **micropuncture.**

The **collecting duct** is made up of several segments, and although there are minimal **morphologic** differences between them, there are important **physiologic** differences. The first segment is the **connecting tubule** and consists of two cell types: **connecting tubule** cells and **intercalated cells.** The transition to the cortical collecting duct is arbitrarily defined by the first appearance of collecting duct cells. The cortical collecting duct is located primarily in the medullary rays of the kidney. At the transition between the cortex and medulla, the tubule is referred to as the **outer medullary collecting duct.** Similarly, the collecting duct in the inner medulla is referred to as the **inner medullary collecting duct.** There are two primary cells in the collecting duct — **collecting duct** or **principal cells** and the **intercalated cells.**

There are important anatomic and, therefore, physiologic relationships between the vascular and tubular elements of the kidney. Thus efferent arterioles of the superficial cortex, and to a lesser extent those in the mid-cortical region, form **peritubular capillary networks** that are closely associated with the proximal and distal convoluted tubules of the parent glomerulus. By contrast, efferent vessels of juxtamedullary glomeruli form loop-type structures, called **vasa recta,** which descend to varying depths in the medulla. Consequently, the postglomerular blood of juxtamedullary nephrons does not perfuse proximal or distal convoluted tubules and therefore cannot be affected by transport-related events in these regions of the nephron. Instead, these proximal and distal tubular segments are perfused with blood from the efferent arterioles of glomeruli that originate in the midcortex.

General Aspects of Urine Formation

The physiologic basis of renal function can be summarized by three primary events: **filtration, reabsorption,** and **secretion.**

Filtration

Filtration takes place only in the glomerulus and depends on the balance between **hydrostatic** and **colloid osmotic pressures** in the glomerular capillary and in Bowman's space. In other words, filtration is regulated by the **Starling forces** governing fluid movement across the capillary wall (see Chaps. 1 and 26 for a review of Starling forces). The rate of filtration in the glomerulus is usually expressed as milliliters per minute or as liters per day.

Reabsorption

Reabsorption represents the **movement of water and solute** from the tubular lumen to the peritubular capillary network. Reabsorption of water is passive, but that of solute may be active or passive depending on the particular solute and nephron segment involved.

Secretion

Secretion represents the **net addition** of solute to the tubular lumen and almost always is an **active transport process.** Secretion is often mistakenly equated with excretion, which merely refers to the solute contained in the final urine.

Renal Clearance

The clearance principle, as applied to the kidney, is exceedingly useful and important for determining several variables of renal function in both the experimental and clinical setting. At first glance, the concept is deceptively simple, yet it is often difficult to fully appreciate the physiologic implications of a clearance value. Therefore, the concept of clearance will be approached by analyzing its definition, its mathematical formula, and the clearance of several solutes, the renal handling of which are well known.

Clearance is defined as the volume of plasma required to supply a given amount of a substance excreted in the urine per unit of time; it also can be defined as the volume of plasma cleared of a given substance per unit of time. In general, for clearance to be measured, the subject must be in a steady-state condition. The **formula for clearance is**

$$C_x = \frac{(U_x)(V)}{P_x}$$

(36-1)

where C_x is the clearance of substance x, U_x is the urine concentration of substance x, V is the urine flow rate, and P_x is the arterial plasma concentration of substance x. To satisfy the condition of a steady-state, the urine and plasma concentrations of substance x and the urinary flow rate must not change during the collection period.

The **units of clearance** are defined by the following equations:

$$C = \frac{(U)(V)}{P}$$

$$C = \frac{(mass / volume)(volume / unit\ time)}{mass / volume}$$

$$C = volume / unit\ time\ (usually\ expressed\ as\ milliliters\ per\ minute)$$

(36-2)

Examples of Clearance

Inulin Clearance

Inulin is a polymer of fructose and is one of the solutes used to measure the volume of the **extracellular fluid** (see Chap. 1). It is an inert substance that freely crosses most capillaries yet does not traverse the cell membrane. Consequently, inulin is freely filtered in the kidney, not reabsorbed or secreted. Given these characteristics, the inulin clearance therefore equals the glomerular filtration rate (GFR), for the reasons illustrated in Fig. 36-3. As this figure shows, the amount of inulin entering the total nephron population per unit of time, in a steady-state, must equal the amount of inulin leaving these nephrons. Because inulin is freely filtered, the inulin concentration in the glomerular capillary plasma equals its concentration in the fluid in Bowman's space, both of which are equal to the inulin concentration in arterial plasma. Therefore, the amount of inulin entering the nephron per unit of time is given by the product of the inulin concentration in arterial plasma timcs the volume flow of fluid entering the nephron — the GFR. In other words:

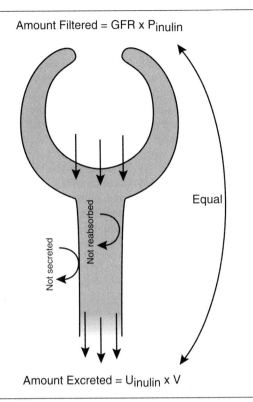

Amount Filtered = GFR x P$_{inulin}$

Not secreted

Not reabsorbed

Equal

Amount Excreted = U$_{inulin}$ x V

Fig. 36-3. This figure represents the sum of all the nephrons. Since inulin is neither reabsorbed nor secreted, the amount of inulin filtered must equal the amount excreted. These facts, coupled with the fact that inulin is also freely filtered, provide the basis for equating the clearance of inulin with the glomerular filtration rate (GFR) (P$_{inulin}$ = inulin concentration in arterial plasma; U$_{inulin}$ = inulin concentration in urine).

$$(GFR)(P_{inulin}) = (U_{inulin})(V)$$
$$\text{or GFR} = \frac{(U_{inulin})(V)}{P_{inulin}} \quad\quad (36\text{-}3)$$

Thus the clearance of inulin, or of any freely filtered, nonreabsorbed, and nonsecreted solute, equals the GFR.

A healthy 20-year-old person who weighs 70 kg has a GFR of about 120 ml/min, or about 70 ml/min/m^2 of body surface area. Males and females with similar weights have similar GFR values. The GFR decreases with aging, such that an average 70-kg, 60-year-old person has a GFR of about 100 ml/min. By contrast, at birth the GFR, corrected for body surface area, is relatively low and averages only

about 20 ml/min/m^2. The GFR reaches the adult value of 70 ml/mm/m^2 by 1 to 3 years of age.

Creatinine Clearance

In the human kidney, besides being freely filtered, a small amount of creatinine (Cr) is secreted into the lumen of the proximal tubule. Consequently, the amount of creatinine excreted slightly exceeds the amount filtered. The difference is relatively small and averages only about 10% in the normal kidney (at low GFR values, the secreted component becomes a larger proportion of the amount excreted). Because creatinine is an endogenous substance and its clearance only exceeds the GFR by approximately 10%, creatinine clearance is an important clinical assessment. Moreover, because the production rate of creatinine is relatively constant (about 1.2 mg/min in a 70-kg person) and is not affected by renal disease, creatinine clearance and the plasma creatinine concentration provide important information regarding the **status of glomerular function.** The usefulness of the plasma creatinine concentration as a predictor of glomerular function is illustrated in the following analysis:

Creatinine production rate = a constant rate (k) of approximately 1.2 mg/min
Creatinine production rate = creatinine excretion rate
Therefore, $k = (U_{Cr})(V) = (GFR)(P_{Cr})$

Given a normal GFR of 120 ml/min, the average plasma creatinine concentration is therefore about 0.01 mg/ml, or 1 mg/dl.

To illustrate the importance of an increasing plasma concentration of creatinine, assume that a patient has an initial plasma creatinine concentration of 1 mg/dl, but several months later this increases to 10 mg/dl. If the patient does not have muscular dystrophy or some other disease that can alter the production rate of creatinine, then the patient's GFR would have decreased to one-tenth of its initial value. In other words, an estimate of the patient's GFR can be obtained by simply determining the plasma concentration of creatinine (it is important to note that following a change in the GFR, 4 to 5 days must elapse before a new steady-state plasma creatinine value can be attained). If the plasma creatinine concentration is elevated, and because the plasma creatinine concentration is only an estimate of the GFR due to the assumptions inherent in creatinine analysis (to be discussed), collection of a timed urine sample (usually for 24 hours) or evaluation of the clearance of an exogenously administered glomerular marker can then be used to verify the status of glomerular function.

As mentioned, there are some qualifications and assumptions regarding the predictive nature of the plasma creatinine concentration as it relates to the GFR. Thus a number of factors affect the plasma creatinine concentration besides the GFR and its endogenous production rate. These factors include the degree of tubular secretion, as well as the dietary intake of creatinine and its extrarenal excretion. Other solutes in plasma also interfere with the chemical assay normally used for creatinine. For these reasons, it is important to measure the renal clearance of creatinine or an exogenous glomerular marker when renal disease is anticipated.

Urea Clearance

Urea is an end product of hepatic protein metabolism. It is routinely measured in blood as the **blood urea nitrogen** (BUN), and its clearance is normally 40% to 50% of the GFR, indicating that there is net passive reabsorption of urea.

The urea clearance (C_{urea}) varies with the urine flow rate; at low flow rates, C_{urea} is about 40% of the GFR but increases to about 60% of the GFR at high rates. Consequently, the BUN is particularly useful as an indicator of extrarenal ECF volume depletion. Since volume depletion results in a greater decrease in urine flow rate relative to the GFR, the BUN will increase more than the plasma creatinine concentration, resulting in a condition referred to as **prerenal azotemia** (BUN/creatinine ratio > 20/1).

The production rate of urea also can vary substantially and will cause related changes in the BUN. For example, the BUN increases with increases in protein intake, during glucocorticoid therapy, and with gastrointestinal bleeding. Nonetheless, the BUN, which is normally about 10 to 20 mg/dl (about 6 mM/liter) does increase as the GFR decreases and, therefore, can be used as a marker for the status of glomerular function in patients.

Clearance of Organic Acids and Bases

The **Fick principle,** a concept discussed in conjunction with the determination of cardiac output (see Chap. 23), also provides the basis for one of the methods used to estimate **renal plasma flow** (RPF). If a solute y is excreted by the kidney but not metabolized and does not enter the lymphatics or red blood cells, then the amount of y entering and leaving the kidney in a steady-state will be the same:

$$(RPF_a)(P_{ay}) = (U_y)(V) + (RPF_v)(P_{vy}) \tag{36-4}$$

where P_{ay} and P_{vy} are the arterial and renal venous plasma concentrations of y, respectively, and a and v are the arterial and venous values, respectively.

Therefore, if RPF_a equals RPF_v, then

$$RPF = \frac{(U_y)(V)}{(P_{ay} - P_{vy})} \tag{36-5}$$

This equation does not yield a clearance but illustrates that RPF can be calculated if the amount of a substance excreted and the difference in the arterial and venous concentrations across the kidney are known. Moreover, a number of weak organic acids and bases (penicillin, uric acid, histamine, serotonin, etc.) are avidly secreted by the proximal tubule, resulting in a very low renal venous concentration of these solutes. One of the most widely studied weak organic acids is **_p_-aminohippuric acid** (PAH). If the concentration of PAH in renal venous plasma is zero, then the preceding equation reduces to a clearance:

$$RPF = \frac{(U_{PAH})(V)}{P_{aPAH}} \tag{36-6}$$

This equation is the clearance of PAH (C_{PAH}). Thus, if a given solute is avidly secreted by the kidney enough that the renal venous concentration of the material is zero, the clearance of that solute will equal the RPF.

If the renal venous concentration of PAH is zero, then the **renal extraction** (E), where E = $P_a - P_v/P_a$, for PAH would be 1.0, or 100%. The renal extraction of all the organic acids and bases is, in fact, less than 100%, with that for PAH averaging about 90%. Therefore, the clearance of PAH is less than the actual RPF by approximately 10%. Some investigators have referred to the clearance of PAH as an indicator of the **effective renal plasma flow.**

The average PAH clearance and extraction values for a healthy 20-year-old person weighing 70 kg are 540 ml/min and 0.9, respectively. Therefore, the average RPF (given by the clearance value of PAH divided by the extraction value) is 600 ml/min. Since the normal hematocrit (hct) is approximately 40%, the RBF is 1000 ml/min (if one neglects the non-red blood cell elements in blood, then RBF = RPF/1 − hct). RPF decreases with age, reaching about 420 ml/min at age 60.

Given that the GFR is normally about 120 ml/min and the RPF is 600 ml/min, only about 20% of the total renal plasma flow is actually filtered. This relationship between RPF and GFR is referred to as the **filtration fraction** (FF) and is equal to the ratio of the GFR to the RPF:

$$FF = \frac{GFR}{RPF} \tag{36-7}$$

The filtration fraction is not a fixed value, and as will be discussed further in Chap. 37, the factors that affect GFR and RPF ultimately affect the filtration fraction.

Glucose and Albumin Clearance

The clearances of glucose and albumin are defined, as previously explained, by the amount of glucose and albumin excreted divided by the plasma glucose and albumin concentrations, respectively. Under normal conditions, virtually no glucose or albumin is excreted, and therefore, the clearance of these solutes is zero. This illustrates one of the **significant limitations** of the clearance approach, namely, that the clearance data alone do not permit firm conclusions to be obtained about the renal handling of a given solute. Thus the clearances of both glucose and albumin are zero, yet, as will be discussed, glucose is freely filtered but avidly reabsorbed by a Na^+-coupled, secondary active reabsorptive process in the early portions of the proximal tubule. By contrast, the **permeability and selectivity** of the renal corpuscle primarily account for the low clearance of albumin. Other methodologies, such as **micropuncture** and **microperfusion** of isolated tubular segments, are used to elucidate tubular events.

Sodium Clearance

The clearance of Na^+ is equal to $(U_{Na})(V)/P_{Na}$. Under normal conditions, the amount of Na^+ ingested is equal to the amount lost from the body (see Chap. 40 for a complete discussion of Na^+ balance). Although the amount of Na^+ ingested varies considerably among individuals, the average person consuming a Western diet ingests about 150 meq/day. Because approximately 95% of this Na^+ (or about 140 meq/day) is excreted in the urine (5% is lost in feces and sweat), and since the plasma Na^+ concentration is about 140 meq/liter, the clearance of Na^+ is roughly 1 liter/day (140 meq/day divided by 140 meq/liter), or only about 0.7 ml/min.

Based on the preceding analysis for Na^+, it is apparent that only a small fraction of the filtered Na^+ load, defined as the product of the GFR and the plasma Na^+ concentration, is actually excreted; that is, most of the filtered Na^+ is reabsorbed. Thus the fractional excretion (FE) of any freely filtered substance x is given by

$$FE_x = \frac{\text{amount of x excreted}}{\text{amount of x filtered}} \tag{36-8}$$

or

$$FE_x = \frac{(U_x)(V)}{(GFR)(P_x)} = \frac{C_x}{GFR} = \frac{C_x}{C_{inulin}} \tag{36-9}$$

The fractional excretion of Na^+ would be less than 1% (140 meq/day excreted compared with approximately 25,000 meq/day filtered).

Summary

The differences in the renal handling of representative solutes translate into a spectrum of renal clearances, differing from one solute to another and varying with the status of renal function. The clearance of a substance such as inulin that is freely filtered and not reabsorbed or secreted is equal to the GFR. In the clinical setting, the clearance of creatinine is especially useful for estimating glomerular function. If a particular solute has a clearance that is greater than inulin's, and if the solute is freely filtered and not synthesized by the kidney, this indicates that the solute undergoes net secretion by the kidney (there could be a combination of active or passive reabsorption in addition to the active secretion). Similarly, if another solute has a clearance less than inulin and is also freely filtered, net reabsorption must predominate (again, a combination of active or passive reabsorption as well as active secretion could occur).

Clearance must represent a virtual (apparent) volume. For example, in the illustration for Na^+, 0.7-ml "packets" of plasma, devoid of Na^+, do not circulate. Rather, it is *as if* 0.7 ml of plasma were completely cleared of Na^+ each minute. In actuality, the excreted Na^+ derives from the entire extracellular fluid or, more precisely, from the total quantity of exchangeable Na^+ in the body. On the other hand, inulin clearance can be equated with an important variable of renal function — the GFR. Similarly, the clearances of PAH and other weak organic acids and bases approximate another important variable of renal function — the RPF.

Bibliography

Beeuwkes, R., III. The vascular organization of the kidney. *Annu. Rev. Physiol.* 42:531–542, 1980.

Kritz, W., and Bankir, L. A standard nomenclature for structures of the kidney. *Am. J. Physiol.* 254:F1–F8, 1988.

37 Renal Hemodynamics and Glomerular Filtration

Robert O. Banks

Objectives

After reading this chapter, you should be able to

List and describe the forces involved in the formation of the glomerular ultrafiltrate

Describe the composition of the glomerular ultrafiltrate

List and describe the physiologic mechanisms involved in the regulation of the glomerular filtration rate and renal blood flow

Explain how autoregulation controls renal blood flow and the glomerular filtration rate and cite possible mechanisms

State the normal adult values for the glomerular filtration rate and renal blood flow in humans

List the major metabolic substrates and describe the unique nature of renal metabolism

Describe the renal handing of low-molecular-weight and high-molecular-weight proteins

---

As noted in Chap. 36, the kidneys represent only about 0.5% of the body weight yet receive approximately 20% of the cardiac output. This relatively large blood flow per gram of tissue (about 4 ml/min/g) is one of the highest blood flow values for any of the organs in the body and undoubtedly reflects the need to support the high filtering capacity of the kidneys rather than to provide for any unique nutrient requirements. The high flow is the result of a relatively low renal vascular resistance. **Renal vascular resistance** is a physiologic variable that is affected by changes in renal sympathetic nerve activity (the kidney is richly innervated); by the influence of a number of hormones, autacoids, and paracrine substances; and by changes in the renal arterial blood pressure (autoregulation of renal blood flow [RBF]).

The profile of the vascular blood pressure values in the renal circulation is illustrated in Fig. 37-1. As noted in Chap. 36 and shown in this figure, the major resistance sites — the vascular regions with the largest decreases in pressure — are located in the afferent and efferent arterioles.

Compared with other capillary beds, the pressure in the glomerular capillary is high. This high pressure accounts for the **net ultrafiltration** pressure in the glomerulus, as will be discussed. In addition, the high vascular resistance of the efferent arteriole produces a relatively low pressure in the peritubular capillaries; this low capillary pressure in the postglomerular vessels favors the reabsorption of solutes and water from the renal interstitial fluid space back into the vascular space.

Approximately 90% to 95% of the total postglomerular RBF perfuses the renal cortex. The remaining 5% to 10% perfuses the renal medulla via the vasa recta, but only a relatively small fraction of this (less than 1%) perfuses the

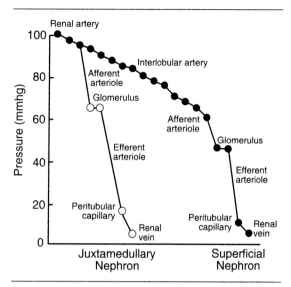

Fig. 37-1. Blood pressure values in arteries, arterioles, capillaries, and veins of the kidney. The largest decreases in pressure, reflecting the highest intrarenal vascular resistance, occur in the afferent and efferent arterioles.

inner medulla. The low inner medullary blood flow helps conserve the **medullary osmolar gradient,** a phenomenon that will be described in Chap. 39.

Glomerular Dynamics

Structure

The glomerular architecture is ideally suited to support its primary function — the formation of an ultrafiltrate of plasma. Each **glomerulus** is composed of 20 to 40 capillary loops with an estimated total surface area of as much as 15,000 cm^2/100 g. A high glomerular **ultrafiltration coefficient** (K$_f$, which is the product of the **hydraulic permeability** and the **filtration surface area**), in conjunction with the favorable net filtration pressure that exists between the glomerular capillary and Bowman's space, results in the ultrafiltration of relatively large volumes of plasma (180 liters/day).

Within the glomerulus, **podocytes** with projected foot processes create **filtration slits** that are about 250 Å wide. These slits may contribute to the **permeability characteristics** of the glomerular unit. However, more recent evidence has demonstrated that **fixed negative charges** (probably afforded by the basement membrane) are also important in determining the glomerular permeability

characteristics. Filtration normally approaches zero for substances with the size and charge of albumin (molecular weight 60,000; diameter 36 Å). The loss of negative charges in the glomerulus may account for the proteinurea often associated with glomerulopathies. Figure 37-2 shows how both the charge and size affect the filtration and subsequent excretion of different sizes of neutral and charged dextran molecules. For any given molecular radius, the fractional clearance of cationic dextran molecules exceeds

Fig. 37-2. The fractional clearance (C$_{dextran}$/C$_{inulin}$) of different-sized neutral, cationic and anionic dextran molecules in normal rats and in rats with experimentally induced nephrotoxic serum nephritis (NSN). (Modified from: Bohrer, M. P., et al. Permselectivity of the glomerular capillary wall. *J. Clin. Invest.* 61:72–78, 1978.)

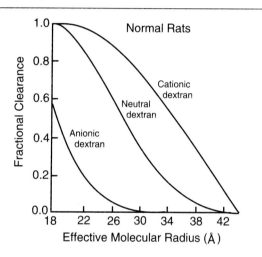

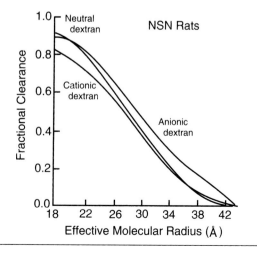

that of neutral molecules, but the fractional clearance of anionic molecules is less. By contrast, in rats with experimentally induced nephrotoxic serum nephritis, the fractional clearance of anionic dextran molecules markedly increases and resembles that of the neutral dextrans; the excretion of neutral dextran molecules is similar in normal and experimental rats.

Physical Forces

As noted in Chap. 36, **glomerular filtration** is determined by the balance of **Starling forces** that exist between the capillary lumen and Bowman's space. Accordingly:

$$GFR = K_f[(HP_{cap} + COP_{BS}) - (HP_{BS} + COP_{cap})]$$
(37-1)

where K_f is the ultrafiltration coefficient, equal to the capillary surface area times the hydraulic (water) permeability coefficient, HP_{cap} is the mean (average) hydrostatic pressure along the length of the capillary, COP_{cap} is the mean (average) colloid osmotic pressure along the length of the glomerular capillary, and HP_{BS} and COP_{BS} are the hydrostatic and colloid osmotic pressures in Bowman's space, respectively (the term **hydrostatic pressure** as used in these equations actually refers to the total pressure, which is the sum of the hydraulic plus the hydrostatic pressure).

Because the **colloid osmotic pressure** in Bowman's space is normally zero, the preceding equation reduces to

$$GFR = K_f[(HP_{cap} - HP_{BS}) - COP_{cap}]$$
(37-2)

or

$$GFR = K_f(\Delta P - COP_{cap})$$
(37-3)

where $\Delta P = HP_{cap} - HP_{BS}$.

The **hydrostatic** and **colloid osmotic pressures** in afferent and efferent arterioles have been measured directly in some species of animals, such as the Munich-Wistar rat and the squirrel monkey, that have glomeruli on the surface of the kidney. Because most animals have glomeruli that originate below the surface of the kidney, afferent and efferent vessels cannot be micropunctured. A typical profile for the hydrostatic pressure difference ($HP_{cap} - HP_{BS}$) and the colloid osmotic pressure along the length of the glomerular capillary in the Munich-Wistar rat is shown in Fig. 37-3A. Since both the hydrostatic and colloid osmotic pressure change along the length of the capillary, the ultrafiltration pressure is constantly decreasing as it approaches

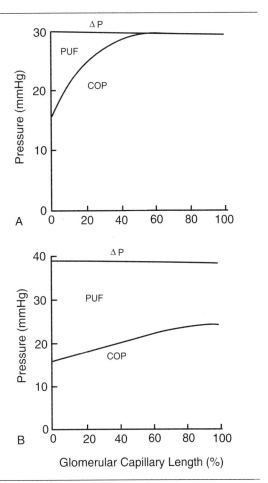

Fig. 37-3. Typical pressure profiles for ΔP and COP along the length of a glomerular capillary of rat (A) and dog (B). (ΔP is the difference in hydrostatic pressure between the capillary and Bowman's space and COP is the colloid osmotic pressure in plasma.) These data depict examples of filtration-pressure equilibrium (A) and disequilibrium (B). Average hydrostatic pressure values in Bowman's space are 11 mm Hg in the rat and 21 mm Hg for the dog. It should be noted that not all investigators have observed filtration-pressure equilibrium in the rat (PUF = net ultrafiltration pressure).

the efferent arteriolar end of the capillary. As is illustrated in Fig. 37-3A, the **net ultrafiltration pressure** (PUF), is delineated by the area between the curves for the net hydrostatic pressure and the colloid osmotic curves along the length of the glomerular capillary. Thus Eq. 37-3 reduces to

$$GFR = K_f(PUF) \qquad (37\text{-}4)$$

Glomeruli characterized by data similar to those illustrated in Fig. 37-3A are said to be in **filtration pressure equilibrium,** whereby the net ultrafiltration pressure is zero at the end of the capillary. Glomeruli that possess this equilibrium have a net ultrafiltration pressure that is highly dependent on the rate of plasma flow through the glomerulus, in that increases in RPF augment the net ultrafiltration pressure. By contrast, in glomeruli exhibiting **filtration-pressure disequilibrium** (Fig. 37-3B), whereby there is a net ultrafiltration pressure remaining at the end of the glomerular capillary, this pressure is less sensitive to increases in RPF.

Values for K_f in the renal vascular bed are one to two orders of magnitude greater than those in other vascular beds, such as in skeletal muscle. A number of factors may affect the K_f and therefore potentially influence the GFR. However, the status of filtration-pressure equilibrium versus disequilibrium determines whether changes in K_f alter the GFR. Specifically, under conditions of **disequilibrium,** increases in K_f augment the GFR but changes in K_f during filtration-pressure **equilibrium** do not markedly affect the GFR.

Regulation of Renal Blood Flow and the Glomerular Filtration Rate

Changes in either the afferent or efferent arteriolar resistance, or both, affect renal hemodynamics and, if there are resultant changes in glomerular capillary pressure, also affect the GFR. Because the glomerulus is a **portal system,** the potential for varying glomerular capillary pressure is great. As discussed previously, depending on whether filtration-pressure dysequilibrium or equilibrium dominates, changes in K_f or RPF also will affect the filtration rate. Finally, as illustrated in Eq. 37-1, the plasma colloid osmotic pressure is one of the determinants of the GFR and any changes will alter the filtration rate.

Hormonal Control

Many endogenous and exogenous substances affect RBF and the GFR, and some of these are listed in Table 37-1.

Administration of vasoconstrictors or activation of the sympathetic nervous system reduces the GFR. By contrast,

Table 37-1. Some Vasoactive Substances and Conditions That Affect Renal Blood Flow

Vasoconstrictors	Vasodilators
Norepinephrine (alpha receptors)	Acetylcholine and other muscarinic agonists
Epinephrine	Bradykinin
Angiotensin-II	Prostaglandins E_2 and I_2
Endothelin	Histamine (H_1 and H_2 receptors)
Vasopressin (V_1 receptors)	Isoproterenol
Serotonin	Dopamine (D_2 receptors)
	Papaverine
	Hyperosmotic solutions (e.g., mannitol)
	Ca^{2+}-channel antagonists
	Adenosine (also induces a transient constriction)
	Sodium nitroprusside
CONDITIONS	
Hemorrhage (mediated by hormones and increased renal nerve activity)	Expansion of the extracellular fluid (mediated by hormones and decreases in renal nerve activity)
Elevated ureteral pressure (chronic)	Elevated ureteral pressure (acute) (may be mediated by histamine and prostaglandins)
Strenuous exercise (mediated by hormones and increases in renal nerve activity)	

most vasodilators cause little or no change in the GFR. This has been attributed to secondary factors that operate during infusions of the vasodilators, such as decreased efferent arteriolar resistance with a resultant increase in tubular pressure, and to agonist-related decreases in K_f.

As discussed in Part IV, "Cardiovascular Physiology," a number of **vasodilators** exert their actions by means of an endothelium-dependent series of events. Although it is more difficult to assess the potential role of the endothelium at the organ level, it is likely that the endothelium dependence of certain vasodilators such as acetylcholine, histamine, and prostaglandins, as well as independence of such agents as nitric oxide and nitroprusside, also applies to vasodilator-induced changes in RBF.

Some of the **vasoactive agents** listed in Table 37-1 also exert direct tubular actions. Thus, for example, angiotensin-II, which is one of the most potent endogenous biologic vasoconstrictors, also stimulates proximal tubular Na$^+$ reabsorption. The **renin-angiotensin-aldosterone** system is important in the control of both vascular reactivity and volume (see Chap. 40).

Another important factor that increases RBF and GFR is **protein intake.** Glomerular hyperfiltration and elevated RBF are deleterious, causing glomerular sclerosis, and are of particular concern when there is reduced renal mass such as exists in various renal diseases. Dietary protein restriction can, under some conditions, offset the progressive loss of glomerular function, and some have advocated this to be an important therapeutic measure in treating renal disease.

Sympathetic Nervous System

Adrenergic postganglionic fibers innervate both vascular and tubular elements in the kidney, including the afferent and efferent arteriole, the proximal tubule, and the loop of Henle. The functional importance of the renal nerves has been the focus of intense investigation for many years. Nonetheless, the role of renal nerves in normal homeostatic functions of the kidney has not been fully elucidated. On the other hand, a number of conditions are associated with activation or inhibition of renal nerve activity and consequently markedly affect renal function. One of these conditions is **hemorrhage.** The loss of vascular volume leads to a decrease in the mean arterial blood pressure and subsequent activation of the carotid sinus and aortic arch reflexes. Heightened renal sympathetic nerve activity activates alpha-adrenergic receptors in afferent and efferent vessels, thereby increasing renal vascular resistance. Both RBF and the GFR decrease in this pathologic condition.

Autoregulation of Renal Blood Flow and Glomerular Filtration Rate

One of the important physiologic variables that does not normally influence renal hemodynamics or the glomerular filtration rate is **renal arterial blood pressure** (RAP). It should be noted that the experimental manipulation used in studies that evaluate the effects of perfusion pressure on renal hemodynamics only affects RAP. This maneuver is generally accomplished by placing an adjustable clamp on the renal artery of an experimental animal. Under these conditions, the mean arterial blood pressure (aortic blood pressure) is constant. As discussed previously, changes in

arterial blood pressure activate the sympathetic nervous system and consequently affect RBF and the GFR. Changing only the RAP avoids changes in the systemic arterial blood pressure and secondary changes in the renal hemodynamics.

Using the preceding methodology, changing RAP from approximately 180 to 80 mmHg causes relatively small changes in RBF and GFR. Typical autoregulatory profiles for RBF and GFR are illustrated in Fig. 37-4. As the RAP is reduced, because flow is constant, there must be a decrease in renal arterial resistance, as illustrated by Ohm's law. Current data indicate that the **afferent arteriole** is the primary site of pressure-induced changes in renal vascular resistance, but under some conditions, the efferent arteriole also may be involved. Thus, as RAP is lowered, there is a relatively large decrease in the afferent arteriolar resistance. Under some conditions, particularly those associated with **high plasma renin concentrations,** such as with low dietary Na$^+$ intake, reductions in RAP also may be associated with small angiotensin-II–mediated increases in efferent arteriolar resistance. As a consequence of afferent, and possibly efferent, arteriolar resistance changes within the autoregulatory range, glomerular capillary pressure remains relatively constant.

Autoregulation can be demonstrated in the isolated, perfused kidney, proving that renal nerves are not required for this phenomenon to occur. Two major theories have been

Fig. 37-4. Typical renal blood flow (RBF) and glomerular filtration rate (GFR) autoregulatory curves in the dog.

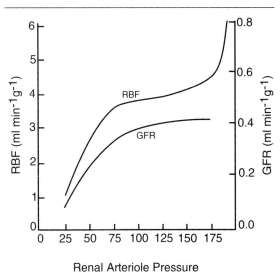

Renal Arteriole Pressure

advanced to account for autoregulation, and either one or a combination of both could be involved. The first is the **myogenic theory,** which proposes that changes in RAP directly affect smooth muscle activity. For example, a decrease in RAP leads to a decrease in stretch of the afferent arteriole causing the smooth muscle to relax and thereby decreasing vascular resistance. The second theory is the **distal tubular feedback theory,** or the so-called tubuloglomerular feedback proposal. It is well established that if the composition or delivery rate of a tubular solute entering the distal nephron is changed, this is detected by some mechanism which in turn changes the resistance of preglomerular elements (the afferent arteriole). If the flow entering the distal nephron is reduced, this causes a decrease in afferent arteriolar resistance, an increase in RBF, and an increase in the net ultrafiltration pressure. The sensor mechanism in the distal nephron appears to be the **macula densa,** but the nature of the triggering signal (changes in concentration of Na^+ or Cl^- or total solute) in the tubular lumen remains unknown. Evidence does not favor a major role for neural factors, adrenergic receptors, or the prostaglandin system. It has been reported that histamine H_1 receptor antagonists block RBF and GFR autoregulation, suggesting that histamine may contribute to this phenomenon. In addition, the increase in efferent arteriolar resistance that may occur when RAP is reduced in Na^+-depleted animals appears to be related to activation of the renin-angiotensin system.

Composition of the Glomerular Filtrate

The ultrafiltrate of plasma that is formed in the glomerulus is about 94% water and 6% solute and is virtually protein-free. **Diffusable nonelectrolytes** (e.g., glucose and urea) have the same concentration in filtrate as in plasma. The **Gibbs-Donnan effects** of charged, impermeant proteins produce small differences in the concentrations of filtered ions between plasma and ultrafiltrate. For example, the concentration ratio of monovalent anions in the filtrate to plasma is about 1.05; it is about 0.95 for monovalent cations.

With regard to **proteins,** the concentration of albumin in plasma is about 40 g/liter. The concentration of albumin in the early proximal tubule of the rat is about 15 mg/liter or less. More than 99% of these small amounts of filtered albumin is reabsorbed by the proximal tubule. Low-molecular-weight proteins (10,000 to 50,000 daltons) are filtered to varying degrees and are also reabsorbed in the proximal tubule.

In **disease states** that primarily interfere with glomerular function, large quantities of high-molecular-weight proteins are filtered and excreted (protein excretion may exceed 20 g/day). However, because low-molecular-weight proteins are filtered to some extent but reabsorbed in the proximal tubule, tubular disorders are more likely to be associated with impaired protein reabsorption and a consequential excretion of larger quantities of low-molecular-weight proteins (a so-called tubular protein-urea).

Metabolism

The metabolic cost of the work performed by the kidney is high. **Oxygen consumption** by the kidney per gram of tissue weight is higher than that for any other organ, primarily because of the large amount of Na^+ that must be reabsorbed (approximately 1 mol of O_2 per 28 eq of Na^+ reabsorbed). Considering the very high blood flow per gram of kidney, the arteriovenous O_2 content difference is very low (approximately 1.7 vol/dl) and is the lowest for any organ.

There is a linear relationship between renal O_2 consumption and the GFR. The reason for this close correlation is that an increase in the GFR is associated with an increase in the filtered Na^+ load and a resultant increase in Na^+ reabsorption. Because Na^+ reabsorption is an energy-dependent process, O_2 consumption by the kidney also increases.

Another unique aspect of O_2 dynamics in the kidney relates to the status of **medullary oxygenation.** Because the **vasa recta** are organized in a countercurrent fashion (see Chap. 39 for details), O_2 diffuses down a partial pressure gradient from the descending into the ascending limb; a CO_2 gradient in the opposite direction reverses the net movement of that gas from the ascending into the descending limb of the vasa recta. These events result in a relatively low medullary partial pressure for O_2 coupled with a relatively high partial pressure for CO_2.

The primary substrates utilized by the kidney are **free fatty acids** (particularly palmitic acid), **citrate,** and **lactate.** The kidney consumes very little glucose, and is in fact a gluconeogenic organ.

Summary

The kidney is a highly vascular organ, receiving approximately 20% of the cardiac output. Thus, under normal conditions, blood flow to the kidneys is about 1 liter/min.

Because the hematocrit is about 40%, the renal plasma flow is roughly 600 ml/min. Of this, approximately 20%, or 120 ml/min, enters Bowman's space in the form of an ultrafiltrate of plasma, which is referred to as the GFR. This ultrafiltrate is formed through the difference in Starling forces between the lumen of the glomerular capillary and Bowman's space. A number of important physiologic variables affect the RBF and GFR. RBF is primarily determined by the vascular resistance in the afferent and efferent arterioles. Because the glomerular capillary is positioned between these two arteriolar units, the glomerular capillary pressure, and hence the GFR, is also affected by the relative balance of afferent and efferent arteriolar resistance. In addition, the GFR is influenced by changes in the colloid osmotic pressure and by changes in the K_f of the glomerular capillary unit. A number of hormones, autacoids, and neural factors influence these physiologic variables, and thereby alter the RBF and GFR. On the other hand, changes in renal arterial pressure in the range of approximately 80 to 180 mmHg, do not markedly alter RBF or GFR, a phenomenon known as autoregulation. The mechanism responsible for autoregulation is unknown but appears to involve both a myogenic component and one that depends on a distal tubule feedback mechanism. The ultrafiltrate normally contains all the small diffusible nonelectrolytes and electrolytes in approximately the same concentrations as in arterial plasma. Because most of the ultrafiltrate is eventually reabsorbed along the nephron by active transport events or by processes that depend on these energy-consuming systems, the metabolic cost to the kidney is relatively large.

Bibliography

Arendshorst, W. J., and Gottschalk, C. W. Glomerular ultrafiltration dynamics: Euvolumia and plasma volume-expanded rats. *Am. J. Physiol.* 239:F171–186, 1980.

Brenner, B. M. Nephron adaptation to renal injury or ablation. *Am. J. Physiol.* 249:F324–F337, 1985.

Brenner, B. M., and Humes, H. D. Mechanisms of glomerular ultrafiltration. *N. Engl. J. Med.* 297:148–154, 1977.

Knox, F. G., et al. Regulation of glomerular filtration and proximal tubular reabsorption. *Circ. Res.* 36–37:I107–I118, 1975.

Navar, L. G. Renal autoregulation: perspectives from whole and single nephron studies. *Am. J. Physiol.* 234:F357–F370, 1978.

Oken, D. E. Does the ultrafiltration coefficient play a role in regulating glomerular filtration in the rat? *Am. J. Physiol.* 256:F505–F515, 1989.

Pollock, D. M., and Banks, R. O. Perspectives on renal blood flow autoregulation. *Proc. Soc. Exp. Biol. Med.* 198:800–805, 1991.

Silva, P. Renal fuel utilization, energy requirements, and function. *Kidney Int.* 32(Suppl. 22):S-9–S-14, 1987.

Wright, F. S., and Briggs, J. P. Feedback control of glomerular blood flow, pressure and filtration rate. *Physiol. Rev.* 59:958–1006, 1979.

38 Proximal Tubule Function

Robert O. Banks

Objectives

After reading this chapter, you should be able to

Distinguish between active and passive transport systems in the kidney

Describe both reabsorptive and secretory transport maximums with examples of each

Calculate the reabsorptive and secretory transport maximums, if given data

Explain renal threshold

Define the significance of a transport maximum value relative to the normal plasma concentration of a given substance

Characterize the renal handling of amino acids

Identify the major events that occur in the proximal tubule, including the nature and quantity of fluid reabsorption (H_2O, HCO_3^-, Cl^-, Na^+, K^+, glucose, amino acids, Ca^{2+}, HPO_4, and so on)

Explain the osmolarity of tubular fluid in the proximal tubule

State the fraction of water and Na^+ reabsorbed in the proximal tubule

Describe the phenomenon of glomerular-tubular balance and the possible mechanisms involved

Interpret the physiologic significance of increases and decreases in tubular fluid to plasma ratios

Major Events in the Proximal Tubule

Sodium Reabsorption

Approximately 60% to 70% of the filtered Na^+ is reabsorbed in the proximal tubule. These and other values for the fractional solute reabsorption in a given segment of the nephron are calculated from the **filtration rate of the single nephron** (the single-nephron glomerular filtration rate [SNGFR]), the tubular fluid to plasma concentration ratio (TF/P ratio) of the solute in question, the TF/P ratio of inulin at that same point, and the tubular fluid flow rate (V). The following analysis illustrates how this is derived.

If f is the fraction of a filtered solute x remaining at any point y along the nephron, because the amount of x at any point y equals $(TF_x)(V_{TF})$ and the amount of x filtered equals $(SNGFR)(P_x)$, then

$$f = \frac{(TF_x)(V_{TF})}{(SNGFR)(P_x)} \tag{38-1}$$

or

$$\frac{TF_x}{P_x} = f\left[\frac{SNGFR}{V_{TF}}\right] \tag{38-2}$$

From Eq. 38-5, it will be seen that

$$\frac{SNGFR}{V_{TF}} = \frac{TF_{inulin}}{P_{inulin}}$$

Therefore,

$$\frac{TF_X / P_X}{TF_{inulin} / P_{inulin}} = f \qquad (38\text{-}3)$$

In other words, the TF/P ratio of a freely filtered solute divided by the TF/P inulin ratio equals the fraction of the initial filtered quantity remaining at a particular point along the nephron. The TF/P Na^+ ratio at all points along the proximal tubule is 1.0. By contrast, the TF/P ratio for inulin at the end of the proximal tubule is 3:1. Thus one-third of the filtered Na^+ remains at this point.

The nature of Na^+ and other solute reabsorption in the proximal tubule is illustrated in Fig. 38-1. **Na^+ reabsorption** accounts for a major portion of the fluid reabsorbed in the proximal tubule (see the section "Volume Reabsorption"). As shown in Fig. 38-1, the driving force for Na^+ reabsorption from the lumen of the tubule into the proximal tubular cell is generated by a favorable electrochemical gradient for Na^+. A low intracellular fluid concentration of Na^+ is maintained by the action of a **Na^+, K^+-ATPase pump** located on the basolateral surface of the proximal tubular cell. The entry of Na^+ into proximal tubular cells is

Fig. 38-1. Some of the major transport-related events in the S_1 segment of the proximal tubule (AA = amino acids; Glu = glucose; PD = potential difference; CA = carbonic anhydrase).

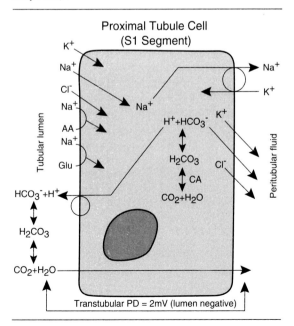

Proximal Tubule Cell
(S1 Segment)

Transtubular PD = 2mV (lumen negative)

accompanied by any one of a number of **secondary transport processes,** including Cl^-, amino acids, and glucose reabsorption, as well as H^+ secretion.

Osmolarity of Proximal Tubule Fluid

Reabsorption in the proximal tubule occurs **isosmotically.** Current evidence indicates that the osmolar concentration of tubular fluid in the proximal tubule may be a few (3 to 5) milliosmoles per liter less than plasma's. Thus, since the water permeability of the proximal tubule is very high, this small osmolar difference is sufficient to account for the large volume of fluid reabsorbed in the segment.

Organic Solute Reabsorption

Most (more than 90%) of the filtered glucose, amino acids, and HCO_3^- is reabsorbed by **Na^+-dependent symport processes** in the early portions of the proximal tubule (see Fig. 38-1). The reabsorption of **glucose** and **amino acids** takes place within the first 20% to 30% of the proximal tubule. Because these nonelectrolytes are reabsorbed with Na^+, the process is **electrogenic,** and this generates a small, lumen-negative, transtubular potential averaging about 2 mV in this region of the nephron. The **reabsorption of HCO_3^-** is secondary to and depends on a Na^+–H^+ antiport process (see Fig. 38-1). The reabsorption of HCO_3^- occurs in the early portions of the proximal tubule and is a preferential process compared with the **reabsorption of Cl^-.** Consequently, the tubular fluid Cl^- concentration increases in the S_1 segment of the proximal tubule. The TF/P Cl^- ratio for the last 75% of the proximal tubule is about 1.2:1. In addition, because the Cl^- permeability of the latter portions of the proximal tubule is relatively high, a small lumen-positive, transtubular potential averaging 2 mV develops in the last 75% of the proximal tubule. Details of HCO_3^- reabsorption and of the factors that influence the reabsorption of this important anion are covered in Chap. 43.

Potassium and Calcium Reabsorption

Roughly 60% to 70% of the filtered K^+ and Ca^{2+} is reabsorbed in the proximal tubule by means of combined active and passive diffusion, including solvent drag-related events mediated by paracellular pathways.

Volume Reabsorption

Approximately 60% to 70% of the filtered volume load is reabsorbed by the time it reaches the end of the proximal tubule. In other words, if the GFR is 120 ml/min, 70%, or 84 ml/min, is returned to the circulation via the peritubular capillaries surrounding the proximal tubule. Consequently, the volume flow entering the loop of Henle is approximately 36 ml/min (120 – 84 ml/min).

Estimates of the fractional volume reabsorption in the proximal tubule are determined from the inulin concentration in samples of tubular fluid taken from segments near the end of the proximal tubule. Because inulin is freely filtered, not reabsorbed or secreted, in the steady-state, the amount of inulin entering a single nephron must equal the amount of inulin passing at any point along that nephron, or

$$(SNGFR)(P_{inulin}) = (TF_{inulin})(V_{TF}) \qquad (38-4)$$

Therefore,

$$\frac{P_{inulin}}{TF_{inulin}} = \frac{V_{TF}}{SNGFR} \qquad (38-5)$$

The P/TF inulin ratio therefore represents the fraction of the initial filtered volume remaining in the nephron at that point. TF/P inulin ratios at the end of the proximal tubule are about 3 : 1. This means that one-third of the initial filtered volume remains and that two-thirds (hence 60% to 70%) was reabsorbed.

Glomerulotubular Balance

Fractional volume reabsorption in the proximal tubule is relatively constant and is independent of fluctuations in the GFR. This phenomenon is referred to as **glomerulotubular (G-T) balance** and serves to minimize large changes in the delivery rate of fluid to the loop of Henle and remaining portions of the distal nephron that would result from changes in the GFR.

The **mechanism of the G-T balance** is unknown but may stem from two factors: (1) increases in **Starling reabsorptive forces** in the peritubular capillaries (this hypothesis depends on there being a greater increase in the GFR than in the RPF such that the colloid osmotic pressure of postglomerular blood would increase and there would be a consequential increase in the reabsorptive force at the level of the tubule) or (2) increases in the **filtered load of organic solute** (glucose and amino acids) that would in turn be reabsorbed in the early portions of the proximal tubule and therefore promote the reabsorption of water.

Possible Mechanisms of Fluid Reabsorption in the Proximal Tubule

Luminal Hypotonicity

The theory of luminal hypotonicity is based on the fact that the water permeability of the proximal tubule is relatively high. Thus, when the osmolality differences between the tubular lumen and renal interstitial fluid space are comparatively small, theoretically, large volumes of water could be reabsorbed. The theory derives from the concept that the **active transport of Na$^+$** across the basolateral membrane (via the Na$^+$, K$^+$-ATPase pump) and the resultant **diffusion gradient** for the entry of Na$^+$ (cotransported with other solutes such as HCO$_3^-$, Cl$^-$, and organic solute) from the tubular lumen into the cell generates tubular fluid that is slightly hypotonic compared to plasma; the osmolality difference may only be 3 to 5 mOsm/kg of H$_2$O. Coupled with the high water permeability of the proximal tubule, this **"trivial" osmolar difference** may be sufficient to account for the relatively large volume of water reabsorbed in this segment of the nephron.

Anion Asymmetry

As noted previously, the preferential reabsorption of HCO$_3^-$ in the early portions of the proximal tubule augments luminal Cl$^-$ concentrations, whereby there is an axial decrease in the HCO$_3^-$ concentration and a corresponding increase in the Cl$^-$ concentration. In addition, the later portions of the proximal tubule become appreciably more permeable to Cl$^-$ than to HCO$_3^-$. Therefore, HCO$_3^-$ in the peritubular fluid becomes an effective **osmotic reabsorptive force** in this region. A favorable concentration gradient for passive Cl$^-$ reabsorption in this segment also causes Na$^+$ and water reabsorption throughout the later segments of the proximal tubule.

Finally, **Starling forces** in the peritubular capillary favor the net reabsorption of fluid from the interstitial fluid space; blood in the peritubular capillary is postglomerular, and therefore has a low hydrostatic pressure and high colloid osmotic pressure.

Reabsorptive and Secretory Transport Maximums

Many substances are reabsorbed or secreted by active transport systems. **Active transport events** are typically characterized by high-energy dependency and saturation kinetics, including both competitive and noncompetitive inhibition.

Reabsorptive Transport Maximums

As already noted, glucose is rapidly removed from the early portions of the proximal tubule (within the first 20% to 30% of the proximal tubule the glucose concentration falls to virtually zero). The Na^+-dependent reabsorptive process for glucose exhibits both competitive inhibition (it displays a reabsorptive transport maximum [T_m]) and noncompetitive inhibition with agents such as the **glucosides.** The **renal handling of glucose** can be partitioned as follows: (1) amount of glucose filtered per unit of time, (2) amount of glucose reabsorbed per unit of time, and (3) amount of glucose excreted per unit of time. Moreover, the amount of glucose excreted (U_{glu})(V) equals the difference between the amount of glucose filtered and the amount of glucose reabsorbed, or

$$(U_{glu})(V) = (GFR)(P_{Glu}) - \text{amount of glucose reabsorbed}$$

or

Amount of glucose reabsorbed =
$(GFR)(P_{Glu}) - (U_{Glu})(V)$

If the **plasma glucose concentration** (P_{Glu}) varies over a wide range, a **glucose "titration" curve** can be plotted, similar to that shown in Fig. 38-2. Several facts are illustrated in this figure. **First,** as the plasma glucose concentration increases, the filtered load of glucose (the product of the plasma glucose concentration and the GFR) increases in a linear fashion; this assumes that the GFR is constant, which, in practice, is difficult to achieve because increases in the plasma glucose concentration are usually associated with changes in the GFR. **Second,** at low plasma glucose concentrations, all the filtered glucose is reabsorbed, such that none is excreted. **Third,** the amount of glucose reabsorbed reaches a maximum value, the so-called $\mathbf{T_m}$ **for glucose** (T_{mG}). In the human, the T_{mG} is 300 to 400 mg/min.

The **renal threshold,** defined as the plasma glucose concentration at which glycosuria (glucose in the urine) is observed, is about 180 to 200 mg/dl. The renal threshold is considerably lower than that calculated because of the phenomenon of **splay.** Thus, given an average T_{mG} of 360 mg/min and an average GFR of 120 ml/min, the predicted renal threshold would be calculated as follows:

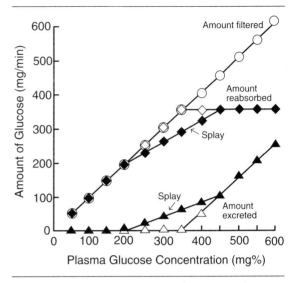

Fig. 38-2. Amounts of glucose filtered, reabsorbed, and excreted are shown as a function of the plasma glucose concentration. The transport maximum for glucose (T_{mG}) is given by the plateau value for the amount of glucose reabsorbed. Splay refers to the fact that glucose is exereted below the plasma value that would be predicted based on the glomerular filtration rate and the T_{mG}.

$$(GFR)(P_{Glu}) = T_{mG}$$
$$(120 \text{ ml/min})(P_{Glu}) = 360 \text{ ml/min}$$
$$P_{Glu} = 3 \text{ mg/ml, or } 300 \text{ mg/dl}$$

There could be a number of factors that influence splay, including a heterogeneity of T_{mG} values in different nephrons. Some nephrons have lower T_{mG} values than others, and consequently, the reabsorptive capacity is exceeded at relatively low plasma glucose concentrations.

At low plasma glucose concentrations the glucose clearance is zero. However, once the renal threshold is exceeded, glucose is excreted and its clearance value can be calculated. As the plasma glucose concentration continues to increase, the clearance increases and approaches the GFR. In other words, at high plasma glucose concentrations, the amount of glucose excreted approaches the amount filtered.

Because the T_{mG} is high relative to the amount filtered, the kidney normally reabsorbs all of the filtered glucose. Thus, the kidney does not participate in regulating the plasma glucose concentration.

Glucosuria can be of **extrarenal origin,** as exemplified by diabetes mellitus. In this disorder, which is due either to a lack of sufficient pancreatic insulin secretion or to resistance to the hormone, the plasma glucose concentration increases, the amount of glucose filtered exceeds the T_{mG}, and the additional glucose is excreted. Glucosuria also can be of **renal origin,** so-called **renal glucosuria.** For example glucosuria is associated with some forms of congenital diseases involving defects in the glucose reabsorptive mechanisms. **Fanconi's syndrome** is one such disorder. Glucosuria is also seen in patients with heavy metal poisoning.

Other substances that have reabsorptive T_m's are amino acids, organic anions, phosphate, and sulfate.

Amino Acids

Amino acids are freely filtered but completely reabsorbed in the early portions of proximal tubules through the mediation of Na^+-dependent processes. Several independent or partially overlapping transport mechanisms exist for the following groups of amino acids: **acidic** amino acids — glutamic and aspartic acids; **iminoglycine** amino acids — glycine, proline, and hydroxyproline; **basic** amino acids — cysteine, lysine, arginine, and ornithine; and **neutral** amino acids — alanine, valine, leucine, isoleucine, methionine, serine, threonine, histidine, tyrosine, phenylalanine, and tryptophan.

The T_m for amino acids is high relative to the filtered load. Consequently, the kidney normally reabsorbs all the filtered amino acids and therefore does not regulate their plasma concentrations.

Organic Anions

Among the **organic anions,** T_m values exist for citrate, acetoacetate, uric acid (undergoes both reabsorption and secretion), and proteins.

Phosphate

In **plasma,** which contains only an **ionized fraction** of phosphate, about 10% to 20% of the total phosphate content is bound to plasma proteins; it is the ionized phosphate in the plasma compartment that is stabilized by renal function.

The major site of **phosphate reabsorption** is in the proximal tubule. Its reabsorption is closely coupled to Na^+ reabsorption. Phosphate has a low T_m (0.1 mM/min 1.73 m^2), such that relatively small changes in the plasma phosphate concentration produce large changes in the amount excreted. In addition, the T_m of phosphate is not fixed. One of the primary factors that affect phosphate reabsorption is **parathyroid hormone** (PTH). PTH inhibits phosphate reabsorption by accelerating the adenylate cyclase activity in

the proximal convoluted tubule, the cortical ascending limb, the distal convoluted tubule, and the branching collecting tubule.

PTH also inhibits Ca^{2+} reabsorption in the proximal tubule, but in the distal nephron it increases Ca^{2+} reabsorption with an attendant decrease in Ca^{2+} excretion. Finally, PTH also activates **renal 25-(OH) D_3-1α-hydroxylase,** the enzyme that converts 25-(OH)D_3 to 1,25(OH)$_2$D$_3$, the biologically active form of vitamin D. The overall regulation and systemic effects of PTH are discussed in Chap. 56.

Sulfate

The normal plasma concentration of inorganic sulfate is 1 to 1.5 mM/liter. The reabsorptive T_m for sulfate is about the same as that for phosphate.

Secretory Transport Maximum

Many weak organic acids and bases are characterized by having secretory T_m values. The rapid uptake of various organic acids by the kidney serves as the basis for their use in renal and urologic evaluations.

The **renal handling of organic acids** can be divided into three phases: (1) amount of organic acid filtered per unit of time, (2) amount of organic acid secreted per unit of time, and (3) amount of organic acid excreted per unit of time. Using PAH as an example, the amount of PAH filtered plus the amount secreted equals the amount excreted.

If increasing amounts of PAH are infused into healthy subjects, a **PAH "titration" curve** can be obtained, similar to that in Fig. 38-3. As this figure shows, given a constant GFR, the amount of PAH filtered increases linearly as the plasma PAH concentration increases. The total amount of PAH excreted exceeds the amount filtered by the amount secreted, but the amount secreted attains a maximum value, the T_m of PAH.

Increasing the plasma concentration of PAH (or of other weak organic acids and bases) reduces the clearance of PAH (or of the other weak acids or bases). As the plasma concentration of PAH increases, the clearance of PAH decreases and approaches the GFR. In other words, because the amount of PAH secreted at high plasma PAH concentrations is constant (it reaches the T_m value) whereas the amount of PAH filtered (and excreted) continues to increase as the plasma PAH concentration increases, the secreted component becomes an increasingly smaller fraction of the total PAH excreted. Thus, at high plasma PAH concentrations, the amount of PAH excreted approaches the amount filtered, and consequently the clearance of PAH approaches the GFR.

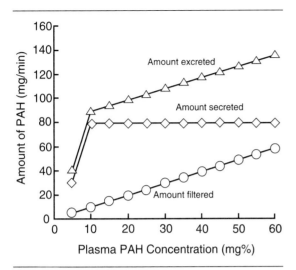

Fig. 38-3. Amounts of *p*-aminohippurate (PAH) filtered, secreted, and excreted are shown as a function of the plasma PAH concentration. The transport maximum for PAH represents the plateau value for the amount of the weak organic acid secreted.

Summary

The largest fraction (about 60% to 70%) of the filtered volume and of the filtered Na^+ is reabsorbed in the proximal tubule. In addition, most of the filtered organic solute (glucose, amino acids, and bicarbonate) is reabsorbed by Na^+-dependent, cotransport processes, primarily in the beginning regions of the proximal tubule. A portion of the Na^+ that is reabsorbed in the proximal tubule is exchanged for intracellular H^+, most of which are reabsorbed as water during the hydrogenation of the filtered bicarbonate. The primary factor that initiates Na^+ reabsorption in the proximal tubule, and consequently, the reabsorption of water and other solutes, is the passive entry of Na^+ into the tubular cell. The Na^+ gradient from the tubular lumen into the cell is generated by the Na^+,K^+-ATPase pump located on the basolateral surface of the tubular cell. Many of the filtered solute molecules, such as glucose, amino acids, sulfate, and phosphate, are reabsorbed by transport processes that have a T_m and consequently display saturation kinetics. Similarly, a number of weak organic acids and bases are actively secreted into the proximal tubule and possess secretory T_m values.

A summary of the major events that take place in the proximal tubule is well illustrated when the TF/P ratios of different solutes are plotted as a function of the fractional length of the proximal tubule (Fig. 38-4). The tubular fluid and *not* the arterial concentration is the variable that changes as a function of distance along the tubule. An understanding of the data illustrated in Fig. 38-4 should further clarify the major concepts underlying proximal tubule function.

Fig. 38-4. Tubular fluid (TF) to plasma (P) concentration ratios for some of the major solutes are plotted as a function of distance along the proximal tubule (PAH = *p*-aminohippurate).

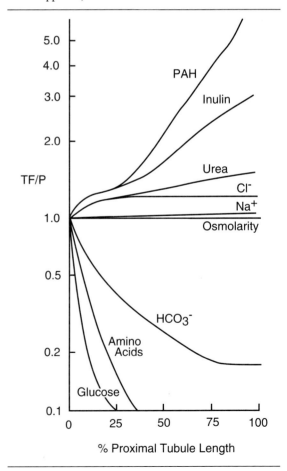

Bibliography

Andreoli, T. E., and Shafer, J. A. Effective luminal hypotonicity: The driving force isotonic proximal tubular fluid absorption. *Am. J. Physiol.* 236:F89–96, 1979.

Knox, F. G., and Haramati, A. Renal regulation of phosphate excretion. In: Seldin, D. S., and Giebisch. G., eds. *The Kidney.* New York: Raven Press, 1985.

Larson, T. S., et al. Renal handling of organic compounds. In: Massry, S. G., and Glassock, R. J. eds. *Textbook of Nephrology.* Baltimore: Williams & Wilkins, 1989.

39 Urinary Concentration and Dilution: Loop of Henle Function

Robert O. Banks

Objectives

After reading this chapter, you should be able to

Describe the transport and permeability characteristics of the descending and ascending loop of Henle and the distal nephron as they pertain to the generation of the medullary osmolar gradient

Explain the role of the vasa recta in maintaining the osmolar gradient

Describe the roles of antidiuretic hormone and urea in the generation of the medullary osmolar gradient

---

The ingestion of solute and water varies widely from day to day, yet the osmolality of the body fluids remains relatively constant at approximately 280 mOsm/kg H_2O. Maintaining constant osmolality of the body fluid depends on the ability of the kidney to excrete urine with a wide range of osmolar concentrations. The human kidney can produce urine with osmolalities ranging from about 50 mOsm/kg H_2O (specific gravity 1.002) to about 1200 mOsm/kg H_2O (specific gravity 1.032). Osmolality is often measured by **freezing point depression** (1 mOsm/kg H_2O decreases the freezing point by 1.86°C) or by **lowering of the vapor pressure. Specific gravity** is not a very precise evaluation of the total solute concentration because it varies with the composition of the solution (e.g., the presence of proteins in a solution markedly affects the specific gravity determination but has little effect on the osmolality of the solution).

Events that take place in the renal medulla, by and large, account for the ability to excrete a urine that can range from about one-sixth the osmolality of body fluids to one that is as much as four times as concentrated.

For many years it has been recognized that an **osmolar gradient** exists between the corticomedullary junction and the tip of the papilla. Tissue samples from the cortex have an osmolality of 280 mOsm/kg H_2O, whereas the osmolality at the tip of the papilla is 1200 mOsm/kg H_2O. This is illustrated in Fig. 39-1, which plots the osmolar constituents in kidneys from dogs following 24 hours of water deprivation. As can be seen, most of the hypertonic fluid in the outer medulla is composed of NaCl, whereas urea contributes significantly to the osmolar gradient in the inner medulla. Tissue samples obtained from the tip of the papilla display an osmolality of about 1200 mOsm/kg H_2O, consisting of approximately 600 mOsm/kg H_2O (300 mM) of NaCl and 600 mOsm/kg H_2O (600 mM) of urea.

Countercurrent Multiplication Without Active Transport in the Thin Ascending Limb

A countercurrent multiplication model with **passive solute reabsorption** in the thin ascending limb of Henle's loop has been proposed to explain the origin of the osmolar gradient. This theory is based on the transport and permeabil-

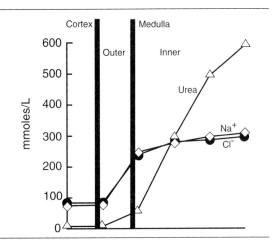

Fig. 39-1. The concentrations of Na^+, Cl^-, and urea are shown in the cortex, outer medulla, and inner medulla of dehydrated dogs. The osmolar gradient in the outer medulla is primarily generated by NaCl, whereas both NaCl and urea contribute to the gradient in the inner medulla. (Adapted from: Ullrick, K. J., and Jarausch, K. H. Untersuchungen zum Problem der Harkonzentrierung und Harnverdünnung *Pflugers Arch. Ges. Physiol.* 262:537–550, 1956.)

ity properties of the descending limb of Henle's loop, the thin ascending limb, the thick ascending limb, the distal convoluted tubule, and the cortical, outer medullary, and inner medullary collecting ducts. To appreciate how this theory might explain the origin of the medullary osmolar gradient, the physiologic properties of each of these nephron segments will be summarized.

Major Permeability and Transport Events

Descending Limb of Henle's Loop

Most studies utilizing perfusion of isolated descending limb of Henle's loop segments from rabbits, rats, and hamsters have shown that this portion of nephron has (1) a **high H_2O permeability,** (2) a very **low solute permeability,** even to urea, and (3) **no active transport.** Because of the low solute permeability of this nephron segment, equilibration between tubular fluid and the renal interstitium takes place by means of water extraction. Therefore, the concentration of NaCl, the major solute entering the loop (leaving the proximal tubule), increases to about 600 mm/liter at the turn (at the base of the loop). Of note, the fluid outside the nephron in the renal interstitium contains 600 mm urea and 300 mm NaCl.

Thin Ascending Limb

Experiments on isolated thin ascending limb segments have shown that this section of the nephron is (1) impermeable to water, (2) moderately permeable to urea, (3) highly permeable to NaCl with evidence of a carrier-mediated, facilitated diffusion of Cl^-, and (4) incapable of active solute transport. There is evidence that a modest degree of **active transport** occurs in the thin ascending limb. Because of these permeability properties of this segment of the nephron and the fact that there is a **favorable NaCl gradient** between the tubular lumen (600 mm NaCl) and the renal interstitium (300 mm NaCl), NaCl passively diffuses into the renal interstitium. Because water cannot follow (this segment of the nephron is always impermeable to water), fluid inside the tubule becomes hypotonic relative to the renal interstitium.

Thick Ascending Limb

The two primary features of the thick ascending limb are that (1) it is **impermeable to water** and (2) it exhibits a large amount of **solute transport.** The cotransport of Na^+–K^+–$2Cl^-$ predominates in this region of the nephron and is illustrated in Fig. 39-2. The transtubular potential is lumen-positive relative to the plasma. This Na^+–K^+–$2Cl^-$ cotransport can be inhibited by ethacrynic acid and furosemide, two of the so-called **loop diuretics.** Because the reabsorption of solute in this region of the nephron initiates the medullary osmolar gradient, if these agents are administered in doses sufficient to block all solute reabsorption in the thick ascending limb, the entire osmolar gradient in the renal medulla is abolished.

The physiologic variables of the remaining nephron segments are also important for an understanding of the countercurrent multiplication model with passive solute reabsorption in the thin ascending limb of Henle's loop and are described in the following sections.

Distal Convoluted Tubule

As a result of the transport-related events in the loop, a hypotonic fluid (about 100 mOsm/kg H_2O) enters the distal convoluted tubule. The distal convoluted tubule is characterized by low water and urea permeability in both the presence and absence of ADH.

Cortical Collecting Duct

The cortical collecting duct has a low urea permeability in both the presence and absence of ADH. Conversely, the water permeability in this segment varies and depends on the presence or absence of ADH. Thus there is a high water permeability when ADH is present but this region is impermeable to water when the hormone is lacking.

Outer Medullary Collecting Duct

The water and urea permeability properties of the outer medullary collecting duct are the same as those of the cortical collecting duct.

Inner Medullary Collecting Duct

The water permeability of the inner medullary collecting duct is also regulated by ADH. In contrast to other segments, however, this segment displays variable urea permeability; it is high in the presence of ADH and low in its absence.

Model for Generation of the Osmolar Gradient Without Active Transport in the Thin Ascending Limb

Incorporating the facts given in the preceding sections, the following analysis reflects some of the sequential phases postulated to occur during the generation of the osmolar gradient, and this is also illustrated in Fig. 39-3. For purposes of this discussion, it is assumed that there is initially no osmolar gradient in the medulla and that there is a high plasma concentration of ADH.

The first stage in the process is the **cotransport of Na⁺–K⁺–2Cl⁻** in the thick ascending limb, a phase that has been referred to as the **single-effect mechanism.** Because the thick ascending limb is not permeable to water, this transport process delivers a hypotonic fluid to the distal convoluted tubule. During this initial phase, the tubular fluid entering the distal tubule would be hypotonic relative to plasma, but not as low as the 100 mOsm/kg H_2O observed in the steady-state condition.

Because of the high titer of ADH in plasma, as the hypotonic tubular fluid progresses through the **cortical collecting duct,** a region of the nephron surrounded by an isosmotic (280 mOsm/kg H_2O) fluid, **tubular fluid equilibrates with the interstitium** through the extraction of water. However, since this segment of the nephron is always impermeable to urea, the concentration of urea in tubular fluid leaving this region is elevated. As the tubular fluid flows into the **outer medullary collecting ducts,** it enters a region of the nephron where it encounters **elevated osmolarity** surrounding the tubule; this is due to the solute extrusion from the thick ascending limb. Since the collecting duct in the outer medulla is also permeable to water when ADH is present, but not to urea, the tubular flow rate is further reduced and the concentration of urea further increased.

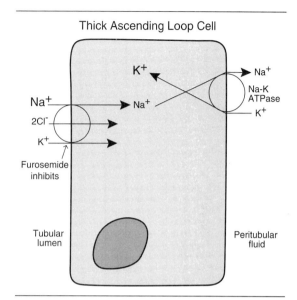

Fig. 39-2. A model illustrating the nature of solute transport in the thick ascending limb.

Tubular fluid then enters **the inner medulla,** a region where the collecting ducts exhibit an ADH-dependent permeability to both water and urea; consequently, urea diffuses into the medullary interstitium.

In the **descending limb of Henle's loop,** the elevated osmolarity in the renal interstitium of the outer medulla also prompts the passive extraction of water from this segment. As tubular fluid in the descending limb enters the inner medulla, it encounters a region where there is an elevated urea concentration in the interstitium, and thus the reabsorption of water continues. Because the fluid at the **end of the proximal tubule** is primarily composed of NaCl, the reabsorption of water in the descending limb promotes delivery of a hypertonic NaCl solution to the turn of the loop. As this tubular fluid enters the **thin ascending limb,** which is permeable to salt but impermeable to water, NaCl passively diffuses out of the nephron and down a **NaCl concentration gradient.** Thus there is **net solute loss** in the thin segment in the absence of active transport. A portion of the **urea** that is cycled into the medullary interstitium diffuses into the ascending limb and therefore is recycled through the distal nephron. This entire process continues until a **steady-state** is reached, wherein the total amount of solute and water entering the medulla equals the total amount leaving the medulla. However, a quantity of solute is trapped in the medulla with a resultant osmolar gradient directed from the outer medulla to the tip of the papilla.

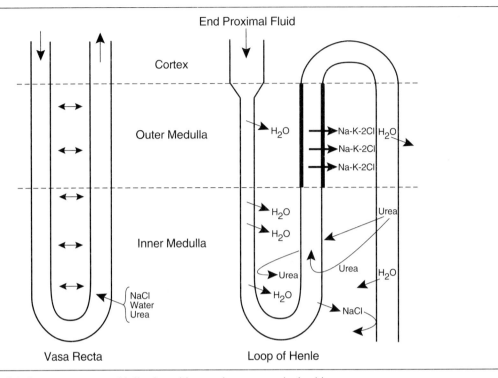

Fig. 39-3. A model of countercurrent multiplication without active transport in the thin ascending limb of Henle's loop. (See text for details.)

Water enters the **medullary interstitium** by means of two sources — the descending limb of Henle's loop and the collecting duct. The effective **osmotic pressure** across the inner medullary collecting duct is a function of the difference in the NaCl concentration between the renal interstitium and fluid in the tubule; urea does not promote water reabsorption because, in the presence of ADH, the collecting duct is permeable to urea. Water entering the medullary interstitium is reabsorbed into the **vasa recta** because the Starling forces in these vascular loops favor net fluid reabsorption; blood in the vasa recta has traversed the glomerulus and the efferent arteriole, and consequently has an elevated colloid osmotic pressure and reduced hydrostatic pressure. **Solute** (primarily NaCl and urea) that enters the capillaries of the vasa recta with water subsequently diffuses down its concentration gradient from the ascending into the descending vascular limb, thereby minimizing solute loss from the medulla; the vasa recta thereby function as passive countercurrent exchangers.

While the **energy input** for generating the osmolar gradient is furnished by the Na^+–K^+–$2Cl^-$ transport in the outer medulla, the system is critically dependent on the subsequent events associated with the cycling of urea. The model explains why, for example, the inner medullary gradient decreases in the absence of ADH or during protein starvation. Both conditions would foster decreased cycling of urea in the system.

There is evidence that the passive movement of solute out of the thin ascending limb of Henle's loop cannot account, quantitatively, for the osmolar gradient in the inner medulla, even under the most optimal conditions with no urea entering the descending limb of Henle's loop. Thus other events also may participate in the generation of the medullary osmolar gradient.

Other Major Reabsorptive Events in the Loop of Henle

Approximately 20% of the **filtered Ca^{2+}** is reabsorbed in Henle's loop through a combination of active (primarily in the thick ascending limb) and passive transport processes.

Parathyroid hormones accentuate the active component of Ca^{2+} reabsorption in the thick ascending loop, whereas the loop diuretics (such as furosemide) decrease Ca^{2+} reabsorption in this region. About 20% of the **filtered K^+** is also reabsorbed in the loop through a combination of passive and active processes. Finally, virtually all the **ammonia** secreted in the proximal tubule is reabsorbed through a combination of active and passive transport processes in the loop (see also Chap. 43 for details).

Summary

The ability to excrete urine with an osmolality ranging from 50 to 1200 mOsm/kg H_2O depends on a number of factors, central to which is the presence of an osmolar gradient in the medulla. The osmolar gradient primarily reflects the reabsorption of Na^+–K^+–$2Cl^-$ in the thick ascending limb and the subsequent transport-related and permeability-related events in the combined distal tubule and collecting duct system. The net effect of this process is that the concentration of urea in the collecting duct increases with a simultaneous cycling of urea into the inner medulla. An elevated urea concentration in the inner medulla fosters water reabsorption from the thin descending limb of Henle's loop and an increased NaCl concentration in the tubular lumen. As tubular fluid enters the thin ascending limb, the elevated NaCl concentration inside the nephron relative to the renal interstitium provides a favorable concentration gradient for NaCl reabsorption; this occurs in the absence of concomitant water flow because the entire ascending limb is impermeable to water under all conditions. The vasa recta function as passive countercurrent exchangers.

Bibliography

Andreoli, T. E., et al. Questions and replies: Renal mechanisms for concentrating and diluting processes. *Am. J. Physiol.* 235:F1–F11, 1978.

Jamison, R. L. The renal concentrating mechanism. *Kidney Int.* 32(Suppl. 21):S-43–S-50, 1987.

Kokko, J., and Rector, F. C., Jr. Countercurrent multiplication system without active transport in inner medulla. *Kidney Int.* 2:214–223, 1972.

Moore, L. C., and Marsh, D. L. How descending limb of Henle's loop permeability affects hypertonic urine formation. *Am. J. Physiol.* 239:F57–F71, 1980.

Stephenson, J. L. Concentration of urine in a central core model of the renal counterflow system. *Kidney Int.* 2:85–94, 1972.

40 The Distal Nephron: Homeostatic Mechanisms

Robert O. Banks

Objectives

After reading this chapter, you should be able to

Describe the factors that are known to influence Na^+ excretion, including the glomerular filtration rate, aldosterone, and third factors such as plasma oncotic pressure, renal arterial pressure, atrial natriuretic factor, and other hormones

Cite the regulatory mechanisms for aldosterone release, the site of aldosterone action, how much of the filtered Na^+ load is controlled by aldosterone, and its mechanism of action

Describe the renin-angiotensin system and the factors that control renin release

Explain how Na^+ is reabsorbed in the distal tubule

Describe the renal handling of K^+, including the factors that affect its distribution between the extracellular and intracellular fluid spaces

---

One of the major functions of the kidney is to **regulate extracellular fluid (ECF) volume** and **osmolality.** Since NaCl is the major osmotic constituent of the ECF, Na^+ balance is a primary determinant of ECF volume. In other words, ECF volume regulation is essentially synonymous with Na^+ regulation, as illustrated by the existence of a **hygienic safety range** of Na^+ intake of approximately 50 to 200 meq/day. A very low salt intake is associated with **hypotension,** particularly orthostatic-induced hypotension, and an **inability to control for volume losses** that arise from sweating or injuries. By contrast, high salt intakes (usually exceeding 250 meq/day) can precipitate Na^+ and volume retention, resulting in **hypertension.** There are also individuals who have a genetic predisposition to salt retention; such people have a reduced ability to excrete salt and develop hypertension at Na^+ intake values that are within the normal range.

Sodium Homeostasis

The total amount of exchangeable Na^+ in the body is about 40 meq/kg of body weight. The amount of Na^+ ingested each day varies widely from individual to individual. When there is very low salt intake (less than 50 meq/day), the kidneys excrete urine that is virtually free of Na^+. However, because the average person consumes about 150 meq/day, to remain in Na^+ balance, 150 meq/day must be lost from the body. Unless large quantities of perspiration are formed, most of this ingested salt is excreted by the kidneys (about 5% is lost in the feces). Consequently, as discussed in Chap. 36, a representative value for Na^+ clearance would be

$$C_{Na} = \frac{(U_{Na})(V)}{P_{Na}} = \frac{140 \text{ meq/day}}{140 \text{ meq/liter}} = 1 \text{ liter/day}$$

(40-1)

where C refers to clearance, U to the urine concentration, V to the urine flow rate, and P to the arterial plasma concentration, all in relation to Na^+.

Given a daily glomerular filtration rate (GFR) of 180 liters/day, the filtered Na^+ load is yielded by: $(GFR)(P_{Na}) = (180 \text{ liters/day})(140 \text{ meq/liter}) = 25,200 \text{ meq/day}$.

Thus, since more than 25,000 meq of Na^+ is filtered each day but only 140 meq/day is excreted, the **excreted**

component represents less than 1% of the filtered Na^+ load, and more than 99% is reabsorbed. In other words,

$$FE_{Na} = \frac{amt.\ Na^+\ excreted = (U_{Na})(V)}{amt.\ Na^+\ filtered = (GFR)(P_{Na})} = \frac{140\ meq/day}{25,200\ meq/day} = 0.01$$

(40-2)

where FE refers to the fractional excretion, in this case, of Na+.

Another equation that illustrates the basis for the fractional excretion of any freely filtered solute x is

$$FE_x = \frac{C_x}{GFR}$$

(40-3)

Approximately 70% of the **filtered Na^+ load** is reabsorbed in the proximal tubule, 20% in the loop of Henle, 5% in the distal convoluted tubule and cortical collecting duct, and 5% in the medullary collecting duct. **Aldosterone,** the primary mineralocorticoid secreted by the adrenal cortex, is one of the major hormones that regulate Na^+ excretion. Aldosterone primarily affects the fraction of the filtered Na^+ load reabsorbed in the cortical collecting duct region of the nephron. Thus, in the absence of aldosterone, roughly 5% of the filtered Na^+ load is excreted; if sufficient amounts of the hormone are present, more than 99% of the filtered Na^+ is reabsorbed.

The quantity of Na^+ regulated by aldosterone is substantial. Given a filtered Na^+ load of 25,000 meq/day, 1260 meq/day (5% of the filtered Na^+ load) would be lost if the mineralocorticoid was lacking. Thus, in the absence of aldosterone, an intake of 1260 meq of Na^+ each day (representing more than 70 g of NaCl) would be required to achieve Na^+ balance. A daily intake of that quantity of Na^+ is not possible, and since the loss of large amounts of salt and water produce profound hypotension, untreated **hypoaldosteronism** is fatal. By contrast, patients with **hyperaldosteronism** retain salt and water, are usually hypertensive and hypokalemic, and suffer from metabolic alkalosis.

Na⁺ Reabsorption in the Aldosterone-Sensitive Region of the Nephron

The paradigm for **solute reabsorption** and **secretion** in the aldosterone-sensitive region of the nephron, the connecting segment, and the cortical collecting duct is illustrated in Fig. 40-1. A significant fraction of the Na^+ reabsorbed in this region is exchanged for intracellular K^+ and H^+. Recent data indicate that the secretion of K^+ and

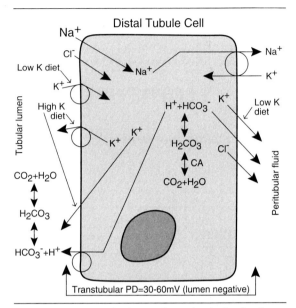

Fig. 40-1. A model of solute reabsorption in the distal tubule (PD = potential difference; CA = carbonic anhydrase).

H^+ may actually take place in different cell types in this region of the nephron. Thus, in principal cells, Na^+ passively enters the intracellular fluid (ICF) compartment, creating a lumen-negative potential. This potential promotes both **Cl^- reabsorption** via a paracellular pathway and **K^+ secretion** across the luminal membrane. By contrast, the **H^+ secretion** occurs in intercalated cells by means of a H^+-ATPase pump situated on the luminal membrane, a process that is not coupled to Na^+ reabsorption (Na^+ is not reabsorbed by the intercalated cells). Both cell types are stimulated by aldosterone. H^+ secretion by intercalated cells is also stimulated by **acidemia.** Thus not only does aldosterone stimulate Na^+ reabsorption but the hormone also enhances the secretion and, therefore, excretion, of K^+ and H^+ as well. Consequently, not only do **fluid volume imbalances** arise with both hyperaldosteronism and hypoaldosteronism, but there are also changes in acid-base and K^+ balance. **Hypoaldosteronism** is usually associated with a metabolic acidosis and hyperkalemia, whereas **hyperaldosteronism** is often characterized by metabolic alkalosis and hypokalemia. Finally, as shown in Fig. 40-1, when K^+ is depleted, a net reabsorption of K^+ occurs in this region of the nephron; this reabsorptive process may be driven by a K^+-ATPase pump located on the luminal surface of intercalated cells.

Mechanism of Action of Aldosterone

When aldosterone is administered to an aldosterone-deficient animal, there is a delay of 30 to 90 minutes before changes in electrolyte excretion appear. The reason for this **delay** is that aldosterone, like other adrenal steroids, modifies the functional activity in its target tissue by changing the rate of a series of metabolic reactions. Aldosterone diffuses down its concentration gradient into cells of the cortical collecting tubule, where it is bound to a cytoplasmic or, more likely, a nuclear receptor protein. The steroid-receptor complex increases RNA transcription and ultimately results in the synthesis of new proteins. Currently, it is unclear how these newly synthesized proteins alter cellular function. They may stimulate the peritubular membrane Na^+,K^+-ATPase pump by furnishing additional energy or may directly facilitate Na^+ entry into the cell by increasing the Na^+ permeability of the luminal membrane; recent studies have indicated that the latter mechanism predominates. Along with the increased Na^+ permeability of the luminal membrane, a process that can be blocked with the diuretic amiloride, there is an increase in the ICF Na^+ concentration and a secondary increase in Na^+,K^+-ATPase activity in the basolateral membrane.

If aldosterone is administered for several days to a healthy subject, the amount of Na^+ excreted initially decreases but then gradually returns to control values within 3 to 5 days, a phenomenon referred to as **aldosterone escape.** Interestingly, K^+ excretion does not escape, and therefore, K^+ depletion develops if the mineralocorticoid infusion is continued. Evidence has been reported that during aldosterone escape, the amount of Na^+ reabsorbed in the pars recta of the proximal tubule or in the loop of Henle is reduced, which offsets the enhanced reabsorption of Na^+ in the aldosterone-sensitive region of the nephron. The reduced reabsorption of Na^+ in the pars recta or loop of Henle may be related to changes in a number of other **nonaldosterone factors** that regulate Na^+ reabsorption. These factors would be activated by the aldosterone-induced expansion of the ECF space (see discussion of third factors at the end of this chapter).

Regulation of Aldosterone Secretion

The secretion of aldosterone from the **zona glomerulosa** in the **adrenal cortex** is regulated by several physiologic variables. The two primary factors are the plasma concentrations of **angiotensin-II** and of K^+; increases in either of these substances stimulate the secretion of aldosterone from the adrenal cortex. **Adrenocorticotropic hormone**

exerts a permissive effect on the zona glomerulosa, in that relatively low levels of it are required for angiotensin-II and K^+ to impose their regulatory actions. Other hormones also affect aldosterone release. For example, **atrial natriuretic factor** (ANF), which will be discussed, inhibits and **endothelin** stimulates aldosterone secretion. Finally, there is evidence that **plasma osmolality** also may directly affect aldosterone secretion; increases in plasma osmolality are associated with decreases in aldosterone secretion.

The Renin-Angiotensin System

Angiotensin-II is the end product of a biologic cascade system initiated by the release of **renin,** a proteolytic enzyme produced by the **juxtaglomerular apparatus** in the kidney. Several factors, all related to arterial blood pressure, participate in the regulation of renin release from the kidney: (1) direct effects of **mean arterial blood pressure,** probably mediated by changes in wall tension in the afferent arteriole (a decrease in mean arterial blood pressure causes a decrease in wall tension of afferent arteriole and an increase in renin release), (2) altered **renal sympathetic nerve activity** (the juxtaglomerular apparatus is richly innervated, and increased sympathetic nerve activity, acting via beta-adrenergic receptors, causes an increase in renin release), and (3) changes related to the **GFR** (a decrease in the GFR prompts a decrease in the Na^+ delivery rate to the macula densa, which in turn is associated with increased renin release).

The renin substrate is a circulating alpha$_2$-globulin, **angiotensinogen** (produced in the liver), and the biochemical product is a decapeptide, **angiotensin-I.** A converting enzyme that exists in relatively large amounts in the lungs but is also found in the kidneys removes two C-terminal amino acids from angiotensin-I, forming the biologically active compound angiotensin-II. Angiotensin-II is degraded to a biologically inactive peptide angiotensin-III by angiotensinase.

Angiotensin-II is one of the primary agonists for **aldosterone release,** though angiotensin-II has a number of other important biologic actions. It serves as a **potent vasoconstrictor,** which is central to its role in the long-term regulation of arterial blood pressure. Angiotensin-II also directly promotes **Na^+ reabsorption** in the proximal tubule. This action complements the effects of aldosterone on Na^+ reabsorption in the cortical collecting duct. In addition, angiotensin-II stimulates the **thirst center.**

Sodium Excretion and the GFR

In addition to the renin-angiotensin-aldosterone system, a second major factor that can influence the excretion rate of

Na^+ is the GFR. Despite glomerulotubular balance, an elevated GFR invariably leads to increased Na^+ excretion. However, whether the GFR functions as a physiologic variable in the regulation of Na^+ excretion is unclear. As has been noted, a number of hormones affect the GFR and therefore potentially regulate Na^+ excretion by means of this mechanism. Certainly, however, adjustments are made in the quantity of Na^+ reabsorbed by the nephron. Because less than 1% of the filtered Na^+ load is normally excreted, relatively small changes in the amount of Na^+ reabsorbed translate into relatively large changes in the amount of Na^+ lost or retained.

Third Factors

Numerous studies have suggested that there are many **non-aldosterone, non-GFR factors** involved in the regulation of Na^+ excretion. These regulatory events are often referred to as **third factors.** Descriptions of some of these factors, which may be interrelated and involve similar mechanisms, follow.

Atrial Natriuretic Factor

Extracts of the atrial, but not ventricular, myocardium contain a potent natriuretic factor referred to as **atrial natriuretic factor** (ANF). The circulating peptide appears to be a 28 amino acid peptide. Bolus injections of ANF elicit a very rapid and transient increase in the **urine flow rate** and **Na^+ excretion.** ANF also suppresses **cardiac output,** with a subsequent period of hypotension. Although ANF relaxes smooth muscle in vitro, it does not cause renal or mesenteric vasodilation (a transient, small increase in RBF has been reported by some investigators following pharmacologic doses of the peptide).

The mechanism by which ANF induces **natriuresis** is still unknown. It has been shown that increases in Na^+ excretion produced by the peptide can be dissociated from changes in the GFR and RBF (high doses of ANF increase the GFR). Therefore, a direct tubular action of ANF has been proposed.

There is evidence that **atrial-stretch activation** of alpha$_1$ receptors and other events stimulate ANF release. ANF receptors have been found in a number of tissues. In the kidney, these receptors reside in the **glomerulus** and **medullary collecting tubule.** There are also receptors in the **adrenal gland** (ANF inhibits aldosterone release) and the **anterior pituitary gland.**

ANF is thought to participate in the natriuretic response to acute changes in plasma or ECF volume. Long-term increases in Na^+ intake do not appear to alter ANF secretion.

Other factors, such as a ouabain-like factor, could be involved in the renal response to elevations in dietary Na^+ intake.

Ouabain-Like Factor

A ouabain-like hormone has been proposed to account for the inhibition of Na^+ reabsorption in the distal nephron (through decreases in Na^+,K^+-ATPase) observed during **chronic volume expansion.** The postulated hormone is often referred to as the **natriuretic hormone.** Extracts of plasma or urine from individuals or animals with expanded ECF volumes contain a natriuretic substance. Indeed, anephric patients have high concentrations of this substance. The factor is often distinguished by its ability to reduce Na^+ transport across isolated epithelial membranes (ANF does not affect Na^+ transport in isolated epithelia). Both a low-molecular-weight (1000 daltons) and higher-molecular-weight (10,000 to 30,000 daltons) substance have been isolated. When the larger-molecular-weight substance is injected into test animals, natriuresis occurs within about 1 hour and lasts for more than 2 hours. By contrast, the low-molecular-weight substance evokes a rapid but short-lived natriuresis. Several reports indicate that this natriuretic factor originates in the brain.

Renal Nerves

The kidney is richly innervated with **sympathetic nerves,** and many physiologic and pathologic conditions have an impact on renal nerve activity. It has been known for many years that cutting the renal nerves produces a "denervation diuresis and natriuresis." Along these lines, there is evidence that **norepinephrine** stimulates Na^+ reabsorption in the proximal tubule and loop of Henle. Conversely, changes in the plasma concentration of hormonal and humoral agents can compensate for the renal nerves, as transplanted, denervated kidneys can function normally.

Pressure Natriuresis and Diuresis

Increases in arterial pressure cause increases in Na^+ and water excretion. The natriuresis and diuresis correlate with increases in renal interstitial fluid pressure (particularly in the renal medulla) and are dependent on an intact renal capsule; intrarenal prostaglandins and/or nitric oxide also may be involved. The inhibition of sodium reabsorption occurs proximal to the thick ascending limb. An abnormal pressure natriuretic and diuretic response to increases in blood pressure may be a major factor contributing to hypertension. Thus, if renal function is normal, it has been argued that hypertension cannot be sustained; that is, an increase in pressure will cause a natriuresis and diuresis, a resulting decrease in vascular volume, and a subsequent decrease in arterial blood pressure. The phenomenon of pressure natriuresis and diuresis may be a critical element in the long-term (day-to-day) regulation of arterial blood pressure.

Physical Forces

Changes in **Starling forces** may be involved in the natriuresis observed in some settings. For example, diminished colloid osmotic pressure may decrease fluid reabsorption along the nephron. Such a mechanism may contribute to the reduced fluid reabsorption observed in the proximal tubule during saline expansion (fractional reabsorption can decrease from a control value of 70% to as low as 50% following expansion).

Changes in the distribution of blood flow or the GFR in the kidney also have been suggested to influence Na^+ excretion. One aspect of intrarenal hemodynamics currently being studied is the possibility that augmented medullary and papillary blood flow reduces the osmolar gradient and hence increases Na^+ excretion, but conclusive evidence that these events are important is lacking.

Other Hormones

There are a number of known hormones or humoral substances with natriuretic properties. These include **antidiuretic hormone** (ADH), **oxytocin, histamine,** and some **prostaglandins.** Whether the natriuretic effect of these substances is physiologic or pharmacologic remains to be determined.

Summary Scheme for Sodium Balance

The kidney varies the amount of Na^+ excreted to ensure a constant circulating blood volume. Thus, depending on the dietary Na^+ intake, Na^+ excretion can range from very low to relatively large amounts. The ingestion of salt heightens body fluid osmolality, and because the primary volume of distribution of NaCl is in the ECF, the increase in osmolality shifts water from the ICF into the ECF. The increase in body fluid osmolality also stimulates the release of ADH from the posterior pituitary gland (see Chap. 41 for details), which in turn activates the thirst center in the hypothalamus. If water is ingested, it is retained until normal osmolality is achieved. This sets up an isotonically expanded ECF, a decrease in colloid osmotic pressure, and an increase in arterial or venous blood pressure, or both. Third factor events are therefore activated, including the pressure natriuretic phenomenon, the release of ANF, and perhaps the ouabain-like natriuretic hormone. In addition, the renin-angiotensin system is inhibited, with a resulting decrease in the aldosterone output from the adrenal glands.

Na^+ excretion rate increases, water returns to the cells, and the ECF volume is reduced isosmotically by a proper plasma concentration of natriuretic factors and ADH.

The adjustments associated with changes in Na^+ intake are rather slow compared with those that occur during changes in water consumption. Several hours (more on a day-to-day scale) must elapse before Na^+-induced changes in ECF volume are manifested, but increases in water intake with accompanying decreases in body fluid osmolality result in changes in renal function that take only minutes to occur (see Chap. 41).

Potassium Homeostasis

The **total body content** of K^+ is about 3500 to 4000 meq (50 to 55 meq/kg). Because the **normal ECF concentration** of K^+ is to 4 to 5 meq/liter, only about 60 meq of the total body K^+ content is in the ECF. High ICF concentrations of K^+ are necessary for many biochemical reactions to take place. In addition, the concentration ratio of K^+-ICF to K^+-ECF is critical for maintaining **resting membrane potentials** and therefore the excitability of nerve and muscle cells.

Distribution of Potassium Between the ECF and ICF

A number of both physiologic and pathologic factors affect the distribution of K^+ between the ICF and ECF and are therefore important in an analysis of K^+ balance. These factors include the acid-base status of the individual, the plasma concentration of several hormones, the activity of the Na^+,K^+-ATPase pump, and the rate of cell breakdown.

Acid-Base Status

During **acidosis,** H^+ shifts into cells in exchange for ICF K^+ (and for some ICF Na^+), and consequently, the plasma K^+ concentration increases. The opposite occurs during **alkalosis.** For every 0.1 pH unit change, there is an approximate 0.6 meq/liter change in the plasma K^+ concentration.

Hormones

Several hormones, including **insulin, catecholamines,** and **aldosterone,** promote the cellular uptake of K^+. Along these lines, it is of interest to note that insulin, in conjunction with glucose plus sodium bicarbonate, is often used for treating acute hyperkalemia. The liver is particularly important in this regulation, since about 70% of the insulin-induced K^+ uptake takes place in this organ.

Disease States

An **increase in cell breakdown,** such as occurs in severe trauma, provokes K^+ release into the ECF and potentially depletes K^+ stores. **Chronic diseases** such as heart failure also lead to decreases in the total body K^+ content. Whether the plasma K^+ concentration is altered depends on subsequent renal adjustments.

Renal Excretion of Potassium

The **dietary intake** of K^+ in a healthy adult is 40 to 120 meq/day. Under normal conditions, most of the ingested K^+ is excreted in the urine (small amounts of K^+ are also lost in feces and sweat). Furthermore, a significant portion of the K^+ excreted derives from K^+ secretion in the combined distal tubule and cortical collecting duct system (about 90% of the filtered K^+ is reabsorbed in the proximal tubule plus the loop of Henle). As a result of these reabsorptive events, the K^+ concentration entering the distal tubule is relatively low (less than 1 meq/liter)

Potassium Regulatory Factors

There are three primary factors that determine the rate of K^+ secretion: the **concentration gradient for K^+** between the cortical collecting duct cell and the tubular lumen, the **transepithelial potential difference** between the tubular cell and the lumen of the nephron, and the **K^+ permeability** of the luminal membrane. Each of these events is summarized below.

The Cell-to-Lumen Potassium Gradient

An increased difference between the K^+ concentration in the cell and the tubular lumen leads to an increase in the K^+ secretion rate, and vice versa. The following factors affect the K^+ concentration in the cell and the tubular fluid.

At least three factors affect the **cell K^+ concentration** in the combined distal tubule and cortical collecting duct; these include the plasma K^+ concentration, the arterial pH, and the plasma concentration of aldosterone.

An increase in K^+ intake will raise the **plasma K^+ concentration** and stimulate Na^+,K^+-ATPase–mediated active transport. This occurs in all cells in the body, including those in the cortical collecting duct, and thereby increases the gradient for K^+ secretion into the tubular lumen.

Since a decrease in **arterial pH** shifts K^+ out of cells, K^+ concentrations in the distal tubular cells drop during acidosis. Consequently, the K^+ gradient between distal tubular cells and the tubular lumen decreases and K^+ secretion diminishes. Although hyperkalemia can develop during the acute phase of metabolic acidosis, K^+ wasting and a resulting hypokalemia normally arise in chronic acidosis. The opposite takes place during alkalosis.

Aldosterone stimulates the peritubular membrane Na^+, K^+-ATPase pump (probably by means of the increased Na^+ entry across the luminal membrane) in cortical collecting cells, thereby enhancing the distal tubular cell concentration of K^+.

The **tubular fluid concentration** of K^+ generally varies inversely with the rate of flow entering the cortical collecting duct. Thus an accelerated distal tubular flow rate increases the K^+ gradient between the cell and the lumen (or the transtubular potential difference, as will be discussed) and results in increased K^+ secretion. Many diuretics (see Chap. 41) enhance K^+ excretion, mediated in part by these mechanisms. Similarly, isotonic expansion of the ECF space reduces fluid reabsorption in the proximal tubule, thereby increasing the distal flow rate and K^+ secretion. Volume depletion has the opposite effect.

The Transepithelial Potential Difference

The transtubular potential in the distal nephron is very high (about 30 to 50 mV lumen-negative relative to plasma) and is related to the transport of Na^+ from the lumen into the plasma. Increases in the transtubular potential difference favor K^+ secretion. Agents that affect the permeability of the luminal membrane to Na^+ alter the transepithelial potential and secondarily influence K^+ secretion. For example, the diuretics **amiloride** and **triamterene** (see Chap. 41) reduce the Na^+ permeability of the luminal membrane, which in turn reduces the transepithelial potential difference and decreases the K^+ secretion rate.

The Potassium Permeability of the Luminal Membrane

Changes in the permeability of the luminal membrane alter the K^+ secretion rate. **Aldosterone** appears to enhance the luminal membrane permeability to both Na^+ and K^+. Thus increases in plasma aldosterone concentrations are associated with augmented K^+ secretion (and excretion).

Calcium Reabsorption in the Distal Nephron

About 10% to 15% of the **filtered Ca^{2+}** is reabsorbed in the distal convoluted tubule and another 5% in the collecting duct. These are both active transport events that are stimulated by parathyroid hormone (PTH) secretion (PTH stimulates Ca^{2+} reabsorption in these regions through the operation of a cAMP-dependent processes). Thus, under normal conditions, about 1% of the filtered Ca^{2+} load is excreted.

Summary

It is essential that Na^+ and K^+ balance is maintained. The importance of balancing the intake and output of Na^+ is primarily dictated by the fact that changes in Na^+ balance markedly affect ECF volume. K^+ balance is critical because of the impact of ECF K^+ concentrations on the resting membrane potential. The amount of Na^+ excreted is largely determined by the amount reabsorbed (or, more accurately, not reabsorbed) from the initial filtered Na^+ load. Under normal conditions, relatively small fractions (less than 1%) of the filtered Na^+ load are excreted. Changes in the Na^+ reabsorption within the aldosterone-sensitive region of the nephron, located primarily in the cortical collecting duct, determine to a large extent the amount of Na^+ excreted. In addition, since most of the filtered K^+ is reabsorbed before it reaches the aldosterone-sensitive region of the nephron, the amount of K^+ secreted in this region determines the amount of K^+ excreted. Aldosterone release from the adrenal gland is regulated primarily by the plasma concentrations of K^+ and angiotensin-II. Angiotensin-II production is controlled by renin output from the kidney, which in turn is elevated by decreases in the renal perfusion pressure, increases in the renal sympathetic nerve tone, or decreases in distal tubular flow rate or any combination of these. Other factors, such as ANF and renal arterial pressure, also participate in the regulation of Na^+ balance.

Bibliography

Anger, M. S., et al. Water and sodium metabolism. In: Massry, S. G., and Glassock, R. J., eds. *Textbook of Nephrology*. Baltimore: Williams & Wilkins, 1989.

Folkow, B. Salt and hypertension. *News Physiol. Sci.* 5:220–224, 1990.

Gottschalk, C. W., Moss, N. G., and Colindres, R. E. Neural control of renal function in health and disease. In: Seldin, D. S., and Giebisch, G., eds. *The Kidney*. New York: Raven Press, 1985.

Guyton, A. C. Renal function curve — A key to understanding the pathogenesis of hypertension. *Hypertension* 10:1–6, 1987.

Sanson, S. C., et al. Potassium homeostasis. In: Massry, S. G. and Glassock, R. J., eds. *Textbook of Nephrology*. Baltimore: Williams & Wilkins, 1989.

41 Water Balance and Diuretics

Robert O. Banks

Objectives

After reading this chapter, you should be able to

State the osmolality of tubular fluid in each major segment of the nephron during dehydration and water diuresis

Cite the fraction of water and Na^+ reabsorbed in each major segment of the nephron

Explain the cellular mechanism of action of antidiuretic hormone

Describe the production and storage site of antidiuretic hormone and the factors that control its release

State the formula for free water clearance

Define osmolar and free water clearance

Give the range of urine osmolality

Describe the significance of positive and negative free water clearance values

Describe the mechanisms of action of various diuretics

Body fluid osmolality is closely regulated by balancing the intake and loss of water. The intake of water is the sum of (1) that contained in the food we eat, (2) that derived from the oxidation of ingested food, or so-called metabolic water, and (3) that which we drink. The amount taken in with drinking can vary substantially from individual to individual, but certain minimum requisite amounts are imposed by (1) insensible water loss, (2) water lost in the feces, and (3) an osmotic ceiling on the urine osmolality. The **thirst center** ensures that this minimum daily intake of water is met.

mental and physical functioning. Problems of dehydration are particularly critical in **infants,** since roughly 70% of an infant's weight is water (compared with 60% in adults). Thus an infant weighing 5 kg contains approximately 3.5 liters of water. Given a fluid intake of about 800 ml/day, this represents a turnover of roughly 25% of the infant's total body water. A 70-kg adult, on the other hand, ingests about 1 to 2 liters of fluid per day, constituting less than 5% of the total body water. Additional water loss in an infant (diarrhea, sweating, or vomiting) more rapidly becomes a life-threatening situation than in an adult.

Water Deprivation

The **maximum water deprivation** that is compatible with life varies among species; the maximum weight loss from desiccation in humans is about 20%; this rises to 40% in dogs and cats and up to 60% in earthworms. A 10% weight loss through desiccation in humans usually compromises

Minimum Daily Water Intake

The following example is an estimate of the **minimum daily intake of water** through drinking necessary for a 70-kg individual. The calculation will vary, depending on such factors as diet, temperature, exercise, and humidity. This example assumes the individual ingests 1.5 kg of food.

Water intake

From food	900 ml
From oxidation of food	400 ml
Total water ingested without drinking	1,300 ml

Water output

Insensible water loss (skin and lungs, or about 0.5 ml/kg · hr)	840 ml
In feces	100 ml
Minimum urine volume	750 ml
Total water lost	1690 ml

The value for the minimum daily urine volume is based on the total osmoles that must be excreted and the maximum urine osmolality. In a **normal diet,** about 150 meq of sodium chloride and 50 meq of K^+ plus anion are ingested daily for a total of 400 mOsm of ions that must be excreted. An additional 500 mOsm of solute, primarily urea, also must be excreted. Assuming a maximum urine osmolality (U_{os}) of 1200 mOsm/kg H_2O, the minimum 24-hour urine volume (V) would be

Total solute excreted = $(U_{os})(V)$ = 900 mOsm/day
$(U_{os})(V)$ = (1200 mOsm/kg $H_2O)(V)$ = 900 mOsm/day
$V = 750 \ ml / day$

For this particular individual, 1690 less 1300 ml, or 390 ml, represents the obligatory water intake that must be ingested by drinking. Most individuals exceed this minimum daily intake, and consequently, the osmolality of urine collected during 24 hours would be less than 1200 mOsm/kg H_2O in these people. The exact value of course depends on the quantity of water consumed but generally ranges between 500 and 800 mOsm/kg H_2O.

Antidiuretic Hormone

The amount of water excreted by the kidney is controlled by **antidiuretic hormone** (ADH), which is also known as **vasopressin.** ADH regulates the water permeability of the **cortical** and **medullary collecting duct system.** If ADH is lacking, this region of the nephron is virtually impermeable to water, and thus water inside the nephron at the turn of Henle's loop would be excreted (the ascending limb of Henle's loop is always impermeable to water).

Mechanism of Action of ADH

The antidiuretic action of ADH is mediated by V_2 **receptors** in the basolateral membrane of the collecting duct. Activation of these receptors stimulates adenylate cyclase activity and consequently increased conversion of ATP to cyclic AMP (cAMP). The mechanism by which cAMP increases water permeability is unclear. cAMP is known to stimulate kinases, and cAMP-induced changes in microtubules and microfilaments also have been reported. cAMP is converted to an inactive form (5′-AMP) by **phosphodiesterase.** These events are summarized in Fig. 41-1.

The preceding series of events can be modulated by different agents at several points. For example, **calcium** can inhibit both the binding of ADH to the V_2 receptor and adenylate cyclase activity. **Prostaglandin E$_2$** and **bradykinin** also suppress adenylate cyclase activity and the ADH-induced **hydroosmotic response** (the effect of bradykinin may be mediated by an increase in prostaglandin E$_2$ synthesis). **Aldosterone** potentiates ADH, probably through inhibition of phosphodiesterase activity. Finally, **parathyroid hormone** also potentiates ADH.

ADH increases **vascular resistance** by activating V_1 **receptors** on smooth muscle cells. The effects of this are coupled to activation of the phosphoinositide pathway.

Fig. 41-1. The major events in the hydroosmotic response to antidiuretic hormone (ADH). (Adapted from: Dousa, T. P., and Valtin, H. Cellular actions of vasopressin in the mammalian kidney. *Kidney Int.* 10:46–63, 1976.)

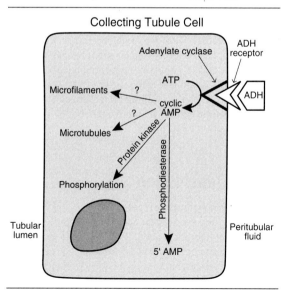

Synthesis of ADH

ADH is a **peptide hormone** synthesized in the **supraoptic** and **paraventricular nuclei** of the hypothalamus and transported down the axons of these cells in association with a larger (10,000 daltons) protein, **neurophysin. Oxytocin** is also produced in this area and undergoes a similar series of events.

ADH is stored in large granules of the posterior lobe of the pituitary gland. With appropriate stimulation and depolarization of these fibers, these granules release their contents by exocytosis into the circulation.

Secretion of ADH

Two major stimuli evoke ADH release: **hypertonicity** of the body fluids and **volume depletion.** A relatively small decrease (about 1%) in the body fluid osmolality below the set point, generally about 280 mOsm/kg H_2O, is associated with a decline in the plasma ADH concentration to virtually undetectable levels (less than 1 pg/ml). By contrast, as the plasma osmolality exceeds 280 mOsm/kg H_2O, the plasma ADH concentration increases, reaching values of about 10 pg/ml at 300 mOsm/kg H_2O.

Volume (pressure) **receptors** that influence ADH release are located in several regions of the circulation. **Low-pressure receptors** in the **left atrium** are among the most important, but input also may derive from baroreceptors in the aortic and carotid regions. Elevated atrial or arterial pressure does not markedly limit ADH secretion, but a decrease in these pressures is a potent stimulus for its release. Many **other factors** also can affect the release of ADH; angiotensin-II, nicotine, and pain stimulate ADH release, while ethanol and glucocorticoids inhibit its release.

ADH has a relatively short half-life of 5 to 10 minutes once it enters the circulation, because it is enzymatically degraded in plasma and rapidly cleared by the kidneys (ADH may be secreted by the proximal tubule).

Quantitation of Water Excretion: Free Water Clearance

One way to quantitate the amount of **solute-free water** that is either excreted or retained by the kidney is to evaluate the **free water clearance.** (The term **solute-free water** refers to the quantity of water that must be added or extracted from a urine sample to render it isosmotic to plasma). Free water clearance (CH_2O) is defined as follows:

$$C_{H_2O} = V - C_{os} \qquad (41\text{-}1)$$

where

$$C_{os} = \frac{(U_{os})(V)}{P_{os}} \qquad (41\text{-}2)$$

All the preceding expressions are given in milliliters per minute. U_{os} refers to osmolality, V to the urine flow rate, C_{os} to the osmolar clearance, and P_{os} to the plasma osmolality.

Free water clearance is, in some respects, a misnomer because it is not an actual clearance but, as this definition illustrates, represents the difference between the urine flow rate and the osmolar clearance. **Osmolar clearance,** a conventional clearance, stands for the volume of plasma completely cleared of total solute per unit of time.

The following examples illustrate the physiologic implications of free water clearance values under three different conditions and are based on the evaluation of the 70-kg subject cited previously in this chapter.

Condition 1: Excretion of Isotonic Urine

In this condition, the individual is producing urine with an osmolality of 280 mOsm/kg H_2O and has a plasma osmolality of 280 mOsm/kg H_2O. Regardless of the urine flow rate, the free water clearance in this condition would be zero. Thus, when the urine osmolality equals the plasma osmolality,

$$C_{H_2O} = V - \frac{(U_{os})(V)}{P_{os}} = 0$$

In other words, this person would be neither excreting nor retaining excess water. Rather a **zero free water clearance** represents an isosmotic reduction in the body fluid volume.

Condition 2: Excretion of Hypotonic Urine

When urine osmolality is less than plasma osmolality, the free water clearance becomes positive. This condition, known as **water diuresis,** arises when ADH release from the pituitary is inhibited; solute-free water, relative to plasma, is thus excreted and body fluid osmolality increases.

If the 70-kg individual were to rapidly ingest (within

5–10 min) 1 liter of water and had an initial plasma osmolality of 280 mOsm/kg H_2O, the plasma osmolality would fall to 273 mOsm/kg H_2O after water absorption (this calculation is based on a total body water content of 60%, or 42 liters, prior to water ingestion). ADH concentrations in plasma would rapidly decline, resulting in the formation of a large volume of hypotonic urine. At peak diuresis, the subject's urine flow rate might be about 12 ml/min with a urine osmolality of 50 mOsm/kg H_2O. Thus the free water clearance at peak diuresis would be

$$C_{H_2O} = V - \frac{(U_{os})(V)}{P_{os}}$$
$$= 12 \text{ ml/min} - \frac{(50 \text{ mOsm/kg})(12 \text{ ml/min})}{273 \text{ mOsm/kg}}$$
$$= 12 \text{ ml/min} - 2.2 \text{ ml/min}$$
$$= +9.8 \text{ ml/min}$$

In essence, the kidney is excreting the solute contained in 2.2 ml of plasma in 12 ml of urine. Thus, in this example, an additional 9.8 ml of solute-free water is excreted each minute.

Solute-free water is generated primarily in the **ascending limb,** but to some degree also in the **distal** and **collecting tubules,** when solute is extracted from tubular fluid without simultaneous water reabsorption. The maximum positive free water clearance is about 15 ml/min.

Condition 3: Excretion of Hypertonic Urine

This calculation will utilize the values given at the beginning of this chapter. Thus urine osmolality is 1200 mOsmoles/kg H_2O with a urine flow rate of 750 ml/day or 0.52 ml/min. The free water clearance would therefore be calculated as follows:

$$C_{H_2O} = 0.52 \text{ ml/min} - \frac{(1200 \text{ mOsm/kg})(0.52 \text{ ml/min})}{300 \text{ mOsm/kg}}$$
$$= 0.52 \text{ ml/min} - 2.08 \text{ ml/min}$$
$$= -1.56 \text{ ml/min}$$

In this example, the free water clearance is negative, and this connotes a state of **dehydration.** In other words, by excreting the solute contained in 2.08 ml of plasma in only 0.52 ml of urine, each minute 1.56 ml of solute-free water is conserved. The total amount of solute excreted is approximately the same as that for the subject in condition 2;

the individual must excrete 900 mOsm/day, or approximately 600 μOsm/min, since the only difference between the two conditions is the amount of water consumed.

A free water clearance of –2 ml/min is approximately the maximum negative free water clearance that the human kidney can produce. Because it can be awkward to deal with negative values, when free water clearance becomes less than zero, the term $T^c_{H_2O}$ is often used and stands for the difference between the osmolar clearance and the urine flow rate. The superscript c indicates that negative free water is formed in the collecting duct.

Pathologic Conditions Associated with ADH Secretion

Excess ADH Excretion

The **syndrome of inappropriate secretion of ADH** is characterized by chronic hypoosmolality and hyponatremia because of the excess water retention and increased Na^+ excretion. Thus elevated ADH concentrations result in a reduced urine output, which in turn provokes increased blood volume and blood pressure with a resulting pressure-induced natriuresis.

The inappropriate release of ADH may be of **pituitary origin** (related to, for example, CNS infections, certain drug treatments, or other endocrine imbalances) or of **nonpituitary origin** (a frequent complication of lung carcinomas). The major symptoms of hypoosmolality are neurologic and stem from the development of **cerebral edema.**

ADH Deficiency

ADH deficiency is a feature of two conditions: **central diabetes insipidus,** in which patients cannot secrete ADH, and **nephrogenic diabetes insipidus,** in which the plasma concentrations of ADH are elevated, but the kidney cannot conserve water because of tubular defects. A number of factors can precipitate the nephrogenic form. The disorder can be inherited (a rare condition), drug related, or a complication of renal disease.

Hyperosmolality and hypernatremia do not develop in diabetes insipidus if water intake is sufficient. The symptoms of hypernatremia are primarily neurologic and range from muscle weakness to convulsions and coma.

Diuretics

Pharmacologic agents are often used to promote the excretion of excess salt and water. Although a complete description of diuretics is beyond the scope of this textbook, Table 41-1 lists some of the major diuretics and gives the site and mechanism of action of these agents.

Carbonic anhydrase is an important enzymatic component in the reabsorption of sodium bicarbonate (see Chap. 43). Agents such as **acetazolamide** that inhibit carbonic anhydrase activity in the tubular lumen elicit a modest diuretic response that involves the excretion of an alkaline urine (sodium bicarbonate). These agents are used primarily to treat edematous patients with metabolic alkalosis.

Osmotic agents, such as mannitol, are often used to reduce intracranial pressure and help prevent acute renal failure. The so-called **loop diuretics,** such as furosemide, inhibit the Na^+–K^+–$2Cl^-$ transport process in the thick ascending limb. These agents are widely used for the treatment of edema. Since more than 20% of the filtered Na^+ is reabsorbed in the loop of Henle, these agents can promote the excretion of relatively large amounts of Na^+ and also K^+. The latter results from inhibition of the Na^+–K^+–$2Cl^-$ transport process and the secondary increase in tubular flow rate through the cortical collecting duct with a subse-

Table 41-1. A Summary of Major Classes of Diuretics

Drug	Major Site of Action	Mechanism	Comments
Acetazolamide (Diamox)	Proximal tubule	Carbonic anhydrase inhibitor (interferes with HCO_3^- reabsorption)	Na^+, HCO_3^-, K^{+*}, and H_2O mainly excreted
Osmotic diuretics (mannitol: glucose in uncontrolled diabetes mellitus)	Primarily loop of Henle, also proximal tubule	Is a non-reabsorbable solute. If infused in sufficient amounts: (1) retains H_2O in the nephron and (2) increases blood flow to the medulla and decreases the osmolar gradient	Excretion of H_2O in excess of NaCl; K^{+*} also excreted; diuresis is not affected by ADH
Loop diuretics (ethacrynic acid, furosemide)	Thick ascending limb	Inhibits Na^+–K^+–$2Cl^-$ reabsorption (can abolish the osmolar gradient; cannot concentrate or dilute urine. Thus lower C_{H_2O} and $T^c_{H_2O}$)	Large amounts of Na^+, Cl^-, and K^{+*} can be excreted (as much as 40% of the filtered Na^+ and H_2O)
Thiazides	Cortical diluting segment (also known as the cortical thick ascending limb) and distal convoluted tubule	May inhibit a Na^+–Cl^- cotransporter on the luminal membrane; lower C_{H_2O} but no effect on $T^c_{H_2O}$	5–8% of the filtered Na^+ excreted. K^{+*}, Cl^-, and H_2O also excreted
Spironolactone	Aldosterone-sensitive region	Aldosterone antagonist	Slow onset of action (12+ hr), Na^+, Cl^-, and H_2O are excreted. K^+ is retained (a K^+-sparing diuretic)
Triamterene and amiloride	Aldosterone-sensitive region	Not aldosterone antagonists: agents block Na^+ entry into CCD cells	Na^+, Cl^-, and H_2O excreted. K^+-sparing diuretics

*Any agent that interferes with Na^+ reabsorption proximal to the site of K^+ secretion will enhance K^+ excretion. In the presence of these drugs, the distal tubular flow rate increases, the lumen concentration of K^+ decreases, or the transtubular potential becomes more negative, thereby favoring the K^+ gradient between the distal tubular cells and the lumen. K^+ secretion (and, therefore, K^+ excretion) increases.
ADH = antidiuretic hormone: C_{H_2O} = free water clearance: $T^c_{H_2O}$ = (see text, p. 448); CCD = cortical collecting duct.

quent increase in K$^+$ secretion (see Chap. 40 for the factors that affect K$^+$ secretion in the cortical collecting duct). Finally, because relatively large amounts of Ca^{2+} are reabsorbed in the loop of Henle, treatment with loop diuretics also markedly augments Ca^{2+} excretion.

The primary diuretic effect of the **thiazides** appears to result from the inhibition of a Na$^+$–Cl$^-$ cotransporter located on the luminal membrane of the distal convoluted tubule. The resulting increase in the tubular flow rate entering the collecting duct also elevates K$^+$ secretion. In contrast to the loop diuretics, the thiazides promote Ca^{2+} reabsorption and therefore reduce Ca^{2+} excretion. The thiazides are used routinely for treating edema and hypertension.

Finally, the **K$^+$-sparing diuretics** represent a class of several agents that cause a modest increase in Na$^+$ and Cl$^-$ excretion without elevating K$^+$ excretion. Examples of these diuretics are spironolactone, amiloride, and triamterene. These agents are generally administered in conjunction with a loop diuretic or a thiazide to prevent the hypokalemia often associated with the loop diuretic or the thiazide.

Summary

Body fluid osmolality (normally about 280 mOsm/liter) is regulated within a relatively narrow range. Water balance is accomplished primarily by means of changes in the amount of water excreted or retained by the kidney and by appropriate increases in the amount of water ingested through stimulation of the thirst center. Decreased body fluid osmolality is rapidly offset by decreased ADH secretion from the pituitary. As ADH concentrations fall, the water permeability of the collecting duct declines, the urine flow rate then increases, and urine osmolality drops. By contrast, water deprivation leads to an increase in body fluid osmolality because of the continued insensible water loss. Consequently, the plasma concentration of ADH increases, water excretion decreases (urine osmolality increases), and the thirst center is stimulated. Water excretion by the kidney can be quantitated by applying the concept of free water clearance, which represents the difference between the urine flow rate and the osmolar clearance. Positive values indicate that the kidney is producing a urine that is diluted (compared with plasma) and is thereby concentrating the body fluids. Negative values are obtained when the kidney elaborates a concentrated urine and is therefore diluting the body fluid osmolality. Finally, a free water clearance of zero signifies that the kidney is neither concentrating nor diluting body fluid osmolality, and an isosmotic urine is being produced.

Bibliography

Abramow, M., Beauwens, R., and Cogan, E. Cellular events in vasopressin action. *Kidney Int.* 32(Suppl. 21):S-56–S-66, 1987.

Robertson, G. L. Physiology of ADH secretion. *Kidney Int.* 32(Suppl. 21):S-20–S-26, 1987.

Suki, W. N. Renal actions and uses of diuretics. In: Massry, S. G., and Glassock, R. J., eds. *Textbook of Nephrology*. Baltimore: Williams & Wilkins, 1989.

42 Acid-Base Balance: Biochemistry, Physiology, and Pathophysiology

John H. Galla and Shahrokh Javaheri

Objectives

After reading this chapter, you should be able to

Describe the overall purpose and burden of acid-base homeostasis

Identify H⁺ concentration as a dependent variable and the major independent variables that determine [H⁺] in biologic solutions: strong ions, weak acids, and partial pressure of CO_2

Explain the difference between the H⁺ concentration and pH

Describe the nature of physiochemical buffers and how they participate in acid-base balance

Describes how CO_2 is an important physiologic buffer and how it behaves in vivo

List the four simple disorders of acid-base balance and describe their pathophysiologic concepts

Describe the concepts of respiratory and metabolic compensation, recognize their presence, and distinguish between simple and mixed disorders

---

In this chapter, acid-base balance is introduced with an overview of its homeostasis followed by discussions of its biochemistry and physiologic and pathophysiologic states.

General Background

Purpose of Acid-Base Homeostasis

The *milieu interieur* of the body is regulated to maintain the **H⁺ concentration** ([H⁺])* of its various compartments within a very narrow range, for the most fundamental reasons. From a biochemical standpoint, the configuration or tertiary structure of many proteins is dependent on the ambient [H⁺]. In particular, the activities of many enzymes are exquisitely sensitive to the [H⁺]. Thus, if [H⁺] is perturbed sufficiently from normal, the structure of fixed or circulat-

ing substances is likely to be altered in such a way that would prevent them from entering into reactions, interacting with receptors, engaging in O_2 exchange, and so on. Thus, without the exquisite regulation of [H⁺], many metabolic processes would rapidly become deranged or cease.

Burden of Homeostasis

The regulation of [H⁺] of the various body fluid compartments is a dynamic process in which [H⁺] is continually perturbed by normal metabolism and promptly corrected to normal. Each day a person consumes carbohydrates, fats, and proteins that produce energy, maintain cellular structure, and restore excreted substances. Most of these substrates are eventually catabolized in mitochondria during normal aerobic metabolism, for example:

$$C_6H_{12}O_6 + 6O_2 \rightarrow 6CO_2 + 6H_2O + heat \quad (42\text{-}1)$$

---

*Square brackets around a substance denote concentration.

451

In all, about 15,000 to 20,000 mmol of CO_2 are generated each day and must be excreted by the lungs to maintain the constancy of the interior milieu, **homeostasis.** The protein consumed, about 1 g/kg of body weight per day, yields about 70 meq of inorganic acid. For example, organic sulfur, a fixed or nonvolatile acid, is oxidized to inorganic sulfate:

$$Cysteine + O_2 \rightarrow urea + H_2O + CO_2 + SO_4^{2-} + 2H^+$$

$$(42-2)$$

Fixed acid is excreted by the kidneys.

Acid-Base Biochemistry

Nature of [H⁺]

The $[H^+]$ in biologic fluids is most commonly expressed by its negative logarithm to the base 10, or **pH.** Because of this logarithmic notation, the changes in $[H^+]$ expressed as pH can be deceptive, since an increase in $[H^+]$ represents a decrease in pH and a small change in pH may indicate a large change in $[H^+]$. Notwithstanding this problem, both expressions are used because of the long-standing and widespread use of pH to denote $[H^+]$.

$[H^+]$ is a **variable** that **depends** on a number of independent variables in any given solution. Thus $[H^+]$ can be described by a set of equations that incorporates these variables and is based on **physicochemical principles,** including the laws of electroneutrality and conservation of mass and the equilibrium reactions. To understand how the $[H^+]$ of a solution is determined, the simplest solution will be considered first, followed by ones of increasing complexity.

In **pure water,** $[H^+]$ is described first by its **dissociation constant** (K_w), which varies directly only according to the independent variable, temperature:

$$[H^+] \times [OH^-] = K'_w \qquad (42-3)$$

where $K'_w = K_w \times [H_2O] = 10^{-14}$. $[H_2O]$ behaves like a constant in this expression; because its concentration is so large (55 M) and changes are minuscule, it is incorporated into K'_w. This relationship, which must always be satisfied, shows that $[H^+]$ and $[OH^-]$ behave in a reciprocal manner.

Second, as in all solutions, **electroneutrality** must be preserved. Thus, for pure water,

$$[H^+] = [OH^-] \qquad (42-4)$$

When Eqs. (42-3) and (42-4) are solved simultaneously, they express the $[H^+]$ for water:

$$[H^+] = \sqrt{K'_w} = 1 \times 10^{-7} \, M \qquad (42-5)$$

Thus, at 25°C, the pH of water is 7.00. As the temperature increases, K'_w increases and, consequently, $[H^+]$.

Effect of Strong Ions on [H⁺]

All biologic solutions contain a wide array of substances, including electrolytes. Those electrolytes which for all practical purposes **dissociate completely,** such as Na^+, K^+, Ca^{2+}, Mg^{2+}, Cl^-, and SO_4^{2-}, are classified as **strong ions.** Some organic anions of sufficiently strong acids, such as lactate, also behave like strong ions. The effect of strong ions can be incorporated into an expression for $[H^+]$. Consider, for example, only Na^+ and Cl^- in a solution. First, electroneutrality must be satisfied:

$$([Na^+] + [H^+]) - ([Cl^-] + [OH^-]) = 0 \qquad (42-6)$$

When solved simultaneously with Eq. (42-3), this yields

$$[H^+] = \frac{\sqrt{K'_w + ([Na^+] - [Cl^-])^2}}{4} - \frac{([Na^+] - [Cl^-])}{2}$$

$$(42-7)$$

Thus $[H^+]$ is dependent on and a function of the strong electrolytes.

The net effect of **all** substances that behave as strong ions is expressed as the **strong ion difference** (SID), which is the sum of all the strong cations minus the sum of all the strong anions in the solution. It is the single most important determinant of $[H^+]$ or $[OH^-]$ in this solution. The essential feature of SID is the **difference in charge** and not the ion species. For example, if Ca^{2+} and SO_4^{2-} are added to the NaCl solution, SID is expressed as

$$([Na^+] + [Ca^{2+}]) - ([Cl^-] + [SO_4^{2-}]) = SID \qquad (42-8)$$

In most body fluids, SID is positive. SID may then be substituted in Eq. 42-7 to yield

$$[H^+] = \sqrt{K'_w + \left(\frac{[SID]}{2}\right)^2} - \frac{[SID]}{2} \qquad (42-9)$$

Because SID in physiologic solutions is several orders of magnitude greater than K'_w, SID dominates the resultant $[H^+]$, as illustrated (Fig. 42-1).

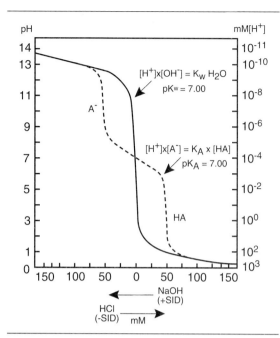

Fig. 42-1. Titration curves for water (*solid line*) and a solution buffered with a weak acid (HA; *dashed line*) (K_w = dissociation constant; pK_w = negative logarithm of K_w; K_a, pK_a = weak acid dissociation constant; SID = strong ion difference).

Titration of water with a strong acid or base, such as HCl or NaOH, shows the dominant effect of strong ions on [H^+] (see Fig. 42-1). In this example, the initial point of addition, indicated by the zero point on the X axis, is arbitrarily set at a [H^+] of 10^{-4} mM (pH 7.00), at the midpoint of the Y axis; the initial point of addition could be set anywhere. The addition of a **strong acid** introduces strong anions and that of a **strong base** introduces strong cations, as shown along the ordinate.

Although H^+ or OH^- (these are not strong ions) is also added to the solution during titration, **equal** changes in strong ions evoke **different** changes in [H^+] and [OH^-], depending on the initial or ambient [H^+] of the solution. For example, if 2 meq of HCl is added at pHs of approximately 12, 10.5, or 1.5, the effect on the final [H^+] is dramatically different, as can be seen by plotting these values on the titration curve (see Fig. 42-1). In a strongly alkaline solution (pH 12), the addition of 2 meq of HCl has a trivial effect on [H^+], whereas in a strongly acidic solution (pH 1.5) [H^+] increases linearly. The reason for this, of course, is that, in solutions of high pH, H^+ reacts with OH^- to form H_2O while the added Cl^- remains an anion. In solutions of

low pH, H^+ does not react with OH^- because virtually none is present and each milliequivalent of H^+ added remains a proton; Cl^- remains an anion. The intermediate effect is observed at pH 10.5 because of the limited availability of OH^- closer to the neutral point for water (pH 7.00).

The impact of titration on changes in pH (see Fig. 42-1, the left scale of the Y axis) can be more difficult to visualize. In contrast to the [H^+], the effect of the 2 meq of HCl on pH is most dramatic at the neutral point but is numerically similar at both high and low initial pHs. This is, of course, simply due to the fact that pH is a logarithmic function that obscures the dramatic difference in the effect of HCl.

Effect of Weak Ions on [H$^+$]

Biologic solutions often contain substantial concentrations of **incompletely dissociated solutes** — "weak" acids or bases. Weak acids, for example, contribute at least three quantities to a solution — HA, A^-, and H^+ for monovalent compounds — as described by the relationship

$$[H^+] \times [A^-] = K_A \times [HA] \tag{42-10}$$

or

$$pH = pK_A + \log\frac{[A^-]}{[HA]} \tag{42-11}$$

where K_A is the weak-acid dissociation constant, also expressed as pK_A; its negative logarithm (HA) is any weak acid, and A^- is its conjugate base. **Proteins** and **phosphates** are the major weak acids in the body.

When a weak acid is considered in solving for [H^+], the relationship described by Eq. (42-10) must be satisfied along with those in Eq. (42-9) and electroneutrality that now includes A^-. The total amount of a weak acid (A_{TOT}) in any solution is described by

$$[A_{TOT}] = [HA] + [A^-] \tag{42-12}$$

which satisfies the law of conservation of mass.

Buffers

Weak acids can act as chemical buffers under the appropriate conditions. A **buffer** is a substance that can give or accept protons in a manner that tends to minimize changes in [H^+] when substances, such as strong ions, which might otherwise produce large changes in [H^+], are introduced into solutions. A buffer exists in solution as a weak acid (proton donor) (HA) and a **conjugate** as a weak base (proton acceptor) (A^-) pair in the relationship

$$[HA] \leftrightarrow [H^+] + [A^-] \tag{42-13}$$

For polyvalent buffers, multiple such relationships exist and in a complex solution:

$$[H_2A] \leftrightarrow [H^+] + [HA^-] \leftrightarrow 2[H^+] + [A^{2-}]; \; H_3A \dots \text{etc.} \tag{42-14}$$

Since the influence of SID on the $[H^+]$ of the solution depends on the ambient $[H^+]$, even more so does the **buffering power.** The effect of adding strong ions to a solution containing a monovalent buffer, HA, with a pK_A arbitrarily set at 7.00 is shown by the dashed curve in Fig. 42-1. At the alkaline end of the titration curve, where only A^- is present, as well as at the acidic end, where only HA exists, the solution behaves like water, as if no buffer were present. However, within about ±1 pH unit of the pK_A (7.00, in this example), the addition of nearly 50 mM of strong ion has little effect on $[H^+]$; the solution is buffered. Figure 42-1 illustrates two important principles regarding buffers:

1. The **pK′** is the pH at which the [HA] equals $[A^-]$, that is, $[A^-]/[HA] = 1.0$.
2. At the pK′, the change in $[H^+]$ elicited by the addition of strong ions is least, or restated, the **most** effective buffering lies in the range of the linear portion (the midpoint) of the titration curve for that buffer.

Isohydric Principle

The **buffering power** of any complex solution (the sum of the effect of all buffers present) also can be determined by titration. When several buffers exist in a solution, all the buffer pairs are in equilibrium at the same $[H^+]$, which in turn depends on the type and concentration of the buffer pairs.

$$\begin{aligned}
pH &= pK_1' + \log \frac{[HCO_3^-]}{[H_2CO_3]} \\
&= pK_2' + \log \frac{[HPO_4^{2-}]}{[H_2PO_4^-]} \\
&= pK_3' \tag{42-15}
\end{aligned}$$

This important principle states that by analyzing one buffer pair, the pH of the system can be determined and hence the status of all other buffer pairs in the solution. This is known as the **isohydric principle.** However, even though $[H^+]$ may be used to determine the status of all buffer pairs, this does **not** mean that $[H^+]$ is an independent variable.

Effect of CO_2 on $[H^+]$

Of particular importance in biologic solutions, the addition of CO_2, a volatile weak acid, to a solution introduces another independent variable and several molecular species:

$$[\text{Dissolved } CO_2] + H_2O \leftrightarrow H_2CO_3 \leftrightarrow H^+ + HCO_3^- \tag{42-16}$$

$$[\text{Dissolved } CO_2] + OH^- \leftrightarrow HCO_3^- \leftrightarrow H^+ + CO_2^{2-} \tag{42-17}$$

The partial pressure of CO_2 (P_{CO_2}) and its solubility coefficient (S_{CO_2}) determine its concentration according to **Henry's law;** S_{CO_2}, in turn, depends on temperature and the other constituents of the solution. Combining these relationships and their dissociation constants algebraically yields two expressions that describe the relationships of all these **molecular species:**

$$[H^+] \times [HCO_3^-] = K_2 \times P_{CO_2} \tag{42-18}$$

$$[H^+] \times [CO_3^{2-}] = K_3 \times [HCO_3^-] \tag{42-19}$$

This expression shows that HCO_3^- is also a dependent variable. The behavior of CO_2 in the physiologic environment will be discussed later.

Summary of Biochemical Considerations

Three independent variables (SID, A_{TOT}, and CO_2) and six variables that depend on them and are pertinent to biologic solutions have now been considered. Plasma SID represents the difference between the sum of all the strong cations and anions; A_{TOT} includes the plasma proteins and phosphates, and P_{CO_2} is set by alveolar ventilation relative to metabolic rate. When the six expressions for these variables (Eqs. 42-3, 42-9, 42-10, 42-12, 42-18, and 42-19, and electroneutrality) are solved simultaneously with the known plasma values for strong ions, total protein content, and the arterial P_{CO_2} ($PaCO_2$) with dissociation constants at 37°C, a fourth-order polynominal yields a value for [H^+] of 40 neq/liter or a pH of 7.40 (Stewart, 1983). This affirms the validity of this approach.

Physiologic pH

Nature and Maintenance of Physiologic pH

These principles of acid-base biochemistry must now be considered in the context of a physiologic system that places certain constraints on the physicochemical system. The normal [H^+] of the mammalian arterial blood at 37°C is 40 nM (10^{-9} M), or a pH of 7.40 with a range of about 7.36 to 7.44. The range of extracellular [H^+] that is compatible with life is roughly 100 to 16 nM (pH 7.00 to 7.80), although patients may survive more extreme transient deviations. Intracellular pH is about 7.00, whereas the neutral pH (when [H^+] = [OH^-]) at 37°C is 6.70; neutral pH is lower with fever because K'_w increases with increasing temperature. Under normal dietary conditions as well as within a broad range of acid or base loads, both **physicochemical** and **physiologic buffering systems** tightly maintain pH in the normal range.

Buffering of CO_2

The enormous CO_2 load produced by normal metabolism enters capillary blood, where it is buffered primarily by hemoglobin in erythrocytes (RBCs) (Fig. 42-2). CO_2 freely enters the RBC, where within milliseconds carbonic anhydrase catalyzes its combination with OH^- to form HCO_3^-. The HCO_3^- is then exchanged for plasma Cl^- through anion antiporters (band 3 protein) in the RBC membrane (the chloride shift). Thus about 80% of the generated CO_2 is transported as HCO_3^- in the plasma en route to the lungs for excretion.

CO_2 is also rapidly and nonenzymatically bound to the alpha-amino groups of deoxyhemoglobin (Hgb) to form carbamino groups, which act as buffers within the RBC:

$$Hgb \cdot R - NH_2 + CO_2 \leftrightarrow Hgb \cdot R - NHCOO^- + H^+$$

$$(42\text{-}20)$$

Hemoglobin has ionized groups with strengths that change in keeping with the state of hemoglobin oxygenation. Thus, when oxyhemoglobin loses its O_2, it can accept H^+, which combines with the NH moiety on the imidazole ring and also forms a buffer:

Fig. 42-2. CO_2 distribution in tissue capillary blood and transport and metabolism in the red blood cells (CA = carbonic anhydrase; Hgb = hemoglobin; Band 3 = anion exchanger; percentages indicate the approximate distributions).

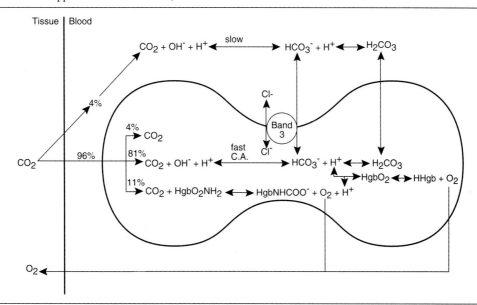

$$O_2 \cdot Fe \cdot Hgb\text{-}NH + H^+ \leftrightarrow O_2 + Fe \cdot Hgb\text{-}NH_2^+$$

$$(42\text{-}21)$$

This buffering allows more CO_2 to react with H_2O and be carried in the plasma as HCO_3^-. Thus, at a constant P_{CO_2}, the CO_2 content of deoxygenated hemoglobin is greater than that of the oxygenated form. This is known as the **Haldane effect.**

Physiologic Buffering

The fixed acids, CO_2/HCO_3^- buffer pair, hemoglobin within RBCs, plasma proteins, and the phosphate buffer systems all participate in the **initial physicochemical buffering** in the blood.

The CO_2/HCO_3^- buffer system has a major role, and its relationship to $[H^+]$ is described by the **Henderson-Hasselbalch equation,** which is a logarithmic rearrangement of Eq. (42-18):

$$pH = pK' + \log\,[HCO_3^-]\,/\,[H_2CO_3]$$

$$(42\text{-}22)$$

in which H_2CO_3 is in equilibrium with dissolved CO_2 and is equal to the $PaCO_2$ multiplied by 0.03, the solubility factor (mM/mmHg CO_2) at 37°C in plasma. Thus, at normal acid-base equilibrium,

$$
\begin{aligned}
pH &= 6.1 + \log\,24\,\text{mM}\,/\,(40 \times 0.03)\,\text{mM} \\
&= 6.1 + \log\,24\,\text{mM}\,/\,1.2\,\text{mM} \\
&= 6.1 + \log\,20 \\
&= 7.40
\end{aligned}
$$

$$(42\text{-}23)$$

where 6.1 is the pK' of the CO_2/HCO_3^- buffer pair, 24 mM is the normal plasma $[HCO_3^-]$, and 40 mmHg is the normal $PaCO_2$.

Based on the characteristics of ideal buffers described earlier in this chapter, the CO_2/HCO_3^- pair should be a poor buffer system because of its pK of 6.1. This paradox is due to (1) the prompt excretion of CO_2 by the lungs and its maintenance at 40 mmHg by the adjustment of ventilation to CO_2 production, (2) its abundance, and (3) the ability of the kidney to regulate $[HCO_3^-]$.

To illustrate physiologic regulation of $[H^+]$, the response to a **fixed acid load** is considered. If a strong acid is added to a closed, unbuffered system, pH plummets, as seen for

water (see Fig. 42-1). In a simplified plasma containing $NaHCO_3$, there is prompt physicochemical buffering of added acid. For example,

$$5H^+ + 5Cl^- + 10Na^+ + 10HCO_3^- \rightarrow 10Na^+ +$$

$$5Cl^- + 5HCO_3^- + 5H_2CO_3$$

$$(42\text{-}24)$$

Although the H_2CO_3 rapidly dissociates to CO_2 and H_2O, the degree of physiologic buffering would be limited if the CO_2 were trapped in a closed system. However, because the physiologic system is open, the excess CO_2 released in the reaction can be excreted by the lungs. As P_{CO_2} decreases and reduces the $[H_2CO_3]$ and $[H^+]$ (Eqs. 42-16 and 42-17), therefore, the $[HCO_3^-]/[H_2CO_3]$ ratio approaches its normal value of 20 (see Eq. 42-23). In addition, the **increased arterial $[H^+]$** rapidly signals the respiratory centers to increase ventilation, which further decreases $PaCO_2$ and brings the $[HCO_3^-]/[H_2CO_3]$ ratio and all other buffer pairs even closer to their normal values.

Within minutes, further physicochemical buffering takes place in soft tissue and bone, where proteins and organic phosphates are the principal participants. Over the course of several hours, the kidney excretes the excess fixed acid, thereby increasing plasma SID and reclaiming HCO_3^- used during initial buffering. At this point, the body $[H^+]$ returns to normal.

Under normal **steady-state conditions** — a diet consisting of 70 g of protein per day which generates about 70 meq of acid — approximately 30 mM H^+ is excreted as titratable acids (PO_4, SO_4, and so on), and the remainder is excreted as ammonium by the NH_4^+/NH_3 urinary buffer system. In the renal response to reclamation of the HCO_3^- expended in the titration of acid loads, the **NH_4^+/NH_3 buffer** pair in the urine is quantitatively more important (see Chap. 43 for details).

Disorders of Acid-Base Balance

When the control mechanisms that maintain acid-base balance either become deranged or are overwhelmed by other pathologic processes, clinical disorders of acid-base balance occur. These can precipitate **acidosis,** an abnormal condition that tends to retain acid or lose base, or **alkalosis,** in which base is retained or acid is lost. These disorders are further classified as either **respiratory,** in which the clearance of CO_2 through the lungs is the primary disturbance, or **metabolic,** in which the extrapulmonary organs are the sites of the primary disturbance.

The primary disorder itself should be differentiated from the actual [H⁺] of the blood. **Acidemia** and **alkalemia** refer to a blood [H⁺] above or below the normal limits, respectively; blood pH, of course, would be the inverse of this. The distinction between, for example, acidosis and acidemia is important because more than one primary disorder can coexist in a patient, resulting in a normal arterial [H⁺]. Multiple coexisting disorders are called **mixed disturbances.** To diagnose these disorders clinically, a more simplified approach than that taken in the foregoing cumbersome theoretical analysis is applied.

Classification

The four basic acid-base disorders can be defined in terms of the perturbations of the variables of the **Henderson-Hasselbalch equation,** all of which are commonly determined by clinical laboratories (Table 42-1). Although the plasma [HCO₃⁻] is a dependent variable, changes in [HCO₃⁻] parallel changes in SID, which would be difficult and cumbersome to calculate.

For respiratory disorders, CO₂ is primarily disturbed, and compensation, reflected in blood [HCO₃⁻], occurs primarily by renal mechanisms. In metabolic disorders, the plasma SID is altered primarily, and the change in the PaCO₂ is compensatory.

Compensation

A primary disturbance in the respiratory system activates a metabolic response that serves to minimize or buffer the magnitude of the disturbed [H⁺] from its normal concentration and vice versa. The net response by the buffer systems that are not primarily disturbed is called the **compensatory response.**

The physicochemical buffering responses occur rapidly in the intravascular, interstitial, and intracellular compartments. These responses are relatively modest. In the respiratory compensation of primary metabolic disorders, changes in plasma [H⁺] and brain extracellular fluid [H⁺] affect the neuronal output from peripheral chemoreceptors (the carotid bodies) and central chemoreceptors (mostly located near the ventral surfaces of the medulla oblongata). These receptors then cause the medullary respiratory centers to stimulate respiratory muscles via the phrenic and intercostal nerves, resulting in increased alveolar ventilation (see details in Chap. 34). This **respiratory response** is complete within minutes.

In contrast to these two rapid responses, the **maximum compensatory metabolic response** by the kidneys for primary respiratory disorders takes up to 2 days to effect changes in SID and HCO₃⁻. Metabolic compensation buffers the change in [H⁺] induced by the rise in PaCO₂. The renal mechanisms involved in this response are covered in Chap. 43.

Because these compensatory responses are physiologic, they are **normal** and **predictable,** in that they can be described in **mathematical** terms. The magnitudes and direction of the responses can and have been obtained only from clinical observations. Widely accepted compensation factors are given (Table 42-2), expressed in terms of the variables of the Henderson equation.

Because both the physicochemical and respiratory buffering responses are rapid, the duration of the metabolic disorder is not considered in clinical circumstances, and only one factor is provided for each disorder (see Table 42-2). In contrast, because the renal compensatory response in the primary respiratory disorders is slow, the duration of the disorder must be considered in order to determine the appropriateness of compensation, making factors for both acute and chronic respiratory disorders necessary. To illustrate the use of these factors, in a simple metabolic acidosis with a serum [HCO₃⁻] of 14 mM, the change in serum [HCO₃⁻] from normal is (–)10 mM (24 – 14 = 10), and the predicted change in PaCO₂ is (–)13 mmHg, or an absolute value of 27 mmHg (40 – 13 = 27).

Table 42-1. Characteristics of Primary Acid-Base Disorders*

Type	pH	[H⁺]	PaCO₂	[HCO₃⁻]	SID
Respiratory acidosis	Decreased	Increased	**Increased**	Increased	Increased
Respiratory alkalosis	Increased	Decreased	**Decreased**	Decreased	Decreased
Metabolic acidosis	Decreased	Increased	Decreased	Decreased	**Decreased**
Metabolic alkalosis	Increased	Decreased	Increased	Increased	**Increased**

PaCO₂ = arterial CO₂ tension; SID = strong ion difference.
*Bold type indicates the primary disturbance (see text).

Table 42-2. Factors for Predicting Compensation in Simple Acid-Base Disorders

Disorder	Compensation Coefficient*
Metabolic acidosis	$(-)$ 13 mmHg $PaCO_2$/ $(-)$ 10 mM $[HCO_3^-]$
Metabolic alkalosis	$(+)$ 6 to 7 mmHg $PaCO_2$/ $(+)$ 10 mM $[HCO_3^-]$
Respiratory acidosis	
Acute	$(+)$ 1 mM $[HCO_3^-]$/ $(+)$ 10 mmHg $PaCO_2$
Chronic	$(+)$ 3.5 mM $[HCO_3^-]$/ $(+)$ 10 mmHg $PaCO_2$
Respiratory alkalosis	
Acute	$(-)$ 2.5 mM $[HCO_3^-]$/ $(-)$ 10 mmHg $PaCO_2$
Chronic	$(-)$ 5.0 mM $[HCO_3^-]$/ $(-)$ 10 mmHg $PaCO_2$

*The use of the coefficient to calculate difference from normal assumes the following normal values: serum $[HCO_3^-]$ = 24 mM and $PaCO_2$ = 40 mmHg.

A composite of these compensatory relationships (Fig. 42-3) is a variant of the pH–HCO_3 diagram popularized by Davenport in which $PaCO_2$ is plotted as isopleths but is preferred because $[H^+]$ is clearly a dependent variable in this format. The isopleths for $[H^+]$ are calculated from the Henderson-Hasselbalch equation. The heavy dashed lines describe a simple effect of respiratory compensation in metabolic acidosis. If the serum $[HCO_3^-]$ decreases from about 26 to 11 meq/liter without respiratory compensation, the arterial $[H^+]$ would be 90 neq/liter (pH 7.05); with respiratory compensation, the $PaCO_2$ falls to 23 mmHg and the resultant $[H^+]$ is 55 neq/liter (pH 7.26). The shaded areas denote the confidence limits for the four basic types of simple disorders; the effect of the duration of both acute and chronic respiratory disorders on compensation is also shown. As a corollary to the compensation relationships, any point that does not fall within the confidence limits for any of the simple disorders represents a mixed disorder (two or more simultaneous disorders).

Clinical Diagnosis of Acid-Base Disorders

In clinical situations, an **arterial blood-gas analysis** provides both $PaCO_2$ and pH or $[H^+]$, from which the plasma $[HCO_3^-]$ may be calculated. In addition, the serum total CO_2 content, which represents the sum of the concentrations of HCO_3^- and the different forms of CO_2 in the blood, the latter normally about 1.2 mM, is usually deter-

mined directly. The application of a few simple steps using these values will yield the correct acid-base diagnosis.

First, the prudent diagnostician should validate the accuracy of laboratory data by comparing the calculated plasma $[HCO_3^-]$ with the directly determined serum total CO_2 concentration. If these values agree within ± 3 mM, the data can be considered accurate; if not, the data are internally inconsistent, and one of the values must be incorrectly determined.

The clinical laboratory data must always conform to the Henderson equation:

$$[H^+]\,(nM) = \frac{24 \times PaCO_2\,(mmHg)}{[HCO_3^-]\,(nM)} \qquad (42\text{-}25)$$

From the foregoing discussion it should be clear that only one independent variable is being measured — PCO_2. However, $[HCO_3^-]$, a dependent variable, conveniently varies directly with SID.

The values for three components of the Henderson-Hasselbalch equation are then examined to determine the dominant type of acid-base disorder (see Table 42-2). For example, predominant metabolic acidosis would be indicated by decreases in plasma $[HCO_3]$, $PaCO_2$, and pH.

Finally, to distinguish between a simple (single) or mixed (multiple) disorder, a simple disorder is assumed, and the expected compensatory response is calculated by applying the appropriate compensation factor. If, in this example of a dominant metabolic acidosis, the predicted compensatory respiratory response is calculated to have a $PaCO_2$ of 20 mmHg and 20 mmHg is measured, a single disorder, metabolic acidosis, is confirmed. If, on the other hand, a $PaCO_2$ of 30 mmHg had been measured, this higher than predicted value would indicate a mixed disorder that includes both a primary metabolic acidosis and a primary respiratory acidosis, since the $PaCO_2$ is higher than predicted. More than two disorders can coexist in a patient, but a consideration of the diagnostic challenge of such cases is beyond the objectives of this text.

Metabolic Acidosis

Metabolic acidoses arise either because of a change in the proportions of the measured anions (Cl^- and HCO_3^-) or accumulation of other strong acids not usually measured in the blood; both represent decreases in SID. When there is a **change in the proportions of these measured anions,** chloride is retained and HCO_3^- is excreted abnormally, as seen in renal tubular acidosis and diarrhea. **Strong acids can accumulate** because of ingestion, excess production beyond the excretory capacity, or impaired excretion per

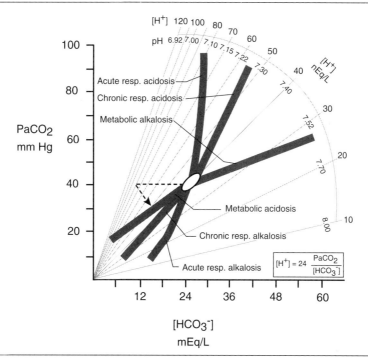

Fig. 42-3. Relationship of arterial CO_2 tension ($PaCO_2$) and HCO_3^- concentration ($[HCO_3^-]$); isopleths for the H^+ concentration ($[H^+]$) are also shown. The darkened lines indicate the ranges of values expected for the compensatory response to the primary acid-base disorders. The changes expected for a metabolic acidosis with and without respiratory compensation are shown. The Henderson equation is given in the lower right.

se, such as caused by ketoacidosis (acetoacetate and beta-hydroxybutyrate), lactic acidosis, uremia, and toxins.

In **lactic acidosis,** for example, the SID decreases because lactate, with a pK of 3, behaves like a strong anion and $[HCO_3^-]$ decreases as it reacts with and buffers the increase in $[H^+]$. In **renal tubular acidosis,** the SID decreases with an increase in plasma $[Cl^-]$ and a direct decrease in $[HCO_3^-]$. Anions (A^-), which buffer the rise in $[H^+]$, decrease to form HA (Eq. 42-12). Respiratory compensation occurs with increased ventilation to excrete CO_2 and lower $[PaCO_2]$, which, as an independent variable, offsets the increase in $[H^+]$.

Metabolic Alkalosis

Metabolic alkaloses are characterized by an **increase in SID** and the **tendency to accumulate base in the extracellular fluid.** In one major group of disorders, the **chloride-depletion alkaloses,** SID becomes more positive

because of the loss of chloride from the body, which leads to retention of base, primarily as HCO_3^-. Loss of gastric fluid and chloruretic diuretic use are examples of conditions that cause this form of alkalosis. In the other major group, the **potassium-depletion alkaloses,** the increase in SID arises from a shift of acid into the intracellular compartment; these disorders usually occur when there is mineralocorticoid excess such as aldosterone-producing adenomas or severe hypertension. In both types of alkalosis, plasma proteins and other buffers release H^+ according to the formula given in Eq. (42-12). With the fall in $[H^+]$, a decrease in ventilation produces respiratory compensation that raises the $PaCO_2$, which in turn ameliorates the initial decrease in $[H^+]$.

Respiratory Acidosis

The central event in respiratory acidoses is **diminished clearance of CO_2** or hypoventilation, which produces hypercapnea, or an elevated $PaCO_2$ (see Chap. 32). Among the main causes of CO_2 retention, the most common are **disorders of the lung parenchyma** that interfere with CO_2 excretion because of ventilation and perfusion mismatch (emphysema, asthma, and adult respiratory distress syndrome). **Neuromuscular diseases,** such as poliomyelitis and Guillain-Barré syndrome, which impair respiratory pump muscles, and **drugs,** such as morphine and anesthetics, which suppress the neuronal circuitry of breathing, cause global hypoventilation and elevate $PaCO_2$.

An increase in PCO_2, as an independent variable, increases [H^+] (Eq. 42-16). However, a number of biochemical reactions are initiated that minimize the rise in [H^+]. Weak acids, such as hemoglobin and proteins, titrate [H^+] according to Eq. (42-13). SID increases (becomes more positive) as Cl^- moves into RBCs in exchange for HCO_3^- (chloride shift) (see Fig. 42-2) and as Na^+ and K^+ move from the intracellular into the extracellular fluid. In **acute respiratory acidosis,** both the rise in SID and the reactive weak acids (fall in A^-) elevate plasma [HCO_3^-] and reduce [H^+].

In **chronic respiratory acidosis,** in which high PCO_2 levels persist for a few days, SID becomes more positive with a further rise in plasma [HCO_3^-] and a further drop in [H^+]. The change in SID is due to an increase in renal Cl^- excretion, which leads to a fall in the plasma [Cl^-] and the generation of new bicarbonate. The excretion of H^+ occurs through the synthesis of NH_3, which forms NH_4^+ (see Chap. 43).

Respiratory Alkalosis

The central event in respiratory alkalosis is the **excess clearance of CO_2** (an increase in alveolar ventilation disproportionate to CO_2 production) which results in reduced $PaCO_2$ (hyperventilation). The most common causes of respiratory alkalosis are **pregnancy, high altitude, lung diseases,** and **liver diseases.** Other causes include endotoxinemia, hysteria, and any condition associated with severe hypoxemia.

As an independent variable, the decrease in $PaCO_2$ lowers [H^+], as the reaction (Eq. 42-16) is shifted to the left by the accelerated CO_2 excretion through the lungs. Compensatory mechanisms mitigate such decreases in [H^+]. SID becomes less positive as Cl^- and lactate move into the extracellular fluid and Na^+ and K^+ move out. Lactate concentration increases because of the heightened activity of certain glycolytic enzymes secondary to intracellular alkalosis. Organic anions and plasma proteins (A^-) increase in accordance with Eq. (42-13). In the face of a **low $PaCO_2$** that persists for more than a few days, renal adaptive mechanisms are maximized that further raise the plasma [Cl^-]. This then elicits a fall in [HCO_3^-] and a rise in [H^+] (see Chap. 43).

Summary

The [H^+] of the body is tightly regulated by and is a function of three independent variables: the SID, the amount and nature of the weak acids (buffers), and PCO_2 set by alveolar ventilation. The simultaneous solution of the expressions for these independent variables and their associated relationships permits calculation of the in vivo [H^+]. For physiologic buffering, nonvolatile (fixed) acids are affected by rapidly responsive physicochemical buffers, mainly proteins and phosphates, in the extracellular and intracellular spaces, and by changes in the alveolar ventilation that adjust PCO_2. CO_2, the major product of catabolism and a volatile acid, is buffered in the blood primarily by hemoglobin and promptly excreted by the lungs. A defect or overload in any of these mechanisms disrupts acid-base balance, and such disorders are classified as acidosis or alkalosis and further defined as respiratory or metabolic, depending on the nature of the defect. These four acid-base disturbances can be understood in terms of the major independent variables.

Bibliography

Davenport, H. W. *The ABC of Acid-Base Chemistry,* 6th ed. rev. Chicago: University of Chicago Press, 1974.

Seldin, D. W., and Giebisch, G. *The Regulation of Acid-Base Balance.* New York: Raven Press, 1989.

Stewart, P. A. Modern quantitative acid-base chemistry. *Can. J. Physiol. Pharmacol.* 61:1444–1461, 1983.

43 Renal Acid-Base Regulation and Micturition

Robert O. Banks

Objectives

After reading this chapter, you should be able to

Describe the role of the kidneys in regulating extracellular pH

Explain the process involved in urinary acidification: the events in both the proximal and distal tubule, formation of titratable acidity, ammonia production, importance of carbonic anhydrase, and production of new HCO_3^-

Define nonionic diffusion and explain how it influences the excretion of ammonium and other weak bases and acids

List the factors that influence HCO_3^- excretion

Compare the renal participation in acid-base balance during acute and chronic alkalosis and acidosis

Describe the process of micturition

A large portion of the diet in many Western countries consists of protein, and persons on such a high-protein diet metabolize some 50 to 100 meq of so-called nonvolatile or fixed inorganic and organic acids per day. In contrast to the H^+ that derives from the hydration of CO_2 and is eliminated through the lungs, the nonvolatile acids must first be buffered by bicarbonate and hemoglobin and then excreted by the kidney. Nonvolatile acid production can increase substantially under both normal and pathologic conditions. Thus lactic acid production is significantly enhanced during heavy exercise and hypoxia. In other conditions, such as uncontrolled diabetes mellitus, the production of nonvolatile acids can increase by as much as tenfold. Diets rich in vegetables and fruits generate nonvolatile products that are alkaline, but these products also must be excreted by the kidney.

The kidney participates in the **overall regulation of acid-base balance** in two ways: (1) it reclaims virtually all of the filtered HCO_3^-, and (2) it excretes acid. **Acid excretion** is accomplished through these routes. The first is excretion of free H^+; because the minimum pH of the urine is about 4.5, this avenue accounts for less than 0.5.% of the

total H^+ excreted per day. The second route is excretion of titratable acid, and the third is ammonia production and the resulting ammonium excretion. Adjustments in the third route of acid excretion primarily explain the increased H^+ excretion seen during a metabolic acidosis. The enhanced production of ammonia by the kidney during acidemia takes 4 to 5 days to reach a maximum (as will be discussed).

Bicarbonate Reabsorption

When the plasma HCO_3^- concentration is less than 26 to 28 meq/liter, virtually all the **filtered HCO_3^- is reabsorbed.** The bulk of this reabsorption occurs in the **early proximal tubule** (within the first 20% to 30% of the total proximal tubule) by means of H^+ secretion (see Fig. 38-1). Most of the H^+ secreted in the proximal tubule derives from **Na^+-H^+ exchange.** However, approximately 20% of the HCO_3^- reabsorption in the proximal tubule can continue following inhibition of Na^+ transport, suggesting that H^+ secretion in the proximal tubule also can be mediated by an **H^+-ATPase electrogenic process.**

461

Secreted H^+ combines with filtered HCO_3^-, thereby generating H_2CO_3. Because the brush border of the proximal tubule contains **carbonic anhydrase,** the H_2CO_3 instantaneously dissociates into CO_2 and H_2O. These products diffuse passively across the luminal membrane and, in the presence of carbonic anhydrase in the cell, are converted back into H_2CO_3 and then to H^+ plus HCO_3^-. The HCO_3^- then moves passively across the peritubular membrane (evidence suggests that this step may be a carrier-mediated, $H^+\text{-}3HCO_3^-$ cotransport process). The net effect of this series of events is the reabsorption of $NaHCO_3$.

The small amount of filtered HCO_3^- that leaves the proximal tubule (about 10% to 20% of the filtered load) is reabsorbed in the **distal tubule** by a similar mechanism (see Fig. 42-1). The major difference, however, is that there is little, if any, carbonic anhydrase in the brush border of the distal tubule (it is only found in the cells of the distal tubule). On the other hand, the luminal pH of the distal tubule can fall as low as 4.5 (versus 7.0 in the proximal tubule) because a H^+-ATPase pump exists on the luminal membrane. This relatively high H^+ concentration shifts the H^+ plus HCO_3^- reaction to the right (to H_2CO_3 and to CO_2 plus H_2O) and therefore promotes reabsorption of essentially all HCO_3^- in the distal tubule. The reabsorption of HCO_3^- across the basolateral membrane in the distal tubule appears to be mediated by a $Cl^-\text{-}HCO_3^-$ exchanger. Thus, on a normal protein diet with 50 to 100 meq of fixed acid formed each day, virtually all the filtered HCO_3^- is reabsorbed (180 liters/day $\times$ 24 meq/liter = 4320 meq/day filtered; 5 meq/day is normally excreted and 4315 meq/day is reabsorbed). It is important to note that 4315 meq of H^+ was secreted in order to reabsorb the 4315 meq of HCO_3^-. This H^+, however, is not excreted. Furthermore, the HCO_3^- consumed during the initial plasma buffering of the fixed acid has not been replaced; instead, HCO_3^- is replaced through the formation of titratable acid and excretion of NH_4^+, as will be discussed.

HCO_3^- reabsorption is affected by a number of factors (Table 43-1). Two of these factors, the plasma HCO_3^- concentration and the extracellular fluid volume, are illustrated in Fig. 43-1. As the plasma HCO_3^- concentration is increased by infusing solutions of $NaHCO_3^-$, there is a resulting increase in the extracellular fluid volume as well as the plasma HCO_3^- concentration. Under those conditions, as is illustrated by the lines marked "expanded" in Fig. 43-1, the amount of HCO_3^- reabsorbed attains a plateau value at high plasma HCO_3^- concentrations. That is, HCO_3^- reabsorption appears to be characterized by a transport maximum. However, when the plasma HCO_3^- is increased with minimal expansion of the extracellular fluid

Table 43-1. Factors Affecting HCO_3^- Reabsorption

Factors That Increase HCO_3^- Reabsorption	Factors That Decrease HCO_3^- Reabsorption	Mechanism
MAJOR FACTORS		
Volume contraction	Volume expansion	Probably via changes in proximal Na^+ reabsorption
Increased filtered HCO_3^- load	Decreased filtered HCO_3^- load	Also may be via proximal Na^+ reabsorption
Hypercapnia	Hypocapnia	Possibly via changes in cell pH
Hypokalemia	Hyperkalemia	Possibly via changes in cell pH
	Carbonic anhydrase inhibition	Carbonic anhydrase is essential for HCO_3^- reabsorption in proximal tubule
MINOR FACTORS		
Hypercalcemia	Hypocalcemia	A combination of direct tubular effects, hemodynamic effects, and external buffering of acid governs the minor factors
PTH deficiency	PTH excess	
Vitamin D	Vitamin D deficiency	
Thyroid hormone	Phosphate depletion	
Glucose	Hypothyroidism	
	Basic amino acids (lysine, arginine)	
	Maleic acid	

PTH = parathyroid hormone.

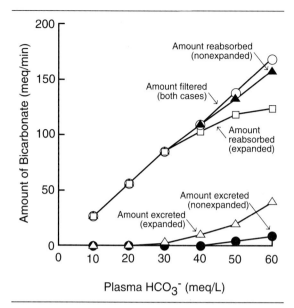

Fig. 43-1. Amounts of HCO_3^- filtered, reabsorbed, and excreted as a function of the plasma HCO_3^- concentration. Data from two groups of rats are illustrated, one group that was volume expanded during the process of increasing the plasma HCO_3^- concentration and a second group that was not. As can be seen, the nonexpanded group reabsorbed virtually all the filtered HCO_3^-, even at high plasma HCO_3^- concentrations. (Adapted from: Purkerson, M. L., et al. On the influence of extracellular fluid volume expansion on bicarbonate reabsorption in the rat. *J. Clin. Invest.* 48:1754–1760, 1969.)

space, as illustrated by the lines marked "nonexpanded" in Fig. 43-1, virtually all the filtered HCO_3^- is reabsorbed, even at high plasma HCO_3^- concentrations. The difference between HCO_3^- reabsorption in the nonexpanded and the expanded states may be related to the fact that reabsorptive events in the proximal tubule decrease during expansion of the extracellular fluid space and increase during volume contraction; these phenomena may be related to changes in the balance of Starling reabsorptive forces between the postglomerular plasma and the renal interstitial fluid space.

Excretion of Titratable Acid

The ability of a weak acid to participate in the formation of titratable acid depends on the quantity of the buffer present and on its weak-acid dissociation constant (pK_a) (maximum buffering occurs within ± 1 pH unit of the pK_a).

HPO_4 (pK_a 6.8) is the major urinary titratable acid buffer. **Uric acid** (pK_a 5.75) and **creatinine** (pK_a 4.97) are present but in smaller amounts. (In uncontrolled diabetes mellitus, the large quantities of ketoacids produced, such as beta-hydroxybutyrate [pK_a 4.8], contribute to the urinary buffering.) The formation of titratable acid is illustrated in Fig. 43-2. It is important to note that the production of titratable acid generates "new HCO_3^-," which is the HCO_3^- that replaces the buffer base consumed in the initial buffering process of the fixed acid.

Ammonia Production and Acid Excretion

The sum of ammonium and titratable acidity minus the amount of excreted HCO_3^- equals the **net acid excretion.** As noted, the net acid excretion for a normal protein diet is about 50 to 100 meq/day. Approximately 30 meq of this H^+ burden is normally excreted as NH_4^+. This NH_4^+ excretion is also advantageous, because it also elicits the generation of "new" HCO_3^-.

As is illustrated in Fig. 43-3, **ammonia** is synthesized in

Fig. 43-2. The formation of titratable acid by tubular cells. During this process, dibasic weak acids (such as HPO_4^{2-}) are converted into the monobasic form. Consequently, Na^+ and newly synthesized HCO_3^- are reabsorbed: the "new" HCO_3^- replenishes that consumed during the initial buffering of the fixed acid (CA = carbonic anhydrase).

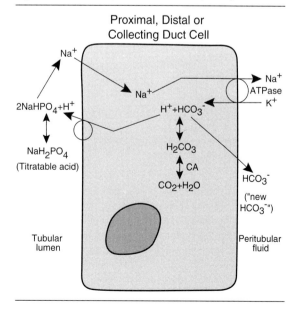

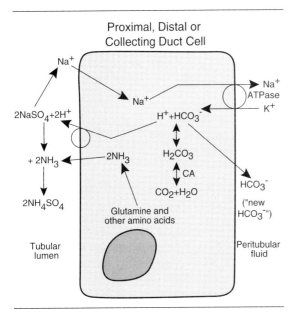

Proximal, Distal or Collecting Duct Cell

Fig. 43-3. The production of ammonia and its subsequent excretion. This process also replenishes the HCO_c^- consumed during the initial buffering of the fixed acid (CA = carbonic anhydrase).

tubular cells in several regions of the nephron. Recent evidence, however, indicates that most is generated in the proximal tubule. Ammonia is derived from the metabolism of amino acids, particularly (but not solely) from **glutamine**. The **biochemical events** that characterize ammonia production via glutamine metabolism are illustrated in the following reaction:

$$\text{Glutamine} \xrightarrow[\text{glutaminase}]{\overset{NH_3}{\uparrow}} \text{glutamic acid}$$

$$\text{Glutamic acid} \xrightarrow[\text{glutamate-dehydrogenase}]{\overset{NH_3}{\uparrow}} \text{alpha-ketoglutarate}$$

Ammonia can readily diffuse into both the tubular lumen and plasma. There is evidence, however, that the transfer of ammonia and ammonium from the cell into the lumen may involve both an **active component** and a component dependent on a Na^+-NH_4^+ **antiport**. In addition, nonionic diffusion contributes significantly to the trapping of ammonia in the lumen of the tubule, as will be discussed. There is also evidence that a substantial portion of

the ammonia secreted in the proximal tubule is reabsorbed (probably as NH_4^+) in the ascending limb of the **loop of Henle**; most of the NH_4^+ excreted appears to derive from subsequent secretion into the collecting duct.

Nonionic Diffusion

The NH_3 molecule is **lipid soluble** and can readily diffuse across the peritubular and luminal membranes, but the charged component, NH_4^+, cannot. This phenomenon is termed **nonionic diffusion.** Because the pH of tubular fluid is lower than that of plasma, there is a preferential movement of NH_3 into the tubular lumen (the reaction $NH_3 + H^+ \rightarrow NH_4^+$ provides a "sink" for the continued movement of NH_3 into the lumen). As noted in Fig. 43-3, the secretion of NH_3 and subsequent excretion of NH_4^+ not only produce the net loss of H^+ but, as indicated, also lead to the generation of "new" HCO_3^-.

Nonionic diffusion is an important phenomenon that affects the excretion of all **weak acids and bases.** These, of course, can be endogenous substances, such as NH_3, or pharmacologic compounds. Thus the rate of excretion of many drugs depends on (and can be regulated by adjusting) the **urinary pH.** For example, the excretion rate of aspirin (pKa 3.0) is relatively low when the urinary pH is between 4 and 5. By contrast, during treatment with acetazolamide (which causes a large increase in HCO_3^- excretion and a resulting urinary pH in the alkaline range), the clearance of aspirin approaches the glomerular filtration rate. In other words, weak acids are trapped in the compartment with the lower concentration of H^+, whereas weak bases are concentrated in the compartment with the higher concentration of H^+.

The major urinary adjustment during chronic **metabolic acidosis** is an increase in ammonia production (Fig. 43-4). As is illustrated in this figure, the production rate of **ammonia** during acidosis can increase markedly; as much as a tenfold increase in ammonia production has been reported. The increase in NH_3 production during acidosis takes 4 to 5 days to reach a maximum. This delay may be due to slow changes in the factors regulating entry of glutamine into the mitochondria or a delayed increase in the enzymatic activity involved in glutamine metabolism. These facts are further illustrated in Fig. 43-5, which shows the net acid excretion in human subjects following ingestion of NH_4Cl. NH_4Cl is converted to ammonia and HCl in the liver, and this precipitates metabolic acidosis. As can be seen, virtually all the additional acid load is excreted through increased ammonia production, a

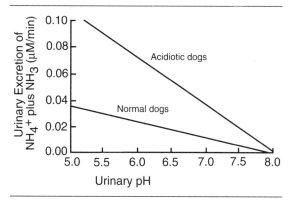

Fig. 43-4. Urinary excretion of ammonia plus ammonium in control and chronically acidotic dogs. The urinary pH in both groups was initially about 5.0 but was rendered progressively alkaline by infusing $NaHCO_3$. (Data from: Pitts, R. F. Renal excretion of acid. *Fed. Proc.* 7:418–426, 1948.)

process that requires several days before a steady-state is reached.

Micturition

Because of the positive pressure exerted in **Bowman's space,** tubular fluid moves along the entire nephron. Once in the ureter, urine is moved into the bladder under the combined influence of **gravitational forces** and **contractions of the ureteral musculature.** Urine is prevented from refluxing into the ureter by a valvular flap at the junction of the ureter with the bladder.

The **capacity of the bladder** can exceed 400 ml. As the bladder is initially distended, the first 30 to 50 ml of urine causes an increase in bladder pressure of about 10 to 20 cmH_2O. Continued filling then produces little change in pressure until the bladder capacity is reached. When the bladder volume is approximately 200 ml, afferent impulses in the pelvic nerves create the sensation of distension and initiate the desire to urinate. Voluntary control can be maintained during continued filling of the bladder, but as filling exceeds 400 ml, pressure can increase to 100 cmH_2O, and involuntary micturition will result.

Initiation of micturition is normally a voluntary act and may be related to the willful relaxation of the external sphincter through inhibition of the pudendal nerves. The subsequent micturition reflex is an **automatic spinal reflex.** Activation of parasympathetic fibers causes stimula-

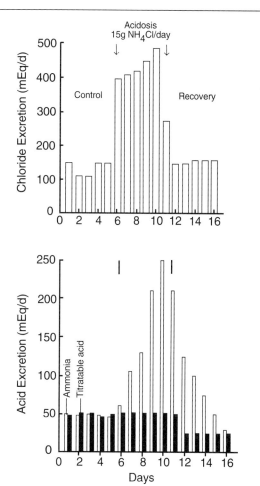

Fig. 43-5. Renal excretion of Cl⁻ and acid (ammonia and titratable acid plotted separately) in human subjects before, during, and after an acid load (15 g of NH_4Cl per day; NH_4Cl is converted to HCl and ammonia by the liver). Cl⁻ excretion increases rapidly but ammonia excretion (the primary urinary buffer that increases in response to the acid load) requires several days to attain a steady-state. (Data from: Pitts, R. F. Renal excretion of acid. *Fed. Proc.* 7:418–426, 1948.)

tion of the detrusor muscle and an increase in intravesical pressure of up to 25 to 50 cmH_2O.

The bladder is also innervated by **sympathetic (hypogastric) fibers,** but their function is not entirely clear. Activation of beta-adrenergic fibers to the fundus causes relaxation whereas activation of alpha-adrenergic fibers in the neck of the bladder and in the urethra causes contraction of those structures.

Summary

Most people who consume a typical Western diet produce 50 to 100 meq/day of so-called nonvolatile or fixed acid, which must be excreted by the kidney. In the process of excreting acid, the kidney reabsorbs virtually all the filtered HCO_3^-. Additional HCO_3^-, so-called new HCO_3^-, is also generated by the kidney as a by-product of acid excretion. Net acid excretion is accomplished both through the formation and excretion of titratable acid and through the secretion of ammonia and subsequent excretion of ammonium (very small amounts of H^+, less than 0.5% of the daily H^+ burden, are excreted as free cations). Under normal conditions, approximately half the acid is excreted as titratable acid and half as ammonium. Eighty to ninety percent of the filtered bicarbonate is reabsorbed in the proximal tubule, and the remaining fraction is reabsorbed in the distal tubule. As H^+ is secreted (either in exchange for Na^+ or via a proton pump), the subsequent combination of H^+ with filtered HCO_3^- generates CO_2 and H_2O. (In the proximal tubule, carbonic anhydrase in the brush border facilitates this process; in the distal tubule, a high luminal H^+ concentration shifts the reaction to CO_2 plus H_2O.) The production of titratable acid (the process of hydrogenation of the conjugate base) is primarily accomplished by a phosphate buffer. Ammonia is produced in tubular cells, principally from glutamine. Ammonia can diffuse into both the lumen of the tubule and the vascular space; however, because of the phenomenon of nonionic diffusion and the presence of a H^+ gradient between the tubular lumen and plasma, larger amounts of the gas are trapped in the lumen as ammonium. During acidosis, the compensatory increase in acid excretion is primarily brought about by increases in ammonia production, but several days must elapse before enhanced synthesis of ammonia achieves a new steady-state.

Micturition is normally a voluntary process that appears to be initiated by the deliberate relaxation of the external sphincter. The desire to urinate is evoked as the bladder fills to about 200 ml. Once initiated, the micturition reflex is an automatic spinal reflex that involves activation of parasympathetic nerves and contraction of the detrusor muscle.

Bibliography

Good, D. W., and Knepper, M. A. Ammonia transport in the mammalian kidney. *Am. J. Physiol.* 248:F459–F471, 1985.

Rector, F. C., Jr. Sodium, bicarbonate, and chloride absorption by the proximal tubule. *Am. J. Physiol.* 244:F461–F471, 1983.

Part VII Questions: Renal and Acid-Base Physiology

1. If the GFR is 120 ml/min and the urine flow rate is 0.5 ml/min, the urine to plasma inulin ratio would be
   A. 10:1.
   B. 24:1.
   C. 100:1.
   D. 240:1.
   E. 1000:1.

2. Based on the following data, which statement is correct?

Oxygen consumption for the whole body = 250 ml/min
Mixed arterial oxygen concentration = 20 ml/dl of whole blood
Mixed venous oxygen concentration = 15 ml/dl of whole blood
RBF/cardiac output = 0.3
GFR/RPF = 0.2
Arterial hematocrit = 0.5
Arterial plasma Na^+ concentration = 140 µeq/ml
Urine Na^+ concentration = 280 µeq/ml
Urine flow rate = 0.75 ml/min

   A. The RBF is 1200 ml/min.
   B. The GFR is 120 ml/min.
   C. The fractional excretion of Na^+ is 2.0%.
   D. The fraction of the filtered Na^+ reabsorbed is 94%.
   E. The urine/plasma inulin concentration ratio is 200:1.

3. The fluid in Bowman's space
   A. contains some protein, but primarily that with a molecular weight greater than 20,000.
   B. would show a fall in pressure if the tubular flow rate in the early distal nephron was increased.
   C. has a glucose concentration higher than that in efferent arteriolar plasma leaving the glomerulus.
   D. has a pressure that is inversely related to the mean arterial pressure.
   E. has a Na^+ concentration higher than that of plasma.

4. With regard to the renal handling of glucose, which of the following statements is true?
   A. The renal extraction of glucose at plasma glucose concentrations well above threshold approaches that of inulin.
   B. The renal threshold for glucose could be calculated if one knew the T_{mG} and the GFR.
   C. At high plasma glucose concentrations, the clearance of glucose approaches the RPF.
   D. Glucose is usually excreted after a high-carbohydrate meal.
   E. The concentration of glucose in the efferent arteriole is higher than that in the afferent arteriole.

5. In the early portions of the proximal tubule,
   A. the TF/P ratio for urea is less than 1.0.
   B. the TF/P Na^+ ratio is 1.2 to 1.3.
   C. the TF/P Cl^- ratio increases.
   D. the TF/P creatinine ratio is less than 1.0.
   E. the TF/P glucose ratio ranges from 1.2 to 1.3.

6. Which of the following statements about the function of long loops of Henle is true?
   A. Fluid entering the loop (leaving the proximal tubule) is hypertonic.
   B. Fluid at the turn is hypertonic compared with the interstitium at that level.
   C. Water permeability of the descending limb is low.
   D. Fluid leaving the loop (entering the early distal tubule) is hypotonic to plasma.
   E. ADH modulates the water permeability of the ascending limb.

7. The following data were obtained from individuals A and B:

	A	B
Urine osmolality (mOsm/kg H_2O)	100	500
Urine flow rate (ml/min)	4.0	0.8
Plasma osmolality (mOsm/kg H_2O)	280	280

Which of the following statements is true?

A. The osmolar clearance is the same in both subjects but the free water clearances differ.

B. The plasma concentration of ADH in person B is probably less than that in person A.

C. Person A could be dehydrated and receiving furosemide.

D. The cAMP concentrations in the collecting ducts of person A are greater than those in person B.

E. The urine creatinine concentration in person B is less than that in person A.

8. Licorice contains an aldosterone-like steroid, glycyrrhizic acid, so individuals ingesting large amounts of licorice would have

A. a reduced inulin space.

B. hyperkalemia (high plasma K^+ concentration).

C. enhanced Na^+ excretion.

D. metabolic alkalosis.

E. hypotension.

9. A comatose patient is seen in the emergency room with an arterial blood pH of 7.20, an $[H^+]$ of 64 nM, a $PaCO_2$ of 72 mmHg, and a plasma $[HCO_3^-]$ of 27 mM. This implies which acid-base disorder(s)?

A. Metabolic acidosis

B. Acute respiratory acidosis

C. Chronic respiratory acidosis

D. Both A and B

E. Data are internally inconsistent.

10. HCO_3^- reabsorption in the proximal tubule

A. occurs primarily in the latter third of this segment.

B. increases during treatment with acetazolamide.

C. increases during volume contraction.

D. increases during hyperventilation.

E. is cotransported with potassium.

VIII Gastrointestinal Physiology

Part Editor

Joseph D. Fondacaro

44 Gastrointestinal Nervous System

Edward S. Redgate

Objectives

After reading this chapter, you should be able to

Identify the principal pathways involved in the sympathetic innervation of the gastrointestinal tract, the responses of target tissue to sympathetic discharges, the neurotransmitters responsible for sympathetic activity, and the distribution of tonic and reflexive sympathetic control

Identify the pathways of somatic and parasympathetic innervation of the esophagus and how they control swallowing and esophageal peristalsis

Explain how vagal excitatory and inhibitory fibers control the circular muscle tone of the lower esophageal sphincter and the receptive relaxation response of the proximal stomach, and their role in the small and large intestines

Describe how the intrinsic innervation of secretory epithelium and external musculature is organized and how this innervation controls the activities of these tissues

The remarkable ability of the gastrointestinal tract to transfer nutrients, salts, and water across the mucosal epithelium is achieved through the coordinated action of several effectors:

1. The **motor apparatus** physically reduces the size of the food particles.
2. The manifold **secretions** of the mucosal epithelium and glands chemically reduce the food particles to more elemental compounds.
3. The **motor apparatus** mixes and propels the resulting **chyme** through the tube.
4. The **vasoconstrictor muscles** direct appropriate changes in blood flow to the above structures.

The coordination of this symphony of events is accomplished by the **autonomic nervous system,** in conjunction with **endocrine and paracrine secretions.** This chapter focuses on the role of the autonomic nervous system, and Chap. 45 examines the role of the gastrointestinal hormones. The autonomic nervous system has two separate outputs to the gut, extrinsic and intrinsic, and these converge on the final common pathway neurons. The **extrinsic innervation** originates at various levels of the cerebrospinal axis and consists of the parasympathetic and sympathetic fibers. The **intrinsic innervation** consists of ganglia located in an intramural plexus called the **enteric nervous system** (ENS). This accounts for the innervation of the segments of the gastrointestinal tract lying between the midesophageal level and the internal anal sphincter but not for the innervation of the upper esophageal musculature and the external anal sphincter. The upper esophagus and the external anal sphincter are composed of striated muscle. The **upper esophagus** is not innervated by the autonomic nervous system but by special visceral efferent fibers in the vagal nerves; the **external anal sphincter** is innervated by sacral somatic efferent fibers in the pudendal nerves.

The **degree of dependence** of various parts of the gastrointestinal system on these sources of innervation varies considerably. For example, at the oral and anal ends of the gastrointestinal tract where the upper esophagus and external anal sphincters are composed of striated muscle, denervation causes a loss of function of the striated muscle. The muscle in the rest of the gastrointestinal tract is smooth muscle innervated by the enteric nervous system, which can continue to function after surgical separation from the central nervous system.

There are two well-established **enteric motor neuron** pathways to gastrointestinal smooth muscle: **cholinergic** and **nonadrenergic noncholinergic** (NANC). This combination of intrinsic nerves and smooth muscle is able to function independently of the innervation by extrinsic nerves, but the degree of independence is not uniform. In certain structures, such as the lower esophageal sphincter, the stomach musculature, and the ileocecal and internal anal sphincters, extrinsic innervation exerts significant control over the motility of the smooth muscle, while in the small intestine the ENS is more important.

In view of these variations in the origin and degree of neural control, the innervation of the gastrointestinal tract will be described starting with the sympathetic and parasympathetic innervation and then proceeding to the intrinsic or enteric innervation.

Extrinsic Innervation

Sympathetic Control

The sympathetic outflow to the gastrointestinal tract originates in the **intermediolateral cell column** of the **thoracolumbar spinal cord.** As shown in Fig. 44-1, the preganglionic neurons project cholinergic fibers into the splanchnic nerves, which converge on noradrenergic neurons in the prevertebral ganglia. In view of species variation and the lack of precise knowledge, it is not possible to be entirely specific in describing the pathways of sympathetic fibers innervating the gastrointestinal tract, but it is clear that most of the sympathetic outflow to it originates in ganglia, as shown in Table 44-1.

Noradrenergic fibers from these prevertebral ganglia decrease blood flow, inhibit secretomotor neurons, relax nonsphincteric circular muscle, and contract sphincteric circular muscle. The prevertebral ganglion cells are the site of convergence of **two inputs:** one from the extrinsic sympathetic preganglionic fibers, as already described, and the other from sensory afferents originating in the muscle coats and mucosa. The influence of the sympathetic system is mainly manifested in a tonic activity in **splanchnic blood vessels** and in the inhibition of **secretions by the mucosal epithelium.** The sympathetic activity on the gas-

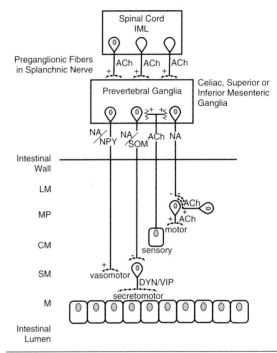

Fig. 44-1. Sympathetic innervation of the intestine in non-sphincter regions. The preganglionic sympathetic neuron output from the thoracolumbar spinal cord innervates ganglion cells in prevertebral ganglia. These postganglionic sympathetic neurons innervate vascular smooth muscle, secretomotor neurons in the submucosal plexus, and motor neurons in the myenteric plexus. The sympathetic output is excitatory to the vascular smooth muscle but inhibitory to the secretomotor and motor neurons (LM = longitudinal muscle; MP = myenteric plexus; CM = circular muscle; ACh = acetylcholine; NA = norepinephrine; SOM = somatostatin; SM = submucosal plexus; M = mucosa; IML = intermediolateral cell column; NPY = neuropeptide Y; DYN = dynorphin; VIP = vasoactive intestinal peptide).

trointestinal blood vessels constricts arterioles and the larger veins, thereby decreasing splanchnic vessel diameter and increasing resistance to blood flow. The vasoconstrictor tone is mediated by the release of **norepinephrine** in combination with **neuropeptide Y** (NPY). Norepinephrine acts at adrenergic receptors, and NPY potentiates the constrictor action of norepinephrine. The tonic activity of the sympathetic innervation mediated by the

Table 44-1. Innervation of the Gastrointestinal System by Postganglionic Sympathetic Fibers

Ganglion of Origin	Destination
Superior cervical	Esophagus
Middle	Esophagus
Stellate	Esophagus
Thoracic	Esophagus
Celiac	Lower esophageal sphincter, stomach, pylorus, proximal duodenum, sphincter of Oddi
Superior mesenteric	Caudal duodenum, jejunum, ileum, ileocecal sphincter, cecum
Inferior mesenteric	Transverse colon, descending colon, sigmoid colon, rectum, internal anal sphincter

adrenergic fibers containing somatostatin acts on the secretomotor innervation of the mucosal epithelial cells to decrease water and electrolyte secretion. Loss of this sympathetic inhibitory control results in increased secretion by the intestinal mucosal epithelium and possibly in diarrhea.

In regard to the sympathetic innervation of the **external muscle layers,** there are only a few sympathetic nerve fibers supplying the smooth muscle of the nonsphincteric regions. In the **sphincteric regions** (lower esophageal, pyloric, ileocecal, and internal anal), noradrenergic innervation is normally more dense than in adjacent nonsphincteric regions. The sphincter muscle is supplied with alpha-excitatory and beta-inhibitory adrenergic receptors. It is the **alpha-adrenergic receptors** of the muscle that are physiologically activated by the release of norepinephrine from adrenergic nerves, causing contraction of the sphincter muscle. There is evidence suggesting that the tonic sympathetic discharge to sphincter muscle originates in the spontaneously active preganglionic neurons of the lumbar spinal cord or in ganglion cells of the prevertebral ganglia. However, if the entire sympathetic chain is removed in laboratory animals, no apparent changes in the digestive process or lasting changes in sphincter activity are observed. From these experimental observations, it appears that the intact parasympathetic innervation and intrinsic reflexes are sufficient and that the sympathetic supply is not essential to the digestive process.

In the **nonsphincteric regions,** the major influence of adrenergic neurons on the motility of the external muscle coats is not exerted directly on the muscle but indirectly by inhibiting the activity of cholinergic ganglion cells in the myenteric plexus which excite muscle contractions. These adrenergic nerve terminals form a dense plexus among the ganglion cells of the myenteric plexus. Norepinephrine acts on presynaptic alpha-adrenergic receptors to suppress release of excitatory neurotransmitters in the intrinsic interneuronal circuitry. While these adrenergic nerves do not discharge spontaneously, they may be induced to discharge reflexly, especially in a protective manner, such as when the muscle wall is threatened by excessive distention or in response to peritoneal irritation. This may lead to a state of **ileus** in which there is no motor activity in the intestinal musculature.

Parasympathetic Control

The role of the parasympathetic innervation of the gastrointestinal tract is different from that of the sympathetic innervation. While excitation of the sympathetic innervation constricts arteries and large veins, inhibits secretion, constricts sphincters, and inhibits nonsphincteric muscle activity, excitation of the parasympathetic innervation not only tends to **oppose all these actions** but also sets in motion coordinated sequences of motility, secretion, and blood flow changes that promote **digestion.** The characteristics of these coordinating actions are unique for each segment of the gastrointestinal tract, so each segment must be considered separately.

Extrinsic Innervation of the Esophagus

The motor fibers innervating the upper striated muscle as well as the lower smooth muscle portion of the esophagus travel in the **vagus nerve,** CN X (Fig. 44-2). The upper striated muscle portion of the esophagus is supplied by **special visceral efferent** fibers in the vagus nerve originating in the **nucleus ambiguus** of the medulla; the lower smooth muscle part is supplied by **general visceral efferent** fibers originating in the **dorsal motor nucleus of the vagus.** The discharge of the vagal motor neurons is controlled by **afferent fibers** of pharyngeal and esophageal sensory receptors that mainly travel in the superior laryngeal branch of the vagus and synapse in the **nucleus of the solitary tract.** There are also **descending polysynaptic pathways** to these nuclei from neurons in the forebrain that also may play a role in initiating swallowing. A **central mechanism** appears to control **swallowing,** and this consists of the nucleus of the solitary tract, the vagal nuclei, and adjacent areas of the medullary reticular formation.

Swallowing takes place when the swallowing center is

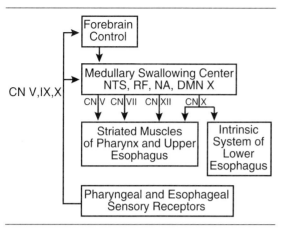

Fig. 44-2. Major neural pathways involved in the control of swallowing. The inputs from pharyngeal and esophageal sensory receptors traveling in cranial nerves V, IX, and X project to centers in the forebrain and medulla oblongata that control swallowing. The output from the medullary swallowing center over cranial nerves V, VII, X, and XII controls striated muscles of the pharynx and upper esophagus (branchiomotor); the output from the dorsal motor nucleus of cranial nerve X (vagus) controls the lower esophagus (CN V = trigeminal nerve; CN VII = facial nerve; CN XII = hypoglossal nerve; CN X = vagus; NTS = nucleus tractus solitarii; NA = nucleus ambiguus; RF = reticular formation; DMN X = dorsal motor nucleus X).

activated by descending signals from the forebrain or reflexly when sensory receptors in spectfic areas of the palate, pharynx, and epiglottis are stimulated. These areas are innervated by the **maxillary branch** of the trigeminal nerve, the glossopharyngeal nerve, and the superior laryngeal nerve (see Fig. 44-2). When the swallowing center is activated, **interneuronal circuits** are triggered to release the programmed sequence of coordinated motor events of primary peristalsis in the upper striated muscle as well as in the lower smooth muscle of the esophagus (Fig. 44-3). Evidence indicates that the **centrally programmed sequence of motor events** of primary peristalsis may be played out without further afferent support. As a result, primary peristalsis may continue without interruption even if the bolus is diverted through an open slit in the esophagus, because it depends on an intact swallowing center and efferent vagal nerves and not on esophageal distension. In contrast, secondary peristalsis consists of a succession of locally initiated reflexes originating in esophageal receptors. It relies on afferent and efferent neural pathways in

the vagal nerves of the upper striated muscle esophagus and on the long vagal reflex pathways plus the local enteric system reflex pathway in the lower smooth muscle esophagus. Since both afferent and efferent pathways are carried in the vagal nerves, the reflex is called a **vagovagal reflex.** Therefore, if a bolus of food descends partway through the esophagus but then deviates through an open esophageal slit, peristalsis of the secondary type ceases below the slit. Peristalsis of the primary type continues to complete its movement to the lower end of the esophagus but is diminished. As a food bolus descends in an intact esophagus, secondary peristalsis reinforces the force and velocity of the primary peristalsis so that the distension created by the bolus produces a larger response than just that from a "dry swallow."

Cervical vagotomy causes loss of function of the striated muscle esophagus because it denervates both the striated muscle innervated by motor neurons of the nucleus ambiguus and the sensory receptors. In contrast, **motor innervation** of the smooth muscle esophagus is supplied by preganglionic fibers originating in the dorsal motor nucleus of the vagus, which terminate in the enteric system of the lower esophagus. While vagotomy severs the preganglionic innervation of the lower esophagus, it does not interrupt the local reflex pathways in the enteric system of the lower esophagus. Secondary peristalsis may be evoked through this local reflex pathway. This information helps us to understand how peristaltic motor events may persist in clinical cases when a neuromuscular blocking agent for skeletal muscle is administered. After **skeletal neuromuscular blockade** (nicotinic cholinergic receptor antagonist), the oropharynx and upper striated muscle esophagus are paralyzed but primary and secondary peristalsis persist in the lower smooth muscle esophagus (muscarinic cholinergic receptors).

Parasympathetic Innervation of the Lower Esophageal Sphincter

Unlike the parasympathetic innervation of other visceral structures, such as that of the heart and bladder, the parasympathetic innervation of the lower esophageal sphincter consists of **two types of preganglionic fibers,** as shown in Fig. 44-4. One set of preganglionic fibers in the vagus nerves is believed to synapse with NANC neurons of the enteric system, which inhibit a permanent myogenic tone of the lower esophageal sphincter smooth muscle and are called **vagal inhibitory fibers** (VIFs). The other set of preganglionic fibers is believed to synapse with cholinergic enteric neurons, which increase tone in the smooth muscle of the sphincter and are called **vagal excitory**

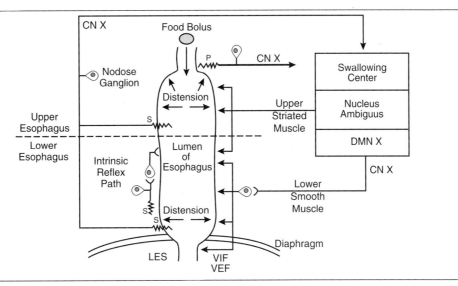

Fig. 44-3. Neural control of upper striated and lower smooth muscle regions of the esophagus. Passage of a food bolus from the pharynx into the esophagus stimulates sensory receptors, initiating primary peristalsis. Local distension of the esophagus initiates secondary peristalsis (VEF = vagal excitatory fiber; VIF = vagal inhibitory fiber; LES = lower esophageal sphincter; *zigzag lines* = mechanoreceptor symbol; p = primary peristalsis; s = secondary peristalsis; CN X = vagus; DMN X = dorsal motor nucleus).

Fig. 44-4. Parasympathetic excitatory and inhibitory fiber innervation of the gastric fundus and gastrointestinal sphincters. The myogenic tone of the lower esophageal sphincter, gastric fundus, gastroduodenal, ileocecal, and internal anal sphincters is controlled by parasympathetic excitatory and inhibitory fibers: these outputs are found in vagal nerves (VEF, VIF) above the transverse colon, and for pelvic nerves (EF, IF) below the transverse colon (DMN X = dorsal motor nucleus X; ACh = acetylcholine; NANC = nonadrenergic, noncholinergic; DRG = dorsal root ganglion; S2 to S4 = sacral spinal segments 2 to 4; NG = nodose ganglion).

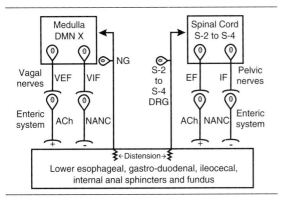

fibers (VEFs). Because both VEFs and VIFs exist in the vagal nerves, sectioning or stimulation of these nerves produces variable results. However, vagotomy may decrease or even abolish the ability to relax the lower esophageal sphincter due to the loss of the VIFs.

Extrinsic Control of the Stomach

When a volume of food passes from the esophagus into the stomach, the intraluminal gastric pressure tends to rise, but this is quickly limited by a reflex relaxation response in the proximal stomach. This response is an extrinsic reflex that relies on vagal afferent and efferent fibers that serve to limit the **intraluminal gastric pressure.** The relaxation response controls the **gastroduodenal pressure gradient,** which tends to expel gastric contents through the pylorus into the duodenum and also reduces the possibility of gastroesophageal reflux.

In the **receptive relaxation response** of the proximal stomach, the VEF and VIF type of preganglionic vagal fibers of the stomach alter their discharge rate reciprocally in a manner similar to that exhibited by the lower esophageal sphincter (see Fig. 44-4). The gastric distension also activates **extrinsic reflexes** mediated by vagal afferent and efferent fibers as well as **intrinsic reflexes,** which increase the mixing and grinding movements of the gastric corpus and antrum.

Duodenal distension activates extrinsic VEF and VIF reflex pathways similar to those that limit the gastroduodenal pressure gradient. In each of the already mentioned pathways, the VEFs synapse with excitatory cholinergic neurons while the VIFs synapse with inhibitory NANC fibers. The reflexes are blocked by vagotomy or by treatment with a ganglionic blocker of the nicotinic type. The **neuromuscular junction** of postganglionic fibers (VEF pathway) is blocked by treatment with a cholinergic blocker of the muscarinic type. When vagotomy blocks the receptive relaxation response, the reservoir function of the stomach is impaired.

Besides the extrinsic reflexes responding to distension that are activated by receptors in the muscular coats, there are extrinsic reflexes responding to **chemical conditions,** such as pH, hypertonicity, or hypotonicity, which involve receptors in the mucosa. Besides controlling gastric motility, extrinsic reflexes also influence the **secretion of HCl** and **pepsinogen** by the gastric secretory epithelium. Proximal gastric vagotomy decreases the secretion of HCl and pepsinogen but preserves antral motility and has been used to manage duodenal ulcers caused by acid secretion mediated by vagal innervation. There are **chemoreceptors** in the duodenum that respond to glucose, pH, fats, fatty acids, and hypertonicity. There are also mechanoreceptors in the muscular layers that react to stretch. Stimulation of these receptors activates vagal reflexes that inhibit gastric emptying. These enterogastric reflexes also appear to employ VEF-type and VIF-type preganglionic vagal fibers and are extinguished by vagotomy.

Extrinsic Innervation of the Small and Large Intestine

The extrinsic parasympathetic innervation of the small and large intestine consists of fibers that travel in the vagus and pelvic nerves (see Fig. 44-4). The **vagal nerves** innervate the small intestine and the ascending and transverse colon; the **pelvic nerves** innervate the descending colon and the rectum. The vagal motor neurons originate in the **dorsal motor nucleus of the vagus,** and the afferent fibers traveling in the vagal nerves have cell bodies in the **ganglion nodosum.** The pelvic nerve motor neurons originate in the **intermediolateral** and **ventral horn areas** of sacral spinal cord segments S2 to S4, and the cell bodies of the pelvic afferent axons are located in the S2 to S4 dorsal root ganglia. The activity of the parasympathetic innervation of the small intestine is believed to resemble that of the esophagus and stomach, in that there is an excitatory cholinergic fiber pathway and an inhibitory NANC fiber pathway, but

the density of preganglionic vagal fibers decreases distally. There are more vagal fibers going to the esophagus and stomach than to the duodenum, and the vagal innervation of the distal small intestine and colon has not been well described. Electrical stimulation or sectioning of the mixture of excitatory and inhibitory fiber pathways in the vagal nerves may elicit inconsistent results. However, evidence suggests that a tonic VEF exists that stimulates intestinal motility.

Extrinsic Innervation of the Colon and Internal Anal Sphincter

The same general pattern of extrinsic nervous control as that described for the esophagus, stomach, and small intestine is seen in the colon and internal anal sphincter (see Fig. 44-4). There are both excitatory and inhibitory fiber pathways in the vagal and pelvic nerve regions of the large intestine, where transmission depends on acetylcholine or NANC signals, respectively. Stimulation of the vagal innervation of the colon elicits contraction of both circular and longitudinal muscles, and stimulation of the pelvic nerve results in relaxation of the internal anal sphincter.

Enteric Nervous System

Intrinsic Innervation by the Enteric Nervous System

The enteric nervous system consists of the **ganglionated plexuses,** which lie in the wall of the gastrointestinal tract and extend from the esophagus to the internal anal sphincter. The two major plexuses of the enteric system are the myenteric and submucosal. As shown in Fig. 44-5, the **myenteric plexus** is located between the longitudinal and circular layers of the external musculature, and the **submucosal plexus** is situated on the submucosal surface of the circular muscle layer. The ganglia of these plexuses are extensively interconnected. These plexuses receive sensory input and contain networks of interneurons that connect with motor and secretomotor neurons. There are **sensory inputs** of mucosal origin that respond to chemical and osmotic stimulation as well as inputs activated by radial stretch of the external musculature. There are also **excitatory** and **inhibitory inputs** from the parasympathetic division of the autonomic nervous system. These inputs synapse with elaborate nerve networks of interneurons that coordinate different patterns of motility and secretomotor activity. These connections are not completely understood, but encouraging progress is being made. It is known that the enteric system contains a **greater number of neurons** — 10^7 to 10^8 — than the spinal cord. In view of this,

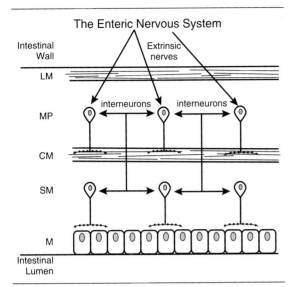

Fig. 44-5. The enteric nervous system contains two main plexuses, the myenteric and the submucosal. The myenteric plexus mainly innervates the external muscle layer and the submucosal plexus, the secretory epithelium. The neurons of each of these plexuses are interconnected and the plexuses are interconnected. The plexuses also receive both sympathetic and parasympathetic extrinsic innervation (LM = longitudinal muscle; MP = myenteric plexus; CM = circular muscle; SM = submucosal plexus; M = mucosa).

the enteric system is considered a major part of the nervous system and one that contains very complex circuits. This view has been reinforced by the discovery of a diversified population of neurons containing many different neurotransmitter and neuromodulator substances, most of which are neuropeptides also found in the CNS.

There are distinct target organs for the two major plexuses. The **major outputs** of the myenteric plexus are directed to the **circular** and **longitudinal muscles.** In certain parts of the gastrointestinal tract, it is possible to distinguish between a plexus innervating the circular muscle and one for the longitudinal muscle. In contrast, the major output of the submucosal plexus is to the **secretory epithelium** and **enteroendocrine cells** (hormone-secreting cells of the mucosa).

Innervation of the Secretory Epithelium

The secretory activity of the intestinal epithelium responds to both neural and hormonal signals. The chemical and osmotic properties of food and distension of the gut activate

neural pathways in the submucosal plexus that control the secretion of the intestinal epithelium. The sensory information is encoded in action potentials that evoke neurotransmitter release in the submucosal plexus. As shown in Fig. 44-6, **acetylcholine** is one of these neurotransmitters, and it acts at nicotinic cholinergic receptors to excite interneurons and secretomotor neurons. The secretomotor neurons also may release acetylcholine, which, in turn, excites muscarinic receptors on epithelial cells, or these secretomotor neurons may release NANC neurotransmitters, such as vasoactive intestinal peptide (VIP), dynorphin, substance P, cholecystokinin, and gastrin releasing peptide, either separately or in combination. The secretomotor neuron activity may trigger the secretion of substances such as pepsinogen, mucus, gastrin, and electrolytes. The activity of the intrinsic secretory pathways is modulated by

Fig. 44-6. The secretory epithelium is innervated by cholinergic and nonadrenergic, noncholinergic (NANC) secretomotor neurons. The activity of these secretomotor neurons is coordinated by sensory receptor input to the enteric system, and by extrinsic sympathetic and parasympathetic innervation. There is a tonic inhibitory sympathetic input and an excitatory parasympathetic input (LM = longitudinal muscle; MP = myenteric plexus; CM = circular muscle; SM = submucosal plexus; M = mucosa).

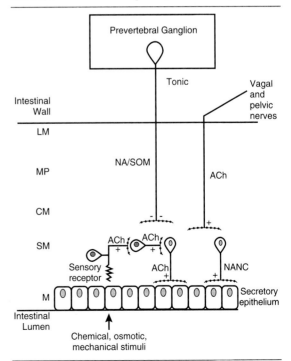

input from both the extrinsic parasympathetic and sympathetic nerves. Stimulation of the sympathetic nerves inhibits neuronal activity in the submucosal ganglia, decreases secretion by the secretory epithelium, and enhances absorption. Removal of the sympathetic input by paralysis or denervation of the sympathetic innervation causes enhanced secretion, reduced absorption, and possibly diarrhea.

Intrinsic Innervation of the External Musculature

Almost all the axons supplying the **circular muscle** originate in the myenteric plexus, and most of the axons supplying the **longitudinal muscle** appear to arise from the myenteric or a closely related plexus. A concept that has emerged from recently acquired information is that the coordination of the longitudinal and circular muscle of the intestine cannot be explained solely by reflex-type activity. Instead, it is proposed that (1) the interneuronal networks in the myenteric plexus contain preprogrammed circuits that selectively activate each of the various motility patterns and (2) with the exception of sphincteric motility, motility patterns such as segmentation, peristalsis, the migrating motor complex, and ileus appear to be generated by circuits in the enteric system and do not depend on long reflex pathways involving the central nervous system.

The preprogramed **patterns of motility** result from the combined function of both the enteric neurons and the external musculature. The circular layer of the external musculature is a **syncytium** that is continuously excited by the rhythmic discharges of pacemaker smooth muscle cells. Its contractile activity generates many of the mechanical forces that mix and propel the luminal contents. The specific intrinsic neural circuits responsible for the motility patterns are not known, but recently acquired information has permitted insight into the neural and muscular mechanisms that generate some of the various patterns of motility. A major function of the intrinsic innervation is inhibition of the spread of smooth muscle pacemaker-initiated excitation throughout the circular muscle syncytium. The intrinsic nerves produce this inhibition, and this effect can be shown when an isolated strip of small intestine is exposed to **tetrodotoxin** (TTX), which blocks Na^+-dependent action potentials. TTX abolishes Na^+ spikes and prevents the release of an inhibitory transmitter (probably VIP or nitric oxide) from inhibitory NANC intrinsic motor neurons. In the absence of the inhibitory transmitter, the strip of external musculature, which prior to TTX treatment was relaxed, develops unpatterned contractile spasms.

The **intrinsic inhibitory motor neurons** exist at all levels of the gut, and in nonsphincteric regions they continuously suppress the myogenic contractile activity of circular muscle. In a sphincter muscle, such as the lower esophageal sphincter, the inhibitory motor neurons do not continuously suppress the myogenic contractile activity of the circular muscle of the sphincter, but are brought into action reflexly during passage of the luminal contents. Inhibitory and excitatory synaptic discharges of intrinsic interneurons maintain control over the inhibitory motor neurons. Inhibitory interneuronal discharges inhibit the inhibitory motor neurons, and this permits increased myogenic contractions of the circular muscle. The process of inhibiting an inhibitory neuron is called **disinhibition.** It is believed that the disinhibition of such motor neurons plays a major role in generating the stereotyped motility patterns of **circular muscle. The longitudinal muscle** differs in this respect. Instead of receiving inhibitory fibers, it is innervated by a cholinergic excitatory pathway.

Since preprogrammed patterns of motility can be evoked by the application of certain putative neurotransmitters to isolated gut preparations, it is believed that the **interneuronal circuits** involved are "hard-wired" programs, comparable to those known to control stereotyped patterns of motor behavior in invertebrates that are evoked by command neurons. For example, in the intestine, **opiate-like substances** evoke segmentation and suppress peristalsis, while serotonin does the opposite. This evidence has been assembled in a model in which opiate-like substances and serotonin activate circuits controlled by command neurons. These **command neurons** cause stereotyped movements by activating certain neuronal networks formed by the enteric nervous system. Other examples of **stereotyped motor behavior** controlled by command neurons are ileus and circular muscle spasm. In the case of **ileus,** the command neurons elicit a continuous discharge of the intrinsic inhibitory motor neurons, causing circular muscle relaxation. Conversely, a **circular muscle spasm** occurs if the intrinsic inhibitory motor neurons are absent or inactive. Inhibitory motor neuron inactivity precipitates the spread of smooth muscle pacemaker-driven contractile activity throughout the circular muscle syncytium.

This model explains the derangements in motility seen in Hirschsprung's disease and achalasia of the lower esophageal sphincter. In these diseases, spasms of contractile activity of circular muscle occur when enteric ganglion cells are lacking in the myenteric plexus. It is believed that the circular muscle spasms are due to the loss of intrinsic inhibitory motor neurons.

Summary

Although our knowledge of gastrointestinal innervation is still far from complete, the properties of certain components of the innervation are beginning to emerge. The major source of innervation is the autonomic nervous system, while the contribution of the somatic nervous system is limited to important controls over the striated muscles involved in swallowing and defecation. With regard to vasomotor and secretomotor control and innervation of the external muscle layers, the effectors from the midesophageal area to the internal anal sphincter receive innervation from the intrinsic and extrinsic parts of the autonomic nervous system. The intrinsic part is called the enteric nervous system and is composed of a diverse array of neurons, most containing neuropeptides. These neurons form an intramural network responsible for producing different coordinated patterns of motor and secretomotor activity.

The extrinsic part of the autonomic nervous system consists of the parasympathetic and sympathetic divisions. The parasympathetic aspect innervates the smooth muscle of the external muscle layers and contains antagonistic outputs consisting of cholinergic excitatory and NANC inhibitory neurons. The circular muscle of the gut is a spontaneously excited electrical syncytium that is activated by pacemaker smooth muscle cells whose contractile activity is held in check by the tonic discharge of inhibitory NANC neurons. Release from this inhibitory tone of NANC neurons, or disinhibition, elicits increased contractile activity. In contrast, the cholinergic innervation of circular muscle is tonically excitatory. These two opposing pathways to circular muscle, one tonically inhibitory and the other tonically excitatory, are extrinsically innervated by preganglionic vagal fibers to that part of the gut orad to the transverse colon. These outputs are the VIFs and VEFs.

Neural control of gut motility is thought to function in the following manner. The extrinsic VIF and VEF pathways control the relaxation and contraction of the lower esophageal sphincter, the receptive relaxation response of the proximal stomach, and the function of the gastroduodenal and ileocecal sphincters. The signals delivered by the parasympathetic VIF and VEF discharges appear to represent a variety of command signals that selectively activate different preprogrammed patterns of gut motility. Other examples of command signals are those which evoke segmentation, peristalsis, the migrating motor complex, and ileus. In addition to the NANC fibers controlling smooth muscle, there are a variety of NANC neurons that function as secretomotor neurons. These NANC secretomotor neurons receive excitatory cholinergic and inhibitory adrenergic input.

The overall activity of the sympathetic division of the autonomic nervous system innervating the gut suppresses digestion. Adrenergic neuron discharges inhibit the excitatory cholinergic input to circular muscle in nonsphincteric regions but excite sphincter muscles to contract, thereby lessening propulsion of intraluminal contents. The inhibition of propulsion, contraction of sphincters, and suppression of secretions transforms the activity of the gut from a propulsive to absorptive mode.

Bibliography

Furness, J. B., and Costa, M. *The Enteric Nervous System.* New York: Churchill-Livingstone, 1987.

Johnson, L. R., ed. *Physiology of the Gastrointestinal Tract,* 2nd ed. New York: Raven Press, 1987.

Schultz, S. G., Wood, J. D., and Rauner, B. B., eds. *Handbook of Physiology,* Sec. 6: The Gastrointestinal System. Bethesda, Md.: The American Physiological Society, 1989.

Wood, J. D. Neurophysiological theory of intestinal motility. *Jpn. J. Smooth Muscle Res.* 23:143–186, 1987.

45 Gastrointestinal Hormones

Edward S. Redgate

Objectives

After reading this chapter, you should be able to

Define endocrine, paracrine, autocrine, and neurocrine

Identify what criteria must be met to establish the endocrine nature of a chemical messenger

Explain the roles of gastrin, cholecystokinin, secretin, and gastric inhibitory polypeptide, and describe the factors controlling their release

Communication between cells in the gastrointestinal tract is subserved not only by the neural reflex pathways described in Chap. 44 but also by a host of chemical messengers. Virtually every function of the gut appears to be influenced by **hormones** produced by specialized cells found throughout the system.

The **study of gastrointestinal peptides** entered a new era with the advent of certain immunologic, genetic. and chemical techniques: immunocytochemistry, radioimmunoassay, methods for studying gene expression and peptide synthesis, and techniques for isolating and culturing functionally intact peptide-secreting cells. Application of these techniques has revealed that significant structural similarities exist among certain gastrointestinal peptides, and these have been grouped into families (Table 45-1), such as the **gastrin** and **secretin** families. As shown in Table 45-1, there is an abundant variety of peptides in the gastrointestinal tract, suggesting the presence of extensive hormonal controls, but at this time the hormonal status of only a few is known. A peptide must fulfill **certain criteria** before it can be considered a true hormone. The following must be demonstrated in order to establish that a gastrointestinal peptide is indeed an endocrine hormone: (1) it is released into the circulation in response to a physiologic stimulus, such as feeding, (2) it produces a response that can be mimicked when the peptide is infused at concentration that are physiologic, and (3) the response to the physiologic stimulus can be antagonized by infusion of a specific antiserum or a selective antagonist. Of the several dozen substances currently being investigated as possible gastrointestinal endocrine hormones (see Table 45-1), only four peptides are known to comply with these criteria: **gastrin, cholecystokinin** (CCK), **secretin,** and **gastrin-inhibitory polypeptide** (GIP).

Gastrin, CCK, secretin, and GIP are found in the **enteroendocrine cells** scattered throughout the mucosa in certain regions of the gut. **Gastrin** is localized in the mucosa of the **gastric antrum,** while **CCK, secretin,** and **GIP** dwell in the mucosa of the **proximal small intestine.** As a rule, the **endocrine cells** releasing the peptide hormones are oriented in the mucosa such that one surface of the cell is exposed to the contents of the gastric or intestinal lumen, where chemicals in the chyme may stimulate or inhibit the cells, and the opposite surface is exposed to interstitial fluid in contact with the gastrointestinal blood vessels and the circulation. The stimulus and response relationships of these four hormones are summarized in Table 45-2.

Table 45-1. Gastrointestinal Peptide Families

Family	Major Members	Principal Biologic Functions
Gastrin	Gastrin	+ Gastric acid, + trophic to mucosa
	Cholecystokinin	+ Pancreozymin, + gallbladder
Secretin	Secretin	+ Pancreas and biliary bicarbonate
	Glucagon	− Intestinal motility
	Vasoactive intestinal peptide	+ Pancreatic and intestinal secretion
	Gastric-inhibitory polypeptide	− Gastric acid
	PHI-27	+ Pancreatic secretion
Pancreatic polypeptide	Pancreatic polypeptide	− Pancreatic secretion
	Peptide YY	− Pancreatic secretion
	Neuropeptide Y	+ Vasoconstriction
Opioids	Enkephalin	− Intestinal transit
	Beta-endorphin	− Intestinal transit
Tachykinin-bombesin	Substance P	+ Smooth muscle
	Substance K	+ Smooth muscle
	Gastrin-releasing peptide	+ Gastrin release
Orphan peptides	Somatostatin	− Gastric acid
	Neurotensin	− Gastric acid

+ = stimulates; − = inhibits.

Table 45-2. Stimulus-Response Relationship of Gut Peptides

Variable	Gastrin	CCK	Secretin	GIP
Stimuli	Feeding, gastric distension, digested protein	Digested proteins and fats	pH 4.5, digested fat	H^+, osmolarity, fats
Cell of origin	G cell	I cell	S cell	GIP cell
Responses	+ Acid, − emptying, + mucosal growth	− Emptying	− Acid −emptying	− Acid, −emptying
Stomach				
Pancreas		+ Enzymes, + bicarbonate*	+ Bicarbonate, + enzymes*	+ Insulin
Liver		+ Bicarbonate*	+ Bicarbonate	
Gallbladder		+ Contraction		

CCK = cholecystokinin; GIP = gastrin-inhibitory polypeptide or glucose-dependent insulinotropic peptide; + = stimulates; − = inhibits; * = CCK + secretin synergism.

Gastrin

Gastrin is a peptide produced by **G cells** of the gastric antrum and duodenum. It is the most potent known stimulant of **gastric acid secretion** by parietal cells. When stimulating gastric acidity, gastrin relaxes proximal gastric stomach muscle, thus retarding gastric acid emptying into the duodenum. There are two major forms of gastrin in plasma, **G-17** and **G-34** (the numbers denote the fact that they are 17 and 34 amino acid polypeptides, respectively). Most of the plasma G-17 originates in the pyloric antral mucosa, while half the plasma G-34 originates in the antrum and half arises from the duodenum. In the pyloric antral region, **G cells** are scattered throughout the pyloric antral glands and are oriented in the typical gut endocrine cell fashion, whereby the **apical border** extends to the gastric lumen and the **basal granule–containing portion** contacts interstitial fluid. When stimulated by feeding, the plasma concentration of gastrin increases within a few minutes, peaks 20 to 30 minutes later, and consists of roughly equal portions of G-17 and G-34.

The **physiologic stimulus** for gastrin release is **feeding.** The mechanisms controlling release are complex and consist of neural reflex pathways with cholinergic and non-adrenergic noncholinergic (NANC) neurotransmission that acts directly on somatostatin cells and G cells, respectively. Direct effects are exerted by **somatostatin** (a paracrine) as well as by the **gastric acidity** and the **amino acid** and **peptide content** of the gastric chyme, as shown in Fig. 45-1.

Neural activity in the vagal pathways to G cells commences with the smell and taste of food and is continued by local and **vagovagal reflexes** elicited by gastric distension when food enters the stomach. In addition, the prod-

Fig. 45-1. Endocrine, neurocrine, and paracrine factors controlling HCl secretion by parietal cells. Parasympathetic innervation of epithelial cells involved in controlling HCl secretion. Parietal cell secretion of HCl is stimulated by a cholinergic vagal pathway. The vagal pathway also excites gastrin (G) release (an endocrine) and inhibits somatostatin (SST) release (a paracrine-inhibiting gastrin release). H^+ feedback increases somatostatin secretion and the presence of amino acids increases gastrin secretion (ACh = acetylcholine; PPD = products of protein digestion; GRP = gastrin-releasing peptide).

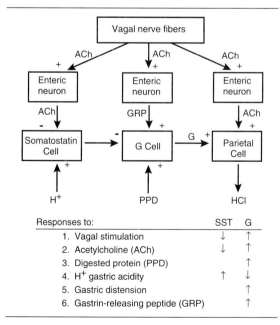

Responses to:	SST	G
1. Vagal stimulation	↓	↑
2. Acetylcholine (ACh)	↓	↑
3. Digested protein (PPD)		↑
4. H^+ gastric acidity	↑	↓
5. Gastric distension		↑
6. Gastrin-releasing peptide (GRP)		↑

ucts of protein digestion act directly on G cells. Undigested protein does not have any particular effect on G cells, but amino acids, especially tryptophan, and polypeptides are potent stimuli and an elevated H^+ concentration is inhibitory below pH 4.5. A model showing the major factors that govern gastrin release is illustrated in Fig. 45-1. The major **neural input** to the G cells is vagal, and the **major chemicals** in the chyme that modulate gastrin release are the **products of protein digestion** and the gastric acidity. **One vagal pathway** to the G cells consists of cholinergic preganglionic fibers to NANC postganglionic fibers in the intrinsic system. This NANC stimulatory pathway releases gastrin-releasing polypeptide (GRP), a member of the bombesin family. The gastrin acts on parietal cells, causing HCl secretion. A **second vagal pathway** to the G cells is indirect. Postganglionic cholinergic fibers activated by the vagal input terminate on somatostatin cells, which are in direct contact with G cells. Release of acetylcholine inhibits somatostatin release. **Somatostatin** is a paracrine hormone that inhibits G-cell secretion. Thus electrical field stimulation of either of these vagal inputs to the G-cell control mechanism stimulates gastrin release: one by releasing an excitatory NANC transmitter (GRP) and the other by inhibiting an inhibitory paracrine hormone (somatostatin). Additional controls arise from the contact of the apical surface of the G cells with the contents of the gastric lumen. The products of protein digestion directly stimulate the G cells to release gastrin, while the H^+ from gastric HCl stimulates somatostatin release, which in turn inhibits gastrin release.

In summary, the evidence indicates that gastrin release is not only the result of excitatory stimulation by NANC neurocrine hormone and the products of protein digestion but also the combined result of the inhibitory action of the paracrine hormone, somatostatin, and gastric luminal H^+ concentration. Finally, gastrin performs an important role in gut function, besides controlling gastric acid secretion. It imposes essential **trophic actions** on the oxyntic (acid-secreting) gastric mucosa, the mucosa of the small and large intestines, and possibly also the exocrine pancreas.

Cholecystokinin

Cholecystokinin (CCK) is a multifunctional endocrine hormone possessing **cholecystokinetic** (stimulating gallbladder contraction), **pancreozymic** (stimulating pancreatic enzyme secretion), and **pancreatic growth–promoting** (trophic) actions. It is the single major factor controlling gallbladder contraction and pancreatic enzyme secretion. The **CCK molecule** is very heterogeneous, consisting of a large group of peptides that are products of preproCCK. Based on current knowledge, CCK-8, CCK-22, and CCK-33 appear to be the dominant forms of CCK in the plasma. Structurally and functionally CCK is related to gastrin but has a **higher affinity** for the receptors that stimulate gallbladder contraction and pancreatic enzyme secretion. CCK is produced by **I cells,** which are distributed in the duodenum and upper jejunum. In their **cholecystokinetic** mode, CCK peptides potently contract gallbladder muscles and relax the sphincter of Oddi so that bile is ejected into the duodenum. CCK also inhibits gastric emptying by relaxing the proximal stomach and stimulating the pyloric sphincter; in this role, CCK acts as an **enterogastrone,** meaning a hormone of intestinal origin that inhibits gastric activity. In their **pancreozymic** function, CCK peptides directly stimulate pancreatic acinar cells to release pancreatic enzymes. The most important stimulus for CCK release is when the products of fat and protein digestion, such as amino and fatty acids, are brought in contact with the mucosa of the upper small intestine.

When the **pancreatic acinar cells** are under the sole influence of CCK, the amount of enzyme secreted is relatively small. However, when another hormone, secretin, is present, enzyme secretion is heightened. This is an example of **potentiation,** in that secretin alone does not stimulate pancreatic enzyme secretion but augments the action of CCK. This potentiation of the action of CCK by secretin is physiologically important for achieving optimal levels of pancreatic enzymes for the digestion of dietary nutrients. The converse is also true, in that CCK potentiates the action of secretin. **Secretin** is a hormone that originates from the duodenal mucosa and regulates hepatic and pancreatic secretion of bicarbonate ion. In the pancreas, CCK enhances the secretin-induced secretion of bicarbonate by pancreatic duct cells but by itself cannot do this.

Secretin

Secretin is the endocrine hormone that exhibits **sequence homology** with several other gastrointestinal peptides, including vasoactive intestinal peptide (VIP), GIP, PHI-27, and pancreatic glucagon. It is secreted by the S cells, which are distributed mainly in the upper small intestine. The major stimulus for secretin release is the **presence of H^+** (as HCl) in the upper small intestine. When gastric chyme is discharged into the initial 2 to 3 cm of the duodenum, the pH of the chyme is often below the threshold (estimated to be 4.5) for stimulating secretin release. Secretin primarily controls the secretion of water and bicarbonate by pancreatic duct cells and potentiates the action of CCK

in stimulating the secretion of enzymes by pancreatic acinar cells. Secretin also stimulates secretion of the aqueous bicarbonate-rich component of hepatic bile.

Secretin and CCK potentiate each other's actions on the exocrine pancreas. By itself, neither secretin nor CCK in the amounts released by a meal is potent enough to substantially stimulate exocrine pancreatic secretion of water and bicarbonate. Secretin also may interact with CCK to delay gastric emptying; that is, it performs the function of an enterogastrone.

Gastric-Inhibitory Polypeptide (GIP)

GIP inhibits **gastric acid secretion** and stimulates **insulin release**. GIP's inhibition of gastric acid secretion accounts for the fact that certain food substances in the small intestine suppress gastric acid secretion. These inhibitory responses are due to duodenal distension or to the presence of gastric acid, fats, or hyperosmolar solutions in the duodenum. It appears that GIP is one of several enterogastrones secreted by the upper small intestine that limit the amount of gastric acid in the intestine. The interactions of these gastrointestinal peptides are complex and may involve mediation by locally released somatostatin.

GIP is one of the hormones secreted by the gastrointestinal tract that participates in the control of **insulin secretion** by the endocrine pancreas. Although plasma glucose levels constitute the most important determinant of insulin release, blood levels of certain amino acids, gastrointestinal hormones, such as GIP, and the autonomic nervous system are also involved. GIP is an **anticipatory type** of controller of insulin secretion, in that GIP is released as gastric chyme enters the duodenum. Because of this, insulin secretion rises earlier and to a greater extent than it would if the plasma glucose level were the only controller.

Summary

The abundance of peptides in the gastrointestinal mucosa suggests that they are extensively involved in the endocrine and paracrine regulation of gastrointestinal function, but only four of these peptides are well-established hormones: gastrin, CCK, secretin, and GIP. Gastrin exists in typical endocrine cells (G cells) scattered in the glands of the antral mucosa and, when released into the circulation, stimulates gastric acid secretion. Feeding activates two types of vagal pathways — cholinergic and NANC —

which stimulate G cells to release gastrin. Food entry into the stomach further modulates gastric acid secretion by evoking local and vagovagal pathway responses to the distension and to the presence of the products of protein digestion (excitatory) and the H^+ concentration (inhibitory). Gastrin also has a trophic effect on the oxyntic gastric mucosa and the mucosa of the small and large intestines. CCK, secretin, and GIP reside in the endocrine cells of the mucosa of the upper small intestine. CCK controls gallbladder contraction, sphincter of Oddi relaxation, pancreatic enzyme secretion, secretion of the aqueous component of bile, and gastric emptying. CCK release is most potently stimulated by the presence of protein and fat digestion products in the upper small intestine. Secretin is mainly released when gastric acid makes contact with the mucosa of the upper intestine. This constitutes an endocrine hormone–controlling secretion of an aqueous bicarbonate fluid by duct cells of the pancreas and liver.

Secretin and CCK interact to potentiate each other. GIP is an enterogastrone secreted by the mucosal endocrine cells of the upper small intestine and inhibits gastric activity when gastric acid, fats, or hyperosmotic solutions are discharged into the small intestine. A major action of GIP is stimulation of insulin secretion.

Bibliography

Del Valle, J., and Yamada, T. The gut as an endocrine organ. *Annu. Rev. Med.* 41:447, 1990.

Johnson, L. R., ed. *Physiology of the Gastrointestinal Tract,* 2nd ed. New York: Raven Press, 1987.

Schultz, S. G., Wood, J. D., and Rauner, B. B. *Handbook of Physiology,* Sec. 6: The Gastrointestinal System. New York: Oxford University Press, 1989.

46 Gastrointestinal Motility

Frank C. Barone and Joseph D. Fondacaro

Objectives

After reading this chapter, you should be able to

Identify the anatomic features of the gastrointestinal tract that provide for motility, specifically the longitudinal and circular smooth muscle layers

Describe the major types of motility patterns seen in the gastrointestinal tract and the primary functions of these patterns

Discuss the motility patterns seen in specific areas of the gastrointestinal tract and the significance of the migrating motor complexes

Describe the various phases of swallowing and the anatomic components (and their role) important to each phase

Explain how the electrical and mechanical events are related to gastric motility.

Describe the pattern of motility unique to the small and large intestines and the mechanisms of defecation

Identify various diseases of gastrointestinal motility

Normally, the human gastrointestinal tract propels nutrients, liquids, other ingested materials, and secretions in an aboral direction from the mouth to anus. Except for the oral phase, this movement, termed **motility,** is involuntary. The term **motility** is also applied to the mechanical contractions of the gastrointestinal tract that are nonpropulsive and that function to mix ingested food with the secretions of mucosal cells. Both the propulsive and nonpropulsive motility patterns are a result of coordinated contractions of discrete sets of longitudinal and circular muscles (the intestinal or visceral smooth muscle). The **mouth, pharynx,** and **esophagus** provide a passageway for ingested materials to enter the stomach, where food is stored and mixed with the various components of gastric juice (including salivary enzymes). Gastric motility provides for "metered" emptying of this now partially digested material into the upper small intestine; this pattern is unique to the stomach and is regulated by both intrinsic and extrinsic nervous and

humoral factors. Intestinal motility allows for nonpropulsive (mixing) and propulsive contractions so that efficient digestion and absorption can occur. Colonic motility, which is normally slower than that exhibited by the small bowel, has both nonpropulsive and propulsive patterns to ensure the maximum absorption of water and salt and the efficient elimination of waste. This chapter reviews the anatomic features of the gastrointestinal musculature, the various specific motor functions of each major organ in the gastrointestinal tract, and some of the clinical manifestations of abnormal motility.

Anatomic Considerations

The basic anatomy of the gastrointestinal wall, including the location of the longitudinal and circular musculature, is illustrated in Fig. 46-1. (This chapter only covers the

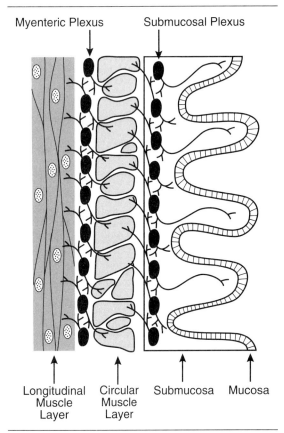

Fig. 46-1. The histologic arrangement of the layers of tissues of the gastrointestinal wall.

neural elements of the gastrointestinal tract. Chapter 44 contains a more detailed description of the gastrointestinal nerves and their role in the regulation of the functions of this system.) The outermost layer of muscle is composed of **longitudinal fibers,** and beneath this is the **circular muscle layer.** Between these muscle layers is the **myenteric nerve plexus,** which is a component of the enteric nervous system and provides for intrinsic modulation of gastrointestinal function. The **submucosal layer** is located beneath the circular smooth muscle and is composed of stromal tissue that contains blood vessels, the submucosal nerve plexus (the other branch of the enteric nervous system), lymphatic channels, and various cell types, including those which comprise the gastrointestinal immune system. Finally, the **mucosal layer** of epithelial cells lines the lumen of the major organs of the tract.

Different motility patterns are exhibited throughout the

gastrointestinal tract. Tonic or sustained contractions are characteristic of the **sphincteric muscle areas** of the gut. The **upper and lower esophageal sphincters,** the **pyloric** and **ileocecal valves,** and the **internal anal sphincter** are all sphincter muscles that maintain a tonic state of contraction. Peristalsis or peristaltic contractions propel luminal contents aborally and are seen in the **esophagus, distal half of the stomach,** the small intestine, and the rectum. **Peristalsis** is characterized by waves of alternating constriction and relaxation such that a band of constriction propels the food bolus from behind and the area in front relaxes, thus facilitating passage of the bolus aborally. This pattern of motility also relaxes sphincteric tone, allowing food to pass from organ to organ within the gastrointestinal tract. After the bolus has passed, sphincteric tone is reestablished in the area of constriction.

In the **colon,** there is a much different pattern of propulsive activity called **mass movement. Peristalsis** is manifested again in the **rectum.** There are also nonpropulsive motor patterns, termed **segmentation,** seen in the small bowel, and **haustrations,** unique to the colon, which serve to mix digested food (small intestine) and feces (colon) with other luminal contents and maximize exposure of material to absorptive surfaces. These mixing, nonpropulsive patterns are absent throughout the gastrointestinal tract during fasting and when the bowel is empty.

Fasting reveals another discrete motility pattern of the gut that migrates from the stomach to the terminal ileum at a speed of about 5 cm/min and occurs about every 90 minutes. Termed the **migrating motor complex,** it consists of little or no activity that changes suddenly to maximum propagated contractile activity and functions to cleanse the lumen of indigestible material.

Motility of the Mouth and Pharynx

Chewing begins the process of gastrointestinal motility but is not necessary for the digestion of food. It is normally voluntary but does have an involuntary component, in that food placed into the mouth of an unconscious person may initiate a chewing reflex. Chewing simply fragments ingested food, mixes it with salivary enzymes, and lubricates it to facilitate swallowing.

Swallowing, or **deglutition,** begins the obvious motility of the gastrointestinal tract and, though initiated voluntarily, becomes completely involuntary within 1 second. Its prime function is to get food or liquid into the stomach without forcing it into the nasopharynx or trachea. Because so many different mechanisms participate in the process, swallowing is separated into three phases: the oral phase, the pharyngeal phase, and the esophageal phase.

In the **oral phase,** the tongue selects a portion of food and pushes it back against the soft palate, which is slightly elevated. As the tongue pushes the food farther back, the soft palate closes the nasopharynx, and food enters the upper pharynx. In the **pharyngeal phase,** the presence of food causes the upper pharyngeal constrictor muscle to contract, ensuring closure of the nasopharynx and initiating a sequential contraction of the middle and lower pharyngeal constrictor muscles. This wave of contraction propels the food toward the esophagus. As food approaches the esophagus, the epiglottis is lowered and the glottis is elevated slightly so that the larynx is covered, preventing food from entering the trachea. At the same time, the upper esophageal sphincter momentarily relaxes, facilitating the entry of food into the esophagus.

During the **esophageal phase,** peristalsis is initiated as the wave of pharyngeal contractions passes through the upper esophageal sphincter. This closes the sphincter behind the bolus of food, and normal peristaltic contractions transport the food down the esophageal tube. As this propulsive wave reaches the lower esophageal sphincter, the area of relaxation preceding the bolus momentarily relaxes the sphincter, and food easily enters the upper stomach. As the propulsive wave passes, sphincteric tone is reestablished in the area of constriction behind the food bolus, and the lower esophageal sphincter closes, preventing reflux of food from the stomach into the esophagus. These three phases ordinarily take about 10 seconds, depending on the consistency of the food consumed. Liquids pass much more quickly.

Esophageal Motility

The esophagus is about 22 cm long. The **extrinsic innervation** of the esophagus involves the vagus nerve synapsing with the myenteric plexus neurons that control peristalsis. These myenteric plexus neurons innervate other myenteric neurons in the outer longitudinal and inner circular smooth muscle layers. The **upper third** of the esophagus is composed of striated muscle that receives direct input from vagal efferent fibers to produce coordinated peristaltic wave. The **middle third** of the esophagus contains mixed smooth and striated muscle with a myenteric plexus that receives vagal input. The intrinsic nervous system receives input from sensory receptors and is also stimulated by stretch (or distension). Consequently, if the

thoracic vagus nerve is cut, normal peristalsis still occurs in the lower two-thirds of the esophagus.

In the **lower esophagus,** which contains only smooth muscle, neuronal impulses pass from the vagus nerves to myenteric neurons. From these, impulses pass to other myenteric cells and to the inner and outer muscle layers that regulate peristalsis. **Primary peristalsis** (swallow reflex) in the esophagus is triggered by swallowing in the pharynx and continues even in the absence of a bolus in the esophageal lumen (dry swallow). **Secondary peristalsis** is stimulated by distension of the esophagus produced by an intraluminal bolus, an event similar to that seen in other parts of the gut (though for shorter distances). Secondary peristalsis is mediated entirely by the **enteric nervous system** and is achieved through the coordinated contraction and relaxation of the muscle layers. The peristaltic reflex is triggered by intraluminal distension, which, in turn, stimulates stretch receptors in the esophageal wall and initiates a progressive neurally mediated sequence. This reflex is also seen in the small intestine. Reflex relaxation (or lack of contraction in an organ such as the esophagus, which has no resting intraluminal tension or tone) precedes the bolus. The simultaneous contraction of circular muscle and relaxation of longitudinal muscle behind the bolus then further propels it forward. As the first portion of circular muscle relaxes, the next portion contracts, and the process is repeated. It has the appearance of a contractile wave that moves slowly (3 cm/sec) down the esophagus.

Figure 46-2 summarizes the roles of the vagus nerve, myenteric nerves, and intrinsic muscle excitability (myogenic response) in the regulation of esophageal motility. **Vagal nerve stimulation** relaxes the upper and lower esophageal sphincters. The lower esophageal sphincter also relaxes immediately when a swallow is initiated in the pharynx or the lower esophagus is distended. These events are mediated by the enteric nervous system. Peristalsis in the esophagus can be elicited by a swallow or by an intraluminal bolus and occurs along the upper esophagus through a direct vagal — hind brain — reflex arc. In the lower esophagus, peristalsis can be independent of the vagus and is mediated by the enteric nervous system. Intrinsic smooth muscle excitability closes the esophageal sphincters and reestablishes sphincteric tone, which is maintained in a tonic state.

Specific diseases can arise because of abnormal esophageal motility. **Gastroesophageal reflux disease,** is caused by incomplete closure of the lower esophageal sphincter (decreased resting pressure) or when there are increased transient relaxations of the sphincter not associ-

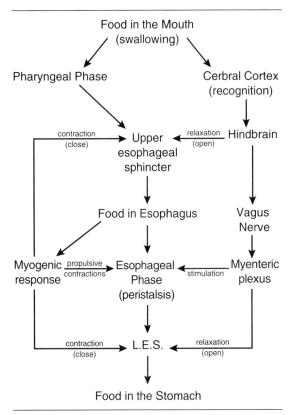

Fig. 46-2. The regulation of esophageal motility and esophageal sphincteric activity (see text for detailed description).

ated with swallowing. **Achalasia** represents a failure of the lower esophageal sphincter to relax completely during swallowing. **Diffuse esophageal spasm** consists of repetitive, high-amplitude contractions that can be painful and produce aperistalsis.

Gastric Motility

The major functions of the stomach are to **store food** temporarily, **continue digestion** by chemically reducing food particle size, and **regulate emptying** into the duodenum. The stomach is divided into three distinct regions: the upper or proximal portion called the **fundus,** the middle region called the **body,** and the lower or distal segment called the **antrum,** which terminates at the pylorus or gastroduodenal junction. The upper portion of the fundus lacks phasic motility but exhibits minimal tonic pressure and a high compliance for storage. Food can accumulate in

the fundus with large volume change but no pressure change. This phenomenon is called **receptive relaxation** and is mediated by the vagus nerves via inhibitory neurons of the myenteric plexus. The body of the stomach displays a motility that mixes and grinds the food with gastric juice and propels the food and liquid toward the antrum and pyloric area for regulated emptying.

Located at approximately the midpoint of the greater curvature of the body of the stomach is an area of rapid spontaneous depolarization known as the **gastric pacemaker.** It establishes the maximum rate of gastric contractile activity for this and the more distal areas of the stomach. The gastric pacemaker generates a well-defined electrical event that can be recorded as intrinsic electrical activity from both the pacemaker area and more distal regions of the stomach. The gastric smooth muscle elicits two types of electrical activity: slow waves and spike potentials (Fig. 46-3). **Slow waves** are slow depolarizations occurring at a frequency of three to six per minute and are often called the **basic electrical rhythm. Spike potentials** are periodic fast waves of depolarization that most often follow a slow wave and, when they do, always initiate contractions of the stomach musculature. Spike potentials are produced by the action of excitatory or disinhibitory enteric nervous regulation. Because muscle contractions always follow spike potentials associated with a slow wave, the slow wave or basic electrical rhythm controls the maximum rate of contraction of the stomach musculature, which is about three to six contractions per minute.

Spike potentials and the subsequent contractions of the gastric musculature are elicited directly by vagal nerve in-

Fig. 46-3. The basic electrical rhythm of the stomach, with slow-wave and spike potential activity illustrating the relationship of spike potentials to muscle contractions.

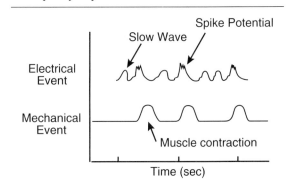

fluence as well as indirectly through the myenteric plexus. Distension of the stomach also evokes spike potential activity. The hormone **gastrin,** released by antral G cells in response to vagal influence and gastric distension, also accentuates the occurrence of spike potentials and contractions. These contractions are primarily peristaltic, with some nonpropulsive contractions manifested during peak digestion. These propulsive peristaltic waves continually move partially digested food toward the pylorus and are the prime mechanism for gastric emptying.

Gastric emptying after feeding takes longer for solids than for liquids — about 3 hours versus 1 hour, respectively — because of the time it takes for the distal stomach to reduce solids to a fluid consistency composed of particles less than 2 mm in diameter. Solid particles of food are broken up by gastric peristaltic contractions that move the particles against a closed pylorus. Only a small amount of partially digested material can move into the duodenum before the pylorus closes. A major portion of this wave rebounds back over the distal stomach and mixes food with gastric secretions, thus promoting further digestion. The **pylorus** limits the size of particles entering the duodenum and appears to prevent the reflux of duodenal contents into the stomach. Indigestible particles remain in the stomach until fasting **migrating motor complexes** move them through the bowel.

Following eating, the primary determinant of emptying is **volume;** the larger the meal volume, the greater is the stretch on the gastric wall and the greater are the force and frequency of gastric contractions. **Isosmotic gastric contents** empty faster than do hypoosmotic or hyperosmotic contents because of the feedback inhibition exerted by duodenal osmoreceptors. In addition, gastric contents with a **low pH** (higher H^+ concentration) empty slowly because of a combined neural and humoral mechanism. Sensory receptors are activated that transmit an inhibitory reflex to the stomach, and **secretin** is released from cells in the duodenum, which reduces the tone of the proximal stomach and decreases antral peristalsis. Intraluminal duodenal nutrients also appear to reduce gastric emptying through the release of hormones. Cholecystokinin release is elicited by proteins and lipids, and **gastric inhibitory peptide** release is evoked by glucose. The two hormones appear to slow gastric emptying by reducing gastric contractions and intragastric pressure. Both hormones are secreted by the duodenal mucosa. An intact **vagal innervation** appears to be important, but not essential, for regulating all aspects of gastric emptying, since loss of vagal integrity modifies the gastric and duodenal neuroneuronal and neurohumoral mechanisms involved. Figure 46-4 illustrates the mechanism of gastric emptying and the feedback regulatory process involved.

Fig. 46-4. The regulation of gastric motility and gastric emptying (CHOs = carbohydrates; GIP = gastric inhibitory peptide; CCK = cholecystokinin; $\oplus$ = stimulation; $\ominus$ = inhibition).

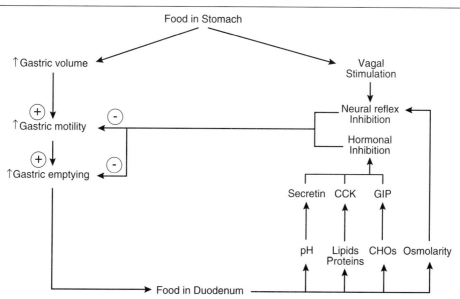

Clinical problems can result from **altered gastric motility.** A **chronic ulcer** in the pyloric channel in an adult may cause scarring, which can narrow the pyloric channel enough to cause obstruction. Its symptoms include vomiting, dehydration, and acid-base and electrolyte imbalances. **Motility disorders** of the stomach typically foster delayed gastric emptying of solid food (termed **gastroparesis**) that is manifested by symptoms of anorexia, persistent fullness after meals, nausea, vomiting, and pain. Delayed gastric emptying is occasionally the primary cause of **gastroesophageal reflux disease.**

Vomiting (emesis), which under some conditions may not be abnormal, is usually infrequent but can indicate a serious disorder. Protracted or frequent vomiting can lead to metabolic alkalosis and electrolyte imbalances. Before vomiting, one senses the inevitable with the feeling of nausea. This reflects a diffuse discharge from both sympathetic and parasympathetic nerves. A patient about to vomit exhibits **sympathetic responses** that include dilatation of pupils, pallor, sweating, cold skin, increased heart rate, and increased respiration. **Parasympathetic responses** consist of increased salivation, more pronounced motor activity in the esophagus, stomach, and duodenum, and relaxation of the upper and lower esophageal sphincters. During vomiting, a person retches, takes a deep breath, and the glottis closes. The pylorus constricts with no gastroesophageal motility, the abdominal muscles contract, and the stomach is squeezed between the diaphragm and the abdominal muscles, thereby rapidly emptying the stomach. The gastric contents are propelled up the esophagus and out the mouth. Emesis is stimulated in the **brain** through sensory stimulation or injury to the viscera or head. It also may be provoked by unusual labyrinth stimulation and by chemical stimulation of receptors on cells in the chemoreceptive trigger zone, located on the floor of the fourth ventricle in or near the area postrema, a circumventricular organ situated outside the blood-brain barrier.

Motility of the Small Intestine

The small intestine is commonly divided into three proximal-to-distal segments: the **duodenum, jejunum,** and **ileum.** It has a total length of approximately 6 to 8 m in the average adult human and functions to absorb water, electrolytes, nutrients, and other nondietary components (such as drugs) necessary to maintain health. To do this, the intestinal contents must be moved in a manner that not only brings them in contact with the intestinal mucosa but also propels them along this tubular organ. Although the **slow-wave** and **spike-potential mechanisms** of contractility as

well as fasting and fed motor patterns resemble those of the stomach, slow waves in the intestine are controlled by several pacemaker areas. Their rate is highest in the duodenum (about 12 per minute), and this is decreased in a graded manner down to the terminal ileum (about 8 per minute).

Propulsive motility in the small intestine is accomplished primarily by peristalsis. The mechanisms involved have been studied more in the small bowel than in any other part of the gut, and the salient features of this reflex are given in the section "Esophageal Motility." Peristaltic contractions do not travel the entire length of the small intestine, except for the propagated contractile waves that arise at certain times during the migrating motor complex. Vagal innervation, which is important for gastric peristaltic amplitude, is not necessary for intestinal peristalsis. Instead, the **enteric nervous system** (mainly the myenteric plexus), **intrinsic smooth muscle excitability,** and certain gastrointestinal hormones modulate the peristaltic activity of the small bowel. The purpose of the fasting pattern or migrating motor complex in the small bowel is similar to the fasting motility patterns in the stomach; it cleanses the bowel of nonabsorbable and indigestible material. During the **fed motility pattern** in the small intestine, a combination of segmental and peristaltic reflex contractions serves to mix chyme with digestive enzymes. **Segmentation,** the nonpropulsive, nonpropagating contractions, allows mixing of nutrients with digestive enzymes and contact of digestive end-products with the mucosal surface to promote absorption. Segmentation appears when alternate contractions and relaxations occur sequentially, moving food back and forth over short segments of small bowel. Segmental contractile patterns are likewise regulated by the enteric nervous system, intrinsic smooth muscle excitability, and gastrointestinal hormones. These controls are absent during the fasting state.

The **biliary tract,** consisting of the hepatic duct, gallbladder, common bile duct, and sphincter of Oddi, exhibits characteristic motility patterns. This system stores and delivers bile to the duodenum during feeding to provide for the efficient digestion and absorption of lipids. The flow of bile to the duodenum is regulated primarily by cholecystokinin, which is released from duodenal mucosal cells by the presence of dietary protein and amino acids. **Cholecystokinin** contracts the gallbladder and relaxes the sphincter of Oddi, thus promoting the flow of bile to the upper small bowel.

Disorders of small intestinal motility can lead to constipation or diarrhea, abdominal distension and pain, or nausea and vomiting. These symptoms appear to be due to altered slow-wave and spike potential changes in extrinsic neuronal or hormonal regulation and to smooth muscle disorders. For example, constipation often arises during **pregnancy** and may be associated with decreased slow-wave frequency produced by elevated progesterone levels. **Hyperthyroidism** increases slow-wave frequency and produces diarrhea, whereas hypothyroidism decreases slow-wave frequency and produces constipation.

Colonic Motility

The ileocecal sphincter (a zone about 4 cm long) is an area of elevated pressure that separates the colon from the small intestine. It possesses those characteristics which qualify it to be a sphincter. That is, it has increased tone that promotes aboral flow, but it can contract to prevent retrograde flow. The colon, or large intestine, is roughly 1.5 m long and is divided anatomically into the ascending, transverse, and descending segments. The colon's function is to conserve water and electrolytes by means of absorption and to form, store, and eliminate waste. Although the basic histologic features of the colonic wall resemble those of the other portions of the gastrointestinal tract (see Fig. 46-1), colonic longitudinal muscle is concentrated in three bundles of taeniae coli. These bundles cause the areas of longitudinal muscle in the large bowel wall to protrude during circular muscle contractions, forming **sacculations** or **haustra.** The function of haustrations or haustral contractions is similar to that of segmentation in the small bowel; they allow mixing of the contents and expose them to the surface mucosa for absorption. Likewise, they are non-propulsive and nonpropagating. Taeniae coli are not found in the sigmoid colon, that area of the intestine between the descending colon and the rectum. At the terminal rectum, the circular smooth muscle coat thickens to form the **internal anal sphincter,** which is surrounded by striated muscle originating from the pelvic floor and forming the **external anal sphincter. Sympathetic innervation** of the colon is furnished via lumbar colonic nerves. **Cranial parasympathetic** (vagal) **innervation** is provided to the right colon, and **sacral parasympathetic innervation** supplies the entire colon via pelvic nerves. Unlike the relatively short **transit time** through the small intestine (several hours), colonic transit is measured in days. Much mixing occurs in the right (ascending) colon, where slow waves of contraction move in an oral direction to delay transit and promote mixing and absorption of water and electrolytes.

The nature of these **slow waves of contraction** in the human colon is controversial. They cannot always be recorded, and when they are, they appear to have a fre-quency of between 3 and 10 per minute. As in the upper gastrointestinal tract, slow waves may be linked to spike potentials that initiate contractions. However, three distinct types of spike activity and related contractile events take place in the colon. **Short spike bursts** arise most frequently; these are associated with a single slow wave and appear to mediate haustral contractions. **Long spike bursts** occur with several slow waves, move in either direction, and appear to accelerate colonic motor patterns, consisting of both haustral activity and propagated, peristaltic-like contractions called **mass movement. Migrating spike bursts** are rapid oscillations of long duration. They are not related to slow waves, which usually begin in the transverse and descending colon and appear to mediate mass movements.

Mass movement constitutes the major propulsive motor activity in the colon. Shortly after eating, when mass movement is usually initiated, a relatively large bolus of stored material in the lower ascending colon, is carried some distance up this colonic area. While haustral contractions keep the bolus firm, a segment may be broken off and, during a subsequent mass movement, be moved rapidly around the hepatic flexure into the transverse colon. Subsequent propulsive activity progressively transports this segment (or a fraction thereof) through the transverse and descending colon into the **sigmoid colon.** There, normal peristalsis is reestablished, which moves the bolus into the **rectum,** where it is stored until defecation. The normal **colonic transit time** in an average adult human is from 1 to 3 days.

In the **ascending colon,** slow waves tend to move in a retrograde direction, which normally retards flow and facilitates the mixing and absorption of water and electrolytes. The **final stages** of fluid absorption and feces formation and storage take place in the descending colon. In the transverse and descending colon, slow waves of contraction move in the expected aboral direction. The lower sigmoid colon, rectum, and anal sphincters collectively provide for defecation and fecal continence.

Defecation is a complex act that involves the colon, rectum, anal sphincters, and striated muscles of the pelvic floor, abdominal wall, and diaphragm. The **rectosigmoid area** stores fecal matter until mechanoreceptors in the wall of the rectum are stimulated. This initiates reflex neuronal impulses, and the internal anal sphincter muscle (an involuntary muscle) relaxes, signaling the urge to defecate. Voluntary contraction of the striated external anal sphincter muscle inhibits the reflex, causing the rectal wall to relax (receptive relaxation) and the internal anal sphincter to contract or close. At the appropriate time and place, the external sphincter is voluntarily relaxed (aided by a sitting or squatting posture), with additional pressure furnished through voluntary contraction of the striated muscles. Propulsive contraction of the rectum and sigmoid colon, coupled with relaxation of both sphincters, forces fecal material out of the anal canal.

Disorders of colonic motility can lead to changes in the consistency and frequency of defecation (including diarrhea and constipation), pain or distension when colonic wall tension is increased, and incontinence. Clinically relevant colonic motor disorders are known to be associated with defects in the intrinsic and extrinsic innervation, slow waves, spike potentials, and smooth muscle functioning. **Irritable bowel syndrome** refers to a condition of altered bowel function and abdominal pain but without any detectable organic disease.

Regulation of Gastrointestinal Motility

Three divisions of the autonomic nervous system innervate the gastrointestinal tract: the **sympathetic, parasympathetic,** and **enteric** divisions. As described in Chap. 44, cell bodies of the enteric division are located in the myenteric and submucosal plexuses within the walls of the digestive tract. Many **postganglionic parasympathetic** motor fibers to intestinal smooth muscle release **acetylcholine,** which increases contractile activity by raising smooth muscle intracellular calcium. **Postganglionic sympathetic** fibers affect the activity of these and other nonparasympathetic cholinergic motor fibers directly by inhibiting their release of acetylcholine, thus inhibiting gastrointestinal motor activity. Neuronal interactions within the enteric nervous system are complex and can involve sensory reflexes and various neurotransmitter systems. These include adenosine, histamine, and serotonin, as well as peptides such as opioids, galanin, substance P, and calcitonin gene–related peptide.

As described earlier, intestinal motor patterns, although influenced by central neuronal input, can occur in the absence of any extrinsic influences. **Nonadrenergic noncholinergic** (NANC) inhibitory motor control can be produced by parasympathetic and local enteric stimulation. In the past, enteric inhibitory motor neurons have been associated with vasoactive intestinal polypeptide or adenosine triphosphate. Recently, it has been demonstrated that **nitric oxide,** released locally on demand by specific synthesizing enzymes in neurons, also inhibits in-

testinal muscle. These substances decrease intracellular calcium, thus reducing muscle contraction and tone causing **relaxation.** Neuronal regulatory processes are very complex in that the removal of these inhibitory stimuli from intestinal muscle can produce a rebound contractile response. In addition, these motor inhibitory substances can function as **neurotransmitters** and **modulators** of enteric neuronal activity.

Summary

The gastrointestinal tract possesses a unique arrangement of smooth muscle layers that are responsible for the distinct patterns of motility observed during and after consumption of a meal. These patterns are both propulsive and nonpropulsive (or mixing) in nature. Propulsive motility patterns move food along and are seen throughout the tract from the mouth to anus. Peristalsis is the major propulsive activity in the esophagus, stomach, small intestine, and rectum, whereas mass movement is the propulsive mechanism in the colon. Segmentation in the small bowel and haustrations in the colon represent the major nonpropulsive force responsible for mixing the intestinal contents with secretions from both the mucosa and the accessory organs of the tract. They also optimize contact of the luminal contents with the absorptive surfaces. Extrinsic and intrinsic nerves, as well as locally released hormones, regulate the motility patterns according to the volume and chemical composition of the intestinal contents. Diseases of motility are quite varied and are determined by which of the many variables regulating motility is compromised.

Bibliography

Brookes, S. J. H. Neuronal nitric oxide in the gut. *J. Gastroenterol. Hepatol.* 8:590–603, 1993.

Camilleri, M., and Phillips, S. F. Disorders of small intestinal motility. *Gastroenterol. Clin. North Am.* 18: 405–424, 1989.

Huizinga, J. D. Electrophysiology of human colon motility in health and disease. *Clin. Gastroenterol.* 15:879–901, 1986.

Johnson, L. R., ed. *Physiology of the Gastrointestinal Tract,* 2nd ed. New York: Raven Press, 1987.

Minami, H., and McCallum, R. W. The physiology and pathophysiology of gastric emptying in humans. *Gastroenterology* 86:1592–1610, 1984.

47 Gastric Secretion

Joseph D. Fondacaro

Objectives

After reading this chapter, you should be able to

Describe the gross and microscopic functional anatomy of the stomach

Identify the various functions of the human stomach

Identify the important cell types of the gastric glands and their secretory products

Explain the transport mechanisms involved in gastric acid secretion

Identify the role of gastric secretory products in the digestive process

Describe the neural and endocrine control of gastric secretion

---

The stomach is a major organ of the gastrointestinal tract and has both physiologic and clinical importance. Functionally, the stomach serves as a storage organ for food. The secretions of the gastric mucosa have some unique roles. Hydrochloric acid secreted by the gastric mucosa kills bacteria in food and is an effective second line of defense against infectious disease. In addition, hydrochloric acid and enzyme secretions initiate the digestive processes, while hormones secreted by the stomach assist in the regulation of gastric function. Also, intrinsic factor secreted by parietal cells is required for the absorption of vitamin B_{12}, which is necessary for proper red blood cell metabolism.

Functional Anatomy

The human stomach is between 10 and 13 cm in length and weighs slightly less than 1% of the body weight. Internally, it is a single-chambered organ with a surface area of approximately 1000 cm². Functionally, the stomach is divided into three regions: the upper **fundus** or cardia, the middle **corpus** or body, and the lower **antrum** or pyloric portion (Fig. 47-1). It is bordered proximally by the **lower esophageal sphincter** and distally by the **pyloric sphincter.** The internal surface area can vary depending on the number and appearance of mucosal folds, called **rugae,** which generally run lengthwise but may be scattered throughout the internal surface of the stomach (see Fig. 47-1). The rugae allow for accommodation and storage of a meal by expanding the inner surface of the stomach, thus increasing the storage capacity of this organ. This process is part of what is referred to as **receptive relaxation** (see Chap. 46).

The mucosal surface is a mixture of cell types, all of which contribute to the unique functions of the stomach. This surface contains many depressions known as **gastric pits** that contain secretory cells of various kinds, all contributing to secretion of gastric juice. These structures are often referred to as **gastric glands** (see Fig. 47-1). At the maximum secretory rate, the human stomach is capable of elaborating nearly 1.0 liters of fluid per day.

The upper third of these glands contain predominantly **neck cells,** which are responsible for the secretion of **mucus.** The lower two-thirds of these glands contain pri-

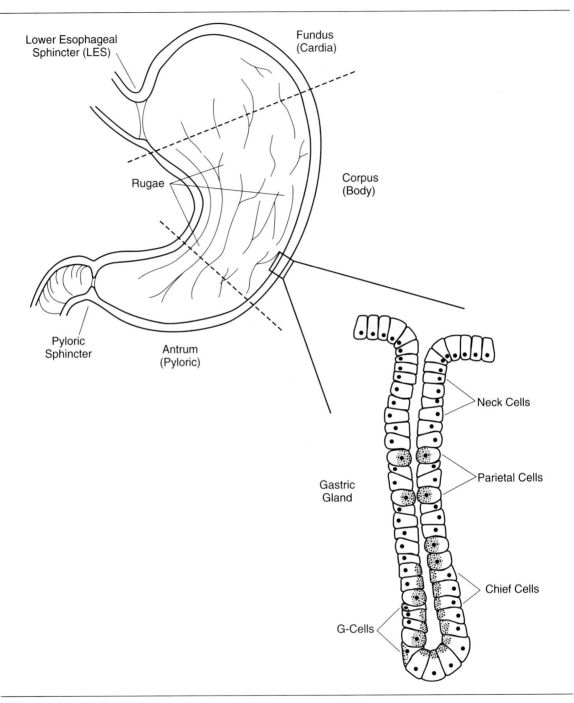

Fig. 47-1. The three anatomic regions of the human stomach indicating the rugae lining the inner surface of the organ. The gastric gland shows the cell types responsible for the major secretory elements in gastric juice (see text).

marily chief cells and parietal cells. The **chief cells** secrete the proteolytic enzyme **pepsin** (in precursor form called **pepsinogen**), while the **parietal cells** are responsible for the production and secretion of **HCl.** In the lower region of the stomach, another important cell type becomes significant within the gastric gland, this being the G-cell. **G-cells** secrete the hormone **gastrin,** which plays a major role in the regulation of gastric function and in mucosal cell growth and differentiation (see Chap. 45).

The **pyloric sphincter** is a specialized area of circular muscle. It remains closed in the resting state and is important in regulating the rate of gastric emptying and in preventing the backflux of partially digested food, called **chyme,** from the duodenum into the stomach.

Gastric Juice

In the normal human stomach at rest and containing little or no food, the basal secretion of the gastric glands consists mainly of water, mucus, and some small amount of HCl. Sodium and potassium ions are present in amounts that are generally isosmolar with plasma, while Cl^- is slightly elevated. At rest, there is measurable basal acid output and usually no pepsinogen secretion. Thus gastric juice in the resting stomach is only slightly hyperosmotic versus plasma, the viscosity is close to that of water, and the pH ranges from 6.5 to 7.0.

However, in the postprandial state, the profile of gastric secretion changes dramatically. With the initiation of feeding (and even before, with the sight and smell of food), the nervous and hormonal mechanisms regulating gastric secretion markedly alter the concentrations of both the organic and inorganic components of gastric juice. As gastric glands are stimulated, gastric secretory rate is increased. **Mucus** secreted from neck cells is enhanced and serves a **cytoprotective** function by lining the gastric mucosa and protecting it from abrasion from food particles and from acid and enzyme digestion. This increases the viscosity of gastric juice. The precursor form (pepsinogen) of the proteolytic enzyme pepsin is secreted from chief cells and is delivered to the gastric lumen along with the other secretions of the gland. As acid is secreted into the stomach, the pH falls, triggering the conversion of pepsinogen to pepsin, the active form of the enzyme. The plasma levels of the hormone gastrin, secreted by G-cells, is also increased. This hormone plays a major role in regulating gastric secretion, which will be discussed later in this chapter.

By far the most striking changes occur in electrolyte concentrations in gastric juice. The Na^+ concentration falls dramatically from approximately 140 meq/liter at rest to less than 10 meq/liter at maximum secretory rate. The H^+ and Cl^- concentrations rise with the increase in stimulation, and this is reflected in the amount of acid secreted during gastric digestion. While the concentration of K^+ in gastric juice is only slightly increased, its role in acid secretion is critical to the normal digestive function of the stomach.

The Parietal Cell and Gastric Acid Secretion

As noted earlier, gastric acid secretion is a function of parietal cells within the gastric glands. Figure 47-2 represents a parietal cell during stimulation and illustrates the specialized subcellular components important to this cell's function. Parietal cells are typically pyramidal-shaped and possess a large number of **mitochondria.** At maximum stimulatory rate, the metabolism of these cells is extremely high. This reflects the enhanced expenditure of energy required for transport processes. As a by-product of metabolism, raw materials are provided for the acid secretory mechanism to function (discussed below). These cells also possess an intricate intracellular network of canals known as **canaliculi.** These canals are open to the extracellular space within the gastric gland and provide a route of exit for acid. Lining these canaliculi are small **tubulovesicles.** These structures are actually outpouchings of the canalicular membrane and contain the acid secretory mechanism, the **H^+,K^+-ATPase,** better known as the **gastric proton pump.** It is into these vesicles that acid is initially secreted before accumulating in the canaliculi for transport to the lumen of the gastric gland.

When the parietal cell is stimulated, several cellular mechanisms are set into motion, resulting in the secreted end-product of hydrochloric acid (Fig. 47-3). As the parietal cell is stimulated, **oxidative metabolism** within the mitochondria increases and yields the usual end-products of **CO_2** and **water.** Through the well-known **hydration reaction** catalyzed by **carbonic anhydrase,** H_2O and CO_2 form **carbonic acid (H_2CO_3),** which at cellular pH quickly ionizes to HCO_3^- and **hydrogen ion.** These H^+ are captured and driven extracellularly in exchange for K^+ by the **proton pump.** This pump is energized by the **hydrolysis of ATP** and requires the presence of H^+ and K^+. As intracellular K^+ accumulates, it diffuses out the cell via specialized K^+ **channels.** The intracellular **HCO_3^-** is exchanged 1 : 1 for extracellular Cl^- at the basolateral membrane by a specialized membrane bound **Cl^--HCO_3^- exchange protein.** Chloride ions are transported through

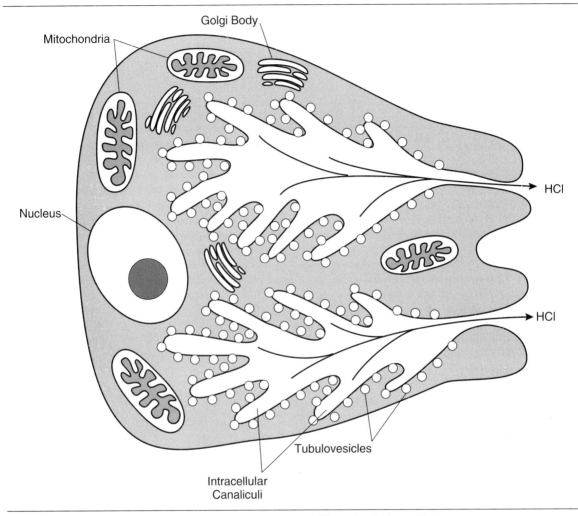

Fig. 47-2. A representation of a parietal cell in the stimulatory state illustrating the intracellular structures important to the acid secretory process.

the cell to the apical membrane, where they exit the cell via a **Cl⁻ channel.** It is believed that the exiting of Cl⁻ is functionally coupled to proton pump activity, resulting in a 1 : 1 release of H⁺ and Cl⁻ (see Fig. 47-3). During maximum acid secretion, excessive amounts of HCO_3^- are released into the **venous blood** of the stomach, elevating the pH locally. This has been referred to as the **alkaline tide.**

Acid secretion by parietal cells is known to be stimulated by several modalities. **Vagus nerve stimulation** and the release of **acetylcholine** locally stimulate the mechanism described above, as does **gastrin** circulating in elevated levels in the blood after a meal and during the entire digestive phase. **Histamine,** released locally by **mast cells,** also stimulates gastric secretion. Actually, the discovery that histamine may be the **final common pathway** for stimulating acid secretion led to a revolution in the treatment of **ulcer disease.** Histamine H_2 receptor antagonists (e.g., cimetidine and ranitidine) were highly successful therapeutic approaches to the treatment of ulcer disease. More recently, the development of selective inhibitors of the gastric proton pump (e.g., omeprazole) has provided physicians with the ultimate pharmacologic approach to treating this disease and other acid-related disorders.

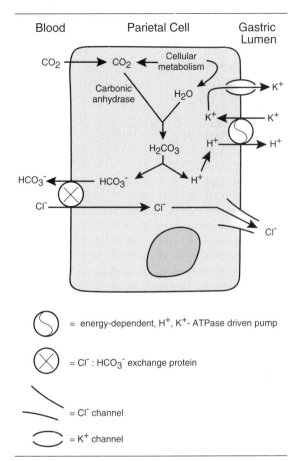

Fig. 47-3. The relationship of the transport and metabolic components of the acid secretory mechanism within a parietal cell.

Legend within figure:

⊘ = energy-dependent, H^+, K^+- ATPase driven pump

⊗ = Cl^- : HCO_3^- exchange protein

= Cl^- channel

= K^+ channel

The Secretion of Pepsin

As the processes of digestion are stimulated, the proteolytic enzyme **pepsin,** the primary digestive enzyme of the stomach, is secreted by **chief cells** of gastric glands. This enzyme is stored in granules of chief cells and is released by the process of **exocytosis.** Pepsin is stored and released as pepsinogen, the inactive precursor form of the enzyme. Once in the stomach, pepsinogen is converted to the active enzyme pepsin in the presence of HCl. Once this occurs, pepsin **autocatalyzes** the conversion of more pepsinogen to pepsin.

Pepsin begins the digestive breakdown of dietary protein. Other enzymes, such as **gastric lipase** and **rennin** (not to be confused with renin), are released into gastric juice but play relatively minor roles in the total digestive process.

Along with these enzymes of gastric origin, **hydrolytic enzymes** found in **saliva** continue their digestive action in the stomach on food as it is swallowed and stored in the stomach. Eventually, the action of salivary enzymes is inhibited by the low pH of the gastric environment. However, the enzymes of gastric origin, which are active optimally at the gastric pH, continue their breakdown of food during most of the storage phase of a meal.

The Secretion of Intrinsic Factor

The parietal cells of the stomach are responsible also for the secretion of an important **mucoprotein** called **intrinsic factor.** Intrinsic factor binds to dietary **vitamin B_{12}** in the stomach and forms a complex that remains intact throughout its transit from stomach to distal small bowel. In the ileum, there are specific carrier molecules on the mucosal membrane of the absorbing cells that sequester the intrinsic factor–B_{12} complex and transport it into the cell and ultimately the circulation.

Vitamin B_{12} is essential for the **proper metabolism of hemoglobin** and functioning of **red blood cells.** In the disease known as **pernicious anemia,** parietal cells are incapable of elaborating intrinsic factor, thus inhibiting the absorption of dietary vitamin B_{12}. Often this is due to the presence of an **antibody** to parietal cells that leads to the depletion of these cells. Thus pernicious anemia is often accompanied by a condition known as **achlorhydria,** or **hyposecretion gastric acid.**

Control of Gastric Secretion

The physiologic regulation of gastric secretion consists of stimulatory and inhibitory components. The entire process can be divided into three phases for convenience of study: the **cephalic, gastric,** and **intestinal phases.**

The stimulatory pathways are illustrated in Fig. 47-4. Before food enters the mouth, recognition of the sight and smell of food by cells in the **cerebral cortex** can **stimulate gastric secretion.** This is referred to as the **cephalic phase** and is mediated by the **vagus nerve.** Vagal efferent fibers release the cholinergic neurotransmitter **acetylcholine** very near gastric glands, thereby stimulating G-cells, parietal cells, and neck cells to secrete their respective products. Gastrin completes the process by stimulating the release of pepsin from chief cells as well as HCl from parietal cells.

Besides food, certain **emotional states** can trigger the

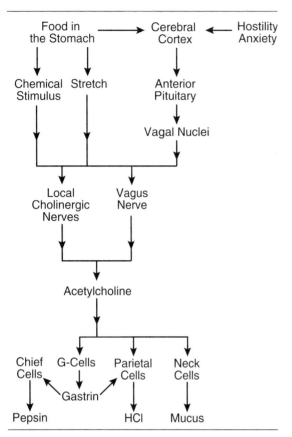

Fig. 47-4. The stimulatory pathways regulating gastric acid secretion.

secretion of gastric juice, in particular **gastric acid.** Anger, hostility, and anxiety can have a stimulatory effect of gastric secretion and are very often **cofactors** in the formation of **peptic ulcers.**

Once food is consumed, two additional stimulatory pathways are triggered. These pathways may be considered to make up the **gastric phase. Stretch** of the stomach wall and chemical stimulation of **chemoreceptors** in the stomach stimulate the release of acetylcholine via **intrinsic nerves** of the stomach. The result is the stimulation of cells in the gastric glands. In addition, **stretch** of the stomach sends signals along **vagal afferent fibers** to the **vagal nuclei.** A **reflex** is initiated (not illustrated) that sends stimulatory impulses down vagal efferent nerves to the intrinsic nerve network enhancing secretion.

As in any physiologic regulatory system, inhibitory factors play an equal role in regulating gastric secretion. Once hunger and appetite have been satisfied by a meal, the inhibitory factors begin to influence the secretory activity of gastric glands. The cephalic phase is no longer involved, and thus vagal impulses are significantly reduced.

The hormone **gastrin** is also part of the inhibitory signal regulating gastric secretion. As the hormone circulates in the blood, it stimulates the release of another hormone, **calcitonin,** from the **thyroid gland.** Calcitonin lowers the blood calcium levels, which, in turn, reduces the secretions of the stomach, particularly acid secretion. Gastric acid itself is involved in a negative feedback role. As the gastric pH falls below 2.0, intrinsic activity signals the release of gastrin, which acts through calcitonin to suppress further acid output.

Finally, as gastric contents are emptied into the **duodenum, partially digested food** and the **acidity** (about pH 4.0) cause the release of two major hormones, **secretin** and **cholecystokinin,** from the duodenal mucosa. Besides their action on the pancreas (see Chap. 48), both of these hormones **inhibit gastric secretion.** Because these inhibitory signals originate in the duodenum, this pathway is referred to as the **intestinal phase** in the regulation gastric secretion.

Summary

The mucosal surface and the musculature of the stomach function to allow the storage of a meal. Rugae permit the expansion of the inner surface of the stomach to accommodate the volume of a normal meal. While the digestion of food by salivary enzymes continues in the stomach, the gastric glands are stimulated to provide a unique profile of secretory products to further break down food. Chief cells provide the enzyme pepsin, which begins the proteolytic digestion of food particles. Pepsin is activated from pepsinogen by gastric acid. Parietal cells secrete gastric acid, which aids the digestive process. Parietal cells possess unique subcellular structure, metabolic pathways, and a number of transport mechanisms that are intricately woven into the acid secretory process. Some of these unique transport processes have provided targets for new drugs designed to treat ulcer disease and other acid-related disorders. Parietal cells also elaborate intrinsic factor, which is important for the normal absorption of dietary vitamin B_{12}. Neck cells secrete mucus, which provides a barrier of protection to the mucosal surface so that auto-digestion does not occur. G-cells in the lower portion of the stomach secrete the hormone gastrin, which is important in the regulation of gastric secretion. This regulation involves the CNS, afferent and efferent vagal nerves, local intrinsic nerves of the gut, acetylcholine, and a variety of hormones from the stomach, duodenum, and thyroid.

Bibliography

Johnson, L. R., ed. *Physiology of the Gastrointestinal Tract,* 2nd ed. New York: Raven Press, 1987.

Schultz, S. G., Forte, J. G. and Rauner, B. B., eds. *Handbook of Physiology*, Sec. 6: The Gastrointestinal System, Volume III. Bethesda, Md.: American Physiological Society, 1989.

48 Pancreatic Exocrine Secretion

Joseph D. Fondacaro

Objectives

After reading this chapter, you should be able to

Identify the important anatomic features of the pancreas

Describe the relationship between the neural, vascular, and cellular components of the pancreas

Discuss the role of the exocrine secretions in normal digestive tract physiology

Explain the action of glycolytic, proteolytic, and lipolytic enzymes on the dietary components of a normal meal

Describe the integral role of pancreatic HCO_3^- secretion in the digestive process, including acid buffering and duodenal mucosal protection

Discuss the neural and hormonal regulation of enzyme and HCO_3^- secretions and the function of second messengers in acinar and duct cells

---

The pancreas is a major component of two physiologic systems: the **gastrointestinal tract** and the **endocrine system.** The exocrine secretions of the pancreas are essential for the normal digestion and absorption of dietary nutrients. Furthermore, a component of pancreatic secretion provides an important protective mechanism for the duodenal mucosa. Thus, given the vital importance of this organ to the normal digestive process, the roles of the pancreas have significant clinical and physiologic relevance. Acute and chronic pancreatitis, pancreatic carcinomas, and cystic fibrosis are major diseases that compromise pancreatic exocrine function, while diabetes mellitus is considered the major metabolic disease caused by loss of pancreatic endocrine secretion. This chapter explores the major anatomic considerations that are important and perhaps unique to the pancreas, the exocrine secretions of this organ and their function, and the intricate role of nerves and humoral agents in the regulation of pancreatic exocrine secretion.

Anatomic Considerations

The pancreas is a **retroperitoneal organ** that can be described as an "accessory" organ of the gastrointestinal tract. It is strategically located between the antral portion of the greater curvature of the stomach and the duodenal bulb and extends horizontally in a tapered fashion almost to the spleen. From this location, pancreatic exocrine secretions are delivered to the **proximal duodenum** such that maximal efficiency can be obtained from their presence in the gut lumen.

The **arterial blood supply** to the pancreas is derived from branches of the celiac and superior mesenteric arteries, the major contributor being the pancreaticoduodenal artery. Arteries and arterioles course through the stroma of the pancreas and terminate in capillary beds adjacent to clusters of exocrine-secreting cells called **acini** (Fig. 48-1). Likewise, arterioles and capillaries surround the **islet of Langerhans** that contains the endocrine-secreting cells of

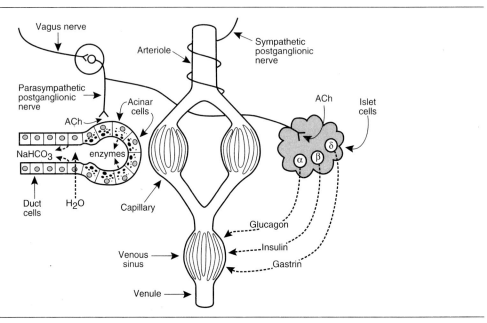

Fig. 48-1. Functional anatomy of the pancreas. The pancreas contains both endocrine- and exocrine-secreting functional units.

the pancreas. Venous blood from the organ drains into the **portal circulation.**

The **efferent motor nerves** to the pancreas are supplied by both sympathetic and parasympathetic branches of the autonomic nervous system. **Postganglionic sympathetic fibers** arise from the celiac and superior mesenteric plexuses and travel to the pancreas along the arterial blood vessels. These adrenergic nerves release **norepinephrine** and are believed to influence pancreatic function mainly through the modulation of arterial blood flow. **Preganglionic parasympathetic fibers** from the vagus nerve terminate in the pancreas. **Postganglionic cholinergic fibers** release **acetylcholine** and are believed to be important in regulating pancreatic function. These fibers terminate on pancreatic acinar and islet cells to regulate their secretion (see Fig. 48-1). Furthermore, **cholinergic muscarinic receptors** have been identified on the acinar cell membrane, supporting the belief that direct parasympathetic influence plays a vital role in pancreatic exocrine secretion.

Recently, important **neurocrine influences** on pancreatic function have been identified that are nonadrenergic noncholinergic nerves and are called the **peptidergic nerves.** These nerves have been shown to directly influence pancreatic acinar and duct cell secretion. They also operate through the modulation of sympathetic and parasympathetic fibers. Cell surface receptors also have

been identified on the end organs. The **peptide neurotransmitters** that are considered important in regulating pancreatic function are vasoactive intestinal peptide (VIP), somatostatin, and enkephalin. **VIP** stimulates the pancreatic secretion of fluid and electrolytes; **somatostatin** inhibits VIP's effect on pancreatic secretion. **Enkephalins** suppress pancreatic fluid and enzyme secretion, most likely by modulating other neural pathways. **Afferent sensory fibers** run from the pancreas to the CNS and are generally nociceptive in nature.

Major Cell Types

There are three major groups of cells that make up the pancreas: acinar cells, duct cells, and the cells of the islets of Langerhans (see Fig. 48-1). The **acinar cells** are the enzyme-secreting cells of the pancreas and are arranged in numerous blind-end glandlike structures called **acini.** Secretions from these cells collect in the acinar duct and travel through a network of converging ducts to the **main pancreatic duct.** From there they are emptied into the duodenum. Acinar cells are characterized by their pyramidal shape and by their dense cytoplasmic granules containing the digestive enzymes to be secreted, many of which are in an inactive precursor form (see Fig. 48-1). Occasionally, a second type of acinar cell, called a **centroaci-**

nar cell, is encountered. Although these cells are somewhat similar in shape to the more peripheral acinar cell, they are located near the center of the acinus and secrete water and electrolytes into the acinar space.

Duct cells are fairly homogeneous, and as their name implies, they line the inner surface of the branching pancreatic ducts (see Fig. 48-1). Somewhat more columnar in shape, these cells are the major contributors of water and electrolytes, the most important of which is HCO_3^-, found in pancreatic juice.

Both the acinar and duct cells are richly supplied with capillaries that supply the raw materials for synthesis and secretion. Abundant **parasympathetic motor nerve pathways** deliver the appropriate stimulation for acinar cell secretion.

Exocrine Secretion

The product of pancreatic exocrine secretion, often referred to as **pancreatic juice,** contains both organic and inorganic components. The **organic components** are those major enzymes necessary for the digestion of dietary nutrients and are synthesized and secreted by acinar cells. HCO_3^- is the chief **inorganic component** and is secreted into pancreatic juice by duct cells. **Water** is also a major component of pancreatic juice and is supplied primarily by the duct cells through an osmotic response to HCO_3^- secretion. The normal adult human pancreas is capable of elaborating approximately 1.5 liters of pancreatic juice per day, which is a remarkable feat for an organ that constitutes barely 0.1% of the total body weight.

Organic Components

The **digestive enzymes** in pancreatic juice are proteins synthesized in acinar cells (see Fig. 48-1). This synthesis takes place in the **ribosomes** lining the **rough endoplasmic reticulum** of these cells. As enzymatic proteins are produced, they are transferred to the lacunae of the rough endoplasmic reticulum and eventually concentrate and bud off as vacuoles. These vacuoles migrate to the **Golgi complex,** where they are enveloped in membranes to form **zymogen granules** containing the inactive precursor (or proenzyme) form of the active enzyme. The **proenzymes** are stored in these granules in the apical portion of the acinar cells until appropriate stimulation of cells triggers secretion by a mechanism known as exocytosis. **Exocytosis** is thought to consist of the following events: (1) migration of the zymogen granule toward the inner surface of the apical membrane, (2) fusion of the granule membrane with that of the cell, a Ca^{2+}-requiring step, and (3) elimination of the bilayers and release of enzyme into the acinar space. This entire secretory process is the result of a series of biochemical events known as **stimulus-secretion coupling.** Utilizing intracellular second-messenger systems, this cascade of events links the stimulation of the acinar cell at the basolateral membrane by specific secretagogues to the release of digestive enzymes at the apical membrane.

Distinct receptors have been identified on the basolateral membrane of the acinar cell as being involved in the secretory process. Separate receptors bind the hormones cholecystokinin and gastrin and the neurotransmitter acetylcholine. Upon binding, receptor-ligand interaction activates phosphatidylinositol hydrolysis, thus elevating the intracellular Ca^{2+} concentration. Ca^{2+}, utilizing either a Ca^{2+}-calmodulin complex or the Ca^{2+}, phosphatidyl serine–dependent protein kinase C, triggers exocytosis. Another receptor on the basolateral membrane of the acinar cell binds the hormone **secretin.** When secretin binds to its receptor, the signal for secretion is communicated by means of the adenylate cyclase–cyclic AMP pathway to the apical cell border, resulting in secretion. Secretin potentiates cholecystokinin's action on enzyme secretion of acinar cell. For all receptors, signal transduction via the second-messenger systems links events at the basolateral membrane to the apical membrane, an intriguing aspect of biochemical regulation.

The **major digestive enzymes** in pancreatic juice are glycolytic, lipolytic, and proteolytic. The **proteolytic enzymes** are secreted in an inactive proenzyme form, which prevents the autodigestion of pancreatic tissue. Once inside the lumen of the duodenum, **enterokinase,** an enzyme secreted by the duodenal mucosa, converts trypsinogen to the active proteolytic enzyme **trypsin** (Fig. 48-2). This conversion sets in motion the conversion of the other three proenzyme forms to their active moieties, as well as the autocatalysis of trypsin on its own precursor (see Fig. 48-2). Finally, because secretion of these enzymes by acinar cells is accompanied by the secretion of water and electrolytes (presumably by centroacinar cells), the substance leaving the acinar space is essentially an ultrafiltrate of plasma.

Pancreatic **alpha-amylase** hydrolyzes 1,4-glycosidic bonds in the dietary carbohydrate molecules. This enzyme does not affect 1,6 linkages or terminal 1,4 bonds. Thus the end-products of pancreatic amylase activity are **maltose** (a disaccharide consisting of two glucose molecules), **maltotriose** (a trisaccharide made up of three glucose molecules), and **alpha limit dextrans** (smaller branch-chain polysaccharides). This is the primary step required for the

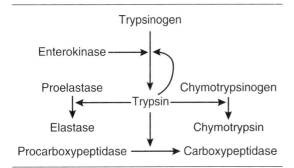

Fig. 48-2. The activation of proteolytic enzymes of the pancreas.

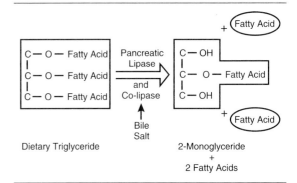

Fig. 48-3. The digestive action of pancreatic lipase and co-lipase on dietary triglyceride.

digestion of **dietary carbohydrates.** However, the resulting molecules are still too large for intestinal absorption, and additional breakdown is needed. This is accomplished by specific enzymes located in the **brush-border membranes** of the small intestinal mucosal cells that reduce these molecules to glucose and other simple sugars.

Pancreatic **lipase** and **co-lipase** reduce dietary triglycerides to simpler molecules to enable their absorption. The **triglyceride molecule** is made up of three fatty acid moieties connected by ester linkages to the glycerol backbone (Fig. 48-3). The lipases preferentially cleave the 1 and 1' ester linkages to eventually yield a 2-monoglyceride and two free fatty acid moieties. Occasionally, the reaction runs to completion and cleaves the ester bond at the 2 position, yielding free **glycerol,** which is readily absorbed. All this lipolytic activity requires the emulsifying action of bile salts in order to solubilize triglycerides in the water environment of the intestinal lumen so that the hydrophilic enzymes can digest the individual molecule. Once liberated, fatty acids and 2-monoglycerides partition readily into **bile salt micelles** and are transported through the aqueous phase of the bowel lumen to the absorbing enterocytes.

Once activated, the **proteolytic enzymes** secreted by the pancreas cleave peptide linkages within the complex structure of dietary protein. **Trypsin** and **chymotrypsin** are endopeptidases that target internal peptide linkages, yielding dipeptides and tripeptides and other small peptide chains. Many of these can be absorbed by the intestinal cells. **Carboxypeptidase** is an exopeptidase that attacks the ends of a peptide chain, liberating free amino acids. In addition, **exopeptidases** secreted by the intestinal mucosa also act on small peptides to yield free amino acids. These simple amino acid molecules are readily absorbed by the intestine (see Chap. 50).

Inorganic Components

As **fluid** leaves the acini and proceeds down the pancreatic ducts, its ionic composition changes. The degree to which it is modified depends on the secretory rate, a phenomenon that will be discussed later in this chapter. The major inorganic components of pancreatic juice are **water** and **electrolytes,** which are furnished mainly by **duct cells.** These cells are somewhat smaller than acinar cells and do not contain zymogen granules. Instead, they possess specific transport mechanisms in their apical and basolateral membranes that facilitate the secretion of certain electrolytes, of which HCO_3^- is the primary constituent.

As pancreatic juice exits from the acinar region and travels down the ducts, the initial concentrations of the major **electrolytes** Na^+, K^+, Cl^- and HCO_3^- reflect that of the extracellular fluid. Upon stimulation of the duct cells, as ordinarily occurs during and immediately after a meal, there are specific changes in the electrolyte composition of the pancreatic juice emptied into the duodenum. The Na^+ and K^+ levels remain relatively constant, but the concentration of HCO_3^- increases significantly and that of Cl^- falls. Thus the pH of the pancreatic juice entering the duodenum is **alkaline** (approximately 7.5 to 8.0). This marked increase in the pH enables pancreatic juice to buffer the extremely acid gastric juice. This **buffering** of gastric juice by pancreatic secretion is considered a major protection against erosion of the duodenal mucosa and the formation of duodenal ulcers.

Another important function of pancreatic HCO_3^- secretion concerns the action of pancreatic **digestive enzymes.** These enzymes have an optimal pH well above that of gastric juice. Thus the buffering of gastric juice optimizes the activity of these enzymes in the small intestine. It has been shown that the increase in pancreatic juice HCO_3^- content is proportional to the rate of stimulation of the pancreas (Fig. 48-4). Thus, as food enters the digestive tract, the intensity of neural and hormonal stimulation of the pancreas increases, resulting in elevated HCO_3^- concentration in pancreatic juice. Furthermore, the Cl^- concentration in the pancreatic juice varies inversely with stimulation of secretion and thus the HCO_3^- concentration (see Fig. 48-4). This suggests a coupling of the transport systems responsible for the duct cell secretion of these electrolytes.

Duct cell HCO_3^- is provided by several different sources (Fig. 48-5). **HCO_3^- dissolved in plasma** is freely diffusible down its concentration gradient through the basolateral membrane of duct cells into the cytoplasm. Carbon dioxide can diffuse from plasma into the cell as well as be produced by cellular metabolism. This carbon dioxide combines with water in the **hydration reaction** catalyzed by carbonic anhydrase to form the unstable carbonic acid, which immediately breaks down into H^+ and HCO_3^-. These **two sources** provide the HCO_3^- that is secreted into the duct lumen by two transport mechanisms. HCO_3^- can **freely diffuse** down its concentration gradient across the apical membrane of the cell into the duct lumen. HCO_3^- also can be exchanged 1 : 1 for luminal Cl^- by an **apical membrane anion exchanger** (see Fig. 48-5). This is thought to represent a specialized apical membrane Cl^--HCO_3^- exchange protein, and its existence accounts for the reciprocal relationship between the luminal Cl^- and HCO_3^- concentrations as the secretory rate increases. Finally, the H^+ produced by the hydration reaction is trans-

Fig. 48-4. Concentration of major ions in pancreatic juice compared to rate of stimulation of secretion. (Modified from: Johnson, L. R. *Gastrointestinal Physiology,* 3rd ed. St. Louis: C. V. Mosby, 1985.)

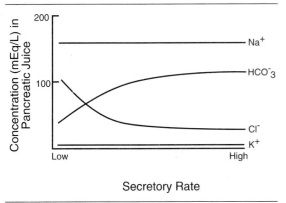

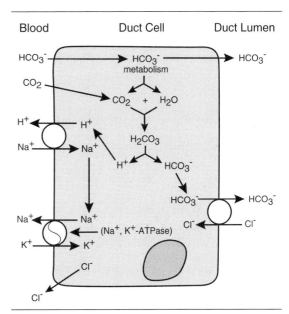

Fig. 48-5. A composite representation of the transport processes involved in pancreatic duct cell bicarbonate secretion.

ported out of the duct cell by a **basolateral cation exchanger,** the Na^+-K^+ exchange mechanism that is energized by the basolateral Na^+,K^+-ATPase–mediated Na^+ pump. The Cl^- that accumulates in the cell from the apical Cl^--HCO_3^- exchange diffuses through the basolateral membrane into the blood. These specialized transport systems of the duct cell membranes ensure that HCO_3^- is efficiently secreted into pancreatic juice. Thus the venous blood leaving the pancreas has a lower pH than the arterial blood entering the pancreas. Water is freely diffusible via paracellular pathways in order to maintain osmotic balance, while the ionic composition of luminally discharged pancreatic juice may vary greatly from that of the ultrafiltrate of plasma first produced by acinar cell secretion.

Control of Pancreatic Exocrine Secretion

The secretion of pancreatic juice is under combined **hormonal** and **neural control. Parasympathetic postganglionic fibers** of the vagus nerve and the gastrointestinal hormones **cholecystokinin** and **secretin** are the major mediators of regulation. It has been useful in our understanding of these processes to divide the **regulation** of pancreatic exocrine secretion into three phases: cephalic, gastric, and intestinal. Although these phases may overlap considerably in time and may actually interact, there are distinguishing features that coincide with the location of food in regions of the gastrointestinal tract.

Cephalic Phase

The cephalic phase of pancreatic secretion is triggered by the CNS recognition and integration of the sight, smell, and taste of food. This phase has been demonstrated in humans when subjects either just see and smell appetizing foods or chew food without swallowing it. These stimuli tend to increase pancreatic enzyme and HCO_3^- secretion. These findings also have been demonstrated in a variety of animal studies. It has been shown experimentally that the degree of enzyme secretion in the cephalic phase is approximately 50% of the maximum response induced by the administration of cholecystokinin and secretin. Furthermore, when duodenal acidification accompanies "sham feeding," the secretory response is markedly enhanced.

The cephalic phase of pancreatic secretion is mediated primarily by the **vagus nerve,** with efferent cholinergic fibers directly and indirectly innervating the pancreatic acinar cells. The vagus also may influence duct cell secretion indirectly by modulating the peptidergic nerves that innervate these cells. Several lines of evidence support the role of the vagus in this phase. **First,** vagal fibers are the **primary source** of CNS cholinergic nerves to the pancreas. **Second,** electrical stimulation of vagal efferent fibers elicits a **pancreatic secretion** that is similar in composition to that produced during sham feeding. **Third,** the exogenous administration of **cholinergic agonists** activates a similar secretory response. **Fourth,** the pancreatic secretory response to sham feeding can be inhibited or abolished by the administration of **anticholinergic drugs.** Sham feeding also has been shown to cause insulin release. Because sham feeding stimulates antral gastrin release and gastric secretion as well, gastric acid emptying into the duodenum and circulating gastrin levels are suspected to enhance the pancreatic secretory response.

Gastric Phase

It is apparent from the preceding discussion that the cephalic and gastric phases overlap considerably. However, physiologic events occur in the stomach that can modulate pancreatic secretion.

Besides vagally mediated gastrin release and gastric acid secretion, **distension** of the stomach stimulates pancreatic secretion. Secretion is inhibited when the anticholinergic agent atropine is administered, but only truncal **vagotomy** produces long-term blockade of the response. The results of these studies suggest that the gastric phase of pancreatic secretion is mediated by a **cholinergic nerve reflex,** most likely involving vagal afferent and efferent fibers (a vagovagal reflex). However, other evidence also suggests the involvement of **gastrin** in this phase. **Distension** of both the proximal and distal portions of the stomach stimulates pancreatic secretion. **Vagotomy** abolishes the response to proximal distension but not that to distal distension, implying that gastrin release elicited by distal distension evokes the pancreatic response. Furthermore, the intravenous administration of an extract of antral mucosa in experimental animals stimulates pancreatic secretion. Although serum gastrin levels have not been examined during these distension studies, it is assumed that the gastric phase is mediated by the combination of a vagally mediated gastropancreatic reflex and antral gastrin release.

Intestinal Phase

The intestinal phase of pancreatic secretion appears to be somewhat more complex than the cephalic and gastric phases because of increasing evidence that certain partially digested dietary substrates, as well as hormones and neural reflexes, participate in this phase. However, studies in the intestine are easier to conduct because a variety of test substances can be perfused or instilled in the small intestine without activating CNS or gastric responses. Gastric acid, monoglycerides, amino acids, peptides, fatty acids, and other substrates individually and in combination stimulate pancreatic exocrine secretion in appropriate amount and composition to promote the efficient digestion of dietary nutrients and the buffering of gastric effluent.

Acidification of the proximal duodenum is a major stimulant of pancreatic exocrine secretion. The major components of acid-induced pancreatic secretion are Na^+, HCO_3^- and water; very little protein is secreted by the pancreas in response to duodenal acidification. Specialized cells of the duodenal mucosa, the **amine precursor uptake and decarboxylation cells,** synthesize and release secretin. Although secretin is the major hormonal mediator of pancreatic HCO_3^- secretion, in the normal response to a meal it is known that cholecystokinin can augment the action of secretin on pancreatic duct cells.

The **duct cell secretory response** to secretin is mediated by cyclic AMP, which serves to increase the production of HCO_3^- by duct cell carbonic anhydrase and to stimulate $Cl\text{-}HCO_3^-$ exchange. The major function of **pancreatic HCO_3^-** is to buffer gastric acid and create an optimal pH environment for digestive enzyme activity. Though some HCO_3^- is contributed by bile and duodenal mucosal cell secretion, these sources provide only about 10% to 15% of the total amount. Thus pancreatic HCO_3^- is the primary source of buffer for neutralizing the gastric acid entering the duodenum.

Within the stomach, the action of gastric acid, pepsin, lingual lipase, and salivary amylase begins the **initial breakdown** of solid food into smaller particles. Once these **partially digested products** are emptied into the duodenum, they become **important stimulants** for the intestinal phase of pancreatic exocrine secretion. Peptides, certain amino acids, fatty acids, monoglycerides, and carbohydrates have all been shown to stimulate pancreatic enzyme secretion. Cholecystokinin, which is released by the specialized amine precursor uptake and decarboxylation cells of the duodenal mucosa, is the mediator of this response. However, plasma cholecystokinin levels are only slightly increased in response to the presence of carbohydrates and fats in the intestinal lumen, suggesting that another mechanism is involved. Some evidence indicates a **neural reflex** involving duodenal and pancreatic cholinergic nerves. Plasma cholecystokinin levels, however, are closely correlated with ingestion of dietary protein. Furthermore, as digestive enzymes, especially trypsin, are released, they down-regulate further release of cholecystokinin, thus creating a negative feedback mechanism in the hormonal regulation of pancreatic enzyme secretion. Recent evidence suggests the presence of a **cholecystokinin-releasing factor** that serves as an intermediate in the cholecystokinin response to food. It has been shown that cholecystokinin-releasing factor is elevated in response to the presence of food in the duodenum and that the supression of cholecystokinin release by trypsin is actually due to the inhibitory effect of trypsin on the cholecystokinin-releasing factor. It remains unclear as to the exact mechanisms that cause these partially digested substances to stimulate the intestinal cells to release hormones and/or initiate neural reflexes.

The cholecystokinin-induced and cholinergic-initiated responses of the acinar cells are mediated by the rise in intracellular Ca^{2+} level that acts as the second-messenger system. Recently, **monitor peptide,** a 61 amino acid peptide expressed in acinar cells, has been discovered in pancreatic juice. Monitor peptide has been shown to increase pancreatic secretion by stimulation of cholecystokinin release. This action of monitor peptide is exquisitely sensitive to extracellular Ca^{2+} in that as extracellular Ca^{2+} is reduced experimentally the influence of monitor peptide on cholecystokinin release is markedly inhibited. It also has been established that secretin can augment the action of cholecystokinin and acetylcholine at the acinar cell through a cAMP-mediated response.

Summary

The pancreas possesses a unique anatomic arrangement of nerves, blood vessels, and exocrine secretory units called acini. This arrangement allows for the efficient delivery of nutrients, which serve as the raw materials required for enzyme synthesis and extrinsic regulatory influences (neurotransmitters and hormones) necessary for the optimal functioning of this organ. Acinar cells synthesize and secrete digestive enzymes with glycolytic, proteolytic, and lipolytic properties. The proteolytic enzymes are secreted in precursor forms and are activated by the pH in the intestinal lumen. Pancreatic duct cells secrete sodium bicarbonate, which osmotically stimulates the movement of water into pancreatic juice and buffers the gastric contents entering the duodenum. Enzyme and HCO_3^- secretion is governed mainly by cholecystokinin and secretin, respectively; these are hormones that are secreted by the duodenal mucosa in response to the presence of food. The parasympathetic nervous system also regulates pancreatic secretion via the vagus nerve.

Bibliography

Johnson, L. R., ed. *Gastrointestinal Physiology,* 4th ed. St. Louis: C. V. Mosby, 1991.

Johnson, L. R., ed. *Physiology of the Gastrointestinal Tract,* 2nd ed. New York: Raven Press, 1987.

49 Liver and Biliary System

James E. Heubi

Objectives

After reading this chapter, you should be able to

Describe the structural and functional relationships of hepatic secretion

Identify the major elements of bile acid and bilirubin handling by the liver

List the principal factors regulating biliary secretion

List the major components of bile

Identify the components of the enterohepatic circulation of bile acids and how bile acid pool sizes are regulated

Discuss how the biliary tract responds to a food stimulus

Explain how gallstones are formed

The functional integrity of the liver is essential for life. The liver is responsible for key components of intermediary metabolism, and its product, **bile,** facilitates fat absorption and cholesterol excretion. Bile consists of varying amounts of water, cholesterol, lecithin, bile salts, bile pigments, protein, and inorganic salts of plasma. It is formed by the liver cells, secreted into the bile canaliculi, and transported to the gallbladder, where it is concentrated and stored until appropriate stimulation initiates its delivery to the duodenum. The excretory products of bile, such as **bile pigments,** are eventually excreted in the feces; other components, such as **bile acids,** are important in the overall digestive and absorptive functions of the intestine. The anatomic and functional aspects of the liver, the formation and components of bile, bilirubin formation and excretion, and the regulation of biliary secretion as it relates to digestion will be the focus of this chapter.

Hepatic Structure

The important microscopic features of the hepatic architecture are shown in Fig. 49-1. The basic unit of hepatic structure is the **lobule.** Within it, the liver cells, **hepato-cytes,** are grouped around a central vein and radiate out in a spokelike fashion. The **sinusoids** extend from the central vein to the portal tracts, or **triads,** which include a portal vein, hepatic artery, and small bile ducts. **Bile canaliculi** lie between adjacent hepatocytes and drain bile into the bile ducts at the periphery of the lobule. The venous sinusoids are not only lined with the usual vascular endothelium but also with specialized cells of the reticuloendothelial system called **Kupffer cells.** Blood flows from the gastrointestinal tract through the **portal vein** to the liver. From the portal tracts, it traverses the short sinusoids between cords of liver cells, one to two cells thick, and the Kupffer cells. Each hepatocyte is in intimate contact with sinusoidal blood. This arrangement promotes the efficient extraction of many compounds from the plasma. Blood is then returned to the general circulation via the **central veins,** which empty into the **hepatic vein.**

The bile **canaliculi** are approximately 1 μm in diameter and are surrounded by hepatocytes. They are closed at the end nearest the central vein and have no membrane or wall (Fig. 49-2). The plasma membrane of the hepatocyte that borders the canalicular lumen serves as the canalicular membrane. Secretions from the hepatocytes are collected

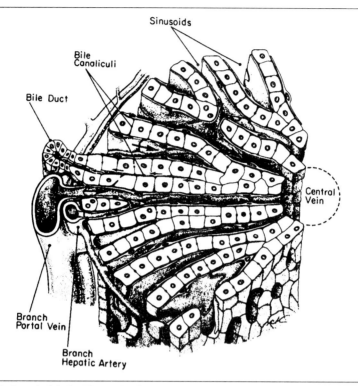

Fig. 49-1. A portion of the hepatic lobule. The cords of hepatocytes radiate out from the central vein. Branches of the portal vein, hepatic artery, and bile ducts located in the periphery make up the portal triad. The *large arrows* show the flow of blood from the portal to central veins, and the *small arrows* indicate canalicular bile flow. (Reproduced with permission from: Bloom, W., and Fawcett, D. W. *A Textbook of Histology,* 10th ed. Philadelphia: W. B. Saunders, 1975.)

Fig. 49-2. The biliary tract. (Reproduced with permission from: Schiff, L., and Schiff, E. R. *Diseases of the Liver,* 6th ed. Philadelphia: J. B. Lippincott, 1987.)

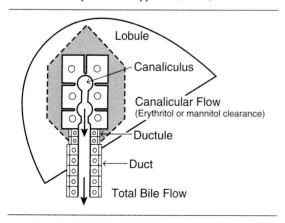

in the canalicular lumen and eventually transported to an intricate system of bile ductules and ducts that are lined by epithelial cells. The ductal system empties bile into the right and left hepatic ducts, which join to form the **common hepatic duct.** The **cystic duct** drains the gallbladder, and the common hepatic duct joins with the cystic duct to form the **common bile duct,** which enters the duodenum at the duodenal papilla, where the **sphincter of Oddi** is located.

Special Aspects of the Structure and Functional Relationships

The bile canaliculus has a high surface-to-volume ratio. The surface area, excluding microvilli, is about 10.5 m². The unidirectional blood flow from the portal to hepatic veins creates a translobular concentration gradient for each of a number of solutes. Likewise, biliary secretion into the canaliculus behaves in a similar fashion. Canalicular bile flows in the direction opposite to sinusoidal plasma flow. Consequently, the concentration of solutes in the canaliculi near the portal venous end is higher than that at the hepatic venous end. This causes bile to contain high concentrations of organic solutes.

Hepatic Function

The liver serves important functions relating to the cardiovascular and immune systems, and it secretes important materials into the gastrointestinal tract. It is pivotal in the regulation of metabolism; these roles include protein synthesis, the storage of vitamins and iron, and the degradation of hormones, drugs, and toxins.

The liver regulates carbohydrate, lipid, and protein metabolism. Glycogen synthesized during glucose excess can be metabolized and released during prolonged fasts, called **glycogenolysis,** to maintain a relatively constant blood glucose concentration. The liver is also capable of synthesizing glucose through the conversion of other substances, including amino acids, referred to as **gluconeogenesis.** Lipids absorbed from the intestine are packaged as **chylomicrons** and carried to the systemic circulation via the lymphatic system. The triglycerides of chylomicrons are hydrolyzed by lipoprotein lipase located on endothelial surfaces. Cholesterol-rich chylomicron remnants are removed by the liver and degraded. The hepatocytes synthesize very low density lipoproteins, which are a major source of cholesterol and triglycerides for use by body cells. Organelles within the hepatocytes are responsible for the beta-oxidation of fatty acids, which provides energy, and their metabolic end-products, **ketone bodies** (acetoacetate, beta-hydroxybutyrate, and acetone). The liver is centrally involved in protein breakdown and synthesis. When proteins are catabolized, their constituent amino acids are deaminated to form ammonia (NH_3). Within the liver, ammonia is converted to urea by metabolism in the urea cycle. Ninety-five percent of all major plasma proteins is synthesized by the liver, including albumin, apoproteins (the protein component of lipoproteins), fibrinogen, and those proteins involved in blood clotting.

Drug, hormone, and toxin degradation is an important hepatic function. The liver participates in the conversion of many compounds to their inactive forms. Conjugation with glucuronic acid, glycine, or glutathione is a common pathway in the degradation or detoxification that occurs in the liver.

Approximately 1400 ml of blood passes through the liver each minute. Of this, nearly 1000 ml comes from the portal circulation, which drains the organs of the gastrointestinal tract and the spleen. The remaining 400 ml consists of arterial blood derived from the hepatic artery. This total blood flow represents about 25% to 28% of the cardiac output. Hepatic arterial blood supplies nutrients to the structural components of the liver, including the biliary tract, and eventually joins the hepatic sinusoids to mix with portal blood. Blood from the hepatic sinusoids eventually drains into the hepatic vein, which empties into the inferior vena cava cephalad to the liver.

The liver performs two major vascular functions: storage and filtration. The liver is somewhat expandable and compressible and can store as much as 500 ml of blood. Two factors influence the amount of blood stored in the liver: right atrial pressure and portal venous pressure. The liver volume can decrease with shock and reduced blood flow. The 1 liter/min of blood delivered to the liver by the portal system filters through the venous sinusoids. The reticuloendothelial cells lining the sinusoids, Kupffer cells, are capable of phagocytizing nearly 99% of the bacteria and other foreign substances in the blood. Thus the liver serves as an important line of defense between the gastrointestinal tract and the systemic circulation that helps to prevent systemic infection and antigen sensitization.

Bile Composition

Inorganic electrolytes exist in bile at concentrations similar to those of plasma. Biliary calcium and bicarbonate concentrations may be higher than in plasma. The major organic components of bile are conjugated bile acids, phospholipids, cholesterol, and bile pigments. There are low levels of proteins and hormones.

The bile acid concentration in bile ranges from 2 to 45 mM. Typically, bile acids are present in the form of glycine or taurine conjugates, with a small fraction existing as free bile acids. Bile acids are amphipathic molecules that form micelles (macromolecular aggregates) above a critical micellar concentration (CMC), which in human bile is approximately 2 to 4 mM. Bile acids in hepatic and gallbladder bile greatly exceed the CMC; therefore, bile acids in bile and in the duodenal and jejunal lumen exist as micelles with small amounts present as monomers.

The phospholipid concentration in human bile ranges from 0.3 to 11 mM, and that for cholesterol is 1.6 to 8.3 mM. Although the levels of organic compounds in bile may vary according to the location in the biliary tract and intestinal lumen (because of reabsorption of inorganic solutes, especially by the gallbladder), the ratios of these compounds remain relatively fixed. Bile acids are especially important for the state of the other two organic compounds for two reasons: (1) hepatocyte secretion of cholesterol and phospholipids relies on bile acid secretion, and (2) the solubility of cholesterol and phospholipids depends largely on bile acids. Because of the formation of mixed micelles containing cholesterol, phospholipid, and bile acids, solubilized concentrations of both cholesterol and phospholipid far exceed their normal aqueous solubilities. In normal humans, bile may be supersaturated with cholesterol during a portion of the day, and cholesterol crystals may precipitate out of bile. In conjunction with compounds that form a nidus (including proteins and calcium), cholesterol crystals may aggregate to foster the development of cholesterol **gallstones.**

The typical concentrations of **bile pigments** range from 0.3 to 3.2 mM. In human bile, about 80% of the total pigments occur as bilirubin diglucuronide, while bilirubin monoglucuronide accounts for 20%. Small quantities of unconjugated bilirubin and other conjugates also may be present but are of minimal importance. Conjugation is essential for the elimination of bilirubin from the body. This process, catalyzed by UDP-glucuronyl transferase, involves esterification of bilirubin to a glycosidic compound,

glucuronic acid. The conjugation of bilirubin, with the resulting formation of glucuronides, makes it more hydrophilic and promotes its excretion in urine and bile while impeding intestinal and gallbladder absorption.

Secretion

Osmotic filtration is considered to be the major bile flow-generating mechanism. Two routes have been proposed for the passage of material from the sinusoids to canaliculi: the transcellular and paracellular pathways. There is clear evidence that the **transcellular pathway** is the principal route, with mounting evidence of a minor role for the **paracellular pathway.**

Bile acid–dependent flow, linked directly to bile acid transport through the hepatocyte and into the canalicular lumen, provides the major impetus for bile flow. The other component, bile acid–independent flow, accounts for a smaller fraction of bile flow.

Taurocholate uptake across the sinusoidal membrane depends on an inwardly directed sodium gradient that may be diminished in the presence of other bile acids, amino acids, ouabain, and furosemide (Fig. 49-3). The sodium gradient is continuously maintained by Na+,K+-ATPase. Once within the hepatocyte, bile acids are bound to cy-

Fig. 49-3. Bile acid (BA⁻) movement across the hepatocyte into the bile canaliculus (BC). Bile acids are transported across the sinusoid membrane by an Na+-dependent transport process. Within the cytosol, bile acids are bound to protein (P) or traverse in vesicles and are carried to the canaliculus, where an Na+- independent or ATP-dependent transport process facilitates movement into the canaliculus. (Adapted from: Sellinger, M., and Boyer, J. L. *Progress in Liver Disease,* Vol. IX. Philadelphia: W. B. Saunders, 1990.)

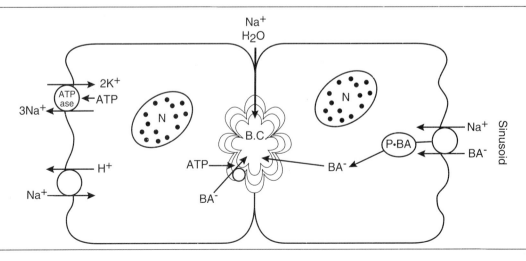

tosolic proteins, the principal one being an oxidoreductase with dihydrodiol dehydrogenase activity. Vesicular transport, which may be affected by microfilament or microtubule inhibitors, may be a major pathway with high bile acid loads. During transcellular passage, unconjugated bile acids are conjugated to taurine and glycine. Canalicular transport carriers facilitate the passage of bile acids into the canalicular lumen. Bile acids are excreted across the canalicular membrane by two independent systems: (1) a sodium-independent process driven by a negative transmembrane potential and (2) an ATP-dependent system. The osmotic activity of transported bile acids promotes the movement of water and other solutes into the canalicular lumen. Movement across the paracellular pathway is poorly understood but also appears to be promoted by osmotic filtration.

A linear relationship has been demonstrated to exist between bile flow and bile acid excretion. At low rates of bile acid excretion, bile flow is called **bile acid–independent flow** that arises from movement of inorganic electrolytes. About 30% to 60% of the basal bile flow can be attributed to either bile acid–dependent or bile acid–independent flow.

Bilirubin uptake and secretion by the hepatocyte merit particular attention. Bilirubin in the serum derives from the breakdown of hemoglobin plus other nonhemoglobin substances. Normally, unconjugated bilirubin is rapidly removed from the circulation by the liver, and serum bilirubin concentrations are less than 1 mg/dl. Bilirubin is complexed with albumin in the systemic circulation. It then dissociates from albumin and is transported into the cell by a carrier-mediated system shared with other organic anions but not with bile acids. In the hepatocyte, bilirubin binds to cytosolic proteins, ligandin, and Z protein. Within the cell, bilirubin is conjugated and thereafter secreted across the canaliculus into bile by a carrier-mediated transport system like the one on the sinusoidal membrane. Bilirubin secretion is enhanced by bile acids, even though it is excreted by a different pathway. Bile salts may form a "micellar sink" in the bile canaliculus that augments passive diffusion of the pigment from the cell into the bile.

Bilirubin glucuronides are deconjugated by bacterial or intestinal glucuronidases. Thereafter, bacteria further metabolize them into urobilinogens and urobilins. Unconjugated bilirubin and urobilinogen undergo an enterohepatic circulation. In the adult, this is of minimal significance; however, in the newborn, absorption of unconjugated bilirubin may contribute to **physiologic jaundice.** Reabsorbed conjugated bilirubin and urobilinogen may be excreted through the kidney. This excretion depends on the size of the fraction of the substances not bound to albumin.

Regulation of Biliary Secretion

Choleresis (the hepatic secretion of bile) is stimulated by increasing the flux of bile acids across the hepatocyte. Bile acid–dependent flow is determined by the number of osmotically active solute particles that exert their effect by passive diffusion and as solvent drag. Pathophysiologic conditions that might accentuate bile acid flux through the hepatocyte and enhance bile flow consist of conditions that increase the bile acid pool size, including alterations in intestinal transit and gallbladder contractility. Additional compounds, including organic anions (bromosulphalein, rose bengal, and indocyanine green), stimulate choleresis by a mechanism similar to that which operates for bile acids. In contrast to the effects described for most bile acids, certain bile acids, including taurolithocholic acid and sulfated forms of lithocholic acid, may inhibit bile flow, presumably through either toxic injury to the hepatocytes, with attendant reduced bile flow, or alteration of bile acid–independent bile glow.

Bile acid–independent bile flow is enhanced by drugs such as phenobarbital and pharmacologic doses of corticosteroids. Inhibitors of sodium transport, including ouabain, ethacrynic acid, and amiloride, all diminish bile acid–independent bile flow. Estrogens suppress bile flow, predominantly by reducing bile acid–independent flow; however, direct effects of estrogens on plasma membranes may contribute to these reductions in flow. Hypothyroidism and the antipsychotic drug chlorpromazine both lead to inhibition of bile acid–independent flow.

Bile Duct Secretion and Absorption

Evidence of ductal secretion, which accounts for 30% of basal bile flow in humans, has derived from studies examining the choleretic effect of secretin. Secretin infusion stimulates increases in flow and changes in bile composition (raised HCO_3^- and pH levels and lowered concentrations of bile acids). The secretory activity of bile ductules and ducts may explain the choleresis that arises in certain diseases that involve an increased number of bile ducts or dilatation of the biliary tree. Bile ductules and ducts are capable of reabsorption. The relative importance of secretion and absorption probably varies during the day and is not well understood.

Biliary Secretion in Humans

In humans, secretion of canalicular bile averages 11μl/μmol of bile acid, and approximately 15μmol of bile acid are secreted each minute, yielding a mean bile acid–dependent flow of 0.15 to 0.16 ml/min. The estimated canalicular bile acid–independent flow is 0.16 to 0.17 ml/min, and ductular secretion is 0.11 ml/min. This gives an estimated bile output of 600 ml/day.

Enterohepatic Circulation of Bile Acids

Bile acids serve at least three major purposes: (1) they enhance bile flow during secretion across the biliary canaliculi, (2) they form aggregates, called **mixed micelles,** in the upper small intestine, which solubilize the water-insoluble products of lipolysis, thereby facilitating their absorption, and (3) they are major regulators of sterol metabolism. In health, the **enterohepatic circulation** is localized to the liver and biliary tract, the intestinal tract, and the portal and peripheral circulations. In disease states, such as cholestasis, the pool shifts from the intestinal and biliary tracts into the liver and peripheral circulation. In the liver, cholesterol is converted to the highly polar bile acids, **cholic acid** (3α, 7α, 12α-trihydroxy-5β-cholanoic acid) and **chenodeoxycholic acid** (3α, 7α-dihydroxy-5β-cholanoic acid), which are termed **primary bile acids** (Fig. 49-4). The initial step of bile acid synthesis involves the 7α-hydroxylation of the sterol nucleus of cholesterol, which is effected by the rate-limiting enzyme of bile acid synthesis, cholesterol 7α-hydroxylase. After hepatic synthesis, bile acids are conjugated with glycine or taurine as *N*-acyl conjugates. All but a small fraction of bile acids are conjugated before excretion by the hepatocyte.

During fasting, most of the bile acid pool is in the gallbladder; however, some bile acids are always entering the intestinal lumen and produce basal intraluminal concentrations plus small but measurable concentrations in the serum because of continuous intestinal absorption. When a meal is consumed, the gallbladder contracts at least once and often twice, whereupon most of the bile salt pool is emptied into the small intestinal lumen (Fig. 49-5). Bile acids are not secreted into the intestine in isolation but rather as mixed micelles containing bile acids, cholesterol, and phospholipids. Within the upper small bowel, bile salts form mixed micelles in combination with the lipolytic products fatty acids and monoglycerides. The lipolytic products are absorbed and bile acids are then reabsorbed by an active transport system localized to the distal ileum, the principal pathway for reabsorption, or by passive transport by nonionic diffusion, which may occur at any location along the length of the small and large intestines.

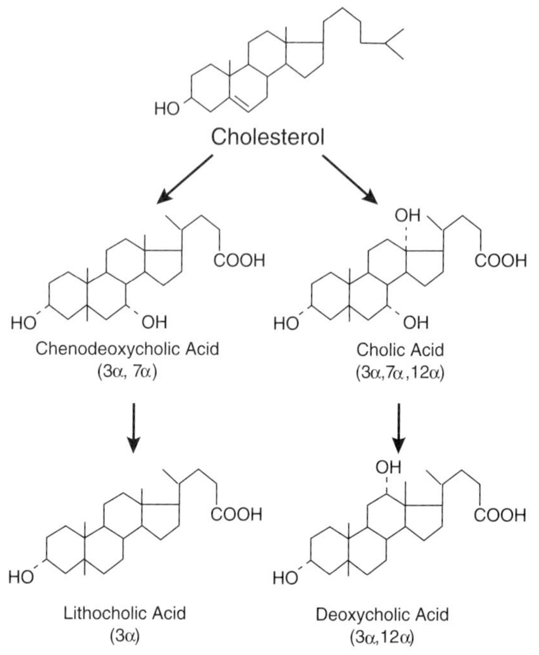

Fig. 49-4. Primary bile acids synthesized in the liver from cholesterol and regulated by the rate-limiting enzyme cholesterol 7α-hydroxylase. Also shown are the secondary bile acids produced by bacterial 7α-dehydroxylation after deconjugation.

Luminal nutrients tend to inhibit passive uptake of bile acids. Only unconjugated bile acids or glycine conjugates of dihydroxy bile acids are absorbed in a significant amount by passive diffusion.

Bile acids absorbed from the intestine are carried to the liver, where transport systems very efficiently remove them from the portal blood. A small fraction of the bile acids in portal blood spills over into the systemic circulation, leading to a predictable postprandial rise in serum bile acids during each of the 6 to 10 enterohepatic cycles of bile acids that occur during a day.

Most of the conjugates of cholic and chenodeoxycholic acid excreted in bile are reabsorbed without intraluminal bacterial alteration. Approximately one-fourth of the primary bile acids are deconjugated by bacteria in the terminal ileum and colon. These free bile acids are reabsorbed and reconjugated in the liver with either glycine or taurine. Additional modifications to the steroid nucleus after deconjugation also may be accomplished within the gut lumen. The most common biotransformation made by bacteria is 7α-dehydroxylation, with the formation of

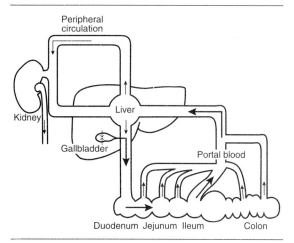

Fig. 49-5. The enterohepatic circulation of bile acids. When the gallbladder contracts, bile acids are expelled into the duodenal lumen. Passive absorption is shown by *small arrows* directed along the entire length of the small and large intestine. The *large arrow* going from the ileum into the portal blood depicts the active transport of bile acids by a carrier-mediated transport system. Bile acids return to the liver via the portal vein. The liver efficiently removes all but a small portion of bile acids that spill over into the systemic circulation. This produces a small but measurable postprandial rise in the serum level of bile acids. A small quantity of bile acids is filtered and excreted by the kidneys.

secondary bile acids. The primary bile acids, cholic and chenodeoxycholic acid, are transformed into the secondary bile acids, deoxycholic acid (3α, 12α-dihydroxy-5β-cholanoic) and lithocholic acid (3α-hydroxy-5β-cholanoic), respectively (see Fig. 49-4). Approximately one-quarter to one-third of the pool of primary bile acids is converted to secondary bile acids each day. Deoxycholic acid is absorbed relatively efficiently and conjugated with either glycine or taurine. The glycine and taurine conjugates are then recycled and reabsorbed with efficiencies similar to the conjugates of chenodeoxycholic acid. Only about one-fifth of the newly formed lithocholic acid is absorbed, because it is very insoluble and adsorbs to colonic bacteria. If reabsorbed, lithocholic acid is also conjugated with glycine or taurine; however, most conjugates are sulfated in the 3 position to form sulfated lithocholate conjugates, which are poorly absorbed.

With efficient recycling and synthesis, biliary bile acids in humans generally comprise cholic (36%), chenodeoxycholic (36%), deoxycholic (24%), and lithocholic (1%) acids

in a ratio of glycine-to-taurine conjugates of 3 to 4 : 1. Depending on diet, normal adults excrete 22 to 650 mg of bile acid per day. Fecal bile acids in healthy humans reflect major bacterial transformation. Most fecal bile acids are unconjugated and lack the 7α-hydroxyl group. Hepatic bile acid synthesis is regulated by feedback inhibition and by the hepatic synthesis of chenodeoxycholic acid and cholic acid that compensates for daily stool losses, thereby creating a steady-state and keeping the primary bile acid pool sizes constant.

Regulation of the Enterohepatic Circulation of Bile Acids

The regulation of bile acid pool size is carefully controlled by the liver through a feedback inhibition system. The rate-limiting enzyme of bile acid synthesis, cholesterol 7α-hydroxylase, is controlled by the return of bile acids to the liver through the portal vein. The bile acid pool size may be depleted, leading to reduced intestinal concentrations of bile acids and impaired fat solubilization, when the enterohepatic circulation is interrupted by ileal disease (Crohn's disease), ileal resection, or small-intestinal bypass. When excess bile acids are lost in the feces, the liver enhances synthesis up to 10-fold in an attempt to maintain a steady bile acid pool size. If the loss exceeds the hepatic ability to synthesize bile acids, the pool will contract. Minor modifications of pool size may result when the small-intestinal transit time is decreased or the gallbladder is surgically removed. In contrast, pool sizes may increase when gallbladder emptying is impaired, as observed in celiac disease or pregnancy, or when the small-intestinal transit time is increased.

Biliary Tract Physiology

The smooth muscle of the common bile duct contracts rhythmically and may enhance bile flow within the biliary tree. The sphincter of Oddi, located at the junction of the common bile duct and duodenum, also undergoes rhythmic contractions. During fasting, bile flows predominantly into the gallbladder because of a pressure gradient created by the contracted sphincter of Oddi. The gallbladder is a saccular organ with a capacity of 15 to 60 ml in adults. The bile collected during the interdigestive phase is concentrated predominantly by the reabsorption of water. Bile acids, bilirubin, cholesterol, and phospholipids are concentrated between 3- and 10-fold in the gallbladder. When a meal is ingested, the gallbladder contracts and the sphincter of Oddi relaxes. Initially, during the cephalic and gastric phases of digestion, this is mediated by cholinergic stimulation mediated by the vagus nerve (see Chap. 48). The greatest gallbladder emptying occurs during the intestinal phase. Products of digestion, especially fatty acids and amino acids, stimulate the release of cholecystokinin (CCK) by the I-cells in the upper small-intestinal mucosa. Circulating CCK causes strong contraction of the gallbladder smooth muscle and relaxation of the sphincter of Oddi. CCK appears to be the major hormone mediating gallbladder contraction; gastrin also may stimulate contraction in doses far exceeding the physiologic range, and secretin has little effect. Intraduodenal acid and alcohol stimulate sphincter of Oddi contraction, as does morphine.

Gallstones

The prevalence of gallstones or cholelithiasis increases with age. Infants and children rarely develop gallstones. There are two major types of gallstones: calcium bilirubinate (pigment) and cholesterol. About 85% of stones in adults in the United States are composed predominantly of cholesterol. A sharp increase in the frequency of cholelithiasis is found in women after puberty, and a gradual increase is noted in males throughout adulthood.

Cholesterol gallstone formation is the consequence of several interrelated events, including (1) hepatic secretion of bile that is supersaturated with cholesterol, (2) nucleation of cholesterol monohydrate crystals, and (3) impaired gallbladder emptying. The bile of virtually all subjects in whom cholesterol stones develop is supersaturated with cholesterol, but many adults without stones have bile supersaturated with cholesterol during at least a portion of the day. Cholesterol supersaturation is commonly found in obese patients, patients with ileal resection, and patients treated with clofibrate, an agent used to treat hyperlipidemia, or estrogens. Unlike normal individuals, those with gallstones exhibit rapid nucleation of cholesterol crystals. A delicate balance appears to exist between the promoters and inhibitors of crystal nucleation, and this determines whether gallstones form. Specific conditions that alter nucleating factors (glycoproteins and mucin) include total parenteral nutrition and cystic fibrosis. Gallbladder stasis, commonly found in patients treated with parenteral nutrition, during pregnancy, and in celiac

disease, allows retention of crystals with subsequent growth into larger calculi.

Most gallstones in childhood are pigment stones that are caused by hemolytic disorders. Pigment stones also can be found with biliary tract infection and alcoholic cirrhosis.

Until recently, the only therapy for symptomatic gallstones was cholecystectomy. Recently introduced alternatives to surgery include sonication (lithotripsy), chemical solubilization with organic solvents infused through biliary catheters, and oral bile acid therapy.

Summary

Hepatic structure and function are closely related. Bile flow is governed principally by the transport of bile acids across the sinusoidal and canalicular membranes. Likewise, bilirubin uptake and excretion are mediated by transport proteins on both the sinusoidal and canalicular membranes. The enterohepatic circulation of bile acids furnishes an efficient means to ensure adequate biliary concentrations of bile acids for solubilizing hydrophobic compounds such as cholesterol and phospholipid (thereby minimizing the risk of gallstone formation). It also ensures adequate intraluminal bile acid concentrations that promote efficient solubilization of the lipolytic products of intraluminal digestion. Meal-stimulated, hormonally mediated (CCK) contraction of the gallbladder and relaxation of the sphincter of Oddi allow delivery of concentrated bile, and this facilitates the formation of intraluminal micelles containing bile acids, fatty acids, phospholipids, monoglycerides, and fat-soluble vitamins.

Bibliography

Erlinger, S. In: Schiff, L., and Schiff, E. R., eds. *Secretion of Bile in Diseases of the Liver,* 6th ed. Philadelphia: J. B. Lippincott, 1987. Pp. 77–101.

Hofmann, A. F. The enterohepatic circulation of bile acids in man. In: Stollerman, G. H., ed. *Advances in Internal Medicine.* Chicago: Year Book Medical Publishers, 1976. Pp. 501–534.

Sellinger, M., and Boyer, J. L. Physiology of bile secretion and cholestasis. In: Popper, H., and Schaffner, F., eds. *Progress in Liver Disease,* Vol. IX. Philadelphia: W. B. Saunders, 1990. Pp. 237–260.

50 Intestinal Absorption

Joseph D. Fondacaro

Objectives

After reading this chapter, you should be able to

Characterize the volume load introduced into the human intestine every 24 hours

Describe how the intestinal mucosa is designed anatomically and functionally to handle this fluid challenge

Describe the mechanisms of intestinal water and electrolyte (especially Na$^+$ and Cl$^-$) transport and absorption and the intracellular pathways that regulate these membrane processes

Discuss the principles of active, energy-dependent, Na$^+$-coupled transport and how the inwardly directed Na$^+$

electrochemical gradient energizes this transport process

Describe the regulatory roles of the autonomic and enteric nervous systems and the influence of various hormones on intestinal absorption processes

Explain the mechanisms of carbohydrate, protein, and lipid digestion and the absorption of the end-products of these digestive processes

Describe the role of bile salts in the digestion and absorption of dietary lipids

---

The mammalian intestine performs several important functions, all of which are integral components of the total digestive process. The intestine, along with the pancreas, secretes digestive enzymes and mixes these enzymes with dietary components, thus providing small, simple molecules for efficient absorption. The intestine, along with the pancreas and the biliary tract, secretes HCO$_3^-$ that buffers the strong acid of gastric juice and thereby protects its delicate epithelium from erosion, damage, and ulceration. In addition, the musculature of the intestine provides for the efficient, coordinated, and timely movement of nonabsorbed substrates in an aboral direction for eventual elimination. One of the most striking aspects of intestinal function is the absorption of water, electrolytes, and dietary nutrients. In the normal-functioning mammalian intestine, nearly all the dietary nutrients and approximately 95% to 98% of the water and electrolytes that enter the

upper small bowel are absorbed. This chapter reviews the major components of intestinal electrolyte and nutrient absorption, those processes whose net result is the movement of electrolytes, water, and metabolic substrates into the blood for distribution and use throughout the body.

Anatomic Considerations

Before exploring how the bowel is equipped functionally to handle the process of absorption, it is important to understand how the bowel is designed anatomically to serve this function. Figure 50-1 is a diagram showing how intestinal structure amplifies the total surface area to promote efficient absorption. If one envisions the small bowel as a **cylinder** with a length of approximately 280 cm and a diameter of about 4 cm, the total internal surface area yielded by these dimensions is approximately 3300 cm^2.

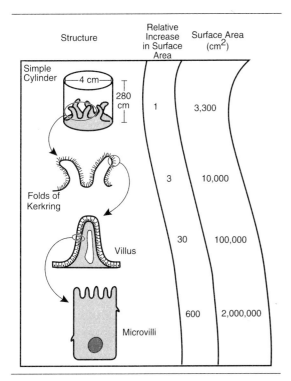

Fig. 50-1. Amplification of intestinal surface area.

Using this as a reference point, **epithelial folds of Kerkring** alone amplify the surface area by a factor of 3 to yield an area of about 10,000 cm². Next, the numerous villi of the intestinal surface further augment the surface area by a factor of 10 to yield an area approximately 30 times that of the reference point, or about 100,000 cm². Finally, the **microscopic surface of the luminal border** of the villous cells contains a microvillar membrane that contributes an additional 20-fold increase in surface area, such that it is 600 times that of the reference standard, or approximately 2 million cm². In graphic terms, the total surface area rendered by the bowel anatomy for the purpose of absorption exceeds the size of a singles tennis court.

Fluid and Electrolyte Absorption

The mammalian intestine is the primary site of fluid and solute absorption within the gastrointestinal tract. The small intestine passively and efficiently absorbs large volumes of fluid by actively transporting smaller quantities of osmotically active solutes. To appreciate the enormous challenge confronting the transport mechanisms of the in-

testine, it is important to consider the total fluid volume handled by the intestines on a daily basis.

Table 50-1 gives a breakdown of the volume of fluid entering the small intestine from all the potential contributors and how this volume is handled. The healthy adult ordinarily consumes approximately 2.0 liters of fluid a day in the diet. In addition, during digestion of dietary substrates, certain organs within the gastrointestinal tract secrete fluid that contains their particular contribution to the digestive process. In a 24-hour period, the salivary glands, stomach, pancreas, biliary system, and the intestine itself secrete about 7.0 liters of fluid. This yields a total fluid volume of roughly 9.0 liters entering the duodenum daily. Ordinarily, the small intestine absorbs about 7.5 liters, or 83% to 85% of this fluid. Combined with the roughly 1.4 liters absorbed by the large bowel, the total fluid absorption represents approximately 98% of total fluid intake, leaving approximately 100 ml of fluid excreted daily from the gastrointestinal tract.

Cellular Transport Process

The transport mechanisms are an integral part of the electrolyte transport process that takes place in the intestine. The wide variety of absorptive and secretory processes exhibited by the intestine are mediated by a single layer of epithelial cells, the **intestinal mucosa,** which lines the entire luminal surface of the intestinal tract. This mucosal layer is made up of finger-like projections or elevations, called **villi,** and pitted areas, called **crypts** (Fig. 50-2). The mucosal cells in these two regions are anatomically different. The **villous cell** has a characteristic microvillous or

Table 50-1. Daily Total Fluid Volume (in liters) Handled by the Intestines

Ingested fluid		2.0
Secreted fluid		
Saliva	1.0	
Gastric juice	2.0	
Pancreatic juice	0.5	
Bile	1.5	
Intestinal secretion	2.0	
Total secretions		7.0
Total fluid input		9.0
Absorption		
Small intestine	7.5	
Colon	1.4	
Total fluid absorbed		8.9
Total fluid excreted		0.1

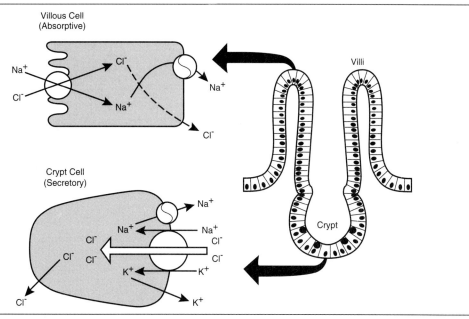

Fig. 50-2. Anatomic and functional differentiation of villous and crypt cells in the intestinal mucous (Modified from: Field, M., Fordtran, J. S., and Schultz, S. G., eds. *Secretory Diarrhea.* Bethesda, Md.: American Physiological Society, 1980.)

brush-border luminal membrane, while the **crypt cell** has no outstanding or distinguishing microanatomic features. Furthermore, these cells are functionally, as well as structurally, different (see Fig. 50-2). The villous cells are almost exclusively **absorptive** and are equipped with the necessary mechanisms to accomplish this task. The crypt cells are primarily **secretory** and possess those mechanisms consistent with this role.

The scientific literature on electrolyte transport and ion-coupled transport processes is enormous. Therefore, it is not possible to give an exhaustive review here, and only the transport of Na^+, K^+, Cl^-, H^+, and HCO_3^- is emphasized in the following discussion.

As just mentioned, the villous cell is the primary site of absorption. There are three basic pathways for **Na^+ absorption** across the intestinal mucosa (Fig. 50-3). It can enter the villous cell at the luminal membrane through an Na^+-conducting pathway, the so-called **Na^+ channel.** This pathway is sensitive to amiloride, and Na^+ entry is energized by an inwardly directed diffusional gradient for the cation. The second mechanism for Na^+ absorption is a **coupled NaCl cotransport process.** This luminal membrane carrier must bind Na^+ and Cl^- before it delivers either ion to the cell interior. The driving force for this

mechanism is again the inwardly directed Na^+ gradient. Finally, Na^+ can be absorbed by **Na^+-solute-coupled cotransport.** The **solutes** known to be cotransported with Na^+ are glucose and amino acids (to be discussed later in this chapter), certain bile acids, and some water-soluble vitamins. Once inside the cell, the solute is freely diffusible down a concentration gradient and through the basolateral membrane of the cell for eventual discharge into the portal bloodstream. The feature common to all these Na^+ absorptive processes is the driving force for Na^+ entry—the **inwardly directed Na^+ gradient**, which is maintained by the basolateral **Na^+ pump.** This Na^+ pump is energized by the hydrolysis of ATP, which is catalyzed by Na^+,K^+-ATPase and exchanges 3 Na^+ out for 2 K^+ in. Thus, following a meal, the intracellular Na^+ concentration is maintained very low relative to the extracellular environment, in particular the intestinal lumen. The movement of electrolytes and the transported solutes causes the concomitant movement of water into the bloodstream in an osmotically obligatory fashion.

Of the three modes of entry, it has been determined that **coupled NaCl cotransport** is the primary contributor to Na^+ absorption. Figure 50-4 illustrates several important features of the NaCl cotransport process. First, the cotrans-

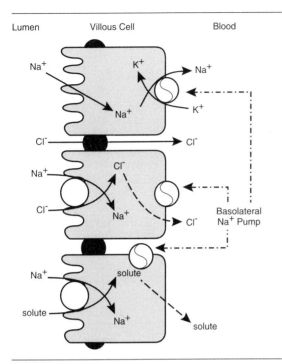

Fig. 50-3. Three pathways for sodium absorption across small-intestinal mucosa.

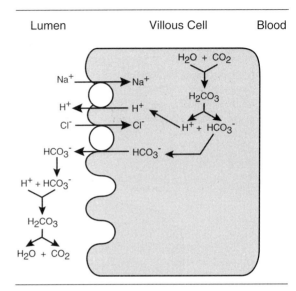

Fig. 50-4. The Na^+-H^+ and Cl^--HCO_3^- exchange mechanisms of coupled NaCl absorption.

port of Na^+ and Cl^- occurs as a result of two separate but functionally parallel exchange processes residing on the luminal membrane: **Na^+-proton** exchange and **Cl^--HCO_3^- exchange.** The absorption of Cl^- into the bloodstream can proceed by two routes: (1) **passive diffusion** from the cell across the basolateral membrane and (2) a paracellular shunt. Finally, the luminal and basolateral membranes may possess a Na^+-proton exchanger, which serves to maintain a constant intracellular pH, since an ion exchanger can function in both directions.

The process of **electrolyte secretion** is a function of the crypt cell. An important transport process is characteristic of cells in the crypt region of the mucosa (Fig. 50-2). These cells are secretory, with Cl^- secretion being the primary event. This is accomplished by the luminal membrane Cl^- conductive pathway, or **Cl^- channel.** Cl^- secretion is believed to be maintained at a **basal rate** under normal physiologic conditions. However, in certain **disease states** marked by **secretory diarrhea,** this Cl^- secretion may be dramatically enhanced in the small intestine. The **outwardly directed Cl^- gradient** is believed to be maintained by a **Na^+-K^+-$2Cl^-$ cotransport** mechanism located on the basolateral membrane (see Fig. 50-2). The

functioning of this cotransport process and the subsequent "loading" of the cell with Cl^- are energized by the inwardly directed Na^+ gradient maintained by the basolateral Na^+ pump. Alterations in the Na^+ pump, the Na^+-K^+-$2Cl^-$ cotransporter, or the basolateral K^+ channel can seriously affect Cl^- secretion. Thus these three basolateral transport processes can be regarded as "functionally" coupled to Cl^- secretion.

Intracellular Regulation of Transport

Like most physiologic events, these transport processes are regulated by both intracellular and extracellular mechanisms. As is true in other systems, the **intracellular regulation** of intestinal electrolyte transport is made up of a complex series of biochemical events. It is well accepted that modulation of the **cyclic nucleotide** pathway, in particular cAMP, and of the intracellular Ca^{2+} concentration alters luminal membrane transport in the villous and crypt cells.

The **adenylate cyclase and cAMP system** plays a major role as second messenger in regulating ion transport (see Chaps. 19 and 51). Protein kinase-A, through phosphorylation, inhibits coupled NaCl absorption in the villous cell and stimulates Cl^- secretion in the crypt cell. Cyclic nucleotide **cGMP** and PK-G are also involved in **villous cell absorption.**

The **signal transduction mechanism** utilizing Ca^{2+} is believed to involve two distinct Ca^{2+} regulatory pathways, both residing within transporting enterocytes (see Chaps. 19 and 51). The **Ca^{2+}-calmodulin** (CMD) and the **Ca^{2+} inositol phospholipid-dependent protein kinase C** (PKC) pathways modulate these transport processes. Both of these pathways are triggered by a rise in intracellular Ca^{2+}, which can be achieved in two ways. The first is via receptors that are linked functionally to receptor operated Ca^{2+} channels. In the second pathway, hormone-receptor interaction stimulates phospholipase C (PLC). PLC accelerates the conversion of phosphatidylinositol to phosphatidylinositol bis-phosphate (PIP_2), which is converted to inositol tris-phosphate (IP_3) and diacylglycerol. IP_3 stimulates the release of Ca^{2+} from intracellular storage sites. In the presence of phosphatidylserine, diacylglycerol and cytosolic Ca^{2+} stimulate PKC, which has a similar effect on the transport of electrolytes. The primary role of CaCAM-PK is regulation of NaCl absorption, while PKC primarily alters Na^+-H^+ exchange and Cl^- secretion.

Finally, important interactions between the membrane **phospholipids** and **arachidonic acid metabolism** have been observed and proposed. In particular, inhibitors of archidonic acid metabolism to prostaglandins have been shown to suppress PKC-mediated secretion. These studies suggest that **prostaglandins,** which are known stimulators of intestinal secretion, are perhaps intimately involved in the combined phosphatidylinositol-PKC regulatory pathway. These regulatory systems are affected in certain disease conditions, such as secretory diarrhea and other transport disorders of the gastrointestinal tract.

Electrolyte and Fluid Absorption in the Colon

The mammalian large intestine plays a vital role in the fluid and electrolyte composition of stool. The colon **absorbs** Na^+, Cl^-, and water and **secretes** small quantities of K^+ and HCO_3^-. The **transport mechanisms** for electrolytes in the colon are similar to those of the small intestine; the colon lacks nutrient transport processes. This poses a potentially serious clinical problem when nutrient absorption in the small intestine is compromised. Unabsorbed dietary substrates entering the colon can provide an osmotic challenge to the movement of fluid across the colonic mucosa, setting in motion a potential diarrheal condition. Fortunately, the colonic epithelium absorbs Na^+ more efficiently than does the small intestinal mucosa. Furthermore, the colon responds more readily to **aldosterone** by increasing Na^+ absorption than does the small bowel.

Although the healthy human colon absorbs approximately 1400 ml of fluid per day, it has the capacity to absorb more than three times this volume, or about 4400 ml. This absorptive "reserve" has been referred to as **colonic salvage** and is of utmost importance in the regulation of fecal water excretion and management of potential diarrheal conditions (Table 50-2). In malabsorptive diseases of the small intestine, the amount of fluid delivered to the colon is markedly increased. In many cases, colonic salvage can compensate for this by absorbing more fluid and preventing diarrhea of small bowel origin. In some cases, such as **cholera,** the fluid volume delivered to the colon (excess fluid from the small intestine) exceeds the absorptive reserve, leading to fluid loss (see Table 50-2). Similarly, in diseases of the colon such as certain **inflammatory conditions,** colonic fluid absorption may be compromised. While the volume of fluid entering the colon may be essentially normal, the absorptive capacity of the colon is markedly reduced, resulting in diarrhea of colonic origin (see Table 50-2).

Fluid absorption in the colon is influenced by the absorption of **electrolytes,** primarily Na^+ and Cl^-. In the colon, **Na^+ absorption** involves electrogenic Na^+ transport (via Na^+ channels) and neutral NaCl cotransport. These

Table 50-2. A Representation of Colonic Salvage and the Failure of This Mechanism in Diarrheas of Small Bowel and Colonic Origin*

	Health	Small Bowel	Disease	Colonic Disease
Fluid volume to the colon	1500	4500	6000	1500
Colonic fluid absorption	1400	4400	4400	700
Stool water	100	100	1600	800
Diarrhea	No	No	Yes	Yes

*All quantities are given in milliliters.

two mechanisms of Na^+ absorption are driven by a **lumen-to-cell Na^+ concentration** gradient, which is maintained by the basolateral Na^+-K^+ pump and resembles that of the small bowel. The resulting accumulation of K^+ in the absorbing cell drives K^+ **secretion** across a luminal membrane K^+ channel. Cl^- **absorption** is accomplished by a passive Na^+-independent diffusional process along an inwardly directed Cl^- gradient and by a Cl^--HCO_3^- exchanger, resulting in HCO_3^- secretion. In the normal colon, electrolyte absorption exceeds secretion, resulting in **net water absorption.**

Neural and Hormonal Regulation of Transport

The various processes of intestinal electrolyte transport are precisely coordinated with the other intestinal functions of motility and secretion to provide an efficient and integrated sequence to the total digestive process. Extrinsic and intrinsic nervous innervation from the autonomic and enteric nervous systems, respectively, along with various hormonal influences, ensures this coordination once food is present in the digestive tract.

The **enteric nervous system** (ENS) resides within the wall of the gastrointestinal tract. The **submucosal plexus** is positioned in the submucosal space between the mucosal layer and the musculature. It mediates **intramural reflex pathways** that regulate electrolyte absorption and secretion. Sensory receptors in the mucosal region detect various characteristics of luminal contents (texture and fluidity). This information is integrated and becomes the afferent signal of the reflex. This signal is sent to the submucosal plexus through the release of acetylcholine, which evokes a rapid excitatory response in the motor neurons innervating the crypt region. This **cholinergic stimulation** of the crypt cells enhances Cl^- secretion, most likely mediated by a Ca^{2+}-phospholipid-PKC pathway.

Extrinsic neural influence also may play a role in this regulatory scheme. These pathways include the **myenteric plexus,** the second component of the ENS, and some external nerves of the autonomic nervous system. The myenteric plexus is located between the inner circular and the outer longitudinal muscle layers of the gastrointestinal tract. The previous discussion described how submucosal nerves can influence Cl^- secretion. However, it is known that other influences may be involved in the secretory

response. Submucosal nerves can be modulated by nerves of the myenteric plexus, which release either **serotonin** (which is stimulatory) or **enkephalins** (which are inhibitory). Furthermore, **extrinsic sympathetic fibers** can influence the activity of enteric, submucosal nerves or provide direct input to the epithelial cells. In this case, **norepinephrine,** the neurotransmitter released by these nerves, has a dual action. Norepinephrine inhibits submucosal nerve activity and reduces Cl^- secretion while directly stimulating villous cells to increase NaCl absorption. This action has been mimicked by alpha 2-adrenergic receptor agonists, which have been proposed as a class of compounds for antidiarrheal therapy. The hormone **somatostatin** also may be a neurotransmitter in the sympathetic neural influence on transport. Somatostatin reduces fluid and electrolyte losses in diarrhea, and a very effective somatostatin analogue has been developed and is effective in treating fluid and electrolyte loss during secretory diarrhea.

It is now well established that several naturally occurring gastrointestinal **hormones** and **paracrine substances** can stimulate electrolyte (NaCl) and fluid absorption (Table 50-3). For the most part, however, the cellular mechanisms that mediate the absorptive response are unknown. In contrast, there are many hormones and paracrine substances within the gastrointestinal tract and elsewhere that promote fluid and electrolyte secretion (see Table 50-3). These secretagogues, generally speaking, alter cyclic nucleotide or Ca^{2+} metabolism within the enterocytes, leading to secretion.

Table 50-3. Endocrines, Paracrines, and Neurocrines that Influence Electrolyte Transport

STIMULATORS OF ABSORPTION	
Aldosterone	Glycocorticoids
Dopamine	Neuropeptide Y
Enkephalins	Norepinephrine
Epinephrine	Somatostatin
STIMULATORS OF SECRETION	
Acetylcholine	Neurotensin
Bombesin	Prostaglandins
Bradykinin	Serotonin
Histamine	Substance P
Leukotrienes	Vasopressin
Motilin	Vasoactive intestinal polypeptide

Carbohydrate and Protein Digestion and Absorption

The digestion and absorption of dietary carbohydrates and proteins take place in the **small intestine**. These are extremely efficient processes; essentially all the carbohydrates and proteins consumed are absorbed.

Carbohydrates

Dietary carbohydrates are either digestible or indigestible (Table 50-4). The common sources of **digestible carbohydrates** are starches (complex sugars), table sugar, fruits, and milk. The **indigestible carbohydrates** are found in legumes in the form of oligosaccharides (e.g., raffinose) and in some vegetables, fruits, and grains as the polysaccharides cellulose, hemicellulose, pectin, and gums. These are often referred to as **dietary fiber** and are valuable to human health.

Starches are complex sugar polymers consisting of long chains of glucose molecules linked by a 1,4-glycosidic bond and branching side chains of glucose connected to the main chain by a 1,6 bond. The **digestion of starch** to simple hexose molecules involves a two-step process: a luminal phase and a brush-border phase (Fig. 50-5). The **luminal phase** begins in the mouth with the action of saliva secreted from three pair of salivary glands: the parotid, submandibular, and sublingual. The watery secretions from the **parotid glands** serve to lubricate food and wash away food particles from the taste buds, allowing taste sen-

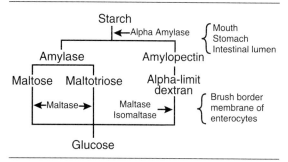

Fig. 50-5. The luminal and brush-border phases of intestinal starch digestion.

sations. This secretion also **buffers** potentially injurious agents, such as hot or acidic liquids, and lubricates the structures of the mouth for clear speech. **Sublingual** and **submandibular glands** secrete a more viscous fluid, which also lubricates food and contains the enzyme **salivary amylase.** This enzyme initiates the digestion of carbohydrates, which is continued in the stomach. Almost 75% of the carbohydrates consumed are digested to disaccharides before reaching the small intestine, where the luminal phase occurs in the upper small intestine as pancreatic alpha-amylase is secreted. The **complex starch polymer** is ultimately reduced to maltose, maltotriose, and alpha-limit dextrans by these enzymes (see also Chap. 48).

In the **brush-border phase,** these three products are dispersed in the **bulk water** and the **unstirred water layers** within the intestine and are eventually exposed to the brush-border membrane of the absorbing enterocyte. These cells secrete disaccharidases and trisaccharidases that reduce these substrates to their simplest form—glucose (see Fig. 50-5). Once in this form, carbohydrates can be absorbed into the enterocyte by mechanisms that will be discussed below and are eventually discharged into the bloodstream.

Sucrose (cane sugar) and **lactose** (milk sugar) are disaccharides that require only the brush-border phase of digestion. Sucrose is reduced to glucose and fructose and lactose to glucose and galactose by the action of the disaccharidases **sucrase** and **lactase,** respectively, which are secreted by the brush-border membrane of the enterocytes. These carbohydrates are now able to be absorbed.

Carbohydrate-induced diarrhea most often results from lactose intolerance because of a genetic deficiency of the brush-border enzyme lactase. This syndrome, called **hypolactasia,** is the most frequent genetic deficiency in

Table 50-4. Important Dietary Carbohydrates

Food Source	Carbohydrate
DIGESTIBLE CARBOHYDRATE	
Starch	Glucose
Milk, milk products	Glucose, galactose
Sugar cane	Glucose, fructose
Vegetables	Fructose
Fruits	Fructose
Honey	Fructose
Corn syrup	Fructose
INDIGESTIBLE CARBOHYDRATE	
Legumes	Raffinose
Vegetables, fruits	Cellulose, hemicellulose pectin, gums

humans and affects approximately one-half the world's population. This is an example of an **osmotic diarrhea,** and thus the primary factor governing the amount of fluid lost is the amount of lactose ingested. These osmotic diarrheas are generally of colonic origin.

Hexose

Glucose, the major hexose derived from carbohydrate digestion, is absorbed by two processes: passive diffusion and active, carrier-mediated transport. The **passive diffusion** of glucose across the intestinal mucosa depends on the concentration of glucose in the intestinal lumen and can occur through the cells as well as by a paracellular route. As long as the glucose concentration in the lumen remains higher than that in the blood, glucose will diffuse down its concentration gradient and be absorbed. Some evidence suggests that the passive diffusion of glucose through the intestinal mucosal cells is carrier-mediated, i.e., **facilitated diffusion** (see Chap. 2). Approximately 80% of luminal glucose is absorbed by diffusion. The remaining 20% is absorbed by an **energy-dependent, carrier-mediated, Na$^+$-glucose cotransport process,** which is maintained for as long as glucose is present in the intestinal lumen. However, following a meal, this active transport of glucose is "masked" by the overwhelming amount of passive diffusion taking place in response to the high luminal glucose concentration. As this luminal glucose concentration falls to about 5 mM and below, active glucose transport becomes dominant and eventually sequesters all remaining glucose in the lumen.

Active glucose transport is an **Na$^+$-coupled, energy-dependent, uphill transport.** Na$^+$ and glucose bind to an apical membrane transport protein and are carried into the cytosol because of a conformational change in the transport protein and because the affinity of the protein for the substrates changes from high to low. Once inside the enterocyte, glucose accumulates to a level that exceeds its concentration in the interstitial space and blood. Glucose then diffuses down this concentration gradient, out of the cell, and into the blood. Following a meal, this cell-to-blood gradient is maintained for some time because the active transport of glucose from the lumen sequesters most, if not all, of the luminal glucose and stimulates villous blood flow, thus preventing glucose from accumulating in the tissue. Cytosolic Na$^+$ is pumped from the interior of the cell by the basolateral Na$^+$,K$^+$-ATPase–mediated Na$^+$ pump. This low intracellular Na$^+$ concentration creates the inwardly directed Na$^+$ gradient and energizes the transport of glucose (and other substrates, as will be discussed). In regard to glucose, this system is often referred to as sec-

ondary active transport, since the active (energy-consuming) step involves Na$^+$ extrusion and energy from the ATPase reaction is not used directly in moving the glucose.

If Na$^+$ is removed from the lumen, active glucose transport is suppressed, and agents that inhibit the Na$^+$,K$^+$-ATPase block glucose transport. Active glucose transport exhibits **saturation kinetics** typical of a carrier-mediated transport process, with a rate of absorption equal to one-half the maximum (the Tm or Km) occurring at about 5 to 10 mM.

Galactose is also actively transported by the glucose carrier system and has been shown experimentally to be a competitive inhibitor of glucose transport. However, the carrier system has a somewhat lower affinity for galactose than for glucose. **Fructose** is not actively transported by intestinal cells but is absorbed by a carrier-mediated, facilitated diffusion system. The distinguishing feature of a faciliated diffusional system is that because it is carrier-mediated, equilibrium is achieved sooner than it would be in a simple non-carrier-mediated, passive diffusion system. Carrier-mediated fructose absorption does not require the input of energy.

Proteins

Like carbohydrates, dietary proteins must be reduced to their simplest forms before they can be absorbed by the intestinal mucosa. This digestive process begins in the stomach, through the action of the gastric enzyme **pepsin,** and is continued in the upper small bowel by the proteolytic enzymes of the **pancreas.** Dipeptidases from the brush border and cytosolic compartments of enterocytes mediate the final breakdown of small peptides into individual **amino acids. Hydrolytic products** of protein digestion (amino acids, dipeptides, and tripeptides) are each capable of being absorbed intact across the luminal membrane of the intestine into the enterocyte and eventually into the bloodstream.

In the intestinal lumen, amino acids are actively transported into the blood by active **Na$^+$-dependent, carrier-mediated** systems similar to those for glucose. These transport systems possess all the characteristics of the glucose system except that they are specific to amino acid transport. Furthermore, there appear to be separate carrier systems specific for certain classes of amino acids, that is, the natural, dibasic, acidic, proline, and phenylalanine-methionine groups. All the characteristics of an active carrier-mediated process exist in these groups, such as competitive inhibition, Na$^+$ dependence, saturation kinetics, and metabolic energy. Some amino acids, such as phenylalanine and the basic amino acids, are absorbed primarily through facilitated diffusion from the lumen to blood.

Lipid Digestion and Absorption

Approximately 95% to 98% of the total dietary lipids consumed are in the form of triglyceride. The remainder is made up of phospholipids, cholesterol, and cholesterol esters. Upon oxidation, lipids yield more than **twice as much energy** per gram than carbohydrates or proteins. Lipids also have a **greater satiety** value than do carbohydrates or proteins, since they tend to remain in the stomach longer and are digested more slowly.

Dietary triglycerides also must be broken down into **simpler molecules** — monoglycerides, fatty acids, and glycerol — to facilitate efficient absorption. A very small fraction of dietary triglyceride is digested in the mouth and stomach by lingual lipase, which is secreted by the salivary glands. However, most triglycerides are digested in the upper small intestine. To accomplish this, **two obstacles** must be overcome. First, the lumen of the upper small bowel consists of an aqueous medium, and triglycerides are not soluble in water. Second, digestive enzymes are proteins and are dissolved in the aqueous environment of the intestinal lumen. Thus triglycerides must be solubilized in the aqueous phase before digestion can occur. This requires a coordinated and efficient series of mechanical and chemical interactive steps that are, for convenience sake, divided into **intraluminal** and **intracellular events.**

Intraluminal Events

Triglyceride is solubilized in the aqueous environment of the lumen by processes shown in Fig. 50-6. This is accomplished by the action of **bile salts,** which are introduced into the lumen by biliary secretion. Bile salts are **amphipathic** molecules, in that they have both hydrophilic and lipophilic properties. Thus they are soluble in both the aqueous and lipid mediums and can solubilize or emulsify lipids in water. Bile salts are also involved in lipid absorption, which will be discussed.

Once triglycerides are emulsified in the aqueous phase, pancreatic lipase catalyzes their further breakdown. **Colipase** serves two important functions: It **complexes** the lipase to the bile salt and the triglyceride to ensure digestion, and it also lowers the **optimal pH** of the enzyme to near the prevailing pH (6 to 7) of the intestinal lumen. The pancreatic lipase cleaves the ester linkage of the fatty acid and glycerol at the 1 and 1′ positions, liberating two free fatty acids and 2-monoglyceride. Occasionally, the ester bond at the 2 position is cleaved, leaving a free glycerol molecule. The resulting lipid substrates are slightly more soluble in the aqueous medium of the lumen than are triglycerides but still require the action of bile salts for complete solubility.

At this point, the **bile salt concentration** in the lumen becomes important. Because of their physiochemical na-

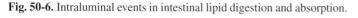

Fig. 50-6. Intraluminal events in intestinal lipid digestion and absorption.

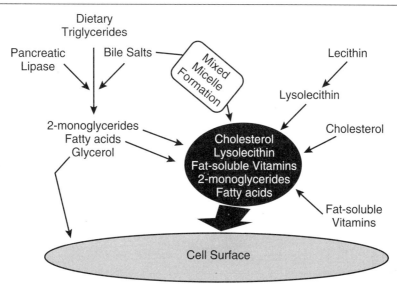

ture, bile salts form **micelles,** which are spherical structures with a diameter of approximately 50Å, above a certain concentration, called the **critical micellar concentration** (CMC). In a micelle, the lipophilic end of bile salt monomers faces inward, creating a **hydrophobic core.** The end-products of triglyceride digestion, namely, the monoglycerides and free fatty acids, are sequestered into the lipid core, which ensures their solubilization in the water medium of the lumen and provides a vehicle for their delivery to the absorbing enterocyte. **Triglycerides** do not partition readily into these micelles and remain in the lumen to be emulsified and digested. **Glycerol,** which is also liberated by triglyceride digestion, does not partition into micelles but is freely dispersed, eventually to be absorbed into the enterocytes by simple diffusion.

Other **dietary lipids** also partition into bile salt micelles. Cholesterol, cholesterol esters, the lipid-soluble vitamins (A, D, E, and K), and the end-products of phospholipid digestion, the lysophospholipids all are sequestered into micelles.

Before discussing lipid absorption and to clarify the integral role bile salt micelles play in this process, certain features of the **aqueous environment** within the lumen of the small intestine will be described. The peristaltic contractions of the intestinal smooth muscle gently move the luminal contents in an aboral direction. In the aqueous environment of the intestine this movement is characteristic of **laminar flow,** in that the flow rate is highest in the center

and lowest near the luminal wall. The centrally moving fluid is referred to as the **bulk-water phase**, while adjacent to the luminal wall, the flow rate is essentially zero and is referred to as the **unstirred water layer.** The thickness of the unstirred water layer varies inversely with the frequency of segmental and propulsive contractions of the intestine. However, it does represent a **diffusional barrier** and slows the movement of absorbable substrates towards the mucosal cell surface. The unstirred water layer would represent a very significant hindrance to lipid absorption in particular, if it were not for the action of bile salts to solubilize absorbable lipids within the micelles. Therefore, lipid-laden micelles gain access to the absorbing surfaces with the same frequency as do other substrates. Through the mixing and churning action created by segmental contractions, micelles contact and adhere to the absorbing cell surface such that lipids freely diffuse out of the lipophilic micellar core and into the lipid matrix of the apical membrane of the enterocyte. Neither bile salt micelles nor any monomeric bile salt molecules diffuse into the cell but are recycled back into the bulk-water phase. The precise mechanisms of micellar adherence, dispersion, and recycling are unknown.

Intracellular Events

The fatty acids sequestered in the apical membrane of enterocytes must be transferred to the cytosol and ultimately

Fig. 50-7. Intracellular events in intestinal lipid absorption.

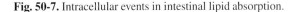

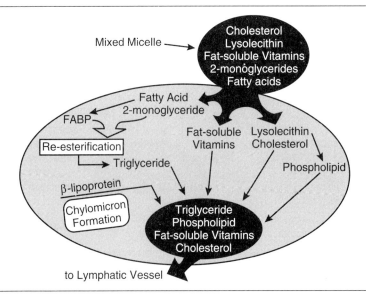

into the bloodstream (Fig. 50-7). Upon entering the cell, an initial event promotes the solubilization of these lipids in the aqueous cytosol. A protein exists in the cytosol of the enterocytes that has a high affinity for these fatty acids. This protein, with a molecular weight of 12,000, is called **fatty acid binding protein** (FABP). It binds fatty acids and transports them into the cytosol, where they are reesterified into triglycerides. Because some fatty acids are known to be toxic in the cytosol, FABP not only transports fatty acids but also protects the cell from any adverse effects. Once fatty acids enter the cell, they are first converted to **acetyl coenzyme A** (CoA), a reaction that requires Mg^{2+}, ATP, and the enzyme acetyl CoA synthetase. In this form, they enter one of two **biosynthetic pathways,** which brings about their reesterification and the resynthesis of triglycerides: the **2-monoglyceride** and the **alpha-glycerol phosphate** pathways. It has been suggested that in humans the 2-monoglyceride pathway is the predominant route of triglyceride resynthesis and the alpha-glycerol phosphate pathway the major route of phospholipid resynthesis.

Before exiting the cell, these re-formed triglycerides, along with cholesterol, cholesterol esters, and various lipoproteins, are packaged into another lipid-carrying particle called a **chylomicron,** which is derived from beta-lipoprotein synthesis in the enterocyte. The phospholipids to be absorbed, along with about 70% of the absorbable free cholesterol, form a monolayer on the surface membrane of the chylomicrons. Chylomicrons vary in size from 700 to 6000 Å depending on how much lipid they contain. The exact mechanism that accomplishes this packaging of lipids in these spheres is unknown. The final intracellular event in **lipid absorption** is the diffu-sion of chylomicrons from the cytosol, through the basolateral membrane, and into the lympathtic channel of the villus, known as the central **lacteal.** From here they are delivered to the systemic circulation through the thoracic duct.

Absorption and Enterohepatic Circulation of Bile Salts

Bile acids are secreted by hepatocytes and collect in the bile canaliculi of liver parenchyma. In the **interdigestive phase,** most bile salts are stored in the gallbladder, and a very small amount leaks into the intestine. During and immediately after a **meal,** the gallbladder empties bile salts into the common bile duct and eventually into the intestinal lumen. In the **small intestine,** bile salts perform their

important actions on lipid digestion and absorption, which are described in the preceding section. Bile salts are eventually absorbed by the small intestine and returned to the liver by means of the **portal circulation.** Upon reaching the **liver,** they are sequestered by **hepatocytes** and recycled through the system. Approximately 95% to 98% of the secreted bile salts are reabsorbed and recirculated in this pathway, called the **enterohepatic circulation.** The remaining 2% to 5% of unabsorbed bile salts enters the colon and is ultimately excreted in the feces. This loss of bile salts is easily replenished by the de novo hepatic synthesis of bile salts. Thus the enterohepatic circulation and hepatic synthesis allow the body to maintain a constant bile salt pool of 3 to 5 g. This pool cycles 5 to 10 times a day; thus it is not unusual for a single bile salt molecule to recycle three times during one meal.

There are **several important factors** that affect the enterohepatic circulation and the maintenance of a bile salt pool. They include (1) the relative impermeability of the upper small bowel to bile salts, (2) the active transport and efficient absorption of bile salts by the terminal ileum, (3) a patent portal blood flow, (4) active sequestration of bile salts from the portal blood by hepatocytes, (5) secretion of bile salts by the liver and storage in the gallbladder, and (6) delivery of bile salts to the intestinal lumen via the biliary system. It is easy to see how a physiologic disturbance in any of these components, such as may result from liver disease or inflammatory bowel disease, will not only seriously affect the bile salt pool but also will markedly compromise lipid digestion and absorption.

The **upper two-thirds of the small intestine** is relatively impermeable to bile salts, and very little absorption takes place there. Thus, although there is still some lipid in this region, more than enough solubilization will be occurring because of the adequate quantities of bile salts, ensuring efficient digestion and the absorption of dietary lipids. As bile salts move into the **lower one-third of the small bowel,** the mucosa becomes more permeable to these substrates, and the monomeric bile salts are absorbed through diffusion, which continues throughout the remaining small intestine. As the luminal concentration falls below the CMC, micelles disperse until all the bile salts exist as monomers. In the **terminal ileum** of humans and most other mammalian species, bile salts are rapidly and efficiently absorbed by an **active Na^+-dependent cotransport system** that is similar to the glucose and amino acid active transport systems operating in the upper small bowel. Thus, by the time a fraction of intestinal contents reaches the ileocecal valve, nearly 98% of the bile salt content has been absorbed into the portal blood.

Vitamins

Lipid-soluble vitamins A, D, E, and K are absorbed with other lipid-soluble nutrients and use the **bile-salt mixed micelle** as a vehicle for their solubilization and transport to the cell surface. The mechanisms involved are the same as those described for lipid absorption. **Water-soluble vitamins** are absorbed by processes similar to those that operate for sugars and amino acids. While few details regarding water-soluble vitamin absorption are available, a few specific mechanisms of absorption of some of these essential substrates are well known.

Vitamin B (thiamine), **vitamin C**, and **folic acid** are absorbed primarily by passive diffusion. At lower concentrations, these vitamins can be actively transported by an active Na^+-dependent process. This process is thought to be carrier-mediated, requiring metabolic energy derived from the hydrolysis of ATP.

Vitamin B_{12} absorption represents a special case. Sufficient absorption requires a glycoprotein called **intrinsic factor,** which is secreted by the parietal cells of the stomach. Once intrinsic factor complexes with vitamin B_{12}, the complex binds to specific receptors on ileal enterocytes and is internalized. Receptor binding of the intrinsic factor–B_{12} complex requires Ca^{2+} or Mg^{2+} and an alkaline pH. The internalization process is not energy dependent and presumably occurs through **pinocytosis.**

A marked decrease in vitamin B_{12} intake or any disease state that diminishes the secretion of intrinsic factor will inhibit or prevent intrinsic factor–B_{12} complexing or binding or will compromise ileal absorption, leading to vitamin B_{12} deficiency. Because this vitamin is important for red blood cell formation and metabolism, if left untreated, vitamin B_{12} deficiency will lead to **pernicious anemia.**

Summary

The human intestine is equipped anatomically and functionally to handle the nearly 9.0 liters of fluid delivered to it daily. The countless numbers of folds and villi endow the human intestine with an absorptive surface area of nearly 2 million cm^2. The epithelial lining absorbs electrolytes through the influence of passive diffusion, ion exchangers, and energy-dependent pumps, creating osmotic gradients for efficient water absorption. Intricate intracellular mechanisms mediated by Ca^{2+} and cAMP precisely regulate these processes. Many, if not most, of these mechanisms are influenced extrinsically by the autonomic nervous network and intrinsically by the enteric nervous system as well as a variety of locally released hormones. Carbohydrates, proteins, and lipids are digested by specific enzymes that are furnished by a variety of sources, including the salivary glands, stomach, pancreas, and intestinal mucosal cells. These many digestive enzymes ensure that dietary nutrients are the right size for efficient absorption. Specific transport mechanisms also exist for the efficient absorption of these digestive end-products. Bile salts play a dual role in lipid digestion and absorption, first by emulsifying triglycerides to facilitate their breakdown by lipases and second by solubilizing free fatty acids, cholesterol, and fat-soluble vitamins for efficient absorption. All the processes described herein are integral components of the total digestive process.

Bibliography

Field, M., Fordtran, J. S., and Schultz, S. G., eds. *Secretory Diarrhea.* Bethesda, Md.: American Physiological Society, 1980.

Fondacaro, J. D. Intestinal electrolyte transport and diarrheal disease. *Am J. Physiol.* 250 (*Gastrointest. Liver Physiol.* 13):G1–G8, 1986.

Fondacaro, J. D. Intestinal absorption of bile acids. In: Kuksis, A., ed., *Fat Absorption.* Boca Raton, Fla.: CRC Press, 1986.

Johnson, L. R., ed. *Physiology of the Gastrointestinal Tract,* 2nd ed. New York: Raven Press, 1987.

Part VIII Questions: Gastrointestinal Physiology

1. The sympathetic innervation of the gut
   A. acts presynaptically to release acetylcholine in the myenteric ganglia.
   B. activates alpha receptors, causing relaxation of sphincter muscles.
   C. tonically relaxes splanchnic vascular smooth muscle.
   D. tonically inhibits secretion by mucosal epithelium.
   E. coreleases NPY which inhibits norepinephrine activity.

2. CCK is a hormone that
   A. stimulates gastric emptying.
   B. inhibits pancreatic bicarbonate secretion.
   C. is pancreozymic.
   D. contracts the sphincter of Oddi.
   E. is released when carbohydrates enter the duodenum.

3. Secretin is a hormone that
   A. is released from the duodenal mucosa by the action of products of protein digestion.
   B. interacts with CCK to inhibit biliary bicarbonate secretion.
   C. acts as an enterogastrone.
   D. causes bile salt secretion.
   E. has growth-promoting effects on the intestinal mucosa.

4. The migrating motor complex
   A. is recorded in the small and large intestines.
   B. occurs randomly throughout the gastrointestinal tract.
   C. is induced by sphincteric relaxation.
   D. is only observed in the fasting state.
   E. is the primary mechanism for moving food throughout the gastrointestinal tract.

5. The basic electrical rhythm of the stomach
   A. is a mechanical force.
   B. determines the slowest rate of peristaltic contractions.
   C. always causes contractions.
   D. determines the maximum rate of peristaltic contractions.

   E. has nothing to do with contractions.

6. Intrinsic factor
   A. forms a complex with dietary vitamin B_{12}.
   B. is secreted by the gastric chief cells.
   C. is essential for absorption of bile salts.
   D. forms a complex with dietary iron.
   E. is required for efficient calcium absorption.

7. The regulation of gastric secretion involves
   A. insulin release.
   B. adrenal glands.
   C. secretions of the duodenum.
   D. bile acids.
   E. ileal receptors.

8. As the rate of pancreatic secretion increases, one would expect the Cl^- concentration in the secretion to
   A. increase.
   B. decrease.
   C. remain unchanged.
   D. parallel the Na^+ concentration.
   E. parallel the K^+ concentration.

9. Which of the following is correct regarding bile acids?
   A. Bile acids are usually present as unconjugated bile acids in bile.
   B. Above a certain concentration, bile acids form macromolecular aggregates called micelles.
   C. Bile acids play a minor role in solubilizing phospholipids and cholesterol in bile.
   D. The ratios between bile acids, phospholipids, and cholesterol in bile vary markedly over broad concentration ranges.

10. Which of the following would be expected to occur in a person with complete lactase deficiency following ingestion of a milk meal?
    A. increased electrolyte and water absorption in the small intestine
    B. decreased sucrose digestion
    C. increased glucose absorption in the colon
    D. the small intestine contents flowing into the colon containing lactose
    E. a decrease in maltose absorption

IX Endocrine Physiology

Part Editor
Lawrence A. Frohman

51 Hormonal and Chemical Transduction of Information

Lawrence A. Frohman

Objectives

After reading this chapter, you should be able to

Distinguish different modes of communication between cellular elements in individual tissues and in different tissues

List the various types of hormones and understand the differences in their modes of biosynthesis

Distinguish how the different classes of hormones are transported through the circulation and the differences in the mechanisms by which they are metabolized

Explain the concept of feedback regulation

Describe the principles of hormone action and distinguish between the action of the various types of hormones

Explain the principle of radioimmunoassay and understand the differences between this assay method and the bioassay and radioreceptor assay in terms of what is actually being measured.

The endocrine system, together with the nervous system, has evolved to provide a means of communication between cells and organs. As single-cell organisms have developed into multicellular organisms, the endocrine system has assumed a critical role in the regulation of many processes crucial to life, including growth and development, metabolic homeostasis, reproduction, and responses to environmental perturbations such as stress. The evolutionary increases in size and complexity of organisms made it impractical for all cells to have direct contact with each other, such as occurs within the nervous system, and thus a hormone signaling system was required.

Endocrine glands are known as the **glands of internal secretion** or the **ductless glands.** A hormone is, in the strict sense, a substance that is secreted by one cell and transported in the circulation to act on other cells.

The classic definition of a hormone has required modification in recent years as substances defined as hormones have been shown to exert actions in multiple settings. Thus the same chemical compound also may function as a neu-

rotransmitter in synaptic clefts (**neurocrine**), by exerting its effects on neighboring cells (**paracrine**), or on itself (**autocrine**). This multiplicity of function underscores an important concept in endocrinology: The same hormone may cause multiple effects by means of separate modes of action which are coordinated with one another, subserving a single homeostatic or reproductive function. For example, norepinephrine, acting as a hormone, inhibits insulin secretion by the pancreatic beta cells and, as a neurotransmitter, enhances hepatic glucose output, both of which result in hyperglycemia. In a similar manner, gonadotropin hormone–releasing hormone, acting as a hypothalamic hormone, stimulates the release of luteinizing hormone and follicle-stimulating hormone from the pituitary and, as a neurotransmitter acting in the brain, stimulates sexual behavior. Thus chemical compounds present in simple organisms and serving as cell-to-cell communicators have been coopted as hormones to reach distant parts of the body via the circulatory system to exert coordinated effects necessary for life.

Hormone Biosynthesis and Secretion

Hormones can be divided into three chemical types: peptides and proteins, steroids, and modified amino acids. The first group includes primarily neuropeptides, pituitary hormones, and gastroenteropancreatic hormones; the second consists of adrenal and gonadal steroids and vitamin D; and the third comprises thyroid hormones and catecholamines.

The biosynthesis of hormones is cell-type specific, though many hormones are synthesized in more than one type of cell. The **protein hormones** are synthesized by stimulation of gene expression, transcription of messenger RNA (mRNA), and ribosomal translation of the mRNA to generate a hormone precursor. The hormone percursor is characterized by an amino-terminal sequence (signal peptide) that contains processing information to ensure that the protein enters the rough endoplasmic reticulum and is enveloped in a secretory granule to facilitate exocytosis (secretion). This multiplicity of events provides many opportunities for variations to occur. For example, a single mRNA precursor may be differentially spliced in individual tissues to provide separate mature mRNA species (e.g., calcitonin mRNA is generated in the C cells of the thyroid, and calcitonin gene–related product mRNA is formed in the brain from the same mRNA precursor). A single protein hormone precursor also may generate one or more hormones (e.g., ACTH and beta-lipotropin, vasoactive intestinal peptide, and peptide histidine-methiodine) and also may give rise to multiple forms of the hormone (e.g., somatostatin[1-28] and somatostatin[1-14]). Finally, **peptide hormones** undergo posttranslational processing in which they are glycosylated (thyroid-stimulating hormone and the gonadotropins) or complexed with metal ions (insulin with the zinc ion). The hormones are packed in secretory granules that migrate to the cell surface while final processing occurs. Thus, under conditions of stimulated secretion, intracellular transit time is shortened and hormone precursors are frequently secreted (Fig. 51-1).

Steroid hormone biosynthesis is initiated by cholesterol side-chain cleavage, the rate-limiting step in steroidogenesis, followed by a cytochrome c P_{450}-linked

Fig. 51-1. Intracellular transport and secretory pathways in a protein-secreting endocrine cell (RER = rough endoplasmic reticulum; SER = smooth endoplasmic reticulum; Golgi = Golgi complex). Proteins are synthesized on polyribosomes attached to the endoplasmic reticulum and directed through the membrane to the cisternal space. Shuttling vesicles are formed from the endoplasmic reticulum and transported to and incorporated by the Golgi complex, where secretory granules are formed. Granules are then transported to the plasma membrane where they fuse with the membrane, leading to exocytosis and resulting in discharge of the granule contents into the extracellular space. Secretion may also occur by transport of secretory vesicles and both immature and mature granules. Some granules are taken up by lysosomes and degraded (crinophagy) without ever being secreted. (From: Gill, G. N. In: Felig, P., Baxter, J. D., and Frohman, L. A., eds. *Endocrinology and Metabolism,* New York: McGraw-Hill, 1995.)

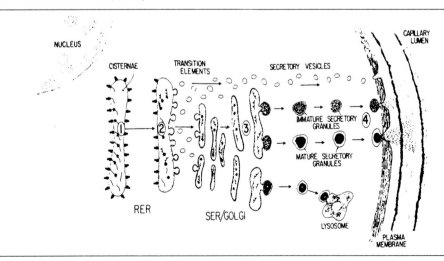

dehydrogenase–isomerase complex and several hydroxy-lases. Biosynthesis requires the shuttling of intermediary compounds between the mitochondria and the endoplasmic reticulum. The cell specificity of certain enzymes explains why various steroid hormones are synthesized only in selected cell types. Vitamin D synthesis, in contrast, requires transport of the precursor between several different organs (skin, liver, and kidney), each of which contains specific enzymes required for biosynthesis. While most steroids are secreted in the biologically active form, further processing to more active forms occurs in some target tissues (e.g., testosterone is converted to 5α-dihydrotestosterone in skin and male reproductive tissues). In contrast to peptide hormones, there is limited storage of steroid hormones in their cells of origin. Thus a stimulus to hormone secretion is intimately linked to new hormone synthesis.

The two distinct categories of **modified amino acid hormones** (monoamines) also have different biosynthetic mechanisms. The catecholamines, consisting of dopamine, norepinephrine, and epinephrine, are derived from the amino acid tyrosine by a series of enzymatic conversions involving a hydroxylase, a decarboxylase, and a methyl transferase. A second set of monoamines, serotonin and melatonin, is derived from the amino acid tryptophan by a similar series of reactions. These hormones are stored in neurosecretory granules in nerve terminals and specialized cell types (pinealocytes and adrenal medulla), from which they are released upon stimulation.

Thyroid hormones are iodinated derivatives of tyrosine. They are formed only in the thyroid gland, by the unique mechanism of iodination of tyrosine residues on a large protein, thyroglobulin. A large storage pool of thyroglobulin, known as **colloid,** exists within the follicular lumen of the thyroid cells. The process of secretion thus requires reabsorption of thyroglobulin, its enzymatic degradation, and release of the two forms of the hormone, thyroxine (T_4) and triiodothyronine (T_3). T_4 is actually a hormone precursor (**prohormone**), since it is much less bioactive than is T_3. An enzymatic mechanism exists for its conversion to T_3 in peripheral tissues.

Hormone Transport and Metabolism

Separate mechanisms exist for transport of the different hormone types in circulation. Many peptide and protein hormones, which are water soluble, do not require transport proteins and exist in their natural state. Others, such as insulin-like growth factors, are almost completely bound

to a carrier protein. These proteins may be present uniquely in circulation or may be similar to tissue hormone receptors (the plasma growth hormone–binding protein is identical to the extracellular domain of the growth hormone receptor).

Steroid and thyroid hormones, in contrast, are tightly bound to specific binding proteins that provide a pool of circulating hormone that, particularly for the thyroid hormones, has a relatively prolonged half-life (several days). Their presence serves to increase the period that a hormone remains in the circulation, thereby providing another readily available reservoir of hormone for biologic action. Protein-bound hormone is in equilibrium with free hormone in the circulation, and it is the free hormone that is the most important determinant of the hormone's biologic activity. Thus individuals with a genetic deficiency of thyroid-binding globulin (TBG) have decreased total T_4 levels in plasma, but their free T_4 levels are normal and they show no evidence of thyroid hormone deficiency. Binding proteins are synthesized in a regulated manner in the liver and may bind multiple hormones (e.g., cortisol-binding globulin also serves as the binding protein for progesterone; testosterone and estrogen both bind to the sex hormone–binding globulin; and both T_3 and T_4 bind to TBG).

Hormones are also metabolized by specific mechanisms. Peptide hormones and some protein hormones are degraded by circulating and tissue peptidases that destroy the hormone's biologic activity by cleavage at critical locations in the molecule. The specific enzymes involved are numerous, though not unique. The half-life of most peptide hormones is on the order of 1 to 20 minutes, and although small amounts of some hormones are recovered intact in the urine, indicating renal clearance, most degradation occurs intravascularly. Some of the bigger protein hormones, particularly those which are glycosylated (e.g., the gonadotropins), are cleared intact by the kidneys and found in large quantities in the urine. Peptide hormones are also metabolized at the site of their action. They are internalized and transported to intracellular lysosomes where they are degraded.

Steroid hormones are metabolized primarily by reduction or hydroxylation, mainly in the liver, to biologically inactive metabolites, which are then often sulfated or glucuronidated before being excreted in the urine. Less than 1% of cortisol, for example, is excreted intact.

Catecholamines and indolamines are metabolized in the synaptic cleft and in circulation primarily by monoamine oxidation and transmethylation. However, termination of action of the monoamines at the synaptic cleft occurs primarily by reuptake into nerve terminals. Thyroid hormones are metabolized in target organ tissues by means of two separate deiodinases, one of which is the same enzyme that converts T_4 to T_3.

Regulation of Hormone Secretion: The Feedback Concept

The control of hormone secretion involves multiple factors, including external neural inputs, endogenous neural rhythmicity, circulating substrate concentrations and hormones, and other products of the target glands on which the hormones act (Fig. 51-2). Each of the various hormone systems (e.g., those mediating growth, metabolic homeostasis, stress, reproduction, and water and electrolyte balance) has its own unique regulatory mechanisms. However, certain

Fig. 51-2. Endocrine gland organization. The signals flow from the central nervous system, through the hypothalamus, the pituitary, and the target glands in order to achieve the desired effect: hormone action on peripheral tissue. A complex feedback system exists that is mediated by any or all of the hormones in the cascade or by the physiologic action mediated by the hormones. Feedback effects may occur at one or more loci, though not all of the possible sites are effective for any particular hormonal system.

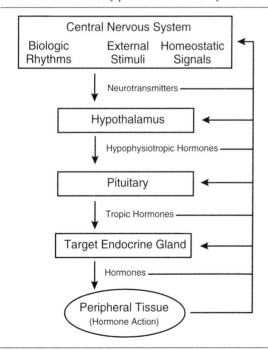

general principles apply. First, the cascade of responses is usually initiated by hypothalamic releasing and inhibiting hormones that are secreted in a pulsatile manner, which reflects neuronal activity. Their half-lives are extremely short, and their concentrations vary considerably within short periods. Second, their effects on the pituitary are greatly influenced by the ambient concentrations of target gland hormones — primarily but not exclusively those in the same hormonal system. Third, levels of circulating target gland hormones change in a smoother manner, with less short-term fluctuation, than do those of hypothalamic or pituitary hormones. Their effects "feed back" on both hypothalamic and pituitary hormone secretion. The acute effects are usually inhibitory and relate to hormone release, while the longer-term effects, which influence hormone synthesis, may be either inhibitory or stimulatory. Thus removal of a target gland will cause elevated levels of the hormones upstream in the particular axis (e.g., adrenalectomy increases the secretion of both corticotropin-releasing hormone and ACTH). These feedback effects are unique for each hormone system, and their disturbances constitute the basis for many endocrine diseases. Knowledge of **feedback concepts** also has formed the basis for diagnostic tests to assess hormone secretory status.

Hormone Receptors and Hormone Action

In order for hormones to act only on their target cells, a specific mechanism of interaction was required and this led to the development of **hormone receptors.** These proteins, to which hormones bind, are present in multiple cell compartments (surface membranes, cytoplasm, and nucleus) and serve two functions. First, they are required for selectivity; they have three-dimensional shapes or conformations that allow them to distinguish the particular hormone that they bind from among the many other substances in the circulation or extracellular environment. Second, they are connected to an effector mechanism; they must transmit a signal to the interior of the cell or compartment to activate the processes that are stimulated by hormones. In many ways, hormone receptors are similar to enzyme systems. Their conformation is changed in response to hormone binding, and this leads to activation of a tightly coupled enzyme system that serves as an amplifier. Several peptide hormone receptors function as enzymes or as substrates for enzymes. In the cytoplasm, multiple "second-messenger" systems have evolved to serve these purposes, while in the nucleus, the hormone-receptor complex binds to DNA and regulates gene expression (Fig. 51-3).

The hormone receptor, therefore, has two important domains: that which recognizes and binds to the hormone and that which couples to the **effector mechanism.** Peptide and monoamine hormone receptors are located on the plasma membrane with the hormone-binding domain located extracellularly and the effector domain located intracellularly. The receptor-binding affinity must be high, since there is frequently competition for hormone binding with plasma-binding proteins. Binding is rapid and reversible. Although there is evidence for internalization of the hormone-receptor complex, this process is not required for the initiation of hormone action after binding and may represent primarily a means of terminating hormone action. The concentration of most receptors is greater than that required for the full biologic effects of the hormone. Thus maximal effects of hormones are generally observed at a receptor occupancy of only 30% to 50%.

The effector domain of the receptor is tightly coupled to the regulatory portion of the effector enzymes and ion channels, which are located on the inner surface of the plasma membrane. These effector systems, in turn, control the production of cyclic nucleotides, the breakdown of phospholipids, membrane transport systems, and ion fluxes. They also may be coupled to high-energy phosphorylation of proteins (including the receptor itself), which mediate other cell processes such as the synthesis,

Fig. 51-3. Target cell activation by hormones acting at membrane receptors (monoamine transmitters, peptide and protein hormones, and growth factors) or cytoplasmic and nuclear receptors (thyroid and steroid hormones). The membrane receptors are coupled by guanine nucleotide regulatory proteins to one of several second-messenger systems for the stimulation of phosphorylation, through which their actions are mediated. The intracellular receptors exhibit a change in conformation after binding to their respective hormones and then bind to specific sites (response elements) on DNA for regulation of gene transcription. Protein hormone and growth factor receptors are often phosphorylated, act as tyrosine kinases, and phosphorylate other intracellular messengers leading to nuclear and cytoplasmic actions (mRNA = messenger RNA; cAMP = cyclic adenosine 5'-monophosphate; IP_3 = inositol triphosphate).

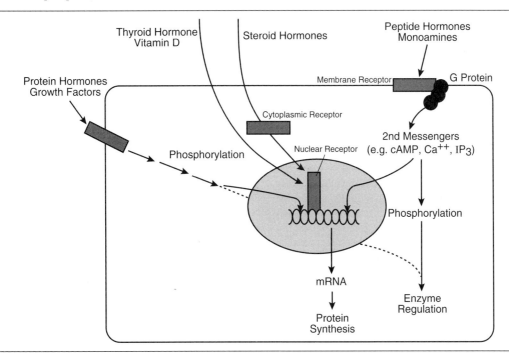

transport, and metabolism of molecules critical for cell viability.

There are numerous **second-messenger systems** associated with plasma membrane receptors, including adenylate cyclase, guanylate cyclase, phospholipase C, protein kinase C, calcium mobilization, ion channel activation, and tyrosine phosphorylation. Many hormone receptors are coupled to multiple mechanisms with a single cell. This interaction is mediated by guanyl nucleotide regulatory proteins. These proteins, which may exhibit either a stimulatory or an inhibitory action, perform a major role in transmembrane signaling that is common to all peptide and monoamine hormone receptors.

Nearly all hormone-regulated cells respond to changes in ambient hormone concentrations by altering the number or affinity, or both, of their cell surface receptors. This phenomenon is most evident when the cell is exposed to high concentrations of the hormone and results primarily in a decrease in receptor-binding sites, leading to a corresponding decrease in the cellular response to the hormone. This decrease is caused both by internalization (endocytosis) of the hormone-receptor complex and by alterations in the dissociation of the complex, making the receptor unavailable for subsequent binding to fresh hormone. Thus exposure of target cells to hormones initiates a local feedback response that limits the cellular effects of the hormone by limiting its ability to initiate the signaling process.

Steroid hormones enter cells by passive diffusion through cell membranes rather than by a transport-mediated process. They bind to specific intracellular receptors that are then translocated into the nucleus. Receptors may exist in the nucleus, even when unbound. Receptor occupation results in a conformational change that increases its affinity to bind to DNA. Specific binding sites are present on regions of genes, frequently upstream from the initiation site of transcription. The binding of the steroid-receptor complex to the specific genomic response element enhances the rate of initiation of mRNA transcription. In addition, effects of the hormone-receptor complex on the other genes can affect the stability of specific mRNAs, thereby enhancing gene expression by an additional mechanism.

Although T_3-binding proteins have been identified in both cytoplasm and mitochondria, the most important actions of T_3 are mediated by nuclear-binding proteins. These receptors, when bound to T_3, attach to a thyroid response element in the gene in a manner similar to that of steroid receptors and result in increased RNA transcription. Many genes have response elements for both T_3 and steroid receptors, and the two systems frequently work in conjunction with one another. Consequently, the amplification of gene expression seen in the presence of both steroid and thyroid hormones can be considerably greater than the sum of the effects of either hormone alone.

Hormone Measurement

The measurement of hormones in tissues and circulating fluids has undergone many changes during the past several decades. Initial assays were based on the biologic properties of the hormones using in vivo tests that were imprecise and insensitive. The ability to label pure hormones and to generate high-affinity antihormone antibodies led to development of the technique of **radioimmunoassay** (RIA), which has become the mainstay of hormone measurements. Concomitantly, more sensitive and precise bioassays evolved, which are also currently in use, though not for routine clinical diagnosis and treatment because of their complexity and expense. Newer techniques based on nonisotopic measurements have been introduced recently. Their concepts, advantages, and pitfalls are described in the next section.

Bioassays

Initial bioassays were based on in vivo animal models, in which graded doses of the hormone were injected and the biologic response quantified. In addition to the large variability created by the imprecision of the techniques, these assay systems were frequently incapable of distinguishing between multiple hormones that had overlapping effects. In vitro culture systems that permit detection of specific biochemical effects of hormone action at the cellular level have a sensitivity comparable with or even greater than what RIA has achieved. This method is generally regarded as the "gold standard" because it measures the hormone's biologic activity rather than its chemical or immunologic reactivity. This is of considerable importance because it is possible to have subtle modifications in the chemical composition of a hormone that are undetectable by any method other than bioassay. One caveat that must be remembered with regard to any bioassay relates to its specificity. While the effects may appear to be specific to all known substances, a yet unidentified compound (hormone) may exhibit similar biologic properties in the particular system and its presence erroneously attributed to the hormone for which the bioassay was designed. A second caveat relates to the nature of the bioassay system. Some substances will exhibit biologic activity in a particular in vitro bioassay system, though not in others or in vivo. Thus extrapolation of in vitro results must be done with caution. One of the current major applications for in vitro bioassays is in screening synthetic hormone analogues for agonist and antagonist properties.

Radioimmunoassays

The concept of RIA was developed nearly 30 years ago by Berson and Yalow and virtually revolutionized the field of hormone measurements. The technique spread rapidly to other disciplines and is currently the most commonly used system for measuring peptide, protein, steroid, and thyroid hormone concentrations, as well as numerous other natural and synthetic compounds. The principle of this technique is based on the competition of a labeled ligand (hormone) with an unlabeled ligand for a fixed number of binding sites on a specific antibody (Fig. 51-4). The quantity of radiolabeled ligand bound is inversely related to the quantity of competing nonradiolabeled hormone and permits the generation of a standard curve from which the unknown samples can be quantified. The most commonly used label is iodine 125. The introduction of chemiluminescent labels has provided even greater sensitivity and has diminished the need for radioisotopes.

The antibodies developed for RIA require a high affinity as well as capacity and have been produced successfully in a variety of species. The binding reaction is reversible and can be performed under both equilibrium and nonequilibrium conditions, with the latter providing greater sensitivity. A number of physicochemical separation methods have been used to separate antibody-bound from free hormone, though the most commonly used technique at present is a coprecipitation reaction using an antibody generated in a second species against immunoglobulins of the species of the primary antibody.

Although the precision and sensitivity of RIAs are generally very high and repeated measurements over short time intervals can be performed readily using small quantities of serum, there are many limitations to the use of RIA, some of which were not initially apparent. The radioiodinated ligand is the most vulnerable component of the assay. If addition of the iodine atom alters the chemical stability or immunologic properties of the hormone, competition between the radioligand and the unlabeled hormone in serum may be altered, yielding incorrect results. Certain sera contain protein components that may alter binding of the ligand to the antibody, artificially elevating or reducing the calculated value. Plasma peptidases may

Fig. 51-4. The principle of radioimmunoassay. Labeled antigen (hormone) competes with unlabeled antigen (endogenous hormone) for binding to a limited number of sites on specific antihormone (anti-IGG) antibodies. A second antibody directed against the primary antibody is then used for precipitation of the bound complex. Other physico-chemical methods of separation of free from bound hormone may also be used. Increasing amounts of unlabeled hormone result in progressive displacement of labeled hormone from antibody. With careful selection of antibodies, labeling techniques, and incubation conditions, sensitivities in the low picomolar range can be readily achieved.

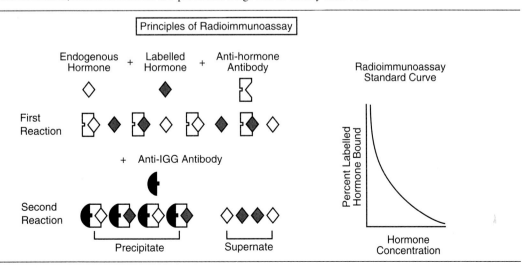

degrade the radioligand or the endogenous hormone during the incubation period, leading to unpredictable results. Circulating hormone fragments that are biologically inactive or other hormones with common sequences may compete for binding with the radioligand. Endogenous antibodies to the hormone (e.g., diabetics receiving insulin) or to the primary antibody species (e.g., animal handlers exposed to rabbits) may markedly alter the ratio of bound to free hormone. Therefore, careful attention must be given to the assay conditions so that the results can be interpreted with confidence. Despite these limitations, however, this technique, more than any other, has contributed to our knowledge of endocrine physiology in experimental animals and in humans.

Radioreceptor Assays

The **radioreceptor assay** differs from the RIA in that a hormone receptor is substituted for the antihormone antibody. This assay has been used primarily for peptide and protein hormone measurement and has the advantage that it measures biologically active hormone. The results of such assays are not always comparable with those of RIAs, since the antibody and receptor may bind different portions of the hormone. The technique is generally less sensitive than RIA, and receptor preparation and storage are technically more difficult. In addition, radioiodination of the peptide may modify its receptor-binding site. However, use of this assay in conjunction with RIA has led to important new concepts related to alterations in the biologic activity of secreted hormones (e.g., the degree of glycosylation of gonadotropins secreted at different times of the menstrual cycle varies, influencing its radioreceptor binding, biologic activity but not its RIA activity).

Summary

Hormones have evolved as the mediators of communication between cells located at great distances in multicellular organisms. They are identical to or derived from chemicals that are used for local cell to cell communication. They function in groups, affecting the major physiologic processes necessary for life, including growth, metabolism, reproduction, and adaptation to the external environment. Their action is initiated by binding to specific cellular receptors that are coupled to second-messenger effector mechanisms, which amplify important cellular cytoplasmic processes, or to nuclear receptors that interact with specific DNA regulatory elements to initiate RNA transcription. Numerous sensitive techniques have been developed for hormone measurement that allow assessment of their storage, secretion, and metabolism.

Bibliography

Baxter, J. D., Frohman, L. A., and Felig, P. Introduction to the endocrine system. In: Felig, P., Baxter, J. D., and Frohman, L. A., eds. *Endocrinology and Metabolism,* 3rd ed. New York: McGraw-Hill, 1995.

Catt, K. J. Molecular mechanisms of hormone action: Control of target cell function by peptide, steroid, and thyroid hormones. In: Felig, P., Baxter, J. D., and Frohman, L. A., eds., *Endocrinology and Metabolism,* 3rd ed. New York: McGraw-Hill, 1995.

Clark, J. H., Schrader, W. T., and O'Malley, B. W. Mechanisms of action of steroid hormones. In: Wilson, G. D., and Foster D. W., eds., *Williams Textbook of Endocrinology,* 8th ed. Philadelphia: W. B. Saunders, 1992. Pp. 35–90.

Gill, G. N. Biosynthesis, secretion and metabolism of hormones. In: Felig, P. A., Baxter, J. D., and Frohman, L. A., eds., *Endocrinology and Metabolism,* 3rd ed. New York: McGraw-Hill, 1995.

Roth, J., and Grunfeld, C. Mechanism of action of hormones that act at the cell surface. In: Wilson, G. D., and Foster, D. W., eds., *Williams Textbook of Endocrinology,* 8th ed. Philadelphia: W. B. Saunders 1992. Pp. 91–134.

52 The Hypothalamus and Neuroendocrinology

Lawrence A. Frohman

Objectives

After reading this chapter, you should be able to

List the different neuroregulatory systems in which the hypothalamus participates and distinguish their differences

Describe the origin of the blood supply to the pituitary and its functional importance

List the hypophysiotropic hormones of the hypothalamus and the pituitary hormones that they regulate

Identify the mechanisms used by hypothalamic hormones to alter pituitary hormone secretion

Describe the individual hypothalamic-pituitary-target gland axes, the hormones involved, and the functions they serve

Characterize the role of cytokines in neuroendocrine activation

---

Considerable regulatory control of hormonal secretion and metabolic processes is exerted by the CNS. The integration of this control occurs in the **ventromedial hypothalamus,** known as the **hypophysiotropic area,** and consists of three major components.

The first is a **neuroendocrine** system involving clusters of peptide- and monoamine-secreting neurons in the anterior and medial (periventricular) ventral hypothalamus, whose products are transported along nerve fibers to terminals in the outer layer of the median eminence. The releasing and inhibiting hormones are secreted into capillaries of the hypothalamic-hypophyseal portal vascular system and transported to the pituitary, where they regulate the secretion of the anterior pituitary hormones.

The second component is a **neurohypophysial pathway** from selected nuclear regions in the anterior hypothalamus that traverses the floor of the ventral hypothalamus and pituitary stalk and terminates in specialized neuronal elements, called pituicytes, located in the posterior pituitary. This system is responsible for **osmoregulation** mediated by the secretion of **vasopressin** (antidiuretic hormone) and for **parturition** and **nursing,** which are mediated by the secretion of **oxytocin.** A more detailed discussion of this system is found in Chap. 54.

The third aspect is a **neurometabolic pathway** with bidirectional fibers that traverses the base of the brain and autonomic nervous system pathways of the spinal cord and terminates in the liver, gastrointestinal tract, pancreas, adrenal medullae, and adipose tissue. The primary effects of this pathway are on **substrate regulation** (e.g., glucose, fatty acids, and amino acids) and on **metabolic homeostasis,** consisting of the control of food intake (satiety), temperature (thermoregulation), and body fat stores (nutrient regulation).

Anatomic

Hypothalamus

The neuronal **perikarya** (cell bodies) of the neuroendocrine system are distributed throughout the mediobasal hypothalamus. Although the hypophysiotropic hormone–secreting neurons receive input from many brain regions in response to external environmental changes, they maintain their secretory activity even in the absence of extrahypothalamic input, indicating that their most important homeostatic signals are derived from the circulation. Neuronal perikarya that secrete thyrotropin-releasing hormone (TRH), corticotropin-releasing hormone (CRH), and somatotropin release–inhibiting factor (somatostatin, SRIF) are located in the **anterior hypothalamus,** in the region of the **paraventricular nucleus.** Those secreting growth hormone–releasing hormone (GRH) are located almost exclusively in the **arcuate nucleus,** which also contains the perikarya of gonadotropin-releasing hormone (GnRH) neurons. Dopamine-secreting neurons arise from the **tuberoinfundibular tract,** and those releasing a recently identified prolactin-inhibiting factor exhibit an identical distribution to those secreting GnRH.

The releasing and inhibiting hormones are **axonally transported** and stored in nerve terminals in the outer layer of the **median eminence,** where their concentrations are many times greater than those in other hypothalamic regions. When stimulated, the nerve terminals release their contents into the **portal capillaries,** which transport the hormones to the **pituitary** (Fig. 52-1). Because portal blood flow is not compartmentalized, the various cell types in the anterior pituitary have access to all the releasing and inhibiting hormones. Thus **specificity of action** is achieved by the presence of specific hormone receptors on individual cell types rather than by anatomic segregation.

Neurons composing the neurohypophysial system are anatomically more distinct, with neuronal perikarya located in the paraventricular and supraoptic nuclei of the **anterior hypothalamus.** The **cell bodies** are large (magnocellular) in contrast to the releasing hormone–secreting cells (parvicellular). The posterior pituitary hormones are synthesized in cell bodies as part of a precursor molecule, which also contains their carrier proteins, known as **neurophysins.** During transport from the hypothalamus to the posterior pituitary, the precursor molecules are converted into mature hormones, and in the pituicytes of the posterior pituitary, they are packaged into **secretory granules,** which are released in response to stimulation of the receptors on the cell bodies in the hypothalamus.

The **neurometabolic functions** of the hypothalamus are closely tied to the sympathetic and parasympathetic components of the **autonomic nervous system.** The hypothalamus is divided into a **medial sympathetic** and a **lateral parasympathetic zone,** though the neuronal perikarya involved with a specific function cannot always be localized to one precise nuclear region. Those neurons participating in the inhibitory **control of food intake** (satiety) tend to be located more medially, while those concerned with the

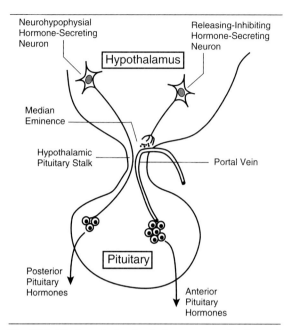

Fig. 52-1. The hypothalamic-pituitary neuroendocrine and neurohypophysial systems.

stimulation of appetite are located more laterally. This distribution helps explain why destructive lesions of the hypothalamus, which frequently occur in the midline, are more likely to cause obesity than anorexia or starvation, because they abolish satiety control. In addition, some fiber tracts from these hypothalamic regulatory centers cross the midline, which protects the organism from interruption of normal regulatory control unless there is bilateral hypothalamic destruction.

Portal Vascular System

The blood supply of the anterior pituitary is distinct from that of the posterior pituitary and the CNS, in that it is not directly connected with the systemic arterial system. All **arterial blood** flows first through the hypothalamic arteries, which give rise to an extensive capillary plexus in the outer layer of the median eminence, juxtaposed to the nerve terminals of the hypophysiotropic hormone–secreting neurons. The **blood-brain barrier** in this region of the brain is incomplete, permitting access of charged particles and proteins in circulating plasma to the interstitial areas of the ventral hypothalamus and nerve terminals in the median eminence. This allows the nerve terminals and their neuronal perikarya to respond to changes in circulating hormones and metabolic signals, in addition to CNS-derived signals. The portal capillaries combine to form a series of portal veins that descend through the portal stalk and reach the anterior pituitary, where they again give rise to a series of capillaries that bathe the pituitary cells. **Venous drainage** from this system enters the posterior pituitary and eventually reaches the systemic veins in the region of the petrosal sinus. Some blood flow travels in a reverse direction, from the posterior pituitary to the anterior pituitary, though the physiologic significance of this circulation with respect to anterior pituitary hormone secretion is unknown. Similarly, some of the anterior pituitary venous drainage seems to ascend the pituitary stalk, though it does not appear to reach the level of the median eminence.

Hypothalamic Hormones

Structure and Synthesis

The hypothalamic hormones that regulate **anterior pituitary hormone** secretion and their overall effects on the individual pituitary hormones are shown in Fig. 52-2. The control of most of the pituitary hormones involves multiple hypothalamic hormones (some of which remain to be identified). In addition, there are stimulatory and inhibitory hypothalamic hormones for several pituitary hormones, and single hypothalamic hormones have effects on multiple pituitary hormones.

Fig. 52-2. Hypothalamic hormone and pituitary hormone relationships. Hormones boxed in interrupted lines have not been fully characterized (CRH = corticotropin-releasing hormone; VP = vasopressin; GnRH = gonadotropin-releasing hormone; GRH = growth hormone–releasing hormone; SRIF = somatostatin; TRH = thyrotropin-releasing hormone; PRF = prolactin-releasing factor; PIF = prolactin-inhibiting factor; DA = dopamine; Prl = prolactin; ACTH = adrenocorticotropic hormone; LH = luteinizing hormone; FSH = follicle-stimulating hormone; GH = growth hormone; TSH = thyroid-stimulating hormone).

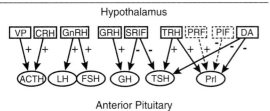

Hypothalamus

Anterior Pituitary

The predominant effect of the hypothalamic hormones on the pituitary, with a single exception, is **stimulatory.** Therefore, disruption of the integrity of the hypothalamic-pituitary interconnection decreases the secretion of pituitary hormones. The control of **prolactin** secretion is the exception; elimination of the hypothalamic input increases hormone release.

All the hypothalamic hormones, again with a single exception, are **single-chain peptides** with sequence lengths ranging from 3 to 44 amino acids (Fig. 52-3). While the smaller peptides (TRH and GnRH) show almost no species variation, each of the larger peptides exhibits either variable chain length (SRIF and GRH) or a small to moderate variation among species (GRH and CRH). Two candidates for prolactin-releasing and prolactin-inhibiting factors are actually contained within the structure of a larger precursor that also gives rise to other neuropeptides. **Vasoactive intestinal peptide** (VIP) stimulates prolactin release and has the same precursor as peptide histidine-isoleucine. A putative prolactin-inhibiting peptide is located on the C-terminal extension of GnRH (GnRH-associated peptide). In addition, a partially characterized peptide in the neurointermediate lobe of the pituitary also exhibits potent prolactin-releasing effects. The single nonpeptide hypophysiotropic hormone is **dopamine.** This catecholamine, besides its important role as a neurotransmitter, is the most important physiologic inhibitor of prolactin secretion.

Each of the peptide hormones is derived from a **precursor molecule.** There is a single copy of the hypothalamic hormone on each precursor (except for TRH, where multiple copies are present), and processing of the precursor is believed to occur in the neuronal perikarya and also during transport along the axon fibers. **Differential processing** of the precursor is believed to account for the generation of those hormones which exist in multiple forms. While the processing enzymes remain to be identified, they are not unique to the specific hypothalamic neurons, since GRH, CRH, TRH, and SRIF have each been observed in nonneural tissue under normal conditions (placenta, pancreatic islets, C cells of thyroid) and in certain pathologic states (ectopic hormone secretion).

Regulation of Secretion: Role of Biogenic Amines and Neuropeptides

The hypothalamic hormone–secreting neurons have been called **transducer cells** because they possess both neural and endocrine characteristics. Although they respond

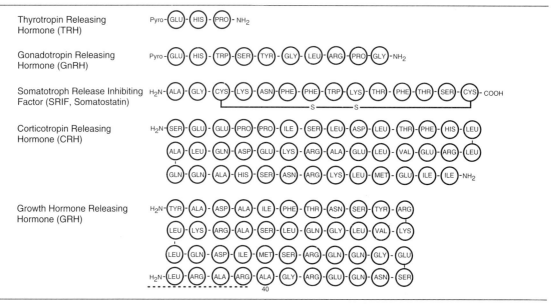

Fig. 52-3. Structures of hypothalamic-releasing and -inhibiting hormones. The sequences of thyrotropin-releasing hormone, gonadotropin-releasing hormone, and somatostatin (somatotropin release–inhibiting factor) are identical in all mammalian species studied. The sequence of human corticotropin-releasing hormone (CRH) has been deduced from that of its complementary DNA and differs by 7 amino acids from ovine CRH. Two forms of growth hormone-releasing hormone have been identified in humans, which differ only by the additional carboxyl-terminal tetrapeptide, indicated by the interrupted line. Sequences in most large mammals show small variations, while those in rodents differ by more than 30 percent. (From: Frohman, L. A., and Krieger, D. T. Neuroendocrine physiology and disease. In: Felig, P., et al., eds. *Endocrinology and Metabolism.* New York: McGraw-Hill, 1987. P. 200.)

to classic neurotransmitter-mediated signals, they release peptide hormones into a regional or, in some cases, systemic vascular system. The neurotransmitter signals used for communication throughout the CNS — monoamines and neuropeptides — also regulate hypothalamic hormone secretion. Their effects may occur at axodendritic interactions and at axoaxonic connections on the releasing hormone–containing nerve terminals. Multiple neurotransmitters and neuropeptides may participate in the release of a single hypothalamic hormone, and intermediary neurons also may be involved.

The **monoamines** participating in the neuroregulation of hypothalamic hormones include catecholamines (dopamine, norepinephrine, epinephrine), indolamines (serotonin, melatonin), acetylcholine, gamma-aminobutyric acid (GABA), histamine, and glutamine. A detailed discussion of their synthesis and action is beyond the scope of this chapter. However, it is important to remember that agents used to modify their function, including synthesis blockers, receptor agonists and antagonists, reuptake inhibitors, and degradative enzyme inhibitors, are all capable of modifying hypothalamic hormone secretion and pituitary function.

Numerous **neuropeptides** have been identified in the hypothalamus and are capable of influencing hypothalamic hormone secretion. They are listed in Table 52-1. Many of these peptides are also widely distributed in extraneural tissue, particularly in the gastrointestinal tract where they exert independent actions. Several can be traced back in evolution to unicellular organisms, underscoring their importance in intercellular communication. Overall, they appear to be crucial in a number of integrative systems relating to homeostatic mechanisms, such as nutrition, growth, and reproduction, and their actions in the CNS complement those exhibited in extraneural tissues. The hypothalamic-releasing hormones themselves are included in this category because they also serve as neurotransmitters and neuromodulators within the CNS.

Pattern of Hypothalamic Hormone Secretion

Hypothalamic hormone levels in portal vessels have been measured in several animal species, and the results have been extrapolated to humans, based on a similarity of responses to the hormones among the various species. There is good evidence for the **pulsatile secretion** of GnRH, GRH, SRIF, and CRH (Fig. 52-4). The pulse frequency varies between species but, at least for GnRH, is closely entrained with the pulsatile pattern of luteinizing hormone (LH) secretion by the pituitary. CRH secretion also appears to be entrained to that of adrenocorticotropic hormone (ACTH), though the interrelationship of GRH and SRIF pulses to growth hormone (GH) pulses is more complex. Alterations in the pulsatile pattern of hormone secretion have been observed in patients with certain types of neuroendocrine disorders, such as **anorexia nervosa.**

Transport and Metabolism of Hypothalamic Hormones

The extremely short distance between the median eminence and pituitary eliminates necessity for carrier or binding proteins for the releasing hormones. There is no physiologic role for the hormones in the peripheral circulation. Reports of their presence there are frequently artifactual (produced by nonspecific factors in the radioimmunoassay), are attributable to cross-reactivity with par-tially metabolized hormones, or are the result of their secretion from extraneural sites. A large number of peptidases exist in plasma that rapidly destroy the releasing hormones. Because of these considerations, the biologic effects of hypothalamic hormones on the pituitary can be regarded as a single-pass phenomenon.

Mechanism of Action of Hypothalamic Hormones

The hypophysiotropic hormones bind to **high-affinity receptors** on anterior pituitary cells and affect both hormone secretion and cellular function through a variety of mechanisms. Pituitary hormone secretion is stimulated through the participation of one or more second-messenger systems; these include adenylate cyclase–cyclic AMP (cAMP), Ca^{2+}-calmodulin, phosphatidylinositol, and protein kinase C. Individual **releasing hormones** appear to utilize multiple mechanisms to release the same pituitary hormone. In addition, the releasing hormones enhance **gene expression** of the hormones, whose release they stimulate, and the effects (where studied) appear to be independent. In the **somatotroph,** this effect is mediated by cAMP. Releasing hormones also stimulate overall cellular growth and mitogenesis.

The mechanism of inhibiting hormone action is less clearly understood but, in part, relates to an inhibition of adenylate cyclase activity, enhanced phosphodiesterase activity, and impaired transmembrane Ca^{2+} transport. In ad-

Table 52-1. Neuropeptides with Effects on Hypothalamic Releasing and Inhibiting Hormones

I. Gastroenteropancreatic peptides 　Cholecystokinin 　Gastrin 　Secretin 　Motilin 　Substance P 　Neurotensin 　Gastrin-releasing peptide 　Insulin 　Glucagon 　Pancreatic polypeptide II. Hypothalamic hormones 　Somatostatin 　Thyrotropin-releasing hormone 　Growth hormone–releasing hormone 　Corticotropin-releasing hormone 　Vasopressin	III. Endorphin/enkephalin peptides 　Methionine/leucine enkephalin 　Dynorphin 　Beta-endorphin 　Alpha melanocyte–stimulating hormone IV. Others 　Neuropeptide PYY 　Neuropeptide PHI/PHM 　Calcitonin 　Calcitonin gene–related peptide 　Angiotensin 　Bradykinin 　Galanin

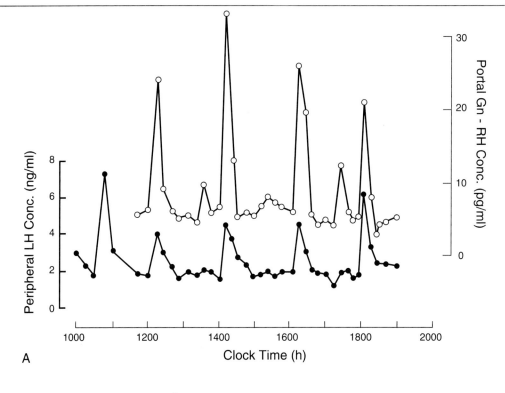

A

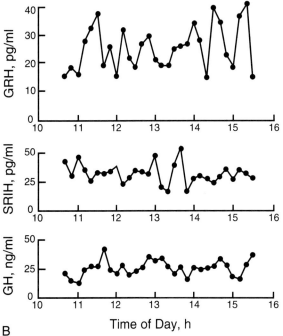

B

Fig. 52-4. Pulsatile patterns of hypothalamic hormone secretion in the unanesthetized sheep. (A) Relationship between gonadotropin-releasing hormone (GnRH) and luteinizing hormone (LH) secretion. (From: Clarke, I. J., and Cummins, J. T. The temporal relationship between gonadotropin-releasing hormone (GnRH) and luteinizing hormone (LH) secretion in ovariectomized ewes. *Endocrinology* 111:1737–1739, 1982. Copyright by The Endocrine Society.) (B) Growth hormone–releasing hormone (GRH) and somatotropin release–inhibiting hormone (SRIH) secretion integrate to generate a more complex pulsatile secretory pattern of growth hormone (GH). (From: Frohman, L. A., et al. Measurement of growth hormone–releasing hormone and somatostatin in hypothalamic-portal plasma of unanesthetized sheep: spontaneous secretion and response to insulin-induced hypoglycemia. *J. Clin. Invest.* 86:17–24, 1990. By copyright permission of the American Society of Clinical Investigation.)

dition, there appear to be other effects in the late stages of hormone secretion, possibly involving exocytosis.

The actions of all hypothalamic hormones are influenced by **target gland hormones,** including glucocorticoids, sex hormones, thyroxine, inhibin, and a number of growth factors. These hormones modify the number of hypothalamic hormone receptors and also exert effects at postreceptor sites.

Individual Hypothalamic-Pituitary Hormone Systems

Each of the hypophysiotropic-pituitary hormone systems consists of closed-loop feedback systems mediated by blood-borne signals, including those from target organs. Superimposed on these feedback systems are open-loop signals that are mostly of CNS origin and mediated by neurotransmitters; these signals reflect alterations in environment (temperature, light), stress (physical and psychic), and intrinsic rhythmicity (ranging from short-term or ultradian to seasonal periodicity). Consequently, both internal and external environmental factors exert major forces on the activity of these systems.

Hypothalamic-Pituitary-Adrenal Axis

CRH is a 41 amino acid peptide whose release is affected by nearly all neurotransmitters. The effect of **stress,** the major external stimulus for CRH secretion, is mediated through **nicotinic cholinergic receptors.** Serotonin also stimulates CRH release, but cholinergic interneurons are involved because atropine can block this response. **Norepinephrine** and **GABA** inhibit cholinergic stimulation of CRH secretion. **Melatonin** and **enkephalins** also inhibit CRH release, and melatonin is likely responsible for the circadian pattern of ACTH secretion that is entrained to the light-dark cycle.

CRH stimulates the release of **ACTH,** which in turn stimulates glucocorticoid and mineralocorticoid secretion by the adrenal cortex. ACTH secretion is inhibited by glucocorticoids through both rapid (minutes) and delayed (hours) feedback mechanisms. Both types of feedback operate at the level of the pituitary and hypothalamus, by inhibiting the response to and secretion of CRH, respectively. Longer-term effects of glucocorticoids include the inhibition of ACTH and CRH gene expression. In addition, ACTH inhibits CRH release by a short-loop feedback effect.

There is considerable interaction between the feedback influence of glucocorticoids and neurotransmitters. For example, **phenytoin,** a membrane stabilizer, decreases CNS sensitivity to glucocorticoid feedback, thereby diminishing the ACTH response to **metyrapone** (an adrenal enzyme inhibitor that reduces circulating glucocorticoid levels), but also enhances pulsatile ACTH secretion, though it does not affect the ACTH response to vasopressin or stress. **Vasopressin** stimulates ACTH release, both directly and through a CNS-mediated mechanism, and also potentiates the effects of CRH.

Hypothalamic-Pituitary-Gonadal Axis

GnRH is a decapeptide (10 amino acids) that stimulates the release of both LH and follicle-stimulating hormone (FSH). **Dopamine** and **serotonin** are the primary neurotransmitters that affect GnRH secretion; the former is stimulatory and the latter is inhibitory. A central inhibitory role of CRH also has been proposed. The regulation of the reproductive hormone axis is complex, varying with age and sex. Prior to **midpuberty,** FSH secretion is greater and is more responsive to GnRH than is LH secretion. After this, the pattern is reversed, concomitant with the development of a greater CNS sensitivity to the inhibitory feedback effects of gonadal steroids. The sleep-related pulsatile secretion of LH and synchronization of LH and FSH pulses begin in the **late prepubertal period** (ages 7 to 9 years) and are responsible for the nocturnal rises in testosterone (boys) and estradiol (girls) that initiate the clinical manifestations of puberty. There is a simultaneous decrease in the sensitivity of the CNS to steroid feedback effects which culminates in the **cyclic preovulatory gonadotropin surge** that results in onset of **cyclic ovulation.** In men, the nocturnal gonadotropin surges are replaced by an irregular pulsatile pattern throughout the day; a more regular 90-minute pattern is observed in mature women.

During **menopause,** when ovarian follicles disappear and the secretion of the major ovarian hormones decreases, FSH and LH secretions are enhanced, though their inherent pulsatility is preserved. A similar increase in gonadotropins is observed in **men in the eighth and ninth decades,** along with decreasing testicular function. **Stress** causes a transitory increase in LH in men, followed by a prolonged decrease and accompanied by reduced testosterone levels. In women, stress is associated with hypothalamic **anovulation.**

Gonadal steroids regulate the tonic secretion of LH and FSH by a negative feedback mechanism that operates at both the hypothalamic and pituitary levels, with testosterone more potent than estrogen. **Inhibin,** a peptide produced by the germinal epithelium, selectively inhibits FSH secretions by impairing the effects of GnRH. The effects of estrogen on cyclic gonadotropin secretion, however, are opposite those on tonic secretion. The rising **estradiol** levels in the preovulatory period are actually responsible for the surge of LH that triggers **ovulation.** These stimulatory feedback effects also occur at both the hypothalamic and pituitary levels, though the pituitary appears to be a more important site of action.

Hypothalamic-Pituitary-Thyroid Axis

TRH is a tripeptide that is the primary regulator of thyroid-stimulating hormone (TSH), though the inhibitory effects of SRIF and dopamine are also of physiologic significance under certain conditions. TRH secretion is stimulated by norepinephrine and dopamine, and inhibited by serotonin. TSH secretion enhances thyroid hormone secretion, and the feedback effects, primarily mediated by triiodothyronine, predominantly affect the pituitary through an inhibition of TRH action. Longer-term effects also take place in the hypothalamus through inhibition of TRH gene expression. A reduction in circulating thyroid hormone levels translates into an acute rise in TSH secretion, for which TRH is not required. However, prolonged and sustained TSH secretion does require TRH. TRH stimulates TSH biosynthesis and release, and in the absence of TRH, TSH glycosylation is altered, resulting in a biologically less potent molecule.

Rapid changes in environmental conditions necessitating increased metabolic activity (e.g., cold exposure) provoke a noradrenergic-mediated CNS stimulus to increased TRH secretion. This effect is readily demonstrable in infants, but not in adults, who possess other more important mechanisms of thermogenesis, such as shivering and the mobilization of free fatty acids through activation of the autonomic system.

Somatostatin inhibits TSH secretion but has a relatively minor role in its physiologic regulation under normal conditions, since it is much less effective in inhibiting TSH than GH secretion. Nevertheless, when SRIF secretion is increased (e.g., because of increased GH levels), TSH production can be suppressed. Dopaminergic inhibition of TSH secretion is most readily demonstrable when TSH secretion is elevated.

Hypothalamic-Pituitary-Somatotroph-Liver Axis

The secretion of **GH** is regulated by a releasing (GRH) and an inhibiting (somatostatin, SRIF) hormone. GRH exists in both 40 and 44 amino acid forms, which have identical biologic activity. The **neurotransmitter regulation** of GRH is extensive, with stimulatory effects from acetylcholine, norepinephrine, and epinephrine (through the alpha-adrenergic receptor), as well as from dopamine, serotonin, and enkephalin. Beta-noradrenergic receptors are inhibitory, and the effect of GABA may be either inhibitory or stimulatory. SRIF secretion is stimulated by dopamine and inhibited by acetylcholine. Within the hypothalamus, GRH and SRIF have a reciprocal influence on each other's secretion. GH secretion is characterized by a pulsatile pattern, frequently beneath the limits of detectable measurement, superimposed on which are occasional surges of secretion that are related to the postabsorptive state and in association with deep sleep (electroencephalograph stages III to IV). GH secretion changes dramatically with age. Extremely high levels are seen neonatally, which decrease within a few weeks of life. Pulses that are indistinguishable from those of adults, except for increased frequency, are seen during puberty. After the fourth decade, GH secretion diminishes, and after the sixth decade, significant pulsatile secretion is uncommon during either waking or sleeping periods.

Nutrient status profoundly affects GH secretion. Increases in amino acid levels, decreases in free fatty acid levels, and hypoglycemia all stimulate GH secretion; hyperglycemia inhibits GH release. GH secretion is stimulated by exercise and stress. **Thyroxine, glucocorticoids,** and **sex steroids** all affect GH secretion, though in a complex manner. In general, both **androgens** and **estrogens** stimulate GH responses to many stimuli, while **glucocorticoids** inhibit the same responses. However, the timing of hormone administration in relation to testing is of crucial importance. GH secretion is sexually dimorphic, in that women generally have higher baseline levels and lower pulse peaks than do men. Thyroid hormone deficiency tends to decrease GH secretion.

A **closed-loop feedback system** also exists for GH secretion and is mediated by both GH itself and the major GH-dependent growth factor, insulin-like growth factor I (somatomedin C, IGF-I). IGF-I and GH both stimulate SRIF release and inhibit GRH release. In addition, IGF-I inhibits basal and GRH-stimulated GH secretion by the pituitary. Each of these effects occurs at hormone levels that are achieved under physiologic conditions. Although most circulating IGF-I originates from the liver, the feedback (and also growth-promoting) effects also may occur through a paracrine action, since IGF-I is produced by many tissues.

Hypothalamic-Lactotroph-Breast Axis

The secretion of **prolactin** is under an inhibitory CNS tone that is chiefly supplied by dopamine. Both TRH and VIP have physiologic prolactin-releasing activity, though their relative importance in the overall control of prolactin is controversial. Serotonin stimulates prolactin release through effects on a prolactin-releasing factor, most likely VIP. Melatonin and histamine have stimulatory effects within the CNS, as do enkephalins and GABA. The effects of these two latter substances are related to their inhibitory role on the tuberoinfundibular dopaminergic system.

The secretion of prolactin is enhanced by **tactile stimulation of the breast** via sensory receptors on the nipple and areola, fibers from which travel through the intercostal nerves to the spinal cord. Prolactin levels increase during pregnancy as a result of estrogen stimulation of the **lactotroph.** The rapid decline in estrogen and progesterone levels after parturition establishes an environment for lactation from the estrogen-primed breast. The suckling stimulation of prolactin secretion is mediated by VIP, though it is not responsible for the **milk letdown reflex,** which depends on **oxytocin.**

Prolactin is also a **stress-responsive hormone,** and increased levels are seen after surgical or emotional stress, exercise, and insulin-induced hypoglycemia. Thyroid hormone exerts an inhibitory effect on prolactin secretion, which is increased in thyroid hormone deficiency.

Neuroimmunoendocrinology

The immune system is one of the major intracellular communication systems. Considerable interaction between the immune and neuroendocrine systems has recently been recognized, as well as the regulatory effects they exert on one another. The regulatory signals of the immune system, the **lymphokines** and **monokines,** affect the hypothalamic pituitary system, and **neuroendocrine peptides** such as ACTH and beta-endorphin have been shown to be produced by immunologically competent cells (lymphocytes). Although an understanding of how these two systems interact is still in its infancy, certain important concepts are recognized.

It is now clear that certain monokines or lymphokines are capable of stimulating the hypothalamic-pituitary-adrenal axis. **Interleukin l** (IL-1), a product of activated macrophages, stimulates CRH secretion from the hypothalamus, both after systemic administration and in vitro. Because IL-1 is released during infection and is believed to serve as an endogenous pyrogen, it is a likely candidate as the mediator (or one of the mediators) of the associated **hypothalamic-pituitary-adrenal stress response.** The mechanisms of a feedback system exist, since activation of this axis increases glucocorticoid production by the adrenals, which in turn suppresses many immunologic functions. The same compound has been shown to stimulate somatostatin release and decrease TSH release by an action imposed at the hypothalamic or pituitary level.

Cytokines other than IL-l also have been reported to affect neuroendocrine function. **IL-6,** another cytokine produced by T cells, monocytes, and endothelial cells, can stimulate the release of GH, prolactin, and LH directly from the pituitary. In addition, a **thymic factor** (thymosin fraction 5) stimulates GnRH release from the hypothalamus and, after systemic administration, ACTH release. Although the role of these agents in neuroendocrine function under normal physiologic conditions remains to be clarified, the interrelationship of the neuroendocrine and immune systems is clearly important and may serve as a vehicle for regulating pathophysiologic responses to stimuli that provoke immunologic mechanisms.

Summary

The CNS regulates the endocrine system through specific neuroanatomic pathways that involve the hypothalamus and a series of specific releasing and inhibiting hormones that control the secretion of the anterior pituitary. Each hormone is involved in a complex integrated feedback system that maintains a level of basal hormone secretion, and the feedback systems are influenced by signals derived from perturbations of the external environment, inherent biologic rhythms, and circulating nutrients. The most important of endocrine functions — growth, reproduction, and the response to stress — all require the integrative functions of this system. In addition, the hypothalamus has a major involvement in non-pituitary-mediated homeostatic mechanisms, including neurometabolic regulation, thermoregulation, autonomic nervous system function, and immunoregulation.

Bibliography

Krieger, D. T., and Hughes, J. C., eds. *Neuroendocrinology.* Sunderland, Mass.: Sinauer Associates, 1980.

Molitch, M. Neuroendocrinology. In: Felig, P., Baxter, J. D., and Frohman, L. A., eds. *Endocrinology and Metabolism,* 3rd ed. New York: McGraw-Hill, 1995.

Reichlin, S. Neuroendocrine-immune interactions. *N. Engl. J. Med.* 329:1246–1253, 1993.

Reichlin, S. Neuroendocrinology. In: Wilson, G. D., and Foster, D. W., eds. *Textbook of Endocrinology,* 8th ed. Philadelphia: W. B. Saunders, 1992. Pp. 135–220.

53 The Anterior Pituitary

Lawrence A. Frohman

Objectives

After reading this chapter, you should be able to

Describe the anatomy and blood supply of the pituitary gland

List the cell types of the anterior pituitary and the hormones they secrete

Cite the families of pituitary hormones and describe their characteristics

List the individual pituitary hormones, their general chemical characteristics, and their target glands

Discuss the major actions of each of the hormones of the anterior pituitary

Describe the types of tests used for evaluating the secretion of the individual pituitary hormones

---

Anatomy

The pituitary gland (0.5–0.7 g) is located in the **sella turcica,** a saddle-shaped cavity at the base of the skull that forms an integral part of the sphenoid bone. It is bounded anteriorly by the midline **tuberculum sellae** and the **anterior clinoid processes,** which project posteriorly from the sphenoid wings. Posteriorly, the sellar boundaries consist of the **dorsum sellae,** the lateral portions of which form the **posterior clinoid processes.** The lateral boundaries of the pituitary consist of the nonosseous medial wall of the cavernous sinus, through which travel the internal carotid artery together with the third, fourth, and sixth cranial nerves. The roof of the pituitary consists of a thickened reflection of the dura mater, the **diaphragma sellae,** which is attached to the clinoid processes. The **pituitary stalk** and its portal blood vessels pass through a foramen in this membrane. The outer layer of the dura mater extends into the pituitary sella (oval to spherical in shape) to form its **periosteum,** thereby making the pituitary extradural and

not in contact with the cerebrospinal fluid. The anterior lobe comprises about two-thirds of the total weight; the remainder comprises the posterior lobe.

The **blood supply** of the pituitary originates from the **internal carotid artery,** through interconnecting branches of the circle of Willis, and the three hypophysial arteries. The branches supplying the stalk and the posterior pituitary are derived directly from these vessels, whereas the anterior pituitary has no direct arterial supply. Rather, its entire vascular supply originates in a portal system that first bathes the outer layer of the median eminence, then coalesces into long and short portal veins that travel through the pituitary stalk, and finally terminates in a dense plexus of sinusoidal capillaries within the anterior pituitary. **Venous drainage** from the anterior pituitary enters the posterior pituitary and from there to the cavernous sinus or the petrosal sinus.

The **nerve supply** of the anterior pituitary is sparse and consists of postganglionic fibers of the sympathetic nervous system that accompany and terminate on arteriolar vessels. They may regulate pituitary blood flow and, in this manner, regulate the extent of exposure of the anterior pituitary to hypothalamic hormones.

Developmental Aspects

The anterior pituitary (adenohypophysis, **pars anterior**) is derived from an ectodermal evagination of the oropharynx, **Rathke's pouch,** that fuses with an outpouching of the third ventricle early in fetal development. The latter eventually develops into the **neurohypophysis (pars nervosa),** or posterior lobe. The posterior portion of Rathke's pouch is less well developed, particularly in humans, and is called the **pars intermedia,** or **intermediate lobe.** Cell types and hormone precursor processing in this lobe differ from those in the anterior lobe. Cells in this region may assume the characteristics of mature anterior pituitary cells and secrete hormones. **Pituitary hormones** exist as early as 4 to 5 weeks of gestation and can respond prenatally to some hypothalamic-releasing hormones. However, the full feedback regulatory system is not fully established until postnatal life.

Cells of the **anterior pituitary** develop the capacity to secrete **adrenocorticotropic hormone** (ACTH), **growth hormone** (GH), **prolactin, thyroid-stimulating hormone** (TSH), **luteinizing hormone** (LH), and **follicle-stimulating hormone** (FSH). Those in the **posterior pituitary** secrete **vasopressin** and **oxytocin,** while cells of the **intermediate lobe** secrete **ACTH, melanocyte-stimulating hormone** (MSH), **beta-lipotropin** (β-LPH), and **endorphins.** Within the anterior pituitary, cells are arranged in a sinusoidal or rosette formation, and all cell types are intermingled. More important, however, is the association seen at the **microscopic level** between somatotrophs and thyrotrophs and between gonadotrophs and lactotrophs. There is evidence for intercellular communication between the various cell types in the anterior pituitary, which may have an important physiologic function.

Pituitary Cell Types

The cells of the anterior pituitary can be divided into several subtypes, based on the class of hormones they secrete. They include the **somatomammotropic group,** responsible for the secretion of GH and prolactin; the **glycoprotein-secreting cells,** which secrete TSH, LH, and FSH; the **corticotroph cells,** which secrete ACTH and the other hormones derived from the **proopiomelanocortin** (POMC) **molecule;** and the **folliculostellate cells,** recently identi-

fied to secrete an endothelial cell growth factor. There are additional cell types, but their function is not known. The individual cell types were originally identified by their **staining characteristics,** based on pH-dependent histochemical stains (acidophils, basophils, and chromophobes). **Morphologic differences** in granule size, when viewed under the electron microscope, also exist among the various cell types. However, precise identification of the cell types is currently determined through the use of immunohistochemical stains that indicate the presence of specific hormones.

Somatomammotropic Family

The somatomammotropic family includes three cell types: somatotrophs, lactotrophs, and somatomammotrophs. The **somatotrophs** were originally identified as acidophilic cells, and their function as GH-secreting cells was based on their predominance in tumors associated with acromegaly and gigantism. They are the most common cell type and are located primarily in the lateral wings of the anterior pituitary. The **lactotrophs** are also acidophilic, though they stain less intensely than do somatotrophs. They are slightly less numerous than are somatotrophs and secrete prolactin. The lactotrophs increase greatly in number during pregnancy, under the influence of estrogen, and may constitute up to 75% of the mass of the anterior pituitary. Lactotropic tumors are associated with increased prolactin secretion. The **somatomammotroph,** which constitutes about 1% to 2% of the anterior pituitary cells, secretes both GH and prolactin and is believed to serve as a precursor cell for both somatotrophs and lactotrophs. Tumors derived from this cell type exhibit hypersecretion of both GH and prolactin.

Glycoprotein Hormone–Secreting Family

The glycoprotein hormone–secreting family consists of two cell types: thyrotrophs and gonadotrophs. The **thyrotrophs** are intensely basophilic, are polyhedral, and tend to be concentrated in the anterior portion of the pituitary, near the midline. They secrete TSH and normally represent about 5% to 6% of the anterior lobe cells, though marked increases in size and number occur after thyroidectomy. A single type of gonadotroph cell secretes both LH and FSH. Although gonadotrophs constitute only 3% to 4% of the anterior lobe cells, they increase in number after castration. They decrease during pregnancy as a consequence of the high levels of circulating steroids secreted by the corpus luteum in response to chorionic gonadotropin production and by the placenta.

Corticotroph Family

There are two types of corticotroph cells. One type is located in the **medial region** of the anterior lobe and the other in the **junctional region** between the anterior and posterior lobes. Anterior lobe corticotrophs are sparsely granulated, in contrast to those in the junctional area, which have large electron-dense granules. Both types produce peptides that are derived from the common POMC precursor. However, the specific peptides found in each of the cell types vary greatly, based on differences in the processing enzymes present. **ACTH,** the most physiologically important member of this hormone family, is secreted primarily by the cells in the anterior lobe. In states of **glucocorticoid insufficiency,** anterior lobe corticotrophs proliferate, while those in the junctional area do not.

Folliculostellate Cells

A small number of cells exhibit a stellate shape and send processes into the perivascular spaces. A peptide hormone, **endothelial cell growth factor,** with mitogenic activity specific for endothelial cells, has recently been isolated from these cells, and they must therefore be added to the list of anterior pituitary hormone–secreting cells.

Anterior Pituitary Hormones

There are three separate families of anterior pituitary hormones: corticotropin-lipotropin, glycoprotein, and somatomammotropin. A comparison of their chemical characteristics is given in Table 53-1. Additional discussion of the neuroendocrine regulation of each of the hormones is provided in Chap. 52.

Table 53-1. Anterior Pituitary Hormones

Class	Members	Molecular Weight	Amino Acids and Carbohydrate
Corticotropin-lipotropin[a]	ACTH	4,500	39
	α-MSH	1,800	13
	β-LPH	11,200	91
	β-Endorphin	4,000	31; C-terminal (amino acids 61 to 91) portion of β-LPH
Glycoprotein[b]	LH	29,000	Alpha subunit, 89; beta subunit, 115; 1% sialic acid
	FSH	29,000	Alpha subunit, 89; beta subunit, 115; 5% sialic acid
	TSH	29,000	Alpha subunit, 89; beta subunit, 112; 1% sialic acid
	Chorionic gonadotropin[d]	46,000	Alpha subunit, 92; beta subunit, 139; 12% sialic acid
Somatomammotropin[c]	Growth hormone	21,800	191
	Prolactin	22,500	198[e]
	Placental lactogen	21,800	191

ACTH = adrenocorticotropic hormone; MSH = melanocyte-stimulating hormone; LPH = lipotropin; LH = luteinizing hormone; FSH = follicle-stimulating hormone; TSH = thyroid-stimulating hormone.
[a]Members derived from a single precursor.
[b]The alpha subunits are nearly identical, and the beta subunit confers biologic specificity.
[c]Single-chain proteins with two or three disulfide bridges.
[d]Of placental origin and included for comparison purposes.
[e]Carbohydrate-containing forms of prolactin have recently been identified.
Adapted from: Frohman, L. A. Diseases of the anterior pituitary. In: Felig, P., Baxter, J. D., and Frohman, L. A., eds. *Endocrinology and Metabolism,* 3rd ed. New York: McGraw-Hill, 1995.

Corticotropin-Related Peptides

ACTH and its related family of peptides are derived from a **single precursor molecule,** POMC. A stepwise processing of this molecule occurs, with cleavage into three major fragments (Fig. 53-1). The amino-terminal end has an uncertain biologic function, the midportion fragment contains ACTH, and the carboxyl-terminal fragment contains β-LPH. ACTH is not further processed in the anterior lobe corticotrophs but is cleaved to α-MSH and corticotropin-like intermediate lobe peptide in the junctional zone cells (and also in the CNS). β-LPH is also further processed in these same cells to other endorphin-related peptides. Although the structures of β-MSH and met-enkephalin are contained within that of β-LPH, each of these compounds has a different mechanism of synthesis, with that for met-enkephalin originating from a separate precursor.

Adrenocorticotropin

ACTH is a 39 amino acid, single-chain peptide with its biologic activity contained in the first 24 residues. Its primary site of action is the **adrenal cortex,** where it stimulates the secretion of glucocorticoids, mineralocorticoids, and androgenic steroids. ACTH binds to specific receptors on the adrenocortical cell plasma membranes and

Fig. 53-1. The posttranslational processing of proopiomelanocortin (POMC), the precursor of adrenocorticotropic hormone (ACTH). After removal of the signal peptide from the POMC precursor (pre-POMC), the glycosylated (indicated by *closed circles*) POMC is further processed in the anterior lobe to an amino-terminal peptide (NT), ACTH, and beta-lipotropin (β-LPH). In the junctional zone, each of these peptides is further cleaved; gamma-melanocyte-stimulating hormone (γ-MSH) is derived from NT; α-MSH and corticotropin-like intermediate lobe peptide (CLIP) are derived from ACTH; and γ-LPH and beta-endorphin (β-END) are derived from β-LPH.

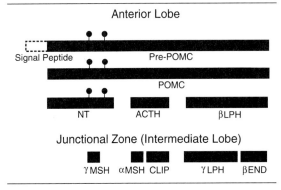

exerts its action by cyclic AMP–mediated effects that enhance cholesterol side-chain cleavage, resulting in its conversion to **pregnenolone.** In addition, ACTH has trophic effects on the adrenal cortex, stimulating DNA and protein synthesis and mitogenesis. ACTH also possesses some **extraadrenal effects** at very high concentrations. ACTH has **pigmenting action** that is of likely physiologic importance in humans in ACTH hypersecretion.

ACTH is measured primarily by **radioimmunoassay** (RIA), and levels in plasma vary from less than 1 pg/ml (less than 0.2 pM) to 80 pg/ml (18 pM). During stress, ACTH levels may reach 200 to 300 pg/ml (45 to 67 pM). ACTH is rapidly cleared from the circulation, with a **plasma half-life** of 3 to 9 minutes. The **daily secretion rate** is approximately 25 μg/day. ACTH secretion is **episodic,** but a diurnal rhythm is also observed, with highest levels in the early morning and lowest levels in the late evening (Fig. 53-2). Pulses of ACTH secretion are coupled to those of cortisol secretion.

Glycoprotein Hormones

The pituitary glycoprotein hormones consist of TSH, LH, and FSH. In addition, there is a placental glycoprotein hormone, **chorionic gonadotropin,** that is structurally similar to LH and exhibits many of its biologic characteristics. The glycoprotein hormones are composed of **two subunits,** alpha and beta, each consisting of a protein core with branched carbohydrate side chains that constitute from 15% to 30% of the hormones' molecular mass. The carbohydrates are essential for the hormones' biologic activity and also markedly influence their stability in plasma. Within a particular species, the alpha subunits of the pituitary glycoprotein hormones are identical, but the beta subunits vary, providing the biologic specificity of action. Even the beta subunits exhibit some homology. It is therefore not surprising that an overlap in biologic function can be demonstrated at extremely high hormone levels. The subunits by themselves do not possess intrinsic biologic activity. The beta subunit of chorionic gonadotropin in particular is identical to that of LH, with the exception of a 30 amino acid extension at the carboxyl terminal. The individual subunits are under separate genetic control, and the rate-limiting step in hormone biosynthesis appears to depend on the expression of the beta subunit gene.

Thyroid-Stimulating Hormone

The actions of TSH on the thyroid cells parallel those of ACTH on the adrenal cortex. TSH binding leads to the **activation of adenylate cyclase,** which mediates a number

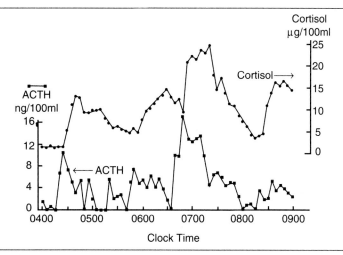

Fig. 53-2. Secretory pattern of adrenocorticotropic hormone (ACTH) and cortisol during a 5-hour, early morning period in a normal man. The more pronounced pulsatility of ACTH is, to a large extent, a consequence of its more rapid disappearance from plasma than is cortisol. (From: Gallagher, T. F., et al., ACTH and cortisol secretory pattern in man. *J. Clin. Endocrinol. Metab.* 36:1058, 1973. Copyright by The Endocrine Society.)

of processes, including iodide transport and binding and thyroglobulin synthesis and proteolysis. TSH also **stimulates RNA** and **protein synthesis,** thus increasing thyroid size and vascularity. TSH is measured by ultrasensitive immunoassays that can distinguish between low, normal, and high levels. **Normal TSH concentrations** in plasma range from 0.5 to 6 μU/ml. In prolonged and severe thyroid hormone deficiency, TSH levels may exceed 100 μU/ml; in conditions of thyroid hormone excess, levels are undetectable (less than 0.1 to 0.15 μU/ml). The half-life of TSH in circulation is approximately 75 minutes, and the daily secretion rate is 100 to 200 mU. Secretion rates of up to 10 times the normal rate may occur in hypothyroidism.

In addition to neuroendocrine control, TSH secretion is also affected by thyroid hormone, glucocorticoids, estrogen, and GH. **Glucocorticoids** suppress both basal and stimulated TSH secretion, and **estrogens** enhance the TSH response to TRH. This is reflected in the higher TSH responses in women as compared with men and during the late follicular phase of the menstrual cycle in women, when estradiol levels are increased.

Luteinizing Hormone and Follicle-Stimulating Hormone

LH and FSH are the two pituitary hormones that regulate **gonadal function. FSH** stimulates ovarian follicular growth, testicular growth, and spermatogenesis. **LH** promotes ovulation and follicular luteinization, stimulates testicular Leydig cell function, and enhances the production of sex steroids from both the ovary and testis. FSH promotes ovarian growth and maturation of the primordial follicle, while LH stimulates the production estrogens by the thecal cells and progesterone by the corpus luteum by enhancing the conversion of cholesterol to pregnenolone. In the testis, FSH acts on Sertoli cells, together with testosterone, to stimulate the production of an androgen-binding protein. The target cell of LH in the testis is the Leydig cell, where testosterone production is stimulated. The androgen-binding protein transports testosterone in high concentrations into the tubular cells to stimulate spermatogenesis. Details of the actions of LH and FSH are provided in Chaps. 59 and 60.

Gonadotropin concentrations are primarily determined by RIA, in which there is some degree of cross-reactivity between the hormone and its subunits, though this is not of practical importance.

Plasma levels of LH and FSH vary with the **menstrual cycle.** Plasma FSH levels rise slightly and then decline during the early follicular phase, at which time LH levels are stable or slightly increasing. Increasing estrogen stimulation at **midcycle** causes an abrupt increase in the LH level, which together with an increase in FSH levels triggers **ovulation.** Both hormone levels decline during the **luteal phase.** In men, FSH and LH levels are similar to those in women during the follicular phase. No identifiable cyclic function exists in either the hypothalamus or testis, and the primary feedback effect on LH secretion is mediated through testosterone, acting at both the hypothalamic and pituitary levels. The negative feedback on FSH secretion in both sexes occurs primarily through gonadally produced **inhibin,** acting at the pituitary. The hormone levels increase in response to age-associated decreases in gonadal function in both sexes. This occurs at menopause in women; in men, it is generally seen after age 70. The half-life of LH in plasma is approximately 50 minutes, whereas that of FSH is 3 to 4 hours and that of chorionic gonadotropin even longer. The difference is attributed to the varying content of sialic acid.

The secretion of LH and FSH is also influenced by **prolactin.** The LH response to gonadotropin-releasing hormone (GnRH) is also inhibited by glucocorticoids.

Somatomammotropic Hormones

The three members of this family are **GH, prolactin,** and a placental hormone, **chorionic somatomammotropin,** also known as **placental lactogen** (PL). Placental lactogen is 83% homologous with GH but also displays considerable homology with prolactin and is believed to be the phylogenic ancestor of the two pituitary hormones. In contrast, GH and prolactin only exhibit 16% homology. Each hormone is a single-chain peptide; prolactin exists in a glycosylated form, with a reduced biologic activity. Despite these differences, each hormone has intrinsic growth-promoting and lactogenic properties. GH and prolactin exist as larger molecules in the circulation. Some of the heterogeneity in size is due to noncovalent homodimerization and binding to proteins.

Growth Hormone

GH has a major role in **promoting linear growth** and in the regulation of **metabolism.** Administration of GH to patients deficient in the hormone produces a positive nitrogen balance, decreased urea production and body fat stores, increased muscle mass, and enhanced carbohydrate utilization. GH produces **biphasic effects** on circulating levels of glucose, amino acids, and fatty acids, with an initial decrease followed by a return to normal levels, or even an increase. At the **cellular level,** GH stimulates the uptake and incorporation of amino acids into protein, enhances RNA synthesis, accelerates glucose uptake, and antagonizes the lipolytic effect of catecholamines. These acute effects disappear within 3 to 4 hours of continuous expo-

sure and are replaced by a series of **insulin antagonistic effects,** including enhanced triglyceride lipolysis, increased sensitivity to catecholamine-mediated lipolysis, and impairment of glucose uptake and utilization. These effects form the basis for the **diabetogenic effects** of GH. In the pancreatic beta cell, GH exhibits multiphasic effects on insulin secretion. An acute direct stimulatory effect is followed by a secondary inhibitory effect and then a prolonged stimulation of insulin secretion, secondary to the impairment of carbohydrate metabolism. The latter effect is of greatest importance in the development of diabetes in states of GH hypersecretion.

GH also stimulates the production of several tissue growth factors, particularly **insulin-like growth factor I** (IGF-I), also known as **somatomedin C.** IGF-I is a peptide that structurally resembles proinsulin and binds to the insulin receptor. Separate IGF-I receptors exist in many tissues. IGF-I can thus be considered a mediator of many GH effects and acts as an **autocrine** or **paracrine growth factor.** It is also released into the circulation, primarily from the liver and kidney, and may act as a true hormone. Many of the actions originally attributed to GH are in fact caused by IGF-I. Furthermore, IGF-I and GH act **synergistically** in cell differentiation and cell growth. GH serves to commit a precursor cell (such as a fibroblast or prechondrocyte) to a specific pathway of differentiation, and IGF-I enhances its growth and replication. In addition, GH enhances the activity of another growth factor, **epidermal growth factor,** by stimulating production of its receptor. Overall, the capacity of tissues such as the liver, heart, and kidney to undergo hypertrophy depends on GH and IGF-I.

Because GH is secreted in an episodic manner, with values ranging from less than 0.1 ng/ml (4.5 pM) to levels of from 30 to 50 ng/ml (1.4 to 2.3 nM), mean values can only be determined by integrating a series of repeated measurements. In adults, mean levels are less than 2 ng/ml (less than 100 pM). About 70% of **GH secretion** occurs during the night in association with deep sleep (Fig. 53-3). Values in women during the reproductive years are slightly greater, both basally and in response to stimuli. The **integrated secretory rate** during the adolescent growth spurt is greater and after the sixth decade is considerably lower. The largest secretory bursts of GH occur at night, in association with deep sleep (electroencephalograph stages III to IV). The episodic pattern of GH secretion is also important in modulating its metabolic actions, as described, since the nearly complete absence of GH effects during trough periods is important in maintaining the anabolic as compared with the insulin antagonistic actions of the hormone on peripheral tissues. GH is cleared from plasma pri-

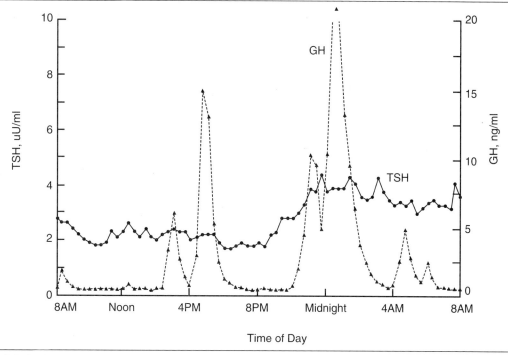

Fig. 53-3. Pulsatile pattern of growth hormone (GH) and thyroid-stimulating hormone (TSH) secretion in a normal man. The largest pulses of GH are seen in association with electroencephalograph stages III to IV sleep (deep sleep). TSH levels, while increased during the night, exhibit a different pattern.

marily by the liver but also by the kidney. The **plasma half-life** of GH is 20 minutes, and the 24-hour secretion rate in adults ranges from 300 to 400 µg/m².

Prolactin

Prolactin stimulates the **synthesis of milk constituents** (e.g., casein, lactalbumin, lipids, and carbohydrates). There are prolactin receptors on the alveolar surface of mammary cells and also in the liver and kidney. Breast development during puberty is not determined by prolactin secretion, and a pathologic increase in prolactin secretion does not, by itself, increase breast size. During **pregnancy,** however, prolactin, together with estrogen, progesterone, and PL, promote breast enlargement and initiate milk production. The abrupt decrease in placental estrogen and progesterone immediately following parturition initiates lactation. Continued prolactin secretion is necessary for maintaining **lactation** in the postpartum period, and the return of prolactin levels to normal is delayed in women who nurse for prolonged periods. Although prolactin displays other effects in lower species, including behavioral (mater-

nal) activity and water metabolism, these activities have not been confirmed in humans.

Normal levels of prolactin are lower than 15 ng/ml (0.7 nM) in men and less than 20 ng/ml (0.9 nM) in women. Prolactin levels do not change significantly during the menstrual cycle, though levels in pregnancy increase to 200 ng/ml (9 nM) at term. The **half-life** of prolactin in plasma is approximately 50 minutes, with removal occurring primarily in the liver and kidney.

Clinical Evaluation of Anterior Pituitary Hormones

The evaluation of anterior pituitary hormones involves the assessment of spontaneous secretion, the pituitary secretory reserve using one or more stimuli, and their ability to respond to suppressive agents. The general endocrine physiologic principle followed is that **stimulation tests** are performed when hormone levels are in the basal state and **suppression tests** are performed when hormone levels are elevated. Measurements of hormones in plasma have replaced urine measurements; however, urine collections still are useful in evaluating overall secretory activity (during a 24-hour period).

ACTH measurements are generally performed in conjunction with those of cortisol. In suspected **primary adrenal insufficiency,** a single plasma ACTH level is often diagnostic, since it will be elevated if the disease originates in the adrenal gland (primary) and normal or low in hypothalamic pituitary disease (secondary). Differentiation of the latter two conditions frequently can be accomplished by testing with corticotropin-releasing hormone (CRH) (which stimulates the pituitary directly) and with **insulin hypoglycemia** (which requires the participation of the combined hypothalamic-pituitary unit). A positive response to CRH, coupled with no response to insulin, points to the CNS as the source of the problem. A single **injection of ACTH** along with the measurement of plasma cortisol levels is also a simple screening procedure for the adequacy of ACTH secretion, since the unstimulated adrenal cortex undergoes atrophy and does not respond normally. The axis also can be tested with **metyrapone,** an inhibitor of adrenal 11-hydroxylase and therefore of cortisol biosynthesis. This reduces the feedback effects on CRH and ACTH, leading to a rise in the ACTH level. However, this type of stimulus differs from that of insulin hypoglycemia, which evaluates stress-induced ACTH release, a pathway largely independent of feedback regulation.

The best assessment of **suspected increased ACTH production** is by measuring the 24-hour urinary cortisol excretion. The suppressibility of ACTH and cortisol by dexamethasone (a synthetic glucocorticoid) is used to determine the integrity of feedback inhibition.

TSH levels are the most useful indicator of TSH secretory capacity when evaluating a patient with **hypothyroidism.** If the disease originates in the **thyroid** (primary), the TSH level will be elevated. If it is of **pituitary** (secondary) or **hypothalamic** (tertiary) **origin,** the level will be low or (inappropriately) normal. Differentiation between hypothalamic and pituitary disease can generally be accomplished by TRH stimulation, which customarily produces an enhanced or prolonged increase in TSH levels in hypothalamic disease and a reduced or absent response in pituitary disease. On occasion, however, the TSH response may not be exaggerated in hypothalamic hypothyroidism. A suspected **autonomous origin** of the elevated TSH levels (caused by a TSH-secreting tumor) can be assessed by suppression with thyroxine, using feedback inhibition. If suppression occurs only at abnormally high thyroxine levels, this indicates a genetic (thyroid hormone–receptor mutation) or drug-induced condition.

LH and **FSH secretions** are assessed by measuring basal levels in conjunction with gonadal steroid levels and in response to GnRH challenge. If there is **generalized gonadal failure,** testosterone or estradiol levels are reduced and LH and FSH levels are elevated. **Selective gonadal failure** (such as Sertoli cell dysfunction with impaired spermatogenesis) will result in a disproportionate increase in FSH levels with only minimal changes in the LH levels. If LH and FSH levels are not elevated in the presence of decreased levels of gonadal steroids, the disturbance is either pituitary or hypothalamic in origin. GnRH stimulation may be useful in distinguishing between the two. Repeated stimulation at frequent intervals (every 3 hours for 5 to 7 days) is often necessary to prime the gonadotrophs to respond.

GH secretion is tested if there is a suspected deficiency in children with growth failure or in patients with destructive lesions (usually tumors) of the pituitary gland. It is also assessed in patients with suspected GH-secreting tumors causing **gigantism** or **acromegaly,** a disorder characterized by the enlargement of hands and feet, coarsening of facial features, soft tissue overgrowth, and metabolic disturbances.

GH overproduction is frequently revealed simply by measuring the basal hormone level in plasma. The inability of GH to be suppressed by hyperglycemia (after ingestion of glucose) indicates autonomous secretion of the hormone, typically seen in GH-secreting tumors.

Prolactin secretion is assessed by measuring hormone levels under basal conditions. Reduced hormone levels are rarely of clinical diagnostic importance, because they appear only in association with panhypopituitarism. **Hyperprolactinemia,** in contrast, is an important problem and is documented by repeated measurement of the hormone on separate occasions (because prolactin is a stress-responsive hormone and may be transiently elevated in anxious patients).

Summary

The anterior pituitary, once called the "master gland," is the primary mediator through which the CNS controls endocrine function. It is composed of several different cell types, each of which produces one or more hormones that stimulate target endocrine glands or other sites, such as the liver, breast, skeletal muscle, or bone. The secretion of each of the pituitary hormones is regulated (1) by hypothalamic-releasing hormones or hypothalamic-inhibiting hormones, or both, and (2) by feedback signals derived from the target glands. Measurement of pituitary hormones in blood is used to assess pituitary function and involves both dynamic and static measurements.

Bibliography

Daniels, G. H., and Martin, J. B., Neuroendocrine regulation and diseases of the anterior pituitary and hypothalamus. In: Braunwald, E., et al, eds., *Harrison's Principles of Internal Medicine.* New York: McGraw-Hill, 1987. Pp. 1694–1717.

Frohman, L. A. Diseases of the anterior pituitary. In: Felig, P., Baxter, J. D., and Frohman, L. A., eds. *Endocrinology and Metabolism,* 3rd ed. New York: McGraw-Hill, 1995.

Thorner, M. O., et al. The anterior pituitary. In: Wilson, J. D., and Foster, D. W., eds. *Williams Textbook of Endocrinology.* Philadelphia: W. B. Saunders, 1992. Pp. 221–310.

54 The Posterior Pituitary

Lawrence A. Frohman

Objectives

After reading this chapter, you should be able to

Discuss the components of the hypothalamic-neurohypophysial system and the hormones they secrete

Describe the mechanisms of biosynthesis, transport, storage, and secretion of the neurohypophysial hormones

List the sites of vasopressin activity, and describe its mechanism of action

Describe the major mechanisms involved in the regulation of vasopressin secretion and their interaction

List the sites and describe the mechanism of action of oxytocin

The posterior pituitary is a component of two independent neuroendocrine systems that produce the hormones vasopressin and oxytocin, each of which has multiple functions. The most important action of vasopressin relates to water conservation; oxytocin is important in uterine contraction at parturition and also in milk secretion. The anatomy, biochemistry, and secretion of these hormonal systems will be considered together, and the mechanism of action and regulation of secretion will be described separately.

Anatomy

The posterior pituitary or **neurohypophysis** is an integral part of the CNS. It extends ventrally from the **median eminence** of the hypothalamus and is attached to the caudal border of the **anterior pituitary.** The intrasellar portion of the neurohypophysis is known as the **pars nervosa,** and the portion above the diaphragma sellae is the **infundibulum.** The **blood supply** of the posterior pituitary is derived directly from the arterial circulation by branches of the in-

tracavernous portion of the internal carotid artery and the posterior communicating arteries. Venous drainage is to the jugular vein via the cavernous and petrosal sinuses.

The physiologic units of the posterior pituitary consist of neuronal cell bodies, the **perikarya,** which are located in two nuclear groups in the anterior hypothalamus: the **paraventricular nucleus** (PVN) and the **supraoptic nucleus** (SON). The perikarya are relatively large and have been termed **magnocellular neurons.** From the perikarya in the SON, axonal fibers travel through the ventral hypothalamus and pituitary stalk and terminate in bulbous extensions called **pituicytes** in the pars nervosa. These neurosecretory cells are responsible for most, if not all, of the vasopressin and oxytocin that is secreted into plasma. A second system originates in the PVN and sends fibers to the median eminence, where the released vasopressin participates in the control of adrenocorticotropic hormone secretion, to the medulla and spinal cord, where it regulates autonomic nervous system function, and to the amygdala, other hypothalamic nuclei, and the wall of the third ventricle, the presumed sites of origin for vasopressin and oxytocin in the cerebrospinal fluid.

Biochemistry, Synthesis, and Secretion

There are multiple neuropeptides in the posterior pituitary that probably have important physiologic functions, though the most well characterized and studied are **vasopressin** and **oxytocin**. Each is a **nonapeptide** consisting of a six-member disulfide-containing ring and a carboxylamidated three-residue tail (Fig. 54-1). The structures of the two peptides differ by only two amino acids. Both are derived from a single precursor present in nonmammalian vertebrates, **arginine vasotocin,** that exhibits similar biologic properties. Extensive structure-function studies of vasopressin have indicated that the arginine in the 8 position is critical to the pressor activity but not to the antidiuretic activity of vasopressin. Substitution of D-arginine in this position, along with removal of the terminal amino group of cysteine (desamino-8-D-arginine vasopressin [DDAVP]) produces a highly potent and long-acting antidiuretic peptide possessing virtually no pressor activity. This agent is the drug of choice in treating disorders of vasopressin deficiency (diabetes insipidus).

Vasopressin and oxytocin are synthesized in the SON and PVN perikarya as a large **prohormone** (molecular weight 21,000 to 23,000) containing an amino-terminal neuropeptide, followed by a **neurophysin** (a binding protein specific for each neuropeptide) with a molecular weight of 10,000, and a **carboxyl-terminal peptide.** The precursor is proteolytically processed, and **neurosecretory granules** are formed that contain the neuropeptide bound to its neurophysin. Although vasopressin and oxytocin are made in separate cell bodies, the biosynthetic processes are similar. The granules are then transported axonally and stored in pituicytes in the posterior pituitary or in nerve terminals in the central nervous system.

Hormone secretion is accomplished through a stimulus-secretion coupling mechanism. The stimulus, which is applied to the perikarya in the SON or PVN, propagates an electrical impulse down the axon, leading to depolarization of the cell membrane; increased calcium permeability, leading to rapid entry of calcium; and exocytosis of the secretory granule. Thus the neurophysin is secreted in equimolar amounts to the neuropeptide. The relatively low binding affinity and pH optimum, however, promote nearly complete dissociation of the complex in plasma.

In addition to vasopressin and oxytocin, **endothelin,** an endothelial cell–derived peptide with potent vasoconstricting properties, has recently been identified in the posterior pituitary and shown to be secreted under conditions that favor vasopressin secretion. Its role in the response to osmotic regulation remains undefined.

Vasopressin

Mechanism of Action

The primary effect of vasopressin is to enhance the formation of **concentrated** (hypertonic) **urine.** It also increases vascular smooth muscle tone, enhances intestinal motility, and stimulates the production of clotting factors, including factor VIII and von Willebrand's factor. Two separate **vasopressin receptors** have been identified, one (V_1) that mediates the pressor effect and a second one (V_2) that mediates antidiuresis and the effects of clotting factors. Mutations in the V_2 receptor are associated with resistance to the action of vasopressin.

In the vasopressin-responsive **renal epithelial cells,** receptor binding is coupled to a guanine-nucleotide regulatory protein (G_s) that stimulates cyclic AMP formation and protein phosphorylation. This heightens water permeability in the collecting duct and the medullary thick ascending loop of Henle. If vasopressin is lacking, the collecting tubules are almost completely impermeable to water. In its presence, there is a concentration-dependent increase in the water-specific channels or pores that accentuates the transport of solute-free water through the luminal membranes. The renal handling of salt and water metabolism is discussed in Chap. 41. A feedback process that modulates the effects of vasopressin is mediated by **prostaglandin E,** the synthesis of which is stimulated by the hormone. Prostaglandin E, in turn, inhibits the effects of vasopressin on adenylate cyclase.

The **pressor effects** of vasopressin in humans are much greater than those necessary for maximal antidiuresis, and there is currently no convincing evidence that the hormone has any physiologic role in regulating blood pressure in humans. Similarly, any physiologically important effects

Fig. 54-1. Chemical structures of vasopressin and oxytocin, the major hormones of the posterior pituitary.

Vasopressin

$$NH_2-Cys-Tyr-Phe-Gln-Asn-Cys-Pro-Arg-Gly-NH_2$$
$$\underline{\hspace{1.2cm}} S-S \underline{\hspace{1.2cm}}$$

Oxytocin

$$NH_2-Cys-Tyr-Ile-Gln-Asn-Cys-Pro-Leu-Gly-NH_2$$
$$\underline{\hspace{1.2cm}} S-S \underline{\hspace{1.2cm}}$$

on intestinal motility and clotting factors have yet to be proved. Nevertheless, the use of vasopressin, or DDAVP, in the treatment of milder forms of **hemophilia** has been valuable in reducing the need for plasma transfusions.

Plasma Levels and Metabolism

Plasma levels of vasopressin in normally hydrated, non-stressed individuals are less than 2 pg/ml. Levels are highest in the early morning and lowest in late afternoon. Most of the peptide is inactivated in the liver, though plasma enzymatic degradation also occurs, particularly during pregnancy, when plasma vasopressinase activity increases. Plasma neurophysin levels are considerably greater than those of vasopressin, because of a much slower metabolic clearance of the protein.

Regulation of Secretion

Osmoregulation

Under physiologic conditions, the most important regulator of vasopressin secretion is the **osmotic pressure of plasma.** This control is mediated by a group of highly specific neurons called **osmoregulators** that are located in the anterior hypothalamus, near but clearly distinct from the SON. There are bimodal inhibitory and stimulatory inputs from the osmoregulatory neurons, although the net result resembles that of a **"set point,"** or threshold, **mechanism.** Plasma osmolality normally fluctuates within a very narrow range of between 275 to 290 mOsm/kg. Within this range, plasma vasopressin levels are near or beneath the lower limit of detection (less than 2 pg/ml). When the osmolality level is exceeded (the critical value varies among individuals), there is a steep and proportionate rise in vasopressin levels such that a 1% change in osmolality triggers vasopressin release by an amount (1 pg/ml) sufficient to alter urine osmolality (Fig. 54-2). The set point, though constant in an individual for long periods, may vary by up to 5 mOsm/kg in conjunction with other factors, such as age, hemodynamic alterations, and pregnancy. The rates of change in vasopressin secretion in response to alterations in osmolality are also constant in individuals and appear to be determined genetically. However, they may be modified if blood volume, blood glucose, or calcium levels are disturbed or by certain drugs, such as lithium. The sensitivity of the osmoregulatory mechanism is also solute-dependent. While **Na+** is the most potent solute and, together with its anions, constitutes 95% or greater of the plasma osmotic pressure, **sugars** such as sucrose and mannitol also have similar stimulatory effects. One exception is

Fig. 54-2. Relationship of plasma vasopressin levels to plasma and urine osmolality in normal adults. A very narrow range of change in the plasma osmolality results in increased vasopressin secretion and near-maximal antidiuresis, even before thirst perception. (From: Robertson, G. L. Posterior pituitary. In: Felig, P., Baxter, J. D., and Frohman, L. A., eds. *Endocrinology and Metabolism,* 3rd ed. New York: McGraw-Hill, 1995.)

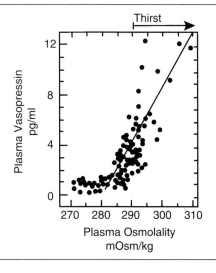
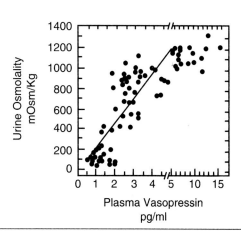

urea, which is almost entirely ineffective in stimulating vasopressin secretion. Osmoreceptors respond to changes in the glucose level, but only when entry of this solute into cells is impaired, such as in uncontrolled diabetes.

Hemodynamic Regulation

Changes in **blood volume** and **blood pressure** profoundly affect vasopressin secretion, independent of osmoregulation. These changes are recognized by **baroreceptors** (pressure-sensitive receptors) in both the low-pressure (cardiac atria) and high-pressure (carotid bifurcation and aortic arch) regions of the circulatory system. They travel via parasympathetic fibers in the vagus and glossopharyngeal nerves, which synapse in the brainstem with fibers that project to the PVN and SON. Their impulses appear to be chiefly inhibitory under nonstressed basal conditions. When blood pressure decreases, the plasma vasopressin level rises exponentially in proportion to the degree of hypotension. A reduction of more than 10% is generally necessary before plasma vasopressin levels are increased; a 20% to 30% decrease in blood pressure elevates levels to many times that needed for maximal antidiuresis. A blood volume decrease of more than 7% is required to increase plasma vasopressin levels, and levels are markedly elevated when there is a 20% decrease. Increases in blood volume or blood pressure produce corresponding decreases in the vasopressin levels.

Because the variation in body water content is very small under normal physiologic conditions, the osmoregulatory mechanisms provide the primary control of vasopressin secretion. However, fluctuations in blood pressure during exercise or stress are enough to provoke baroreceptor regulatory input that is comparable with that of the osmoreceptor in regulating vasopressin secretion (Fig. 54-3). Yet these two mechanisms are distinct, as shown by individuals with disturbed baroreceptor activation of vasopressin secretion, who respond normally to stimulation of the osmoreceptor.

Neuroregulation

The most potent neurogenic stimulus for vasopressin secretion is **nausea.** This pathway originates from the **area postrema** in the medulla and is mediated by **dopaminergic fibers.** Antidopaminergic agents that are effective in alleviating nausea also inhibit vasopressin secretion. Many physiologic and pathologic processes associated with increased vasopressin secretion and antidiuresis, such as vasovagal reactions, acute motion sickness, and acute hypoxia, are probably mediated by their associated emetic stimuli.

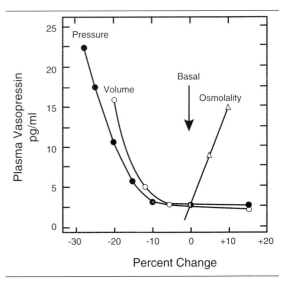

Fig. 54-3. Stimulus-response relationship between plasma vasopressin levels and percentage change in osmolality, blood volume, and blood pressure in normal adults. (From: Robertson, G. L. Posterior pituitary. In: Felig, P., Baxter, J. D., and Frohman, L. A., eds. *Endocrinology and Metabolism,* 3rd ed. New York: McGraw-Hill, 1995.)

Stress and **increased temperature** also enhance vasopressin secretion, though it is not clear whether these effects are primary or are mediated by associated changes in blood pressure or the effective blood volume. Clinically, high fevers may be associated with vasopressin secretion that is osmotically inappropriate. **Severe hypoxemia** also may stimulate vasopressin secretion, even in the absence of nausea. **Central glucopenia** is another potent stimulus for vasopressin secretion. Although the stimulus is not specific for vasopressin, it may be physiologically important, for example, in diabetics who are receiving excessive amounts of insulin. **Pain** also constitutes a stimulus for vasopressin release, but the response is not specific.

Angiotensin

Angiotensin-II is a potent stimulus for vasopressin secretion. It has a **central site of action** and also stimulates the **thirst mechanism.** The nature of this stimulation is not known, though its role is believed to be physiologic because angiotensin antagonists inhibit vasopressin release, implying the presence of an endogenous stimulatory tone.

Oxytocin

Mechanism of Action

The biologic activity of oxytocin in **females** is confined to the **uterus** and **breasts.** There are specific myometrial receptors that bind the hormone, leading to membrane depolarization and myometrial contraction. These effects are enhanced by estrogen and are important during parturition. Although the initiation of labor is largely independent of oxytocin, the hormone appears to participate in the final expulsion of the fetus and placenta when the cervix is fully dilated.

Oxytocin also produces contraction of the myoepithelial cells of the **breast alveoli,** causing expulsion of milk from the secretory channels into the large sinuses connected to the nipple. Although oxytocin does not participate in milk production, which is largely regulated by prolactin, it is critical to the secretory process and was originally called the "milk letdown" factor.

In **males,** oxytocin participates in the process of **sperm ejection** into semen upon stimulation of the reproductive organs, though the importance of this action is uncertain. The hormone also exhibits slight antidiuretic activity (about 0.5% to 1%), but it is doubtful that this represents a physiologic role.

Regulation of Secretion

The regulation of oxytocin secretion is less well understood than that of vasopressin. The major stimulus appears to be **suckling,** which is mediated through nerve fibers in the nipple. **Distension of the female genital tract,** particularly during parturition, also serves as possible stimulus for oxytocin release. Estrogen administration heightens the secretion of the oxytocin-associated neurophysin and was originally believed to elevate oxytocin release as well. However, the specificity of assays used to demonstrate these effects has recently been questioned, and the possibility of another, yet unidentified, posterior pituitary hormone has been raised. **Pain** is also a stimulus for the secretion of oxytocin, though this response is not specific.

Bibliography

Baylis, P. H. Vasopressin and its neurophysin. In: DeGroot, L. J., et al., eds. *Endocrinology.* Philadelphia: W. B. Saunders, 1989. Pp. 213–229.

Reeves, W. B., and Andreoli, T. E. The posterior pituitary and water metabolism. In: Wilson, J. D., and Foster, D. W., eds. *Williams Textbook of Endocrinology.* Philadelphia: W. B. Saunders, 1992. Pp. 311–356.

Robertson, G. L. Posterior pituitary. In: Felig, P., Baxter, J. D., and Frohman, L. A., eds. *Endocrinology and Metabolism,* 3rd ed. New York: McGraw-Hill, 1995.

55 Thyroid Physiology

Nelson D. Horseman

Objectives

After reading this chapter, you should be able to

Describe the metabolic pools and pathways for iodine metabolism

Outline the pathways for thyroid hormone biosynthesis, secretion, regulation, and circulatory transport

Describe the actions of thyroid hormones on metabolism in the whole organism

Explain how thyroid hormones act at the cellular and molecular levels

Describe the physiologic basis of disease during thyroid hormone hypersecretion and hyposecretion

---

The enlargement of the thyroid gland, referred to as **goiter,** has, since ancient times, been one of the most recognizable symptoms in human disease. Thyroid tumors, Graves' disease, and thyroid autoimmune destruction are relatively common adult endocrine diseases. The fact that thyroid hormones are key regulators of metabolism and development accounts for the broad range of symptoms associated with these disease states.

The thyroid gland develops from the pharyngeal enteric epithelium very early in embryonic development and secretes thyroid hormone in the fetus. Fetal thyroid hormone is important for neural development. Within the thyroid gland, two cell types produce hormones; follicular cells produce thyroxine and triiodothyronine (generically referred to as **thyroid hormones**), and C-cells produce calcitonin.

The thyroid gland develops as an endodermal evagination from the pharynx. It grows to form a bilobed structure connected across the midline of the trachea by the thyroid isthmus. The mature thyroid is situated just below the larynx. The bulk of the thyroid mass consists of thyroid follicles, comprised of a single follicular epithelium cell layer surrounding a colloid-filled lumen. The follicular epithelial cells have a clearly polarized structure consisting of a basal surface in contact with the blood vessels, connective tissue, and intersticium surrounding the follicles and an apical surface facing the lumen. The parafollicular C-cells are derived embryonically from the ultimobranchial bodies and migrate into the mammalian thyroid during embryogenesis. The parathyroid gland, which produces parathyroid hormone, is a distinct organ that is attached to, or embedded within, the dorsal surface of the thyroid gland.

Iodine Metabolism

Thyroid hormones, their precursors, and their metabolic products are the only iodinated organic compounds of the body. Therefore, the intermediates of thyroid hormone synthesis are found only in the thyroid follicles. Thyroid hormones are iodinated metabolites of the amino acid tyrosine. Essentially all the iodine secreted from thyroid cells is in the form of three products. These are thyroxine (T_4, 3,5,3',5'-tetraiodothyronine), which represents about 90% of secreted iodine; 3,3'5'-tridothyroine (T_3), about 10% of iodine; and reverse T_3 (3,5,3'-T_3, or rT_3), which is hormonally inactive and accounts for less than 1% of secreted iodine. Because iodine metabolism is inextricably linked with thyroid function, it is important to understand it thoroughly. Also, because of its exclusive association with the synthesis of thyroid hormones, iodine metabolism is probably the most simple and well-understood nutrient metabolism system in the body. Therefore, it provides an excellent opportunity to study how nutrient metabolism operates. The basic principles of nutrient flux through various pools and storage sites are the same for other, more complicated metabolic systems (Fig. 55-1).

A typical dietary iodide intake is about 500 μg/day, and essentially all of this is absorbed by the gastrointestinal tract. The iodide absorbed from the diet contributes to the circulating extracellular fluid pool, and from this, iodide disappears rapidly (within a few hours) by either excretion in the urine or uptake into the thyroid gland. Use by the thyroid gland is relatively stable (100–150 μg/day) in normal individuals. The remainder of absorbed iodide is ex-

creted in the urine. In addition to ingested iodide, two other routes contribute to the circulating pool of iodide. These are leakage of iodide from the thyroid gland and release of iodide from deiodination of thyroid hormones in peripheral tissues. These routes contribute something in the neighborhood of 40 and 60 μg of circulating iodide each day, respectively.

One very important aspect of iodide metabolism and thyroid gland function is the relationship of thyroid hormone storage to the daily secretion of thyroid hormones. Follicular cells release about 75 μg of iodine per day in the form of thyroid hormones. In contrast, the gland stores about 7500 μg of iodine in the follicular colloid as iodinated hormone. Therefore, the gland has at least 2 months of hormone in reserve under normal conditions. In addition to this reserve of glandular hormone, there is about 600 μg of iodine in the form of thyroid hormones in the circulation at any given time. This represents about 7 or 8 days of hormone reserve, most of which is bound to circulating carrier proteins. When thyroid hormones are taken up from the circulation, the iodine contained in them is either released by deiodination and returned to the circulation (about 60 μg/day) or removed in the feces by way of the liver's bile secretion (15 μg/day).

Iodide in the Thyroid Gland

Iodide is "trapped" by follicular cells (Fig. 55-2). This iodide trapping mechanism requires that iodide is actively transported against a concentration and electrochemical gradient such that follicular cell iodide is about 30 times higher than plasma iodide. This iodide transport mechanism can be competitively inhibited by the transport of various other anions such as thiocyanate, perchlorate, and pertechnitate. However, there is no significant competition from other halides such as Cl⁻ ions. This high specificity for iodide, compared with other halides, is extremely important from a physiologic point of view, since chloride ions are present in the circulation at concentrations many orders of magnitude higher than iodide.

The iodide trapping system provides one of the most useful diagnostic methods for thyroid medicine. Either radioiodide or radiolabeled technetium (Tc) (as pertechnitate) is administered, and the pattern of thyroid radiolabeling is observed by fluorimetry or photometry. The radiolabel distribution may indicate tumors, nodules, diffuse enlargement of the gland, regions that do not take up iodide, or other conditions.

In addition to its diagnostic value, the iodide uptake mechanism is exploited therapeutically. Radioisotopic de-

Fig. 55-1. The metabolic pathways for iodine in the human. Daily average intake of 500 μg is indicated at the top of the chart. The intake can vary substantially among individuals, but chronic intake of substantially lower amounts leads to goiter. The arrows indicate the pathways from one nutrient pool to another. The numbers within the parentheses are average amounts within each pool, whereas the numbers associated with the arrows represent daily fluxes.

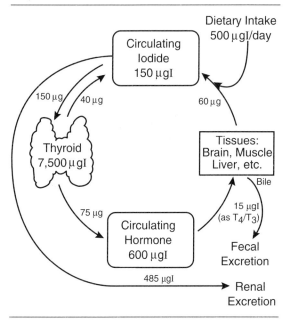

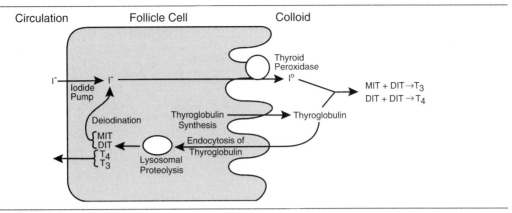

Fig. 55-2. Thyroid follicular cell physiology. Iodide is actively taken up exclusively by the thyroid gland and is converted to iodine or iodinium ions by thyroid peroxidase. Thyroglobulin, which is synthesized in follicular cells and secreted into the colloid space, is iodinated on tyrosine residues to produce monoiodotyrosine and diiodotyrosine. These intermediates are then coupled to produce thyroid hormones. After being taken back into the follicular cells, thyroglobulin is broken down to release the thyroid hormones and intermediates, which are recycled. More details of these functions are described in the text.

struction of thyroid tumors or a hyperactive thyroid in Graves' disease is relatively simple if the trapping mechanism is active in the follicular cells. Moderate doses of radioiodide are administered systematically and highly concentrated in the thyroid gland, where the cells are killed by ionizing radiation. This treatment modality, while specific to thyroid cells, destroys both normal and diseased thyroid cells. This necessitates long-term therapy with exogenous thyroid hormones after initial treatment of the disease.

After being taken up at the basolateral surfaces of follicular cells, iodide is rapidly moved to the apical surface. Here, either in apical vesicles or on the luminal surfaces of the follicular cells, iodide is oxidized to atomic iodine (I^0) and iodinium ions (I^+). Thyroid peroxidase is the enzyme responsible for oxidation of iodide. Thyroid peroxidase uses H_2O_2 as a source of oxidizing potential.

Thyroglobulin: Organification of Iodide and Thyroid Hormone Release

Thyroglobulin is an exceptionally large protein, with a molecular mass of about 670,000 daltons. It is found exclusively within thyroid follicles. Thyroglobulin is secreted directionally into the lumina of the follicles, where it accumulates as a colloidal solution. Tyrosine residues

within the thyroglobulin molecule are iodinated and coupled together to produce thyroid hormones. The iodination and coupling reactions are depicted in Fig. 55-3. The process of covalently binding iodine to tyrosine residues in thyroglobulin is called **organification,** and it occurs exclusively in the thyroid gland. This set of reactions is controlled by factors from outside the thyroid gland, such as thyroid-stimulating hormone, and by factors within the thyroid gland cells, such as the intracellular concentration of iodide.

The coupling reaction is believed to be catalyzed by thyroid peroxidase, but the exact mechanisms and intermediates are not fully understood. Thyroglobulin consists of two identical peptide chains (molecular weights of approximately 330,000 each). A tyrosine residue at the 5th position from its amino-terminus is the preferred site of iodination and coupling. Other tyrosines in thyroglobulin are also used less frequently.

The secretion of thyroid hormone is accomplished by a paradoxical mechanism. Stimulation of thyroid follicular cells by **thyroid-stimulating hormone** (TSH) causes thyroglobulin to be taken up from the colloid by endocytosis. Lysosomes fuse with the colloid vesicles formed by endocytosis, and lysosomal proteases break down thyroglobulin, liberating the iodinated thyroid hormones. These freely diffuse out of the cell because of their lipid solubility. Therefore, unlike protein hormones that follow a Golgi apparatus–exocytosis pathway of secretion, thyroid hor-

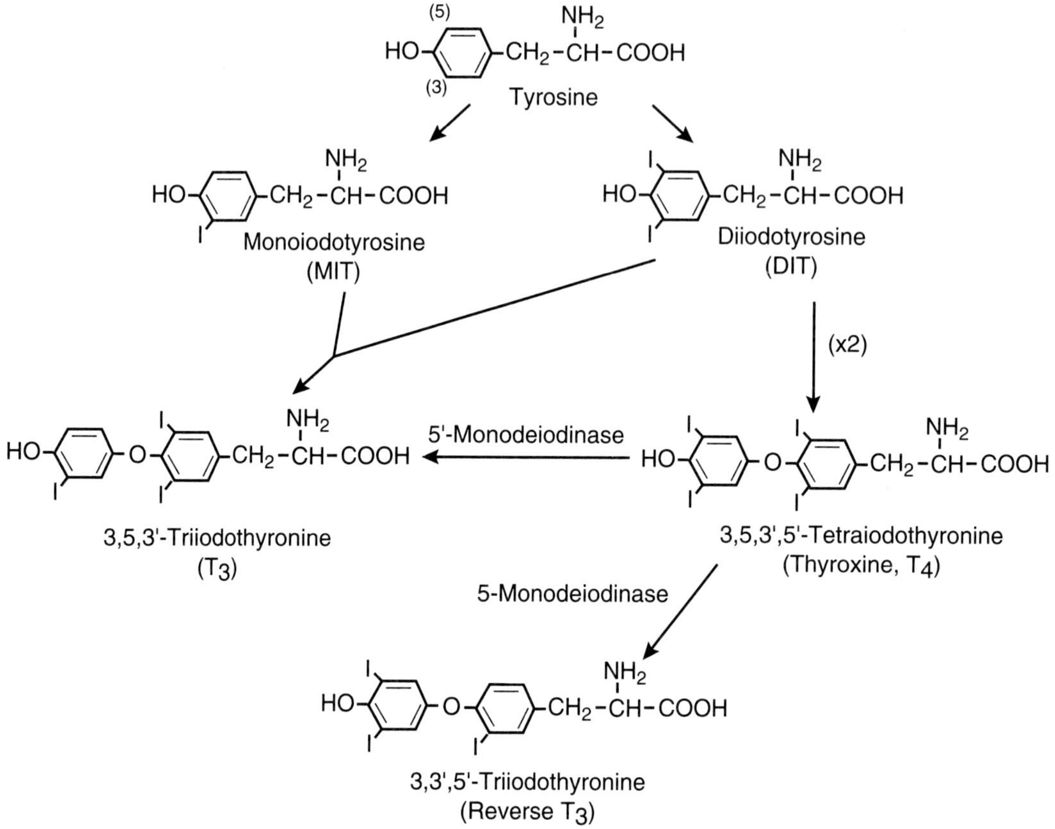

Fig. 55-3. The thyroid hormone biosynthetic pathway. Remember that the reactions involved in synthesis of T_3 and T_4 take place within the context of the thyroglobulin molecule, whereas the deiodination reactions take place primarily in peripheral tissues.

mones are released as a consequence of traffic through the lysoendosomal pathway.

The intermediate precursors of thyroid hormones, **monoiodotyrosine** (MIT) and **diiodotyrosine** (DTT), are also released by proteolysis of thyroglobulin. However, these precursors are not lipid soluble, so they do not diffuse out of the cell. Therefore, they are rapidly deiodinated, and the iodine and tyrosine are recycled into the new synthesis of hormones.

Regulation of Thyroid Hormone Secretion

The most important physiologic regulator of thyroid function is thyroid-stimulating hormone (TSH, or thyrotropin) from the anterior pituitary (Fig. 55-4). TSH is released

from thyrotropes in the anterior pituitary in response to thyrotropin-releasing hormone (TRH). TRH is a 3 amino acid peptide that is secreted into the hypothalamic-pituitary portal system. It circulates to the pituitary and binds to receptors on thyrotropes. Cold stress is a strong stimulator of TRH and TSH release. In addition to the rapid secretory stimulation from TSH, there is a longer-term elevation of thyroid function caused by TSH. TSH stimulates growth and proliferation of thyroid follicular cells, increased thyroid blood flow, and increased iodide trapping. TSH causes rapid increases in thyroglobulin endocytosis and hydrolysis, leading to T_4 and T_3 release.

T_3 is a potent inhibitor of TRH release and therefore suppresses TSH secretion. In addition, T_3 also causes a marked increase in the release of somatostatin, which inhibits both TSH and growth hormone secretion. A lack of T_3 or defective conversion of T_4 to T_3 leads to markedly el-

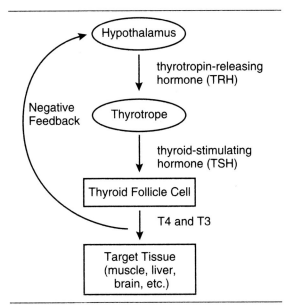

Fig. 55-4. The regulatory relationships of the hypothalamic-pituitary-thyroid axis.

evated TSH secretion (Fig. 55-5). Because TSH secretion is absolutely linked to the feedback effects of thyroid hormones, the level of TSH will define thyroid status. The euthyroid state is represented by balanced thyroid function and normal TSH levels. The hyperthyroid individual will present low TSH levels, depressed by the increased feedback of thyroid hormones. Conversely, in hypothyroidism, TSH levels are high because of insufficient thyroid hormones to suppress the hypothalamus and pituitary.

Thyroid hormone has a very long circulating half-life. T_4 half-life is about 7 days, and T_3 is about 1 day. Therefore, thyroid hormone levels change very slowly over time. Normal levels are about 8 mg/dl.

TSH acts through a G_s protein–coupled membrane receptor. Binding of TSH to its receptor increases cyclic AMP (cAMP) synthesis in the follicular cell. cAMP can mimic all the known effects of TSH on thyroid cells, so it is probably the sole second messenger for thyroid stimulation. cAMP phosphodiesterase converts the active cAMP into inactive AMP, thereby desensitizing the thyroid cells.

Iodide is itself a regulator of follicle cell iodide trapping and thyroid hormone synthesis. This autoregulatory action is called the **Wolff-Chaikoff effect.** In this intrinsic regulatory mechanism, high intrafollicular iodide inhibits iodide trapping and lowers thyroid hormone synthesis. The precise molecular targets that sense follicular cell iodide levels are unknown.

Fig. 55-5. Thyroid hormone feedback mechanisms. The two sites of feedback regulation of the thyroid axis are the pituitary and hypothalamus. The major effect is on the hypothalamus, as depicted in Fig. 55-4. In the hypothalamus, T_3 (either from the circulation or from deiodination of T_4) causes both decreased thyrotropin-releasing hormone (TRH) secretion and increased somatostatin (SRIF) secretion. Both these effects tend to decrease secretion of thyroid-stimulating hormone (TSH) from the anterior pituitary.

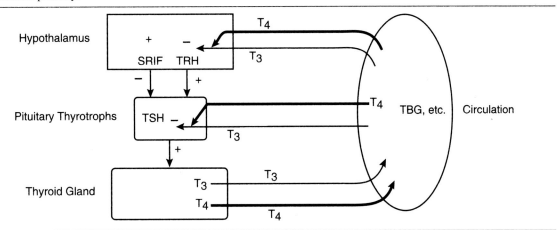

Immediately after birth there is large increase of TSH and thyroid hormone synthesis. This is probably associated with development of homeothermy in the infant.

Thiourea and propylthiouracil (PTU) are **antithyroid compounds** that block thyroid hormone synthesis primarily by blocking iodide organification. PTU has the additional effect of inhibiting the activity of **5'-deiodinase** in thyroid hormone target tissues. By decreasing deiodination, PTU decreases the conversion of T_4, which is relatively weak, to T_3, which is much more active. Because circulating T_4 has such a long half-life, decreasing its biopotency by inhibiting conversion to T_3 is a valuable way to rapidly relieve some of the symptoms of hyperthyroidism.

Thyroid Hormone Metabolism

T_3 is the most active form of thyroid hormones, about 4 times more active than T_4. Reverse T_3 (rT_3) is essentially inactive. These variations in potency are based entirely on the relative affinities of each hormone for the thyroid hormone receptor, which is often referred to as the **T_3 receptor** because T_3 is the most important form of the hormone in terms of receptor activation. In the circulation, 99.9% of T_3 and T_4 are bound to plasma proteins. **Thyroxin-binding globulin** (TBG) is a high-affinity carrier for both T_4 and T_3, but it circulates at low concentrations. Therefore, it only carries about 60% of thyroid hormones. **Thyroid-binding prealbumin** (TBPA) is a lower-affinity carrier for T_4. It normally carries approximately 30% of T_4 but no appreciable amount of T_3. **Albumin** is a low-affinity carrier for more than 30% of T_3. It also binds a small amount of T_4 with low affinity.

The **T_3-resin uptake (T_3-RU) test** is a useful clinical means of determining the status of circulating free and bound thyroid hormones (Fig. 55-6). In this test, serum is mixed with radiolabeled T_3 and a resin that selectively binds free thyroid hormones. The radiolabeled T_3 binds to either the resin or TBG, depending on the relative amounts of thyroid hormones and TBG in the patient's serum. When the resin-bound radiolabel is determined, the results can be interpreted to establish the relative levels of hormone and carrier. It is necessary to simultaneously know the level of total T_4 and T_3 in the circulation to establish a value for the free thyroid index.

The T_3 receptor has about a 5 to 10 times higher affinity for the hormone than does TBG. There is, therefore, a small soluble pool of T_3 that is in equilibrium with the receptor- and carrier-bound pools. For T_4 there is a much smaller difference in affinities between TBG and the re-

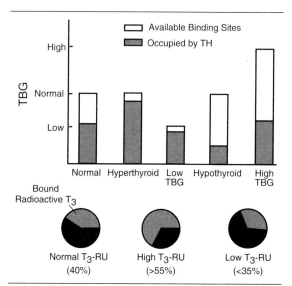

Fig. 55-6. The T_3-resin uptake (T_3-RU) test and its interpretation. In the histogram the total height of the bars represents the total serum thyroxine-binding globulin (TBG) capacity and the stippled portion represents that which is occupied by circulating thyroid hormones. In the T_3-RU test, radioactive T_3 is added to a serum sample along with a resin that will bind whatever fraction of the T_3 that does not bind to serum TBG. In the pie charts at the bottom, the stippled area represents the fraction of radiolabeled T_3 bound to the resin and the darkly shaded portion represents that bound to serum TBG. Therefore, higher than normal T_3-RU could indicate elevated thyroid hormone secretion or low TBG. Conversely, low T_3-RU would indicate decreased serum thyroid hormones or elevated TBG.

ceptor, so the equilibrium is less favorable for binding to the receptor, even though total circulating T_4 levels are higher than T_3.

As noted previously, T_4 is activated by 5'-deiodinase to form T_3, which is the main active hormone. The circulating concentration of T_4 is about 60 times higher than that of T_3; therefore, most T_3 is derived from 5'-deiodination of T_4 within the tissues of the body. T_3 released from the thyroid gland represents only a small fraction of the active T_3.

Deiodination of the 5 (inner ring) rather than 5' (outer ring) position (see Fig. 55-3) is catalyzed by **5-deiodinase.** This reaction is inactivating, since the product, reverse T_3, does not bind to the T_3 receptor. Most of the turnover of thyroid hormones goes through this pathway before excretion (see Fig. 55-1). A small fraction of active hormone is eliminated by the gut without being deiodinated at the 5 position.

Whole-Body Actions of Thyroid Hormone

In the adult, the most obvious action of thyroid hormones in the whole body is to increase basal metabolism and oxygen consumption and to increase heat production. The latter effect is termed the **calorigenic action** of thyroid hormones. At the clinical extreme, resting O_2 consumption (which is sometimes referred to as the **basal metabolic rate**) can be as low as 150 ml/min in severe hypothyroidism. This is about 40% below the normal metabolic rate. In hyperthyroidism, the O_2 consumption may reach as much as 400 ml/min, or 180% of normal. During these large changes in metabolism, the **respiratory quotient (RQ)** is not affected. This indicates that both glucose oxidation and fatty acid oxidation are increased simultaneously. If glucose were preferentially used, one would expect that the RQ (CO_2 produced per O_2 consumed) would be closer to 1.0, whereas fat utilization would result in an RQ significantly below 1.0.

Cardiac output increases in hyperthyroidism. These increases can be traced to changes in peripheral resistance, heart rate, and myocardial contractility. Most of these effects on cardiac output are probably a consequence of elevated sensitivity to catecholamines. Beta-adrenergic receptors are elevated in tissues of individuals with hyperthyroidism, leading to sympathetic nervous system hypersensitivity.

Elevated thyroid hormone levels also increase intestinal glucose absorption and the mobilization of nutrients from liver, adipose, and muscle stores. Another effect of elevated thyroid hormones is hyperperistalsis of the gut. This effect leads to frequent defecation, which can be mistaken for diarrhea.

Many actions of thyroid hormone on the whole body are secondary to the increased sensitivity to sympathetic nervous system catecholamines. The combined effects of metabolic elevation caused by the calorigenic effect of thyroid hormones and neural hypersensitivity lead to a generalized syndrome of hyperactivity.

In moderate to severe thyroid hormone hypersecretion, the synergism between thyroid hormones and beta-adrenergic sensitization can lead to acute, life-threatening "**thyroid storm.**" This condition cannot be predicted on the basis of thyroid hormone levels alone, since there is a hormone–nervous system interaction. The only way to alleviate the symptoms of thyroid storm is to use drugs that block the actions of the sympathetic nervous system. The reduction of thyroid hormone level is a much longer-term process because of the long half-life of thyroxine.

Thyroid hormones are necessary for normal development of nervous, reproductive, cardiovascular, and skeletal systems during both infancy and childhood. If there is a deficiency of thyroid hormones during early infancy, the child develops cretinism. This syndrome includes severe retardation and numerous other developmental deficiencies. In the United States and other developed countries, infants are always tested for thyroid hormones as neonates. Provided they are treated in the first few days of life, there are no long-term problems, except the need to continue thyroid therapy indefinitely.

Cellular and Molecular Actions of Thyroid Hormones

The receptor for T_3, and T_4, is in the nucleus of most cells of the body. After binding the hormone, the receptor stimulates the synthesis of mRNA from those genes that contain a DNA sequence known as a T_3 **response element** (TRE). This system is similar in most respects to the steroid hormone mechanism of action (see Fig. 57-3). In fact, the T_3 receptor is a member of the same family of proteins as the steroid hormone receptors and the vitamin D receptor, all of which directly interact with sequences generically called **hormone response elements** (HREs) within the genes of target tissues. Genes that are stimulated by thyroid hormones include mitochondrial proteins, malic enzyme, Na^+,K^+-ATPase, growth hormone, and others. Malic enzyme is involved in fat mobilization. Na^+,K^+-ATPase consumes large amounts of metabolic energy, and its stimulation may be the most important determinant of the calorigenic action of thyroid hormones.

Clinical Manifestations

The most common form of thyroid hormone hypersecretion is **Graves' disease.** Graves' disease is a consequence of autoantibodies called **thyroid-stimulating immunoglobulins** (TSIs), which were called **long-acting thyroid stimulators** (LATS) in the older literature. Because TSIs are not regulated by normal feedback mechanisms, there is a tendency to gradually increase thyroid hormone levels. This causes increased metabolism, loss of weight and muscle mass, edema, cardiomyopathy, and a characteristic eye protrusion called **exophthalmos.** The exophthalmos is associated with periorbital edema. At high thyroid hormone levels, mental agitation and anxiety can result. These latter effects are probably due to sympathetic hyperactivity. The development of Graves' disease is usually gradual and insidious. As TSI levels increase, the level of secretion of thyroid-stimulating hormone from the pituitary will undergo a compensatory decrease. Therefore, the early preclinical stages of the disease are hidden by the efficient nature of the feedback regulatory system.

The question of whether mild forms of hypothyroidism might contribute to obesity is still controversial and unproven. True clinical hypothyroidism is most often a result of gland atrophy following a severe autoimmune reaction. The most common form of thyroid destruction by autoimmune attack is called **Hashimoto's thyroiditis.** Its symptoms include lethargy and fatigue and a characteristic puffiness of the face and lower eyelids called **myxedema.** Prior to the development of hypothyroidism, many individuals will undergo a phase of hyperthyroidism as the thyroid hormone stored in the colloid of the gland is dumped into the circulation due to glandular damage.

Summary

The thyroid gland synthesizes two hormones, T_4 and T_3, that are important for both developmental and metabolic control. These hormones are iodinated metabolites of the amino acid tyrosine, and their synthesis is the product of a highly specialized set of metabolic adaptations of the thyroid gland. The active transport and organification of iodine lead to trapping of large amounts of iodine exclusively in the thyroid gland. The thyroid hormones are carried in the plasma by a set of both specific and generalized carrier proteins, the most important of which is thyroxine-binding globulin. This protein-bound circulating pool of thyroid hormones is in equilibrium with a small pool of free hormone, which can diffuse into cells and bind to the thyroid hormone receptor. The thyroid hormone receptor, like the steroid hormone receptors, is a ligand-dependent transcription factor. That is, after binding the proper hormone, the receptor can bind to and stimulate transcription of specific genes within target tissue cells. One of the genes stimulated by thyroid hormones is Na^+,K^+-ATPase, which consumes large amounts of energy and contributes to the calorigenic (heat-producing) effects of thyroid hormones. Other enzymes that are synthesized in response to thyroid hormones are involved in proper development and fat metabolism. Thyroid hormones are regulated by thyroid-stimulating hormone, which is secreted in response to hypothalamic stimulation of the pituitary thyrotrope cells.

Bibliography

DeGroot, L. J., et al., eds. *Endocrinology,* 3rd ed. Philadelphia: W. B. Saunders, 1995.

Goodman, H. M. *Basic Medical Endocrinology,* 2nd ed. New York: Raven Press, 1994.

Greenspan, F. S. *Basic and Clinical Endocrinology,* 3rd ed. Norwalk, Conn.: Appleton and Lange, 1991.

56 Calcium and Phosphate Homeostasis

James P. Hughes

Objectives

After reading this chapter, you should be able to

Explain the importance of calcium and phosphate in cell structure and cell function

Describe the distribution of calcium and phosphate within the intracellular and extracellular fluid spaces

Describe the steps in the synthesis, secretion, and metabolism of parathyroid hormone, calcitonin, and vitamin D

Describe the mechanisms by which parathyroid hormone, calcitonin, and vitamin D alter cellular function

List the important biologic actions of parathyroid hormone, calcitonin, and vitamin D

Describe the mechanisms by which parathyroid hormone, calcitonin, and vitamin D regulate calcium and phosphate homeostasis

---

The physiologic importance of calcium and phosphate can be divided into two categories, structural and functional. A large proportion of body calcium and phosphate is found in bone. Both substances are necessary for bone mineralization and consequently for maintaining the structural integrity of the skeletal system. Chronic depletion of calcium and/or phosphate reduces the mineral content in bone and increases the risk of fracture. Phosphate, in the form of phosphoproteins and phospholipids, is also a vital constituent of cellular structure. Soluble calcium and phosphate are critical for many regulatory and metabolic functions. Extracellular calcium plays a crucial role in regulating proteolytic processes (e.g., blood coagulation) and membrane potential (e.g., neuromuscular function). Low serum calcium (**hypocalcemia**) causes profound increases in neuromuscular excitability, while elevated calcium (**hypercalcemia**) depresses excitability. Intracellular calcium mediates the actions of many signaling agents, including hormones, and is a critical factor in the activity of numerous enzymes, including kinases and ATPases. Phosphate is an essential component of regulatory phosphoproteins, en-zyme cofactors, nucleic acids, and molecules that store chemical energy such as adenosine triphosphate (ATP). Phosphorylation and dephosphorylation are common mechanisms for modifying protein activity; thus phosphate as well as calcium plays a role in intracellular signaling. It is obvious that calcium and phosphate are not only important for the integrity of the skeleton but also for maintaining the structure and function of every cell in the body.

Calcium and Phosphate Distribution

A 70-kg adult contains approximately 1300 g of calcium and 700 g of phosphate. Most calcium (99%) and phosphate (86%) exist in bone as **hydroxyapatite** $[Ca_{10}(PO_4)_6OH_2]$. Therefore, only about 1% of calcium and 15% of phosphate are found in extraskeletal sites, including extracellular fluid (ECF) and cytoplasm. ECF calcium accounts for 0.1% of body calcium.

In plasma, approximately 43% of the calcium is ionized, 47% is bound to albumin and other proteins, and the remainder is complexed to bicarbonate, phosphate, citrate, and other anions. It is the ionized calcium that participates directly in most physiologic processes, and it is the ionized fraction that is tightly regulated by **parathyroid hormone (PtH), vitamin D,** and **calcitonin (CT).** In contrast, only about 13% of plasma phosphate is protein-bound, while 52% is ionized and 35% is complexed with various cations. Plasma phosphate concentration is less tightly regulated than calcium concentration and may vary by up to 50% within a day.

The basal concentration of calcium in the cytoplasm ($\sim 0.1 \mu M$) is 10,000-fold less than that in serum. Most intracellular calcium is sequestered in the mitochondria in association with phosphate, but a small portion is bound to the inner surface of the plasma membrane and endoplasmic (sarcoplasmic) reticulum. Low cytoplasmic calcium is maintained by at least two types of Ca^{2+} transporters, an Na^+-Ca^{2+} exchanger driven by the transmembrane sodium gradient and an energy-requiring transport system involving Ca^{2+}-ATPase enzymes. Sudden rises in cytoplasmic calcium occur when ion channels allow calcium to move down its gradient from sources such as the ECF, endoplasmic (sarcoplasmic) reticulum, and mitochondria. Changes in cytoplasmic calcium characterize some signal-transduction mechanisms such as the phosphatidylinositol system that mediates some of the actions of parathyroid hormone and calcitonin. Phosphate is not subject to the steep concentration gradients that characterize cytoplasmic calcium. Nevertheless, the phosphate concentration in the mitochondria is about fivefold greater than that in the cytoplasm, and the cytoplasmic phosphate concentration is about half that of plasma.

The first priority of calcium and phosphate homeostasis is to maintain a normal ECF ionized calcium concentration. Calcium homeostasis in the ECF depends on a continuous exchange among the gastrointestinal tract, kidney, and bone (Fig. 56-1). Calcium absorbed from the lumen of the gut must balance losses due to intestinal secretion and renal excretion. A continual exchange with bone also helps to maintain ECF calcium and bone remodeling. Disturbances in calcium and phosphate in the ECF disrupt many critical processes in the body and can lead to life-threatening changes in neurologic, cardiovascular, and renal functions. It is not surprising, therefore, that complex hormonal systems have evolved to regulate calcium-phosphate exchange and that the gastrointestinal tract, kidney, and bone are major targets for these hormones. The most important hormones for day-to-day regulation are PtH, secreted by

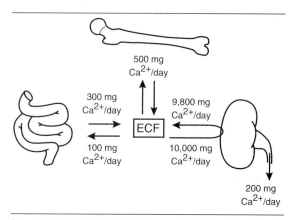

Fig. 56-1. Calcium balance in a normal adult. There is a net absorption of 200 mg of calcium from the intestine that is balanced by renal excretion. Calcium exchange between bone and the ECF shows no net gain or loss.

the parathyroid glands, and the active form of vitamin D, produced by the kidneys. Calcitonin also regulates calcium and phosphate metabolism, but the physiologic importance of this hormone is unclear at this time.

Parathyroid Glands
Embryology, Anatomy, and Histology

Two pairs of parathyroids develop from the endoderm of the third and fourth branchial pouches and migrate caudally to associate with the capsule covering the dorsolateral portion of the thyroid. The **superior pair** of parathyroids, which develop from the fourth pouch, remains almost stationary and locates near the isthmus of the thyroid. Developing from the third pouch in association with the thymus, the **inferior parathyroids** migrate a greater distance and generally assume a position at the lower poles of the thyroid. However, the inferior parathyroids may migrate anomalously and be found with the thymus in the anterior mediastinum or at other locations.

In the adult, the parathyroids are oval and measure about 6 mm in length and 4 mm in width. Each gland weighs approximately 40 mg, but normal glands may weigh as much as 70 mg. Usually there are four parathyroid glands, but additional glands may be present in as many as 6% of normal individuals. In most cases, the parathyroids are supplied by the inferior thyroid artery.

The parathyroids are encapsulated by a fibrous connective tissue. The glandular parenchyma is partitioned into lobules, and these lobules are formed into cords by a highly vascular fibroconnective tissue stroma that also contains nerves, lymphatics, and fat cells. The **chief cell** is responsible for PtH secretion. Active chief cells contain a well-developed endoplasmic reticulum for hormone synthesis as well as a prominent Golgi apparatus for hormone packaging. Unlike some endocrine cells (e.g., somatotrophs), chief cells contain few secretory vesicles. Oxyphil cells appear in the gland after puberty. These cells are characterized by a sparse endoplasmic reticulum and a poorly developed Golgi apparatus. The function of these cells is unknown.

Parathyroid Hormone

Biosynthesis and Metabolism

The principal form of PtH secreted by the parathyroid gland is a single-chain polypeptide consisting of 84 amino acids. Its molecular weight is about 9300. In humans, there is a single PtH gene located on the short arm of chromosome 11. The gene codes for messenger RNA (mRNA) that is translocated from the nucleus to the cytoplasm, where it associates with ribosomes of the rough endoplasmic reticulum. A **prepro-PtH** composed of 110 amino acids is synthesized and simultaneously translocated into the lumen of the endoplasmic reticulum. The 25-amino acid signal peptide is cleaved upon translocation to yield **pro-PtH.** This prohormone is transferred to the Golgi apparatus, where it is cleaved to generate the form composed of 84 amino acids that is packaged into secretory vesicles. The amino-terminal third of PtH is critical for the primary actions associated with the hormone. Polypeptides containing the first 34 amino acids express full activity in several biologic assays. This portion of PtH is highly conserved among PtHs from different species, and the basic features of this sequence also are conserved in the **PtH-related peptide (PtHrP)** that binds to the PtH receptor. The circulating half-life of PtH is relatively brief (minutes) because the hormone is rapidly metabolized by the liver and kidney yielding fragments of various sizes. Most of the circulating fragments are devoid of the biologic actions primarily associated with PtH. It is possible, however, that some of these fragments exert actions through novel receptors.

Another substance secreted by chief cells is **parathyroid secretory protein,** a glycosylated protein that is similar or identical to chromogranin-A in the secretory granules of the adrenal medulla. Parathyroid secretory protein is secreted along with PtH, but it has no known function.

Regulation

PtH synthesis and secretion primarily are regulated by serum ionized calcium concentrations, but other factors such as vitamin D and neurotransmitters play a role. Decreases in serum calcium stimulate PtH secretion, and increases inhibit secretion. The precise mechanism whereby calcium regulates secretion has not been firmly established. However, regulation by calcium may be mediated in part through a cell-surface receptor that is coupled to a GTP-binding protein (G protein). Binding to the **calcium receptor** is postulated to activate the phosphatidylinositol system, thereby elevating intracellular levels of inositol trisphosphate (IP_3) and DAG and activating protein kinase C (PKC). Along with increasing IP_3 and PKC activity, calcium decreases intracellular levels of cAMP. This latter action also may mediate some of the inhibitory effects of calcium, because agents that decrease cAMP generally inhibit PtH secretion. The signaling pathways activated by calcium appear to regulate transcriptional and posttranscriptional processes. Chronic hypocalcemia increases PtH mRNA levels and stimulates chief cell hyperplasia, whereas elevated calcium promotes degradation of intraglandular PtH and decreases PtH mRNA. Although serum ionized calcium is the major regulator, other factors may affect PtH secretion. For example, 1,25-dihydroxyvitamin D_3 decreases PtH mRNA and inhibits secretion. Chronic hypomagnesemia also inhibits PtH secretion, but an acute decrease in serum magnesium stimulates secretion. Beta-adrenergic agonists such as epinephrine can stimulate PtH secretion, probably by increasing intracellular levels of cAMP. It is important to note, however, that the physiologic importance of 1,25-dihydroxyvitamin D_3, magnesium, and beta-adrenergic agonists has not been established.

Receptor/Mechanism of Action

Bone and kidney, the principal target organs for PtH, express cell-surface receptors that bind PtH and PtHrP with high affinity. **PtH/PtHrP receptors** also have been identified in a variety of other tissues, but the physiologic relevance of these receptors is unclear at this time. The PtH/PtHrP receptor (Fig. 56-2) is a member of a subfamily that includes receptors for calcitonin, secretin, vasoactive intestinal peptide, glucagon, glucagon-like peptide, and growth hormone–releasing hormone. A single gene appears to code for the receptors in bone and kidney; however, tissue-specific PtH/PtHrP receptors may be produced by alternative splicing of the initial mRNA transcript or by

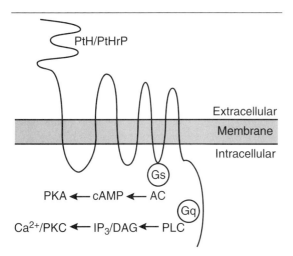

Fig. 56-2. Structure of the PtH/PtHrP receptor. The receptor contains seven transmembrane domains and interacts with two separate G proteins, G_s and G_q. G_s is linked to adenylyl cyclase, an enzyme that activates protein kinase A (PKA) by increasing cAMP. G_q may be linked to phospholipase C, an enzyme that generates inositol trisphosphate (IP_3) and diacylglycerol (DAG). IP_3 increases intracellular calcium, while DAG and calcium activate protein kinase C (PKC).

as yet undiscovered genes. The cloned receptor contains seven transmembrane domains, characteristic of receptors that signal through G proteins. Studies suggest that distinct intracellular domains of the PtH/PtHrP receptor interact with two separate G proteins, G_s and G_q. Through G_s, PtH is coupled to adenylyl cyclase and stimulates cAMP formation and activation of protein kinase A (PKA). Acting via G_q, PtH stimulates phospholipase C, which activates the phosphatidylinositol pathway. This latter pathway produces IP_3, raising intracellular calcium and DAG, and increases protein kinase C activity. It is likely that many actions of PtH require the integrated activation of both pathways; however, a single pathway may predominate in some situations. Stimulation by PtH of calcium uptake in the distal renal tubules is an example of an action that requires activation of both PKA and PKC.

Two determinants in the amino-terminal portion (amino acids 1–34) of PtH and PtHrP appear to participate in binding to the receptor. This is consistent with the fact that the first 34 amino acids of PtH retain full biologic activity in assays measuring increases in serum calcium, stimulation of cAMP, or urinary phosphate excretion. Studies have shown, however, that portions of PtH inactive in the preceding assays as well as PtHrP exert other activities. Therefore, some actions of PtH and PtHrP may be mediated through unknown receptors.

Actions on Target Tissue

Maintenance of calcium and phosphate homeostasis by PtH involves direct effects on bone and kidney and indirect effects on intestine. Regulation is complex, because PtH exerts multiple actions in both bone and kidney. One thread that ties many of the actions together is that PtH inevitably increases the level of ionized calcium in the ECF.

In the kidney, PtH stimulates reabsorption of calcium, inhibits reabsorption of phosphate, and stimulates the enzyme that generates the active form of vitamin D_3. PtH-stimulated **calcium reabsorption** occurs primarily in the distal renal tubules. Evidence suggests that PtH opens voltage-sensitive **calcium channels** in the apical (luminal) membranes of distal tubule cells, allowing calcium to enter the cells. Channel opening is a result of membrane hyperpolarization that occurs when PtH increases chloride conductance across the apical membrane. PtH also may regulate insertion of apical calcium channels and modulate Ca^{2+}-ATPase activity. The Ca^{2+}-ATPase transports calcium into the ECF against concentration and electrical gradients. As indicated earlier, the actions of PtH in the distal tubule cells probably require activation of both adenylyl cyclase (cAMP, PKA) and phospholipase C (IP_3, DAG, PKC). In addition to stimulating calcium reabsorption, PtH inhibits proximal tubular reabsorption of phosphate, sodium, potassium, and bicarbonate. The primary targets for PtH are a sodium-phosphate cotransport system that is a rate-limiting step for proximal phosphate reabsorption and a sodium-hydrogen exchanger involved in bicarbonate reabsorption. It is unclear which signaling system mediates inhibition of phosphate transport. The kidney also is the principal site for generation of the active form of vitamin D_3 (1,25-dihydroxyvitamin D_3). PtH increases synthesis of 1,25-dihydroxyvitamin D_3 by stimulating 1α-hydroxylase activity in the proximal renal tubules. Through its effects on 1α-hydroxylase, PtH indirectly stimulates intestinal absorption of calcium. Activation of PKC seems to play a major role in stimulation of 1α-hydroxylase. The net effect of PtH on the kidney is increased reabsorption of calcium and excretion of phosphate (phosphaturic effect). Ionized calcium increases in the ECF because more is returned and less is bound to phosphate.

As discussed earlier, bone is the chief reservoir of calcium within the body. It is not surprising, therefore, that bone is a major target of PtH. The primary action of PtH is to stimulate osteoclastic bone resorption and inhibit osteoblastic activity. Current evidence suggests that PtH does not directly increase osteoclastic activity, since osteoclasts express few, if any, receptors for the hormone. Rather, PtH acts on **osteoblasts** and osteoblast precursors to induce factors that increase osteoclastic activity (Fig. 56-3). The factors responsible for **osteoclast** activation are largely uncharacterized; however, **cytokines** such as **tumor necrosis factor** and **interleukin 6** (IL-6) may play important roles. Osteoclastic activation is marked by an increase in carbonic anhydrase activity (H^+ production) and activation of hydrogen-potassium ATPase (H^+ pump), creating an acidic environment for solubilization of **hydroxyapatite crystals.** Degradation of organic bone matrix (osteoid, primarily type I collagen) is facilitated by the release of acidic hydrolases and collagenase. The net effect of PtH on bone is release of calcium and phosphate into the ECF. It must be remembered, however, that bone resorption is somehow coupled with bone formation. PtH may play a role in this coupling process, because there is substantial evidence that PtH exerts anabolic actions on bone. The anabolic actions may be mediated through stimulation of growth factors, including **insulin-like growth factors** (IGFs). Coupling factors also may include agents such as

Fig. 56-3. Actions of PtH on bone. PtH indirectly activates osteoclasts by stimulating osteoblasts and osteoblast precursors to induce factors that increase osteoclastic activity. Although the factors induced by PtH are largely uncharacterized, prostaglandins (PG) and cytokines such as interleukin 6 (IL-6) may play important roles.

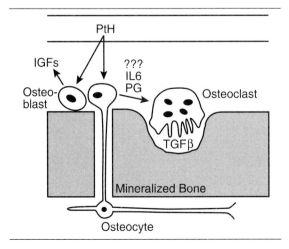

transforming growth factor beta (TGF-β) that are liberated from the bone matrix.

Increased intestinal absorption of calcium and phosphate is an indirect effect of PtH. In the kidney, PtH stimulates 1α-hydroxylase, the enzyme that converts 25-hydroxyvitamin D_3 to the active metabolite 1,25-dihydroxyvitamin D_3. Activated vitamin D_3 directly increases intestinal absorption of calcium and phosphate.

Parathyroid Hormone–Related Protein (PtHrP)

PtHrP originally was identified in tumors, often malignant, that promote hypercalcemia. Sequencing studies showed that the first 13 amino acids of PtHrP and PtH exhibit considerable homology but that the rest of the molecules are different. Despite the structural differences between PtHrP and PtH, both are bound with high affinity by the PtH/PtHrP receptor. Accordingly, PtHrP can exert all the actions that are associated with the 1–34 region of PtH. Unlike PtH, PtHrP is produced by many tissues in the body. For this reason, it is believed that PtHrP functions primarily as an **autocrine** or **paracrine regulator** rather than entering the systemic circulation. The wide distribution of PtHrP and the fact that its structure is highly conserved among species suggest that this agent plays important physiologic roles. Its importance is further underscored by the fact that "knockout" of the gene for PtHrP or its receptor is lethal. One factor causing fetal death is restriction of the rib cage due to poor development of the ribs. Physiologic functions postulated for PtHrP include roles in growth and development, gestation and reproduction, smooth muscle relaxation, and transepithelial calcium transport. Under normal circumstances in the adult, PtHrP probably does not play a major role in regulating calcium in the ECF. In the fetus, however, PtHrP increases calcium levels in the circulation by stimulating maternal-to-fetal calcium transport across the placenta. Many of the actions of PtHrP probably are exerted through receptors in tissues other than bone and kidney. Studies have shown that PtH/PtHrP receptors are present in many "nonclassic" tissues, making it likely some are intended for locally produced PtHrP rather than systemic PtH. Furthermore, receptors specific for PtHrP may be present. This may be true in the placenta, where PtHrP, but not PtH, stimulates calcium transport. Additional studies are needed to define the true physiologic roles of PtHrP.

Parafollicular or C Cells

Embryology, Anatomy, and Histology

Parafollicular or C cells of the **thyroid** gland produce **calcitonin** (CT). The parafollicular cells arise from the neural crest and migrate to the fifth branchial pouch. In nonmammalian vertebrates, the fifth branchial pouch gives rise to a distinct structure, the **ultimobranchial body.** In mammals, cells of the fifth branchial pouch become embedded in the lateral lobes of the thyroid. Parafollicular cells comprise about 0.1% of the mass of the thyroid, occurring singly or in small clusters.

Calcitonin (CT)

Biosynthesis and Secretion

Calcitonin is a 32-amino acid, single-chain polypeptide with a 7-residue disulfide ring at the amino-terminus and a prolineamide at the carboxy-terminus. Its molecular weight is approximately 3400. Unlike PtH, the CT molecule must be virtually intact to exert significant biologic activity. The gene for CT resides on the short arm of chromosome 11. Alternative splicing of the initial RNA transcript can produce mRNAs that code for different proteins. Parafollicular cells primarily produce an mRNA that codes for CT and a 21-amino acid peptide known as **katacalcin.** The physiologic importance of katacalcin is unknown. In the CNS and other tissues, splicing produces an mRNA that codes for **calcitonin gene–related peptide** (CGRP) rather than CT.

Regulation

Secretion of CT increases when circulating calcium levels rise (**hypercalcemia**) and declines when calcium falls (**hypocalcemia**). It is unclear, however, whether calcium concentrations normally found in the circulation significantly alter CT secretion. Gastrointestinal hormones such as **cholecystokinin** and **gastrin** stimulate CT secretion in some species, leading to speculation that CT plays a role in retention of ingested calcium. However, it has not been demonstrated that gastrointestinal hormones are significant secretagogues for CT in humans. Other factors that influence CT secretion include estrogen and 1,25-dihydroxyvitamin D_3. Taken together, the data suggest that CT is not a primary factor in acute regulation of calcium concentration in the ECF. Rather, the major role of CT may be protection of skeleton during times of calcium

stress such as growth, pregnancy, and lactation. Circulating levels of CT increase in these situations.

Receptor/Mechanism of Action

As discussed earlier, the **CT receptor** is closely related to the PtH/ PtHrP receptor. Like the PtH/PtHrP receptor, the CT receptor contains seven transmembrane domains and appears to be linked to adenylyl cyclase and phospholipase C. CT receptors appear to be expressed in a wide variety of tissues, including kidney, osteoclasts, brain, spinal cord, bone marrow, stomach, ovary, testis, skeletal muscle, and uterus.

Actions on Target Tissue

Lowering of serum calcium is the principal physiologic action of CT. This **hypocalcemic effect** is not dependent on a functioning gastrointestinal tract, kidney, or parathyroid gland, suggesting that the primary effect of CT is to **decrease bone resorption.** By decreasing bone resorption, CT also decreases serum phosphate concentration (**hypophosphatemia**). CT directly inhibits **osteoclastic activity** at hormone concentrations normally found in the circulation. Accordingly, CT may exert a tonic influence on osteoclastic activity. In kidney, the actions of CT are similar to those of PtH. CT increases calcium reabsorption in distal tubules and inhibits phosphate reabsorption in proximal tubules. The phosphaturic effect of CT contributes to hypophosphatemia. Like PtH, CT increase 1α-hydroxylase activity and increases production of 1,25-dihydroxyvitamin D_3.

Calcitonin Gene–Related Peptide (CGRP)

At high levels, CGRP can exert CT-like actions, but these probably do not represent the physiologic actions. CGRP is present in high concentrations in perivascular nerves, and it possesses potent **vasorelaxant effects**. It has been postulated, therefore, that CGRP regulates regional blood flow and may be important in volume-overload states and in heart failure. The distribution of CGRP in the CNS suggests that the peptide has neuromodulator or neurotransmitter functions other than vasoregulatory effects. High concentrations of CGRP are found in the dorsal horn of the spinal cord, suggesting involvement in **transmission of sensory impulses**. CGRP is present in the circulation. Although the parafollicular cells secrete some CGRP, it is likely that most of the circulating peptide is released by nerves. More research is needed to establish the physiologically important roles of this interesting peptide.

Vitamin D

Biosynthesis and Metabolism

Vitamin D is not a true vitamin because it can be synthesized in the body as well as being obtained through the diet. The term **vitamin D** is used to refer to either vitamin D_3 (**cholecalciferol**) or vitamin D_2 (**ergocalciferol**). The latter substance is derived from ergosterol, a plant sterol, while vitamin D_3 occurs naturally in animals. Both vitamin D_2 and vitamin D_3 are added to milk and other foods and can be metabolized along the same pathways to produce active metabolites. In animals, vitamin D_3 is produced primarily in the epidermis of the skin by irradiation of its precursor **7-dehydrocholesterol** (Fig. 56-4). Vitamin D_3 is actually a prohormone that must undergo hydroxylation to become biologically active.

Vitamin D produced in the skin or obtained in the diet is transported in the circulation to the liver, where it is hydroxylated at C-25, forming 25-hydroxyvitamin D_3. The 25-hydroxylase occurs in both the microsomal and mitochondrial fractions of the liver. Although a weakly active form of the vitamin, 25-hydroxyvitamin D_3 is probably biologically inert at physiologic concentrations. 25-Hydroxyvitamin D_3 must be transported to proximal tubules of the kidney, where it is hydroxylated at C-1 by the mitochondrial enzyme 1α-hydroxylase. Hydroxylation at C-1 produces the fully active hormone, **1,25-dihydroxyvitamin D_3**. As one might expect, 1α-hydroxylase is tightly regulated by multiple factors, including PtH. The proximal tubules of the kidney also can hydroxylate vitamin D at C-24, producing 24,25-dihydroxyvitamin D_3. In most cases, 24,25-dihydroxyvitamin D_3 exhibits weak activity similar to that of 25-hydroxyvitamin D_3. Both 1α-hydroxylase and 24-hydroxylase are present in other tissues, but it is unlikely that extrarenal hydroxylases play a significant role in hydroxylating vitamin D under normal conditions.

Vitamin D is a **fat-soluble secosterol** that is only sparingly soluble in aqueous solutions. Although the hydroxylated metabolites are more polar than the parent vitamin D, they also have limited solubility in aqueous solutions. Accordingly, a large proportion of vitamin D, and to a lesser extent its hydroxylated metabolites, partitions into adipose tissue. In the circulation, vitamin D and its metabolites associate with a vitamin D–binding protein (**transcalciferin**), an alpha-globulin with a molecular weight of approximately 55,000. This binding protein probably protects vitamin D and its metabolites, increases their solubility in serum, and acts as a reservoir. The binding preference of transcalciferin is for 25-hydroxyvitamin D_3 = 24,25-

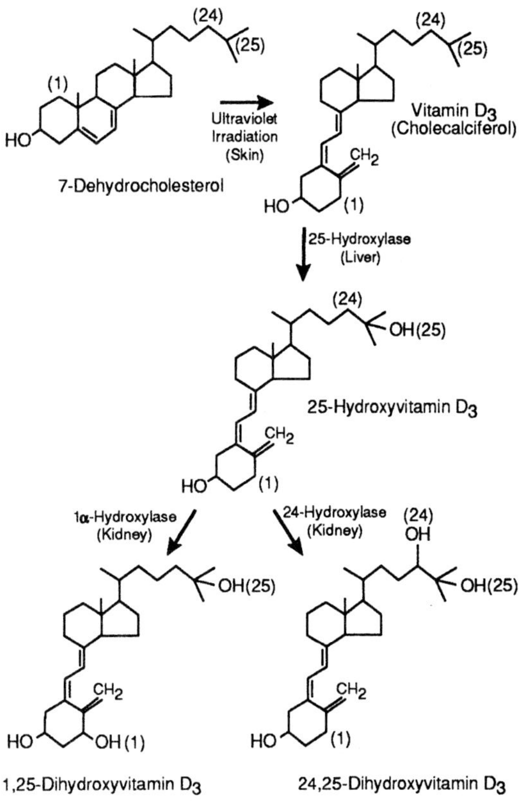

Fig. 56-4. Biosynthesis of vitamin D_3 and its metabolites. Vitamin D_3 is produced primarily in the epidermis of the skin by irradiation of its precursor 7-dehydrocholesterol. In the liver, vitamin D_3 is hydroxylated at C-25, forming 25-hydroxyvitamin D_3. In the kidney, hydroxylation of 25-hydroxyvitamin D_3 at C-1 produces the fully active hormone, 1,25-dihydroxyvitamin D_3, whereas hydroxylation at C-24 produces a weakly active metabolite.

dihydroxyvitamin D_3 1,25-dihydroxyvitamin D_3 >> vitamin D. Transcalciferin's high affinity for 25-hydroxyvitamin D_3 accounts in part for the longer circulating half-life of 25-hydroxyvitamin D_3 (15 days) in comparison with that for of 1,25-dihydroxyvitamin D_3 (0.2 days). It also helps to maintain circulating 25-hydroxyvitamin D_3 at a level 1000-fold higher than that of 1,25-dihydroxyvitamin D_3. Despite the higher concentration of 25-hydroxyvitamin D_3, 1,25-dihydroxyvitamin D_3 is responsible for most of the vitamin D activity.

Hydroxylated vitamin D metabolites are primarily cleared by side-chain oxidation in the liver, with excretion in the bile. Enterohepatic recirculation reclaims 5% to 30% of these metabolites.

Regulation

Under normal conditions, 25-hydroxyvitamin D_3 is present at relatively high concentrations, so the major control step in synthesis and secretion of 1,25-dihydroxyvitamin D_3 is hydroxylation at the C-1 position. PtH acts on the **proximal tubules** of the kidney to increase 1α-hydroxylase activity. **Hypocalcemia** also stimulates this enzyme, but the effects of low blood calcium are mediated through increased release of PtH. **Hypophosphatemia** increases 1α-hydroxylase activity, and unlike hypocalcemia, low blood phosphate acts through mechanisms independent of PtH. Both PtH and hypophosphatemia inhibit the activity of the 24-hydroxylase. 1,25-Dihydroxyvitamin D_3 also is an important regulator of synthesis and secretion. The active metabolite of vitamin D is a potent inhibitor of 1α-hydroxylase activity, and it stimulates 24-hydroxylase activity. Other hormones that directly or indirectly stimulate 1α-hydroxylase activity include growth hormone, estrogen, and prolactin. Before vitamin D_3 and D_2 were added to milk and other foods, exposure to ultraviolet radiation and ingestion of foods naturally rich in vitamin D were important concerns in the United States. Today, these are major concerns only in less developed countries.

Receptor/Mechanism of Action

Vitamin D receptors (VDRs) are expressed in intestine, bone, and kidney, the "classic" target tissues for active vitamin D. Other tissues also express VDRs, including skin, bone marrow, thymus, breast, brain, and endocrine glands. The receptor for 1,25-dihydroxyvitamin D_3 (VDR) is a member of the steroid/thyroid superfamily of hormone receptors. Members of this family of receptors contain a conserved DNA-binding domain and a carboxy-terminal ligand–binding domain.

Regulation of gene transcription by vitamin D involves a complex series of events. Like steroid and thyroid hormones, 1,25-dihydroxyvitamin D_3 enters target tissues and is **translocated to the nucleus** by a poorly defined process. VDR bound to ligand resides almost exclusively in the nucleus of the target cell, but it is unclear whether all or only part of unliganded receptor is in the nucleus. VDRs regulate transcription by binding to specific DNA elements in the promoter regions of hormone-responsive genes. The sequence of the **vitamin D–responsive element** (VDRE) differs among genes but contains imperfect direct repeats

of the consensus hexanucleotide motif GGGTGA separated by a three-nucleotide spacer (Fig. 56-5). Unlike steroid receptors that form homodimers, VDRs preferentially bind to the VDRE as a heterodimer with the **retinoid X receptor** (RXR) or sometimes with the retinoic acid receptor (RAR). Thus 1,25-dihydroxyvitamin D_3 binds to the VDR and facilitates its interaction with unliganded RXR. The VDR-RXR complex binds to the VDRE and, through interactions with additional proteins, regulates RNA polymerase II activity. The natural ligand for the RXR, 9-*cis*-retinoic acid, may inhibit the VDR-RXR interaction by promoting the formation of RXR homodimers.

Actions on Target Tissue

Similar to PtH, vitamin D's primary physiologic function is to maintain **calcium and phosphate homeostasis**. The principal target tissues for vitamin D in regulating calcium and phosphate are intestine and bone and to a lesser extent kidney. Vitamin D also exerts additional actions, including regulation of cell growth and differentiation in hematolymphopoietic tissue and other tissues.

In the intestine, 1,25-dihydroxyvitamin D_3 stimulates large increases in fractional absorption of calcium and lesser increases in absorption of phosphate. The mechanisms whereby 1,25-dihydroxyvitamin D_3 increases transepithelial transport of calcium have not been fully characterized, but a model based on current data has been developed (Fig. 56-6). At the apical (luminal) membrane, 1,25-dihydroxyvitamin D_3 increases movement of calcium into intestinal cells by **opening calcium channels**. Channel

Fig. 56-5. The vitamin D receptor (VDR) and retinoid X receptor (RXR) bind as a heterodimer to the vitamin D response element (VDRE). The VDRE is comprised by direct nucleotide repeats (*arrows*) separated by three nucleotides (NNN).

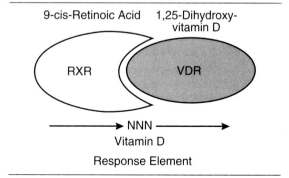

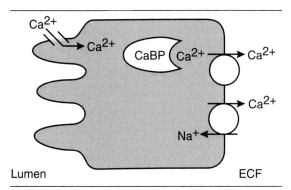

Fig. 56-6. Model for transepithelial transport of calcium across an intestinal cell. Calcium enters through channels in the apical membrane (*left*), is translocated across the cell by a calcium-binding protein (CaBP), and is transported into the ECF by a Ca^2-ATPase or Na^+-Ca^{2+} exchange (*right*).

opening in response to 1,25-dihydroxyvitamin D_3 occurs via a poorly defined process that appears to be independent of gene transcription. Active metabolites of vitamin D also stimulate expression of a **calcium-binding protein** (CaBP). The CaBP, also called **calbindin,** probably facilitates entry of calcium and movement from the apical membrane to **calcium pumps** in the **basolateral membrane**. At the basolateral membrane, 1,25-dihydroxyvitamin D_3 increases the concentration and activity of an ATP-dependent calcium pump (Ca^{2+}-ATPase) that transports calcium into the ECF against calcium and electrical gradients. Phosphate uptake in response to 1,25-dihydroxyvitamin D_3 appears to occur through mechanisms independent of calcium absorption. Although the process is poorly defined, stimulation of phosphate uptake also involves movement of phosphate across apical membranes and active transport into the ECF.

Vitamin D exerts seemingly paradoxical actions in bone in that it directly stimulates **bone resorption** but promotes **bone mineralization**. The resorptive effects are mediated in large part through increased **osteoclastic activity**. 1,25-Dihydroxyvitamin D_3 stimulates fusion and differentiation of hematopoietic precursors into osteoclasts and may increase the activity of mature osteoclasts. These actions lead to mobilization of mineralized bone and elevate circulating levels of calcium and phosphate. Nevertheless, vitamin D can promote bone mineralization and is important in preventing disturbances in bone ossification that occur in **rickets**. The positive effects of 1,25-dihydroxyvitamin D_3 on bone mineralization may be due in large part to increased **intestinal absorption** of calcium and phosphate. Increased intestinal absorption elevates the levels of cal-

cium and phosphate in the ECF, producing concentrations suitable for mineralization of osteoid. There also is evidence that 1,25-dihydroxyvitamin D_3 exerts anabolic actions on osteoblast-like cells.

The effects of vitamin D on the kidney are less well defined. Nonetheless, there is evidence that 1,25-dihydroxyvitamin D_3 stimulates calcium reabsorption in the distal **renal tubules**, probably though mechanisms similar to those described for intestinal uptake. As discussed earlier, 1,25-dihydroxyvitamin D_3 also acts on **proximal tubules** to inhibit 1α-hydroxylase activity and stimulate 24-hydroxylase activity.

Hormonal Regulation of Calcium and Phosphate Homeostasis

PtH and the active forms of vitamin D are the principal regulators of calcium and phosphate homeostasis. Calcitonin also contributes to the regulatory process under some conditions, but it is unlikely that this hormone plays a major role. The first priority of each of these hormones is to maintain calcium homeostasis in the ECF. Phosphate homeostasis, though important, is more of a secondary consideration because phosphate deficiency in the absence of specific organ dysfunction is unlikely. Under normal circumstances, adjustments in intestinal absorption or renal reabsorption are sufficient to maintain calcium balance. There is a **constant exchange of calcium** between bone and the ECF, but only severe stresses cause a net loss of bone mass.

PtH is the principal regulator of calcium (Fig. 56-7). The parathyroids are particularly sensitive to changes in the extracellular ionized calcium concentration, and secretion of PtH correlates inversely with calcium levels. **Hypocalcemia** produces a prompt rise in PtH secretion, and the hormone has several important effects on the kidney. It stimulates calcium reabsorption in the distal tubules, inhibits phosphate reabsorption in the proximal tubules (**phosphaturic effect**), and increases production of 1,25-dihydroxyvitamin D_3 in proximal renal tubules. 1,25-Dihydroxyvitamin D_3 produced in response to PtH increases intestinal absorption of calcium and phosphate. In addition, PtH and 1,25-dihydroxyvitamin D_3 act in concert to increase release of calcium and phosphate from bone. The phosphaturic action of PtH in the kidney eliminates excess phosphate and indirectly increases levels of ionized calcium by decreasing formation of calcium-phosphate complexes. Normalization of ionized calcium, a direct result of the preceding actions, suppresses PtH secretion.

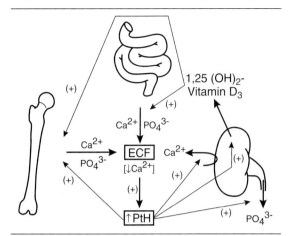

Fig. 56-7. Regulation of calcium and phosphate homeostasis by PtH and vitamin D. A decrease in calcium in the ECF increases the secretion of PtH. In turn, PtH regulates calcium and phosphate handling by bone and kidney and stimulates production of 1,25-dihydroxyvitamin D_3. The latter metabolite of vitamin D increases intestinal absorption of calcium and phosphate and acts in concert with PtH in stimulating bone resorption.

Production of 1,25-dihydroxyvitamin D_3 is suppressed by declining levels of PtH, increased levels of phosphate, and active metabolites of vitamin D.

Disorders of Calcium and Phosphate

Disorders of calcium and phosphate lead to neuromuscular, renal, and skeletal abnormalities, as well as to other problems. Common causes of these disorders include problems with hormonal secretion (e.g., hypo- or hyperparathyroidism), diet or intestinal absorption, organ dysfunction (e.g., renal failure), drugs, and malignancies. Some specific abnormalities and causes are discussed below.

Hypercalcemia

Hypercalcemia often is caused by **hyperparathyroidism** but may be the result of a malignancy (e.g., PtHrP secretion), increased intestinal absorption (e.g., granulomatous diseases that elevate 1α-hydroxylase activity), increased renal reabsorption (e.g., thiazide diuretics), or other factors. Elevated serum calcium decreases neuromuscular excitability, leading to slow mentation, poor memory,

depression, emotional lability, and **muscular weakness.** Easy fatigability is one of the most common symptoms. Renal excretion of excess calcium increases urine volume (polyuria) and the formation of kidney stones. Hypercalcemia secondary to hyperthyroidism is characterized by increased bone resorption and a decrease in bone mass (**osteoporosis** or osteopenia).

Hypocalcemia

Hypoparathyroidism and **vitamin D deficiency** are two of the most common causes of hypocalcemia, but PtH resistance, chronic renal failure, acute hyperphosphatemia, and other abnormalities reduce calcium levels in the ECF. Low serum calcium increases neuromuscular excitability causing neuromuscular irritability, including tetany/muscle cramps, paresthesias (numbness and tingling) of the extremities, seizures, and cardiac arrhythmias. Symptoms of fatigue, anxiety, and depression also are common. Severe manifestations include laryngospasm, which fixes the vocal cords in the midline and interferes with breathing. Clinical signs of neuromuscular excitability include Chvostek's sign and Trousseau's sign. **Chvostek's sign** is elicited by tapping the facial nerve just anterior to the ear to produce ipsilateral contraction of the facial muscles. **Trousseau's sign** is a carpal spasm that occurs when a blood pressure cuff is used to induce pressure ischemia of the nerves of the upper arm. Chronic hypocalcemia, secondary vitamin D deficiency, or other factors result in a failure of the bone to mineralize normally. This condition is referred to as **osteomalacia** in adults and **rickets** in growing children.

Hyper- and Hypophosphatemia

Pathologic changes in serum phosphate are less common than changes in calcium. The most common cause of hyperphosphatemia is **renal failure** leading to uremia. Many of the symptoms of acute hyperphosphatemia are attributable to depletion of ionized calcium. Chronic hyperphosphatemia leads to **calcification** of the kidney and other soft tissues. Hypophosphatemia generally does not develop from deficiencies in natural diet. Phosphate is abundant in available foods, and absorption is efficient even in the absence of vitamin D. More commonly, it arises from an organ dysfunction such as **excess renal excretion** of phosphate, perhaps secondary to hyperparathyroidism. Symptoms of acute hypophosphatemia include muscle weakness, paresthesias, depressed reflexes, cranial nerve palsies, tremor, and confusion, due in large part to impairment of cellular energy metabolism. Chronic hypophosphatemia alters mineral and bone metabolism.

Aging and Bone Loss

Peak bone density is achieved in the third or fourth decade; thereafter, bone density declines throughout life. Bone loss occurs in both men and women; however, bone loss accelerates in women after menopause. A woman can easily lose 15% to 20% of her trabecular bone during the 5 years following menopause. **Osteoporosis** resulting from the bone loss increases the risk of a fracture, usually a vertebral compression fracture or a fracture of the wrist, hip, ribs, pelvis, or humerus. The primary factor responsible for postmenopausal bone loss is estrogen deficiency. Estrogen decreases bone resorption, in part by antagonizing the bone-resorptive actions of PtH. It also has been suggested that estrogen regulates calcium handling by the intestine and kidney and production of PtH, 1,25-dihydroxyvitamin D_3, and calcitonin. Estrogen replacement is an effective treatment for postmenopausal loss, particularly if used in conjunction with regular exercise, calcium supplements, and perhaps calcitonin.

Summary

Calcium and phosphate play critical roles in cellular function and in mineralization of the skeleton. Accordingly, a highly integrated and complex hormonal system involving PtH, vitamin D, and calcitonin has evolved to regulate calcium and phosphate levels. The first priority of this system is to ensure calcium homeostasis in the ECF.

Bibliography

Aurbach, G. D., Marx, S. J., and Spiegel, A. M. Parathyroid hormone, calcitonin and the calciferols. In: Wilson, J. D., and Foster, D. W., eds. *Textbook of Endocrinology,* 7th ed. Philadelphia: W. B. Saunders, 1992. Pp. 1397–1476.

MacDonald, P. N., Dowd, D. R., and Haussler, M. R. New insight into the structure and functions of the vitamin D receptor. *Semin. Nephrol.* 14:101–118, 1994.

Nissenson, R. A., Huang, Z., Blind, E., and Shoback, D. Structure and function of the receptor for parathyroid hormone and parathyroid hormone-related protein. *Receptor* 3:193–201, 1993.

57 Physiology of the Adrenal Gland

Lawrence M. Dolan

Objectives

After reading this chapter, you should be able to

Describe the significance of the anatomic relationship between the adrenal cortex and the medulla

Define the major branch points in steroid hormone synthesis and their significance

List the major hormones produced by each section of the adrenal gland

Define the major factors that regulate the production and release of each adrenal hormone

State the action of each adrenal hormone

Describe the degradation of each adrenal hormone

Compare the known differences in steroid hormone receptors

Apply the general principles of adrenal function tests to the diseases described

---

The **adrenal glands** are paired structures located superior to the upper pole of each kidney and lateral to the lower thoracic and upper lumbar vertebrae. Each gland is composed of an **outer cortex** that completely encircles the **inner medulla.** The cortex and medulla are distinct structural units.

Three groups of **arteries** perfuse each gland. The **superior group** arises from the inferior phrenic artery, the **middle group** directly from the aorta, and the **inferior group** from the renal artery. These arteries enter the **adrenal capsule** and form a **thin plexus.** Blood vessels from the plexus form a **sinusoidal circulation,** which nurtures the cortex. After traversing the cortex, the blood vessels reunite to form the **plexus reticularus** at the cortical-medullary junction. A few arterioles pass directly through the cortex to supply the plexus reticularus. Thus the blood flow to the medulla includes not only arterial sources but also blood that has traversed the cortex. Blood from the plexus reticularus then bathes the cells of the medulla. The complex blood supply to the adrenal glands protects

the glands from infarction and provides the appropriate milieu for the production of epinephrine.

Embryology

Two separate germ lines contribute to the formation of the adrenal gland. The **cortex** arises from mesoderm found medial to the genital ridge and is present by the fourth week of gestation. The **medulla** is of ectodermal origin and evolves from neural crest cells that invade the "cortical" mesoderm during the fourth week of gestation. Thus the intimate anatomic association between the cortex and medulla is established early in development.

Histology

The **fetal adrenal cortex** consists of three concentric layers. The outer layer, the **true cortex,** is beneath the connective tissue capsule. The middle layer, the **fetal cortex,** constitutes 80% of the adrenal gland at birth. The fetal cortex involutes during the first 3 weeks of life, leaving only a remnant of connective tissue surrounding the inner layer, the **medulla.**

After the first month of life, the true cortex dominates and comprises approximately 90% of the adrenal gland's weight. The **true cortex** is composed of three concentric layers. Directly beneath the capsule is the **zona glomerulosa,** which constitutes 15% of the cortex. The **zona fasciculata,** immediately below the zona glomerulosa, makes up 75% of the cortex. The **zona reticularis,** the inner layer of the adult cortex, surrounds the medulla. The medulla occupies approximately 10% of the adrenal gland. The cortex produces three types of **steroid hormones:** mineralocorticoids, glucocorticoids, and androgens. The medulla manufactures **catecholamines.**

Steroid Hormones

Synthesis

Cholesterol is the common precursor of cortical steroid hormones. A unique cascade of biochemical alterations within each cortical zone produces steroid hormones with different biologic properties (Fig. 57-1). The **zona glomerulosa** synthesizes aldosterone. **Aldosterone,** the primary **mineralocorticoid,** contributes to sodium retention and K^+ and H^+ excretion by the kidney, gastrointestinal tract, and salivary and sweat glands. The **zona fasciculata** synthesizes cortisol, a **glucocorticoid. Cortisol** plays a major role in metabolic homeostasis of cells. It also helps to maintain the circulating blood sugar level by diminishing peripheral glucose use and increasing hepatic glucose production from amino acids and free fatty acid precursors. It also participates in the response to physical and emotional stress and facilitates macrophage, B-cell, and T-cell functions. The **zona reticularis** manufactures **androgens** and physiologically insignificant amounts of estrogens. **Dehydroepiandrosterone** (DHEA), **dehydroepiandrosterone sulfate** (DHEA-S), and **androstenedione** are the major androgens. The androgens contribute to **virilization** (pubic and facial hair development) and **somatic growth.**

The adrenal cortex does not store a large concentration of any of the steroid hormones. Therefore, an increased demand for steroid hormones requires a readily available supply of **cholesterol.** The adrenal gland has three sources of cholesterol: (1) increased uptake from circulating low-density and high-density lipoproteins, which is the primary source, (2) endogenous synthesis by the gland, and (3) hydrolysis of stored cholesterol esters.

The rate-limiting step in the production of cortical steroid hormones is the conversion of cholesterol to **pregnenolone** (see Fig. 57-1). Subsequent alterations in the activity of the enzymatic pathways dictate the type and concentration of steroid hormone produced.

Figure 57-1 details the production of aldosterone in the zona glomerulosa. The unique features of the mineralocorticoid enzymatic pathway are the presence of 18-hydroxylase and the absence of 17α-hydroxylase. This lack of 17α-hydroxylase prevents the zona glomerulosa from synthesizing glucocorticoids, androgens, or estrogens. 18-Hydroxylase catalyzes the final step in aldosterone production but is not found in other cortical layers. This special enzymatic milieu makes the zona glomerulosa the sole source of aldosterone.

The presence of 17α-hydroxylase in the zona fasciculata and reticularis permits both pregnenolone and progesterone to enter the glucocorticoid and androgen pathways. The subsequent enzymatic conversion of these substances results in the production of cortisol, DHEA, DHEA-S, and androstenedione, as well as the estrogens. Figure 57-1 documents the details of the biochemical pathways involved.

Secretion and Metabolism

Mineralocorticoids

The renin-angiotensin system and changes in the serum concentrations of potassium, sodium, and adrenocorticotropin hormone (ACTH) regulate aldosterone secretion. The **renin-angiotensin system** is the major factor governing aldosterone synthesis and secretion. **Renin,** a proteolytic enzyme, is synthesized, stored, and secreted by the **juxtaglomerular apparatus** of the kidney. It is released in response to reduced systemic pressure and increased sympathetic nervous system activity. Conversely, a rise in systemic blood pressure, decreased sympathetic nervous system activity, or increased angiotensin-II concentrations suppress renin release.

Renin cleaves **angiotensinogen,** an alpha$_2$-globulin produced by the liver, to form the decapeptide, **angiotensin-I** (Fig. 57-2). Angiotensin-I is converted to **angiotensin-II** by a **converting enzyme** that removes two amino acids from the carboxyl terminal of angiotensin-I. The converting enzyme is found in numerous organs, including the lung, kidney, and liver, as well as throughout the systemic vascular bed. Amino-terminal cleavage of angiotensin-II by aminopeptidases produces **angiotensin-III.**

Angiotensin-II has two major functions. It is one of the

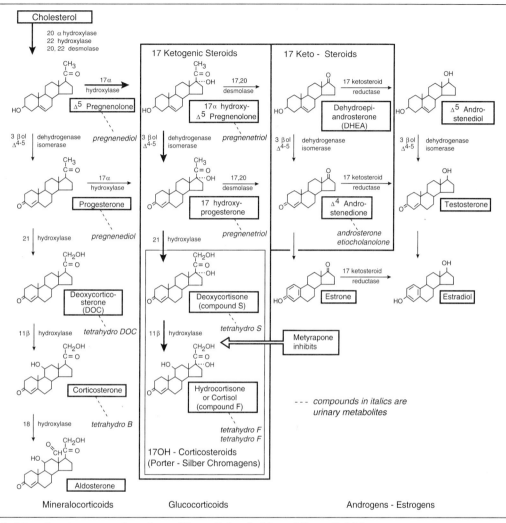

Fig. 57-1. Adrenal cortex enzymatic pathway. (From: Dolan, L. M., and Carey, R. M. In: Vaughan, E. D., and Carey, R. M., eds. *Adrenal Disorders.* New York: Thieme Medical Publishers, 1989. P. 85; with permission.)

most potent vasoconstrictors found in mammals, and it stimulates the **production and secretion of aldosterone** from the cells of the zona glomerulosa. Angiotensin-II has two known influences on the **mineralocorticoid enzymatic pathway.** It increases the conversion of cholesterol to **pregnenolone** and the conversion of corticosterone to **aldosterone** (see Fig. 57-1). Angiotensin-III is only 25% as effective as its parent compound, both as a vasoconstrictor and as a stimulator of aldosterone secretion. The role of angiotensin-III in steroidogenesis is unclear.

Angiotensin-II binds to a surface-cell receptor and this initiates its biologic action. The exact intracellular messenger for angiotensin-II has not been identified, but there is mounting evidence that a rise in intracellular calcium concentration is the second messenger. Intracellular calcium concentration can be altered by directly affecting the calcium flux across membranes or by varying the activity of phospholipase C. **Phospholipase C** (a membrane enzyme) catalyzes the breakdown of phosphoinositol-4,5-bisphosphate (a membrane phospholipid) to form both inosi-

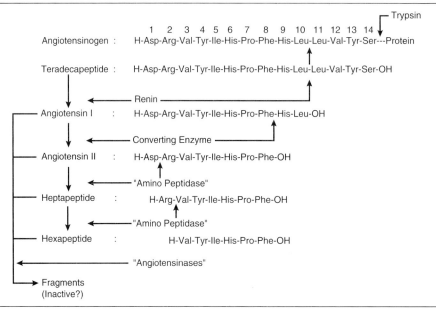

Fig. 57-2. The renin-angiotensin system. (Adapted from: Genest, J. *Hypertension.* New York: McGraw-Hill, 1977. P. 141.)

tol-tris-phosphate (IP$_3$) and diacylglycerol (DAG). IP$_3$ promotes calcium flux from the endoplasmic reticulum to the intracellular space. DAG enhances calcium binding to protein kinase C, and this enhances protein kinase C activity. Activation of protein kinase C is associated with the phosphorylation and dephosphorylation of other intracellular proteins that are believed to mediate the biologic effect of angiotensin-II. The intracellular messenger for angiotensin-III has not yet been determined.

Angiotensin-II and angiotensin-III are both inactivated by cleavage to smaller peptides by **angiotensinases,** endopeptidases, and carboxypeptidases. These **peptidases** are found in serum and the vascular beds of the kidney, liver, and lung.

Other factors that directly regulate aldosterone secretion include serum potassium, sodium, and ACTH concentrations. Small alterations in the serum potassium level (0.1 meq/liter) and large changes in the serum sodium concentration (greater than 10 meq/liter) can affect aldosterone secretion. In both instances, there is an inverse relationship between the electrolyte concentration and the rate of aldosterone secretion.

The final known mediator of aldosterone secretion is **ACTH.** In normal individuals, an acute injection of ACTH results in a prompt increase in the serum aldosterone con-

centration. Continuous infusion produces a rise in the serum aldosterone level, which is maintained for 24 hours. Subsequently, the concentration falls to preadministration levels despite the continued administration of ACTH.

Aldosterone is poorly bound to serum proteins and has a serum half-life of 20 to 30 minutes. Aldosterone is metabolized by the liver, primarily to **tetrahydroaldosterone.** Tetrahydroaldosterone, which comprises 30% to 40% of the aldosterone excreted, and an **18-glucuronide** byproduct are the major metabolites.

Glucocorticoid

ACTH, a 39-amino acid polypeptide secreted by the pituitary gland, exerts a major influence on adrenal cortical function. It stimulates cortisol release, increases the uptake of cholesterol from serum lipoproteins, preserves and enhances the ability of the enzymatic cascade to produce cortisol, and maintains the adrenal cortex through a trophic action.

The serum **cortisol** concentration increases within 3 minutes of the administration of ACTH. Because only a small amount of cortisol is stored in the adrenal gland, the rise in its serum concentration is primarily achieved by increased hormone production. ACTH appears, however, to be a **regulator** rather than an initiator of cortisol synthesis and secretion. This concept is supported by the following evidence. Low serum cortisol concentrations are found in subjects who have undergone total hypophysectomy, and the serum cortisol concentration does not increase after an acute administration of ACTH in such subjects. In this situation, priming with an infusion of ACTH for 48 to 72 hours is required before the serum cortisol concentration increases.

ACTH also has a trophic action on the **adrenal gland.** When administered to both intact and hypophysectomized animals, it causes adrenal cortical hypertrophy. Cortical atrophy develops after total hypophysectomy. If one of the adrenal glands is removed, the remaining adrenal gland exhibits compensatory hypertrophy. In hypophysectomized animals, compensatory hypertrophy is not observed unless exogenous ACTH is administered.

ACTH secretion is regulated by an inherent circadian rhythm, stress, and the circulating cortisol concentration. The morning serum cortisol concentration varies between 8 and 25 μg/dl, with an approximate 50% decrease by late afternoon. The **circadian rhythm** is established shortly after infants begin sleeping through the night. The serum cortisol concentration also rises in response to **physical or emotional stress.** Both the diurnal rhythm and the stress response of ACTH are mediated by the release of a hypothalamic peptide, **corticotropin-releasing hormone** (CRH). The **cerebral cortex** and **brainstem** regulate the release of CRH from the hypothalamus. Increased serum cortisol concentration inhibits the release of both CRH and ACTH.

ACTH binds to a surface-cell receptor to initiate ACTH's biologic effect. The exact intracellular mechanism whereby ACTH stimulates cortisol synthesis and release is unknown. The administration of ACTH, however, activates adenylate cyclase with attendant increased production of cyclic AMP (cAMP). cAMP subsequently activates protein kinase A, resulting in the phosphorylation of specific proteins. The rise in cAMP levels precedes heightened steroidogenesis. cAMP derivatives can also stimulate steroid production. These associations suggest that the generation of cAMP is intimately involved in glucocorticoid production.

At physiologic concentrations, 80% of cortisol is bound to corticosteroid-binding globulin (CBG), 15% to albumin, and the remaining 5% to other serum glycoproteins. Physiologic and pharmacologic changes alter the CBG level. **Pregnancy** and **hyperthyroidism** increase its concentration, while **liver disease** and **nephrotic syndrome** lower the concentration. These conditions cause a change in the total serum cortisol concentration but do not signifi-

cantly influence the **free cortisol concentration,** which is the metabolically active component.

The half-life of serum cortisol is 60 to 120 minutes, and the primary site for cortisol metabolism is the **liver.** To do this, the double bond in the cholesterol ring (see Fig. 57-1) is reduced, and this forms the inactive compound, dihydrocortisol. Sixty to seventy percent of the metabolites of cortisol are **conjugated to glucuronide,** while a small fraction is bound to sulfates. The addition of glucuronide and sulfate increases the solubility of the metabolites and enhances **renal excretion.**

Androgens

DHEA, DHEA-S, and **androstenedione** are the principal androgens secreted by the adrenal cortex, but the production and release of these compounds are not well understood. Acute administration of ACTH elicits a rise in DHEA. Serum DHEA concentration mimics the **circadian variation** seen in serum cortisol concentration. Prolonged ACTH administration raises both the DHEA and DHEA-S concentrations.

ACTH is not the only regulator of androgen secretion. The circulating DHEA-S concentration increases at **adrenarche,** which occurs 1 year before the onset of puberty, and is unassociated with significant changes in ACTH or cortisol secretion. This dissociation of adrenarche both from puberty or a change in cortisol secretion makes it unlikely that either the gonadotropins or ACTH mediate adrenarche. Investigators have suggested two regulators of adrenarche: (1) a **maturational shift** in the pathway of adrenal steroid biosynthesis (increased activity of 17,20-desmolase activity [see Fig. 57-1]) or (2) increased secretion of a yet to be isolated hormone, referred to as **adrenal adrenarche–stimulating factor.** Investigators have suggested both a pituitary and an extrapituitary source of this factor.

Circulating androgens are weakly bound to circulating proteins. The androgens have several potential metabolic fates. **Degradation** primarily takes place in the liver but can also occur in the kidney. DHEA and androstenedione are converted principally to sulfate or glucuronide conjugates and then excreted in the urine. DHEA can, however, be directly excreted in the urine.

Receptors

In contrast to the peptide hormone receptors, which are found on the surface of the cell membrane, steroid hormone receptors are found in either the **cytoplasm** or **nucleus** (Fig. 57-3). The lipophilic properties of the steroid hormones allow their passage through the cell membrane

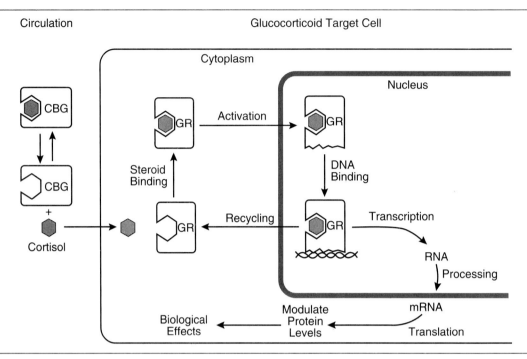

Fig. 57-3. Activation of the glucocorticoid receptor (GR) (CBG = corticosteroid-binding globulin). (Adapted from: DeGroot, L. *Endocrinology,* 2nd ed. Philadelphia: W. B. Saunders, 1989. P. 1558.)

and access to the receptor. After the hormone binds to the receptor, the receptor undergoes a **conformational change** that reveals a **DNA-binding site.** If the receptor-hormone complex is in the cytosol, it translocates to the nucleus. In the nucleus, the receptor-hormone complex binds to chromatin by means of the DNA-binding site. This process initiates or inhibits the transcription of specific genes producing messenger RNA (mRNA). mRNA is then translated into specific proteins. Changes in the concentrations of induced proteins mediate the biologic effect of the steroid hormone. When transcription is completed, the receptor-hormone complex dissociates from the chromatin and each other. The receptor returns to its original environment (nucleus or cytoplasm) and configuration (hidden DNA-binding site).

Mineralocorticoid Receptor

The gene for the human mineralocorticoid receptor is present on **chromosome 4.** This receptor has been cloned and sequenced, revealing a 984 amino acid protein with a molecular weight of 107,000. The mineralocorticoid receptor is found primarily in the **cytoplasm.** The specific intracel-

lular messengers that mediate the biologic action of the mineralocorticoids have not been defined.

Recent work with the mineralocorticoid receptor has revealed some intriguing data. In vitro, the receptor binds aldosterone and certain glucocorticoids at physiologic concentrations with a high affinity. These data are consistent with the significant homology that exists between the mineralocorticoid and glucocorticoid receptors at their steroid hormone–binding sites. However, in vivo experiments using tissues responsive to mineralocorticoids demonstrate binding of mineralocorticoid but not glucocorticoid to the mineralocorticoid receptor. These data suggest that the tissue response to mineralocorticoid is dictated by factors other than the mineralocorticoid receptor alone. Two possible mechanisms have been suggested. First, CBG does not bind aldosterone but may selectively inhibit the binding of glucocorticoid to the mineralocorticoid receptor in mineralocorticoid-responsive tissues. Second, 11β-hydroxysteroid dehydrogenase, an enzyme that converts cortisol to its 11-keto analogue, may be present in the mineralocorticoid-responsive tissues. The 11-keto analogue of cortisol does not bind to the mineralocorticoid receptor. Thus degradation of glucocorticoid may take place locally in tissues that are mineralocorticoid responsive. Further work is required to clarify these issues.

Glucocorticoid Receptor

The human glucocorticoid receptor gene is found on **chromosome 5.** The receptor, a 777 amino acid protein, has a molecular weight of 94,000 and is found in both the **cytoplasm** and **nucleus.** The significant homology between the glucocorticoid and mineralocorticoid receptor and its possible physiologic significance have been discussed. The specific intracellular proteins generated after mRNA translation that mediate the biologic actions of glucocorticoids have not been identified.

Androgen Receptor

The gene for the androgen receptor is found on the X chromosome, and the human form of the receptor has a molecular weight of 98,000. Human androgen receptors are found in both the **nucleus** and **cytoplasm.** The specific intracellular proteins that mediate the biologic actions of androgen have not been identified.

Catecholamines

Synthesis

Catecholamines are naturally occurring compounds consisting of a catechol (3,4-dihydrophenyl) nucleus linked to an amine (Fig. 57-4). The catecholamines are synthesized by the sequential conversion of dietary tyrosine to epinephrine. **Tyrosine hydroxylase** is the major regulator of catecholamine production (see Fig. 57-4). **Dopamine, norepinephrine,** and **epinephrine** are the catecholamines found in humans. Each is stored in high concentrations in separate vesicles.

During **gestation** and the **newborn period,** the primary end-product of the adrenal medulla is norepinephrine. With **advancing age,** there is a dramatic decline in the norepinephrine-to-epinephrine ratio, associated with a marked rise in **phenylethanolamine-N-methyl transferase** (PNMT) activity, the enzyme that catalyzes the conversion of norepinephrine to epinephrine (see Fig. 57-4). PNMT activity requires high local concentrations of **glucocorticoid.** Thus the production of epinephrine by the medulla is linked to the anatomic and vascular relationship between the cortex and medulla, which ensures that the medullary cells are bathed with a high concentration of cortisol.

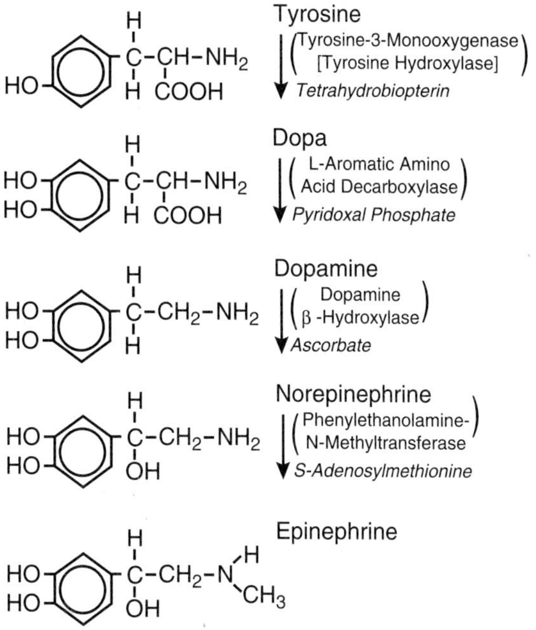

Fig. 57-4. Enzymatic pathway and cofactors for catecholamine synthesis. (Adapted from: *Goodman & Gilman's The Pharmacological Basis of Therapeutics,* 8th ed. New York: Pergamon, 1990. P. 102.)

Secretion and Metabolism

The major stimulus for catecholamine release from the adrenal medulla is **preganglionic sympathetic nervous system activation.** Stress, change in posture or temperature, asphyxia, hypotension, low blood sugar levels, and sodium depletion are all factors that activate the sympathetic nervous system. Direct stimulation of the medullary cells by histamine, acetylcholine, and angiotensin-II also produces catecholamine release, but the physiologic significance of these factors is unknown.

Serum catecholamines are rapidly removed from the circulation and have a serum half-life of less than 20 seconds. This brief half-life is the combined result of rapid uptake of catecholamines by tissues and inactivation in the vascular system and liver. The major process of catecholamine inactivation is believed to be uptake by tissues. The process has been divided into two categories: uptake$_1$ and uptake$_2$. **Uptake$_1$** consists of the removal of serum catecholamines, primarily norepinephrine, by postganglionic sympathetic neurons, with subsequent sequestration in neuronal storage vesicles. **Uptake$_2$** principally involves the accumulation of epinephrine by extraneuronal tissues. Epinephrine is then degraded by catecholamine-*O*-methyltransferase and monoamine oxidase to form inactive metabolites. The primary metabolites are vanillylmandelic acid, metanephrine, normetanephrine, and their glucuronide and sulfate derivatives.

Receptors

The catecholamine receptors consist of several similar, but distinct, types of surface-cell receptors defined by their physiologic action and pharmacologic specificity. The subtypes include alpha$_1$, alpha$_2$, beta$_1$, and beta$_2$ adrenergic receptors. In general, norepinephrine and epinephrine have an equipotent effect on the alpha$_1$, alpha$_2$, and beta$_1$ receptors. Epinephrine has a more potent effect on the beta$_2$ receptor.

The **alpha$_1$ receptors** are primarily found on vascular smooth muscle, and their activation results in **vasoconstriction.** The alpha receptor activates phospholipase C, a membrane enzyme, and this leads to the generation of intracellular second messengers, DAG and IP$_3$ (see the section on mineralocorticoid secretion and metabolism for details). Both products enhance the intracellular calcium concentration.

The **alpha$_2$ receptors** are found principally on presynaptic nerve terminals. Activation inhibits the production of cAMP and attenuates norepinephrine release by the sympathetic nervous system. Postganglionic alpha$_2$ receptors are also found in gastric smooth muscle cells and the beta cells of pancreatic islets. Stimulation causes **decreased gastric motility** and **attenuated insulin secretion.**

The **beta$_1$ receptors** are found primarily on cardiac pacemakers and muscle cells. Stimulation increases cAMP production with increased **chronotropic** and **inotropic function.**

The **beta$_2$ receptors** are found principally on respiratory smooth muscle cells, uterine smooth muscle, salivary glands, and the liver. Stimulation increases cAMP production, with resultant respiratory and uterine smooth muscle dilatation, increased secretion by the salivary glands, and enhanced glycogenolysis and gluconeogenesis.

Major Clinical Disorders

The major clinical disorders of the adrenal gland can be defined as pathologic states reflecting either an excessive or deficient production of the adrenal hormones. Following are examples of diseases involving each hormone.

Mineralocorticoid

Primary **hyperaldosteronism,** a rare cause of mild to moderate hypertension, is the result of the autonomous, unilateral, and excessive secretion of aldosterone by a tumor. **Hypokalemia** is a cardinal sign. Total-body potassium depletion results in excessive H$^+$ secretion by the cortical collecting duct, resulting in metabolic alkalosis. Diagnostic tests reveal autonomous mineralocorticoid secretion. Surgical removal of the tumor is required for effective treatment.

Deficient aldosterone production can result from a number of enzymatic deficiencies in steroidogenesis (see Fig. 57-1) or from destruction of the zona glomerulosa or the adrenal cortex (Addison's disease). Isolated **mineralocorticoid deficiency** causes intravascular volume depletion, hyponatremia, hyperkalemia, and shock. In **Addison's disease** (mineralocorticoid and glucocorticoid deficiency), the patient also exhibits signs of insufficient cortisol production (to be discussed). The lack of aldosterone response to ACTH (see the section "Adrenal Function Tests") is diagnostic. Effective treatment requires exogenous mineralocorticoid replacement.

Glucocorticoid

Cushing's disease is characterized by the inability of physiologic concentrations of serum glucocorticoid to suppress ACTH secretion, resulting in excessive cortisol secretion. The signs and symptoms include growth failure, cutaneous hyperpigmentation (ACTH excess), moon facies, purple striae, mild hypertension, trunkal obesity, and thin skin. Diagnosis requires the suppression of glucocorticoid secretion by a pharmacologic, but not physiologic, dose of glucocorticoid. Treatment usually requires the surgical removal of the pituitary lesion.

Glucocorticoid deficiency can result from an enzymatic deficiency in steroidogenesis (congenital adrenal hyperplasia) or destruction of the adrenal cortex (Addison's disease). Decreased glucocorticoid production provokes excessive ACTH secretion. Although five types of congenital adrenal hyperplasia have been described, the most common is **21-hydroxylase deficiency.** The position of the deficient enzyme in the steroidogenic cascade dictates the steroid hormones produced and the accompanying clinical signs and symptoms. The **clinical picture** can include hyperpigmentation, shock due to cardiac dysfunction, mineralocorticoid deficiency, and excessive virilization of a genetic female or undervirilization of a genetic male. **Addison's disease** is characterized by glucocorticoid deficiency (cardiac dysfunction, anorexia, fatigue, weakness) and mineralocorticoid deficiency (as previously described). Treatment of congenital adrenal hyperplasia and Addison's disease requires the administration of glucocorticoid and mineralocorticoid.

Androgen

Excessive androgen production is characterized by premature or exaggerated virilization. This can result from certain forms of congenital adrenal hyperplasia (as described) or an adrenal tumor. This latter condition requires surgical removal of the tumor.

An isolated deficiency of adrenal androgen production has no known clinical consequence.

Catecholamines

A prime example of excessive catecholamine production is a **pheochromocytoma.** The typical symptoms of this rare cause of intermittent hypertension are headaches, palpitations, excessive perspiration, and paroxysm (pallor, anxiety, nausea, and weakness). Surgical removal is the standard form of therapy.

Epinephrine plays a secondary role in the acute response to **hypoglycemia.** Some individuals with diabetes mellitus do not produce enough epinephrine, and are thus at risk for asymptomatic, prolonged hypoglycemia.

Adrenal Function Tests

Diagnostic tests that assess adrenal integrity document either basal or dynamic function. Baseline tests employ single or serial measurements of the circulating concentration of a hormone or a timed urine collection. The former test assesses a single moment or series of moments in time. The latter gives an integrated view of baseline function over a longer period. Either method can only be used as a screening process, but baseline tests are not very sensitive for diagnosing adrenal insufficiency.

Dynamic adrenal function tests attempt to either stimulate or suppress the basal level of the adrenal hormone of interest. Stimulation tests are required when decreased production is suspected. Suppression tests are in order if the converse is entertained.

The interpretation of both baseline and dynamic tests must take into consideration the clinical status of the patient. Dietary sodium intake and the patient's posture significantly affect mineralocorticoid metabolism. Stress can prevent glucocorticoid suppression. **Androgen tests** are

influenced much less by the clinical status of the patient. **Catecholamines values,** however, are significantly influenced by exercise, stress, posture, and a number of medications. Before performing any adrenal function tests, the patient's clinical status should match that of the reference population to avoid the risk of misinterpretation of the results.

Mineralocorticoid

Basal serum aldosterone concentrations yield little useful diagnostic information. **Hypokalemic metabolic alkalosis** can be an early clue to excessive aldosterone production. Manipulation of aldosterone secretion is, however, an effective diagnostic tool. The most useful stimulation test exploits the response to ACTH administration. If the adrenal gland is present and the enzymatic cascade intact, there is a prompt rise in aldosterone secretion following the acute administration of ACTH. If excessive aldosterone production is suspected, suppression tests are used, including oral and intravenous sodium loading and mineralocorticoid and glucocorticoid administration.

Glucocorticoid

Basal glucocorticoid function tests give some insight into the status of the CRH-ACTH-adrenal axis. A low 8:00 AM serum cortisol value raises the question of glucocorticoid deficiency. Lack of a circadian rhythm or increased urinary concentrations of free cortisol, 17-hydroxycorticosteroids, 17-ketogenic steroids, or metabolites of a precursor of cortisol (see Fig. 57-1) suggest either excessive ACTH production or autonomous activity in the zona fasciculata. Only dynamic testing can identify the pathologic process.

Three **stimulation tests** are commonly employed: stress, metyrapone, and ACTH. **Insulin-induced hypoglycemia** is the most widely used stress test. An appropriate rise of serum cortisol in response to hypoglycemia documents an intact CRH-ACTH-adrenal axis. A subnormal response fails to identify which part of the axis is deficient. Because of the risks associated with hypoglycemia, **metyrapone** is preferred by some to evaluate the CRH-ACTH-adrenal axis. Metyrapone inhibits the final step in the production of cortisol, rendering the patient glucocorticoid deficient (see Fig. 57-1). A normal response is an increase in ACTH and the immediate precursor of a cortisol, deoxycortisone. As with insulin-induced hypoglycemia, a subnormal response does not identify the specific part of the axis that is defective.

A normal response to **exogenous ACTH** documents a

functionally intact adrenal gland that has been primed with endogenous ACTH, but the test does not directly document CRH and ACTH sufficiency.

Suppression tests exploit the response to different doses of **dexamethasone** (an extremely potent glucocorticoid) to identify the source of either excessive ACTH (pituitary, ectopic) or cortisol production. In normal individuals, endogenous glucocorticoid production is suppressed with low-dose dexamethasone. In subjects with excessive ACTH production of pituitary origin, cortisol production is inhibited only with high-dose dexamethasone. Individuals who show no suppression with either low or high doses of dexamethasone have either an ectopic (nonpituitary) source of excess ACTH production or autonomous production of cortisol by the adrenal gland. The concentration of basal circulating ACTH and radiographic studies can help to differentiate ectopic ACTH production from an adrenal tumor.

Androgen

Androgen function tests are principally employed to identify individuals with excessive androgen production caused by a physiologic (enzymatic defect in steroidogenesis, increased production of ACTH by the pituitary) or autonomous (tumor) process. Elevated basal serum levels of DHEA-S, androstenedione, or 17-ketosteroids can be used to screen individuals with suspected excessive production (see Fig. 57-1). The dexamethasone suppression test differentiates between physiologic and autonomous processes.

Medulla

Baseline medullary function tests can be used to identify individuals with excessive catecholamine production. Both single-serum and 24-hour urine concentrations are employed.

Dynamic tests include the administration of glucagon, phentolamine, or clonidine. **Glucagon** stimulates the catecholamine release. A patient with excessive catecholamine production will exhibit a rapid and dramatic increase in blood pressure. The **phentolamine** test blocks the alpha$_1$-adrenergic effect of catecholamines. Subjects synthesizing an excessive quantity of catecholamine will display a fall in systemic pressure. **Clonidine** inhibits centrally mediated adrenergic function. As a result, a subject with autonomous catecholamine production will not show decreased sympathetic nervous system activity or serum catecholamine concentration.

Summary

The basic anatomic and physiologic relationships within the adrenal cortex and between the adrenal cortex and medulla have been described. This chapter also highlights the important physiologic branch points in steroidogenesis. The characteristics of adrenal hormone receptors have been described and compared. Finally, selected diseases have been briefly described and tests of adrenal function discussed to help the student place the basic anatomy and physiology of the adrenal gland into a clinical context.

Bibliography

Bondy, P. K. Disorders of the adrenal cortex. In: Wilson, J. D., and Foster, D. W., eds. *William's Textbook of Endocrinology,* 7th ed. Philadelphia: W. B. Saunders, 1985. Pp. 816–890.

DeQuattro, V. Catecholamines and adrenal disorders. In: DeGroot, L. J., ed. *Endocrinology,* 2nd ed. Philadelphia: W. B. Saunders, 1989. Pp. 1717–1800.

Dolan, L. M., and Carey, R. M. In: Vaughan, E. D., and Carey, R. M., eds. *Adrenal Disorders.* New York: Thieme Medical Publishers, 1989. Pp. 81–145.

58 The Physiology of Fuel Nutrients and Pancreatic Hormones

Nelson D. Horseman

Objectives

After reading this chapter, you should be able to

Describe the physiology of fuel metabolism as it relates to carbohydrate, protein, and fat catabolism

Identify the secretory functions of the cells of the endocrine pancreas

Describe the actions of insulin on whole-body fuel metabolism

Describe the cellular mechanisms of insulin action

Compare and contrast the actions of the four counterregulatory hormones that increase blood glucose concentrations

Describe the basic pathology and etiology of each type of diabetes mellitus

Overview of Fuel Metabolism in the Human

Because all cells must have a steady energy-producing fuel supply, the ability to store and dispense nutrients in a regulated fashion is essential to life and health. In contrast with herbivorous animals such as cattle and other ruminants, which have a relatively constant nutrient intake, the human nutrient intake pattern is meal-oriented. In addition, over long evolutionary times the human nutrient intake pattern has been highly dependent on seasons of plenty and scarcity. This pattern has required the human species to use an endocrine system that promotes nutrient storage during times of feast and dispenses nutrients carefully during times of famine. In species such as the human that experience highly variable nutrient flux, the pancreas dominates fuel metabolism. This evolutionary fact contributes greatly to many modern disease issues, such as obesity, cardiovascular disease, and diabetes. The regulation of fuel metabolism is dominated by three basic principles. Understanding these basic ideas will allow one to have an overall perspective on metabolic regulation that makes several aspects of these complex systems easier to understand.

Principle 1: Nutrient storage is promoted by a single hormone, **insulin,** which is highly sensitive to circulating levels of glucose and amino acids. The lack of redundancy in the regulation of fuel storage makes diabetes mellitus a common and life-threatening disease.

Principle 2: Four separate hormones — glucagon, epinephrine, cortisol, and growth hormone — stimulate the release of fuel substrates from storage. The roles played by each of these **counterregulatory** hormones are different in important ways that will be described later. Adequate blood glucose is absolutely essential for the functions of certain essential tissues such as the brain, renal medulla, and red blood cells. The redundancy of counterregulatory hormones ensures that the glucose supply is not interrupted.

Principle 3: There are four major fuel nutients: glucose, glycogen, proteins, and fats. Each type of fuel nutrient plays a different role in the energy balance of the human body. The endocrine factors that control metabolism of each of the fuel sources optimize the utilization of these foods. In this way, both homeostasis and long-term growth and development can be supported by the available fuel nutrients.

Glucose is easily oxidized by all cells to yield energy (ATP) and is the only useful fuel nutrient for most neural cells. It provides almost 4 kilocalories (Cal) per gram. Since the average human (70 kg) uses about 2200 Cal/day, one would need about 550 g (over a pound) of glucose to survive each day. This amount of glucose must be diluted in over 10 liters (about 25 lb) of water so as not to exceed the osmolarity of cells. It is therefore impractical for the body to carry glucose as a storage form of fuel. Glucose is used as a readily transported substrate, with about 20 g (enough for 1 hour of metabolism) in the circulation at any given time.

Glycogen is a highly polymerized form of glucose (animal starch) that is stored as hydrated crystalline deposits in liver and skeletal muscle. On a molar basis, glycogen is not more efficient than glucose as a form of energy storage. However, because of its crystalline nature, it requires only about 5% as much water for storage. Therefore, it needs only about 0.5 liter to accommodate 550 g. Normally, the body stores about 300 g of glycogen (less than 1 day's total energy needs).

Proteins can be metabolized as a fuel substrate, and the large depot of body (especially muscle) protein (10–15 kg) is a major resource during prolonged starvation. However, metabolism of proteins leads to the production of large amounts of nitrogenous wastes (i.e., ammonia, urea) and sulfur-containing wastes. These create significant detoxification costs that are not generated by carbohydrate fuels. In addition, the loss of muscle mass is an obvious cost of using protein as a fuel substrate.

Fats are by far the most concentrated fuel substrate available (at 9 Cal/g), and because they do not require additional water for storage, they can be stored more efficiently than either carbohydrates or proteins. About 250 g (1/2 lb) of triglyceride provides sufficient energy for an entire day's metabolism. Carbohydrates are converted to fats for storage once the glycogen resources are filled, but this conversion is only about 75% efficient (25% of energy is lost to heat). Fatty acid beta-oxidation requires oxygen (i.e., mitochondrial aerobic metabolism). Therefore, certain tissues such as red blood cells and the renal medulla, which have no mitochondria, cannot use fatty acid for energy. These tissues remain dependent on anaerobic glycolysis even during starvation. The storage of energy in the form of fats has been highly adaptive during human evolution, but in modern society, the efficiency of this system contributes to cardiovascular disease and obesity.

Once glucose has been converted to fatty acids, it cannot be converted back into glucose. Therefore, since the CNS and certain other tissues require glucose, alternative pathways are necessary so that the conversion of glucose to fatty acids does not deprive those tissues. The most important of these pathways are glycogen breakdown (glycogenolysis) and gluconeogenesis from amino acids.

Blood Glucose Regulation

Blood glucose homeostasis is essential. If the blood glucose level falls beneath about 30 mg/dl, brain function is threatened, and coma and death can occur. It follows that blood glucose concentration is a major determinant of hormone secretion. It is important to begin with a general understanding of how blood glucose is regulated before delving into the specifics of each relevant hormone.

Blood glucose is held within a very narrow range (±10% to 20% of normal) despite large variations in dietary intake and metabolic use (Fig. 58-1). This narrrow range is maintained by two opposing activities: insulin-induced glucose storage and glucose replenishment. The liver is the major source of glucose during normal intermeal fasts. Liver glycogen is used immediately, and hepatic gluconeogene-

Fig. 58-1. The upper graph depicts the plasma insulin and glucose responses of a normal individual to eating a 500-Cal (mixed nutrients) meal. Note that the scales are different on the graphs for glucose and insulin. While glucose rises about 30%, the level of plasma insulin increases by nearly 500%. The lower graph shows the results of oral glucose tolerance tests in diabetic and normal subjects. Not only are resting glucose levels higher in the diabetics, the change after glucose intake is significantly higher and more prolonged. (Modified from: Greenspan, F. S., *Basic and Clinical Endocrinology,* 2nd ed. Norwalk, Conn.: Appleton and Lange, 1991.)

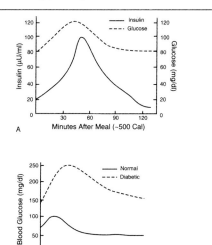

sis from amino acids contributes to the longer term. Gluconeogenesis is very important for continual replenishment of depleted hepatic glycogen stores.

Insulin is the major hormone that causes decreased blood glucose. It stimulates glucose uptake into muscle and adipose tissues and the ultimate conversion of glucose to fatty acids. Insulin also inhibits hepatic glucose release (glycogenolysis).

The short-term elevation of blood glucose is caused by the actions of glucagon and epinephrine (also norepinephrine to a smaller extent), which stimulate glycogenolysis and gluconeogenesis in the liver. They also stimulate adipose lipolysis, thereby providing an alternate fuel source so that glucose utilization is spared.

Long-term maintenance of blood glucose is controlled primarily by cortisol and growth hormone. Cortisol's main action is to increase gluconeogenesis from amino acids, thereby maintaining adequate glycogen stores. Growth hormone's main action is to stimulate lipolysis. Both cortisol and GH have other important effects, and other hormones and local growth factors play important long-term roles.

The Functions of the Endocrine Pancreas

The endocrine functions of the pancreas are the responsibility of small groups of cells called the **islets of Langer-** **hans,** which comprise only about 20% of pancreatic cell mass. The islets are comprised of four cell types: (1) alpha cells, which are glucagon-secreting and make up about 25% of the islet cells, (2) beta cells, which secrete insulin and account for 60% of islet cells, (3) delta cells, which secrete somatostatin and represent 10% of the cells, and (4) pancreatic peptide cells, which secrete a 36-amino acid peptide that controls the exocrine pancreas (the pancreatic peptide cells represent the remaining 5% of islet cells).

Insulin Chemistry and Synthesis

Insulin is a 51-amino acid protein with a molecular weight of about 6000. It consists of the A chain, which is 21 amino acids long, and the B chain, which is 30 amino acids long. The A and B chains are linked by two disulfide bridges.

Insulin is synthesized as a larger precursor molecule called **proinsulin** (Fig. 58-2). In the Golgi apparatus, proinsulin is cleaved by specific proteases to remove the connecting peptide (C-peptide) between the A and B chains. C-peptide is stored along with the processed insulin in secretory granules and released at the same time as mature insulin. There are no known receptors for C-peptide, and it has no apparent biologic action. The concentration of C-peptide in the circulation is often measured as a diagnostic index of insulin secretion. The advantage to

Fig. 52-2. Diagram of the human proinsulin structure indicating the elements contained in the mature insulin molecule (A and B subunits) and the C-peptide. The dipeptide linkages are the sites at which proteolytic cleavage of the precursor takes place.

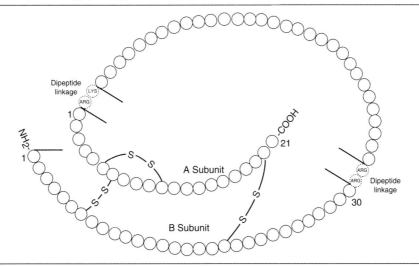

measuring C-peptide is that it is not taken up by receptor-mediated endocytosis, and therefore, it does not undergo variations in clearance, such as those which can affect the plasma concentrations of insulin itself.

Regulation of Insulin Secretion

Insulin is stored as a zinc-containing, quasi-crystalline deposit within beta-cell secretory granules. It is released upon fusion of the secretory granule membranes with the plasmalemma of the beta cell. The feedback loop for insulin secretion is fundamentally a function of nutrient intake and storage (Fig. 58-3). Elevated nutrient concentrations in the plasma stimulate insulin secretion, and insulin lowers circulating nutrient concentrations by stimulating their uptake and storage. Glucose is the primary stimulant for insulin secretion. An elevation of the plasma glucose concentration is followed by both a rapid release of stored insulin and a slower release of newly synthesized insulin.

The glucose effect is a consequence of glucose metabolism within the beta cells. Unmetabolizable glucose analogues do not increase insulin. The final signal for insulin secretion is the increase of ATP and NADPH that occurs after glucose uptake (Fig. 58-4). The level of glucokinase activity in beta cells is closely coupled to insulin secretion, and it is believed that this enzyme may be the **"glucose sensor"** that couples glucose metabolism to insulin release.

Fig. 58-3. The regulatory relationships between insulin secretion and nutrient storage in the human. The circulating factors that (directly and indirectly) cause increased insulin secretion (glucose, amino acids, ketoacids, potassium ions, and free fatty acids) are stored in the muscle, liver, and adipose tissue in response to insulin secretion.

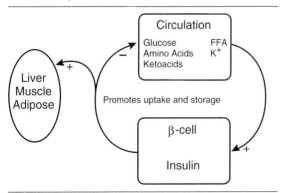

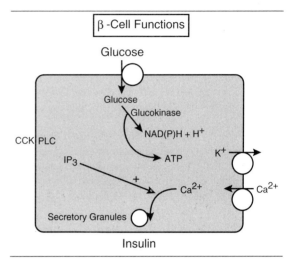

Fig. 58-4. Intracellular mechanisms regulating insulin secretion. The metabolism of glucose, presumably by glucokinase, produces metabolic intermediates such as ATP and NADPH + H$^+$, which affect the activity of K$^+$ and Ca^{2+} channels. The elevation of intracellular Ca^{2+} is the final signal for insulin secretion. Hormones such as cholecystokinin (CCK) that increase the level of insulin secretion in concert with glucose appear to act by the phospholipase C (PLC) inositol trisphosphate (IP$_3$) pathway.

Insulin secretion is greater after oral glucose intake than after intravenous infusion of an equivalent amount of glucose. This is a result of a synergistic stimulation of insulin secretion by gastrointestinal peptides such as gastrin, secretin, and CCK, all of which increase insulin secretion and all of which are secreted in response to the meal. Growth hormone from the pituitary gland causes an increase in basal insulin secretion. This effect of GH is important for maintaining nutrient supply during growth stimulation.

After a meal or glucose infusion, there is a rapid pulse of insulin release followed by a sustained release (see Fig. 58-1). This pattern is a consequence of the release of a pool of presynthesized insulin that can be rapidly mobilized, followed by synthesis and release of new insulin. Because insulin is a small protein and not bound to a larger carrier protein, it is excreted and catabolized rapidly. The insulin half-life in the circulation is normally 5 to 10 minutes. The maintenance of elevated circulating insulin levels by the slow-release mechanism promotes conversion of glucose to lipids after the initial down-regulation of plasma glucose levels. Insulin secretion is also stimulated by circulating amino acids; arginine and lysine are the most potent amino acids that cause insulin release. By contrast, fatty acids have little or no direct effect on insulin release.

The normal plasma glucose concentration in the human is about 80 mg/dl. When the plasma concentration of glucose falls below 50 mg/dl, there is essentially no insulin secretion. Insulin levels increase to half maximum at about 150 mg glucose per deciliter and are maximal at all glucose levels above 300 mg/dl. In obesity, insulin levels are consistently higher than normal, and the postprandial (after meal) peak is much exaggerated.

Whole-Body Metabolic Actions of Insulin

Insulin is secreted in response to elevated nutrient (especially glucose and amino acid) supply, and its overall action is to provide for storage and utilization of those nutrients. The liver, skeletal muscle, and adipose tissues are the main sites of insulin's actions. In the liver, glucose utilization is increased, resulting in glycogen synthesis. In skeletal muscle, both glucose and amino acid transport are stimulated, and these nutrients are used for glycogen and protein synthesis, respectively. In the adipose cells, glucose and fatty acid uptake are stimulated, and triglyceride synthesis is increased. Glucose may be used in part for fatty acid synthesis. In humans, there is little or no fatty acid synthesis in adipose cells, so this effect is less important than in other animals. Glucose uptake in adipose tissue of humans is important for supplying glycerol, which is used in the esterification of fatty acids to make triglycerides.

Simultaneous with increased glucose, amino acid, and fatty acid utilization, there is a decrease of nutrient breakdown in response to insulin. This action occurs in all the major insulin targets (liver, skeletal muscle, and adipose tissue). Gluconeogenesis from proteins is inhibited by insulin in liver and muscle. Insulin is a potent suppresser of the hormone-sensitive lipase in adipose tissue. This is the main enzyme that releases fatty acids from the triglycerides that are stored in fat cells. Because insulin suppresses fatty acid release from adipose tissues, it lowers the availability of substrates for hepatic fatty acid beta-oxidation. Therefore, it diminishes ketoacid generation by liver.

Cellular Actions of Insulin

Insulin binds to a plasma membrane receptor that is a very large (about 270,000 Da) protein consisting of two alpha subunits and two beta subunits (Fig. 58-5). The alpha subunits are entirely extracellular and are mainly responsible for hormone binding. The beta subunits span the membrane. The alpha subunits are linked together by disulfide bridges, and the beta subunits are linked to the alpha chains by disulfide bridges. The intracellular region of the insulin receptor beta subunits contains tyrosine kinase activity. This kinase is activated after hormone binding and serves as the first step of the receptor's signal transduction.

There are two main intracellular effects of insulin: (1) rapid activation of a specific subclass of glucose transporter proteins (called **GLUT4**), and (2) slower alteration of transcription for various genes that encode metabolic enzymes.

Glucose transporter protein activation does not require new protein synthesis. In the absence of insulin, the transporters are contained in the membranes of cytoplasmic vesicles; insulin stimulates fusion of these membranes with the plasma membrane so that the transporters become

Fig. 58-5. Diagramatic representation of the insulin receptor structure. S-S represents disulfide bond and the branching lines represent glycosylations. (Modified from: Goodman, H. M., *Basic Medical Endocrinology,* 2nd ed. New York: Raven Press, 1994.)

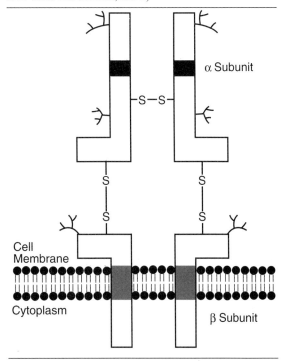

functional. There are several different types of glucose transporters in the human. The GLUT4 transporter is present in skeletal muscle and adipose cells and is responsible for the rapid insulin-dependent uptake of glucose after a meal. Other forms of the glucose transporter are present in tissues such as brain, which requires glucose even at times when circulating insulin levels are low. These other transporter isoforms are not insulin dependent and transport glucose less rapidly than does the GLUT4 transporter.

Numerous metabolic enzyme genes are affected by insulin. Two prominent examples are glucokinase, which is stimulated in muscle and promotes glycogen synthesis, and phosphoenolpyruvate carboxykinase (PEPCK), which is repressed, thereby inhibiting gluconeogenesis from amino acids.

Glucagon and Other Counterregulatory Hormones

The actions of insulin are opposed by at least four separate hormones. Glucagon and epinephrine are the rapidly acting antihypoglycemic hormones. Growth hormone and cortisol (a glucocorticosteroid) are slow acting. Each of these opposes the hypoglycemic actions of insulin so as to prevent low plasma glucose levels. Because the brain and nervous tissues are almost completely dependent on glucose but do not store glucose or glycogen, sufficient plasma glucose must be maintained on a minute-to-minute basis. The redundancy of the counterregulatory hormones is therefore easily understood from an evolutionary perspective.

Glucagon is a single-chain polypeptide of 29 amino acids (molecular weight 3500). Glucagon is structurally related to vasoactive intestinal peptide, gastric inhibitory peptide, secretin, and growth hormone–releasing hormone. The secretion of glucagon is integrated to maintain normoglycemia. It responds in an opposite manner to insulin. Like insulin, its regulation by glucose is a function of glucose metabolism. Increased alpha-cell glucose metabolism causes reduced glucagon secretion.

Insulin amplifies the effects of glucose on glucagon secretion, so elevation of both insulin and glucose is greatly suppressive for glucagon secretion. This situation would arise after a high-carbohydrate meal. On the other hand, a high-protein meal is a potent stimulus for glucagon secretion. This is mediated primarily by arginine and alanine absorption. The combined effect of protein and carbohydrate in a normally balanced meal results in relatively constant intermediate levels of plasma glucagon. Prolonged

fasting (3 days and more) leads to elevated glucagon secretion. Intensive exercise is a very potent stimulus for glucagon secretion.

Gluconeogenesis is stimulated by glucagon in the liver. Therefore, elevation of amino acids (a high-protein meal) increases glucagon and the consequent conversion of amino acids to glucose. This completes a feedback loop because glucose is a suppressor of glucagon secretion.

The metabolic actions of glucagon are to stimulate gluconeogenesis, ketogenesis, and glycogenolysis. Glycogenolysis and gluconeogenesis contribute directly to increasing circulating glucose availability. Ketogenesis contributes β-OH-butyrate and acetoacetate (ketone bodies) that are useful fuels primarily for muscle and secondarily for some nervous tissue. The metabolism of ketoacids by muscle is important for glucose sparing, especially during prolonged fasts. It is also very important in aerobically trained individuals, because they are more efficient at ketogenesis and ketone metabolism.

Epinephrine is an important insulin counterregulator in skeletal muscle. Its main action is to stimulate glycogenolysis. Under normal circumstances, it is derived from sympathetic nerve terminals, and under more severe stresses, it is secreted from the adrenal medulla in physiologically important quantities.

Growth hormone (GH) from the anterior pituitary and cortisol from the adrenal cortex induce long-term changes in the expression of genes that elevate glucose production. Growth hormone's most important actions are to inhibit the response of target tissues to insulin and increase lipolysis in the adipose tissues. Unlike glucagon, GH does not stimulate gluconeogenesis from amino acids. GH-stimulated lipid metabolism spares both glucose and proteins. Therefore, GH can prevent some of the muscle wasting that would otherwise occur during glucose starvation. Cortisol acts primarily by inducing protein catabolism and gluconeogenesis from amino acids. Unlike glucagon, cortisol does not induce glycogenolysis.

Diabetes Mellitus

There are two broad categories of diseases responsible for the essential symptom of diabetes mellitus (sugar in the urine). The least common, and most life-threatening, is type I diabetes, in which there is an absolute deficiency of insulin secretion. The more common type II diabetes mellitus is characterized by a relative insensitivity to insulin. In type II diabetes, the actual levels of insulin secreted may be normal, or either higher or lower than normal, but the insulin in circulation is biologically ineffective.

Type I (Juvenile) Diabetes Mellitus

Type I diabetes is characterized as hyposecretion of insulin. It normally begins in childhood. This early-onset form of diabetes is generally believed to result from autoimmune reactions to insulin or other islet cell proteins. These events result in destruction of the islet beta cells or in exhaustion of their function. The onset of type I diabetes may be triggered by viral infections or by other circumstances wherein the immune system is highly activated.

Type I diabetics are insulin-dependent. That is, they cannot survive without administering exogenous insulin. In the absence of insulin secretion, a combination of hyperglycemia and exaggerated metabolism of nonglucose fuel substrates (fats and proteins) leads to acute **diabetic ketoacidosis** (Fig. 58-6), which can be fatal if not quickly resolved. The primary symptoms of type I diabetes are hyperglycemia (elevated blood glucose) and glucosuria (urinary glucose). Secondary to elevated urinary glucose, there is osmotic diuresis (polyuria). Excess circulating fatty acids are oxidized in the liver and produce ketones (acetoacetic acid and β-OH-butyric acid) that circulate, resulting in metabolic acidosis and ketonuria.

The acute morbidity and mortality from type I diabetes is the result mainly of the renal consequences of excreting fluid along with glucose. This results in dehydration and mineral imbalance, leading to cardiovascular impairment. These acute causes of illness are relatively uncommon since most patients have access to insulin, but they can obviously occur if such access is denied by any circumstance.

The chronic effects of type I diabetes are the most important aspects of the disease in modern societies. These include atherosclerosis, renal disease, eye damage (dia-

Fig. 58-6. The pathophysiology of acute diabetic ketoacidosis.

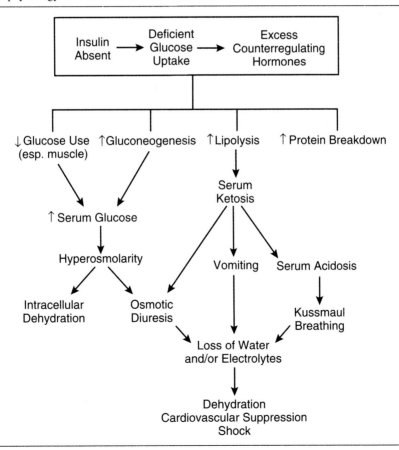

betic retinopathy), and peripheral neuropathies. Most of the chronic complications of type I diabetes are believed to result from excessive glycosylation of proteins of the cytoskeleton and extracellular matrix. This is abnormal glycosylation, not mediated by the normal enzymatic intracellular mechanisms. This leads to loss of membrane elasticity and thickening of membranes. Other disease mechanisms include inappropriate cell growth that is an indirect consequence of poor glucose homeostasis. Unless extremely well controlled, these chronic effects shorten life span and cause problems with childbearing.

Therapy for type I diabetes is based mainly on insulin administration. It includes the use of a wide variety of animal-derived insulins and insulin produced commercially by recombinant DNA techniques. The various insulin preparations have specific pharmacokinetic properties such as rapid action or long circulating half-life. When combined properly, these forms can mimic the physiologic patterns of insulin secretion reasonably well. Recent studies of large populations of diabetics show that careful control of glucose prevents the development of the chronic disease complications. Therefore, close medical monitoring is now understood to be both necessary and highly effective for the disease.

Type II Diabetes

Type II diabetes is also referred to as **non-insulin-dependent diabetes mellitus** (NIDDM) because those afflicted secrete insulin and are therefore not dependent on exogenous insulin. Type II diabetes is characterized by resistance to the hypoglycemic effects of insulin. It normally begins later in life, and there is a large genetic component of predisposition in the development of the disease.

The symptoms of type II diabetes are similar to type I. However, there is generally a slower development of type II disease because elevated insulin secretion can compensate for much of the loss of hormone sensitivity. During this phase of prediabetic insulin resistance, the individual may be unaware of the disease progression. Since type II diabetes usually has a later onset than type I, the development of chronic morbidity is postponed proportionately.

Therapy for type II diabetes includes dietary management and drugs. Two classes of drugs are commonly used.

These include the sulphonylureas, which enhance insulin action, and the biguanides, which inhibit intestinal glucose absorption.

Obesity is often associated with insulin resistance and ultimately with type II diabetes. The causal relationships between obesity and insulin resistance are not clear. Since both are determined in part by genetic predisposition and in part by nutrition, they may be correlated without having any direct causal connections.

Summary

The concentration of circulating blood glucose is normally maintained within very narrow boundaries by the actions of insulin and a set of counterregulatory hormones that oppose the actions of insulin. Glucose is a universal fuel nutrient for all tissues, but it is not an efficient chemical form for nutrient storage. Some tissues, in particular the brain, require a constant source of glucose for energy, whereas most others can utilize fats, proteins, and glycogen as well as glucose. Insulin, secreted from the pancreatic beta cells, lowers blood glucose by stimulating glucose uptake into muscle and adipose tissues and promoting the conversion of glucose to glycogen and fatty acids in the muscles or liver. The plasma glucose concentration regulates insulin secretion via the metabolism of glucose in the beta cell. There are four hormones that increase plasma glucose concentrations to counter hypoglycemia, which might result from fasting or elevated insulin secretion. These include glucagon and epinephrine, which act rapidly, and cortisol and growth hormone, which act over longer periods of time. The mechanisms that are responsible for maintaining blood glucose are elevation of gluconeogenesis, lipolysis, and glycogenolysis.

Bibliography

DeGroot, L. J., et al., eds. *Endocrinology,* 3rd ed. Philadelphia: W. B. Saunders, 1995.

Goodman, H. M. *Basic Medical Endocrinology,* 2nd ed. New York: Raven Press, 1994

Greenspan, F. S. *Basic and Clinical Endocrinology,* 3rd ed. Norwalk, Conn.: Appleton and Lange, 1991.

Part IX Questions: Endocrine Physiology

1. Which one of the following statements concerning RIAs of hormones is true?
   A. The assays are capable of measuring circulating levels of most hormones.
   B. The limiting reagent in the assay is the radioactive hormone.
   C. Assay values indicate biologically active hormone.
   D. The assay is uninfluenced by endogenous antihormone antibodies.
   E. Assays must be performed under equilibrium conditions to be accurate.

2. The tonic influence of the CNS is stimulatory for all of the following pituitary hormones except
   A. corticotropin.
   B. FSH.
   C. GH.
   D. prolactin.
   E. TSH.

3. The secretion of all of the following is increased during stress except for
   A. GH.
   B. TSH.
   C. IL-1.
   D. ACTH.
   E. prolactin.

4. Included among the effects of growth hormone are all except which one of the following?
   A. Stimulation of insulin secretion
   B. Enhanced amino acid uptake
   C. Enhanced glucose uptake
   D. Enhanced triglyceride lipolysis
   E. Increased conversion of amino acids to glucose

5. All of the following are important in the control of vasopressin secretion under physiologic conditions except
   A. plasma osmolality.
   B. blood volume.
   C. blood pressure.
   D. blood urea.

6. Thyroid peroxidase activity is necessary for the
   A. synthesis of thyroglobulin.
   B. iodination of tyrosines.
   C. lysosomal degradation of thyroglobulin.
   D. induction of cAMP by TSH.
   E. Wolff-Chaikoff effect.

7. The hormone that primarily reacts with nuclear receptors is
   A. 1,25-dihydroxyvitamin D_3.
   B. PtH.
   C. Both
   D. Neither

8. The unique enzymatic cascade for promoting aldosterone synthesis by the zona glomerulosa includes
   A. the presence of cortisol reductase.
   B. the presence of 17,20-desmolase.
   C. The absence of 17α-hydroxylase.
   D. the presence of tyrosine hydroxylase.

9. After depletion of hepatic glycogen stores (as the result of fasting), blood glucose levels are maintained by
   A. all tissues of the body utilizing fatty acids as their major energy source rather than glucose.
   B. increasing gluconeogenesis and an increased utilization of fatty acids and ketoacids by some tissues (especially muscle).
   C. increasing insulin secretion.
   D. by decreasing urinary excretion of glucose.
   E. by preventing protein catabolism in all tissues of the body.

10. Shortly after consumption of a high-protein meal in normally fed individuals, blood levels of
    A. insulin would increase and glucagon would decrease.
    B. glucagon would increase and GH would decrease.
    C. insulin would decrease and glucose would increase.
    D. cortisol and epinephrine would increase.
    E. insulin and glucagon would increase, with little change in glucose.

X Reproductive Physiology

Part Editor

Andrew R. LaBarbera

59 Sexual Differentiation, Development, and Maturation

Andrew R. LaBarbera

Objectives

After reading this chapter, you should be able to

Identify the factors that determine gonadal sex

Identify the factors that determine phenotypic sex, that is, the sex of the internal and external genitalia

Describe the extent of prenatal gametogenesis in females and males

Explain the role of steroid hormones in the differentiation of the reproductive tract in males and females

Explain the role of steroid hormones in the sexual differentiation of the brain

Describe the origin of breasts in males and females, including prenatal and postnatal breast development

Describe the changes in the secretion of hypothalamic, pituitary, and ovarian hormones during puberty

---

Functionally, the reproductive system includes the **gonads,** the **internal genitalia** of the reproductive tract, the **external genitalia,** and the **hypothalamic-pituitary unit.** Differentiation of the reproductive systems of both females and males commences early in fetal life. Development of the primary sex organs, the gonads, including the germ cells, begins before the secondary or accessory sex organs start to develop, but development of primary and secondary sex organs is not completed until puberty. The control mechanisms in the hypothalamic-pituitary unit, though functional during childhood, remain quiescent until puberty.

Early Development of the Gonads

The embryonal gonad consists of three elements, each with a different origin. First, the germ cells are derived from the primitive ectodermal cells of the inner cell mass. **Primordial germ cells** can be identified as early as the

fifth day of gestation in the **blastocyst.** The supporting cells of the coelomic epithelium form the second element of the embryonic gonad. These epithelial cells give rise to the **Sertoli cells** of the testis and the **granulosa cells** of the ovary. Stromal or interstitial cells that are derived from the original mesenchymal cells of the gonadal ridge constitute the third element of the embryonic gonad. The formation of the early embryonic gonad is complete by the fifth to sixth week of gestation. At the end of the sixth week, the gonad of either sex is still both indifferent and bipotential. In other words, the gonad is neither male nor female and can develop in either direction as determined by the chromosomal composition.

Genetic Determination of Gonadal Sex

Chromosomal sex determines gonadal sex, which in turn determines the phenotypic sex (Fig. 59-1). The presence of

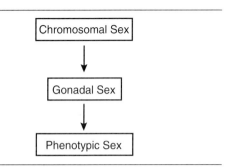

Fig. 59-1. Genetic determination of the sex of the offspring.

a Y chromosome determines whether testes will develop. Regardless of the number of X chromosomes that exist, if there is a Y chromosome, or at least the segment of the Y chromosome containing the sex-determining genes, testes will develop at least partially; if a Y chromosome is not present, ovaries will develop. All the **testis-determining genes** must be present in order for testes to develop completely. These genes normally are located on the short arm of the Y chromosome near the centromere.

Complete sexual differentiation and development require either two normal X chromosomes for genetic females or one X chromosome and one normal Y chromosome for genetic males. Normal sexual differentiation also requires certain autosomal genes in both genetic males and females. The testis-determining genes prevent activation of the autosomal genes for ovarian development during gestation. If there are two X chromosomes in addition to a Y chromosome, then testes will develop but spermatogenesis will be impaired. In the absence of a Y chromosome, the phenotype will be female regardless of the number of X chromosomes, but two X chromosomes are necessary for the complete differentiation and function of ovaries. Sexual anomalies can occur when the X and Y chromosomes fail to segregate completely during meiosis. Some of the most common disorders of sexual differentiation are summarized in Table 59-1. Disorders such as Turner's syndrome and Klinefelter's syndrome result from the abnormal segregation of sex chromosomes during meiosis. Individuals with disorders such as male or female pseudohermaphroditism possess normal complements of sex chromosomes but have defects of sex hormone synthesis or action.

Table 59-1. Disorders of Sexual Differentiation

Gonadal dysgenesis (Turner's syndrome)
Karyotype	45,XO (loss of second sex chromosome)
Phenotype	Female
Manifestation	Short stature, primary amenorrhea, sexual infantilism, elevated gonadotropins

Klinefelter's syndrome
Karyotype	XXY (extra sex chromosome)
Phenotype	Male
Manifestation	Small, firm testes, azoospermia, gynecomastia, elevated gonadotropins, mental and social impairment

Male pseudohermaphroditism
Karyotype	XY (normal)
Phenotype	Male/female
Manifestation	Testes present, deficiencies of either androgen biosynthesis, androgen action (androgen insensitivity), or mullerian-inhibiting hormone formation result in failure of virilization

Female pseudohermaphroditism
Karyotype	XX (normal)
Phenotype	Female/male
Manifestation	Ovaries present, normal reproductive tract, excess androgen production (congenital adrenal hyperplasia) results in virilization

Differentiation and Development of the Gonads

In the seventh week of gestation, gonadal development in males and females diverges. In males with a normal XY chromosomal complement, the primitive sex cords do not degenerate. Rather, the primitive sex cords continue to develop under the influence of the testis-determining genes. In normal females with two X chromosomes, the ovaries begin to develop around the twelfth week of gestation. The epithelial cells of the cortical cords later develop into the cells of the ovarian follicle.

Prenatal Gametogenesis

Human somatic cells normally contain 46 chromosomes. **Oocytes** (female gametes) and **spermatozoa** (male gametes) must each contain only half the normal complement of chromosomes (N or haploid number) so that after fertilization the **zygote** will contain the normal diploid, or 2N, number of chromosomes. The number of chromosomes is reduced from the 2N number in the primordial germ cells to the N number in the mature gametes by **meiosis,** a process of chromosomal reduction division unique to germ cells. During meiosis, genes derived from the maternal chromosomes are exchanged with genes derived from paternal chromosomes prior to segregation of chromosomes into daughter cells. Thus the mature gamete contains genes from both the mother and father.

Oogenesis

The production of female germ cells begins during embryonic life and is completed during the adult reproductive period (Fig. 59-2). In the female, **oogenesis,** the process by which a primordial germ cell develops into an ovum, begins soon after the primordial germ cell arrives in the gonad during embryogenesis. The primordial germ cells undergo numerous mitotic divisions so that by the end of the third month of gestation the fetal ovary contains clusters of **oogonia** derived from a single germ cell and surrounded by a layer of epithelial cells. During the fourth month, oogonia begin to differentiate into the larger **primary oocytes,** replicate their DNA, and enter the prophase of the first meiotic division. At this time, the primary oocytes have 4N quantity of DNA. Oogonia continue to divide so that by the fifth month of gestation the ovary contains the maximum number of primary oocytes, approxi-

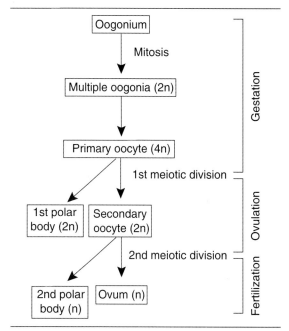

Fig. 59-2. Oogenesis.

mately 7 million. Meiosis in all the female germ cells begins during prenatal development, is arrested at the dictyotene stage of prophase of the first meiotoic division, and does not resume until shortly before ovulation in individual oocytes.

Degeneration of many primary oocytes and oogonia by **atresia** commences during the fifth month of gestation, while development continues. Most of the oogonia degenerate by the seventh month. Individual surviving primary oocytes, however, are surrounded by the flat epithelial cells, thus forming the primordial follicles. At birth, the ovary contains between 700,000 and 2 million primordial follicles. During childhood, most of the oocytes become atretic so that at puberty only approximately 40,000 oocytes remain in the ovary. Throughout this entire period, the oocytes remain arrested in the first meiotic division.

Spermatogenesis

Only the initial stages of germ cell production occur during embryonic life in the male (Fig. 59-3). Unlike the female, in whom meiosis begins during fetal life, meiosis in male germ cells does not begin until puberty and then continues throughout life. At birth, the primitive sex cords of

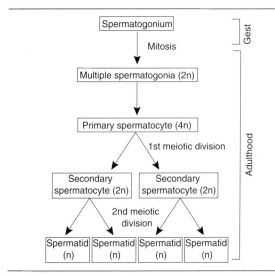

Fig. 59-3. Spermatogenesis.

the testis contain large **spermatogonia** surrounded by supporting cells, which become the Sertoli cells. The maturation divisions of male germ cells differ from those of the female germ cells in that a **primary spermatocyte** gives rise to four **spermatids,** whereas a primary oocyte results in a single mature oocyte and two nonfunctional polar bodies. **Spermatogenesis,** the process of differentiation of the primordial germ cells in the male, does not begin until puberty. Differentiation of male germ cells in the testis occurs in the Sertoli cells, which are epithelial cells lining the lumen of the seminiferous tubules.

Differentiation and Development of the Reproductive Tract

Until the eighth week of gestation, the urogenital tracts and external genitalia of both males and females are indifferent and indistinguishable (Fig. 59-4). Initially, each sex

Fig. 59-4. Differentiation of the reproductive tract.

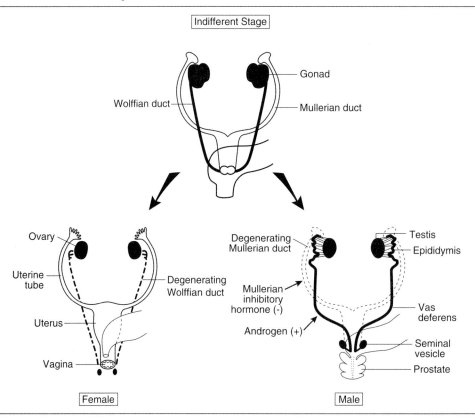

has a dual paired duct system consisting of a **mesonephric duct** and a **paramesonephric duct** within each mesonephric kidney. The mesonephric, or **wolffian,** ducts terminate in the urogenital sinus, the lower portion of which eventually contributes to formation of the external genitalia. Each paramesonephric, or **mullerian,** duct develops at approximately 6 weeks as an evagination in the coelomic epithelium on the anterolateral surface of the urogenital ridge. This evagination becomes tubular and is associated with the wolffian duct at the caudal end.

Male

Shortly after the testes begin to differentiate in the sixth to seventh weeks of gestation, the mullerian ducts begin to regress in response to **mullerian-inhibiting hormone** (MIH), a large dimeric glycoprotein of approximately 140,000 molecular weight that is produced by the Sertoli cells of the fetal testes. As the number of Leydig cells in the fetal testes increases, increasing amounts of the androgenic hormone **testosterone** are produced in response to **human chorionic gonadotropin,** which is synthesized and secreted by the **placenta. Androgens** are not necessary for regression of the mullerian duct; rather, they independently stimulate development of the wolffian duct system with virilization of the urogenital sinus and external genitalia. Androgen production peaks at 12 to 13 weeks of gestation and then slowly declines. The capacity of the fetal testis to produce androgen corresponds to the induction of the 3ß-hydroxysteroid dehydrogenase enzyme system. Androgens cause the differentiation of the epididymis, vas deferens, seminal vesicle, prostate, and ejaculatory duct. The crucial role of testicular secretions in male sexual differentiation is summarized in Fig. 59-5. Development of the external genitalia, including the penis and the scrotum, is androgen dependent and occurs primarily during the first trimester of pregnancy. The testes descend into the scrotum much later in development.

Cells of some androgen-responsive tissues in the male fetus, such as the rete testis, epididymis, vas deferens, and seminal vesicles, have testosterone receptors and respond to testosterone. Testosterone binds to the receptors in target cells and modulates expression of genes necessary for growth and differentiation of these tissues. Other androgen-responsive tissues, such as the urethra, prostate, scrotum, and penis, contain an enzyme, **5α-reductase,** that converts testosterone to **dihydrotestosterone** (DHT). These tissues contain receptors for DHT. A deficiency of 5α-reductase and consequently, an inability to convert

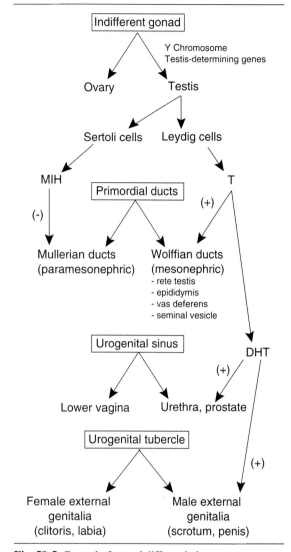

Fig. 59-5. Control of sexual differentiation.

testosterone to DHT, results in incomplete differentiation of the male internal and external genitalia.

Female

Due to the absence of fetal testes that secrete testosterone, the wolffian ducts of the female regress automatically near the end of the second month of gestation. The mullerian ducts differentiate into the genital ducts of the female, including the fallopian tubes, uterus, and vagina. The external genitalia, including the clitoris, the labia majora, and the labia minora, also differentiate in the absence of testosterone.

It is not known whether **estrogens** are involved in the differentiation of the external genitalia in the female. The fetal ovary is capable of producing estrogen early in gestation. However, estrogens in the fetal circulation are derived from the mother, the placenta, and the fetal adrenal cortex and ovary. Thus removal of the fetal ovaries by castration would not eliminate the principal source of estrogens. The cells of the primitive sex accessory structures do possess androgen receptors so that excessive androgen production does cause profound virilization of the external genitalia of the female. Exposure to progestins that possess androgenic activity results in varying degrees of virilization, depending on the androgen activity of the particular progestin.

Sexual Differentiation of the Brain

Gonadal steroid hormones are important in the regulation of sexual behavior. Besides directing differentiation of the reproductive tract, steroids appear to play a role in the differentiation of the neural systems that regulate both sexual function and behavior in the adult. Receptors for estrogens and androgens have been identified in the anterior pituitary, hypothalamus, midbrain, amygdala, and cerebral cortex of adult females and males, respectively. The neural consequences of estrogen or androgen binding have not yet been determined.

The hypothalamic-pituitary unit of the adult female produces hormones, called **gonadotropins,** that stimulate the gonads in a cyclic pattern, with a periodicity of approximately 28 days. This cyclicity is determined by the changing sensitivities of the hypothalamic-pituitary unit to estrogens and progestins (see Chap. 60). Gonadotropin secretion in the male differs from that in the female in that it is not cyclic.

Evidence obtained in laboratory animals indicates that androgens secreted by the testes during the periods of fetal and neonatal development are responsible for the acyclic pattern of gonadotropin secretion characteristic of males. Administration of testosterone to neonatal female rats produces acyclic gonadotropin secretion and sterility or **masculinization** when they become adults. Conversely, castration of neonatal male rats eliminates androgen production, and the adults exhibit cyclic female gonadotropin secretion. In some species, testosterone is first converted to estradiol before exerting its effects, and in these species, administration of estradiol to neonatal males also produces masculinization of the hypothalamic-pituitary axis.

Breast Development

The development of breasts is identical in males and females before puberty. **Mammary glands** begin as bilateral mammary lines that are bandlike thickenings of the ectodermal epidermis. The mammary lines disappear shortly after formation, except for a single small portion on each side in the thoracic region. These remaining mammary buds penetrate the underlying mesenchyme and remain virtually unchanged until the fifth month of gestation. Each mammary bud then gives rise to 15 to 25 separate sprouts, which form small outbuddings. The epithelial sprouts proliferate and canalize throughout the remainder of gestation to form the lactiferous ducts, while the small outbuddings form the small ducts and alveoli of the mammary glands. The lactiferous ducts open into a small epithelial pit, which develops into the nipple connecting the lactiferous ducts to the outside.

Just before birth, the breast undergoes a brief period of growth, but then the mammary glands regress because of low levels of estrogens and progestins. The breast remains quiescent until puberty. Further growth is proportional to the growth of the remainder of the body.

With the increased concentrations of estradiol and progesterone associated with puberty in females, the breasts grow and develop. The areolae enlarge and become more pigmented. The amount of connective tissue and, more significantly, the amount of adipose tissue increase, and the glands become more vascularized. The ducts enlarge to form rudimentary lobules, and alveolar structures enlarge. Fully developed **alveoli,** however, only appear during pregnancy.

The growth and function of the mammary glands in the nonpregnant state depend primarily on estrogens and progestins, but growth hormone, thyroid hormones, and adrenal corticosteroids have permissive effects. Progesterone by itself has little effect on the mammary gland. Ductal breast tissue alternately proliferates and regresses during each menstrual cycle. Proliferative changes are maximal late in the luteal phase, after exposure to peak concentrations of progesterone. Breast development and function during and after pregnancy are discussed in Chap. 62.

Neuroendocrine Control and Puberty

The reproductive systems of males and females appear to remain dormant during childhood. The hypothalamic-pituitary-gonadal axis is at least partly functional during this period. Removal of the gonads, which produce small amounts of steroid hormones, produces a rise in plasma gonadotropin levels. Moreover, administration of very small amounts of steroid hormones suppresses the already low levels of gonadotropins. Thus the small amounts of steroid hormones produced by the gonads during childhood are able to suppress the secretion of gonadotropins by the hypothalamic-pituitary unit. This mechanism is referred to as **negative feedback.**

Males, at approximately 10 years of age, and females, at approximately 11 years of age, begin to undergo puberty, which is the transition from the juvenile state to adulthood. Puberty generally lasts 2 to 4 years. In females, puberty culminates in the onset of menstruation between the ages of 11 and 16. During puberty, the sexually immature child is transformed into a sexually mature adolescent. The hypothalamic-pituitary-gonadal axis gradually begins to function in an adult manner so that the pituitary secretes increased amounts of the gonadotropins, **follicle-stimulating hormone** (FSH), and **luteinizing hormone** (LH). Increased gonadotropin secretion causes increased secretion of sex hormones by the gonads. As a result, secondary sex characteristics appear and mature, the adolescent growth spurt occurs, fertility is achieved, and profound psychological changes are observed. These changes constitute sexual maturation. The signal for puberty is unknown, but the timing of this transitional state may be related to general bodily growth.

Sexual maturation is characterized by an increase in gonadal hormone secretion, referred to as **gonadarche.** However, the first recognizable hormonal change associated with puberty is elevated adrenal androgen production, referred to as **adrenarche.** The signal for adrenarche has not been identified. The source of increased gonadal activity seems to reside in the brain and hypothalamus, since both the anterior pituitary gland and the gonads are capable of adult function during childhood if appropriately stimulated. The transformation from an immature to a mature state is due to maturation of the neural mechanisms in the brain that modulate secretion of **gonadotropin-releasing hormone** (GnRH) by the hypothalamus. This hormone stimulates the anterior pituitary gland to secrete gonadotropic hormones. During puberty, secretion of GnRH by the hypothalamus increases. The control of GnRH secretion is thought to reside in a GnRH oscillator or **pulse generator,** which is the central neural regulator of GnRH secretion. The GnRH pulse generator has not been identified. However, the absence of steroid receptors on GnRH-secreting neurons suggests that the GnRH pulse generator neurons are distinct from GnRH-secreting neurons.

Changes in Gonadotropins During Prenatal and Postnatal Development

Puberty can be considered the final phase of development of the hypothalamic-pituitary-gonadal axis that begins during fetal life. The concentrations of the gonadotropins, FSH and LH, in the fetal circulation of both males (Fig. 59-6) and females increase markedly around the middle of pregnancy. Peak concentrations are achieved at between 100 and 150 days of gestation and then decline as the hypothalamic-pituitary unit becomes very sensitive to the negative feedback inhibition by gonadal steroids. The magnitude of the rise in fetal concentrations of FSH and LH is more dramatic in females than in males, probably because the hypothalamic-pituitary unit is much more sensitive to the negative feedback effects of circulating androgens than to those of circulating estrogens.

FSH and LH in fetal blood are secreted by the fetal pituitary gland, apparently in response to GnRH released by the fetal hypothalamus. The fetal pituitary does respond to exogenous synthetic GnRH. Moreover, the hypothalamic-hypophyseal circulation and the hypothalamic nuclei exist in midgestation. The bell-shaped time course of gonadotropin secretion by the fetus (see Fig. 59-6) is thought to be due to the maturation of hypothalamic GnRH and pituitary FSH and LH secretory capacities (increased gonadotropins) before the hypothalamic-pituitary unit matures and is able to respond to the negative feedback effects of fetal and placental androgens and estrogens (decreased gonadotropins). Immediately after birth, neonatal gonadotropin concentrations rise temporarily because of the sudden absence of inhibitory placental sex steroids (see Fig. 59-7). FSH and LH are elevated in the plasma of male infants to levels that equal or exceed those seen during prepubertal development; elevated gonadotropin secretion is associated with elevated testosterone levels. Plasma LH levels in female infants resemble those in male infants, but plasma FSH levels remain elevated for several years, often in the range of those seen in castrated adult females. This sex-related difference is thought to indicate that the hypothalamic GnRH pulse generator in female infants operates at a slower frequency than that in the adult. Gonadotropin levels decline, and the hypothalamic-pituitary unit, though seemingly mature in both males and females, remains quiescent until the beginning of puberty.

Male

The testis grows very little during childhood. At the onset of puberty it begins to increase from a volume of approxi-

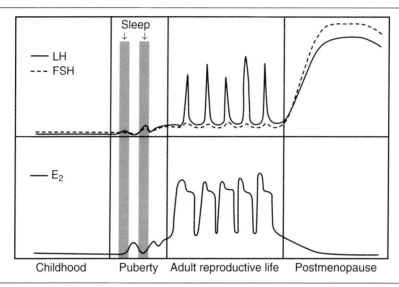

Fig. 59–7. Plasma levels of estradiol (E$_2$), luteinizing hormone (LH), and follicle-stimulating hormone (FSH) during postnatal life of the female.

Fig. 59-6. Plasma levels of testosterone, luteinizing hormone (LH), and follicle-stimulating hormone (FSH) during prenatal and postnatal development in the male.

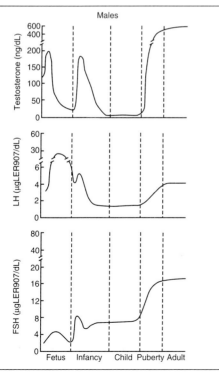

mately 2 ml to the adult volume of 12 to 25 ml. The Leydig cells, which synthesize and secrete testosterone, increase dramatically in number, with a consequential increase in the circulating testosterone levels. Daytime concentrations of testosterone in plasma increase from 0.2 ng/ml before puberty to approximately 6 ng/ml after puberty. The seminiferous tubules increase in diameter and in tortuosity, due to the differentiation of Sertoli cells and proliferation of spermatogonia. Pubertal changes in males include an increase in muscle mass, broadening of the shoulders, and thickening of the vocal cords, which results in the voice breaking.

Female

During childhood, the ovary increases linearly in size. Some follicles continue to grow, but all that do grow become atretic by the time the antrum develops. The growing follicles are capable of steroidogenesis since estradiol concentrations in ovarian venous blood are higher than those in the peripheral circulation. Between the ages of 8 and 10 years in girls, morning estradiol concentrations in serum begin to reach those seen in adult women during the follicular phase of the menstrual cycle; the secretion of androgens, such as **dehydroepiandrosterone,** by the adrenals and ovaries also increases. In this early pubertal period, labial hair appears due to increased androgen levels, and the breasts enlarge due to increased estrogen levels. In middle to late puberty, the pituitary acquires the ability to secrete a burst of gonadotropins in response to GnRH after exposure to elevated levels of estradiol. This ability of estrogen to amplify the pituitary responsiveness to GnRH, which occurs just before ovulation, is termed **positive feedback.** Development of this control mechanism is gradual. As positive feedback develops, the female begins to experience cyclic reproductive function, the menstrual cycle. The first menstrual period, menarche, usually takes place between the ages of 12 and 13, but the first ovulation generally does not occur until at least 6 months later. Regular ovulatory menstrual cycles commence up to several years later. During the transition period, the female experiences anovulatory cycles in which no ovum is released. Pubertal changes in the female include rapid growth of the pelvis and increased formation of fat over the shoulders, pelvis, buttocks, and thighs.

Summary

The reproductive system includes the gonads, the internal genitalia of the reproductive tract, the external genitalia, and the hypothalamic-pituitary unit. The development and differentiation of the male and female reproductive systems commences in utero. Phenotypic sex, or the sex of the internal and external genitalia, is determined by the sex of the gonad, which, in turn, is determined by the chromosomal sex or the complement of X and Y chromosomes. The reproductive tracts differentiate from a bipotential system consisting of two paired duct systems, the mullerian ducts and the wolffian ducts. Breast development prior to puberty is similar for males and females but diverges at puberty, when estrogens and progestins stimulate further development in females. Puberty, the period during which the sexually immature child is transformed into a sexually mature adolescent, results from the maturation of central neural positive and negative feedback mechanisms that regulate the hypothalamic secretion of GnRH, which, in turn, regulates secretion of the anterior pituitary hormones, FSH and LH.

Bibliography

Knobil, E., Neill, J. D., et al., eds. *The Physiology of Reproduction.* New York: Raven Press, 1988.

Sadler, T. W. *Langman's Medical Embryology.* Baltimore; Williams and Wilkins, 1985.

60 The Female Reproductive System

Andrew R. LaBarbera

Objectives

After reading this chapter, you should be able to

List the general functions of the female reproductive system in the nonpregnant state

List the components of the female reproductive system and their specific functions

Describe the hormonal control of the development of ovarian follicles, mature ova, and corpora lutea

Explain the synthesis, secretion, and effects of ovarian steroid hormones

Explain how positive feedback and negative feedback effects of steroids control gonadotropin secretion

Describe the physiologic basis of the menstrual cycle and the coordinated cyclic changes in the functions of the hypothalamus, pituitary, ovaries, and reproductive tract

Explain how sexual function facilitates transport of spermatozoa through the reproductive tract

Identify the cause and effects of menopause, the beginning of reproductive senescence

---

The reproductive system of the female functions to produce offspring. It produces germ cells for sexual reproduction; provides an environment for the transport of the male germ cells, the spermatozoa, to the fallopian tubes for fertilization; provides an appropriate environment for the development of the embryo; and produces milk for the nourishment of the young offspring. Although the reproductive organs are established during the embryonic and fetal periods, they do not reach full maturity until puberty. The active reproductive period begins with **menarche,** the first menstruation, at puberty and lasts until **menopause,** which is the cessation of reproductive function when the supply of ovarian follicles is exhausted.

Approximately once a month throughout the reproductive period of the female, the ovary cyclically produces a **follicle** containing a mature gamete, or ovum. The cycle, which is referred to as the **menstrual cycle,** is controlled by gonadotropic hormones secreted by the pituitary gland in response to the hypothalamic hormone gonadotropin-re-

leasing hormone (GnRH). Secretions of the hypothalamic-pituitary unit are modulated by both positive feedback and negative feedback signals from the ovaries. The components of the reproductive system undergo simultaneous cyclic changes, and each cycle begins with the shedding of the vascularized luminal epithelium of the uterus, called **menses.** The functions of the hypothalamus, pituitary, ovary, reproductive tract, and mammary glands in the nonpregnant and pregnant states are integrated and controlled by neural and hormonal signals. Female reproductive function during the pregnant and postpartum states is discussed in Chap. 62.

Ovary

The ovary serves four functions critical to reproduction: (1) the cyclic production of gametes, (2) secretion of hormones that prepare the reproductive tract to receive and nurture the conceptus and influence the development of secondary sexual characteristics, (3) secretion of hormones that participate in conditioning the mammary glands for lactation, and (4) feedback regulation of hypothalamic-pituitary secretion.

Follicle

The basic functional unit of the ovary is the **follicle,** which consists of an immature female gamete, the **oocyte,** surrounded by one or more layers of specialized follicular cells. These cells secrete autocrine, paracrine, and endocrine factors that modulate the functions of the oocyte and other cells within the follicle, affect the structure and function of the female accessory sex organs, and modulate the actions of the hypothalamic-pituitary unit. The structure of each follicle is related to its stage of development. Follicular growth and differentiation are mediated by the two anterior pituitary gonadotropins, **follicle-stimulating hormone** (FSH) and **luteinizing hormone** (LH), although FSH is capable of stimulating complete development of the follicles by itself. The ovary contains both nongrowing and growing follicles; the nongrowing follicles greatly outnumber the growing ones throughout most of the female life span.

The onset of puberty and the consequential increase in the secretion of GnRH by the hypothalamus and of FSH and LH by the pituitary mark the beginning of ongoing development beyond the primary stage. Follicles do not begin to progress to the preovulatory stage until several months after menarche, however. In each menstrual cycle, several follicles are recruited to develop into secondary follicles. Normally, only a single follicle in each cycle becomes dominant, completes the process of differentiation and maturation, and is then ovulated. The remainder undergo degeneration, called **atresia.**

Evidence from other species indicates that folliculogenesis, beginning with the recruitment of primordial follicles into the pool of developing follicles to formation of the dominant follicle, is a continuous process that appears to span three to four menstrual cycles. During the first cycle, follicles develop to the secondary preantral stage; during the second and third cycles, they become tertiary antral follicles; and during the third and fourth cycles, they become mature preovulatory follicles. Follicular development requires physiologically effective levels of gonadotropins, since development beyond the primordial follicle stage is rarely seen in hypogonadotropic hypogonadal women.

In the early reproductive years, most of the follicles in the ovary are nongrowing primordial follicles. Beginning

in fetal life and continuing throughout childhood, individual primordial follicles start to enlarge and develop by mitosis of the epithelial cells but then degenerate through atresia. This appears to be a random process. The oocyte is maintained in the arrested dictyotene stage of the first meiotic prophase by a putative oocyte maturation inhibitor, presumably secreted by the epithelial/granulosa cells. Recruitment and atresia of follicles continue throughout the reproductive life span so that the pool of available follicles continually decreases.

Early in the developmoent of a follicle, the oocyte and surrounding epithelial cells grow in tandem to become a primary follicle. A glycoproteinaceous material forms the **zona pellucida** around the oocyte. The epithelial cells acquire the cuboidal shape of granulosa cells, and the number of FSH receptors in the membranes of these cells increases, enabling them to respond to FSH.

Under the influence of FSH, granulosa cells continue to proliferate. The oocyte reaches its maximal size of 120 μm. When there are two to three layers of granulosa cells, mesenchymal cells migrate to the basal lamina and align themselves in parallel around the entire follicle to form the beginnings of the theca interna and theca externa. Capillary networks form around these theca cells. These are secondary follicles. The oocyte has the capacity to complete the first step of meiotic maturation, consisting of germinal vesicle breakdown and progression to metaphase I.

As the follicle enlarges, fluid accumulates among some of the granulosa cells, forming the **antrum,** which is a cavity filled with follicular fluid. At this stage, the follicle is a tertiary antral follicle. The number of granulosa cells increases a further 100-fold to 1000-fold. Theca cells have LH receptors, enabling them to repond to LH. LH induces synthesis of the **cholesterol side-chain cleavage 3β-hydroxysteroid dehydrogenase/Δ^{5-4}isomerase** and **17α-hydroxylase** enzyme complexes in theca cells, resulting in increased production of **androstenedione** and testosterone, the obligatory androgen precursors for estrogen biosynthesis. FSH acts on granulosa cells to induce synthesis of the **aromatase** enzyme complex, which converts androgens to estrogens, resulting in increased plasma concentrations of estrogen. The effects of FSH on granulosa cells are amplified by **insulin-like growth factor I** (IGF-I), a peptide that is produced in granulosa cells as well as other bodily tissues. Estrogen acts within the follicle to enhance the responsiveness of granulosa cells to FSH. It also progressively sensitizes the pituitary gland to GnRH, accounting for the positive feedback effect of estrogen on the hypothalamic-pituitary unit.

As the granulosa cells proliferate further under the influence of FSH and estradiol and the volume of follicular fluid increases, the follicle enlarges to become a preovulatory **graafian follicle.** The granulosa cells lining the follicle aromatize androgens synthesized in the theca to estrogens in increasing amounts. Consequently, plasma concentrations of estradiol continue to increase exponentially. FSH induces a 20-fold to 100-fold increase in LH receptors as well as an increase in LH-responsive adenylyl cyclase activity in the granulosa cells, thus preparing them to respond to the preovulatory surge of LH. The theca-interstitial cells in the theca interna continue to proliferate until there are approximately eight layers of theca-interstitial cells in a mature graafian follicle. As the follicle matures, these cells produce increasing amounts of androgen under the influence of LH. The oocyte of a mature graafian follicle has the capacity to proceed to metaphase II of meiosis and to complete meiotic maturation after fertilization. Normal oocyte maturation requires adequate levels of estradiol in the follicle. It appears that an increase in the ratio of androgen to estrogen and an increase in the ratio of LH to FSH are associated with the disorder **polycystic ovarian syndrome** (PCO). In this disorder, follicles become very large (cysts) but do not differentiate normally and do not produce normal ova.

Usually, only a single follicle survives to the graafian follicle stage in humans. Follicles require FSH to develop. As they develop, they secrete increasing amounts of the hormone **inhibin,** which partially suppresses FSH secretion by the pituitary, causing FSH levels in the blood to decline. Only the most mature follicle, the **dominant** one, is able to survive with the diminished FSH levels.

Follicular Fluid

The composition of the fluid in the follicular antrum changes as the follicle develops and the granulosa and theca cells mature. Initially, antral follicles contain a solution of proteoglycans, predominantly chondroitin sulfate, which is rapidly diluted by fluid derived from plasma. The osmolality and electrolyte composition of follicular fluid are nearly identical to those of plasma. The protein content ranges from 50% to 100% of that of serum. FSH and LH levels reflect those of serum. Steroid hormone and precursors levels are determined by the rates of synthesis and diffusion from the theca and granulosa cells as well as concentrations of steroid-binding proteins, which heighten steroid levels relative to plasma. Numerous enzymes have been detected in follicular fluid, including peptidases, phosphatases, nucleotidase, hyaluronidase, plasmin, and collagenase. **Plasmin** and **collagenase** are thought to be involved in weakening the follicle prior to rupture, or **ovulation.**

Corpus Luteum

The preovulatory surge in the plasma level of LH, which is initiated by GnRH after the pituitary gonadotropes have been sensitized to GnRH by high levels of estradiol, causes expulsion, called **ovulation,** of the cumulus-oocyte complex. Prior to ovulation, the granulosa and theca cells lining the follicle begin a process of cytodifferentiation, called **luteinization.** After ovulation, a fibrin clot fills the empty cavity of the follicle. This clot is gradually replaced by the luteinizing cells of the corpus luteum. An unidentified angiogenic factor appears to participate in the vascularization of the corpus luteum. Luteinization is maximal 5 to 6 days after ovulation, when the corpus luteum becomes maximally functional.

The primary function of the corpus luteum appears to be to secrete progesterone, which is necessary for preparing the uterine **endometrium** to accept the blastocyst for **implantation** and for maintaining the fetal-placental unit during early pregnancy. If fertilization of the ovum and implantation of the blastocyst do not occur, the corpus luteum degenerates through the process of **luteolysis,** which is evident histologically 8 days after ovulation. Progesterone production begins to decline around the tenth day after ovulation.

Low levels of LH are necessary for luteal function. Administration of LH during the luteal phase increases plasma progesterone levels and can prolong the life span of the corpus luteum for at least several days. Conversely, administration of antiserum to LH during the luteal phase can cause premature menstruation. The effects of LH on luteal cells are mediated by LH receptors coupled to adenylyl cyclase. Although both LH receptors and LH-responsive adenylyl cyclase activity decline after the LH surge through the processes of down-regulation and desensitization, respectively, they reappear during the early luteal phase and become maximal in the midluteal phase.

Regulation of the corpus luteum in humans is poorly understood. The human corpus luteum produces androstenedione and estradiol as well as progesterone and 17α-hydroxyprogesterone. LH can increase both progestin and estrogen production, but FSH, whose receptors are maximal in the early luteal phase, increases only estrogen production. Plasma estrogen levels and luteal aromatase activity both increase prior to luteolysis. Furthermore, exogenous estrogen inhibits luteal progesterone production. Although **prostaglandin $F_{2\alpha}$** (PGF$_{2\alpha}$) can cause luteal regression in primates, removal of the uterus, a principal source of PGF$_{2\alpha}$, has no effect on the lifespan of the corpus luteum in humans. Luteal cells contain receptors for **oxytocin,** a peptide of the posterior pituitary, but the role of oxytocin in regulating luteal function has not been established.

Secretory Products

The ovary produces several substances that regulate ovarian function itself, control the hypothalamic-pituitary secretion of gonadotropins, and condition the accessory reproductive organs for pregnancy. These include steroid hormones, inhibin, growth factors, prostaglandins, proteoglycans, and proteolytic enzymes.

Secretion of **steroid hormones** is a principal function of the follicle, interstitial cells, and corpus luteum of the ovary. The follicle produces progestins, androgens, and estrogens, whereas the corpus luteum produces mainly progestins and some estrogen. The steroid hormones are synthesized from **cholesterol** (Fig. 60-1), which is derived

Fig. 60-1. Sources of ovarian cellular cholesterol.

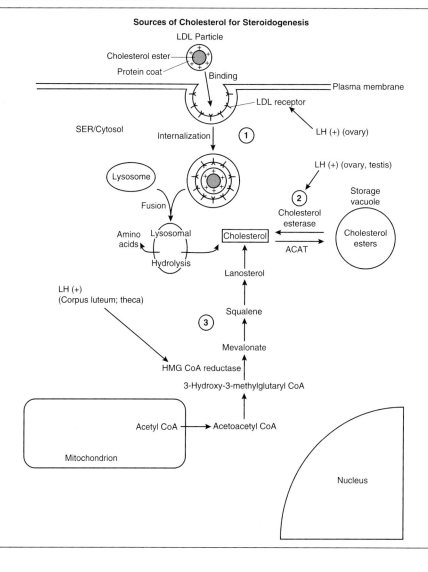

Sources of Cholesterol for Steroidogenesis

from three sources: (1) **circulating low-density** (LDL) and **high-density** (HDL) **lipoproteins,** (2) **preformed cholesterol** stored within the ovarian cell, and (3) de novo synthesis from acetate within the ovarian cell. In the avascular antral and preovulatory follicles, cholesterol is probably synthesized de novo, since the basement membrane of the follicle excludes cholesterol-carrying LDL from the granulosa cell layer. After vascularization associated with luteinization, luteal cells use circulating LDL as the primary source of cholesterol. LH increases the number of LDL receptors in luteal cell membranes, leading to increased uptake of cholesterol from the LDL. Cholesterol is stored in lipid droplets in ovarian cells as esters of long-chain fatty acids. Intracellular concentrations of free cholesterol are maintained by three enzymes that are regulated by hormones: (1) **cholesterol ester synthetase** (acyl coenzyme A:cholesterol–acyl transferase, or ACAT), which esterifies free cholesterol, (2) **cholesterol esterase** (sterol ester hydrolase), which catalyzes the release of cholesterol, and (3) **HMG CoA reductase** (3-hydroxy-3-methylglutaryl coenzyme A-reductase), which is the rate-limiting enzyme in cholesterol biosynthesis. LH increases luteal cell cholesterol concentrations by increasing both HMG CoA reductase and cholesterol esterase activities.

Progestin

Progesterone is a 21-carbon steroid that is the most potent of a class of steroids called **progestins.** It is synthesized to varying degrees in all steroid-producing tissues, but the principal secretory organs are the corpus luteum of the ovary and the placenta of pregnancy. Pregnenolone is the most important progestin as a precursor for other steroid hormones.

The biosynthesis of progesterone is outlined in Fig. 60-2 and can be summarized as follows: (1) Cholesterol is converted to pregnenolone in the mitochondria by the action of the C_{27} side-chain cleavage cytochrome P_{450} (20,22-hydroxylase/20,22-desmolase). This enzyme complex is usually referred to as **side-chain cleavage P_{450} or $P450_{scc}$.** In the ovary, it is induced in theca cells by LH and in granulosa cells by FSH and by LH. This enzyme is the rate-limiting step in steroid biosynthesis. (2) Pregnenolone diffuses to the smooth endoplasmic reticulum (SER), where it is converted to progesterone by the sequential actions of 3β-hydroxysteroid dehydrogenase and Δ^{5-4}isomerase. It is not clear whether these two activities are a single enzyme or distinct enzymes. However, they function together and are induced in theca cells by LH and in granulosa cells both by FSH and by LH.

In the female, progesterone is produced by both the

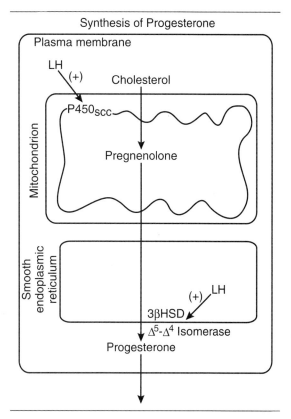

Fig. 60-2. Biosynthesis of progesterone.

adrenals and gonads. Production varies during the menstrual cycle, being approximately 10-fold greater in the luteal phase (10–40 mg/day) than in the follicular phase (1–3 mg/day). During the follicular phase, approximately 60% of plasma progesterone is synthesized in the adrenal cortex and approximately 40% in the ovary; during the luteal phase, greater than 90% is synthesized in the ovary (corpus luteum). Plasma progesterone levels are lowest in the follicular phase (0.05 µg/dl) and peak (0.5–2.5 µg/dl) in the midluteal phase.

Progesterone circulates in the blood bound primarily to **albumin** and secondarily to **corticosteroid-binding globulin** (CBG). Only a small fraction circulates free or unbound to plasma proteins, but this is the most important fraction because the free hormone is able to interact with target cells. The bound and free forms are in equilibrium. Progesterone in the plasma is metabolized and conjugated to yield a water-soluble product that is excreted in the urine with a plasma half-life of approximately 60 minutes. Approximately 10% of the total progesterone in the circulation is excreted as the conjugated metabolite **pregnane-diol glucuronide.**

Progesterone acts on the reproductive tract, the mammary glands of the breast, and the hypothalamic-pituitary unit and exhibits the following actions. During the luteal phase of the menstrual cycle, progesterone promotes active secretion by the mucosa of the fallopian tubes and by the glands of the uterine endometrium in preparation for possible implantation of a blastocyst. It also decreases the frequency of contractions of the uterine myometrium to minimize expulsion of the ovum. The prolonged elevated progesterone levels during pregnancy cause the smooth muscle of the uterine myometrium to relax and the uterus to expand. Progesterone also changes the secretory activity of the cervix, causing the cervical mucus to decrease in volume and become thicker in consistency. This thickening provides a barrier against the penetration by other spermatozoa. In the breast during pregnancy and postpartum lactation, progesterone synergizes with estrogen and the lactogenic hormones, **placental lactogen** and **prolactin,** to stimulate development of the lobuloalveolar system. Progesterone plays an important role in regulating FSH and LH secretion by the hypothalamic-pituitary unit. It decreases secretion of the gonadotropins, primarily by decreasing the frequency of hypothalamic GnRH pulses.

The effects of progesterone are mediated by specific high-affinity intracellular receptors located at the nuclear membrane of the cell. Receptor binding makes the receptor capable of binding to nuclear acceptor sites associated with DNA and nuclear proteins. Binding of progesterone-receptor complexes to DNA heightens the synthesis of the messenger RNAs (mRNAs), which direct the numerous biosynthetic processes.

Estrogen

Estradiol-17β is an 18-carbon steroid that can be distinguished from the other types of steroids by the presence of the aromatic A ring. On the basis of quantity and potency, estradiol is the most important of the class of compounds called **estrogens.** Estradiol is approximately 10 times as potent as estrone. The aromatic ring by itself is not necessary for activity, since the synthetic estrogen diethylstilbestrol (DES) has no aromatic rings. Estradiol is synthesized and secreted primarily by the ovarian follicle and corpus luteum.

The two-cell theory of the follicular biosynthesis of estradiol is outlined in Fig. 60-3 and can be summarized as follows: (1) Cholesterol is converted to pregnenolone in the mitochondria of the theca cell by the action of side-chain cleavage cytochrome P_{450}. (2) Pregnenolone diffuses

to the SER, where it is converted to 17α-hydroxypregnenolone by the action of 17α-hydroxylase cytochrome P_{450} (P450$_{C17}$). (3) 17α-Hydroxypregnenolone is converted to dehydroepiandrosterone (DHEA) by the 17,20-desmolase activity of the P450$_{C17}$ in the SER. (4) DHEA is converted to Δ^4-androstenedione by the sequential actions of 3β-hydroxysteroid dehydrogenase and Δ^{5-4}isomerase in the SER. (5) Δ^4-androstenedione diffuses out of the theca cell, across the basement membrane, and into the granulosa cell, where it is converted to estrone by the action of aromatase cytochrome P_{450} (reversible) in the SER. (6) Estrone is converted to 17β-estradiol by 17β-hydroxysteroid dehydrogenase or 17-ketosteroid reductase in the SER. LH increases expression of cholesterol side-chain cleavages 3β-hydroxysteroid dehydrogenase and 17α-hydroxylase in theca and luteal cells; FSH increases expression of aromatase enzyme in granulosa cells.

Estrogens are produced at different rates during the menstrual cycle. As ovarian follicles grow in the early follicular phase of the menstrual cycle, estrone and estradiol are secreted in nearly equal amounts, 60 to 170 μg/day. As the **dominant follicle** enlarges in the latter half of the follicular phase, secretion of estradiol increases to 400 to 800 μg/day, resulting in plasma estradiol concentrations of 25 to 40 ng/dl. The corpus luteum secretes about 250 μg of estradiol per day, which is approximately four times the secretion of estrone. Only 2% to 3% of circulating estradiol is free, that is, not bound to plasma-binding proteins. Approximately 38% is bound to testosterone estradiol–binding globulin (TeBG), a beta-globulin produced in the liver with a higher affinity for testosterone than for estradiol. The remaining 60% of circulating estradiol is bound to albumin.

Numerous metabolites of estrogens are excreted in both the urine and bile. The **liver** plays a major role in the metabolism and excretion of estrogens. Most of the metabolites of estrogens are sulfated, conjugated, or both to glucosiduronic acid in the liver. The two major metabolites of both estradiol and estrone are **estrone glucuronide** and free unconjugated estriol, but catechol estrogens are also excreted in the urine. Physiologically, estradiol is more than 10 times as potent as estrone and more than 80 times as potent as estriol. The metabolic clearance rates of estradiol and estrone are 1350 and 2210 liters/day, respectively. The half-life in the plasma is less than 20 minutes.

Estrogen has numerous and diverse effects on the organs and tissues of the reproductive system (Table 60-1). These effects are observed during the follicular phase of each menstrual cycle and are reversed during the luteal phase. Estrogen stimulates cellular proliferation and growth of

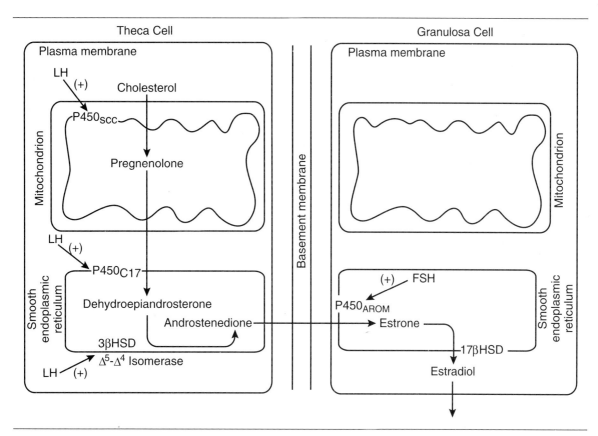

Fig. 60-3. Biosynthesis of androstenedione and estradiol in the follicle.

tissues of the reproductive tract. At puberty, estrogen causes an increase in size of the fallopian tubes, uterus, vagina, and external genitalia; conversely, estrogen deprivation results in atrophy of these organs. In the fallopian tubes, estrogen increases proliferation of cells of the mucosal lining, including the ciliated epithelial cells, which promote movement of the ovum toward the uterus. The endometrium of the uterus is profoundly affected by estrogens, which cause thickening due to proliferation of the stromal cells, endometrial glands, and blood vessels. Estrogens also increase the number of progesterone receptors in endometrial cells; endometrial sensitivity to progesterone requires prior exposure to estrogen. The lining of the cervix produces copious amounts of a thin, watery mucus after exposure to estrogen, and the cells lining the vagina proliferate, transform from cuboidal to stratified, and become more secretory.

Animal studies suggest that within the ovary, estrogen enhances its own production and amplifies the effects of

FSH on granulosa cell function and follicular development. It is not clear whether this is true in humans. Estrogen synthesized in the granulosa cells can inhibit synthesis of androgen in the theca cells, thereby coordinating production of substrate and product. In the breasts, estrogen causes deposition of fat and growth of stromal tissues and ducts. Estrogen is responsible for breast enlargement but not for milk production.

Estrogens cause deposition of fat in subcutaneous tissues other than those of the breast. This effect, which is most pronounced in the buttocks and thighs, results in a lower specific gravity of the female body than the male body. Estrogens have dual effects on the skeleton. They augment osteoblastic activity, leading to rapid growth at puberty, but they also cause closure of the epiphyseal plates, which prevents further growth of the long bones. Estrogen receptors have been identified in osteoblastic cells.

Ovarian function is regulated indirectly by estrogens by

Table 60-1. Actions of Estradiol

AT PUBERTY
1. Cause enlargement of the fallopian tubes, uterus, vagina, and external genitalia to adult size (deprivation leads to atrophy)
2. Increase growth of the mammary ducts
3. Increase growth and closure of the epiphyses by increasing osteoblastic activity
4. Increase fat deposition in the buttocks and thighs

DURING ADULTHOOD
1. Increase general protein anabolism (to a lesser degree than androgens)
2. Increase synthesis of plasma proteins, e.g., TeBG, in the liver
3. Moderately increase retention of Na^+, Cl^-, and water in the kidney

DURING THE FOLLICULAR PHASE OF THE MENSTRUAL CYCLE
1. Increase growth of ovarian follicles by amplifying the effects of FSH
2. Increase growth and cellular proliferation of the uterine endometrium (increase protein synthesis, proliferation of glands, blood supply)
3. Increase contractility of the uterine myometrium and fallopian tubes due to increase in contractile proteins
4. Increase progesterone receptors in the endometrium
5. Increase quantity and decrease viscosity of cervical mucus (thin, watery)
6. Increase thickening (cornification) of the vaginal epithelial mucosa

AT PARTURITION
1. Increase growth and differentiation of stromal tissues and mammary ducts (breast enlargement but not milk production)
2. Increase sensitivity of the myometrium to oxytocin to promote contractility

ON THE HYPOTHALAMIC-PITUITARY UNIT
1. Increase GnRH receptors in gonadotropes
2. Increase pituitary content of FSH, LH, and prolactin
3. Decrease GnRH pulse amplitude

means of their positive feedback and negative feedback effects on the hypothalamic-pituitary unit. Estrogen suppresses the pituitary secretion of FSH and LH by the hypothalamic-pituitary unit, and the gonadotropins are maintained at a relatively low level by this negative feedback effect. Decreased plasma estradiol levels, such as occur after menopause or removal of the ovaries, result in greatly elevated plasma gonadotropin levels. The mechanism of this negative feedback effect of estrogen on the hypothalamic-pituitary unit has not been established definitively. However, it is thought that estrogen decreases the amplitude of GnRH pulses, since estrogen decreases the amplitude of pituitary LH pulses. Paradoxically, rising estrogen levels also cause the surge of LH and FSH in the late follicular phase prior to ovulation. As the dominant follicle grows and secretes increasing amounts of estrogen, plasma levels of estrogen rise. Elevated estrogen concentrations progressively sensitize the pituitary gland itself to the relatively constant pulsatile hypothalamic GnRH secretion, culminating in the preovulatory LH surge. This positive feedback effect of estrogen is due both to increased pituitary receptors for GnRH and to increased contents of FSH and LH in the gonadotropes. The paradoxical

positive feedback and negative feedback effects of estrogens are related to the plasma levels and the duration of exposure to these steroids.

Estradiol, like progesterone, binds to specific high-affinity receptor proteins that are only loosely associated with the nucleus of the target cell. Binding of estradiol to its receptor transforms the estradiol-receptor complex to a form that binds tightly to nucleoprotein acceptor sites associated with DNA. Estradiol thus regulates gene transcription leading to the synthesis of mRNAs, which direct the formation of specific proteins responsible for estrogenic effects.

Androgen

Androgens are 19-carbon steroids that are synthesized in both the ovaries and adrenals of females. Ovarian androgens are important in females as substrates for estrogen biosynthesis in granulosa cells. Adrenal androgens are important for the development of female axillary and pubic hair that occurs at adrenarche, which is maturation of adrenal function at puberty. Androstenedione and testosterone, which are secreted by theca and interstitial cells, are the most important ovarian androgens. Androstenedione production in adult females averages 3 mg/day. Only approximately half the circulating androstenedione is produced by the ovary; most of the remainder is produced by the adrenal cortex. Concentrations of androstenedione in follicular fluid are 100 to 500 times greater than those in plasma and reach a maximum of approximately 74 μg/dl during the midfollicular phase, after which they decline. The androstenedione concentration in plasma is between 40 and 240 ng/dl, with higher concentrations during the luteal phase than during the follicular phase.

In the human ovary, the preferred pathway for androgen biosynthesis is from pregnenolone to dehydroepiandrosterone, which is converted to androstenedione. In premenopausal females, androstenedione production (3 mg/day) predominates over testosterone production (300 μg/day); in postmenopausal females, more testosterone than androstenedione is produced. Androstenedione and testosterone are metabolized to 17-ketosteroids and excreted in the urine as conjugated steroid glucuronosides. Androstenedione functions primarily as the substrate for estrogen biosynthesis in the granulosa cells. However, the mechanism by which it traverses the basement membrane to the granulosa cells has not been established. Androgens also appear to modulate steroidogenesis in the human ovary. Androstenedione and testosterone can both inhibit progesterone biosynthesis in the granulosa cells. Furthermore, atretic follicles have higher levels of androgens in the follicular fluid than do normally developing follicles.

Inhibin

Inhibin is a glycoprotein with an apparent molecular weight of 32,000 and consists of two dissimilar subunits that are covalently linked by disulfide bonds. The larger α subunit has an apparent molecular weight of 20,000. The smaller β subunit, which has an apparent molecular weight of 13,000, exists in two forms, β_A and β_B. Both $\alpha\beta_A$, known as **inhibin A,** and $\alpha\beta_B$, known as **inhibin B,** are synthesized in ovarian granulosa cells. Both FSH and testosterone stimulate granulosa cells to synthesize and secrete inhibin. In males, inhibin is produced by Sertoli cells in the testis. The initial half-life of inhibin in the circulation is approximately 15 minutes. Two β (A or B) subunits can combine to form the molecule **activin,** which amplifies the effects of FSH in the follicle and enhances FSH secretion in the pituitary. Its physiologic significance has not been established.

Inhibin preferentially suppresses the synthesis and secretion of FSH by gonadotropes in the anterior pituitary. Circulating FSH levels are inversely related to circulating inhibin levels. Inhibin production, which is low at the beginning of the menstrual cycle, increases late in the follicular phase, reaches a peak prior to the midcycle surge of LH and FSH, decreases slightly, and then increases further in the midluteal phase to levels approximately twice the levels at midcycle. As the corpus luteum declines late in the luteal phase, inhibin levels decrease and FSH levels increase at the same time as the onset of the next menstrual cycle.

Neuroendocrine Regulation of the Ovaries

Regulation of ovarian function occurs through the secretion of two gonadotropic hormones synthesized in the anterior pituitary gland in response to hypothalamic stimulation (Fig. 60-4). The structurally similar glycoproteins FSH and LH are the most important reproductive peptide hormones produced by the anterior pituitary in the nonpregnant state. Synthesis and secretion of FSH and LH are regulated by hypothalamic and ovarian hormones. Prolactin, which is also produced in the anterior pituitary, and oxytocin, which is secreted by the posterior pituitary, are important during and after pregnancy and are discussed in Chap. 62.

Follicle-Stimulating Hormone

FSH is a heterodimeric protein with a molecular weight of 32,600. It consists of two dissimilar subunits strongly associated by noncovalent interactions. The α subunit is identical to the α subunit of LH, thyrotropin (TSH), and human chorionic gonadotropin (hCG) and confers species specificity on the hormone. The β subunit confers hormonal specificity on FSH. Each subunit has two N-linked branched oligosaccharide moieties that are involved in the receptor-mediated activation of adenylyl cyclase. These carbohydrate side chains of FSH have terminal sialic acid (N-acetylneuraminic acid) residues that prolong the half-life of the gonadotropin in the circulation.

Specialized cells, **gonadotropes,** in the anterior pituitary gland synthesize, store, and secrete both FSH and LH. The peptides are synthesized in the endoplasmic reticulum and glycosylated in the Golgi apparatus. Synthesis of FSH is regulated primarily by GnRH and inhibin. GnRH has a permissive effect on the synthesis of the β subunit of FSH. Synthesis of the β subunit is rate-limiting for the production of FSH, whereas synthesis of the α subunit occurs at a relatively constant rate. GnRH also stimulates secretion of mature, fully glycosylated FSH from secretory

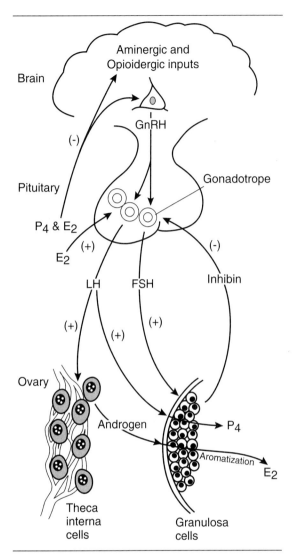

Fig. 60-4. Neuroendocrine control of ovarian function.

granules. Inhibin, whose secretion varies during the menstrual cycle, opposes the effects of GnRH; it inhibits both the synthesis and release of FSH.

Circulating levels of FSH reflect a steady-state determined by rates of secretion and disappearance. FSH is secreted by the pituitary in a pulsatile manner in response to pulses of GnRH, though discrete pulses of FSH in the circulation are difficult to discern because of the relatively long half-life of FSH in the circulation. The initial half-life of FSH is between 3 and 4 hours. Both the liver and kidney are important in the clearance and excretion of FSH. FSH

in the pituitary is turned over once per day, and this accounts for the amount secreted and metabolized. Both FSH synthesis and secretion are inhibited by a direct action of inhibin on pituitary gonadotropes.

The effects of FSH on follicular granulosa cells are mediated by membrane-bound receptors that are coupled functionally to the membrane-bound adenylyl cyclase enzyme system. Activation of the cyclase in response to stimulation by FSH involves the interaction of the FSH-receptor complex with a stimulatory guanine nucleotide regulatory protein (G_S) that must bind both magnesium and guanosine triphosphate in order to be activated. Cyclic AMP (cAMP), which is generated from ATP by the action of cyclase, activates one or more cAMP-dependent protein kinases, which catalyze the phosphorylation of proteins. Theoretically, FSH could exert its effects by regulating either the enzyme activities or substrate levels.

FSH stimulates numerous processes associated with differentiation in the granulosa cells, leading to growth and development of the ovarian follicles. These include increased lactic acid production; induction of aromatase, the enzyme complex that catalyzes conversion of androgens to estrogens; induction of the cholesterol side-chain cleavage enzyme, which is rate-limiting in the synthesis of pregnenolone, a precursor of progesterone; induction of LH receptors; induction of LH-sensitive adenylyl cyclase; increased activity of plasminogen activator; enhanced synthesis of proteoglycans; and increased synthesis of inhibin.

Luteinizing Hormone

Structurally, LH is very similar to FSH. It is a heterodimeric protein with a molecular weight of 29,400 and consists of two dissimilar, noncovalently associated subunits. The α subunit, which is identical to that of FSH, confers species specificity on the hormone. The β subunit confers hormonal specificity on LH. LHβ has a single N-linked, branched oligosaccharide moiety and less than half the sialic acid content of FSH, so the half-life of LH in the circulation is much shorter than that of FSH.

LH is synthesized, stored, and secreted by the same gonadotropes of the anterior pituitary gland that produce FSH, though some gonadotropes may produce only LH or only FSH. Synthesis, glycosylation, cisternal packaging, and storage of LH resemble those for FSH, except that the terminal sialic acid–galactose disaccharide of FSHβ is replaced by sulfated N-acetyl-D-galactosamine in LHβ. Synthesis of LH is regulated primarily by GnRH and estrogens. GnRH increases the number of translatable mRNAs for the β subunit so that synthesis of the β subunit, which is rate-limiting for production of the hormone, is enhanced. GnRH also stimulates secretion of mature, fully glycosylated LH from secretory granules. Estrogens increase the pituitary content of LH and potentiate gonadotrope responsiveness to GnRH. The effect of the rising plasma estrogen concentrations on the pituitary response to GnRH in the late follicular phase of the menstrual cycle accounts for the dramatic increase in LH secretion prior to ovulation, referred to as the **midcycle LH surge.** LH is secreted in a pulsatile manner in response to pulses of GnRH. Progesterone indirectly inhibits secretion of LH by decreasing the GnRH pulse frequency. This effect is evident during the luteal phase of the menstrual cycle (Fig. 60-5).

The **liver** and the **kidney** are involved in the clearance and excretion of LH. Because LH contains less sialic acid than FSH, LH is cleared from the circulation more rapidly than FSH. The initial half-life of LH is approximately 20 minutes. The rapid clearance of LH from the circulation contributes to the pronounced pulsatile nature of plasma concentrations of the hormone.

The effects of LH on follicular granulosa cells, theca cells, and interstitial cells are mediated by membrane-bound receptors that are coupled functionally to cAMP-dependent protein kinase by the intracellular mediator cAMP, which is produced through activation of the membrane-bound adenylyl cyclase enzyme system. As with other cyclase systems, the LH-responsive production of cAMP is modulated by magnesium and guanosine triphosphate by means of a guanine nucleotide regulatory (G_S) protein.

LH is a major regulator of steroid biosynthesis in the ovary. It stimulates androgen production in the theca and interstitial cells throughout follicular development, as well as estradiol and progesterone production in mature, differentiated granulosa cells of preovulatory follicles and the corpus luteum. LH regulates the availability of steroidogenic substrates by enhancing the mobilization, transport, and metabolism of cholesterol. LH increases the activity of the cholesterol ester hydrolase, an enzyme which deesterifies cholesterol and provides free cholesterol for steroidogenesis. In addition, LH increases the side-chain cleavage P_{450}, 17α-hydroxylase P_{450}, and 3β-hydroxysteroid dehydrogenase enzymes.

Gonadotropin-Releasing Hormone

Secretion of FSH and LH by the gonadotropes of the anterior pituitary gland is controlled by neurons with cell bodies in the **mediobasal hypothalamus** (MBH), particularly the **arcuate nucleus–median eminence** region. These neurons secrete GnRH into the extracellular space. The hormone diffuses into the **hypothalamic-hypophysial portal vessels,** which carry it to the anterior pituitary gland. Either surgical separation of the MBH from the remainder of the CNS or ablation of the arcuate nucleus causes an abrupt decline in circulating levels of both FSH and LH.

GnRH, which is sometimes referred to as **LH-releasing hormone,** is a decapeptide (10 amino acids) with a molecular weight of 1182 that stimulates both the synthesis and release of FSH and LH by gonadotropes of the anterior pituitary. It is synthesized in neurons that form loose net-

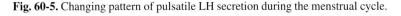

Fig. 60-5. Changing pattern of pulsatile LH secretion during the menstrual cycle.

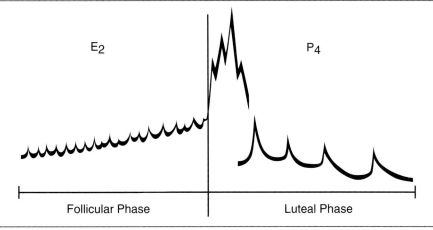

E₂   P₄

Follicular Phase   Luteal Phase

works, rather than distinct nuclear clusters, in the MBH, which contains the arcuate nucleus and the periventricular structures adjacent to it. Release of GnRH from nerve endings in the median eminence and diffusion into the portal circulation are pulsatile; secretion of pituitary gonadotropins is correspondingly pulsatile. The initiation of each LH pulse is synchronous with a marked increase in multiunit activity, the pulse generator, in the MBH. The relationship between the vollies of electrical activity and the initiation of LH pulses is absolute. The GnRH pulse generator, which has not been identified, can be suppressed by alpha-adrenergic and antidopaminergic blocking agents, as well as by morphine and the endogenous opiate beta-endorphin. Inhibition of LH secretion by beta-endorphin can be reversed by administration of the opiate antagonist naloxone. Opioid peptides appear to mediate stress-induced inhibition of reproductive function. GnRH pulse frequency, as indicated by the frequency of LH pulses in peripheral plasma, is more rapid in the estrogen-dominated follicular phase of the menstrual cycle than in the progesterone-dominated luteal phase. It is thought that estrogen exerts its negative feedback effect on gonadotropin secretion by decreasing the amplitude of GnRH pulses. Progesterone is thought to exert its negative feedback effect by decreasing the frequency of GnRH pulses. In the absence of the ovaries, artificial reduction of the GnRH pulse frequency below the physiologic rate leads to increased plasma FSH and decreased plasma LH levels, probably because the gonadotropin pulses are larger when the GnRH stimulation occurs more slowly.

Menstrual Cycle

During the reproductive life span of the adult female, between menarche and menopause, the reproductive system cyclically undergoes a series of structural and functional changes that result in gamete production and preparation of the reproductive tract for implantation of a fertilized zygote, should fertilization occur. This recurring menstrual cycle usually lasts 28 to 32 days. By convention, timing of the cycle begins either with menses or with the ovulatory surge of LH (Fig. 60-6). During the menstrual cycle, a single ovarian follicle develops to maturity, ovulates, and then luteinizes to form a corpus luteum. The cells of the follicle and the corpus luteum secrete different amounts of the steroid hormones estradiol and progesterone, which produce characteristic changes in the reproductive tract. The absence of cyclic reproduction function coupled with failure to menstruate is called **amenorrhea.**

Follicular Phase

The follicular phase, which begins with the onset of menstrual bleeding, is signaled when a single ovarian follicle becomes dominant and matures and the cells of the uterine endometrium rapidly proliferate. It is also referred to as the **preovulatory** or **proliferative phase.** At the beginning of this phase, estradiol and inhibin production is low. The GnRH pulse generator produces a pulse of GnRH approximately once every 90 minutes. Pituitary gonadotropes respond to each pulse of GnRH by releasing a pulse of either LH, FSH, or both. The plasma FSH level begins to rise late in the luteal phase of the previous menstrual cycle and continues into the early follicular phase, due to a decline in inhibin secretion. Plasma LH levels are low during the early follicular phase. LH and FSH are carried by the circulation to the ovary where (1) LH stimulates the theca-interstitial cells to differentiate and produce increased androgen and (2) FSH stimulates the granulosa cells to proliferate and then differentiate.

As multiple follicles enlarge and the granulosa cells differentiate under the influence of FSH and estrogen, increasing amounts of thecal androgen are aromatized to estrogen, causing plasma levels of estradiol to rise. The estrogen has a negative feedback effect on the hypothalamus, thereby modulating the amplitude rather than the frequency of LH and FSH pulses. FSH secretion is also negatively modulated by inhibin. However, inhibin levels do not rise until the late follicular phase. Thus the midfollicular phase decline in FSH secretion primarily may reflect the negative feedback effect of estrogen. Alternatively, the pituitary may become progressively sensitized to inhibin. Estrogen acts within a follicle to sensitize granulosa cells to FSH so that a follicle producing large quantities of estrogen can continue to develop despite declining plasma FSH levels. In this way, the most mature follicle appears to become the dominant follicle. As the follicle grows and matures, plasma estrogen concentrations increase exponentially with time. In the late follicular phase, plasma levels of androgens and the progestin 17α-hydroxyprogesterone increase. The uterine endometrium increases in size and vascularity, and the pituitary gland gradually becomes sensitized to estrogen. After plasma estradiol concentrations have exceeded 150 to 200 pg/ml for approximately 36 hours, the negative feedback effect of estrogen is reversed, and the pituitary secretes a surge of LH and FSH. This preovulatory surge of gonadotropins appears to be due to the direct effects of estrogen on pituitary gonadotropes rather than to a change in the GnRH pulse frequency or amplitude.

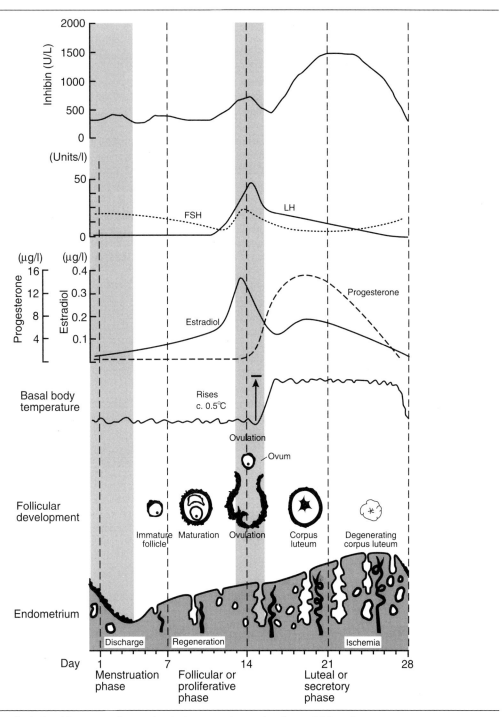

Fig. 60-6. Temporal relationship among changes in pituitary, ovarian, and endometrial function throughout the menstrual cycle. The beginning of menses is considered day 0.

Ovulation

The preovulatory surge of LH in plasma, which lasts approximately 48 hours from onset to the return of presurge levels, induces several profound, cAMP-mediated changes in the graafian follicle. Maturation of the oocyte resumes so that by the time the ovulated oocyte reaches the fallopian tube, meiosis will have reached the stage of extruding the first polar body. As the granulosa and theca cells begin to luteinize in response to LH-induced increases in the intracellular cAMP content, they secrete increased amounts of estradiol and progesterone. As a result, plasma concentrations of estradiol rise sharply, and plasma progesterone levels continue to increase. The follicular cells also secrete **plasminogen activator,** which increases the activity of the proteolytic enzyme **collagenase** in the follicular fluid. Collagenase digests collagen fibers in the follicular wall, which increases distensibility. In response to LH, secretion of prostaglandins PGE_2 and $PGF_{2\alpha}$ by granulosa and theca cells is augmented. PGE_2 enhances plasminogen activator production. Histamine (from mast cells), norepinephrine (from noradrenergic neurons in the follicular wall), and $PGF_{2\alpha}$ appear to facilitate rupture of the follicle by increasing vascular permeability, hyperemia, and consequently, intrafollicular pressure. The combined effect of decreased tensile strength of the follicular wall and an intrafollicular pressure of 15 to 20 mmHg triggers follicular rupture, with expulsion of the cumulus-oocyte complex. Ovulation occurs 1 to 2 hours before the plasma progesterone levels peak or 34 to 35 hours after the onset of the LH surge.

Luteal Phase

After ovulation, a fibrin clot forms in the cavity of the ruptured follicle. The granulosa and theca cells lining the wall of the follicle continue to luteinize, and as the corpus luteum forms, plasma progesterone and estradiol concentrations continue to rise. The life span of the corpus luteum determines the length of the luteal phase of the menstrual cycle. The luteal phase is more constant than the follicular phase and usually lasts approximately 14 days. Progesterone decreases the frequency of GnRH pulses so that the frequency of LH pulses decreases, but the concomitant increase in LH pulse amplitude causes little change in the mean plasma concentrations of LH. Continued secretion of progesterone, which prevents maturation of follicles, requires LH.

The excitability of the uterine myometrium decreases, and the secretory activity of the endometrium increases, both in response to progesterone. This altered intrauterine environment facilitates implantation of the blastocyst.

Menses

If the cycle is nonfertile and pregnancy does not ensue, the corpus luteum ceases to function, degenerates, and involutes in a process of luteolysis. This process usually begins 14 to 15 days after ovulation. Progesterone levels decline to levels seen during the follicular phase of the cycle. Three days following the initiation of luteolysis, the endometrial lining of the uterus is shed in menstruation. Approximately 1 day before menstruation, plasma FSH levels rise and folliculogenesis resumes. Menses, which consists of endometrial vasospasm and ischemic necrosis culminating in desquamation and bleeding, usually lasts 1 to 4 days. Approximately 35 ml each of blood and serous fluid are usually lost.

Reproductive Tract

The reproductive tract, which is the duct system consisting of fallopian tubes, uterus, cervix, and vagina, facilitates (1) reception and transport of the spermatozoa, (2) reception and transport of an ovum, (3) fertilization of the ovum by a single spermatozoan, (3) embryogenesis and fetal development, and (4) delivery of an infant. The components of the reproductive tract cyclically undergo a series of dramatic structural and functional changes. During the proliferative follicular phase of the cycle, the reproductive tract is dominated by estrogen; during the secretory luteal phase, by progestin.

Fallopian Tubes

The fallopian tube serves as a conduit for the ovulated ovum and the spermatozoa and as a source of nutrients for the gametes and early pre-embryo. It is the normal site of fertilization. The ciliated cells at the open fimbriated end (ostium) of the oviduct direct the ovum into the infundibulum and down through the ampulla toward the isthmus. Estrogens promote growth, proliferation, and ciliogenesis in the epithelium of the fallopian tubes during the follicular phase of the menstrual cycle. In addition, estrogens increase the number of progesterone receptors. Estrogen and progestin together condition the cells of the muscular layers to contract in a coordinated manner to promote transport of the ovum to the uterus.

The composition of **oviductal fluid** is regulated by the secretory epithelial cells, which secrete fluid against a pressure gradient. Sodium is the principal cation and chloride the principal anion, and the concentrations of both are higher than those in plasma. In addition, oviductal fluid is enriched in potassium so that the ratio of potassium to sodium is higher than that in plasma. Electrolyte concentrations fluctuate during the menstrual cycle, with the sodium and chloride concentrations decreasing when the estrogen content is lowest. The protein concentration is highest in the immediate postovulatory period. For metabolism, human oviductal epithelial cells utilize the glycolytic pathway and produce lactic acid, which is present at concentrations of 1.0 to 8.4 g/dl, compared with concentrations of only 1.6 to 3.6 mg/dl for glucose. Bicarbonate ion, which stimulates oxygen uptake by the spermatozoa, has concentrations of 110 to 220 mg/dl. Both lactic acid and bicarbonate are important for the cleavage of zygotes in the fallopian tubes.

Uterus

Endometrium

The endometrium plays a major role in prepregnancy reproductive function. Its secretions affect the spermatozoa en route through the uterine cavity to the oviducts and provide nutrients to the zygote during the days prior to implantation. The endometrium must be appropriately conditioned and highly vascularized in order for implantation to occur. The endometrial layer of the uterus contains secretory glands, stromal tissue, blood vessels, and an epithelium that covers the luminal surface.

The endometrium undergoes a characteristic sequence of changes in response to ovarian steroid hormones during each menstrual cycle. Optimal growth and maturation of the endometrium require sequential exposure to these ovarian hormones in definite ratios. During the proliferative phase, when plasma estrogen levels are increasing, the thickness of the endometrium increases to 3 to 5 mm because of the proliferation of glandular and superficial epithelium, stroma, and blood vessels. The stroma becomes edematous, and the glands become very tortuous. During the secretory phase after ovulation, when both progesterone and estrogen are secreted by the corpus luteum, the thickness of the endometrium increases to 4 to 6 mm. Glycogen-containing vacuoles appear at the base of the glandular epithelial cells, and lipid and glycogen accumulate in the stromal cells. The glandular cells secrete fluid into the glandular lumina. The stroma becomes loose and more edematous, facilitating implantation of the blastocyst. In the latter part of the secretory phase, lymphocytes invade the stroma. If implantation does not occur, levels of ovarian hormones drop precipitously, polymorphonuclear leukocytes migrate into the stroma, and the secretory phase is followed by desquamation of the endometrium

and menses, the genital bleeding due to sloughing of the endometrial lining of the uterus. Only a thin layer of endometrial stroma remains after menstruation. New epithelial cells appear on the luminal surface of the endometrium within 3 to 7 days after the beginning of menstruation, and the proliferative phase ensues. If implantation does occur, the endometrium gives rise to the decidua (see Chap. 63).

Myometrium

Contractions of myometrial smooth muscle fibers are crucial in the expulsion of the fetus at parturition. It is important that the uterus not contract prematurely during either the preimplantation or postimplantation phases of pregnancy. Progesterone directly influences myometrial contractility. It increases the membrane potential and the liminal stimulus required to elicit contractions of the myometrial smooth muscle. Thus, during the secretory phase of the menstrual cycle when implantation would occur, the myometrium is quiescent. If implantation takes place and pregnancy ensues, the high plasma levels of progesterone maintain the myometrium in a quiescent state so that the developing embryo and fetus are not expelled. After the thirty-eighth week of pregnancy, progesterone levels fall and the electrical activity of the myometrium increases.

Cervix

The cervix consists of an endocervical canal that communicates with the uterus via the internal os and with the vagina via the external os. The epithelium of the endocervical canal consists of tall, secretory columnar cells that respond to estrogens by increasing in height and by accumulating columns of cervical mucus at their apical end. After ovulation, a portion of the endocervical cell is sloughed off.

The mucus secreted by the endocervical cell is rich in glycogen, glycoproteins, and glycosaminoglycans. Both before and after ovulation, the cervical mucus is highly viscous and sparse. Around the time of ovulation, however, the mucus becomes thin and increases sevenfold to facilitate the rapid transport of sperm to the fallopian tubes.

Vagina

The vagina is the outermost section of the female reproductive tract. The cells of the vaginal mucosa proliferate from mitoses in the cells of the basal layer. Estrogens, androgens, and progestins enhance this thickening of the vaginal epithelium, although estradiol is the most potent steroid. The cells transform from cuboidal to stratified, making the lining of the vagina much more resistant to infection and trauma than that of a non-estrogen-primed epithelium. Progestins also bring about desquamation of the superficial layers of epithelial cells.

Sexual Function

Female sexual function promotes the reception and transport of spermatozoa in the female reproductive tract. The physiologic processes of the female sexual act are influenced both by psychic factors that are not well understood but are responsible for the sex drive and by reflexes that involve the local stimulation of components of the reproductive organs. Neuronal signals triggered by local stimulation, such as massage or irritation, of the perineal region, the genitalia, and the urinary tract are transmitted via the pudendal nerve and sacral plexus to the brain. The clitoris is especially sensitive to physical stimulation.

The female sexual response consists of two physiologic reflexes: (1) the **vasocongestive reflex** and (2) the **orgasmic reflex.** These reflexes, which begin at puberty and are amplified by estrogens, can occur throughout an adult female's life even in estrogen-deficient females. The sexual response can be divided into four phases. The first phase, **excitement** or arousal, occurs in response to psychogenic or neurogenic stimulation and includes (1) **erection** due to gradually increasing vasocongestion and muscular tension in the genitalia and (2) **lubrication** of the vagina. During this phase, parasympathetic efferent signals transmitted from spinal cord segments S2 to S4 via the sacral plexus cause arteriolar dilatation and venous constriction in the erectile tissues that surround the introitus and project into the clitoris. As a result, blood rapidly accumulates in the erectile tissue, enabling the introitus to tighten around the male penis. At the same time, parasympathetic signals to the bilateral Bartholin's glands beneath the labia minora lead to increased secretion of mucus into the vagina. This mucus, along with other vaginal secretions, provides lubrication during sexual intercourse so that the sexual act produces a satisfactory massaging sensation in the female rather than irritation. This massaging sensation is necessary for the female to progress to the second phase of the sexual response, the plateau phase. Continued satisfactory stimulation causes excitement to increase in intensity to a **plateau,** where a high state of sexual sensitivity and receptivity is maintained. The length of this phase can vary greatly among individuals. The plateau phase culminates in **orgasm,** the third phase of the sexual response.

Orgasm occurs when the sexual organs receive appropriate psychic signals from the brain at the same time that they are receiving local stimulation of maximum intensity.

Because psychological and physical intensities are maximal, orgasm is referred to as the **climax.** The perineal muscles contract rhythmically at a frequency of 0.8 per second in response to sympathetic efferent impulses transmitted from spinal cord segments T10 to L2 via the hypogastric plexus. At the same time, intense sexual signals transmitted to the thalamus via the spinothalamic tracts and then distributed to the limbic system lead to increased muscular tension throughout the body. Orgasm culminates in rapid release from the developed vasocongestion during intense muscular tension, and it may be accompanied by secretion of copious amounts of vaginal fluid. The fourth phase of the sexual response, **resolution,** is often characterized by relaxation and sleep. Many females, however, return to the first phase of arousal, remain responsive to sexual stimulation, and may experience plateau and orgasm repeatedly with no refractory period.

Menopause

Menopause, defined as the last menstrual period, signals the cessation of reproductive function in females and marks the end of a gradual diminution of the number of follicles in the ovary. It usually occurs around the age of 51. About 7 years before menopause, the menstrual cycle length begins to be more variable as the follicular phases shorten and ovulations do not occur. Long, short, normal, and anovulatory cycles can be interspersed during the perimenopausal period.

Nearly complete loss of oocytes is a major factor in the onset of menopause. Exhaustion of the supply of primordial follicles leads to cessation of ovarian follicular production of estrogen and progestin, as well as of inhibin, and a consequential decrease in the plasma levels of these hormones. The hypothalamic-pituitary unit also becomes less sensitive to the negative feedback effects of estrogen. Consequently, plasma FSH levels rise severalfold to levels seen in castrated females because of elimination of negative feedback. The excessive secretion of LH associated with menopause is thought to be due in part to the altered microheterogeneity of the hormone, causing secretion of forms of LH with relatively low biologic activity. The neuroendocrine mechanisms that control FSH and LH secretion remain intact, since surges of FSH and LH, similar to normal preovulatory surges, can be induced by the administration of estrogen and progestin. The pituitary response to GnRH is not impaired by menopause, although artificially induced hypersecretion of GnRH can lead to depletion of pituitary stores of the hormone.

Certain physiologic changes eventuate from the decreased secretion of ovarian steroid hormones. These include hot flashes or flushes, atrophy of the genitourinary tract, atrophy of the epithelial glands and ducts of the breasts, and bone loss. Tissues that depend on estrogen and progestin regress after menopause. Bone loss, or **osteoporosis,** results from both direct and indirect effects of estrogen on bone but is not solely a function of plasma estrogen concentrations. Similarly aged males, who normally have much lower plasma estrogen levels than females, also experience a certain degree of bone loss. Estrogen appears to have permissive effects on calcium absorption and to enhance the proliferation and differentiation of osteoblasts, the cells responsible for bone formation.

Hot flashes, which are irregularly occurring thermogenic episodes that cause peripheral vasomotor dilatation and sweating, are associated with transient elevations in the plasma levels of GnRH, LH, and catecholamines. Although the cause of hot flashes is unknown, administration of estrogen prevents them. In some females, hot flashes subside within 5 years of menopause; in others, they continue unabated for many years.

Genital atrophy encompasses the vulva, vagina, urethra, uterus, and fallopian tubes. With estrogen depletion, the size of these organs, their vascularity, and their secretions diminish. Administration of estrogen, however, will not reverse atrophy of the external genitalia, though it can reverse atrophy of the internal genitalia.

Summary

The reproductive system of the female consists of paired ovaries, the reproductive tract or internal genitalia, external genitalia, and the breasts. The ovaries produce germ cells containing the haploid number of chromosomes. Ovarian cells of the follicle, corpus luteum, and interstitium produce hormones that condition the reproductive tract to receive the male germ cells and to provide a beneficial environment for fertilization, implantation of the blastocyst, and pregnancy. Reproductive function begins at puberty when the hypothalamic-pituitary unit matures functionally. During the reproductive period, a mature ovum is produced by the ovary each month. The cyclic production of a female gamete and the concomitant changes in the reproductive tract are called the menstrual cycle. The cyclic reproductive processes are controlled by interacting neural and hormonal signals originating from the hypothalamic-pituitary-ovarian axis. As the pool of primordial follicles in the ovary is depleted, reproductive function declines and ceases at menopause.

Bibliography

Becker, K., Bilezikian, J. P., Bremner, W. J., et al., eds. *Principles and Practice of Endocrinology and Metabolism.* Philadelphia: J. B. Lippincott, 1990.

Knobil, E., Neill, J. D., et al., eds. *The Physiology of Reproduction.* New York: Raven Press, 1988.

Odell, W. D., and Moyer, D. L. *Physiology of Reproduction.* St. Louis: C. V. Mosby, 1971.

Yen, S. S. C., and Jaffe, R. B., eds. *Reproductive Endocrinology: Physiology, Pathophysiology, and Clinical Management,* 2nd ed. Philadelphia: W. B. Saunders, 1986.

61 The Male Reproductive System

Andrew R. LaBarbera

Objectives

After reading this chapter, you should be able to

List the components of the male reproductive system and their functions

Describe the synthesis, secretion, and effects of testosterone

Explain how the hypothalamus and anterior pituitary gland regulate male reproductive function

Explain how negative feedback by gonadal steroid hormones and inhibin modulates gonadotropin secretion

Describe spermatogenesis and maturation of spermatozoa

Explain how the reproductive tract functions to deliver mature spermatozoa to the female reproductive system

---

The male reproductive system, which consists of the paired **testes,** the reproductive tract or **internal genitalia,** and the **external genitalia,** functions to produce germ cells for sexual reproduction and to deliver them to the female reproductive tract. The organs of the male reproductive system, which are established during gestation, reach full maturity during puberty. Production of **spermatozoa,** the male germ cells, differs from that in the female in two major respects: (1) development beyond the primordial germ cell stage does not occur until puberty in the male, and (2) beginning at puberty, the development of spermatozoa is continuous. **Spermatogenesis,** the process by which primordial germ cells form into spermatozoa, and the production of androgens, the male sex hormones, both occur in the testes and are controlled by the hypothalamic-pituitary unit. Gonadotropin secretion and at least some spermatogenesis usually continue until death in the male, although testosterone secretion begins to decline between the ages 40 and 50.

Testis

The paired testes serve at least three functions critical to successful propagation of the species: (1) production of

gametes, (2) secretion of hormones that cause differentiation of the brain and reproductive tract during fetal and neonatal development, maintain the structure and function of the reproductive tract in the sexually mature adult, participate in the regulation of metabolism and skeletal growth, and promote development of secondary sexual characteristics, and (3) feedback regulation of hypothalamic-pituitary hormone secretion. The testes consist primarily of the seminiferous tubules that are separated by interstitial tissue. Each testis is surrounded by a thick fibrous capsule, the tunica albuginea, and is located outside the body in the scrotal sac. If the testes do not descend into the scrotum properly (**cryptorchidism**), usually during the seventh to ninth month of gestation, spermatogenesis is not normal. While the cause of cryptorchidism is not known, the disorder can be associated with abnormal fetal testicular androgen production.

Interstitial Cells of Leydig

The spaces between the seminiferous tubules are filled with interstitial tissue composed of connective tissue stroma, blood and lymph vessels, nerves of the testicular parenchyma, mast cells, macrophages, and the interstitial cells of Leydig, or Leydig cells. The principal function of the Leydig cells appears to be to produce androgens, although some estrogen is also secreted.

Leydig cells differentiate and begin to secrete androgens during the seventh week of fetal life in response to chorionic gonadotropin (hCG), which is produced by the placenta. During childhood, when gonadotropin secretion is low, the Leydig cells regress to an undifferentiated state. When plasma LH levels rise again at puberty, the Leydig cells differentiate again and acquire the characteristics of steroid-producing cells. They are maintained by LH during adulthood.

Androgen

Androgenic steroid hormones are the male sex hormones. They perform numerous functions throughout the body (Table 61-1). These include (1) differentiation of the male reproductive tract and brain during fetal life, (2) stimulation of testes descent during the last 3 months of gestation, (3) stimulation of maturation and maintenance of the reproductive tract, including the internal and external genitalia, at puberty and during adulthood, (4) maintenance of spermatogenesis in the adult testes, (5) negative feedback regulation of LH secretion by the pituitary, and (6) facilitation of sexual drive and aggressive behavior. Androgens also stimulate development of the male secondary sexual characteristics, including (1) growth of facial, chest, axillary, and pubic hair, as well as hair recession and balding, (2) hypertrophy of the laryngeal mucosa causing enlargement of the larynx and deepening of the voice, (3) development of increased musculature due to increased protein deposition and nitrogen retention, and (4) enhancement of

linear growth through stimulation of bone growth. Androgens and growth hormone cause the growth spurt at puberty. Androgens are very potent **anabolic hormones** that accelerate metabolism.

Testosterone is the major androgen synthesized by the Leydig cells and secreted at a rate of approximately 6 to 7 mg/day. Ninety-five percent of plasma testosterone in men (600–700 ng/dl) is secreted by the testes. Other potent androgens produced by the testes include 5α-dihydrotestosterone (DHT, 0.3 mg/day) and androstenedione (2.4 mg/day), which serves mainly as a precursor for estrogen biosynthesis. DHT and androstenedione are present in plasma at concentrations of 50 to 60 and 150 ng/dl, respectively.

Testosterone is synthesized from cholesterol, which is preferentially derived from circulating low-density lipoproteins (LDL) but which can be synthesized de novo from acetate in the Leydig cell (Fig. 61-1.). Cholesterol derived from LDL is stored in lipid droplets in the cytoplasm. It is transported to the mitochondria, where it is converted to pregnenolone through the action of the C_{27} side-chain cleavage P_{450} enzyme. Pregnenolone is transported to the microsomal compartment (smooth endoplasmic reticulum). In humans, pregnenolone is converted to testosterone preferentially via the Δ^5-pathway, involving the intermediates 17α-hydroxypregnenolone and dehydroepiandrosterone. The conversion of pregnenolone, which is a C_{21} steroid, to dehydroepiandrosterone, which is a C_{19} steroid, occurs through the action of the C_{21} side-chain cleavage P_{450} enzyme, which possesses both 17α-hydroxylase and C17,20-lyase activities. LH enhances androgen biosynthesis primarily by stimulating transport of cholesterol from the outer to the inner mitochondrial

Table 61-1. Actions of Androgens

1. Stimulate differentiation of the male reproductive tract
2. Stimulate sexual differentiation of the male brain
3. Stimulate maturation of the external genitalia
4. Increase size of larynx and thickness of vocal cords
5. Increase hair growth (facial, axillary, pubic) and hair recession (balding)
6. Increase libido and sexual potency
7. Increase aggressive behavior
8. Maintain spermatogenesis in conjunction with FSH
9. Maintain male reproductive tract and accessory sex glands
10. Decrease LH, and to a lesser extent FSH, secretion by hypothalamic-pituitary unit
11. Stimulate growth of bone and closure of epiphyses
12. Increase protein anabolism (increase protein synthesis, decrease protein catabolism) leading to increased linear body growth, nitrogen retention, and muscular development

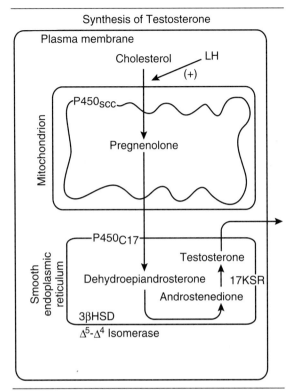

Fig. 61-1. Biosynthesis of testicular androgens in Leydig cells.

membrane. LH also may increase the amounts or activities of the steroidogenic enzymes.

Testosterone, which has a low solubility in an aqueous medium, is transported in the blood bound to **plasma proteins.** The principal androgen transport protein is **testosterone-estradiol–binding globulin** (TeBG), a 94,000 molecular weight glycoprotein with one steroid-binding site per molecule. Thirty percent of the testosterone in plasma is bound to TeBG, 67% circulates bound to albumin and other plasma proteins, and only 3% is free. Testosterone bound to TeBG does not appear to be available for metabolism or for uptake by target tissues, since the rate of testosterone metabolism correlates directly with the amount of free plus albumin-bound testosterone. The biologically relevant testosterone is that which is free; many species do not have TeBG. The plasma concentration of TeBG is enhanced by both estrogen and thyroid hormone, whereas testosterone itself decreases plasma TeBG.

Testosterone has a plasma half-life of approximately 15

minutes. It can be metabolized either to active compounds in specific target tissues or to inactive compounds that are excreted. Examples of the first instance include (1) aromatization to estradiol in the brain, breast, and other tissues, (2) conversion by the enzyme 5α-reductase in the prostate, urethra, scrotum, and penis and in skin to DHT, a more potent androgen than testosterone, and (3) conversion by 5β-reductase to compounds that possess little androgenic activity but that stimulate production of red blood cells in bone marrow. In the second situation, androgens are metabolized to inactive sulfates and glucuronide conjugates in the liver and then are excreted in either the bile or urine. The mean metabolic clearance rate for testosterone is approximately 1000 liters/day.

Testosterone diffuses from the plasma into target cells, where it either binds immediately to an intracellular receptor or is first converted to DHT or estradiol. Testosterone and DHT bind to specific high-affinity intracellular androgen receptors that appear to be loosely associated with the nuclear membrane. Estradiol also binds to specific high-affinity receptors similarly situated within the cell. The androgen-receptor complex interacts with specific nuclear acceptor sites on chromatin. This binding to chromatin triggers increased RNA synthesis, which in turn leads to increased synthesis of the proteins necessary for growth and differentiated function.

Seminiferous Tubules

Each mature testis contains 20 to 25 m of highly convoluted, anastomosing seminiferous tubules per gram of tissue. The ends of these tubules open into the rete testis, a network of intercommunicating channels that link the seminiferous tubules with the efferent ducts. The cytoarchitecture of the tubular epithelium is characterized by a basement membrane lined with sustentacular (**Sertoli**) cells and **spermatogonia.** The Sertoli cells are surrounded by spermatogonia, which are progressively more developed going from the basement membrane to the tubular lumen. The luminal surface of the Sertoli cell surrounds spermatids that are maturing into spermatozoa.

Sertoli Cells

The Sertoli cells, which are tall, columnar cells that extend centripetally from the basement membrane to the lumen, constitute the nongerminal component of the epithelium of the seminiferous tubule. These cells are linked by tight junctional complexes to form the **blood-testis barrier,** which limits the movement of fluid and nutrients between the interstitial space of the testis and the lumen of the seminiferous tubule. Lipid-soluble substances, such as steroids, are able to traverse the barrier and enter the lumen of the seminiferous tubule at a rate that is related to their lipid solubility. Presumably, lipid-soluble substances diffuse passively through the Sertoli cells. Glucose is transferred across the barrier by facilitated diffusion. The significance of the blood-testis barrier is unknown, but it may serve to prevent the body's immune system from recognizing the haploid germ cells. If the barrier is interrupted, as happens in vasectomy, the male can become immune to his own spermatozoa. Findings from animal studies indicate that the barrier does not form until puberty. The shape, volume, and ultrastructure of Sertoli cells change to accommodate the changing size and shape of the surrounding germ cells at various stages of development.

Sertoli cells have several functions: (1) provision of nutrients to the germ cells, (2) synthesis of multiple proteins that are secreted into the luminal fluid and are also present in the plasma, including ceruloplasmin, acidic glycoprotein, and transferrin, (3) synthesis of estrogen, (4) production of androgen-binding protein (ABP), (5) phagocytosis of damaged germ cells, and (6) synthesis and secretion of inhibin.

Inhibin

Sertoli cells synthesize and secrete inhibin, a heterodimeric protein that selectively inhibits the synthesis and secretion of follicle-stimulating hormone (FSH) by pituitary gonadotropes and apparently is identical to the inhibin synthesized by granulosa cells. The structure and synthesis of inhibin and the related molecule, activin, by ovarian granulosa cells are discussed in Chap. 60. The concentrations of FSH and inhibin in the circulation are in a dynamic equilibrium. FSH stimulates Sertoli cells to produce inhibin, which, in turn, negatively modulates further FSH production. If one or both testes are removed, or if the seminiferous tubules are damaged, the plasma FSH concentrations rise and can only be partially suppressed by administration of testosterone.

Androgen-Binding Protein

ABP is a dimeric protein that binds androgens with high affinity. The two protomers have molecular weights of 48,000 and 46,000. ABP is found in both the luminal fluid and the plasma and is structurally very similar to the serum transport protein TeBG, also referred to as **sex hormone–binding globulin** (SHBG). Because ABP is concentrated in the luminal fluid and in the epididymis, its putative

physiologic role is to carry testosterone within the Sertoli cell and from the testis to the epididymis in order to maintain high testosterone concentrations within these androgen-dependent tissues.

Estrogen

The principal estrogens in the plasma of adult males are estradiol and estrone. Only 10% to 20% of circulating estrogens are synthesized by the Sertoli cells in the testes, however. The remainder originate through the extragonadal conversion of testosterone and androstenedione by means of cytochrome P_{450} aromatase, which is present in numerous tissues. The ratio of estrogens to androgens appears to be more important than the absolute levels of the steroids, because decreased plasma testosterone levels with normal plasma estrogen levels result in feminization.

Spermatogenesis

Development of the male germ cells occurs continuously and repeatedly in the epithelium lining the seminiferous tubules of the mature testis. Areas of active spermatogenesis are interspersed with resting epithelia so that areas of progressively more developed germ cells succeed each other along the length of the tubule. As the germ cells develop, they move from the outer wall to the luminal surface so that the least developed cells line the walls of the tubule and the most developed cells line the tubular lumen. Spermatogonia are the least differentiated cells of the germ cell population. They are derived from primordial germ cells and divide by mitosis both to form the pool of cells that will undergo meiosis and also to replenish themselves. FSH enhances the mitotic proliferation of spermatogonia such that if FSH secretion is suppressed, spermatogenesis will be greatly reduced.

Spermatogonia give rise to the primary spermatocytes. Prior to prophase of the first meiotic division, primary spermatocytes double the DNA content of their 46 chromosomes so that they have 92 daughter chromatids with the 4N DNA content. DNA replication in primary spermatocytes represents the final synthesis of DNA in spermatogenesis.

Primary spermatocytes undergo the first meiotic division to yield two secondary spermatocytes, each with the N, or haploid, number of chromosomes; each chromosome has two chromatids, so the secondary spermatocyte has the 2N DNA content. Secondary spermatocytes have a short lifespan. They rapidly undergo the second meiotic division, during which the chromatids of each chromosome separate to the two daughter cells by processes similar to those of mitosis. The final result of these divisions is four spermatids, each with 23 unpaired chromosomes, the N, or haploid, number. Each spermatid has 22 autosomes and either an X or a Y chromosome.

Spermiogenesis

The spherical **spermatids,** which are considerably smaller than the secondary spermatocytes, mature into spermatozoa through the process of spermiogenesis. Neither mitosis nor meiosis is involved in the transformation of the spermatid into an oval-shaped, highly organized cell. Spermatids are located near the luminal surface of the seminiferous tubule. During the early phase of spermiogenesis, they become engulfed by Sertoli cells.

During spermiogenesis, both the cytoplasm and nucleus of the spermatid differentiate to form the head and the tail. The shape changes from spherical to oval. The Golgi apparatus aligns itself on one side of the cell nucleus and begins to form small vesicles that appear as dense bodies (proacrosomic granules). These granules coalesce to form the head cap and acrosome. In the nucleus, basic proteins such as histones and protamine combine with DNA to produce a semicrystalline chromatin structure. The nucleoplasm fills with tightly packed dense granules. The midpiece and flagellum form from the centrioles on the sperm head opposite the site where the acrosome forms. Most of the cytoplasm migrates to the area around the midpiece, forms a residual body, and pinches off from the cell.

Mature Spermatozoon

The mature spermatozoon consists of (1) a head, which is ovoid and flattened anteriorly and is composed of the **nucleus** and **acrosome,** and (2) a tail, which is composed of the **neck, midpiece, principal piece,** and **endpiece.** The condensed nuclear elements from the spermatid are located in the head. The acrosomal portion of the head contains Golgi elements and enzymes that are responsible for penetration of the ovum, such as **hyaluronidase** and **acrosin.** Hyaluronidase, which is located on the outer surface of the acrosomal membrane, facilitates penetration of the cumulus cells surrounding the female oocyte by digesting hyaluronic acid. Proacrosin, the precursor of acrosin, is located inside the acrosome. It must be converted to the active acrosin, which is a serine protease that facilitates penetration of the zona pellucida by digesting zona proteins. The acrosome also contains glycosaminoglycans and the enzymes acid phosphatase and nucleoside phosphatase. The mitochondria from the spermatid form a mitochondrial sheath around the axial filament complex in the mid-

piece. Ultrastructurally, the axial filament complex of the tail, which extends from neck to end, resembles that of cilia with the same number and arrangement of longitudinal tubules. The flagellum has some additional coarse actin fibers. The centrioles, which are involved in spindle formation in the fertilized ovum, are located in the neck of the tail.

Fully developed but nonmotile mature spermatozoa are released from the Sertoli cells into the tubular lumen. Most of the testicular fluid produced by the Sertoli cells is absorbed in the first segment of the epididymis, the **caput,** thus generating a fluid flow that washes the spermatozoa out of the tubules and into the rete testis and then into the epididymis. Spermatozoa achieve full maturation and fertilizing potential in the epididymis, where they remain for 4 to 10 days. They also acquire the capacity for motility, although they remain immotile until after ejaculation. Spermatozoa from the caudal epididymis or even ejaculated spermatozoa cannot fertilize oocytes. Spermatozoa must first undergo an as yet unidentified biochemical change, referred to as **capacitation,** in the female genital tract. Capacitation can be achieved in vitro by incubating spermatozoa in a medium containing agents such as calcium, serum albumin, and hyaluronic acid.

The **spermatogenic cycle,** the frequency with which spermatogenesis begins in a given section of the seminiferous tubule, is 16 days in humans. **Spermatogenesis,** from the time a spermatogonium begins to replicate its DNA to the time mature spermatozoa are released from the Sertoli cells into the tubular lumen, requires 70 to 74 days, or approximately 4.5 cycles.

Maintenance of spermatogenesis requires testosterone. Androgen production, in turn, is regulated by the anterior pituitary hormone luteinizing hormone (LH), which formerly was referred to as **interstitial cell-stimulating hormone** (ICSH). FSH is required for development of the seminiferous epithelium and initiation and maintenance of the mitotic phases of spermatogenesis.

Neuroendocrine Regulation of the Testes

Adult testicular function is controlled by the hypothalamic-pituitary unit through the action of the gonadotropins FSH and LH on the testes (Fig. 61-2). In the male, unlike the female, FSH and LH act on different cell types whose secretions have separate negative feedback effects on the secretion of the corresponding gonadotropins. Gonadotropin-releasing hormone (see Chap. 60), a hypothal-

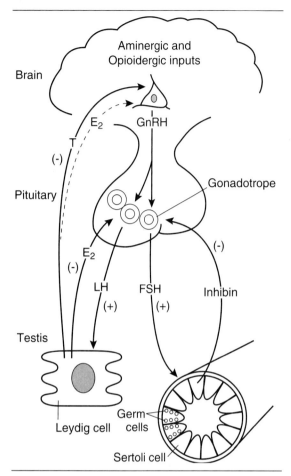

Fig. 61-2. Neuroendocrine regulation of testicular function.

amic hormone, stimulates pituitary gonadotropes to secrete FSH and LH. Because GnRH is secreted in a pulsatile manner, FSH and LH also are secreted in a pulsatile manner. FSH stimulates Sertoli cells, which produce inhibin, which, in turn, specifically inhibits FSH secretion; LH stimulates Leydig cells, which produce testosterone, which, in turn, specifically inhibits LH secretion. Inhibin has a negative feedback effect on the pituitary gonadotropes, whereas testosterone appears to exert its negative feedback effect primarily in the hypothalamus. When plasma testosterone drops, the frequency of pulsatile GnRH secretion increases. Thus plasma FSH and LH are maintained in a dynamic equilibrium with plasma inhibin and testosterone, respectively. In contrast with testosterone, estradiol appears to exert a negative feedback on

LH secretion by decreasing the amplitude of the pituitary discharge of LH.

Follicle-Stimulating Hormone

The structure, synthesis, and secretion of FSH are discussed in Chap. 60. FSH is secreted by the basophilic cells of the anterior pituitary gland in response to stimulation by the hypothalamic hormone gonadotropin-releasing hormone. Secretion of FSH in males neither fluctuates much during the day nor shows the cyclic variation seen in females. Testosterone, the principal male sex steroid, only partially suppresses FSH secretion. Rather, the primary negative modulator of FSH production is inhibin, a product of the Sertoli cell that is stimulated by FSH.

The role of FSH in adult testicular function is not understood completely. It is clear, however, that FSH and testosterone must be present for development of the seminiferous epithelium. Once the tubules are established, FSH is not absolutely required, although spermatogenesis is markedly reduced if FSH secretion is suppressed. If the epithelium regresses, FSH must be administered with testosterone in order to restore it. FSH enhances production of a number of Sertoli cell proteins in culture, including transferrin (an iron-binding protein), plasminogen activator, fibroblast-growth factor, and insulin-like growth factor I (somatomedin C). Chronic administration of pharmacologic doses of testosterone or androgenic steroids, such as those used by body builders, will suppress FSH secretion to the extent that spermatogenesis will cease.

The effects of FSH on Sertoli cells are mediated by membrane-bound receptors. The FSH receptor, a high-molecular-weight multimeric complex containing sialylated glycoprotein, is coupled to adenylyl cyclase, the membrane-bound enzyme that catalyzes the conversion of ATP to cAMP. Cyclic AMP regulates protein kinases, which in turn regulate the expression of genes for enzymes and substrates involved in Sertoli cell function.

Luteinizing Hormone

The structure, synthesis, and secretion of LH are discussed in Chap. 60. LH, like FSH, is secreted in a pulsatile manner by basophilic cells in the anterior pituitary gland in response to pulsatile stimulation by GnRH. Unlike FSH, synthesis and secretion of LH are under the negative feedback control of testosterone, which is produced by the Leydig cells in response to stimulation by LH. Testosterone inhibits pituitary LH secretion by reducing the frequency of LH pulses, presumably by decreasing the frequency of hypothalamic GnRH pulses. Estradiol also decreases LH secretion, but it appears to act by reducing pituitary sensitivity to GnRH. Inhibin has no effect on synthesis or secretion of LH.

The physiologic role of LH is to maintain testosterone production by Leydig cells. The effects of LH can be achieved by administration of testosterone, which alone is necessary for maintenance of spermatogenesis in the differentiated seminiferous epithelium. As in the ovary (see Chap. 60), the effects of LH on the Leydig cell are mediated by specific high-affinity membrane-bound receptors that are coupled to the membrane-bound enzyme adenylyl cyclase. LH stimulates steroidogenesis in the Leydig cell by enhancing the activity of cholesterol ester hydrolase, or cholesterol esterase, which results in increased stores of cholesterol for androgen biosynthesis in the Leydig cell. It also enhances transport of cholesterol into mitochondria.

Gonadotropin-Releasing Hormone

Both FSH and LH are synthesized and secreted in response to GnRH, which is secreted in a pulsatile manner similar to that in females (see Chap. 60). In males, the rate of secretion of GnRH increases and hypothalamic GnRH content decreases after castration, which interrupts the negative feedback effects of steroids. Treatment with either testosterone, DHT, or estradiol reverses the effects of castration, indicating that secretion of GnRH is modulated both by testosterone and by estradiol. As in females, GnRH secretion also is modulated by input from higher centers in the brain. Thus neurogenic and psychogenic influences such as stress can decrease the secretions of the hypothalamic-pituitary unit and, consequently, testicular function.

Prolactin

The anterior pituitary of men secretes prolactin. The significance of prolactin secretion is not clear, however. Men with excessively elevated prolactin levels (**hyperprolactinemia**) frequently have abnormally low gonadal function (hypogonadism). Prolactin does cause a reduction in the conversion of testosterone to dihydrotestosterone, so it is possible that the hypogonadism results from decreased 5α-reductase activity.

Reproductive Tract

The male reproductive tract is a duct system with associated secretory glands. It stores spermatozoa, transports spermatozoa from the testes to the urethral opening in the penis, and supplies the fluid portion of the ejaculate. Each testis has an individual duct system consisting of efferent or collecting ducts, the epididymis, the vas deferens, and the ejaculatory duct. The ejaculatory ducts from the two testes drain into the urethra. The secretory glands include the seminal vesicles, the prostate gland, the bulbourethral or Cowper's glands, and the glands of Littré. The efferent ducts, epididymis, vas deferens, and seminal vesicles develop from the wolffian ducts and thus share a common mesonephric origin with the kidneys. In the reproductive tract, spermatozoa mature, and the composition of the seminal fluid is altered to enhance survival of the spermatozoa after ejaculation.

The rete testis drain into 15 to 20 efferent or collecting ducts that penetrate the tunica albuginea at the upper portion of the testis. Each efferent duct passes upward and becomes highly coiled to form a compact, cone-shaped structure. These multiple coiled tubules are surrounded by connective tissue and form the head, or caput, of the epididymis.

The efferent ducts, which develop under the influence of testosterone but not of DHT, consist of a thin layer of smooth muscle, a basement membrane, and an epithelial layer lining the lumen. The epithelium of the efferent ducts is thought to absorb some of the fluid entering from the rete testis. Particulate matter is removed from the fluid in the ducts by endocytosis.

Epididymis

The transit time from caput to cauda appears to be 4 to 10 days in humans. During this time, spermatozoa acquire both the ability to fertilize ova (capacitation) and the potential for motility. Spermatozoa do not actually become motile until **ejaculation** and exposure to oxygen or lactic acid. They are capable of surviving longer in the epididymis than in any other segment of the reproductive tract, and the cauda is the major site of storage of spermatozoa in the duct system.

The **tall cells,** which have nonmotile stereocilia, secrete ions, nutrients, proteins, glycoproteins, enzymes, and other substances necessary for both survival and maturation of spermatozoa. As in the efferent ducts, the cells of the epithelium of the caput of the epididymis absorb large quantities of fluid. Epididymal fluid is enriched in potassium compared with whole semen. It also contains high concentrations of glycerylphosphorylcholine, which must be metabolized to glycerylphosphate by glycerophosphorocholine esterase in order to be utilized as an energy substrate by spermatozoa. The luminal fluid gradually becomes acidified as it moves from the rete testis to the cauda epididymis.

The epididymis is an androgen-dependent tissue. The epithelial cells lining the adult male epididymis contain the enzyme 5α-reductase and abundant androgen receptors, which bind DHT preferentially. Removal of the testes causes atrophy of the epididymis.

Vas Deferens

The vas deferens, or ductus deferens, is a continuation of the epididymis. This duct, whose luminal epithelium has important absorptive and secretory functions, begins where the epididymis straightens and reverses direction to ascend along the posterior border of the testis toward the inguinal canal. Inside the abdominal cavity, the vas deferens is associated with blood vessels and nerves to form the spermatic cord, which remains outside the peritoneum, however. The vas deferens enlarges to form the ampulla just before it enters the prostate gland. The ampulla serves as a secondary storage site for spermatozoa.

Ejaculatory Duct

The portion of the vas deferens just beyond the point at which the seminal vesicle empties into it is termed the ejaculatory duct. This duct, which is a common duct of both the testis and the seminal vesicle, penetrates the upper surface of the prostate gland and traverses the gland to join the urethra.

Urethra and Penis

The urethra continues through the prostate on its way from the bladder to the penis. The urethra opens at the end of the penis. Ordinarily, the penis is flaccid. Erotic influences, however, elicit involuntary autonomic reflexes that cause the penis to increase in size and become erect. This phenomenon, termed erection, enables the penis to perform the male sexual act.

Secretory Glands

Seminal Vesicles

At the back of the urinary bladder, an outcropping of the vas deferens forms the seminal vesicle, which appears to be a blind, lobulated, elongated sac. In man, each seminal vesicle is a coiled tube approximately 15 cm long and having little storage capacity. The seminal vesicle is comprised of three layers: (1) an outer, fibrous connective tissue coat containing elastic fibers, (2) a middle muscular layer, and (3) an inner mucous membrane that is highly folded, greatly increasing the surface area of the epithelium. The epithelial lining consists mainly of tall columnar cells.

The secretions of the seminal vesicles are alkaline and are rich in fructose, inositol, sorbitol, 19-hydroxylated prostaglandins, and reducing substances. Most of the fructose in semen is secreted by the seminal vesicles to be used as an energy source for motility by the spermatozoa after ejaculation. The fluid also is rich in potassium (20 mM) but poor in sodium, and it contains ascorbic acid, inorganic phosphorus, and acid-soluble phosphorus. The seminal vesicles secrete the proteins, including fibrinogen, that are responsible for clotting of the semen after ejaculation.

Prostate Gland

The prostate gland is a multilobular organ that surrounds the urethra as it emerges from the urinary bladder and the two ejaculatory ducts. It is firm and surrounded by a thin capsule containing both smooth muscle fibers and connective tissue. The prostate gland is comprised of numerous individual glands that are made up of alveoli lined primarily with tall columnar epithelial cells. The individual glands are embedded in the stroma of the organ, which consists of smooth muscle and fibrous connective tissue.

The prostate gland is sensitive to and dependent on the androgen DHT, the principal regulator of growth, differentiation, and function of the prostate gland. If the testes are removed, the secretory cells of the prostate gland shrink. Prostatic cells contain the enzyme 5α-reductase, which converts testosterone to DHT.

The secretion of the prostate gland in man is a slightly acidic (pH 6.5), colorless, thin liquid. It contains acid phosphatase, magnesium, calcium, citric acid, spermine, and fibrinolysin, as well as several strong proteolytic enzymes. Digestion of fibrin by fibrinolysin results in liquefaction of coagulated semen within approximately 20 to 30 minutes after ejaculation. Fructose is not secreted by the prostate gland. Sodium, rather than potassium, is the main cation, and large quantities of zinc are secreted.

Semen

Semen is comprised of spermatozoa and seminal plasma and has a milky appearance. The seminal plasma consists of fluid secretions of the vas deferens, epididymis, seminal vesicles, prostate gland, and mucous glands. Too high or too low of a concentration of spermatozoa in the semen can result in decreased motility. The volume of the normal human ejaculate is 2 to 6 ml; spermatozoa normally are present at concentrations of 20 to 100 million/ml. Seminal plasma is enriched in potassium, zinc, citric acid, fructose, phosphorylcholine, spermine, amino acids, prostaglandins, and the enzymes acid phosphatase, diamine oxidase, lactic dehydrogenase, beta-glucuronidase, alpha-amylase, and seminal proteinase. The pH normally is 7.2 to 8.0 because the prostatic secretions partially neutralize the more basic secretions of the other segments of the reproductive tract.

In the average ejaculate volume of 2 to 3.5 ml, the major contributions to the seminal plasma volume are seminal vesicles, 1.5 to 3 ml; prostate gland, 0.5 ml; and bulbourethral glands and glands of Littré, 0.1 to 0.2 ml. During emission and ejaculation, the secretions of these glands are released sequentially with the mucous secretions of the bulbourethral glands first and the secretions of the seminal vesicles last.

Male Sexual Function

Fertility in the male refers to the at least occasional ability to produce enough semen at ejaculation containing a sufficient number of normal, healthy spermatozoa to result in fertilization of a fertile female. **Potency** refers to the ability to engage in **intercourse,** which depends on erection of the penis. As in the female, the male sexual response consists of two physiologic responses: the vasocongestive response controlled by the parasympathetic nervous system, followed by the tonic, muscular contractions controlled by the sympathetic nervous system. These responses usually are divided into three events: **erection, emission,** and **ejaculation.**

Sexual function is controlled by spinal reflexes on which are superimposed inputs from higher centers in the brain. The CNS processes tactile stimuli from the organs of the reproductive tract as well as psychic, optic, and olfactory stimuli. In males, mere thoughts of the sexual act can result in erection, emission, and ejaculation.

Erection

Erection is defined as penile rigidity or tumescence. In adult males, the penis contains erectile tissue located in three corporal bodies, the two dorsal corpora cavernosa and the single ventral corpus spongiosum through which passes the urethra. Erection involves filling of the cavernous spaces of the three corpora with blood in response to psychic and tactile stimuli. **Parasympathetic impulses** transmitted to the penis from the sacral plexus simultaneously cause dilatation of the arteries and constriction of the veins in the penis. Consequently, arterial blood fills the erectile tissue under high pressure causing the penis to become hard and elongated.

The glans penis has a network of sensory end-organs that transmit sexual sensations to the CNS via the **puden-**

dal nerve and the **sacral plexus.** The **glans penis** is very sensitive and important for initiation and maintenance of erection before and during the male sexual act. Impulses from the anal epithelium, scrotum, and other perineal structures and from internal organs of the genitourinary tract such as the prostate, bladder, urethra, and seminal vesicles aid in amplifying sexual sensation.

The parasympathetic impulses also cause secretion of a small amount of mucus by the glands of Littré and the bulbourethral (Cowper's) glands. The mucus aids in lubrication of the penis during intercourse, although most lubrication is provided by secretions of the female reproductive tract. The pain sensation that can result from inadequate lubrication can lead to loss of erection.

Emission

Emission is defined as the deposition of seminal fluid components from the vas deferens, seminal vesicles, and prostate gland into the posterior urethra. When sexual stimulation reaches a maximum, **sympathetic impulses** originating in the spinal cord and passing through the hypogastric plexus first cause contractions of the epididymis, vas deferens, and ampulla to expel the sperm into the urethra. These contractions are followed rapidly by contractions of the muscular layer of the prostate gland and then by contractions of the seminal vesicles. The contractions cause expulsion of prostatic and seminal fluids, forcing the sperm forward. The sperm and the prostatic and seminal secretions mix with the mucus secreted by the bulbourethral glands to form the semen.

Ejaculation

Ejaculation is the passage of semen through the urethra and its expulsion from the urethral meatus. It occurs because filling of the urethra with semen leads to transmission of sensory signals through the pudendal nerves to the spinal cord, which, in turn, causes transmission of nerve impulses to the skeletal muscles surrounding the erectile tissue of the penis. These rhythmic nerve impulses stimulate rhythmic, wavelike contractions of the muscle that increase the pressure and expel the semen from the urethra.

After semen is ejaculated, prostatic clotting enzymes convert fibrinogen (seminal vesicles) to fibrin, and the semen rapidly coagulates. Fibrinolysin of prostatic origin slowly digests the fibrin so that the coagulum dissolves and the semen liquefies. After ejaculation, spermatozoa normally survive only for 24 to 72 hours, although they can live for weeks in the male reproductive tract.

Summary

The reproductive system of the male consists of paired testes, the reproductive tract or internal genitalia, and external genitalia. Male germ cells, or spermatozoa, containing the haploid number of chromosomes are produced in the seminiferous tubules. Interstitial cells produce the male sex hormones, or androgens, that maintain the structure and function of the internal genitalia. Reproductive function begins at puberty when the hypothalamic-pituitary unit functionally matures. Production of spermatozoa differs from production of ova in the female in two major respects: (1) development beyond the primordial germ cell stage does not occur until puberty in the male, and (2) beginning at puberty, development of spermatozoa is a continuous process. Testicular function is controlled by the gonadotropic hormones FSH and LH. FSH stimulates Sertoli cells, which nurture the developing germ cells, whereas LH stimulates the interstitial cells of Leydig, which synthesize and secrete testosterone, the principal androgen. Male reproductive function is controlled by interacting neural and hormonal signals of the hypothalamic-pituitary-testicular axis.

Bibliography

Ham, A. W. *Histology,* 7th ed. Philadelphia: J. B. Lippincott, 1974.

Knobil, E., Neill, J. D., et al., eds. *The Physiology of Reproduction.* New York: Raven Press, 1988.

Odell, W. D., and Moyer, D. L. *Physiology of Reproduction.* St. Louis: C. V. Mosby, 1971.

Yen, S. S. C., and Jaffe, R. B., eds. *Reproductive Endocrinology: Physiology, Pathophysiology, and Clinical Management,* 2nd ed. Philadelphia: W. B. Saunders, 1986.

62 Fertilization, Pregnancy, and Lactation

Andrew R. LaBarbera

Objectives

After reading this chapter, you should be able to

Explain how spermatozoa travel through the female reproductive tract to the fallopian tubes, the usual site of fertilization

List the cellular events in fertilization of the ovum and early development of the zygote and pre-embryo

Explain how the blastocyst implants in the endometrial lining of the uterus

Characterize the development and function of the placenta in nurturing the fetus

Describe the regulation of maternal and fetal metabolism during pregnancy

Explain how parturition is initiated and proceeds to expel the fetus

Describe the processes of lactation and postpartum changes in maternal function

---

Gamete Transport in the Female Reproductive Tract

Fertilization, which is the fusion of a male gamete (**spermatozoon**) and a female gamete (**ovum**), usually takes place in one of the oviducts, or **fallopian tubes**, of the female reproductive tract. Therefore, spermatozoa must be delivered into the female tract and must travel to the site of fertilization. The ovulated egg likewise must travel from the ovary to the site of fertilization.

Ovum

As discussed in Chaps. 59 and 60, the adult ovary contains primary oocytes that are arrested in the dictyotene stage of prophase of the first meiotic division. In this state, a primary oocyte has replicated its DNA so that it contains the diploid (2N) number of chromosomes, 44 autosomes and 2 sex chromosomes, but the 4N quantity of DNA because each chromosome has two daughter chromatids. The oocyte increases in size during childhood, but the nucleus

remains unchanged. Meiosis resumes in the primary oocyte of the mature graafian follicle at the time of the preovulatory surge in plasma luteinizing hormone (LH), approximately 36 hours prior to ovulation. The first meiotic division, which is completed several hours prior to ovulation, results in two daughter cells. The larger cell is the secondary oocyte, and the smaller cell is the first polar body, which lies between the zona pellucida and the vitelline membrane of the secondary oocyte. Each cell has the haploid (N) number of chromosomes and the 2N quantity of DNA. Further nuclear maturation in the secondary oocyte is halted unless fertilization occurs. Simultaneously with the resumption of oocyte maturation, the cells of the **cumulus oophorus** secrete copious amounts of proteoglycan rich in hyaluronic acid, and the cumulus expands.

After ovulation, the ovum and its surrounding mass of cumulus oophorus cells are transported along the surface of the ovary and through the **ostium**, the opening at the fimbriated end of one of the fallopian tubes. This transport, which requires several minutes, is facilitated by the beating motion of the cilia lining the fimbria. Contractions of

649

the oviductal musculature direct the ovum into the ampulla, where it remains for approximately 3 days. The ovum is kept in the ampulla primarily by constriction of the **ampullary-isthmic sphincter.**

Spermatozoa

During **coitus,** which usually occurs within 10 minutes of **intromission** in the human, semen is ejaculated into the vagina close to the external os of the cervix. The alkaline semen buffers the acidic (pH < 5.0) vaginal fluid to provide a temporarily favorable environment for the spermatozoa, which must undergo **capacitation**, a sequence of incompletely defined spontaneous biochemical changes, in order to be able to fertilize an ovum.

Within 1 minute following ejaculation, the seminal plasma coagulates. The coagulum, which keeps the spermatozoa in the vagina until they become hypermotile, subsequently is broken down during the next 20 to 30 minutes by proteolytic enzymes in the ejaculate. Usually the spermatozoa are maximally motile and the coagulum is completely liquefied within 1 hour of ejaculation.

Motile sperm migrate through the cervical mucus at a rate of 2 to 3 mm/min. Sperm are propelled through the female reproductive tract due to their own motility, which is the result of flagellar action, as well as to the combined effects of vaginal and uterine contractions and the negative vaginal pressure after orgasm. The contractions may be amplified by the copious amounts of 19-hydroxylated prostaglandins present in semen. The first sperm reach the fallopian tubes within 5 minutes of ejaculation, but the number of sperm in the tubes does not reach a maximum until 4 to 6 hours after ejaculation. The uterotubal junction is a major barrier to the ascent of the spermatozoa, which must reach the ampulla of the fallopian tube where fertilization occurs. Fewer than 200 of the 20 to 500 million motile sperm are present in the fallopian tubes at any one time. Spermatozoa traverse the tubes and continue out the infundibular end into the peritoneal cavity. Motile sperm usually are present in the female reproductive tract for 48 to 60 hours but have been found for up to 85 hours after intercourse.

Fertilization

Mature ova remain fertile for only up to 15 to 18 hours after ovulation. The ovum degenerates if fertilization does not occur. An ovum is often fertilized by a spermatozoon that preceded it into the ampulla of the fallopian tube. Capacitated spermatozoa lose their potential to fertilize ova within approximately 24 hours after intercourse.

When a spermatozoon encounters the cumulus-oocyte mass in the fallopian tube, the structure of the outer plasma membrane of the acrosome breaks down, and the outer acrosomal membrane becomes fenestrated in a process termed the **acrosome reaction.** This process appears to be induced by contact with the zona pellucida. It requires a high extracellular Ca^{2+} concentration that favors a massive Ca^{2+} influx. The hydrolytic enzymes such as acrosin that are released during the acrosome reaction digest the zona pellucida, permitting the spermatozoon to penetrate to the membrane of the ovum.

After penetrating the zona pellucida, the spermatozoon lies in the perivitelline space adjacent to the plasma membrane of the ovum. The plasma membrane of the equatorial portion of the sperm head fuses with the oolemma of the ovum, and microvilli of the ovum membrane surround the sperm head. The putative "sperm receptor" on the oolemma has not been identified. Fusion of the two gamete membranes causes activation of the ovum, which results in a series of biochemical events characterized by exocytosis of cortical granules and resumption of meiosis. Release of the contents of the cortical granules is followed by hardening of the zona pellucida, which may prevent **polyspermy,** the penetration of the ovum by more than one spermatozoon.

Fertilization causes the egg nucleus, which was arrested at metaphase of the second meiotic division, to complete maturation. The resulting female pronucleus and the second polar body, which is extruded into the perivitelline space, both have the haploid number of chromosomes and the haploid quantity of DNA. The sperm nucleus embedded in the cytoplasm of the ovum swells and decondenses to form the male pronculeus. DNA synthesis proceeds synchronously in both pronuclei of the zygote to duplicate the chromosomes. Fertilization is complete when the membranes of the pronuclei, which are in close contact with each other, break down, the chromosomes mingle, and mitosis and cleavage of the 1-cell zygote to a 2-cell pre-embryo occur, approximately 24 hours after fertilization.

Preimplantation Development

The zygote is the same size as the unfertilized ovum, approximately 100 to 125 μm in diameter, and still is invested by the zona pellucida. Development through the early cleavage stages progresses as the pre-embryo descends through the fallopian tube aided by ciliary motion and muscular contraction. The cryptoid surface of the oviductal lining and the spastic contractions of the estrogen-dominated isthmus portion of the tube impede movement of the pre-embryo into the uterus so that the pre-embryo is retained in the fallopian tube for approximately 3 days. Rising plasma progesterone causes the tone of the smooth muscle in the oviductal wall to decrease so that the isthmus relaxes and the pre-embryo is able to pass through the uterotubal junction into the uterus.

During the time in the fallopian tube, the pre-embryo undergoes cleavage division. The cells, or **blastomeres**, of the 2-cell, 4-cell, and 8-cell pre-embryos all are **totipotential.** In other words, at these stages of development, each cell is capable of developing into a complete human being. At the 8-cell stage, the cells undergo compaction in which the individual blastomeres become less prominent and begin to display polarity. Cells around the periphery develop microvilli on their outer surfaces. At the 16-cell **morula** stage, the cells on the inside of the pre-embryo begin to develop into the inner cell mass, which eventually develops into the fetus; the cells on the outside begin to develop into the trophectoderm, which gives rise to the extra-embryonic tissues, including the placenta and membranes. Six days after conception, when the morula consists of approximately 64 cells, a cavity, or **blastocoele**, begins to appear opposite the inner cell mass. As cells surrounding the blastocoele degenerate, the cavity enlarges and becomes filled with fluid. At this stage, termed the **blastocyst**, the inner cell mass is clearly distinguishable from the trophectoderm, which is comprised of a single layer of cells. The trophectodermal cells form giant cells that have tight junctions capable of excluding large molecules and which completely encircle the blastocyst.

Implantation of the Blastocyst

Approximately 7 days after fertilization, the blastocyst, which consists of approximately 200 cells, loses the zona pellucida in a process termed **hatching** and implants in the wall of the uterus. **Implantation**, also termed **nidation**, depends on prior conditioning of the endometrium by progesterone, which causes the stromal cells to swell and accumulate glycogen, protein, and lipids intracellularly. Administration of antiprogestins prevents implantation. The blastocyst is capable of secreting chorionic gonadotropin (hCG), which stimulates cells of the corpus luteum to produce progesterone.

The blastocyst attaches at its embryonic pole to the wall of the uterine fundus, and the microvilli of the trophecto-

dermal cells interdigitate with the microvilli on the luminal surface of the endometrial cells. The trophectodermal, or trophoblast, cells then invade through the basement membrane underlying the endometrial epithelium aided by proteolytic enzymes secreted by the blastocyst and establish an implantation site in the endometrial stroma. The stromal cells then **decidualize**; that is, they enlarge, become transcriptionally active, and surround the blastocyst. The decidual response of the uterine endometrium also involves an increase in vascular permeability around the nidation site that is thought to be mediated via local production of histamine and prostaglandins. After implantation, the embryo rapidly develops to form distinct placental and fetal structures.

Development and Function of the Placenta

The trophoblast differentiates into two layers within 11 days of fertilization. The inner layer, the **cytotrophoblast**, consists of numerous individual cells. The outer layer, the **syncytiotrophoblast**, is much thicker and resembles a continuous mass of cytoplasm containing many nuclei. This syncytium contains small spaces, or **lacunae.** The lacunae enlarge and become continuous. Early in pregnancy, the lacunae form sinuses that contain blood from the maternal uterine veins and venous sinuses eroded by the trophoblast. As the lacunae enlarge, the strands of trophoblast left between them form finger-like projections termed **villi.** Each villus consists of a core of cytotrophoblast covered with an irregular layer of syncytiotrophoblast cells. The villi become vascularized by fetal blood vessels so that the fetal capillary endothelium is in close proximity to the trophoblast cells, and fetal blood flows by the sixteenth day after fertilization. Later in pregnancy, the trophoblast erodes the maternal spiral arteries so that maternal blood flows into the intervillous spaces surrounding the villi. The placenta forms a barrier that permits exchange of nutrients, gases, and metabolic wastes without maternal blood and fetal blood ever mixing.

At term, the placenta is a disk-shaped, ovoid structure approximately 18×20 cm in diameter and 2 cm thick. It consists of (1) the inner **amnion**, which consists of a single layer of ectodermal epithelium completely enclosing the embryo, (2) the middle **chorion**, which surrounds the amnionic sac and includes the villi and trophoblast, and (3) the **decidua** of the maternal endometrium. The umbilical cord, which arises from the center of the disk, carries fetal blood between the fetus and the chorionic villi.

Transfer of Nutrients and Gases

The placenta functions principally to provide a barrier that allows nutrients to diffuse from the maternal blood supply to the developing fetus and excretory products to diffuse from the fetal blood supply to the maternal blood supply. The placenta also provides a protective barrier against microorganisms. The two principal elements in transplacental transfer of substances are (1) the maternal-facing trophoblast microvillus membrane and (2) the fetal-facing basal trophoblast membrane. These membranes regulate transfer of glucose, lactate, certain amino acids, oxygen, carbon dioxide, electrolytes, and several minerals between mother and fetus.

The net transfer of a substance from the maternal circulation to the fetal circulation is the net transplacental flux J_{net}, which follows the **Fick principle** and can be defined as

$$J_{net} = J_{mf} - J_{fm} \qquad (62-1)$$

where J_{mf} is the flux from the maternal compartment to the fetal compartment and J_{fm} is the flux from the fetal compartment to the maternal compartment. The unidirectional fluxes in each direction for a particular substance are complex processes because they are affected by (1) the rate of delivery of the substance to the placenta via the circulation, (2) the difference in the concentrations of the substance between the maternal and fetal circulations, (3) the interaction of the substance with different components of the placental barrier, and (4) the relationship of the maternal and fetal blood flows to each other.

Maternal uteroplacental blood flow increases as pregnancy progresses. The increased blood flow is due mainly to progressive vasodilation. **Nitric oxide**, which is produced abundantly in uterine and placental vascular endothelial cells as well as in syncytiotrophoblast cells, may mediate the vasodilation, since it is a potent vasodilator (see Chap. 26). It has been suggested that disorders of pregnancy such as preeclampsia, pregnancy-induced hypertension, and fetal growth retardation may be the result of decreased uteroplacental blood flow, due perhaps to defective nitric oxide synthase activity.

Small Organic Molecules

D-Glucose is transferred from mother to fetus by facilitated diffusion. There is a small but significant difference between the maternal (4.4 mmol/liter) and fetal (3.6 mmol/liter) plasma glucose concentrations. The fetal arterial plasma glucose concentration is a function of the maternal arterial or venous plasma glucose concentration up to approximately 20 mmol/liter, at which concentration the transfer mechanism becomes saturated. Glucose transfer kinetics are complicated by active glucose metabolism in the placenta itself. Moreover, some of the glucose that is metabolized in the placenta is supplied by the fetus.

Transfer of L-lactate across the placenta occurs by facilitated diffusion. Presumably transfer of lactate occurs as lactic acid, since there is evidence of cotransport of hydrogen ion. An artificially induced gradient of hydrogen ions can cause net transfer of lactic acid against its concentration gradient. Carriers that bind lactate have been demonstrated on both the maternal and fetal sides of the placenta. Pyruvic acid competes with lactic acid for the carriers. The placenta produces lactate, which is released primarily into the maternal circulation at midgestation. Near term, placental lactate is released into both the maternal and fetal circulations so that there is no net transplacental transfer of lactate.

Many amino acids are transferred across the placenta by energy-dependent active transport. It appears that amino acids are transported actively across the maternal-facing plasma membrane of the trophoblast cell. Subsequently, they diffuse across the fetal-facing plasma membrane into the fetal circulation. Neutral amino acids are transported by three systems. The A (alanine) system transports alanine, glycine, proline, serine, threonine, and glutamine. The L (leucine) system transports leucine, isoleucine, valine, and phenylalanine, as well as alanine, serine, threonine, and glutamine. The ASC (alanine-serine-cysteine) system preferentially transports alanine, serine, threonine, and glutamine. Transport mechanisms for basic and acidic amino acids have not been demonstrated. Measurements of human fetal umbilical venous-arterial plasma concentration differences indicate that there is net uptake by the fetus of at least alanine, glycine, leucine, isoleucine, phenylalanine, and histidine. In contrast to other amino acids, glutamate does not cross the placenta at physiologic concentrations. Moreover, it is removed from the fetal circulation even though concentrations of glutamate in umbilical venous plasma are greater than those in maternal plasma. The placenta releases glutamine into the umbilical circulation. Glycine and leucine appear to be produced in the placenta, since they are secreted into the umbilical circulation but removal from the maternal circulation is undetectable.

The human placenta is permeable to free fatty acids and ketones. Maternal concentrations of most free fatty acids are greater than fetal concentrations, and they appear to cross the placenta by simple diffusion. Arachidonic acid, however, is found in higher concentrations in fetal plasma than in maternal plasma. Free fatty acids that are transferred from mother to fetus rapidly are esterified to triglycerides in the fetal liver. Triglycerides do not cross the placenta. Cholesterol, which is carried in lipoprotein particles in the circulation, is transferred from mother to fetus via uptake of low-density lipoprotein particles by trophoblast cells. High-density lipoprotein is not taken up by these cells. The total concentration is lipoprotein-bound cholesterol in maternal venous plasma (230 mg/dl) is approximately 4 times that in mixed umbilical plasma (60 mg/dl) at term.

Ions

Transfer of ions and minerals between mother and fetus varies greatly both among the solutes and among species. In humans, it appears that the placenta transfers most sodium from the maternal circulation (135 mmol/kg H_2O) to the fetal circulation (137 mmol/kg H_2O) by passive diffusion. A small amount of sodium may be transported actively by cotransport with other solutes. The concentration of potassium is higher in the fetal circulation (5.7 mmol/kg H_2O) than in the maternal circulation (3.8 mmol/kg H_2O) but the transfer mechanism is not understood well. Chloride appears to be able to diffuse across the placenta with concentrations in maternal plasma (107 mmol/kg H_2O) resembling those in fetal plasma (109 mmol/kg H_2O). Both calcium and phosphorus concentrations in fetal plasma exceed those in maternal plasma, and evidence suggests that both are transferred across the placenta by active transport.

Vitamins

Most water-soluble vitamins are thought to be transferred across the placenta via specialized transport mechanisms. Lipid-soluble vitamins, in contrast, appear to diffuse freely across the placenta. In humans, transport of water-soluble vitamin C is energy-dependent and requires sodium and Na^+,K^+=ATPase activity. It is not clear whether fetal plasma concentrations of vitamin C are significantly higher than maternal plasma concentrations. Vitamin D_3 and its metabolites are present in higher concentrations in the mother than in the fetus. Administration of large quantities of 1,25-dihydroxycholecalciferol (1,25-OHD, or vitamin D) leads to elevations in fetal concentrations, but there does not appear to be net transfer of 1,25-OHD, since the placenta itself is capable of converting 25-hydroxycholecalciferol to 1,25-OHD. Vitamin B_{12} is present in higher concentrations in the fetus than in the mother and is transferred across the placenta by active transport. Other water-soluble vitamins that are present in higher concentrations in fetal plasma than in maternal plasma and which

appear to be transferred by active transport include vitamin B_6, biotin, folate, nicotinate, pantothenate, riboflavin, and thiamine.

Maternal plasma concentrations of lipid-soluble vitamin A (retinol) are more than 2.5 times those in fetal plasma at term. Retinol appears to diffuse passively through the placenta due to its lipophilicity and then to bind to retinol-binding protein (RBP). RBP also crosses the placenta but to a lesser extent than retinol itself. Since more than 90% of retinol in human fetal serum is complexed with either RBP or prealbumin, the fetal-maternal transfer rate of retinol is only one-fifth the maternal-fetal transfer rate across the placenta.

Proteins

The placenta is relatively impermeable to proteins, with the exception of certain immunoglobulins and RBP. Proteins such as albumin and small peptide hormones are not able to cross the placenta, suggesting that permeability of the placenta to hydrophilic molecules is limited by small pore size. Protein hormones such as chorionic gonadotropin and chorionic somatomammotropin (hCS) are produced by trophoblast cells and secreted into the maternal circulation. The fact that hCS and most other hormones are low in or absent from the fetal circulation indicates the existence of a barrier between placenta and fetus. Fetally produced **alpha-fetoprotein** normally is present in maternal plasma at low concentrations, indicating that it is able to cross the placenta at least to a small extent. It appears that the placental capillary wall is the effective barrier to transplacental transfer of large or medium-sized molecules, whereas the fetal surface of the trophoblast is limiting for small proteins.

Immunoglobulin G (IgG) is transferred from mother to fetus in quantitatively important amounts. Fc receptors for IgG are present on the microvillous membranes of trophoblast cells. IgG, but not other classes of immunoglobulins, is taken up by trophoblast cells by the process of **endocytosis.** Maternal antibodies can have both beneficial and deleterious effects on the fetus.

Respiratory Gases

Exchange of oxygen and carbon dioxide between mother and fetus across the placenta occurs by simple diffusion, as it does in the lungs. Oxygen dissolved in maternal blood in the placental sinuses diffuses through the cells of the villi and placental capillaries and into the fetal blood because the P_{O_2} of maternal blood in the placental sinuses is approximately 50 mmHg, whereas the P_{O_2} of blood in the umbilical vein leaving the placenta is only approximately 30 mmHg. The fetus is able to obtain sufficient oxygen at such a low oxygen tension because (1) fetal blood has approximately 50% more oxygen-carrying hemoglobin than maternal blood, (2) at a given partial pressure of oxygen (Po_2), fetal hemoglobin can carry 20% to 30% more oxygen than adult hemoglobin so that at pH 7.4 fetal hemoglobin is 80% saturated at a Po_2 of 34 mmHg (Fig. 62-1), and (3) hemoglobin can carry more oxygen at a low partial pressure of CO_2 (Pco_2) than at a high Pco_2 (Bohr effect). Transfer of oxygen and carbon dioxide is dependent in part on rates of blood flow in the uterine and umbilical circulations and the geometric relationships between these two circulations. Carbon dioxide exchange also is affected by the equilibrium between carbonic acid and bicarbonate. The Fick principle can be utilized to determine oxygen uptake by the uterus. Uterine blood flow F (ml/min) and the oxygen contents (at standard temperature and pressure, STP) of blood simultaneously drawn from a maternal artery A (ml_{STP}/ml blood) and from the uterine vein V (ml_{STP}/ml blood) are measured, and O_2 uptake by the uterus is calculated by the formula

$$O_2 \text{ uptake} = (A - V) \times F \qquad (62\text{-}2)$$

Fig. 62-1. Oxyhemoglobin dissociation curves for maternal and fetal blood at pH 7.4.

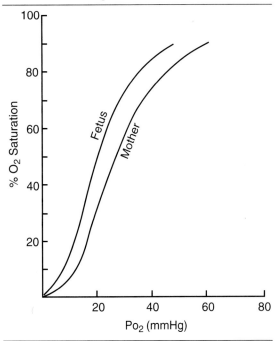

Maternal uptake by the uterus of the pregnant sheep is approximately 48 ml_{STP}/min. Similarly, oxygen uptake by the fetus can be determined by measuring umbilical blood flow f (ml/min) and the oxygen contents of blood simultaneously drawn from the umbilical artery a (ml_{STP}/ml blood) and the umbilical vein v (ml_{STP}/ml blood). O_2 uptake by the fetus is given by the formula

$$O_2 \text{ uptake} = (a - v) \times f \qquad (62\text{-}3)$$

In the pregnant sheep, O_2 uptake by the fetus is 26.5 ml_{STP}/min. It is not possible to make all the preceding measurements during pregnancy in humans. However, maternal blood flow rates to the human placenta (124 ml/min/kg uteroplacental unit) are much lower than those to the sheep placenta (288 ml/min/kg uteroplacental-fetal unit). Fetal blood flow to the placenta both in humans (120 ml/min/kg fetus) at 35 weeks of gestation and in sheep (256 ml/min/kg fetus) is similar to maternal blood flow.

Carbon dioxide formed from metabolism of oxygen must be transported via the maternal circulation to the lungs, where it is eliminated. The placental barrier membrane is highly permeable to carbon dioxide. In order for carbon dioxide to diffuse from fetus to mother, the Pco_2 of the fetal circulation must be higher than that of the maternal circulation. The Pco_2 of umbilical arterial blood is approximately 48 mmHg compared with a Pco_2 of 40 mmHg in maternal arterial blood. Thus carbon dioxide is able to diffuse across the placenta along a pressure gradient. Alterations in maternal respiration, and consequently in maternal arterial Pco_2, rapidly are reflected in the fetal circulation.

Endocrine Control of Maternal and Fetal Metabolism

Since the fetus must be nourished by the mother, the placenta secretes factors that regulate the maternal and fetal environments. Placental factors include **chorionic gonadotropin** (hCG), **chorionic somatomammotropin,** estrogens, progestins, growth factors, and a number of peptides that are either identical or similar to peptides of the hypothalamic-pituitary unit. At least, hCG, estrogens, and progestins are required for maintenance of pregnancy. In addition, secretion of anterior pituitary hormones increases to such an extent that the pituitary gland enlarges by approximately 50% during the first trimester of pregnancy and by more than 100% by term. Pituitary hormones include prolactin, adrenocorticotropin, and thyrotropin. Changes in maternal plasma concentrations of hormones are illustrated in Fig. 62-2. The importance of these hormones in maintaining pregnancy is discussed below.

Chorionic Gonadotropin

hCG is a glycosylated heterodimeric protein with a molecular weight of 38,600 produced by the syncytiotrophoblast. The α subunit synthesized in the placenta is nearly identical to the α subunits of FSH, LH, and TSH synthesized in the pituitary. The β subunit of hCG is considerably larger than the β subunits for the other hormones, consisting of 145 amino acids and having a molecular weight of 24,000. hCGβ also differs from the β subunits of FSH, LH, and TSH in the type of carbohydrate residues and its lack of sulfation. Deglycosylation of hCG increases receptor-binding potency approximately twofold, with concomitant inhibition of hCG's ability to activate adenylyl cylase.

As with FSH and LH, a single copy of the gene for the α subunit is located on chromosome 6. In striking contrast to LH, there are seven genes or pseudogenes for hCGβ on chromosome 19. Only one of the genes is transcribed, however. Translation of the mRNAs for the α and β sub-

units appears to be similar to that for the pituitary gonadotropins, since placental cells contain free α subunits and intact hCG, but little, if any, free hCGβ. Synthesis, glycosylation, and packaging occur by similar mechanisms described in the pituitary. Synthesis and secretion of hCG by the syncytiotrophoblast appear to be enhanced by gonadotropin-releasing hormone synthesized in the cytotrophoblast.

Recent evidence suggests that one of the fragments of hCGβ, termed the β **core fragment**, which is detected in both plasma and urine, may be secreted by the placenta and by hCG-producing neoplasms. The clinical utility of this peptide in monitoring treatment of hormone-producing neoplasms is under investigation.

hCG is detectable in the circulation within 8 days of conception. Peak plasma concentrations of 1000 to 2000 IU/dl are achieved around the fourteenth week of pregnancy. Fetal plasma concentrations are much lower, approximately 3 IU/dl. hCG-stimulated luteal progesterone secretion peaks around the fourth week after conception, much earlier than the peak of hCG, suggesting that the corpus luteum becomes at least partially refractory to stimulation by hCG. During early pregnancy, the placenta gradually becomes capable of secreting sufficient quantities of progesterone so that the corpus luteum no longer is needed. Consequently, hCG levels decline and the corpus luteum regresses, since by the twentieth week of pregnancy the placenta is fully developed as a steroidogenic organ.

hCG is secreted during the first trimester of pregnancy to stimulate the corpus luteum to produce progesterone, 17α-hydroxyprogesterone, and relaxin. If fertilization and implantation occur, hCG prevents decline of the corpus luteum during the menstrual cycle so that progestins can by synthesized and secreted by the corpus luteum until the placenta can assume this function. Exogenous hCG can prolong the life of the corpus luteum if fertilization and implantation do not occur. An exponential increase in hCG during the first few weeks of pregnancy is an indicator that the placenta is developing normally.

hCG stimulates progesterone biosynthesis in the fetal testes, if present. Maximal levels of testosterone in the blood of male fetuses occur during the eleventh to seventeenth weeks after conception, coinciding with peak concentrations of hCG. Moreover, hCG stimulates testosterone synthesis and DNA synthesis in fetal testes obtained during this period, thus providing androgens that stimulate male sexual differentiation, which occurs around this time.

Regulatory roles for hCG in other tissues have been suggested but not definitively proven. These include regula-

Fig. 62-2. Maternal serum concentrations of hCG, hCS, PRL, progesterone, cortisol, estrone (E_1), estradiol (E_2), and estriol (E_3) throughout pregnancy.

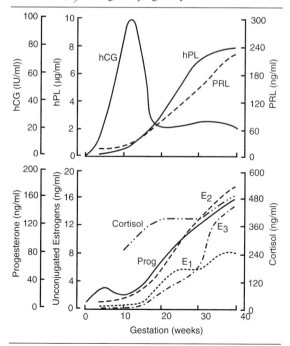

tion of steroidogenesis in both the fetal adrenal and the placenta. By virtue of its structural similarity with LH, hCG can interact with LH receptors and exert LH-like effects when administered artificially. hCG only has physiologic significance during pregnancy, however.

Metabolic clearance of hCG from the maternal circulation, is dependent on the liver and kidney. The hormone has a relatively long, biphasic rate of disappearance on the order of 24 to 36 hours, with a first component of 6 to 8 hours. The long half-life has been attributed to its high content of sialic acid and to the glycosylated carboxyterminal peptide. In contrast to intact hormone, the half-life of free α subunits is approximately 13 minutes, whereas the half-life of the free β subunits is approximately 41 minutes. Completely desialylated hCG has a plasma half-life of just a few minutes and low biologic activity in vivo because of rapid hepatic uptake.

hCG binds to specific membrane-bound receptors in cells of the corpus luteum. Since luteal cells result from luteinization of granulosa cells, the hCG receptor is identical to the LH receptor of preovulatory granulosa cells. hCG receptors gradually appear on the surface of luteal cells after disappearance, i.e., down-regulation, of LH receptors induced by the midcycle surge of LH. Signal transduction for hCG is nearly identical with that for LH, with only minor quantitative differences in the characteristics of hCG–receptor–G_s–adenylyl cyclase interactions.

Chorionic Somatomammotropin

Chorionic somatomammotropin (hCS), also referred to as **placental lactogen** (hPL), is a single-chain polypeptide consisting of 191 amino acids and having a molecular weight of 23,279 that is synthesized and secreted by the syncytiotrophoblast. Structurally, it closely resembles both growth hormone (somatatropin) and prolactin. The genes for hCS are located on chromosome 17. The hormone is present in syncytiotrophoblast by the second week after conception and is detectable in maternal plasma as early as the fourth week of gestation (0.7–0.9 μg/dl). Unlike hCG, the concentration of hCS increases throughout pregnancy in direct proportion to the weight of the placenta. Expression of hCS mRNA in syncytiotrophoblast does not change during pregnancy, suggesting that the progressive increase in hCS secretion is due to the increase in the number of syncytiotrophoblast cells. At term, plasma concentrations in the mother normally range from 0.5 to 1.5 mg/dl. hCS concentrations in the fetal circulation are very low, averaging only approximately 0.003 mg/dl. Following delivery of the placenta, hCS disappears from the maternal circulation in 10 to 12 minutes.

hCS is one of the principal regulators of maternal homeostasis during pregnancy. It causes alterations in maternal intermediary metabolism that increase the availability of glucose to the fetus. hCS enhances insulin secretion by the pancreas in response to a glucose load; however, it also increases insulin resistance; that is, it diminishes the effects of insulin on tissues such as liver. The net result is impaired glucose tolerance and elevated plasma levels of glucose. hCS also enhances lipolysis. Thus it increases concentrations of nonesterified fatty acids, ketones, and glycerol in the blood. Finally, hCS may inhibit secretion of growth hormone by the pituitary, which is depressed during pregnancy. Although the hormone has lactogenic properties and may have mammotropic effects, it does not appear to be involved in milk production in humans.

No secretagogues that regulate hCS secretion by human placental cells have been identified. However, arachidonic acid and phospholipase A_2, which catalyzes cleavage of arachidonic acid from membrane phospholipids, stimulate (1) intracellular calcium mobilization, (2) hydrolysis of phosphoinositides to diacylglycerols and inositol phosphates, and (3) release of hCS. Diacylglycerols increase protein kinase C activity and the synthesis and secretion of hCS, and inositol triphosphate mobilizes calcium. Thus arachidonic acid might mediate stimulation of synthesis and secretion of hCS by an unidentified secretagogue by causing hydrolysis of phosphoinositides to diacylglycerols and inositol phosphates, which, in turn, increase protein kinase C activity and calcium mobilization leading to increased synthesis and secretion of hCS.

Steroid Hormones

Throughout gestation from implantation to parturition, progestins, androgens, and estrogens are important to both the mother and the fetus. Steroid hormones are synthesized, metabolized, and excreted by mechanisms that involve the mother, the placenta, and the fetus (Fig. 62-3).

Progesterone is synthesized by the maternal-placental unit. Maternal plasma concentrations of progesterone and urinary excretion of its metabolite pregnanediol do not change following fetal death in utero, indicating that progesterone biosynthesis is independent of fetal steriodogenesis. Maternal plasma progesterone concentrations range from 4 μg/dl during the first trimester to 16 μg/dl during the third trimester. At term, approximately 90% of the 250 mg produced each day by the placenta is secreted into the maternal circulation and 10% into the fetal circulation. During the first 6 weeks of gestation, maternal plasma progesterone is produced by the corpus luteum. During the eighth to ninth weeks, progesterone production shifts

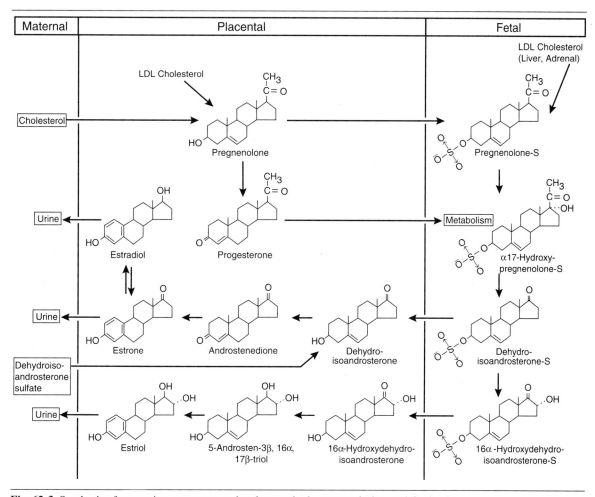

Fig. 62-3. Synthesis of progestins, estrogens, and androgens in the maternal-placental-fetal unit.

(luteal-placental shift) to the placenta. As in the corpus luteum, progesterone is synthesized from cholesterol obtained by uptake of low-density lipoprotein by trophoblast cells. Cholesterol is converted to pregnenolone through the action of cytochrome P_{450} enzyme–dependent side-chain cleavage and hydroxylation by mitochondrial enzymes. Pregnenolone is converted to progesterone by the microsomal enzymes 3β-hydroxysteroid dehydrogenase and $\Delta^{5,4}$-isomerase. Progesterone synthesis is stimulated by beta-adrenergic agonists, whose effects are mediated via cAMP and are inhibited by GnRH. Since the placenta does not possess the 17-hydroxylase enzyme, maternal plasma concentrations of 17α-hydroxyprogesterone are very low in midpregnancy. In early pregnancy, maternal 17α-hy-

droxyprogesterone is produced in the corpus luteum. After the thirty-second week of pregnancy, maternal plasma concentrations of 17α-hydroxyprogesterone increase due to production by the fetal adrenal gland.

Progesterone has several actions crucial to initiation and maintenance of pregnancy: (1) It prepares the uterine endometrium for implantation, (2) it promotes decidualization of the endometrial cells to provide nourishment for the early embryo, (3) it acts synergistically with relaxin to reduce uterine contractility and sensitivity to oxytocin during pregnancy, and (4) it promotes development of the mammary glands prior to lactation.

Androgens are synthesized by the maternal and fetal adrenal glands but not by the placenta, which lacks the 17-

hydroxylase and 17,20-desmolase enzymes necessary to convert C_{21} steroids (progestins) to C_{19} steroids (androgens). The placenta takes up both dehydroepiandrosterone (DHEA; also known as **dehydroisoandrosterone**) and dehydroepiandrosterone sulfate (DS) from the maternal and fetal circulations. Sulfate is cleaved from the latter to yield DHEA, which, in turn, is converted to androstenedione (A) and testosterone (T). Maternal plasma levels of DS and DHEA remain virtually unchanged throughout pregnancy, whereas levels of A and T increase two- to threefold. A and T serve as substrates for aromatase, which converts the androgens to estrogens.

Esterone (E_1) and estradiol (E_2) are synthesized in syncytiotrophoblast cells from A and T via the action of the cytochrome P_{450}–dependent aromatase enzyme. Estradiol concentrations in maternal plasma increase throughout pregnancy, reaching levels of 2 to 3 µg/dl. Estriol (E_3) is not formed from estradiol or estrone because the placenta lacks 16-hydroxylase. However, copious amounts of E_3 are formed from 16α-hydroxydehydroepiandrosterone of fetal adrenal origin. Concentrations of E_3 in maternal plasma are very low during the first trimester but then are similar to E_1 levels for the duration of pregnancy. Estrogens are very important in the mother during pregnancy. They promote relaxation of the pelvic ligaments and elasticity of the public symphysis so that the fetus can pass through the birth canal at parturition. Estrogens also are necessary for enlargement of the breasts and for growth of the ductule system and lobule-alveolar tissue of the breasts. Finally, estrogens cause enlargement of both the uterus and of the external genitalia of the mother.

Other Placental Factors

Several peptides that are identical to hypothalamic peptides are present in placenta. Gonadotropin-releasing hormone (GnRH) is synthesized in cytotrophoblast, which is close to the syncytiotrophoblast, the site of synthesis of hCG and hCS. GnRH is able to stimulate placental production of hCG. Synthesis of GnRH in the placenta may be inhibited by inhibin, which also is present in cytotrophoblast.

Both adrenocorticotropin (ACTH) and corticotropin-releasing hormone (CRH), as well as the ACTH-related pro-opiomelanocortin-derived peptides such as beta-lipotropin, alpha-melanocyte–stimulating hormone, and beta-endorphin, are synthesized in the placenta. The presence of placental ACTH in the maternal circulation contributes to the mother's relative resistance to negative feedback suppression of ACTH by glucocorticoids. Levels of ACTH in maternal plasma are similar in the first and third trimesters, whereas levels of CRH in both maternal and fetal plasma rise progressively during pregnancy.

The human placenta produces both a chorionic thyrotropin (hCT) and thyrotropin-releasing hormone (TRH), whose physiologic importance has not been established. Somatostatin- and growth hormone–releasing hormone-like activities have been identified in placenta.

Prolactin

Prolactin (PRL) is a single-chain polypeptide produced by specialized cells (**lactotropes**) of the anterior pituitary gland. In humans, the hormone also is synthesized in the decidua but not in the placenta. Structurally, PRL is very similar to growth hormone and hCS. The glycosylated form has a molecular weight of 25,000, whereas the non-glycosylated form has a molecular weight of 23,000. The gene that encodes the mRNA for PRL is located on chromosome 6. Preprolactin, the precursor form of PRL, is synthesized on ribosomes in the endoplasmic reticulum, processed to the mature form, and then stored in secretory granules.

Prolactin is secreted in males and in both pregnant and nonpregnant females. During pregnancy, maternal plasma PRL concentrations gradually begin to rise in the first trimester and by term reach levels 10 times nonpregnant levels, or approximately 12 µg/dl. This increase is coincident with increased plasma estrogen concentrations. After parturition, basal plasma PRL concentrations return to nonpregnant levels.

Synthesis and secretion of PRL by pituitary lactotropes are regulated by hypothalamic factors and by estrogen. The hypothalamus secretes **dopamine**, a neurotransmitter, that inhibits pituitary but not decidual PRL secretion. There is substantial physiologic evidence for a PRL-releasing factor (PRF), but it has not yet been identified. Thyrotropin-releasing hormone (TRH) stimulates prolactin secretion. Thus individuals with primary hypothyroidism (elevated TRH and TSH) can have hyperprolactinemia. Estrogens enhance PRL production by increasing the amount of preprolactin mRNA. Estrogen also increases the size (hypertrophy) and number (hyperplasia) of lactotropes in the pituitary. In both nonpregnant and pregnant states, maternal PRL secretion is pulsatile, with the magnitude of the pulses being greater during sleep. Chronic excessive secretion of prolactin (hyperprolactinemia) in nonpregnant women can lead to abnormal production of mild (galactorrhea) and absence of menses (amenorrhea).

The fetal pituitary also synthesizes, stores, and secretes PRL beginning early in gestation. Secretion is highest, however, late in gestation, when PRL levels in fetal plasma exceed those in maternal plasma. Although the physiologic role of PRL in the fetus is unknown, evidence suggests that it promotes fetal lung maturation by increasing levels of pulmonary lecithin, a component of surfactant. PRL is present in very high concentrations in amniotic fluid, which has PRL concentrations 5- to 10-fold greater than those in maternal serum. Decidual prolactin synthesis can account for the PRL in amniotic fluid. PRL is not synthesized in the trophoblast or amnion. Since experimental intraamniotic injection of PRL in monkeys can cause a 50% decrease in amniotic fluid volume, PRL may be an osmoregulator in the amniotic fluid compartment of the fetal-placental unit. Prolactin promotes growth of the mammary glands, initiates postpartum milk delivery, and maintains milk secretion during lactation.

Maternal Physiology

During pregnancy, maternal physiology is reorganized to simultaneously accommodate the metabolic demands of the fetus and prepare the mother for delivery of the fetus and postpartum nourishment of the neonate. Reorganization of maternal function occurs first in response to maternal reproductive hormones and then in response to hormones of the fetal-placental unit. Major changes occur in water and electrolyte balance, cardiovascular function, respiration, and metabolism.

Maternal blood volume expands by approximately 40% during pregnancy. Plasma volume begins to increase early in pregnancy and then more rapidly during the second trimester; it increases only slightly during the third trimester. Increased plasma is required to supply the utero-fetal-placental unit with an adequate blood supply and to protect the mother against the blood loss associated with delivery. A human mother loses an average of 500 ml of blood during a vaginal delivery. Expansion of maternal blood volume appears to be due to retention of both water and minerals by the kidneys. During the course of pregnancy, an extra 500 to 900 meq of sodium, 300 meq of potassium, and 30 meq of calcium are retained above normal. Since a proportionately greater amount of water, 4 to 6 liters, is retained, the sodium concentration in the maternal circulation decreases during pregnancy. Although the mechanism of pregnancy-induced electrolyte and water retention has not been defined precisely, estrogens and progesterone both increase plasma concentrations of aldosterone, the adrenal cortical hormone that promotes sodium retention, and increase total-body water. Red blood cell volume in the maternal circulation begins to in-

crease during the second trimester, with the greatest increase occurring in the third trimester.

Cardiac output increases during pregnancy in order to maintain arterial blood pressure and achieve adequate uterine blood flow in the face of decreased peripheral vascular resistance due to vasodilation. Maternal resting cardiac output reaches a peak by the twentieth week of pregnancy, at which time it has increased an average of 40%, from 5 to 7 liters/min. Increased cardiac output is due both to increased heart rate and to increased stroke volume. The increase in cardiac output is necessary to compensate for the proportionately greater decline in peripheral vascular resistance, which reaches its lowest level in midpregnancy.

Blood flow to the uterus increases as pregnancy advances and has been estimated to approach 1200 ml/min, or 17% of maternal cardiac output, in humans near term. Since uterine blood flow increases more slowly than the size of the fetal-placental unit, the rate of oxygen extraction from uterine blood increases during pregnancy.

Maternal oxygen consumption increases during pregnancy to meet the energy requirements for maternal and fetal metabolism and synthesis of new tissue. The maternal metabolic rate is higher at term than in the nonpregnant state. Basal oxygen consumption increases by approximately 51 ml O_2 per minute, or 20% of the total maternal oxygen uptake at term. Oxygen uptake is achieved via an increase in minute ventilation, which is increased, in turn, by an increase in tidal volume without an increase in respiratory rate. Plasma bicarbonate concomitantly is reduced to offset the respiratory alkalosis that would result from this hyperventilation.

The average net energy cost of pregnancy has been estimated to be 77,000 kcal. It is comprised of (1) the caloric value of maternal and fetal tissues formed during pregnancy, (2) the energy required for the biosynthetic processes themselves, (3) the energy required to maintain newly formed tissues, and (4) the energy required for transport and exchange of nutrients and gases among the mother, placenta, and fetus. Maternal metabolism fulfills these energy requirements not only for pregnancy itself but also to provide the fetus with adequate energy stores to survive during the immediate postnatal period and to provide the mother with adequate energy to nourish the fetus in the event of diminished food intake.

Parturition

A mature fetus is expelled from the uterus, normally at term, by a process referred to as **parturition.** The mechanism of parturition in humans is not understood completely. The lack of understanding is due, in part, to the major differences among mammalian species in the types and quantities of hormones that are secreted near term. It is clear that initiation of parturition, or **labor**, is not a function of the maturity of the fetus itself, since labor frequently occurs before (**preterm**) the fetus is fully developed. Rather, it appears to result from maturation of a complex system of communication among various endocrine organs.

Regulatory Factors

Parturition is the culmination of processes that occur throughout pregnancy to prepare the reproductive tract for expulsion of the fetus. Near term, the uterus becomes progressively more excitable. Rhythmic contractions of the uterus increase in frequency and intensity to the level where the fetus is forcefully expelled from the uterus. **Estradiol**, **progesterone**, **relaxin**, **prostaglandins**, **oxytocin**, and **catecholamines** all play roles in the chronic and/or acute regulation of cellular processes prior to parturition. In contrast with other species, in humans, adrenal glucocorticoids do not appear to play a major role in parturition. The primary signal for initiation of parturition has not been established.

Estradiol and Progesterone

Estradiol and progesterone have opposite permissive effects on uterine contractility. The plasma concentrations of both hormones increase during the first 7 months of pregnancy. During the last 2 months, however, progesterone concentrations stabilize, whereas estrogen concentrations continue to increase. As a woman approaches term, levels of estrone sulfate, which can be converted to estradiol and estrone in chorion and decidua, increase in amniotic fluid. Estrogens themselves inhibit synthesis of progesterone from pregnenolone. Thus the estrogen-progesterone ratio increases during the 2 months preceding parturition.

Estrogens also promote parturition in part by inhibiting production of PGI_2, an inhibitory prostaglandin, and enhancing production of stimulatory prostaglandins such as PGE_2 and $PGF_{2\alpha}$ in the decidua. Estrogens increase the concentration of oxytocin receptors in the myometrium, resulting in increased myometrial sensitivity to oxytocin in late pregnancy. They also promote formation of gap junctions between myometrial cells, leading to increased electrical coupling among cells.

Relaxin

During pregnancy, a 23,000 molecular weight polypeptide is produced in the corpus luteum, the placenta, and the de-

cidua of the uterus. This polypeptide, **preprorelaxin**, is processed by proteolytic enzymes to yield the active relaxin molecule, which has a molecular weight of 6300. Structurally, it resembles insulin in that it consists of two dissimilar chains with some homology with insulin and insulin-like growth factors. The two relaxin chains are held together by disulfide bonds located in similar positions as those in the insulin molecule. The mRNA for the preprorelaxin molecule is encoded by two genes located on the short arm of chromosome 9, though only one of the genes is known to be actively transcribed during pregnancy.

The corpus luteum in the ovary is the major source of relaxin in the peripheral circulation during pregnancy. Uterine decidual tissue and placental tissue produce lesser amounts of the hormone that may act locally within the uterus. Peripheral blood levels of relaxin are elevated throughout most of gestation, but they are highest near the end of the first trimester, reaching concentrations of greater than 0.1 µg/dl and then declining to and remaining stable at less than 0.05 µg/dl during the twenty-fifth to thirty-ninth weeks of gestation. Corpora lutea produce relaxin in response to hCG. Circulating levels of relaxin are directly related to the amount of circulating hCG and to the number of corpora lutea present in the ovary. Relaxin is not detectable in plasma in the nonpregnant state.

Relaxin has several effects on the reproductive tract, although its importance in humans has not been established as well as its role in other mammalian species. Relaxin first appears to inhibit myometrial contractility throughout pregnancy in order to maintain the uterus in a quiescent state so that the fetus is not expelled prematurely. Second, it causes relaxation of the pelvic ligaments, leading to separation of the pubic symphysis. In women, pubic separation is detectable by the end of the first month of pregnancy, is near maximal by the fifth to seventh months, and then is relatively constant during the last 2 to 3 months. Third, relaxin is one of the factors that enhances softening of the cervix in preparation for passage of the fetus. This softening, or "ripening," of the cervix involves an increase in water content, a decrease in collagen content, and an increase in total glycosaminoglycan content, which includes a decrease in sulfated glycosaminoglycans. The effects of relaxin on the pubic symphysis and on the cervix require prior sensitization by estrogen.

Oxytocin

Oxytocin is a nonapeptide (9 amino acids) that stimulates secretion of the prostaglandins PGE_2 and $PGF_{2\alpha}$ from the decidua. It is synthesized by neurons whose cell bodies are located in the supraoptic and paraventricular nuclei of the hypothalamus. The hormone is transported through the axons bound to the protein neurophysin I to nerve endings in the neurohypophysis, or posterior pituitary gland, where it is secreted. Since it is undetectable in plasma until after the beginning of parturition, its function probably is to enhance rather than to initiate parturition. Uterine responsiveness to oxytocin is enhanced by estrogen, which could account for the 12-fold increase in myometrial oxytocin receptors that occurs between the thirteenth and seventeenth weeks of pregnancy and term.

Prostaglandins

Prostaglandins, also termed **eicosanoids**, are thought to comprise the most important signal for parturition because (1) they increase in concentration in amniotic fluid at parturition, (2) administration of prostaglandin synthase inhibitors such as aspirin suppresses uterine activity and prolongs pregnancy, and (3) the myometrium is very sensitive to exogenous prostaglandins. Prostaglandins E_2 and $F_{2\alpha}$ can increase myometrial contractility throughout pregnancy. They appear to modulate calcium fluxes in myometrial smooth muscle fibers. $PGF_{2\alpha}$ inhibits calcium uptake by the sarcoplasmic reticulum so that cytoplasmic calcium concentrations increase. Increased intracellular calcium leads to activation of **myosin light-chain kinase** (MLCK), a critical enzyme in myometrial contraction. MLCK catalyzes phosphorylation of the myosin light chain. The high-energy phosphate bond of phosphorylated myosin is hydrolyzed, providing the energy for cross-linking of myosin and actin that results in shortening of the myometrial smooth muscle cell.

PGE_2 is synthesized in both amnion and decidua; little, if any, PGE_2 is synthesized in chorion. $PGF_{2\alpha}$ can be formed from (1) PGE_2 from amnion, (2) arachidonic acid released from amnion, and (3) de novo synthesis of **arachidonic acid** in decidua. Arachidonic acid is liberated from its intercellular esterified storage form by the action of phospholipase A_2, a lysosomal enzyme whose regulation by a variety of stimulators is only beginning to be understood.

Mechanism

Delivery of the fetus, or labor, is the result of sustained, rhythmic, and coordinated contractions of uterine smooth muscle and can be divided into three phases. The first phase extends from the first uterine contractions to complete dilatation of the cervix. The second phase extends from complete cervical dilatation to birth of the infant. The third phase extends from delivery of the infant to delivery of the placenta. The three phases last a total, on average, of 14 hours for a woman's first delivery.

Unlike other muscular contractions, uterine contractions of labor are painful. Contractions occur approximately 10 minutes apart during the first stage of parturition; the interval decreases to as little as 2 minutes during the second stage. Each contraction typically lasts 60 seconds. During labor, the cervix shortens in length and dilates so that the diameter of the external cervical os, the opening to the uterus, increases from a few millimeters to approximately 10 cm. As labor progresses, the fetal membranes rupture, and amniotic fluid is released. Delivery of the infant follows as the upper portion of the uterus thickens and continues to contract strongly.

Lactation

Postpartum growth, development, and survival of the newborn require nourishment, which is provided for a variable period of time by the mother's milk. Milk is produced in the mammary glands of the appropriately conditioned breasts. It is delivered to the infant in response to the mechanical and neural stimuli that constitute the suckling reflex.

Development of the Breasts and Mammary Glands

Throughout gestation, the mammary glands grow and develop in response to the coordinated actions of pituitary, ovarian, thyroid, and adrenal hormones. During the first and second trimesters, estrogens, growth hormone, and glucocorticoids synergize to stimulate growth of the mammary ductal system. Stromal tissue increases, but there is some loss of interstitial adipose tissue. The terminal portions of the mammary glands enlarge, the breasts become more vascularized, and the nipples enlarge. During the second and third trimesters of pregnancy, the lobuloalevolar epithelium of the mammary gland differentiates and acquires the capacity to synthesize milk in a process termed **lactogenesis.** Lobuloalveolar development requires estrogen, progesterone, and prolactin. Lactogenesis during pregnancy is minimal, however, and lactation is absent because estrogens and progesterone inhibit actual formation of milk.

Synthesis and Secretion of Milk

In the final month of pregnancy, the parenchymal cells of the mammary glandular alveoli hypertrophy due to intracellular accumulation of a hyaline, eosinophilic, proteinaceous, low-fat secretion termed **colostrum.** It has the following composition: 87% water, 1.3% fat, 3.2% lactose, 7.9% protein (principally alpha-lactalbumin, lactoferrin, and immunoglobulin A), and 0.6% mineral-containing ash. Colostrum has a higher protein content but a lower carbohydrate content than mature human milk. Within 2 to 3 days after parturition and the decline of estrogens and progesterone in maternal plasma, the fat content of the mammary secretion increases abruptly, and it becomes milk.

Human milk is an emulsion of fat in water that is isotonic with plasma. It has the following composition: 87% water, 4.5% fat, 6.8% lactose, 0.9% casein, 0.4% lactalbumin and other proteins, and 0.2% mineral-containing ash. It has an energy content of 60 to 75 kcal/dl. Milk is not secreted before parturition because estrogen and progesterone secreted by the placenta block the lactogenic effects of prolactin and hCS. At birth, the mammary glands are released from the inhibitory effects of the estrogen and progesterone. The lactogenic effects of prolactin result in synthesis of milk rather than colostrum by the mammary glands. Other hormones such as glucocorticoids, growth hormone, and thyroid hormone appear to be important in regulating the composition of milk. Production of milk can reach 1.5 liters/day.

Prolactin

Prolactin stimulates several important biochemical processes in milk synthesis and thus is the most important hormone for lactogenesis. Prolactin stimulates cells of the mammary glandular epithelium to synthesize the milk proteins casein and alpha-lactalbumin. Administration of the dopamine agonist 2-bromo-α-ergocryptine in the immediate postpartum period causes prolactin levels to drop and breast engorgement and lactation to cease. The first step in the interaction of prolactin with target cells is binding to cell surface receptors, which leads to increased expression of genes for milk proteins and RNA synthesis. However, the intermediate steps in prolactin action are not known. Similarly, it is not known how estrogens and progesterone block the stimulatory effects of prolactin on lactogenesis.

Basal prolactin levels in maternal plasma gradually return to nonpregnant levels within several weeks after birth. Stimulation of the nipples by the infant's suckling, however, causes a transient 10-fold increase in prolactin secretion that lasts approximately 1 hour each time suckling occurs. These repeated prolactin surges provide the stimulus for continued lactogenesis. If the prolactin surges are blocked or absent, they disappear within a few days. Thus, if the mother does not nurse, prolactin surges gradually disappear, and lactogenesis ceases.

Suckling and Milk Ejection

Milk is continuously synthesized and secreted into the lumina of the aleveoli. Milk does not flow readily from the alveoli to the duct system so that milk does not leak out of the nipple. The 12 to 20 lactiferous ducts, or **galactophores**, leading into the nipple are dilated to form sinuses. Most milk, however, is stored in the alevoli. Milk is ejected from the alveoli, or let down, only in response to suckling by the infant. The mammary glands contain contractile tissue consisting of (1) myoepithelial cells surrounding the alveoli and small ducts and (2) smooth muscle surrounding the larger milk ducts and blood vessels. The myoepithelial cells generate the major expulsive force during milk ejection.

The suckling reflex that controls milk ejection involves neurogenic and hormonal signals including the hormone oxytocin (Fig. 62-4). Mechanical stimulation of the nipple generates impulses that are transmitted to the spinal cord through the dorsal roots of the spinal nerves. The neural pathways terminate in the paraventricular and supraoptic nuclei of the hypothalamus. Oxytocin synthesized by neurosecretory cells in these nuclei and secreted from the posterior lobe of the pituitary gland stimulates myoepithelial cells surrounding each alveolus to contract, thus expelling milk. Milk ejection usually occurs within 30 seconds to a minute after a baby begins to suckle. Although milk ejection occurs primarily in response to suckling, it can be conditioned. For example, sight of the infant, crying by the infant, or breast preparation can cause milk ejection, whereas embarrassment or pain can inhibit it.

Postpartum Changes in the Mother

The 4- to 5-week period between delivery and resumption of ovulation and menstruation is referred to as the **puerperium.** It begins immediately after delivery of the placenta. The uterus rapidly involutes and decreases in size as a result of frequent strong myometrial contractions. Within a week, it has decreased in size by 50% and by 6 weeks it has decreased almost to its nonpregnant size. By the sixteenth day, the endometrium resembles that of the nonpregnant uterus in the proliferative phase of the menstrual cycle. The placental site of the endometrium requires several more weeks to recover. In gross appearance, the cervix resembles that in the nonpregnant state within 1 week postpartum, although involution continues until at least 6 weeks. The vagina returns to its normal nonpregnant state in 6 to 10 weeks postpartum.

Ovulatory function returns only gradually after parturi-

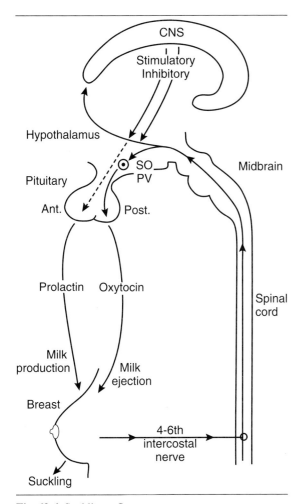

Fig. 62-4. Suckling reflex.

tion. The mechanism for postpartum amenorrhea is unknown. However, gonadotropin secretion, which is necessary for ovarian function, is minimal for 2 to 3 weeks after delivery. The initial ovulation can occur as early as 27 days after delivery. In nonlactating women, the initial ovulation occurs at a mean of 10 weeks; in nursing women, the initial ovulation occurs at a mean of 17 weeks. Women who breast-feed for less than 28 days ovulate at approximately the same time as women who do not breast-feed at all. In nonlactating women, the mean time to the first postpartum menses is 7 to 9 weeks, with 70% having menstruated within 12 weeks. In lactating women, the time of the first postpartum menses increases as the duration of lactation increases. Prolactin, which is secreted in response to suckling, inhibits ovarian function either directly or indirectly via inhibition of the hypothalamic-pituitary unit.

Maternal metabolism generally, but not always, returns to normal within 6 to 8 weeks after parturition. Cardiac output and blood volume, which increase greatly during pregnancy, and peripheral vascular resistance, which decreases during pregnancy, return to baseline within 6 weeks after delivery. Most of the regression in parameters of cardiovascular function, such as heart rate, blood pressure, oxygen consumption, and total-body water, occurs during the first 2 weeks. Parameters of renal function, such as renal plasma flow, glomerular filtration rate, and serum creatinine clearance, increase during pregnancy and return to normal levels by 6 weeks postpartum. Liver function, which is altered by rising levels of estrogens during pregnancy, appears to be normal within 3 weeks of delivery.

Summary

Fusion of male and female gametes and subsequent development of the offspring occur in the reproductive tract of the female. Spermatozoa are delivered from the penis of the male into the female reproductive tract through the vagina during coitus, the sexual act. If conception, or fertilization of an ovum by a spermatozoon, occurs, the resulting zygote begins to undergo a series of profound changes that enable it to develop into a full-term fetus. The conceptus, which develops in the uterus, regulates its environment via specific humoral signals. During the developmental period, which usually lasts approximately 39 weeks and is termed gestation or pregnancy, maternal metabolism is reoriented toward providing nutrients to the conceptus. Pregnancy culminates in parturition, the process by which the fetus is expelled from the uterus. Further development and maturation of the infant, or neonate, occur outside the body of the mother. For several months after birth, the neonate receives nutritional support in the form of breast milk from the mother. Development and maturation of the offspring are not completed until puberty.

Bibliography

Creasy, R. K., and Resnik, R., eds. *Maternal-Fetal Medicine: Principles and Practice.* Philadelphia: W. B. Saunders, 1989.

Knobil, E., Neill, J. D., Ewing, L. L., et al., eds. *The Physiology of Reproduction.* New York: Raven Press, 1988.

Sadler, T. W. *Langman's Medical Embryology.* Baltimore: Williams and Wilkins, 1985.

Steven, D. H., ed. *Comparative Placentation: Essays in Structure and Function.* New York: Academic Press, 1975.

Part X Questions: Reproductive Physiology

1. The mullerian-inhibiting hormone is
   A. required for differentiation of the wolffian (mesonephric) ducts.
   B. synthesized and secreted by Sertoli (sustentacular) cells.
   C. synthesized and secreted by Leydig (interstitial) cells.
   D. secreted in response to human chorionic gonadotropin.
   E. a small-molecular-weight decapeptide.

2. LH and FSH levels in the fetal circulation increase around the middle of pregnancy because
   A. the hypothalamus of the mother secretes increased amounts of GnRH.
   B. the fetal pituitary is sensitive to the positive feedback effects of steroid hormones.
   C. the fetal hypothalamic-pituitary unit is able to secrete gonadotropins but is not yet sensitive to the negative feedback effects of steroid hormones.
   D. the placenta has acquired the capacity to synthesize LH and FSH.
   E. All of the above

3. Which of the following is *not* a precursor in the synthesis of 17β-estradiol in the ovary?
   A. Androstenedione
   B. Testosterone
   C. Cholesterol
   D. Pregnenolone
   E. Estriol

4. FSH and LH
   A. both are required for development of ovarian follicles.
   B. secretions by the anterior pituitary gland are modulated by inhibin.
   C. are glycosylated heterodimeric proteins that bind to membrane-bound receptors.
   D. concentrations in the plasma reach peak levels during the early follicular phase of the menstrual cycle.
   E. None of the above

5. Inhibin is a male hormone that
   A. is a lipophilic steroid.
   B. is synthesized in the interstitial cells between the seminiferous tubules.
   C. suppresses production of FSH but not of LH.
   D. reduces the frequency of pulsatile secretion of GnRH by the hypothalamus.
   E. is produced in response to testosterone.

6. In the male, FSH
   A. binds to receptors on primary spermatocytes, causing them to enter meiosis.
   B. concentrations in plasma are independent of hypothalamic GnRH secretion.
   C. stimulates Sertoli cells to synthesize inhibin and androgen-binding protein.
   D. concentrations in plasma decrease after removal of the testes (castration).
   E. All of the above

7. Biosynthesis of steroid hormones during pregnancy
   A. involves conversion of progestins to androgens by the placenta.
   B. involves a shift of progesterone production from the corpus luteum of the ovary to the chorion during the eighth to ninth weeks of gestation.
   C. is regulated by chorionic somatomammotropin (hCS).
   D. involves rapid 16-hydroxylation of estradiol to estriol in syncytiotrophoblast cells of the placenta.
   E. is inhibited by dehydroepiandrosterone and dehydroepiandrosterone sulfate of maternal and fetal origin.

8. Which of the statements is *incorrect*?
   A. The human fetus secretes hormones that initiate parturition when it has reached maturity.
   B. Placental synthesis and secretion of chorionic gonadotropin (hCG) reach a maximum around the twelfth week of gestation and then decline.
   C. Estrogens promote parturition by increasing myometrial sensitivity to oxytocin and by enhancing production of prostaglandins E_2 and $F_{2\alpha}$.
   D. Relatively little prostaglandin E_2 is formed in the chorion.
   E. None of the above

XI Adaptation and Exercise Physiology

Part Editor

Ernest C. Foulkes

63 Physiologic Compensation and Adaptation

Ernest C. Foulkes

Objectives

After reading this chapter, you should be able to

Distinguish between compensation and adaptation

Describe the extent to which humans can respond to environmental challenges

Describe the difference between physiologic and behavioral responses

Discuss the physiologic responses to heat, cold, high altitude, high pressure, and microgravity

---

Intact organisms, and especially **homeotherms** like mammals, can within limits **compensate** for, or **adapt** to, considerable changes in the environment and thereby continue to maintain **steady-state** (**homeostasis**). Humans, for example, respond to environmental challenges such as heat and cold, pressure, partial anoxia, absence of gravity, physical exercise, dietary changes, environmental pollution, and others. Physiologic responses to acute exposures differ from those elicited by chronic exposures; they may consist of metabolic changes like synthesis of new proteins (e.g., the so-called stress proteins, including the metal-binding metallothionein, new enzyme molecules, etc.) or of some of the many functional changes listed below under the subheading, "Specific Adverse Conditions."

The concept of challenge and response has proven useful in many fields of study. Within the present context, the ability to maintain homeostasis by adapting to or compensating for an environmental challenge is restricted to limited exposure ranges. If these limits are exceeded, pathologic consequences such as hypothermia, heat shock, acute mountain sickness, etc., may supervene.

The discussion here focuses on human physiologic compensation, a rapid short-term process, and slower but longer-lasting **physiologic adaptation** to selected environmental challenges. On the other hand, **cultural, psycho-**

logical, and **behavioral adaptations**, such as the institution of a siesta during the hottest part of the day, lie beyond the scope of this chapter. Nor will the chapter refer to genetic adaptation of whole populations to adverse environments.

The ability to compensate or adapt to a new environment may be limited by internal or external factors. For instance, the normal response to heat is abolished in the absence of adequate salt and water intake. Under suitable conditions, and as discussed in more detail in the appropriate chapters, function of many systems in the body can respond to environmental changes and thus help maintain homeostasis. Thus the kidney conserves water during dehydration. The intestine responds to hypoglycemia or an increased oral carbohydrate load by increased rates of sugar absorption; this rise in glucose transport does not reach maximal levels for 1 to 2 weeks after increased loading. Physiologic responses to selected environmental challenges are discussed below under separate subheadings.

Compensation

When facing acute environmental challenges, organisms must respond rapidly in order to maintain homeostasis. Appropriate **physiologic compensation** such as an acute sweating response thus permits survival for a limited time at the temperature of the dry sauna (100°C or above). Reflex compensation is characterized by rapid onset and by its cessation as soon as the stimulus disappears and/or any deviation from the normal steady-state has been corrected. Hyperventilation, for instance, continues after strenuous exercise until any O_2 debt that may have been incurred has been discharged.

Table 63-1 illustrates how compensation represents the attempt to maintain, or to return to, a preset steady-state. Here a normal subject is shown whose core body temperature after strenuous exercise had risen to 39°C (transient exercise hyperthermia). The second subject is a patient with fever of 39°C. Both subjects are at rest at an ambient temperature of 31°C; this represents the **neutral temperature** (see under subheading "Heat," below) for the control subject but lies below that of the feverish patient. The feverish patient therefore attempts to conserve heat by vasoconstriction and may even shiver to produce heat. In contrast, the control subject dissipates by vasodilation and sweating what in this instance represents excess heat.

Renal function, respiration, the cardiovascular system, and others all compensate for changes in the environment in such a way that the body can either maintain steady-state or at least rapidly return to it at the end of the stimulus. Compensation in each case is characterized by rapid onset and by cessation as soon as the steady-state has returned to normal at the end of the stimulus or soon thereafter. There is little memory effect; i.e., repetition of the stimulus will elicit the same response as the first one.

Adaptation

Adaptation to a sustainable environmental stress differs from compensation: It is a gradual process, influenced by earlier experience, leading after relatively prolonged exposure to improvement in the efficiency of compensation. This result may involve achievement of new steady-state levels. For instance, prolonged exposure to the low P_{O_2} of high altitudes stimulates production of erythropoietin and synthesis of red cells, as well as other responses; the increased steady-state hematocrit helps counteract effects of partial anoxia.

The hematocrit does not immediately fall to control values upon return to sea level; i.e., there is a definite memory effect. Loss of adaptation (deadaptation) resembles adaptation. Both are slow processes triggered by prolonged or frequently repeated changes in the environment. Table 63-2 documents the fact that several years were required after the introduction of protective diving suits before Korean sponge divers had finally lost their ability to enter water colder than 29.9°C (the critical temperature for unadapted controls) without shivering; note the somewhat more rapid fall of the basal metabolic rate to control levels.

Even though most adaptive changes occur over periods much shorter than that shown in Table 63-2, they do require time. Climbers in the Himalayas routinely prepare for high altitudes by several weeks' acclimation at intermediate levels. Acclimation is possible up to 6000 m of altitude. At higher altitudes, the stress becomes excessive, and deterioration sets in.

Table 63-1. Thermal Response During Fever and Physiologic Hyperthermia*

Variables	Exercise Hyperthermia	Fever
Body temperature		
Actual	39	39
Steady-State	37	39
Environmental temperature		
Actual	31	31
Neutral	31	33
Responses		
Sweating	+	0
Vasoconstriction	0	+
Reflex heat production	0	+

*The two individuals were resting at 31°C. All temperatures are given in degrees Celsius. + = increased; 0 = no response.

Table 63-2. Loss of Cold Adaptation in Korean Diving Women

Years	Basal Metabolic Rate (% of control)	Critical Water Temperature (°C)
1960–1977	130	25.9
1977 — Introduction of Wet Diving Suits		
1980	100	27.9
1981	100	28.9
1982	100	29.7
1983	100	29.9

Critical water temperature is the temperature at which shivering could first be observed in absence of diving suit — that for nondivers was 29.9°C.

From: S. K. Hong. *News Physiol. Sci.* 2:79, 1987.

No significant adaptation occurs when exposure is too short, i.e., when the challenge falls below some limiting level. This is illustrated in Fig. 63-1. Here sweat rates (in grams per square meter) were determined by weight loss at the stated body temperatures during successive daily heat exposures of 0.5 as contrasted with 2 hours. Individuals were quickly heated to the stated oral temperatures. Note on day 1 that, as expected, the higher the body temperature, the more the subjects sweated. If daily exposure was restricted to only 1/2 hour, sweat rates remained relatively constant. If, however, daily exposure was continued for 2 hours, sweat production increased from day to day. In other words, there is a clear memory effect, the response to each exposure being influenced by preceding exposures.

Fig. 63-1. Sweat loss during repeated heat exposure. Individuals were quickly heated to the stated oral temperatures. Sweat production was then measured at that temperature for 2 hours (A) or 0.5 hour (B). (Modified from: Fox, et al. *J. Physiol.* 166:530, 1963.)

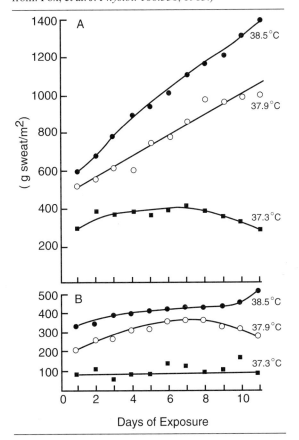

The end result of this adaptive process is that the adequately exposed subjects dissipate heat more effectively after than before adaptation.

Usage has, in some cases, established the term **adaptation** to mean no more than compensatory response to an altered environment. The eye, for instance, is said to adapt to darkness. Other than rapid responses to changes in light intensity by altering the size of the pupil, the process is relatively slow, requiring as long as 30 minutes. However, there is no evidence to suggest that the efficiency of this "adaptation" improves with experience, and it should therefore more correctly be included under compensation.

Heat

Mechanisms of temperature control were discussed in Chap. 13. The more core temperature exceeds the desired steady-state value, the more active become the compensatory mechanisms (sweating, vasodilation). Reducing the temperature to the set point abolishes these processes, provided passive heat loss balances basal metabolic heat production; under these conditions, there is no need for any temperature compensation. The ambient temperature where this balance is achieved is defined as the **neutral temperature.** For healthy humans, this temperature lies at approximately 31°C. The concept is illustrated in Fig. 63-2.

The compensatory response to heat consists primarily of circulatory adjustments (e.g., peripheral vasodilatation) and activation of the sweating response. For limited periods of time, humans can maintain body temperature in dry heat as high as 130°C. At that temperature, sweat is lost at a rate of liters per hour.

After more gradual exposure to heat, the body begins to adapt (see Fig. 63-1). The resulting increased work efficiency in a hot environment is illustrated in Table 63-3. Here, young men before and after adaptation carried out a standard external workload of 50 Cal/hour at an ambient temperature of 40°C. Heat load consisted of total caloric output (T) calculated from O_2 consumption, minus external work performed (W), plus the heat gained from radiation (R) and conduction (C). Increased sweating after adaptation lowered the skin temperature to 35.6°C, at the cost of increasing R and C. The unadapted core temperature rose to 39.5°C, a level associated with rapidly developing exhaustion. However, the core → skin temperature gradient was lower before than after adaptation (2.5 versus 2.9°C); i.e., each liter of blood flowing from core to pe-

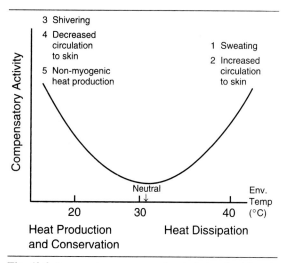

Fig. 63-2. Temperature compensation in hot and cold environments. At the neutral temperature, the temperature gradient from skin to environment permits the basal metabolic heat production to be dissipated primarily by conduction. Over the environmental temperature range shown, compensation permits maintenance of core body temperature at close to 37°C.

Table 63-3. Adaptation to Work in a Hot Environment

	Nonadapted	Adapted
Energy exchange (Cal/hr)		
T	565	580
W	−50	−50
R	20	30
C	30	40
Heat load	565	540
Temperatures (°C)		
Core	39.5	38.5
Skin	37.0	35.6
Core-to-skin gradient	2.5	2.9
Thermal blood flow (liters/min)	3.1	

T = total caloric output; W = external work performed; R = heat gain by radiation; C = heat gain by conduction.
Based on Belding, H. S. In: Yousef, M. K., ed. *Physiological Adaptation*. New York: Academic Press, 1972.

riphery could discharge 2.5 Cal before but 2.9 Cal after adaptation. Accordingly, peripheral blood flow required for heat dissipation fell from $565/(2.5 \times 60) = 3.7$ liters/min to $540/(2.9 \times 60) = 3.1$ liters/min. In summary, adaptation consisted primarily of an increased sweating response (see Fig. 63-1) and thereby raised the efficiency of work performance; both core temperature and work-related cardiac output remained lower after adaptation. There is evidence that this adaptive response represents to a significant extent a local training effect at the level of the sweat glands rather than stimulation of central activity.

Circulatory changes (increased extracellular and circulatory volumes and peripheral vasodilation) and improved salt retention also contribute to heat adaptation. As in the case of other environmental stresses, the response thus involves a variety of mechanisms and is influenced by external factors such as salt and water intake, as well as by intrinsic factors such as age, physical fitness, and others.

Cold

The processes permitting compensation to cold exposure are shown in Fig 63-2. Physiologic adaptation to cold environments is also well documented. Table 63-2, for instance, illustrates gain and loss of cold adaptation in Korean sponge divers. Fully adapted divers immersed in water started shivering only when the water temperature dropped to 25.9°C; the critical water temperature for nondivers was 29.9°C. Another example is that of fishermen from the Gaspe Peninsula. Vasoconstriction, as measured by heat transfer from an immersed finger to water, is lowest during the period spent indoors in winter and then gradually increases during the fishing season with the unavoidable exposure, especially of the hands, to cold water. It has been observed, however, that in various cold-adapted primitive populations, blood flow to the extremities is better maintained than in unadapted individuals. This may result, in part, from genetic selection rather than physiologic adaptation. It is important to emphasize in this connection that the Eskimo is superbly adapted to life in the cold, but this adaptation rests largely on clothing, diet, housing, and other nonphysiologic factors. The skin temperature of Eskimos under their clothing differs little from that of inhabitants of more temperate zones.

The main factors involved in adaptation to the cold are circulatory adjustments and metabolic changes. Basal metabolic rate may rise (see Table 63-2), especially under the influence of increased thyroid activity. Metabolic acclimation of humans to cold has been reported to require about 6 weeks. However, even when working at the maximum rate that can be supported for prolonged periods (total caloric expenditure about 200 Cal/m²/hr), cold-adapted humans are unable to maintain a normal temperature below approximately 10°C. Below that temperature, survival will depend on protective clothing.

High Altitudes

Adaptation to high altitudes primarily represents the response to low partial pressures of O_2; contributing to this environmental stress is cold exposure. A major adaptive response to partial anoxia is the gradual rise in hematocrit referred to earlier. Hyperventilation will produce respiratory alkalosis, with a consequent shift of the O_2 dissociation curve to the left, i.e., toward increased O_2 saturation of hemoglobin. Initial rises in cardiac output, stroke volume, and heart rate tend to be transient, and these physiologic variables return to normal. The net result of adaptation is an increased mechanical efficiency of work at high altitudes. This is illustrated in Fig. 63-3.

Fig. 63-3. Adaptation to high altitudes. Mechanical efficiency was measured at sea level (SL); after 2, 7, and 12 days at about 4000 m of altitude (atmospheric pressure 453 torr); and after return to sea level. (Modified from Yousef, M. K., and Horvath, S. M. *Physiological Adaptations.* New York: Academic Press, 1972.)

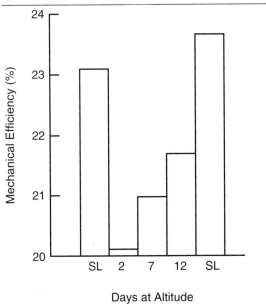

Note the immediate fall in work efficiency, followed by a gradual return toward normal. This adaptive response, which presumably included general physical conditioning, was not lost immediately upon return to sea level (SL).

High Pressure

Humans are exposed to high pressures primarily while diving or during underwater construction; each 10 m of depth corresponds to an increase of 1 atm of pressure. Successful diving involves considerable learning and behavioral adaptation, but there is evidence also for physiologic changes. Chief among these is the respiratory system. Thus development of increased respiratory work capacity and vital capacity and of decreased residual volumes has been described in professional divers.

Another well-documented effect of diving is an increased tolerance to CO_2. Although the adaptive advantage of this effect may not be entirely clear, it gradually develops after repeated exposures and slowly disappears after cessation of diving. In diving instructors, for instance, the respiratory response to 5% CO_2 returned toward its normal high sensitivity over a period of 3 months. To this extent, this represents a typical adaptive response.

Weightlessness (Microgravity)

With the beginning of space exploration about 30 years ago, humans have spent considerable periods under conditions of relative weightlessness or microgravity. This elicits a variety of early effects, including sensory-motor disturbances and an increase in central blood volume. Within a few days, the body establishes a new steady-state; i.e., it adapts to weightlessness. The relatively rapid adjustment to the new environment is followed by more gradual changes such as muscle wasting, bone resorption, and an extensive deconditioning of the cardiovascular system. These changes have proven reversible upon return to ground level and can be prevented to some extent by suitable exercise in space. As a result, space missions have been extended successfully for many months.

The changes occurring near the beginning of exposure and permitting the reversal of the overt early effects of microgravity over a period of days may presumably be ascribed to adaptation. There is no direct evidence, however, for this conclusion. Testing for an adaptive "memory" would require rapidly repeated space flights, before the traveler has undergone deadaptation. In the few cases of repeat flights by one individual, a second exposure led to symptoms similar to those experienced on the first flight. The ability to prevent or at least to slow down the development of gradual deterioration in space by appropriate exercises constitutes behavioral rather than physiologic responses.

Summary

This chapter defines the difference between physiologic compensation and adaptation when an individual is challenged, within certain limits, by environmental stress. Physiologic responses must be distinguished from behavioral responses such as changes in clothing, diet, search for shelter, etc. or from genetic adaptation of whole populations.

Compensatory changes set in rapidly and cease as soon as normal steady-state has been reestablished after the end of exposure. In contrast, adaptation is generally a much slower and more long-lasting process. Provided adaptation has not been lost because of passage of time (deadaptation), the response to an environmental challenge is influenced by previous exposures.

Humans can adapt physiologically to a wide variety of environmental stress factors. This is illustrated here specifically by reference to a selected group of environments, including heat, cold, high altitudes, high pressure, and microgravity.

Bibliography

Dill, D. B., ed. *Adaptation to the Environment: Handbook of Physiology*, Sec. 4, Washington, D.C.: American Physiological Society, 1964.

Samueloff, S., and Yousef, M. K., eds. *Adaptive Physiology to Stressful Environments*. Boca Raton, Fla.: CRC Press, 1987.

64 Exercise Physiology

Barbara N. Campaigne

Objectives

After reading this chapter, you should be able to

Name the primary physiologic systems involved in exercise

Identify the three energy systems brought into use during exercise

Describe the determinants of O_2 use by the exercising muscle

List the components and discuss the function of the respiratory response to exercise

Name the three primary forms of input to the control of respiration during exercise

Identify the major component of the circulatory system that limits maximal O_2 consumption

Describe the neuroendocrine response to exercise

Outline and discuss the adaptation of the systems attributed to physical training

---

Exercise represents an integration of all physiologic systems and processes involved in preserving a constant internal environment. A physiologic **steady-state** is reached when supply meets demand. An example of this is the delivery and use of O_2 and metabolic substrates to meet the demand of working muscle during exercise. In addition, steady-state involves the maintenance of a relatively stable body temperature, pulse rate, blood pressure, and respiratory rate for a given period (see Chap. 13). This chapter examines independently several of the systems involved in the response to acute exercise and the adaptation to physical training. This chapter is not all-inclusive but will cover such aspects as the metabolic basis of the exercise response, involvement of the respiratory and circulatory systems, and a short section on the neuroendocrine response to exercise. Exercise-induced changes in sleep, the immune system, gastrointestinal function, and the psychoneuroendocrine system are not discussed.

Systems Involved

The **skeletomuscular systems** are the primary ones involved in **movement.** However, the respiratory, circulatory, and neuroendocrine systems also directly participate.

The **respiratory response** involves the lungs, as well as gas transport and exchange. The **circulatory response** to exercise involves the heart and its function as a muscle pump. The hemodynamics of blood flow and vascular response are of prime importance during muscular activity. The **neural response** to exercise, including the organization of this response, will be described in this chapter as well. The **endocrine system** is intimately involved in fuel homeostasis, which is of major importance during exercise. The hormones involved in exercise also will be considered, along with their action. Finally, the **acute response** and the **long-term adaptation** to exercise will be compared. Short-term single bouts of muscular activity (acute effects) require immediate responses from the systems involved. When exercise is performed repeatedly over time at regular intervals, certain aspects of the physiologic systems adapt. This is the process of adaptation (chronic effects), and it will be discussed in the concluding portion of each section.

The Metabolic Basis of Exercise

The supply of biologic energy for physiologic activity, known as **bioenergetics,** is the basis for exercise. According to the **first law of thermodynamics,** energy can be neither created nor destroyed but only transferred from one form to another or from one place to another. Accordingly, energy from the system, **cellular energy,** is needed for exercise to take place, and with the exhaustion of this energy, new energy has to be made available. Because the mechanical efficiency of muscle performing external work averages only around 20% (see Chap. 63), most of the energy used is released as heat that must be eliminated from the body.

During exercise, three different energy systems come into play. **High-energy phosphate compounds** supply energy for the systems. Exercise that lasts only a few seconds uses several sources of immediate energy. During forceful exercise lasting from a few seconds to a minute, energy is primarily obtained from **glycolytic or nonoxidative sources.** The third energy system is **aerobic or oxidative** and is used for muscle contraction that lasts 2 minutes or longer, referred to as **endurance.** Figure 64-1 illustrates the use of the three energy systems as a function of duration of activity (see also Fig. 17-8). As Fig. 64-1 shows, no activity relies solely on one system; however, one will predominate during activity of a particular intensity and duration.

The **oxidation of fuel** is the primary pathway for energy generation and subsequent heat production during exercise. During sprinting or brief high-intensity exercise, glucose stored in the form of **muscle glycogen** is the major fuel source. Continuing exercise makes use of substrates carried in the blood in the form of glucose and free fatty acids. Prolonged exercise that lasts longer than 2 hours depletes glycogen stores, and free fatty acids become the dominant fuel source. The greatest source of potential energy in the body is fat. Fat reserves account for about 90,000 to 110,000 Cal of energy. In contrast, energy available in the form of carbohydrates constitutes less than 2000 Cal. About 1500 Cal (375 g) of glycogen is stored intramuscularly; 400 Cal (100 g) exists as liver glycogen, and 80 Cal (20 g) of carbohydrate is available in the form of glucose in the extracellular fluids. **Protein** can serve as an important source of energy during prolonged exercise,

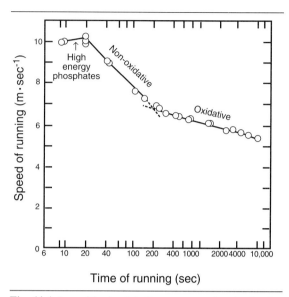

Fig. 64-1. Logarithmic plot of average speed maintained versus time of event for men's world records in running. The presence of three curve components suggests the use of three energy systems. (Modified from: McGilvery, R. W. *Biomedical Concepts.* Philadelphia: W. B. Saunders, 1975.)

such as marathons or ultraendurance events. However, it must be broken down to specific amino acids for energy release and is thus a less efficient form of fuel.

Physical fitness is most often defined as an individual's maximal ability to use O_2, given in liters per minute ($\dot{V}O_2$max). $\dot{V}O_2$max is determined by cardiac output (heart rate [HR] × stroke volume [SV]) and the arteriovenous O_2 difference [(a–v)O_2], expressed as milliliters per 100 ml of blood, as represented in the **Fick equation:** $\dot{V}O_2 = (HR \times SV) \times (a–v)O_2$. Often the intensity of exercise performed is defined as a percentage of $\dot{V}O_2$max. The effect of exercise intensity on fuel utilization has been studied, and it has been shown that at 50% of $\dot{V}O_2$max or less, glycogen accounts for less than 50% of the muscle substrate and only small amounts of blood glucose are used. When exercise is performed above 50% $\dot{V}O_2$max, carbohydrate use increases, leading to depletion of glycogen stores. At 70% to 80% of $\dot{V}O_2$max, the muscle glycogen store is depleted at exhaustion, which occurs approximately 1½ to 2 hours after initiation. During exercise at extremely high intensity (90% to 100% $\dot{V}O_2$max), glycogen use is highest, but depletion does not occur with exhaustion. At these high intensities, the intracellular pH and the buildup of metabolites, rather than fuel availability, appear to limit performance.

The Respiratory System

Ventilation

Pulmonary ventilation requires work to expand the lung and overcome the resistance to movement of the lung tissue and the gas in the lung airways. The **work of breathing** can be obtained by calculating the area enclosed by the curve of the pressure-volume relationship. During exercise, both the respiratory rate and tidal volume increase, thus elevating the minute volume. There is an initial rise in tidal volume that may reduce the work performed by the lungs because of decreased flow resistance. At very high workloads with tidal volumes exceeding 50% of the vital capacity, the pulmonary work against elastic forces is heightened. Thus, during greatly increased workloads, breathing frequency continues to increase with no further change in the tidal volume. This markedly increases the work of breathing. During exercise, the anatomic dead space ventilation increases slightly, and because tidal volume rises markedly, the ratio of the two decreases. This lower ratio represents a more efficient gas exchange brought about by an increase in the volume of air available to the alveoli for ventilation.

During the first few minutes of **submaximal exercise,** ventilation increases exponentially and remains nearly constant during the remainder of the exercise session. It has been demonstrated that the minute volume during a 2½-hour marathon is almost 70% of the maximal exercise ventilation.

Diffusion

Gas exchange between the alveoli and the pulmonary blood is known as the **diffusing capacity,** which is the volume of gas diffusing through the respiratory membrane at a pressure difference of 1 mmHg each minute. During each breath, O_2 diffuses into the pulmonary capillaries through the alveolar membrane. Diffusion of O_2 through the alveolar membrane is directly proportional to the partial pressure difference of O_2 (Po_2) between the alveolus and capillary and the cross-sectional area of the surface for gas exchange (see Chap. 32). With exercise, both the cross-sectional area and Po_2 gradient increase, permitting increased diffusion of O_2 across the alveolar-capillary membrane. The increased alveolar ventilation also produces a lower alveolar CO_2 and an increased diffusion pressure gradient for CO_2 from the capillaries into the alveolus and, therefore, into the atmosphere. An increase in the effective alveolar-capillary membrane area results

from the opening of additional capillaries in the lung, as well as dilatation of capillaries and alveoli (Fig. 64-2). Consequently, the capacity for diffusion increases almost threefold with exercise.

The pulmonary circulation (cardiac output) during exercise increases to match the increased ventilation. Pulmonary vascular resistance decreases but the increase in cardiac input is greater, and therefore, pulmonary arterial pressure rises. This augmented pulmonary blood flow decreases the amount of time the red blood cell (RBC) spends in the pulmonary capillaries. Under resting conditions, it takes the RBC about 0.75 second to travel through the pulmonary capillary; during heavy exercise, the transit time is only 0.3 to 0.4 second. However, even though the actual time in the alveolar capillary is reduced, the equilibration of gases between the capillary blood and the alveolus can still be accomplished, as proved by the fact that, during exercise, the arterial blood of healthy individuals remains fully oxygenated. The blood normally (at rest) stays in the lungs about three times longer than required for it to be fully oxygenated.

Fig. 64-2. The stages of oxygen uptake. (Modified from: Frontera, W. R., and Adams, C. Endurance exercise: Normal physiology and limitations imposed by pathological processes, part 1. *Phys. Sports Med.* 14(8):96, 1986.)

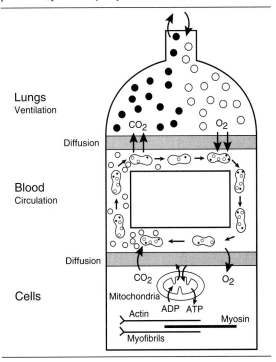

Control

There are a minimum of three documented **primary afferent inputs** that control the output of the medullary inspiratory neurons. The first of these primary afferents are the **descending influences** from the CNS relative to locomotor activity. In a feed-forward manner, the motor cortex sends signals to the respiratory center to increase the rate and depth of breathing in a cognitive response to exercise. The second primary afferent consists of the **ascending influences** from exercising skeletal muscle. At the muscle level, afferents include the muscle spindle, Golgi tendon organs, and skeletal joint receptors. These send signals to the sensory cortex, which relays information to the respiratory center. The third primary afferent is the **humoral input** relative to the increasing production of CO_2. The central and peripheral chemoreceptors sense a change in the partial pressure of CO_2 (P_{CO_2}) and pH, and signal the respiratory center to increase respiration. The amount of neural input to inspiratory muscles is proportional to the rising metabolic demand. The mechanisms that control respiration during exercise are very effective. During all but very heavy exercise, the arterial P_{O_2}, P_{CO_2}, and pH remain almost the same. **Peripheral chemoreceptors** also may play a role in the ventilatory response to exercise. During exercise, arterial pH does decrease, and arterial P_{O_2} is maintained or decreases slightly. These factors may stimulate the carotid bodies during exercise, which then send signals to the medullary respiratory center. The variation in arterial P_{O_2} occurring with exercise may increase the CO_2 and H^+ sensitivity of the carotid bodies.

During exercise, an important function of the respiratory control system is to minimize the effort of respiratory muscle. Although respiratory control mechanisms are poorly understood, there is evidence that, during exercise, the respiratory control system is "aware" of and responds to the mechanical needs of the chest wall.

Adaptation to Physical Training

In contrast to the anatomic changes in the lung that accompany chronic stressful situations, such as hypoxia, the lung shows only very minor adaptation as the result of physical training. However, maximum ventilatory performance may be improved, such that a trained athlete can achieve and sustain a higher percent (75%) of the **maximal ventilatory volume** than can a nonathlete (68%). Athletes also have been shown to maintain a maximal ventilatory volume following exhaustive exercise, while nonathletes show reduced volumes under similar circumstances. These

enhanced maximal ventilatory responses may result from specific respiratory muscle training. The major non-pulmonary-related effect of physical training on the pulmonary system is the reduction in ventilatory response to heavy, short-term, submaximal exercise. This is most likely induced by a decreased ventilatory drive, primarily attributable to decreased lactic acidosis, as well as to decreased levels of circulating catecholamines. During prolonged exercise, trained individuals also show enhanced **heat dissipation,** resulting in lower core body temperatures (see Table 63-3), and this reduces the ventilatory response. This is not seen in untrained individuals, though both trained and untrained individuals have elevated temperatures during exercise. It has not been established which humoral stimulus, if any, is responsible for increased ventilation during exercise. The decreased respiratory rate that occurs in trained athletes during submaximal exercise associated with physical training may reflect a decreased neural-induced recruitment of locomotor and respiratory muscles brought about by delayed muscle fatigue.

Pathophysiologic Limitations

Under pathologic conditions, such as chronic obstructive pulmonary disease, interstitial lung disease, and asthma, exercise capacity may be limited as a consequence of the pulmonary dysfunction. In such individuals, exercise may be limited because of abnormal pulmonary mechanics, impaired gas exchange, ventilatory muscle fatigue, or a combination of these factors. These problems are manifested as abnormal exercise responses, including dyspnea, arterial O_2 desaturation, and the development of respiratory acidosis during work. In fact, exercise can be used as a diagnostic procedure in the early stages of certain diseases. Pulmonary patients who have a low cardiovascular work capacity may be good candidates for exercise training programs that improve the physical work capacity.

The Circulatory Response to Exercise

Muscle demand for metabolic fuel increases during exercise, and this demand is met by an increased supply of blood carrying necessary O_2 and metabolic substrates to the muscle. The changes in cardiovascular function that take place during exercise depend on both the type and intensity of exercise. **Dynamic-type activity** that involves the large muscle groups, such as running, swimming, and cycling, places the greatest demand on the circulatory system. Large increases occur in both the cardiac output (heart rate and stroke volume) and systolic blood pressure. The diastolic pressure tends to fall, so the mean arterial pressure remains fairly constant. This indicates a match of the increase in cardiac output to the decrease in vascular resistance. **Static-type exercise,** such as weight lifting, which uses little muscle mass, causes moderate increases in cardiac output and heart rate, with accompanying increases in systolic, diastolic, and mean blood pressure caused by increases in sympathetic activity (norepinephrine release).

Cardiac Output and Heart Rate

The increase in cardiac output during exercise is partially mediated by a **decrease in vascular resistance** combined with an **increase in the venous-filling pressure gradient.** The **sympathetic nervous system** also plays an important role in determining cardiac output during exercise. During **dynamic exercise,** the cardiac output increase is accomplished by increases in both heart rate and stroke volume. Heart rate rises in conjunction with O_2 consumption and workload. As $\dot{V}O_2max$ is reached, cardiac output attains a plateau value in order to match lung perfusion to ventilation. The increase in cardiac output and heart rate depends on the type of exercise as well as on the individual's fitness, age, and sex. When **work output** is submaximal, cardiac output and heart rate rise and then plateau as O_2 transport requirements are met. **Exercise heart rate** is influenced by a host of **environmental factors,** such as anxiety (which also affects resting heart rate), dehydration, ambient temperature, and altitude. These environmental factors may not always be linked to changes in cardiac output, due to the inverse relationship between heart rate and stroke volume when "afterload" and "preload" factors are constant (nonexercise settings).

As mentioned previously, heart rate is not only affected by the intensity and duration of exercise but also by the type of exercise performed. At the same percentage of $\dot{V}O_2max$, cycling elicits a higher heart rate than does treadmill running. This may be attributable to the workload placed on the muscles in relation to the size of the muscle group used. Another example of such a response is exhibited by work that involves only the arms, which causes a 10% greater heart rate response than does cycling at the same workload. Smaller muscle groups, such as the arms, seem to be used at a higher percentage of their maximum capacity during activity than are the larger muscle groups, such as the legs during walking or running. In general, the heart rate is lower during exercises such as weight lifting.

Thus heart rate rises in response to the percentage of maximal contraction of the muscle mass involved as well as to the amount of muscle used.

The heart rate responds to the exercise changes during the **adaptive process** of physical training. In general, heart rate after physical training is lower than that in untrained subjects at any absolute submaximal workload. However, the heart rate response at a submaximal workload relative to the newly attained heart rate remains unchanged after training. During maximal exercise, heart rate is usually unchanged or somewhat lower in individuals who have undergone physical training than in those who have not.

Cardiac Output and Stroke Volume

Stroke volume appears to be the variable that responds most to the increased cardiac output demand during exercise. For example, the cardiac output of a trained athlete during maximal exercise may be as high as 38 liters/min as compared with a sedentary individual whose maximal cardiac output is 23 liters/min. Both groups may respond to a similar workload with a heart rate of 195 beats per minute but with different stroke volumes. The trained athlete will have a stroke volume on the order of 195 ml and the sedentary individual's will be 118 ml. One physiologic mechanism responsible for the greater stroke volume, both during exercise and at rest in trained athletes, is an **increased ventricular filling** during the diastolic phase of the cardiac cycle (due to a higher venous pressure gradient from the body periphery to the heart). The enhanced end-diastolic volume stretches the fibers of the myocardium, and this strengthens contraction, with a resulting more powerful ejection. This response is described as **Starling's law of the heart.** Another mechanism that elicits a greater stroke volume during exercise is the **increased systolic emptying** of the heart. This is due to the actions of epinephrine and norepinephrine, which increase during exercise. **Decreased systemic vascular impedance** also contributes to greater emptying of the left ventricle, as does direct **myocardial autonomic nervous system** stimulation.

Blood Flow and the Distribution of Cardiac Output

The distribution of cardiac output to different organs is in general directly related to and regulated by the **metabolic activity** of the tissue (Table 64-1). Under resting conditions in a comfortable environment, about 1 of the 5 liters of cardiac output perfuses skeletal muscle, while most of

Table 64-1. Distribution of Cardiac Output Expressed as Blood Flow to Various Tissues, at Rest and During Light, Moderate, and Maximum Exercise

Tissue	Resting Blood Flow, ml/min (% of total cardiac output)	Exercise Blood Flow, ml/min (% of total cardiac output)		
		Light	Moderate	Maximum
Splanchnic	1350 (27%)	1100 (12%)	600 (3%)	300 (1%)
Renal	1100 (22%)	900 (10%)	600 (3%)	250 (1%)
Cerebral	700 (14%)	750 (8%)	750 (4%)	750 (3%)
Coronary	150 (3%)	350 (4%)	750 (4%)	1000 (4%)
Muscle	750 (15%)	4500 (47%)	12,500 (71%)	22,000 (88%)
Skin (cool environment)	300 (6%)	1500 (15%)	1900 (12%)	600 (2%)
Other (lungs, bone, etc.)	650 (13%)	400 (4%)	400 (3%)	100 (1%)
Total	5000	9500	17,500	25,000

Modified from: Anderson, K. L. The cardiovascular system in exercise. In: Falls, H. B. *Exercise Physiology.* New York: Academic Press, 1968.

the remaining 4 liters is distributed to the digestive tract, spleen, brain, kidneys, and liver. During brief, intense exercise, the blood flow to the working muscles increases progressively with increasing intensity of work, while the fractional blood flow to the organs and skin decreases (see Table 64-1). Implications of this flow redistribution for heat dissipation have been discussed in Chap. 13.

O₂ Extraction Reserve

The heart uses about 75% of its O_2 supply at rest. Because of the greater demand on the heart during exercise, both the coronary blood flow and O_2 supply must increase. The four- to fivefold increase in cardiac output that occurs during exercise is accompanied by a similar increase in coronary circulation.

Oxygen Transport

In general, 1 liter of blood contains about 200 ml of O_2 when saturated. O_2 consumption at rest is about 250 ml/min in both trained and untrained individuals, but about 1000 ml/min is potentially available if all the O_2 in the cardiac output is consumed. Thus, at rest, O_2 extraction is 25% and reserve is 75%.

O_2 is extracted more effectively during exercise in the trained individual than it is in an untrained subject. Sedentary individuals have a higher cardiac output during submaximal exercise than do trained athletes. The greater O_2 requirement of exercising muscle is thus primarily supplied by an increased O_2 extraction during submaximal exercise. At rest, skeletal muscle consumes about 5 ml of O_2

per minute of the total 20 ml of O_2 that is available from the 100 ml of capillary blood supplied: $(a-v)O_2 = 5$ vol%. During submaximal exercise, the $(a-v)O_2$ increases to 15 vol%, both in sedentary individuals and in trained athletes. After physical training, the $(a-v)O_2$ increases by about 2% to 3%, causing about 80% of the O_2 to be extracted during submaximal exercise (Table 64-2). Because the capacity to increase $(a-v)O_2$ is limited, an increase in the stroke volume during maximal exercise, as well as increased density of muscle capillaries and mitochondria, contribute to the increased $\dot{V}O_2$max that occurs following physical training.

Pathophysiologic Limitations and Application

Exercise training has been found to reduce ischemia and improve ventricular function and aerobic capacity in men

Table 64-2. Arteriovenous Oxygen Difference Under Various Conditions

Condition	Arterial O_2 (ml/100 ml blood)	Venous O_2 (ml/100 ml blood)	Arteriovenous Oxygen Difference (%)
Rest	20	15	25
Submaximal exercise	20	5	75
Submaximal exercise (after physical training)	20	4	80

with stable coronary heart disease (CHD), though stroke volume and cardiac output are only slightly affected. However, the ability of skeletal muscle to receive and use O_2 can be improved, resulting in a greater (a–v)O_2 after training. Such patients can thus exercise at a given submaximal level with a lower cardiac output or perform higher workloads at a cardiac output similar to the pretraining one. Regular exercise thus reduces symptoms such as angina during submaximal efforts. Changes in heart function are modest in most cases, however. Marked increases in blood pressure occurring with heavy weight lifting should be avoided by those with CHD, due to the large oxygen demands placed on the myocardium.

Microcirculatory Changes

The microcirculation in muscle is also improved with physical training. Specifically, in endurance-trained muscle there is an increase in capillary density (number of capillaries per muscle fiber). Such an adaptation improves muscle fiber contact with the blood supply, which enhances the exchange of substrates and metabolic products. The (a–v)O_2 is also increased following training due to an increase in the metabolic capacity of muscle cells. For instance, mitochondrial size and number increase and there is increased oxidative enzyme activity. These changes improve aerobic ATP production without increasing lactate formation.

Neuroendocrine Response During Exercise

The physiologic response necessary to maintain blood glucose homeostasis (approximately 90 mg/dl) during exercise is coordinated by two systems: the **autonomic nervous system** and the **endocrine** (hormonal) **system.** By means of chemical mediators, these systems coordinate the responses that maintain blood glucose concentration within the normal range during exercise. One example of the endocrine response to exercise is the decrease in insulin secretion as glucose levels fall. The declining plasma insulin concentration causes a decrease in the rate of glucose uptake while promoting fat utilization; these events contribute to the maintenance of normal blood glucose levels during exercise. The action of the autonomic nervous system includes sympathetic stimulation of cardiac contractility and frequency of contraction as well as the mobilization of fuels such as free fatty acids and glucose. At rest, the parasympathetic component of the autonomic nervous system permits fuel storage and reduces heart rate.

Control

Both the intensity of exercise and physical training affect the autonomic nervous system response to exercise. **Moderate exercise** has minimal effects on circulating blood catecholamine levels. As the intensity of exercise increases to 50% to 70% of $\dot{V}O_2$max, blood catecholamine levels rise markedly. The release of catecholamines into the bloodstream during exercise is diminished following physical training because the exercise workloads impose less stress and cause diminished catecholamine release (Fig. 64-3).

Glucose and carbohydrate metabolism during exercise are affected greatly by epinephrine. By activating the beta receptors in muscle, **epinephrine** increases adenylate cyclase activity, intracellular free calcium levels, and, as a result, stimulates **glycogenolysis,** which is the breakdown of stored glycogen to form glucose. Glycogenolysis in the liver is also stimulated by catecholamines and to a greater extent by **glucagon** also increases with exercise and in response to decreasing blood glucose levels. However, during high-intensity exercise, the large increase in blood catecholamine levels suffices to stimulate hepatic glycogenolysis and elevate blood glucose concentrations. In addition, epinephrine indirectly affects glucose and glycogen metabolism by mobilizing free fatty acids from adipose tissue. At the onset of exercise, epinephrine released into the blood from the adrenal medulla quickly initiates **lipolysis** by stimulating hormone-sensitive lipase; this is followed by a slower, prolonged effect of growth hormone, which in turn maintains lipolysis. Other hormones that are important in fuel homeostasis during exercise are: **corti-**

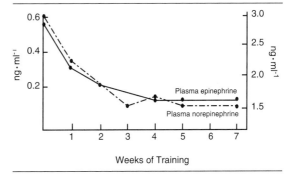

Fig. 64-3. Plasma norepinephrine (right axis) and epinephrine (left axis) concentrations decrease in response to exercise of a given submaximal intensity, as a result of endurance training. (Modified from: Winder, W. W., et al. Time course of sympathoadrenal adaptation to endurance exercise training in man. *J. Appl. Physiol.* 45:370, 1978.)

sol, thyroid hormone, and antidiuretic hormone. Figure 64-4 illustrates how hormones mobilized during exercise influence the cellular energy systems such as glycolysis, lipolysis, and the Krebs' cycle. For example, as shown, a decrease in insulin and increase in glucagon bring about increased availability of glucose to the working muscle by means of glycogenolysis. This same combination of hormonal changes that occurs with exercise enhances lipolysis, thus making free fatty acids available as a fuel source for the working muscle.

Adaptation to Physical Training

Just as the neuroendocrine response is used to maintain glucose homeostasis during exercise, after physical training it also ensures "near normal" glucose levels. In general, following physical training, exercise of a given absolute or relative intensity imposes less metabolic stress and elicits a lower neuroendocrine response. Thus resting insulin levels are lower after physical training. It has been found that exercise enhances insulin sensitivity and may result in lower insulin requirements in insulin-dependent diabetics. An increase in cellular glucose transport following exercise has also been documented.

Pathologic Limitations

In disease states that affect the autonomic or central nervous systems the normal neuroendocrine response to exercise is limited. The autonomic response to exercise may be impaired in **autonomic neuropathy,** one of the complications associated with diabetes. Diabetic individuals with

Fig. 64-4. The hormones mobilized during exercise and their influence on fuel supply to the muscles by means of several metabolic pathways within the muscle tissue, including glycolysis, lipolysis, and the Krebs' cycle (Acetyl-CoA = acetyl coenzyme A). (Modified from: Frontera, W. R., and Adams, C. Endurance exercise: Normal physiology and limitations imposed by pathological processes, part 2. *Phys. Sports Med.* 14(8):111, 1986.)

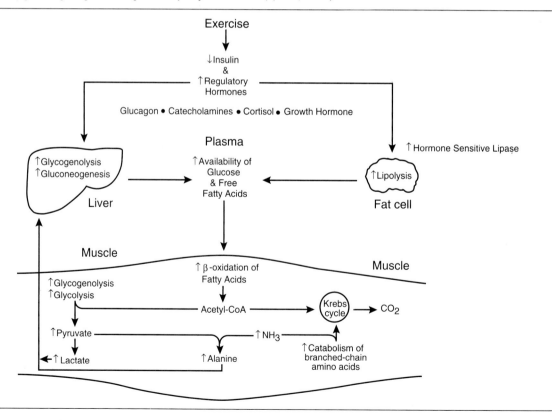

autonomic neuropathy may have an altered norepinephrine and epinephrine response. This may be attributed to a reduced catecholamine release and possibly to lower clearance. Although the catecholamine response is blunted in patients with diabetes who are in poor glucose control, the adrenergic response to exercise may be elevated. Whether physical training alters these abnormal responses to exercise has not been studied thoroughly.

Summary

The physiologic response to exercise consists of a more or less efficient attempt to adjust to a new, high steady-state, even during heavy exercise. Thus there are circulatory and respiratory adjustments, with neural and hormonal inputs acting as stimulating mechanisms to meet the added fuel demand of working muscle. While providing for the increased metabolic needs of the working muscle, the systems exquisitely sustain the basal requirements of the nonexercising tissues and organs for as long as possible. The efficiency of the homeostatic response to exercise is generally improved by physical training, in that the circulatory, neuroendocrine, and, to a lesser extent, respiratory systems adapt during training. Pathophysiologic limitations may alter the response to exercise and need to be carefully considered when exercise is recommended.

Bibliography

Brooks, G. A., and Fahey, T. D. *Exercise Physiology: Human Bioenergetics and Its Applications.* New York: John Wiley and Sons, 1984.

Dempsey, J. A., Aaron, E., and Martin, B. J. Pulmonary function and prolonged exercise. In: Lamb, D. R., and Murray, R., eds. *Perspectives in Exercise Science and Sports Medicine,* Vol. 1: *Prolonged Exercise.* Indianapolis: Benchmark Press, 1988. Pp. 75–119.

Guyton, A. C. *Textbook of Medical Physiology,* 5th ed. Philadelphia: W. B. Saunders, 1976.

McArdle, W. D., Katch, F. L., and Katch, V. L. *Exercise Physiology: Energy, Nutrition, and Human Performance,* 2nd ed. Philadelphia: Lea & Febiger, 1986.

Saltin, B., and Karlsson, J. Muscle glycogen utilization during work of different intensities. In: Pernow, B., and Saltin, B., eds. *Muscle Metabolism During Exercise.* New York: Plenum Press, 1971. Pp. 289–300.

Part XI Questions: Adaptation and Exercise Physiology

1. Indicate the one answer that correctly describes the relationship between physiologic adaptation and compensation.
   A. Adaptation is faster than compensation.
   B. Adaptation is restricted to the same feedback loops as compensation.
   C. Eskimoes survive in their native environment because of adaptation and not compensation.
   D. Unlike compensation, adaptation may lead to changes in the physiologic steady-state levels.
   E. The process of adaptation is reversed, just as compensation stops, as soon as the inducing stress is removed.

2. The neutral temperature defines
   A. the point of minimal BMR.
   B. an invariable temperature characteristic for each individual.
   C. the optimal temperature for doing heavy work.
   D. the point where resting O_2 consumption is minimal.
   E. the point where heat production equals heat loss.

3. After physical training, the $(a-v)O_2$ at submaximal exercise
   A. increases from pretraining values.
   B. is the same as at rest.
   C. is unchanged.
   D. decreases from pretraining values.
   E. is the same as at maximal exercise.

4. The distribution of cardiac output during exercise goes mainly to the
   A. brain.
   B. kidneys.
   C. skeletal muscle.
   D. skin.
   E. cardiac muscle.

Appendixes

Appendix I

Normal Values of Electrolytes, Metabolic Variables, and Hormones in Whole Blood, Plasma, or Serum

Constituent	Traditional Units	SI Units
Acetoacetate plus acetone (S)	0.3–2.0 mg/dl	3–20 mg/liter
Aldosterone (S)	3–20 ng/dl	83–277 pmol/liter
Ammonia (B)	12–55 µmol/liter	12–55 µmol/liter
Amylase (S)	4–25 units/ml	
Bilirubin (S)	Conjugated (direct) up to 0.4 mg/dl	Up to 7 µmol/liter
Calcium (S)	8.5–10.5 mg/dl; 4.3–5.3 meq/liter	2.1–2.6 mmol/liter
Carbon dioxide content (S)	24–30 meq/liter	24–30 mmol/liter
Carotenoids (S)	0.8–4.0 µg/ml	1.5–7.4 µmol/liter
Chloride (S)	100–106 meq/liter	100–106 mmol/liter
Cholesterol (S)	120–220 mg/dl	3.1–5.7 mmol/liter
Cortisol (S)	5–25 µg/dl	0.14–0.69 µmol/liter
Creatinine (S)	0.6–1.5 mg/dl	53–133 µmol/liter
Estradiol (PO)	Women: basal, 20–600 pg/ml	74–221 pmol/liter
	Ovulatory surge: >200 pg/ml	>735 pmol/liter
	Men: <50 pg/ml	<184 pmol/liter
Glucose (B)	70–110 mg/dl	3.9–5.6 mmol/liter
Insulin (fasting) (P)	5–15 µU/ml	22–67 pmol/liter
Iron (S)	50–150 µg/dl	9.0–26.0 µmol/liter
Lactic acid (B)	0.6–1.8 meq/liter	0.6–1.8 meq/liter
Lipase (S)	Up to 2 U/ml	4.5–10 g/liter
Magnesium (S)	1.5–2.0 meq/liter	0.8–1.3 mmol/liter
Osmolality (S)	280–296 mOsm/kg H_2O	
P_{CO_2} (arterial) (B)	35–45 mmHg	
pH (arterial)	7.35–7.45	45–35 nmol/liter
Phosphatase, alkaline (S)	13–39 IU/liter (adults)	2.9–5.2 mmol/liter
Phosphorus, inorganic (S)	3.0–4.5 mg/dl	
P_{O_2} (arterial) (B)	75–100 mmHg	
Potassium (P)	3.5–5.5 meq/liter	
Progesterone (P)	Men and preovulatory and	
	postmenopausal women: >2 ng/ml	>6 nmol/liter
	Women, luteal peak: <5 ng/ml	<16 nmol/liter
Protein		
Total (S)	6.0–8.4 g/dl	60–80 g/liter
Albumin (S)	3.5–5.0 g/dl	35–50 g/liter
Globulin (S)	2.3–3.5 g/dl	23–35 g/liter
Sodium (S)	135–145 meq/liter	135–145 mmol/liter
Testosterone (P)	Men: 300–1000 ng/dl	10–35 nmol/liter
	Women: <80 ng/dl	<2.8 nmol/liter
Thyroid-stimulating hormone (P)	0.5–4 µU/ml	
Thyroxine (P)	5–12 µ/dl	64–154 nmol/liter
Triiodothyronine (P)	70–190 ng/dl	1.1–2.9 nmol/liter
Transaminase (SGOT) (S)	7–24 U/liter	0.12–0.45 µmol/sec/liter
Urea nitrogen (BUN) (B)	8–25 mg/dl	2.9–8.9 mmol/liter
Uric acid (S)	3.0–7.0 mg/dl	0.18–0.42 mmol/liter

B = whole blood; P = plasma; S = serum.
Modified from: Scully, R. E. Case records of the Massachusetts General Hospital. *N. Engl. J. Med.* 314:39–49, 1986.

Appendix II

Measurement of Cardiac Output

Cardiac output is a clinically important measure that integrates ventricular performance with the metabolic needs of tissues. Although there are a number of techniques for measuring cardiac output, methods based on the Fick principle and indicator-dilution techniques are generally employed in the clinical setting.

The **Fick principle** is based on the law of conservation of mass, and states that the quantity of a substance produced or consumed by an organ is equal to the product of blood flow to that organ and the difference in arterial and venous concentration of that substance. Therefore, flow is equal to the amount of substance produced or consumed divided by the arteriovenous difference of the substance.

In clinical practice, oxygen is used as the substance consumed (Vo_2); arterial and mixed venous (pulmonary arterial) blood is sampled and the arteriovenous oxygen difference $[a–v(O_2)]$ is computed. Thus pulmonary blood flow (Q) is calculated, which, in the absence of an intracardiac shunt, equals systemic blood flow. Lung oxygen uptake is assumed to equal tissue oxygen consumption. Thus $Q = Vo_2/(a–v)O_2$. This method requires right-heart catheterization and careful spirometry, as well as steady-state conditions during the measurement process.

An **indicator-dilution curve,** which plots the concentration of indicator against time, also can be used to determine cardiac output. The indicator-dilution method is actually an application of the Fick principle. The indicator substance can be introduced either by continuous infusion or by a single injection. A given volume of indicator (e.g., indocyanine green) is injected into a peripheral or central vein and arterial blood is withdrawn at a constant rate for analysis. A mixing (cardiac) chamber is necessary, and any recirculation of the indicator needs to be corrected for. Before the indicator recirculates, the decline of indicator over time is exponential (Fig. A-1, *top*). The curve is corrected for recirculation by extrapolation of the exponential portion of the curve (Fig. A-1, *bottom*). The area under the corrected indicator-dilution curve divided by the duration of the dye curve represents the mean concentration of the indicator. After correcting for a 1-minute interval, one gets the cardiac output:

$$\text{Cardiac output} = \frac{60I}{ct}$$

where I is the amount of indicator added, c is the mean concentration of indicator, and t stands for time. Indicator-dilution methods have the advantage of only minimally interfering with the circulation. However, they are inconvenient and their use in measuring cardiac output in humans has largely been replaced by the thermodilution method.

Thermodilution cardiac output methods use temperature as an indicator. Cold saline solution is injected into

Fig. A-1. (Top) Indicator-dilution (time-concentration) curve. One milliliter of indocyanine green is injected into the pulmonary artery at time zero. Blood is withdrawn continuously through a densitometric curvette to derive an instantaneous concentration of dye. The dye first appears at A, peaks at B, and recirculates from C. (Bottom) The time-concentration curve is replotted on semilogarithmic paper. The exponential decline (B–C) is a strait line. Extrapolation of this line to baseline corrects for recirculation. (From: Grossman W., ed. *Cardiac Catheterization and Angiography.* Philadelphia: Lea & Febiger, 1986.)

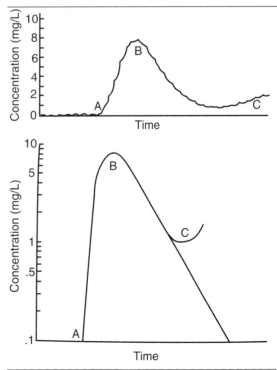

the central veins; it then mixes in the right ventricle and the change in blood temperature is detected by a sensor located in the pulmonary artery. The cardiac output is computed from the time-dependent temperature change. Cardiac output may be overestimated in low-flow states, because of loss of indicator ability as the injectate warms during slow passage from the injection to the measuring sites. Although blood withdrawal and arterial puncture are unnecessary for this method, right-heart catheterization is required.

Answers

Part I: Cellular Physiology

1. C. Cell membranes are permeable to urea. Therefore, the infused urea, and consequently the infused water, will distribute throughout the ECF and ICF.

2. A. The cell membrane is impermeant to both sucrose and NaCl. Because the total osmolarity of the solution is 300 mOsm, the solution is isotonic (i.e., no net water flow into or out of cells will occur with this solution).

3. C. Secondary active transport involves an uphill movement of a solute molecule powered by the downhill movement of another solute molecule. Such transporters include cotransporters (symporters) and exchangers (antiporters). Channels do not mediate active transport. The movement of solutes through channels is only downhill (down an electrochemical gradient).

4. D. An electrogenic transporter mediates net charge movement. Of the examples given, only the movement of 3 "+" charges into a cell in exchange for the efflux of 1 "2+" results in the net inward movement of one "+" charge.

5. B. When $[K]_0$ is equal to $[K]_1$, E_K is zero and the resting potential is zero.

6. E.

$$E_m = +60 \text{ mV} \log \frac{[Cl]_1}{[Cl]_2}$$
$$= +60 \text{ mV} \log \frac{100 \text{ mM}}{1 \text{ mM}}$$
$$= +60 \text{ mV} \log 100$$
$$= +60 \text{ mV} (2.0)$$
$$= +120 \text{ mV}.$$

7. D. At the threshold voltage and above (more positive or greater depolarization), there is a net inward current. Therefore, the inward Na^+ current must exceed the outward K^+ current, and there is further depolarization (rising phase of action potential).

8. D. The fast Na^+ current spontaneously inactivates because the I-gate (or h-gate) of the fast Na^+ channel closes after a delay of 1 to 2 msec. The fast Na^+ current turns on quickly and is responsible for the rising (depolarizing) phase of the action potential.

9. D. Propagation velocity increases with smaller membrane capacitance, shorter time constant, longer length constant, and lower (more negative) threshold potential. Cooling slows most chemical and physical reactions, including propagation of APs.

10. B. The myelin sheath *decreases* the effective capacitance (because of capacitors in series), *increases* the length constant (because of the effective increase in membrane resistance due to resistors in series), and causes the saltatory (jumping) conduction. Myelination has relatively little effect on the time constant (τ_m) because the increase in membrane resistance (R_m) is offset by the decrease in membrane capacitance (C_m): $\tau_m = R_m \times C_m$.

Part II: Neurophysiology

1. D. The EPSP is associated with net inward current carried by Na^+ ions, which depolarized the neuronal membrane.

2. D. The stretch reflex is important in maintaining postural muscle tone. Interruption of the reflex arc by section of the dorsal root causes the affected muscle to become hypotonic.

3. C. Bradykinesia is a characteristic sign in Parkinson's disease that results from dysfunction of the basal ganglia.

4. C. Experimental decerebrate rigidity is produced by transection of the neuraxis at the intercollicular level, resulting in overactivity of the facilitatory reticular formation and overfacilitation of the alpha and gamma neurons to the extensor (antigravity) muscles.

5. E. Enkephalin is a major inhibitory transmitter, and its release in the dorsal horn inhibits transmission of pain to higher centers.

6. B. The visual cortex is organized in columns that contain simple and complex cells that have the same orientation and directional sensitivities.

7. E. The difference in the size of the surface areas of the tympanic and oval window can produce 2.5×

amplification. Answer B is the definition of CF. Answer C, the lateral inhibition causes sharp tuning curves. Answer D, there is direct projection from the superior colliculus.

8. E. A and B are incorrect because each olfactory receptor and each neuron in the olfactory system responds to many odorants. C and D are incorrect because in the taste system each neuron responds to all four tastants but has a low threshold for only one type of tastant.

9. B. By interacting with the medullary centers, in particular the solitary tract nucleus, hypothalamic centers modulate short- and long-term feeding behavior. A and C are incorrect because hunger can be induced by activation of other hypothalamic and cortical areas. D is incorrect because dryness of the mouth and an increase in the level of angiotensin-II are strong signals for thirst.

10. A. Habituation occurs because the synaptic efficacy decreases.

Part III: Muscle Physiology

1. A. At long muscle lengths (sarcomere lengths greater than 3.6 μm), there is no overlap between thin and thick filaments, and hence no possibility for active force development. Therefore, the increases in total force are ascribable to the passive elastic behavior of muscle.

2. C. Relaxation is associated with lowering the intracellular Ca^{2+} concentration by the SR to the point where Ca^{2+} dissociates from troponin and there is subsequent restoration of the inhibition of tropomyosin on actin-myosin interaction.

3. D. ATP plays two roles: it dissociates the actin-myosin complex, and its hydrolysis provides the energy for contraction; however, only one ATP per crossbridge cycle is hydrolyzed.

4. A. Oxidative metabolism can sustain sufficient levels of ATP for moderate muscle activity. High levels of activity, however, would quickly exhaust the available phosphocreatine stores and normally depend on the glycolysis pathway to furnish ATP relatively rapidly. An increase in muscle lactate levels is a consequence of heavy activity.

5. A. Phosphorylation of the myosin light chain by the Ca^{2+}-dependent enzyme myosin light-chain kinase is an obligatory step in the activation of smooth muscle. Relaxation involves the dephosphorylation

of the light chains, catalyzed by myosin light-chain phosphatase.

6. A. Slow-twitch fibers are more oxidative, with higher levels of myoglobin to facilitate diffusion of oxygen. They are slower, and this is paralleled by the decreased T-tubule–sarcoplasmic reticulum junctional surface area, which reflects slower speeds of activation and relaxation.

7. B. The Ca^{2+}-release channels of the SR are activated by Ca^{2+}, known as *Ca^{2+}-triggered Ca^{2+} release,* and by IP_3, produced by phosphatidylinositol metabolism. The drugs caffeine and ryanodine bring about Ca^{2+} release from the SR, but they are not physiologic compounds.

8. B. In the reverse mode of operation, the exchanger swaps one extracellular Ca^{2+} for three intracellular Na^+, and is therefore electrogenic. A significant amount of Ca^{2+} influx into the myocardial cell may occur by this mechanism for excitation–contraction coupling during the long-duration cardiac AP plateau.

Part IV: Cardiovascular Physiology

1. D. A mechanical function of the pericardium is to prevent the heart from overdistention and to anchor it in the chest cavity; it also protects the heart against the spread of inflammation and infection from the lungs.

2. C. The inward current during the AP plateau is carried by the Ca^{2+} current.

3. A. (See the second paragraph of the section "Terminology of the ECG.")

4. B. The force-velocity relationship is an inverse hyperbolic curve that relates afterload to the initial velocity of shortening. The X intercept (P_o) is the load at which muscle cannot shorten; the extrapolated Y intercept (V_{max}) is the theoretical rate of shortening of an unloaded contraction. An increased inotropic state causes an increase in both P_o and V_{max}.

5. A. The Frank-Starling relationship states that increasing left ventricular end-diastolic volume (preload) increases stroke volume in ejecting beats and increases peak left ventricular pressure in isovolumic beats.

6. D. Because myocardial oxygen extraction from coronary artery blood is near maximal at rest, the

major mechanism by which oxygen supply is augmented to match increased demand is through increased coronary blood flow.

7. A. When energy (ATP) use increases, the relative concentration of ATP metabolites increases. Adenosine, a potent vasodilator, is the final product of the breakdown of ATP to ADP and then AMP. Adenosine-mediated vasodilation results in increased coronary blood flow, and thus more oxygen delivery and augmented washout of adenosine so that flow is readjusted as the energy balance is restored with the synthesis of more ATP.

8. E. An increase in vascular compliance means that the blood vessels will accommodate a larger volume of blood and that blood pressure will either not change or will decrease.

9. D. Increases in mean arterial pressure have little involvement in increasing capillary pressure. Only about one-tenth of the arterial pressure increase is transmitted into the capillary. Thus moderate increases in central venous pressure can readily cause systemic edema, but moderate increases in arterial pressure do not. Increases in capillary pressure are caused mainly by increases in venous pressure.

10. C. Muscular activity produces vasoactive metabolites, increased local oxygen flux and potassium release, and changes in H^+ flux. These factors produce local vasodilation and increased blood flow to the working muscle and through the coronary arteries to supply the myocardium. There are also systemic circulatory adjustments, but these local factors redistribute a disproportionate amount of the increased cardiac output to the working tissues, where vascular resistance is lowest.

Part V: Hemostasis and Blood Coagulation

1. B. These are the normal reactions that occur when platelets come in contact with collagen.

2. B. This is the only correct statement concerning vitamin K.

3. D. Because a bleeding time, PTT, and clot solubility test were not performed, the defects in A, B, C, and E are still possible and would yield the test profile given. However, vitamin K deficiency would yield a prolonged PT and therefore could be ruled out as a possible diagnosis.

4. D. The values are approximately normal. The platelet turnover is 250,000 platelets/μl/10 days, or 2.5 × 10^4 platelets/μl/day.

Part VI: Respiratory Physiology

1. E. By definition, the maximum volume of air that can be exhaled after a maximum expiration is the VC.

2. E. 0.6 liter/3 cmH_2O/2.5 liters = 0.08 cmH_2O.

3. B. Patients with emphysema lose lung elastic tissue. Consequently, they have increased lung volume with a given change in intrapleural pressure, which, by definition, is an increase in compliance.

4. B. Rearrange the simplified alveolar gas equation and solve for $PACO_2$, such that (120 mmHg – 100 mmHg) × 0.8 = 16 mmHg.

5. E. 65% of the CO_2 in blood is transported in the plasma as bicarbonate.

6. E. As in the vascular smooth muscle of systemic smooth muscle, acetylcholine vasodilates the pulmonary vasculature. (Recall that acetylcholine vasoconstricts the smooth muscle of the airways.)

7. D. The millions of intraalveolar vessels located between alveoli provide the greatest cross-sectional area in the pulmonary circulation. At high lung volumes, these vessels are compressed. Thus, at high lung volumes, the highest pulmonary vascular resistance is in the intraalveolar vessels.

8. C. The central chemoreceptors and other brain cells may actually be depressed by hypoxemia. Irritant receptors are stimulated by chemical substances in the intraluminal airway and not by hypoxemia. Pulmonary stretch receptors are mechanoreceptors.

9. B. At the base of the lung, pulmonary blood flow exceeds alveolar ventilation, resulting in a reduced $\dot{V}_A/\dot{Q}$ ratio.

10. A. In low $\dot{V}_A/\dot{Q}$ units, ventilation is reduced relative to blood flow. This hypoventilation lowers the P_{O_2} and elevates P_{CO_2} in the blood, leaving the low $\dot{V}_A/\dot{Q}$ units.

Part VII: Renal and Acid-Base Physiology

1. D. Calculated using the clearance formula:

$$C = \frac{(U)(V)}{(P)}$$

2. E. This calculation is based on the Fick principle, the fraction of the cardiac output perfusing the kidneys and the clearance of inulin.

3. B. Increases in the distal tubular flow rate cause an increase in afferent arteriolar resistance and therefore reduce the GFR and tubular pressure in Bowman's space.

4. A. Because the clearance of glucose approaches the GFR at high plasma glucose concentrations, the renal extraction of glucose approaches the renal inulin extraction.

5. C. The TF/P Cl^- ratio increases from 1.0 to 1.2 in the early segments of the proximal tubule (due to preferential organic solute reabsorption with Na^+) and remains elevated in the S_2 and S_3 portions of the tubule.

6. D. Samples of tubular fluid in the early segments of the distal tubule are, under normal conditions, markedly hypotonic (about 100 mOsm/liter) to plasma.

7. A. The osmolar clearance, given by $(U_{os})(V)/P_{os}$, is the same in both individuals.

8. D. Aldosterone and aldosterone-like drugs stimulate H^+ secretion, and therefore can foster metabolic alkalosis.

9. B. From Equation (42-25), $24 \times 72/64 = 27$ mM, which makes the data consistent. From Table 42-1, the increases in $[H^+]$, $PaCO_2$, and plasma $[HCO_3^-]$ conform to the pattern for respiratory acidosis. The small 3-mM increment in plasma $[HCO_3^-]$ for the 32-mmHg increment in $PaCO_2$ conforms to the predicted compensation for an acute respiratory acidosis. This is expected because full metabolic compensation for respiratory disorders requires many hours to take effect. The data are consistent with a simple disorder.

10. C. The volume of the extracellular fluid is one of the major factors affecting HCO_3^- reabsorption; there is an inverse relationship between the two.

Part VIII: Gastrointestinal Physiology

1. D. The sympathetic innervation of the gut acts presynaptically to inhibit acetylcholine release in the myenteric ganglia, activates alpha receptors, causing contraction of sphincter muscles, tonically constricts blood vessels, and inhibits secretion. NPY potentiates norepinephrine.

2. C. CCK is an enterogastrone and is pancreozymic; it relaxes the sphincter of Oddi and is released when the products of fat and protein digestion are present in the duodenum.

3. C. Secretin is released from S cells in the duodenal mucosa in response to gastric and fatty acids. It acts as an enterogastrone, potentiates the action of CCK, stimulates biliary bicarbonate and not bile salt secretion, and has a growth-promoting effect on the pancreas.

4. D. The migrating motor complex is only recorded in the small intestine and represents an orderly (not random) occurrence. The complex is independent of sphincteric activity and is not considered to represent the primary motor pattern for propelling food following a meal. It is only observed in the fasting state.

5. D. Peristaltic contractions of the stomach always result when a spike potential is generated. In turn, a spike potential is always associated with a slow wave of the basic electrical rhythm. Because of this interdependency, the basic electrical rhythm determines the maximum rate of peristaltic contractions in the stomach. In this regard, it does influence contractions. The basic electrical rhythm is an electrical, not mechanical, event, but it does not always cause contractions, as do spike potentials.

6. A. Intrinsic factor is secreted by parietal cells and complexes with dietary vitamin B_{12}. This complex is required for absorption of the vitamin.

7. C. Secretions of the duodenal mucosa (namely, secretin and cholecystokinin) are involved in the intestinal phase of the regulation of gastric secretion. Insulin release, adrenal gland secretions, bile salts, and ileal receptors play no role in this process.

8. B. Because HCO_3^- secretion by pancreatic duct cells is energized by a $Cl^--HCO_3^-$ exchanger, the luminal Cl^- concentration would decrease as the rate of pancreatic secretion increases. Na^+ and K^+ concentrations remain relatively constant.

9. B. Bile acids form macromolecular aggregates called micelles when a critical concentration is reached and are essential for solubilizing phospholipids and cholesterol.

10. D. A person lacking lactase will be unable to digest the milk sugar lactose. Thus the undigested lactose from a milk meal would likely enter the colon undigested in such a person. Water absorption also would be decreased. The digestion of sucrose and

maltose and the absorption of glucose and electrolytes are all essentially unaffected.

Part IX: Endocrine Physiology

1. A. The RIA measures the presence of the epitope on the hormone against which the antibody is directed. This may be present on both biologically active hormones as well as inactive precursors or metabolites. RIAs can also be performed under nonequilibrium conditions, which actually increase the sensitivity of the assay. The rate-limiting reagent is the antihormone antibody. Endogenous antihormone antibodies can bind with native and labeled hormone and give spurious results.

2. D. Loss of hypothalamic control of prolactin secretion of the anterior pituitary results in increased secretion. Thus transection of the pituitary stalk produces hyperprolactinemia together with diminished secretion of all other pituitary hormones.

3. B. TSH secretion is not stimulated during stress. It is frequently inhibited, probably because of increased glucocorticoid secretion.

4. E. GH has many metabolic effects on carbohydrate metabolism that regulate the uptake and use of substrates such as glucose. It does not, however, participate in gluconeogenesis.

5. D. Even though urea penetrates the blood-brain barrier very slowly, it is a poor stimulator of vasopressin. This observation strongly implies that the osmoreceptor is located outside the blood-brain barrier.

6. B. Thyroid peroxidase is associated with the luminal membrane of follicular cells and catalyzes the oxidation of iodide, which is a required step in the iodination of tyrosine and the eventual synthesis of T_3 and T_4.

7. A. Vitamin D is a sterol hormone that interacts primarily with nuclear receptors.

8. C. The absence of 17-hydroxylase limits steroidogenesis in the zona glomerulosa to aldosterone production.

9. B. Gluconeogenesis replenishes glycogen stores and provides glucose for immediate use. Ketoacids are an important alternative energy source for some but not all tissues.

10. E. The amino acid content of a high-protein meal is a potent stimulus for both insulin and glucagon secretion. Glucose levels are relatively unchanged because of the counterbalancing actions of insulin on glucose uptake and of glucagon on glycogenolysis and gluconeogenesis.

Part X: Reproductive Physiology

1. B. Mullerian-inhibiting hormone is a large-molecular-weight glycoprotein synthesized and secreted by Sertoli cells of the testis.

2. C. LH and FSH levels in the fetal circulation increase around the middle of pregnancy because at that time the fetal hypothalamic-pituitary unit is able to secrete gonadotropins but is not yet sensitive to the negative feedback effects of steroid hormones.

3. E. Estriol is a metabolite of estradiol.

4. C. FSH and LH both are glycosylated heterodimeric proteins that bind to membrane-bound receptors.

5. C. Inhibin suppresses synthesis and secretion of FSH but not of LH.

6. C. In the male, FSH stimulates Sertoli cells to synthesize inhibin and androgen-binding protein.

7. B. Involves a shift of progesterone production from the corpus luteum of the ovary to the chorion during the eighth to ninth weeks of gestation termed the luteal-placental shift.

8. A. Parturition is independent of the stage of development of the fetus itself.

Part XI: Adaptation and Exercise Physiology

1. D. Adaptation is slower to develop than compensation and may involve different mechanisms, as, for instance, with the thyroid in cold environments. Different loops may therefore be involved in the two processes. The normally high skin temperature of the Eskimoes shows that, to a significant extent, their adaptation to the cold is cultural and behavioral, rather than physiologic. The maintenance of normal oxygen supplies to tissue at high altitudes requires a raised steady-state value of the hematocrit. Adaptation is often noted long after the initial stimulus has been removed.

2. D. There is a minimum metabolic rate, and therefore O_2 consumption, but the definition of BMR excludes the existence of maximal or minimal values. During work, the extra heat produced can be lost by passive conduction more efficiently at lower than at

higher temperatures, without the need for evaporative heat loss. The neutral temperature is not invariable; for example, it is raised under the influence of pyrogens. At any steady-state, heat production equals heat loss.

3. A. As shown in Table 64-2, the $(a–v)O_2$ rises after physical training. Because of greater O_2 extraction by the muscle, the venous O_2 level is lower after physical training.

4. C. During light, moderate, and maximum exercise, the cardiac output to the skeletal muscle is 47%, 71%, and 88%, respectively, of the total cardiac output. Any single tissue or organ receives no more than 15%, depending on the intensity of exercise.

Index

Page references followed by an *f* refer to figures; those followed by a *t* refer to tables.